CLINICAL DECISIONS IN THERAPEUTIC EXERCISE
PLANNING AND IMPLEMENTATION

John Nyland, PT, EdD, SCS, ATC, CSCS, FACSM

University of Louisville
Department of Orthopaedic Surgery
Louisville, Kentucky

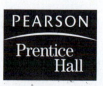

PEARSON
Prentice
Hall

Upper Saddle River, New Jersey 07458

Library of Congress Cataloging-in-Publication Data

Clinical decisions in therapeutic exercise : planning and implementation / [edited] by John Nyland.
 p. ; cm.
 Includes bibliographical references and index.
 ISBN 0-13-048036-3 (alk. paper)
 1. Exercise therapy.
 [DNLM: 1. Exercise Therapy. 2. Biomechanics. 3. Planning Techniques.
WB 541 C6406 2006]   I. Nyland, John.
 RM725.C57 2006
 615.8'2—dc22

                                                                   2005011757

Publisher: Julie Levin Alexander
Publisher's Assistant: Regina Bruno
Executive Editor: Mark Cohen
Associate Editor: Melissa Kerian
Editorial Assistant: Jaquay Felix
Developmental Editor: Annette Ferran
Director of Marketing: Karen Allman
Senior Channel Marketing Manager: Rachele Strober
Media Editor: John J. Jordan
Director of Production and Manufacturing: Bruce Johnson
Managing Production Editor: Patrick Walsh
Production Liaison: Julie Li
Production Editor: Mike Remillard
Manager of Media Production: Amy Peltier
New Media Project Manager: Stephen J. Hartner
Manufacturing Manager: Ilene Sanford
Manufacturing Buyer: Pat Brown
Senior Design Coordinator: Christopher Weigand
Cover Designer: Christopher Weigand
Cover Photo: Getty Images
Composition: Pine Tree Composition, Inc.
Printer and Binder: The Banta Companies, Harrisonburg VA
Cover Printer: Coral Graphics

Pearson Education LTD., *London*
Pearson Education Australia PTY, Limited, *Sydney*
Pearson Education Singapore, Pte. Ltd
Pearson Education North Asia Ltd., *Hong Kong*
Pearson Education, Canada, Ltd., *Toronto*

Pearson Educación de Mexico, S.A. de C.V.
Pearson Education–Japan, *Tokyo*
Pearson Education Malaysia, Pte. Ltd
Pearson Education, Upper Saddle River, New Jersey.

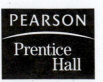

10 9 8 7 6 5 4 3 2 1
ISBN 0-13-048036-3

To my parents John and Betty for everything.

Brief Contents

Contents

Chapter 5   Training for Muscular Strength, Power, Endurance
and Hypertrophy   **171**
J.A. Brosky, Jr. and Glenn A. Wright

Chapter 6   Training for Joint Stability   **231**
Timothy F. Tyler and Michael Mullaney

Part II   Therapeutic Exercise Program Implementation: Introduction to Client Cases

Legends for Items on the Student CD-ROM

Preface

Rehabilitation clinicians are constantly challenged to match the therapeutic exercises they prescribe with the needs and desires of the individual client on a number of different health levels (physical, social, emotional, mental, etc). As we acknowledge the importance of evaluating existing research evidence and understanding its applicability to our clientele, we must not forget that client outcomes are largely determined by compliance with the mutually agreed upon therapeutic exercise program and its goals. Generic, off-the-shelf, therapeutic exercise interventions often attain less than optimal functional outcomes because they do not sufficiently comprehend the importance of learning about the client as a person, not merely someone who has a disease, dysfunction, or movement impairment. By effectively combining the weight of existing research evidence with a more comprehensive, holistic understanding of the individual, we can greatly improve our likelihood of attaining success with therapeutic exercise program intervention.

This textbook was designed to provide a contemporary evidence-based overview of topics that influence the rehabilitation clinician's decisions regarding therapeutic exercise program development. In Section I, the reader is taken through the effects of immobilization and disuse on body system function, the physiology of neuromuscular activation, stretching for musculotendinous extensibility and joint flexibility, and various methods of therapeutic exercise intervention and volume determination guidelines. Methods of therapeutic exercise intervention include training for muscular strength, power, endurance and hypertrophy, cardiopulmonary and cardiovascular fitness, joint stability, proprioception and kinesthesia, neuromuscular coordination and re-education, balance and agility. Following this, alternative movement-based exercise therapies are discussed. The final part of Section I attempts to "Put It All Together" by addressing issues related to patient/client psychobehavioral issues, education, compliance/adherence, designing plan of care algorithms, considerations regarding return to play readiness, and the measurement of therapeutic exercise program effectiveness. The final and most essential section of this textbook involves the ten illustrative client cases in Section II. The reader will be presented with ten very unique and diverse clients who require therapeutic exercise program intervention. From an initial history, the author of each case will ask the reader to make decisions on how best to manage the individual client. The author of each case will guide the reader with comments regarding their perception of an effective therapeutic exercise program intervention for their client, providing evidence-based support for the decisions they make along the way. Each case author has also provided an algorithm that provides a synopsis of his or her decision-making process. Differing opinions between the case authors and the reader should be used to stimulate class discussions with applicable evidence supporting assertions. Illustrations are provided throughout the textbook to enable the reader to visualize essential elements of each chapter. Illustrations of client case models are intended to provide the reader with a sense of familiarity with the individual (perhaps knowing someone like the person described in the case) and they are encouraged to discuss how and why the individual that they know might respond differently to the intervention described by the case author.

An instructional package is also offered to accompany Clinical Decisions in Therapeutic Exercise. The Instructor's Resource Manual contains a wealth of material to help faculty plan and manage their course. It contains chapter outlines, discussion questions, learning objectives and more for each chapter. The Instructor's Resource CD-ROM provides many resources in an electronic format. First, the CD-ROM contains the complete test bank, which allows instructors to create customized exams and quizzes. Second, it includes a lecture package in PowerPoint format. The lectures contain discussion points and embedded images from the textbook to help infuse an extra spark into the classroom experience. Instructors may use this presentation system as it is provided or they may opt to customize it for their specific needs.

This textbook includes two Student CD-ROMs. The CD provides a variety of specific therapeutic exercise interventions in both line drawing and computer graphic forms. This book is our first attempt at a project of this magnitude. Any feedback from readers with constructive ideas of how to improve the text would be appreciated.

John Nyland
2005

Acknowledgments

I thank each contributor for his or her dedication and commitment to this project. Thanks to my wife Robin. Thanks also to my teachers, colleagues, mentors, students and clients for their encouragement and support. Special thanks to Annette Ferran for her editorial assistance throughout book development. Thank you to the reviewers:

John Bartholomew, MS, ATC, CSCS
Head Athletic Trainer
Department of Athletic Training
Graceland University
Lamoni, Iowa

Elizabeth Chape, PT, MS
Coordinator/Instructor
Physical Therapist Assistant Program
Sacramento City College
Sacramento, California

Robert H. Fuchs, PT, MA, ATP, CSCS
Assistant Professor
Physical Therapy Education
University of Nebraska Medical Center
Omaha, Nebraska

Burke Gurney, PT, PhD
Assistant Professor
Department of Physical Therapy
University of New Mexico
Albuquerque, New Mexico

Christopher Hughes, PT, PhD, OCS, CSCS
Professor
School of Physical Therapy
Slippery Rock University
Slippery Rock, Pennsylvania

Christine Kasinkas, MS, PT
Assistant Professor
Department of Physical Therapy
Quinnipiac University
Hamden, Connecticut

James Laskin, PT, PhD
Assistant Professor
Department of Physical Therapy
The University of Montana
Missoula, Montana

Heather Levering, MS
Assistant Athletic Trainer and Instructor
Department of Health, Physical Education and Recreation
Henderson State University
Arkadelphia, Arkansas

Robert Manske, Med, MPT, ATC, CSCS
Assistant Professor
Department of Physical Therapy
Wichita State University
Wichita, Kansas

Thomas Mohr, PT, PhD
Professor and Chairman
Department of Physical Therapy
University of North Dakota
Grand Forks, North Dakota

Jaime C. Paz, MS, PT
Associate Clinical Specialist
Department of Physical Therapy
Northeastern University
Boston, Massachusetts

Rosalyn Pitt, EdD, PT, SPE
Department Head
Department of Physical Therapy
Tennessee State University
Nashville, Tennessee

Nicholas Quarrier, MNS, PT, OCS
Clinical Associate Professor
Department of Physical Therapy
Ithaca College
Ithaca, New York

Contributors

Kent J. Adams, PhD, FACSM, CSCS
Associate Professor
Department of Health Promotion
Physical Education and Sport Studies
College of Education and Human Development
University of Louisville
Louisville, Kentucky
Client Case 9

Claudia Angeli, PhD
Gait Laboratory Director
Frazier Rehabilitation Institute
Adjunct Associate Professor
Department of Mechanical Engineering
University of Louisville,
Clinical Assistant Professor
Division of Physical Medicine and Rehabilitation
University of Louisville
Adjunct Professor, Department of Physical Therapy
Bellarmine University
Chapter 9: Training for Agility and Balance

Timothy J. Brindle, PT, PhD, ATC
Post Doctoral Research Physical Therapist
Physical Disabilities Branch
National Institutes of Health
Bethesda, Maryland
*Chapter 8: Training for Neuromuscular Coordination
and Re-Education*

Joseph A. Brosky Jr., PT, MS, SCS
Associate Professor
Department of Physical Therapy
Lansing School of Nursing and Health Sciences
Bellarmine University
Louisville, Kentucky
*Chapter 5: Training for Muscular Strength, Power,
Endurance and Hypertrophy*

Angela M. Corio, MPT
Staff Physical Therapist
Florida Orthopaedic Institute
Tampa, Florida
Client Case 2

Tony English, PT, MS Ed
Associate Professor
Division of Physical Therapy
Department of Rehabilitation Sciences
University of Kentucky
Lexington, Kentucky
Client Case 4

Jason Gauvin, PT, MS, SCS, ATC, CSCS
Senior Physical Therapist
Duke Sports Medicine Physical Therapy
Duke University Health System
Durham, North Carolina
Client Case 6

Andrea Gallagher Hoff, PT, MS, OCS
Senior Physical Therapist
Duke Sports Medicine Physical Therapy
Duke University Health System
Durham, North Carolina
Client Case 1

Barbara Hoogenboom, PT, MHS, SCS, ATC
Assistant Professor
Program in Physical Therapy
College of Health Professions
Grand Valley State University
Grand Rapids, Michigan
Client Case 7

Theresa J. Kraemer, PT, PhD, ATC
Assistant Professor
Department of Physical Therapy
Arizona School of Health Sciences
A.T. Still University
Mesa, Arizona
*Chapter 10: Complementary and Alternative
Approaches to Movement and Exercise*

Thomas W. Miller, PhD, ABPP
Professor and Head
School of Allied Health
Department of Health Promotion and Allied Health
  Sciences
University of Connecticut
Storrs, Connecticut
*Chapter 11: Therapeutic Exercise Program Design
Considerations: "Putting It All Together"*

Michael J. Mullaney, MPT
Senior Physical Therapist
Research Assistant
Nicholas Institute of Sports Medicine & Athletic Trauma
Lenox Hill Hospital
New York, New York
Chapter 6: Training for Joint Stability

J. Timothy Noteboom, PT, PhD, SCS, ATC
Associate Professor
Department of Physical Therapy
Rueckert-Hartman School for Health Professions
Regis University
Denver, Colorado
Chapter 2: The Physiology of Muscle Activation
Chapter 3: Stretching for Musculotendinous Extensibility and Joint Flexibility

John Nyland, PT, EdD, SCS, ATC, CSCS, FACSM
Assistant Professor
Division of Sports Medicine
Department of Orthopaedic Surgery, School of Medicine
University of Louisville
Frazier Rehabilitation Institute
Adjunct Professor, Bellarmine University
Louisville, Kentucky
Chapter 1: Effects of Immobilization and Disuse on Body System Function
Chapter 11: Therapeutic Exercise Program Design Considerations: "Putting It All Together"

William K. Ogard, PT, PhD
Assistant Professor
Department of Physical Therapy
School of Health Related Professions
The University of Alabama at Birmingham
Birmingham, Alabama
Chapter 7: Training for Proprioception and Kinesthesia

Christine Price, PT, MMSc, CWS
Associate Professor
Department of Physical Therapy
Lansing School of Nursing and Health Sciences
Bellarmine University
Louisville, Kentucky
Chapter 1: Effect of Immobilization and Disuse on Body System Function

Mark F. Reinking, PT, PhD, SCS, ATC
Assistant Professor and Assistant Chair
Department of Physical Therapy
Doisy College of Health Sciences
Saint Louis University
Saint Louis, Missouri
Chapter 4: Introduction to Training for Cardiopulmonary and Cardiovascular Fitness

Tom Squires, PT, ATC, MBA
Director of Rehabilitation
South Bend Orthopaedic Associates
South Bend, Indiana
Client Case #3

Ann M. Swartz, PhD
Assistant Professor
Department of Human Movement Sciences
College of Health Sciences
University of Wisconsin-Milwaukee
Milwaukee, Wisconsin
Client Case #8

Laura Lee (Dolly) Swisher, PT, PhD
Assistant Professor
School of Physical Therapy
College of Medicine
University of South Florida
Tampa, Florida
Client Case #5

Timothy F. Tyler, PT, MS, ATC
Clinical Research Associate
Nicholas Institute of Sports Medicine and Athletic Trauma
Department of Orthopaedics
Lenox Hill Hospital
New York, New York
Chapter 6: Training for Joint Stability

Harvey Wallmann, PT, DPTSc, SCS, ATC, CSCS
Associate Professor and Chair
Department of Physical Therapy
University of Nevada, Las Vegas
Las Vegas, Nevada
Chapter 3: Stretching for Musculotendinous Extensibility and Joint Flexibility
Chapter 4: Introduction to Training for Cardiopulmonary and Cardiovascular Fitness

Rick W. Wilson, PT, PhD
Assistant Professor
School of Physical Therapy
Member, H. Lee Moffitt Cancer Center & Research Institute
College of Medicine
University of South Florida
Tampa, Florida
Client Case #10

Wendy Wormal, MS, LMT, CSCS
Pro-Formance Fitness and Training
Louisville, Kentucky
Chapter 11: Therapeutic Exercise Program Design Considerations: Putting It All Together

Glenn A. Wright, PhD, HFI, CSCS
Assistant Professor
Director, Graduate Program in Human Performance
University of Wisconsin-LaCrosse
LaCrosse, Wisconsin
Chapter 5: Training for Muscular Strength, Power,
Endurance and Hypertrophy

Jerrad Zimmerman, MD
Director of Sports Medicine
Carle Clinic
Team Physician
University of Illinois
Champaign-Urbana, Illinois
Chapter 1: Effects of Immobilization and Disuse on Body
System Function

PART I

Foundations of Therapeutic Exercise Program Planning

1

Effects of Immobilization and Disuse on Body System Function

JERRAD ZIMMERMAN
CHRISTINE PRICE
JOHN NYLAND

Objectives

The reader will be able to:

- Identify the indications and contraindications for prolonged bed rest and immobilization.
- Explain the physical and emotional consequences of bed rest and immobilization.
- Develop better therapeutic exercise interventions using knowledge of the deleterious effects of bed rest and immobilization.

- Identify specific consequences of bed rest and intervene in preventing further loss at an earlier point in therapeutic exercise program development.
- Describe disability models and explain how they improve and modify patient-client care.
- Describe the contraindications to therapeutic exercise interventions and modifications that may enable their use.

Outline

INTRODUCTION

Case Scenario

Virgil is a 49-year-old cattle rancher who was trapped by a 1-ton beef bull when working with his cowherd. The otherwise healthy farmer sustained a pubic rami fracture of his pelvis in addition to a non-displaced tibia fracture of his right leg. Virgil was transported to the local emergency room for treatment and was found to have no other major soft tissue or bony injuries. He was treated in a local hospital by the orthopedic surgeon with a long leg cast on the right leg and bed rest for the pelvic fracture (**Figure 1.1**). Virgil was hospitalized three days for observation before being discharged to home with a prescription for oral pain medication. Virgil was advised that he would need to wear the cast for six to eight weeks and maintain bed rest for the same period of time for the pubic rami fracture. Virgil's wife Alice and son Donny live on the farm with him and will help support him during his recovery. Although cattle ranching is both Virgil's "vocation and his vacation," he also enjoys fly-fishing for trout and playing basketball with his friends and son.

This chapter will discuss the effects of immobilization and disuse on body system functions, and the use of disability models to guide the rehabilitation clinician as they design therapeutic exercise programs. The chapter will also discuss the use of disability models to guide rehabilitation clinicians as they design therapeutic exercise programs. Immobilization has many detrimental effects on the human body, ranging from well known deleterious effects on muscle mass and strength to lesser-understood psychological effects. The idea of bed rest for treatment of medical conditions originated from the observation that

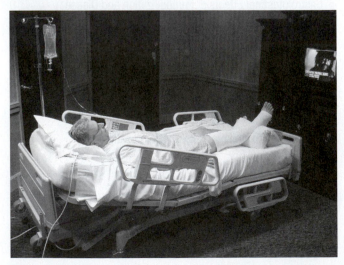

Figure 1.1   49-year-old farmer "Virgil" recovering in hospital room following the farm accident described during the case.

sleep is required for normal daily functioning. When people become ill they get weak and want to do little other than sleep. These observations are believed to have led to the first thoughts that bed rest may actually benefit ill patients. Hippocrates was quoted as saying, "In every movement of the body, whenever one begins to endure pain, it will be relieved by rest."[1]

The use of immobilization in the treatment of many different illnesses is often overlooked in today's health care environment. Most hospital rooms are equipped with a hospital bed, bedside table on wheels, a firm chair, television, and bathroom. When walking through a hospital you notice that most patients with any type of illness spend most of their day in a hospital bed unless they are undergoing a particular therapeutic or diagnostic procedure. For many of these patients, bed rest is not a specific order, but a system consequence.

> ## Key Point:
> Bed rest and prolonged disuse may not be a specific order, but rather a health care system consequence.

Despite many research studies showing the deleterious effects of bed rest, the health care community continues to be slow to accept change. A 1998 study showed that 80 percent of neurologic units in the United Kingdom had standing orders of bed rest following a routine lumbar puncture.[2] What makes this interesting is that data obtained in the United Kingdom 17 years earlier showed no therapeutic benefit of bed rest following a routine lumbar puncture.[3] In a review of 39 randomized controlled trials of bed rest versus early mobilization for treatment of a medical condition or procedure, Allen et al.[4] reported that for 24 trials investigating the effects of bed rest following a medical procedure, no outcome improved significantly, and eight worsened significantly. In 15 trials that investigated bed rest as a primary treatment, no outcomes improved significantly and nine worsened significantly.

Patients generally are instructed to immobilize a body segment or assume bed rest status for three main reasons: 1) because of the patient's own weakness as a result of his or her physical illness, 2) to relieve pain symptoms, and 3) to speed recovery. As health care providers become more aware of the true indications for immobilization or full bed rest they will be more effective in managing their patients.[1] The detrimental effects of immobilization and bed rest on many different organ systems will now be discussed. We will also identify some preventative measures that can be taken to limit these deleterious effects.

Effects of Immobilization and Disuse on the Musculoskeletal System

Muscular Consequences

Disuse and immobilization affect the musculoskeletal system in many ways. We will begin by discussing the effects of immobilization on muscles specifically. It has been well documented that disuse of muscles results in decreased muscle mass and strength, which begin within a matter of days and progressively worsen with increasing duration of disuse or immobilization (**Figure 1.2**). The decrease in muscle mass and strength as a result of bed rest is a result of two key factors: lack of normal weight bearing forces acting on bones in the upright position, and a decreased number and/or magnitude of muscle activations.

> ## Key Point:
>
> A lack of normal weight bearing forces acting on bones in an upright position and a decrease in the number and magnitude of muscle activations contribute to the decreased muscle mass and strength loss associated with bed rest.

Immobilization by application of a plaster or fiberglass cast or the use of a suspension system such as a sling produces much greater and more rapid muscle mass and

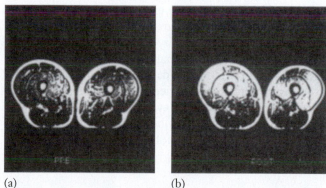

(a)   (b)

Figure 1.2   Magnetic resonance images of left and right legs mid-thigh, (a) is at baseline, (b) is taken after five weeks of suspension of the left lower extremity (appears on the right of each image). Left lower extremity suspension results in unloading of weight bearing forces. The image on the right shows a decreased muscle cross sectional area of the left lower extremity after suspension. (Image courtesy of G. A. Dudley and L. Ploutz-Snyder in *Med Sci Sports Exerc.* 1997:29 197–206.)

strength reductions than bed rest alone.[5–8] Veldhuizen et al.[7] studied eight healthy volunteers (six males, two females, 19–26 years of age) during a four week period of non–weight bearing knee immobilization in a long leg cast. They reported a 21 percent reduction in quadriceps femoris area, a 16 percent reduction in muscle fiber diameter, a 29 percent decrease in mean cross-sectional fiber area and a 52 percent and 26 percent deficit in knee extensor and flexor torque, respectively.[7]

Using a combination of magnetic resonance imaging with spectroscopy, isokinetic and isometric muscle testing, and simple functional tests, Vandenborne et al[8]., studied the effects of eight weeks of ankle immobilization in a short leg cast following a closed bimalleolar fracture and open reduction-internal fixation (four weeks non–weight bearing, four weeks weight bearing as tolerated), followed by 10 weeks of physical therapy intervention. By eight weeks of immobilization lateral gastrocnemius, medial gastrocnemius, and soleus cross sectional areas were reduced by 32.4 percent, 22.9 percent, and 20 percent, respectively. During the first week of therapeutic exercise plantar flexor strength was decreased by approximately 50 percent. By 10 weeks post-therapeutic exercise intervention all changes were reversed with the exception of a remaining 5.5 percent deficit in total muscle cross-sectional area.[8] In an evaluation of six non-impaired males (21.5 ± 1.4 years of age) who underwent 21 days of wrist and elbow joint immobilization in a long arm cast, Kitahara et al.[9] reported no changes in forearm circumference; however, maximum grip strength decreased by 18 percent and phosphocreatine recovery after submaximal exercise performance was prolonged.

During both bed rest and immobilization the muscle's nerve source is still intact and the muscle is capable of performing at least isometric contraction without any appreciable changes in joint position.[2] Muscular changes following immobilization or disuse has been intensively researched. The amount of nitrogen excreted in the urine begins increasing shortly after the initiation of immobilization, with significant increases noted by the fifth day.[10] This is important because urinary nitrogen levels serve as an important indirect measurement of protein or muscle degradation. Peak urinary nitrogen excretion occurs during the second week of bed rest or immobilization.[2]

Cross sectional limb muscle mass has also been studied using biopsy and microscopy techniques following both bed rest and immobilization using limb suspension. Suspension casting of an arm for as brief as a nine day period invoked a 4 percent decrease in the cross sectional area of the forearm muscles.[5] Different muscle groups respond to disuse at different rates and amounts: "For example, the ankle plantar flexors are more affected by bed rest than the ankle dorsiflexors in both cross sectional area and strength[11,12], while the psoas muscle, a hip flexor and low back stabilizer displays very little or no atrophy following prolonged bed rest. (**Figure 1.3**).

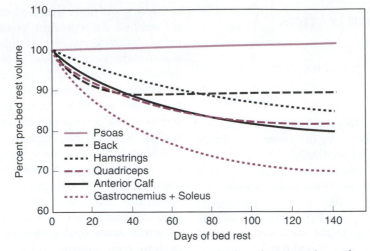

Figure 1.3 Percent pre–bed rest muscle volume vs. days of bed rest using magnetic resonance imaging quantitation. (From LeBlanc A, et al. *Int J Sports Med.* 1997;18:S283–S285.)

The primary muscle fibers affected most by immobilization or bed rest varies with the duration of the disuse and with which studies are reviewed. Immobilization studies using animal models have shown that slow twitch muscle fibers generally display more atrophy than fast twitch muscle fibers; however, in humans the opposite is true. This difference may be explained by the relative size of the muscle fibers prior to immobilization. In animals like rats the muscles with the largest fiber diameters are the slow twitch fibers. In humans, the largest muscle fibers are the fast twitch fibers. This may explain the difference between the muscle fiber atrophy that has been observed between human studies and studies which have relied on animal models.[13] The muscle fiber cross sectional area at baseline is an important determinant of the magnitude and location of atrophy.[13] Perhaps the larger fibers, whether slow twitch or fast twitch, experience the greater relative decrease in daily loading during bed rest and therefore atrophy relatively more. In humans the larger, fast twitch muscle fibers are more likely to be affected by immobilization. The important point to remember from this muscle fiber discussion is that if fast twitch muscle fibers are more affected than slow twitch muscle fibers during disuse in humans, then therapeutic exercise programs may need to be focused not only on specific muscle groups, but also on specific muscle fiber types.[2]

Body fluid shifts during prolonged bed rest also contribute to muscle mass reductions. Intramuscular fluid volume increases in the upper extremities during prolonged bed rest and decreases in the lower extremities. This fluid shift helps explain why lower extremity muscle mass tends to atrophy more quickly than upper extremity muscle mass during bed rest.[5]

As expected given the decreased muscle mass and cross sectional area following disuse, strength is also negatively affected. Bed rest for 30 days decreases knee extensor strength by about 20 percent, while knee flexor strength shows a non-significant decrease.[14] It has been documented multiple times that extensor muscles are weakened more by bed rest than their corresponding flexor muscles. The upper extremity musculature generally experiences less strength loss than the lower extremities during disuse. For up to 60 days of bed rest the upper extremity musculature experiences little strength loss.[2] In stricter immobilization, however—especially casting—the upper extremity musculature begins weakening within the first nine days following immobilization.[5]

> **Key Point:**
> The lower extremities are generally affected more by prolonged immobilization, bed rest, and disuse than the upper extremities, and the extensor muscles of the lower extremity are generally affected more than the flexors.

> **Key Point:**
> In humans, larger fast twitch muscle fibers are generally affected more by immobilization and disuse; therefore, therapeutic exercise programs may need to prescriptively target these fibers.

The maximal instantaneous power that a muscle or muscle group can produce also decreases following bed rest.[6] This measurement was taken by using a force platform to measure the force created while the subject attempted to perform a vertical jump. The maximal instantaneous muscular power should theoretically decrease proportionately to the rate at which muscle strength and mass decrease. However, this is not the case. Decreases in muscle mass alone may not completely explain maximal instantaneous muscular power decreases following disuse. Some investigators believe the lower extremity power decreases are a result of a change in the muscle unit's mechanical properties, while others hypothesize that the decreasing power is a result of a change in calcium levels within the muscle fiber. Another group of researchers believe that it could be caused by changes at the neuromuscular junction. All of these concepts warrant further research to help better explain the excessive muscular power loss observed during disuse or bed rest.[6]

Following bed rest, cellular changes to the ultrastructure of the muscle fibers also occur. Some of these changes include Z-line streaming and myofibrillar protein disorganization (**Figure 1.4**).[13] These changes along with cellular edema and occasionally mitochondria observed within

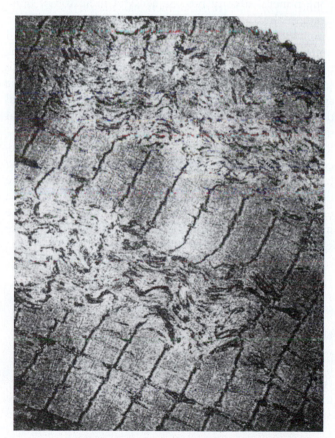

Figure 1.4   Microscopic changes seen in the ultrastructure of muscle cells taken from a healthy male soleus muscle after 30 days of bed rest. Note the Z-line streaming and myofibrillar protein disorganization. (Photograph courtesy of R. S. Hikida published in *Med Sci Sports Exerc.* 1997;29:197–206.)

the extracellular space suggest a disruption of the muscle sarcolemma or outer wall following extended bed rest or disuse.[2] What these findings suggest and how they affect muscle functioning after prolonged bed rest is yet to be determined.

The rate at which muscle strength, mass, and power return to baseline following cessation of bed rest, immobilization, or disuse differs by muscle group and the training method used. Dudley et al. reported a 92 percent knee extensor strength recovery within 30 days following bed rest cessation when subjects followed an unsupervised exercise regimen.[14] Following an average of five weeks of immobilization, Sale et al.[15] reported thenar muscle strength return at 18 weeks following resistance training initation. Some studies have relied on intense therapeutic exercise regimes, while others have relied more on a progressive resumption of normal functional activities of daily living. An important point to remember is that you do not have to worry about restoring something that was never lost. Rehabilitation clinicians should stay current with innovative new methods of preventing the loss of muscle mass, strength, and power despite the need for bed rest and/or immobilization and relative disuse. The best current proven way is to limit the length of bed rest and immobilization to the minimum needed to safely care for the client.[10]

The influence of disuse or bed rest on muscle function warrants consideration when designing a therapeutic exercise program. The rehabilitation clinician must remember that extensor muscle groups are generally more affected than flexor muscle groups, lower extremity muscle groups generally decrease in size and strength faster than upper extremity muscle groups, and casted or suspended limbs suffer more loss than non-restricted muscle groups during prolonged bed rest.[5,11,12,14] The therapeutic exercise program should also consider ways to manage the associated muscle power decreases and possibly which muscle fiber type the rehabilitation clinician should focus on. The therapeutic exercise program must also consider the functional activities the client deems important and tap into them in a manner that might best contribute to the neuromuscular recovery of the target muscle groups. In Virgil's case this includes, but is not limited, to the muscle strength and power to perform ranch activities, interact with his family and friends, play basketball, fly fish, etc.

Bony Consequences

Bloomfield[16] reported that dramatic decreases in lower extremity muscle mass occur within four to six weeks of bed rest, accompanied by 6-40 percent decreases in muscle strength. Appropriately designed therapeutic exercise intervention can reverse these changes. However, simultaneous decreases in lumbar spine, femoral neck, and calcaneous bone mineral density may not be reversed even after six months of normal weight bearing activities. This combination of muscle mass and strength restoration in combination with decreased bone mineral density increases fracture risk. Simply reducing normal activity levels represents the first component of a spectrum of disuse which is further compounded by bed rest and reduced weight bearing, with extreme effects following spinal cord injury.[16,17]

The major effects of immobilization and bed rest or disuse on the bony skeleton do not occur as quickly as the previously described muscular changes. Nishimura et al.[18] studied the effects of 20 days of bed rest on nine healthy subjects between 19 and 29 years of age (six males, three females). They suggested that during the early stages of immobilization bone matrix might be partially resorbed without any activation of osteoclasts, resulting in rapid decalcification of vertebral and cortical bones without any discernible changes in anatomical structure. As bone remodeling occurs more rapidly in spongy or cancellous bone than in cortical bone, the cancellous bone may be more sensitive to a cessation of mechanical loading. This would imply that bony weakening secondary to disuse predominantly occurs in the trabecular part of the weight bearing skeleton.[18]

Dietary calcium absorption is generally decreased during bed rest. Schneider et al.,[19] in a study of healthy volunteers who underwent 20 weeks of bed rest reported that 50 percent of the subject's negative calcium balance was due to fecal calcium loss. The remaining calcium loss was from urinary calcium excretion, which will be discussed later. Fecal calcium loss is a direct result of decreased intestinal calcium absorption. LeBlanc et al.,[17] reported that subjects who underwent four months of bed rest experienced intestinal calcium absorption decreases from 31 percent of ingested calcium to 24 percent.

Intestinal calcium absorption is regulated by the parathyroid gland. Parathyroid hormone stimulates the conversion of inactive 25-hydroxyvitamin D to active 1,25-dihydroxyvitamin D by the kidney, which then directly stimulates gastrointestinal calcium absorption. Bergmann et al.[20] reported that clients with spinal cord injury had low 1,25-dihydroxyvitamin D and parathyroid hormone serum levels, explaining their decreased calcium absorption. In healthy subjects undergoing prolonged bed rest, decreased[21] or slightly increased[17,22] parathyroid hormone serum levels have been reported. The complete mechanism of decreased calcium absorption during bed rest is not completely understood and further research is needed. Studies have shown that increasing dietary calcium intake to 1000 mg a day during periods of bed rest can decrease the negative calcium balance.[23]

Urinary calcium excretion increases as early as seven days after beginning bed rest.[2] Calcium released in urine is taken from the bony skeleton or elsewhere in the body. Schneider et al.,[19] in a study of healthy bed rested male subjects, showed a 60 percent increase in urinary calcium levels after 20 weeks of bed rest, with the amount of urinary calcium loss peaking at five to seven weeks after bed

Key Point:

Dietary calcium supplementation of 1000 mg/day during bed rest can help minimize the effect of a negative calcium balance, thereby helping prevent bone degradation.

rest initiation. Bergmann et al.[20] reported that in clients with spinal cord injuries the amount of calciuria is two to four times greater than what is seen in healthy, bed rested subjects and the condition sometimes persists for up to 12 months post-injury. This increased calcium loss might best be explained by clients with spinal cord injuries having more complete immobilization than clients who undergo bed rest with intact neuromuscular units capable of muscle activation.[2]

Studies of clients undergoing bed rest show decreased mineral density primarily at weight bearing bones. Volumetric quantitative computerized tomographic scans of bone mineral density provide a useful indicator of bone strength. In a study of clients with lumbar disc disease who were treated with bed rest and traction, Krolner and Toft[24] reported a one percent per week reduction in lumbar spine bone mineral density. In a study of healthy male subjects who underwent four months of bed rest, lumbar spine, femoral neck, tibia and calcaneous bone mineral density decreases were observed, but radius bone mineral density did not change (**Figure 1.5**).[25] Even during prolonged space flight, radius bone mineral density reportedly does not change substantially.[26] This finding during both bed rest and space flight can best be explained by the decreased daily loading of the lower extremities and spine during both bed rest and space flight. The radius bone mineral density is likely not affected during bed rest or space flight because it is not a weight bearing bone.[2]

Key Point:

Weight bearing bones undergo demineralization more quickly and to a greater extent than non–weight bearing bones during immobilization, disuse or prolonged bed rest.

Researchers are trying to explain whether the decrease in bone mineral density is a result of increased bone resorption (osteoclast activity), decreased bone formation (osteoblast activity), or both by examining bone biopsies following bed rest in healthy subjects. Most human bone biopsies have been performed at the iliac crest region because a bone biopsy directly from a weight bearing bone

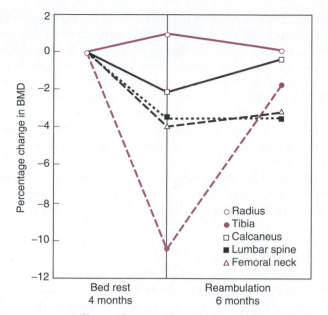

Figure 1.5 Effects of 4 months of bed rest on bone mineral density with six-month reambulation period in healthy young men. Bone mineral density is represented in percent change in bone mineral density from the start of the trial. (Data is from LeBlanc A, et al. *J Bone Min Res.* 1990:5:843–850. Graph obtained from *Med Sci Sports Exerc.* 2001;29:197–206.)

will result in an increased fracture risk for the volunteer in the study. Microscopic examination of iliac crest biopsies of 20 healthy males taken before and after 120 days of bed rest has revealed a 51 percent increase in bone resorption and a 26 percent decrease in the mineralization of newly formed bony matrix.[27] The total bone mass was unchanged and the amount of non-mineralized newly formed bony matrix was not significantly different from baseline levels. Once again these findings following bed rest are different from those reported following spinal cord injury. Following a spinal cord injury bone volume decreases as a result of increased bone resorption and decreased bony matrix formation which results in a decreased baseline bony volume by approximately six months post-injury.[28] In primate studies, tibial bone mineral density decreases 31 percent following six months of being restricted to a chair.[29,30]

Biochemical bone resorption markers have also been studied to explain the decrease in bone mineral density observed following bed rest. Following only four days of head down bed rest biochemical markers of bone resorption including pyridinoline, deoxypyridinoline, and hydroxyproline all significantly increased from baseline.[31] This increase only lasted until approximately day 20 of bed rest then returned to normal. Further study is needed to determine the significance of these findings.

The recovery of bone mass and density is much slower than the rate at which it is lost and also slower than the

> ## Key Point:
> Bone mass and mineral density recover at a much slower rate following cessation of bed rest, immobilization or disuse than muscle strength and mass.

rate at which muscle strength and mass is regained. In a study of subjects who experienced 17 weeks of bed rest, lumbar spine and femoral neck bone mineral density returned to baseline after six months of regular ambulation.[25] However, calcaneus bone mineral density may remain decreased for up to five years after space flight. As we age, decreased osteoblast activity occurs naturally, implying that the older the client undergoing bed rest, the slower their bone mineral density will return to baseline.[32] This fact, and the fact that bone mineral density baseline decreases with age, suggests that prevention of bone weakening following injury is vital. Every bone has a specific "fracture threshold," meaning the bone mineral density at which it is at a significant risk of fracturing with minimal trauma.[33] In a recumbent position, longitudinal compression forces on the spine and long bones are virtually eliminated.[34]

> ## Key Point:
> In relationship to its functional significance, each bone has a specific "fracture threshold" or bone mineral density that it must maintain to avoid fracturing with minimal trauma.

Health care providers must be aware of their client's bone mineral density prior to bed rest or prolonged disuse to help minimize the risk of fractures. For example, a healthy 20-year-old male is at much less risk of reaching his fracture threshold after bed rest or disuse than an 86-year-old female with osteopenia.[2]

Bony changes following bed rest or immobilization are very significant. Calcium absorption decreases and excretion increases during bed rest with the client undergoing a concurrent reduction in bone mineral density.[2] This information reinforces the importance of proper calcium intake and early protected mobilization after any trauma or injury. These changes are even more important to remember when dealing with fractures of elderly clients that are a result of osteoporosis or osteopenia.

Elderly clients may have already reached their fracture threshold and each day of bed rest lowers their bone mineral density further below that point. Luckily in Virgil's case, he is a relatively healthy man with no existing

> ## Key Point:
> Appropriate dietary calcium intake and early protected mobilization are essential to maintain or improve bone mineral density values.

problems associated with osteopenia or osteoporosis. The rehabilitation clinician must consider how he or she might modify the therapeutic exercise program if the client in question was, for example, a 90-year old woman with osteoporosis.

LIGAMENT AND TENDON EFFECTS OF IMMOBILIZATION AND DISUSE

Whether they are examined anatomically, physiologically, or biomechanically, immobilization or disuse is deleterious to all joint structures. Convincing evidence from controlled experimental and clinical trials suggest that controlled mobilization is superior to immobilization for musculoskeletal soft tissue injuries.[35] This holds true not only in the primary treatment of acute injuries (albeit with considerable respect for pain and inflammation), but also in their post-operative management.[35] Wren et al.[36] reported that in mature animals, immobilization causes a drastic decrease in the loading, and consequently the strain stimulus, experienced by a tendon or ligament (see Chapter 3). This reduced strain stimulus leads to a rapid loss of cross sectional area, modulus, and strength. When loading is restored through therapeutic exercise, the strain stimulus is elevated and the properties rapidly recover, leading to increases in both the geometric and material properties.[36]

Obvious changes in the mechanical properties of ligaments from immobilization have been demonstrated in the collateral knee ligaments in a time-dependent manner, including reductions in the mechanical and structural properties, and a decrease in cross sectional area.[37] Immobilization reportedly increases the rate of periarticular connective tissue collagen turnover with an increased rate of both collagen synthesis and degradation.[38] Regarding the time-dependent effect of immobilization, Amiel et al.[39] reported that degradation produced minor net decreases in total collagen mass (2 percent) after nine weeks of immobilization, but a large decrease in total collagen mass (27 percent) was observed by the end of 12 weeks. The mechanical properties and morphology of tendons and ligaments change in response to mechanical demands. During stress deprivation the mechanical properties of these tissues rapidly and substantially decrease in a time- and dose-dependent manner.

Tendon is a highly organized connective tissue that is approximately 85 percent collagen. Like muscles and liga-

ments, tendons need to transmit tensile forces. Compared with muscle, however, the metabolic turnover of tendon tissue is many times slower due to poorer vascularity and circulation. Therefore, the adaptive responses of tendons to training or therapeutic exercise intervention are also slower than those in muscles.[40] The early application of tensile forces across a healing tendon helps to orient the healing collagen fibers and increase the ultimate strength of the repair. Montgomery and Steadman[41] recommended that immobilization, when used following knee surgery, should be confined to less than three weeks in duration and applied exercises initiated following the use of immobilization should be limited and gradually increased in volume and intensity. Tipton et al.[42] suggested that endurance exercise training enhanced the strength between ligament–bone and tendon–bone junctions. Using a canine model to evaluate the influence of early motion, delayed motion and immobilization on healing canine flexor tendons at 12 weeks following surgery, Gelberman et al.[43] reported that the immediate mobilization group produced 95 percent ± 10 percent of the control joint motion while the immobilized group displayed only 19 percent ± 2 percent of the control joint motion. They concluded that early, protected passive mobilization augments the physiologic processes that ultimately determine the strength and excursion of the repaired flexor tendons. In a later study that compared flexor tendon immobilization to a protected passive mobilization regimen, Gelberman et al.[44] reported that repaired flexor tendons that received protected passive mobilization displayed accelerated changes in peritendinous vessel density and increased repair site total deoxyribonucleic acid (DNA) content, while immobilized tendons displayed adhesions that obliterated the space between the tendon surface and the tendon sheath. In evaluating the effects of controlled passive range of motion on healing canine flexor tendons, Takai et al.[45] reported that biomechanical tendon properties were superior in the group that received 12 motion cycles/minutes for five minutes/day compared to the group that received one cycle/minute for 60 minutes/day. In comparing the effect of continuous passive motion versus short-term immobilization (three weeks) on the biochemical and biomechanical properties of rabbit tibialis anterior tendons, Loitz et al.[46] reported that cyclic tensile loading by continuous passive motion lessened the harmful effects of immobilization.

Although having the "green light" to intervene with early mobilization is an exciting possibility for the rehabilitation clinician, these decisions must be closely coordinated with the referring physician. Although all musculoskeletal tissues can respond to repetitive loading, they vary in the magnitude and type of response to specific patterns of activity. Furthermore, this responsiveness may decline with increasing age. Early motion and loading of injured tissues is not without risks, however.[47] The level of protection, limitations of range of motion and force applications will vary based on the age and tissue integrity of the individual client, the method of surgical fixation, and the desires of the surgeon based on their experiences.

> ## Key Point:
> Although early mobilization has been shown to benefit tendon healing, the level of protection, safe applied forces and range of motion will vary based on age, tissue integrity, method of surgical fixation, and the desires of the surgeon.

Using a rabbit model to attempt to evaluate the combined beneficial effects of immobilization with protected function using functional casting following surgical Achilles tendon repair, Stehno-Bittel et al.[48] reported that functional casting resulted in a 60 percent greater increase in total collagen content and a 20 percent increase in maximum load at failure compared to rigid casting. In a similar study using a rabbit model, Pneumaticos et al.[49] reported that early mobilization of Achilles tendon repairs appeared to restore tendon functional properties more rapidly than continuous immobilization of an identical surgical repair.

ARTICULAR CARTILAGE EFFECTS OF IMMOBILIZATION AND DISUSE

Immobilization and disuse negatively influence the articular cartilage of synovial joints. Articular cartilage is the fibrous tissue that coats the bone surface within a joint. Articular cartilage is made by chrondrocytes on the bony surface. Immobilization causes the chondrocytes to decrease production of articular cartilage and cartilage matrix, resulting in less functional articular cartilage within the joint capsule. Repetitive muscle stimulation of an immobilized joint will slow articular cartilage degeneration, but both loading and motion are required to fully maintain articular cartilage integrity.[47,50–52] Degenerative processes can be explained by a breakdown of the normal load-bearing capacity associated with the mechanics of improper fluid flow. Factors which may lead to this breakdown include direct trauma, obesity, immobilization, and excessive repetitive loading.[52]

Osteoarthritis is a generally progressive loss of normal structure and function of articular cartilage resulting from the mechanical environment, biologic behavior, and aging.[51,53,54] As the disease progresses, the surface irregularities become clefts, and more of the articular joint surface becomes rough and irregular, with fibrillations extending deeper into the articular cartilage until they reach the subchondral bone.[55]

Animal model studies have reported altered articular cartilage between six days and six weeks following immobilization.[56–58] Alterations include decreased synthetic activity of chondrocytes, reduced proteoglycan concentrations, and decreased cartilage thickness.[51,56,57] Using a canine model, Olah and Kostensky[58] reported a 41 percent decrease in articular cartilage proteoglycan synthesis following six days of immobilization, a loss of proteoglycan aggregates by three weeks, and decreased glycosaminoglycan concentrations following 40 days of immobilization. Presumably, there is interference with cellular nutrition, which is dependent on the cyclic compression and expansion of articular cartilage that normally occurs with intermittent loading.[60]

> ## Key Point:
> Articular cartilage health requires regular, controlled loading and unloading.

Canine studies have revealed significantly decreased articular cartilage thickness, hyaluronic acid content, and proteoglycan content following six weeks of cast immobilization. These changes reversed with simple ambulation after three weeks. Research has shown that intense and frequent loading after immobilization can both prevent and worsen the condition of the articular cartilage following immobilization. The rehabilitation clinician should be careful when working with a previously immobilized joint by mobilizing the joint enough to improve the condition of the articular surface, while not stressing the joint excessively, thereby causing further articular cartilage damage.[50,51] Unfortunately the precise formula for mixing therapeutic exercise volume components such as intensity and frequency are currently not well understood, so the rehabilitation clinician should proceed guardedly, particularly with older clients who have undergone prolonged bed rest or immobilization.

Long periods of immobilization can cause irreversible joint damage. Following prolonged disuse the joint space and articular cartilage will be replaced with fibro-fatty tissue leading to fibrous ankylosis. Once fibro-fatty tissue invades the joint space, any forceful attempt to move the affected joint will result in trauma and tearing of the remaining joint lining. This will result in further scarring and worsening function of the already debilitated joint. Animal studies have revealed that the time needed to cause irreversible joint surface damage may be as little as one month of immobilization.[50,51]

Prolonged joint immobilization causes articular cartilage damage in two main ways. The first way, *compression necrosis*, is the result of continuous pressure being placed on an immobilized articular surface preventing the synovial fluid within a joint from bathing the compressed articular cartilage. The lack of synovial fluid flowing over the compressed articular cartilage results in necrosis because the cartilage is unable to extract needed nutrients from the synovial fluid to remain healthy.[50,51]

Key Point:

Joint movement creates a pumping action to deliver nutrients to and remove waste from the articular cartilage. Compression removes fluids and metabolic wastes and unloading allows for the articular cartilage matrix to resorb nutrient-rich synovial fluid to support metabolic needs.

The second method of articular cartilage damage during prolonged immobilization has been termed *obliterative degeneration*. This occurs when an articular surface of a joint is no longer in contact with an opposing articular surface for a prolonged period of time, resulting in the articular surface being in constant contact with the synovial membrane within the joint. Research has found that constant contact between the synovial membrane and articular cartilage results in the two tissues becoming adherent to one another. This adherence also prevents the bathing of the articular cartilage with synovial fluid. The articular cartilage then becomes necrotic from a lack of nutrients it normally extracts from regular contact with synovial fluid.[50,51]

One of the most commonly seen examples of articular cartilage dysfunction secondary to immobilization or disuse occurs at the glenohumeral joint of the shoulder in association with adhesive capsulitis. This condition commonly occurs following prolonged use of a sling to treat a rotator cuff tear, acromioclavicular joint separation, or clavicle fracture. Adhesive capsulitis is more common in older clients and those with other chronic conditions such as diabetes mellitus. With this condition, decreased glenohumeral joint range of motion leads to progressive articular cartilage degeneration. If left untreated, the joint condition progressively deteriorates. Early treatment is mobilization of the affected joint. If this does not improve the functional status of the shoulder, the final therapy is mobilization under anesthesia.

Therapeutic exercise following short-term immobilization has been shown to reverse its adverse effects.[56,57] The duration of the immobilization,[57,61] the type of immobilization used,[56] the joint involved[47] and the post-immobilization therapeutic exercise intensity[59] have all been shown to influence the ability of the articular cartilage to return to a normal state following immobilization. Using a canine model, Palmoski and Brandt[59] reported that low intensity therapeutic exercise following immobi-

lization restored normal articular cartilage more effectively than high intensity running exercise. Their results suggest that alternative periods of unloading and loading should be used, and, in the early stages of therapeutic exercise programs, unloaded periods should be longer than loaded periods and quick movements should be employed.[53] Jurvelin et al.[57] reported that 15 weeks of therapeutic exercise following 11 weeks of immobilization improved canine articular cartilage, but was unable to completely restore its original mechanical properties. Suh et al.[62] reported that both active and passive joint motion after articular cartilage injury may facilitate healing as long as the shear forces are minimized. Articular cartilage can withstand compressive loads, but shear forces can create lesions at the interface between the calcified and uncalcified layers.[63] Continuous passive motion has been shown to be beneficial in the repair of animal articular cartilage defects,[50] with one study recommending six hours of continuous passive motion per day to maximize articular cartilage repair.[64] Using a rabbit model, Shimizu et al.[64] reported that eight hours continuous passive motion helped to facilitate articular cartilage repair; however, if its application was delayed by one week immobilization, it was ineffective. In animal studies, passive range of motion is reportedly effective at promoting a high quality of tissue during the early recovery of articular cartilage lesions that also involved subchondral bone.[47,65] Shear stress in combination with compression of articular cartilage may adversely affect healing, but controlled compression alone may prove beneficial.[62]

NEUROMUSCULAR EFFECTS OF IMMOBILIZATION AND DISUSE

Immobilization or disuse invokes many responses at the neuromuscular junction. The first change seen shortly after initiation of disuse is a decrease in the electrical efficiency within the muscle. This decreased electrical efficiency leads to an increased amount of electromyographic activity within the motor neuron to achieve the same level of force. Decreased neuromuscular junction efficiency has been seen following a short, seven day space flight.[66] This change in neuromuscular efficiency could be the result of a motor neuron not being able to activate as many functioning motor units following disuse. Five weeks of cast immobilization of the human thenar muscles results in a 57 percent decrease in maximal voluntary isometric contraction force, a 29 percent reduction in the number of functioning motor units, and decreased reflex activation; however, these changes are reversed following 18 weeks of strength or resistance training.[67]

After immobilizing the human thumb for six weeks in a plaster cast following forearm fracture, Duchateau and Hainaut[68] reported a 55 percent amplitude decrease in maximal adductor pollicis muscle voluntary isometric contractions and a 33 percent decrease in electrically evoked maximal *tetanic contractions* (sustained contraction of a whole muscle without intervals of relaxation). Decreased maximal tetanic contraction levels are associated with an increased maximal rate of tension development and a decreased maximal rate of relaxation (**Figure 1.6**). These results suggest that immobilization not only modifies the peripheral neuromuscular processes associated with contraction, but they also change the central and/or peripheral neural command of the contraction.[68] They proposed that changes in intracellular contraction processes played the major role in the contractile impairment observed during immobilization.[68]

The relationship between mean motor neuron firing rate and mean submaximal voluntary muscle force levels of human thenar muscles both before and after immobilization have also been studied. Both during and immediately following immobilization the mean motor neuron firing rate needed to elicit a specific sub-maximal voluntary muscle force is decreased, while the twitch force is increased.[69] Reasons for these neuromuscular changes are not fully understood. Decreased voluntary muscle forces may simply be explained by atrophy. The increased *muscle twitch* strength (a brief contractile response of a skeletal muscle elicited by a single maximal volley of impulses in the motor neurons supplying it) at submaximal force levels could be a result of slower re-uptake of calcium by muscle sarcoplasmic reticulum following immobilization. This may result in an adaptation of the excitation-contraction coupling of the neuromuscular unit. Reduced mean maximum motor neuron firing rate may also partially explain some of the muscle weakness, but why and how this develops needs to be studied further.[69] During bed rest and immobilization, the functional level of the neuromuscular unit changes. Why and how these changes occur are not completely understood and warrant further research.

Following lower leg fracture, White and Davies[70] reported that the contractile properties of human calf muscles displayed 51 percent and 46 percent reduced maximal tetanic contractions at 10 and 20 Hz, respectively, and the force of maximal voluntary isometric contraction was decreased by 50 percent. Since the injured leg displayed a faster time to peak tension, they surmised that greater type I (slow twitch) muscle fiber atrophy may have occurred.[70] Booth[71] reported that decreased muscle protein synthesis rates begin during the initial six hours following immobilization and after several weeks of immobilization slow twitch muscle fibers began to develop properties that resembled fast twitch muscle fibers.[71] In evaluating the effects of strength training and limb immobilization on human thenar muscles, Sale et al.[67] reported that five weeks of immobilization resulted in a 42 percent decrease in voluntary isometric muscle strength, a 37 percent reduction in reflex amplitude, 25 percent decreased twitch tension, and an 8 percent decreased contraction time. They concluded that both neural and muscular adaptations occurred in response to immobilization, and that strength training prior to immobilization provided a reserve of neuromuscular function that helped to attenuate the effects of immobilization.[67]

MacDougall et al.,[72] in studying the effects of strength training and immobilization on human muscle fibers using tissue biopsies, reported that five to six weeks of upper extremity immobilization in elbow casts resulted in atrophy at both fast twitch (33 percent) and slow twitch (25 percent) muscle fibers.

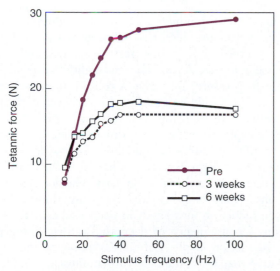

Figure 1.6   The effects of immobilization on the stimulus frequency–force relationship. Note how the tetanic force achieved at each stimulus frequency is reduced following three and six weeks of bed rest. (From Seki K, et al. *J Physiol.* 2001;530.3:507–519.)

Because short-term limb immobilization produces selective adaptations in the neuromuscular system that probably interact with the task-dependent expression of muscle fatigue, Yue et al.[73] studied the effects of elbow joint immobilization on the ability of human subjects to sustain low and moderate submaximal isometric muscle forces. They reported that four weeks of immobilization resulted in a significant reduction in biceps brachii cross sectional area and volume as measured by magnetic resonance imaging, and a decline in maximum voluntary isometric contraction amplitude and force of the elbow flexor muscles.[73] Immobilization had a task-dependent effect on muscle fatigue, with a substantially increased endurance time (less fatigue) at a low (20 percent maximum voluntary isometric contraction) force and no effect at a moderate (65 percent maximum voluntary isometric contraction) force. Despite atrophy, biceps brachii muscle twitch force elicited by electrical stimulation was increased following immobilization. This selective fatigue resistance improvement for the low force contraction suggests that immobilization induced adaptations included an improved efficiency of some excitation-contraction processes, supporting the role of these mechanisms in determining muscular endurance time during relatively low force, long duration contractions.[73]

> ## *Key Point:*
> Immobilization-induced neuromuscular adaptations may include improved efficiency of some excitation-contraction processes during relatively low force, long duration contractions.

Duchateau and Hainaut,[74] in studying the effect of six to eight weeks of immobilization on human adductor pollicis and first dorsal interosseous muscle contractile properties and motor unit activation characteristics, reported that both low threshold (slow twitch) and high threshold (fast twitch) motor units showed proportional twitch tension magnitude decreases and timing delays. Although more high-threshold motor units were recorded as a percentage of maximal voluntary isometric contraction in disused muscles than in control muscles, and maximal firing or activation rate was decreased for both motor unit types, this decrease was greater in the low threshold motor units.

CARDIOVASCULAR EFFECTS OF IMMOBILIZATION AND DISUSE

Bed rest evokes both central and peripheral changes in the cardiovascular system. One of the first changes seen during bed rest is a decrease in the client's plasma volume. This decrease is associated with a 5–25 percent decrease in red blood cell mass. The reduced red blood cell mass is not associated with a significant decrease in a client's hemoglobin or hematocrit because of the above mentioned decrease in plasma volume. This decrease in plasma volume and red blood cell mass seen during bed rest are generally not identified on a complete blood count and for that reason are largely overlooked.[75]

Decreased cardiac stroke volume is associated with bed rest. Cardiac stroke volume is the amount of blood pumped from the left ventricle with each beat into the peripheral circulation. Some of this can be explained by the decrease in plasma volume during bed rest changing the left ventricular filling pressure. This decreased filling pressure would decrease cardiac stroke volume as described in the *Frank-Starling curve.* The Frank-Starling curve is the cardiac stroke volume response to different filling pressures. As filling pressure increases, stroke volume increases, and as filling pressure decreases, stroke volume decreases. The change in filling pressure only partially explains the reduced left ventricular stroke volume. When clients who undergo bed rest are compared to control subjects with similar filling pressure, the cardiac stroke volumes of the bed rest clients are still significantly lower even when corrected for the left ventricular end diastolic volume. This suggests that bed rest causes an unexplained decrease in left ventricular blood inflow, resulting in a decrease in left ventricular stroke volume.[76,77]

> ## *Key Point:*
> Prolonged bed rest results in decreased inflow into the left ventricle, resulting in decreased left ventricular stroke volume.

The decreased filling pressure alone does not completely explain the decreased left ventricular stroke volume observed during bed rest. It is believed that a decrease in cardiac *distensibility* (the ability to expand in response to pressure) may play a role in decreased stroke volume. This would best explain the shift seen in the pressure–volume relationship displayed in **Figure 1.7.** One possible explanation for the postulated decreased cardiac distensibility is cardiac remodeling. Following both bed rest and space flight, researchers have found a 5 to 12 percent decrease in cardiac muscle mass. The decrease in cardiac mass may be attributed to many things. Plasma volume reduction may result in decreased cardiac muscle mass as a consequence of decreased cardiac filling pressure. Reduction in physical activity reducing the cardiac workload may also stimulate cardiac muscle remodeling. Similar cardiac muscle remodeling has been observed with increased cardiac muscle mass following increased exercise or increased cardiac filling pressure as a result of diastolic hypertension.[76]

Maximal oxygen uptake (VO_{2max}) is a measure of oxygen delivery to peripheral tissue and is a measurement of

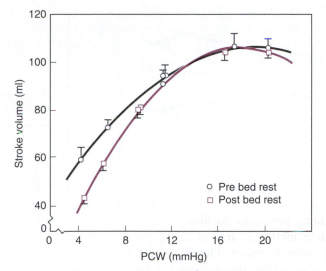

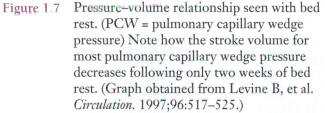

Figure 1.7   Pressure–volume relationship seen with bed rest. (PCW = pulmonary capillary wedge pressure) Note how the stroke volume for most pulmonary capillary wedge pressure decreases following only two weeks of bed rest. (Graph obtained from Levine B, et al. *Circulation.* 1997;96:517–525.)

cardiovascular function. The maximal oxygen uptake measurements of clients following bed rest are not as decreased as expected from decreased left ventricular stroke volume because of a compensatory increase in both maximal and submaximal heart rate following bed rest.

This significant increase in heart rate does not completely compensate for the decreased stroke volume, but it does improve *cardiac output* because cardiac output is the product of cardiac rate multiplied by stroke volume. The increased heart rate seen after bed rest is believed to be a result of increased sensitivity of beta-adrenergic cardiac receptors and increased sympathetic secretion of norepinephrine. This is supported by the findings that there is increased norepinephrine levels at maximal exercise following bed rest, and the heart rate response to isoproterenol, another beta receptor agonist, is increased following bed rest.[72] Maximal oxygen uptake studies have also revealed that the more *cardiac reserve* (capacity for increasing volume or activation rate under differing stress levels) the client has, or the greater their level of physical fitness, the greater his or her percent loss of cardiac output.[75]

> ## Key Point:
> Prolonged bed rest creates increased maximal and submaximal heart rates.

The cardiovascular effects of bed rest include decreased stroke volume and increased heart rate. These changes

may be more significant to remember in clients who have cardiac conditions that limit function, such as coronary artery disease, congestive heart failure, cardiomyopathies, or cardiac valve disorders. These cardiac conditions all can cause decreased baseline cardiac stroke volumes and limits on heart rate. The rehabilitation clinician needs to find out about the baseline cardiovascular status of the client prior to bed rest to establish a baseline for the cardiac changes that occur due to bed rest. In Virgil's case, for example, the therapeutic exercise program would require modification if he had also suffered from a cardiac valve defect or congestive heart failure.

PULMONARY EFFECTS OF IMMOBILIZATION AND DISUSE

The effects of immobilization on the pulmonary system can be devastating (**Figure 1.8**). McGuire et al.,[78] in a 30-year study of five healthy subjects, reported that three weeks of bed rest when these subjects were 20 years of age had a more profound impact on their capacity for physical work than did three decades of aging. Decreased pulmonary capacity and secretions that are not mobilized effectively set the stage for pneumonia and *atelectasis* (a shrunken or airless state affecting all or part of the lung). Immobilized clients spend most of their time in the supine position or some variation thereof. This is especially the case with dependent clients who are not on a regular turning schedule imposed by a health care worker or caregiver. In supine position, the abdominal contents press on the diaphragm; the diaphragm moves upward, limiting lung expansion and *tidal volume* (the amount of air inhaled and exhaled with each breath); and the respiratory rate increases to compensate, but breaths tend to be shallow.[79] The normal *functional residual capacity* in the lungs (the volume of air that remains in the lungs between breaths) is reduced by an average of 800 cc in the supine position.[80]

Gravity also plays a role, shunting blood flow and secretions to dependent areas in the lung. The shallow breaths described above cause most of the air exchange to occur in the top of the lungs, where there is the least blood flow. Dependent pulmonary edema occurs secondary to the shift of blood and fluids in the lung, increasing the risk of severe dyspnea and even pulmonary emboli. These positional factors cause a decrease in PO_2 (partial pressure of arterial oxygen) and oxygen saturation in the blood. The client may become hypoxemic even at rest.[79,81,82]

The horizontal position of bed rest affects lung function; however, it is not the only factor. Respiratory muscles are underused and lose strength with immobilization. Weak respiratory muscles make it more difficult for the client to breathe deeply and effectively. Chest wall expansion decreases. Tidal volume is decreased, even when the

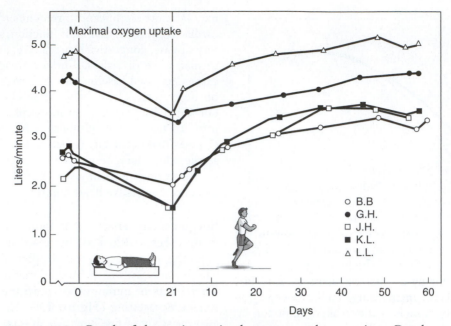

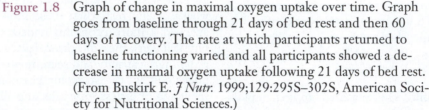

Figure 1.8   Graph of change in maximal oxygen uptake over time. Graph goes from baseline through 21 days of bed rest and then 60 days of recovery. The rate at which participants returned to baseline functioning varied and all participants showed a decrease in maximal oxygen uptake following 21 days of bed rest. (From Buskirk E. *J Nutr.* 1999;129:295S–302S, American Society for Nutritional Sciences.)

client is positioned with the head of the bed elevated. Weak respiratory muscles, dependence on a supine position, and pain all contribute to a weak and ineffective cough with bed rest. A weak cough hampers the ability to effectively clear secretions.

> ## *Key Point:*
> Weak respiratory muscles, the amount of time spent in a supine position and pain all contribute to a weak and ineffective cough during prolonged bed rest.

An inability to clear secretions is a problem because retained secretions can occlude air passages. Occluded air passages may cause alveoli to collapse, resulting in atelectasis and hypoventilation. Hypoventilation reduces the exchange of oxygen and carbon dioxide, leading to *hypoxia* (low arterial oxygen levels) and *hypercarbia* (elevated arterial carbon dioxide levels). Retained secretions also increase the risk of developing pneumonia, a common cause of death in immobilized clients.[82,83]

The effects of immobilization on the liver and cardiovascular system can have serious effects on the lungs. Immobilization interferes with normal liver function and coagulation and sets the stage for thrombophlebitis and deep venous thrombosis (DVT). The obvious risk to the pulmonary system is the possibility of a thrombus traveling to the lungs and lodging in a pulmonary artery as a pulmonary embolus. The risk of a pulmonary embolus is increased in clients, like Virgil, who are recovering from fractures of the pelvis, hip, or leg.[84]

The hypoxemic effect of immobilization reduces the oxygen available to cells, impairing cellular function. Oxygen is necessary for collagen synthesis, and an inadequate supply of oxygen to the cells will hinder tissue repair.

> ## *Key Point:*
> Having sufficient oxygen available at the cellular level is vital to tissue repair.

The irony is that many clients, including Virgil, are immobilized following an injury or surgery to enhance tissue repair, but immobilization is creating a state of *hypoxemia* (low arterial blood oxygen concentration) that impedes the ability of tissues to heal. The rehabilitation clinician should consider the pulmonary effects of immobilization on the tissue-healing rate and include deep breathing, trunk excursion exercises, and effective coughing in the treatment plan. Clients should be taught to breathe deeply and cough throughout the day, not just during therapeutic exercise sessions. The importance of these simple activities in promoting healing and decreasing the risk of pulmonary edema and pneumonia should be emphasized to clients and their caregivers.

HEMATOLOGICAL EFFECTS OF IMMOBILIZATION AND DISUSE

In conjunction with decreased cardiac output, prolonged bed rest also affects peripheral blood flow. Doppler flow studies of multiple major vessels have shown a decrease in blood flow to the abdominal aorta and femoral arteries following bed rest. In the same subjects, flow in the common carotid arteries was unchanged after bed rest. These findings suggest that the body adapts to the decreased cardiac output by decreasing blood flow to less important organs while maintaining blood flow to the heart and brain.

> ## Key Point:
> The body adapts to decreased cardiac output from prolonged bed rest by decreasing blood flow to areas other than the heart and brain.

These findings may need to be further studied, and other discoveries could change the therapies currently used to treat peripheral vascular disease with non-healing ulcers that many times involve bed rest, anticoagulation medication, and no weight bearing.[85]

Clients undergoing bed rest are at increased risk of developing deep venous thrombosis and pulmonary embolism. Deep vein thrombosis is the development of a blood clot in a peripheral deep vein, most commonly in the leg. Pulmonary emboli occur when a deep vein thrombus travels through the blood stream and lodges within the pulmonary vasculature, negating blood flow in the area of the lung distal to where it lodges. The larger the clot is, the more effect it has on blood oxygenation. A large pulmonary embolus can be fatal. Some common signs of a pulmonary embolus are tachycardia, tachypnea, chest pain, and hypoxia.

> ## Key Point:
> Common signs of a pulmonary embolus are tachycardia, tachypnea chest pain, and hypoxia.

As discussed earlier in the chapter, plasma volume decreases during bed rest. This results in increased blood viscosity and a hypercoagulable state. Not only are immobilized clients in a hypercoagulable state—they also have increased venous stasis in their lower extremities.[86] This is a result of a decrease in muscle pumping in the lower extremities, forcing blood return back to the heart. The signs and symptoms of a deep vein thrombosis are displayed in **Figure 1.9.**

INTEGUMENTARY EFFECTS OF IMMOBILIZATION AND DISUSE

Integumentary effects of immobilization and disuse are many times overlooked. Increased *turgidity* (swollen beyond the natural state) and atrophy of the skin may occur with immobilization, increasing fragility and risk of injury. Limitations in mobility and activity are the primary risk factors for pressure ulcers. The prevalence of hospitalized clients with pressure sores ranges from 3.5 percent to 29.5 percent, with the highest number being among those with long-term disability or being cared for in an intensive care unit. Clients with musculoskeletal injuries have an especially high risk of integumentary problems associated with prolonged immobilization, disuse, or bed rest. Clients hospitalized for fractures are at a higher risk than those who are admitted for elective procedures. Elderly clients hospitalized for femoral fractures are in the highest risk group, with a 66 percent incidence of pressure ulcers reported.[87–89] It is reported that 8–25 percent of hospitalized clients undergoing three weeks of bed rest or restricted chair activity develop pressure ulcers. Additionally, up to 20 percent of home care clients develop pressure ulcers, also called pressure sores.[90] Pressure sores are very important to health care providers not only because of cost, but also because nursing home clients with pressure ulcers have a two to six times higher mortality rate than those who do not.[91]

A pressure ulcer is defined as a localized area of soft tissue injury resulting from compression of an external surface by a bony prominence. Pressure ulcers are divided into four different stages. A stage one pressure ulcer is identified as an area of soft tissue with non-blanching erythema. In highly pigmented skin, stage one pressure ulcers may be characterized by purple discoloration and

> Pain
>
> Edema
>
> Warmth
>
> Palpable thrombus cord in calf or thigh
>
> Pain with ankle flexion

Figure 1.9   Common clinical markers (signs and symptoms) of a deep venous thrombosis.

local warmth and induration. A stage two pressure ulcer develops when there is partial-thickness skin loss, and presents as a shallow crater or blister. When the ulcer extends through the entire skin thickness and into the subcutaneous tissue it is a stage three pressure ulcer. A stage four pressure ulcer is present when the tissue damage extends beyond the fascia to muscle, bone, tendon, joint capsule, or other supporting structures. A pictorial representation of different stages of pressure ulcers is presented in **Figure 1.10.** Allman et al.[92] reported that non-blanchable erythema, lymphopenia, immobility, dry skin, and decreased body weight are independent and significant risk factors for pressure ulcer development among hospitalized clients whose activities are restricted to bed or chair.

In healthy clients, capillary filling pressure is about 32 mm Hg. When a client undergoing bed rest exerts a pressure > 32 mm Hg over any soft tissue the result is hypoxia. This hypoxia results in the formation of pressure ulcers. Tissue damage can be observed after only one to two hours of 60 mm Hg applied to a soft tissue. This is important because clients lying in a hospital bed have sacral soft tissue pressure measurements as high as 100–150 mm Hg. In the seated position the pressure can be as high as 300 mm Hg. Studies have shown that clients who move spontaneously 50 times a night or who are turned by health care staff every two hours are at significantly lower risk of developing pressure ulcers. Other methods of pressure ulcer reduction include the use of special mattresses or pads placed on the client to further protect the skin.[91]

Pressure ulcers are also the result of shear force, friction, moisture, and chemical irritants. Rehabilitation clinicians must limit the shear force and friction a client's skin is exposed to. Shear force and friction are the forces placed on the skin when a client slides in bed and the moving skin rubs against a stationary object. Friction of the skin across rough sheets most often results in superficial injuries: abrasions, blisters, and skin tears. Shearing forces are more serious and contribute to deep ulcers that may not be noticed until they reach stage three. Shearing is especially problematic over the sacrum when the head of the bed is elevated. With the head of the bed elevated 30° or more (**Figure 1.11**), a high coefficient of friction keeps the skin and superficial fascia over the sacrum fixed against the bed linens, while gravity pulls deep fascia and the skeletal frame toward the foot of the bed. The shearing forces between tissue layers produce torsion in the blood vessels between these tissues, resulting in blood supply occlusion and tissue ischemia. This, in combination with loose skin due to atrophy of the underlying musculature, may further exacerbate the problem. The semi-Fowler's position, as depicted in **Figure 1.11,** may be most comfortable, but the Agency for Healthcare Research and Quality recommends keeping the head of the bed at the lowest possible level consistent with medical conditions and other restrictions to prevent pressure ulcers.[93]

Moisture and chemical irritants increase the risk of pressure ulcers. The most common sources of chemical irritants are the client's urine, stool, or sweat. Prolonged

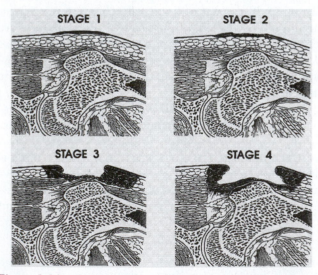

Figure 1.10   Pressure ulcer classification. Stage 1, non-blanchable erythema. Stage 2, partial-thickness skin loss. Stage 3, full thickness skin loss. Stage 4, full thickness skin loss with underlying tissue destruction and damage. (Redrawn from Smith D. *Annals Int Med.* 1995:123:433–442.)

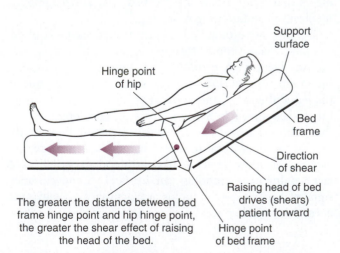

Figure 1.11   Semi-Fowler position and pressure ulcer development. (Redrawn from Sussman C, Bates-Jensen B. *Wound Care: A Collaborative Practice Manual for Physical Therapists and Nurses,* 2nd ed. Gaithersburg, MD: Aspen Publishers, 2001.)

> ### Key Point:
> If possible, given the client's medical condition and other restrictions, the head of the bed should be maintained at the lowest possible level to prevent pressure ulcer formation.

contact with moisture causes skin to become macerated. Macerated skin is more fragile than dry skin, and will break down with less force and in less time than dry skin. All of these risks for developing pressure ulcers can be minimized by following proper care guidelines about moving clients and keeping them clean.[91]

Skin breakdown is often overlooked in a client with multiple medical problems. The skin is a barrier to the outside world. Pressure ulcers create an opening for infections that can lead to serious health consequences for a client who is immobilized or bed ridden. The health care team must focus on daily skin care in bed-ridden clients to reduce the risk of pressure ulcer formation.[94] Every client whose mobility is limited to bed or chair, even temporarily, should be assessed for risk of skin breakdown. Risk assessment tools, such as the Braden Scale or Norton Scale, only take a minute or two to complete.[95] An example of the Braden Scale is shown in **Table 1.1.**

GASTROINTESTINAL EFFECTS OF IMMOBILIZATION AND DISUSE

The inactivity and positional restrictions associated with immobilization contribute to decreases in gastrointestinal motility and gastric secretions. Nausea, loss of appetite, and constipation are commonly experienced. These problems can increase the client's discomfort, and more critically, can negatively affect the rate of healing. Clients who are immobilized following an injury or surgery must have an adequate intake of calories and fluids for tissue repair to occur. Unfortunately, immobilized clients often restrict their food and fluid intake secondary to the loss of appetite, nausea, and gastrointestinal discomfort.

> ### Key Point:
> Adequate hydration and intake of calories are necessary for tissue repair to occur; however, immobilized clients often restrict their food and fluid intake secondary to loss of appetite, nausea, and gastrointestinal discomfort.

Food and fluid intake may also be decreased because of mechanical difficulties associated with the immobilized body part. Swallowing is difficult in the recumbent position and is awkward even when the head of the bed is elevated. Taste and smell may be impaired by immobilization and by prescribed drugs, further decreasing appetite. Gastric secretions are also decreased by immobilization. Consequently, whatever food the client does take in may not be sufficiently digested. The catabolic processes from immobilization result in a negative nitrogen balance as early as the sixth to tenth day and can cause anorexia.[82]

The physiological fluid shifts associated with immobility, especially in the first few days, can also result in nausea and constipation. The client may lose 600 cc of fluid in the first two days, and 15 to 20 percent of their fluid volume within two weeks of bed rest.[96] This loss of fluid by *diuresis* (secretion of large amounts of urine) compounds problems associated with the previously mentioned inadequate fluid intake. Supplemental intravenous fluids may be used to offset this loss during a hospital stay, but may be impractical for the client who is recovering at home.

Inactivity decreases the accustomed external compression from the abdominal muscles on the intestines. The recumbent position also eliminates the gravitational force on the gut. The loss of these external forces conspires to decrease peristalsis, or bowel motility. Constipation and discomfort from intestinal gas (*flatus*) often occurs. Decreased fluid intake and the physiological fluid shift discussed above increases the problem with constipation. Prolonged, severe constipation can lead to fecal impaction requiring medical intervention. *Paralytic ileus* is an extreme variation of decreased gastrointestinal motility, and may occur if the reason for immobilization is major trauma or surgery.[82] Oral intake is restricted until *peristalsis* (smooth muscle contractions propelling foodstuffs distally through the gastrointestinal system) recurs, which can augment the negative nitrogen balance and impair healing. Our client Virgil can avoid or counteract the decrease in gastric mobility by performing isometric abdominal and pelvic stabilization exercises that increase compression on the gut. His family and the rehabilitation clinician should encourage Virgil to eat and drink frequently during the day to ensure that he takes in enough calories to heal, and enough fluids to maintain normal hydration and avoid constipation.

URINARY EFFECTS OF IMMOBILIZATION AND DISUSE

The effects of immobility and disuse on the urinary system begins with an initial increase in diuresis and can escalate to urinary distension, loss of the sensation to void, urinary stasis, frequent infections, a decreased glomerular filtration rate, and renal calculi formation.[97]

The early increase in diuresis occurs as a result of an extracellular-to-intracellular fluid shift triggered by adopting a primarily recumbent position. Immobility triggers

Key Point:

Immobility and disuse may increase diuresis, urinary distention, loss of sensation to void, urinary stasis, frequent urinary tract infections, renal calculi formation and decrease glomerular filtration rate.

release of a surge of aldosterone, boosting the renin-angiotensin cycle that regulates the excretion of sodium and water.[84] Activation of renal and hormonal receptors results in the loss of approximately 600 cc of extracellular fluid volume by the second day of immobilization. The client may lose 15 to 20 percent of their fluid volume within two weeks of bed rest.[96]

This physiological fluid shift causes an initial increase in urine production, requiring clients to void more frequently. Unfortunately, this early immobilization period frequently coincides with the early post trauma or post surgical period when mobility is most restricted and clients have the most difficulty using bedpans or urinals independently. Urinary catheters can be useful for dealing with this increase in urine production, but are not practical in the home setting. Early discharge to home may result in clients needing to deal with bedpans and urinals when they are still in the increased diuresis phase.

Immobilized clients often avoid urination because they are embarrassed to use a bedpan or urinal, or to ask a family member to empty it. This avoidance of urination causes over-distension of the detrusser muscles of the bladder, and, over time, to a decreased sensation to void. Clients who do not feel, or who suppress or ignore, the need to void can develop additional problems with urinary retention, difficulty voiding, overflow incontinence, stasis, *post void residuals* (the amount of urine that remains in the bladder after urination), and an increased risk of urinary tract infections.

Non–weight bearing status can affect the urinary system as well. The demineralization of calcium and phosphorus that occurs when long bones do not receive normal weight bearing forces was addressed earlier in this chapter. The excessive amounts of calcium and phosphorous released from the bones into the blood is filtered by the kidneys, and can predispose clients to the formation of renal calculi (kidney stones).[82]

METABOLIC EFFECTS
OF IMMOBILIZATION AND DISUSE

The metabolic effects of bed rest are beginning to be studied more closely. A study of 14 healthy subjects who underwent 20 days of bed rest with consistent daily caloric intake revealed that lean body mass, body fat percentage, and levels of total cholesterol, high density lipoproteins

(HDL), low density lipoproteins (LDL), triglycerides, and free fatty acids did not change. However, it is speculated that during longer periods of bed rest the HDL cholesterol (good cholesterol) may decrease as a result of a decrease in apolipoprotein-AI seen during 20 days of bed rest. Apolipoprotein-AI is contained within HDL cholesterol particles.[98]

Glucose tolerance testing of clients has revealed no change in serum glucose concentration following oral glucose loading during or after bed rest. Research has proven that insulin sensitivity decreases and the peak insulin concentration following an oral bolus of glucose is delayed during bed rest. It is believed the reduced insulin sensitivity is due to inactive muscles responding less efficiently to insulin. This hypothesis is not completely proven and further research is ongoing.[98]

There have been conflicting reports on the effects of bed rest on basal metabolic rate. Some studies report a slight decrease in basal metabolic rate during bed rest and others report no change. *Basal metabolic rate* is the measurement of the body's oxygen consumption at basal or resting conditions. It is very difficult to measure basal metabolism and for this reason no definitive answer on the effects of bed rest has been developed. It is postulated that basal metabolic rate decreases and many studies now support this notion. Further research is needed to solidify this hypothesis.[98] When appetite eventually returns, the combination of a decreased metabolic rate, prolonged bed rest or immobilization, and reduced lean body mass would contribute to the client having a relative increase in percent bodyfat, placing them potentially at risk for conditions associated with obesity.[99]

Clients with confounding metabolic disorders such as diabetes mellitus can have severe metabolic consequences from bed rest and immobilization if the condition is not addressed appropriately. Other metabolic changes described above, if not addressed, may also lead to poor client health.

PSYCHOSOCIAL CONSIDERATIONS

Psychosocial concerns have a significant effect on healing and rehabilitation. Some important aspects to consider include the client's insurance, family support, and return to work issues. The impact of changes in function or inde-

Key Point:

The impact of changes in functional status or independence affects how clients view themselves, their role and interaction with family members, friends, and co-workers.

pendence, short term or long term, affects how the client views him- or herself, and his or her role and interactions with family, friends, and work cohorts.[100]

Virgil has been a physically active cattle rancher. His family is believed to be supportive, but what is the extent of their ability to assume Virgil's responsibilities in addition to their own? Who is caring for the cattle and assuming responsibility for all aspects of his farm business? Can Virgil's wife and son take over the care of the cattle until Virgil is able to do so? If not, who is, and at what cost? Concerns about the business impact of his injury and rehabilitation may be an overriding concern for Virgil, and could impact his decisions about participating in a therapeutic exercise program. Attempting to rush the process by weight bearing too soon, too much, or too often, or attempting physical farm activities before he has regained the strength, endurance and flexibility required for these activities may result in re-injury and prolonged disability. Virgil's physician and rehabilitation clinician must emphasize that he will need to recover strength, coordination, and agility before he will be able to safely resume many of his routine daily activities. A sequenced return may be possible and advantageous for Virgil's "peace of mind."

DISABILITY AND QUALITY OF LIFE

The health care industry has recently shifted its focus more from treating various diseases and conditions to health promotion and disease prevention.[100,101] This provides goals of preventing disease, morbidity, and mortality rather than previous goals of health care oriented towards treating conditions once they occur. In turn, the health care industry has spent millions of dollars on health screening programs and health promotion. This trend in health promotion and prevention must now take the next step and encompass not only healthy individuals, but clients with disabilities and chronic illnesses as well. Some of the major secondary conditions that clients with disabilities face are obesity, hypertension, and pressure sores. Many clients with disabilities are bed ridden and experience the ill effects of bed rest described earlier in this chapter as a result (**Table 1.2**).[101]

The state of a client's health shifts back and forth on a continuum. This is true for both clients with disabilities and those who are considered healthy. For example, a client with spastic cerebral palsy will always have some disability. Prevention includes adequate nutrition, prevention of pressure sores, regular medical check ups, and therapeutic exercise program intervention to help keep the client at his or her personal peak of health. Denial of these treatments results in poorer health and most likely a lesser quality of life. Clients with permanent disabilities start at a lower point on the health continuum and therefore may actually need more health promotion and prevention than healthy individuals. This is because a minor illness in a disabled client may compromise his or her functional mobility and independence in daily living to a greater extent. The same illness in an individual with no disability may have little to no effect on his or her daily life.[101]

Key Point:

Individuals with permanent disabilities may need more health promotion and prevention than healthy individuals. Even a minor illness in a disabled client may compromise his or her functional mobility and independence in daily living.

In the document *Healthy People with Disabilities 2010*, the definition of health promotion for clients with disabilities is outlined. The first part is the promotion of healthy lifestyles and a healthy environment. The second is the prevention of further health complications. Third, health care providers should strive to prepare a disabled client to be able to understand and monitor their own health care needs if possible. Finally, health care professionals should promote opportunities for disabled clients to participate in common life activities.[101]

The future goal of the health care industry in preventing further disability has many barriers. Some of the barriers include cost, lack of energy or enthusiasm, lack of knowledge, lack of transportation, and lack of availability. Health care providers must consider these issues when developing a comprehensive strategy and find ways to provide needed services to clients in a timely and cost effective manner. When designing therapeutic exercise programs, the barriers that clients perceive as affecting their ability to effectively participate must be taken into consideration.[101]

In the case described at the outset of this chapter, the client's acute injury had major implications in his ability to function in society until his leg and pelvis were healed. In the model of disability, the goal of all health care providers involved in his care would be to heal his injury as fast as possible. Health care providers must also prevent any further decrement in Virgil's overall health. This would include limiting his health consequences from prolonged bed rest and arranging for health care once the client is discharged from the hospital, taking into account all of the barriers to health care described above. Finally, the goal would be to get the client as far to the right ("healthy" end) along his own individual health continuum as soon as possible without risking his safety.

Definitions of Disability

The concept of *disablement* refers to the impact of health conditions on the function of specific body systems, basic human performance, and the performance of usual,

TABLE 1.1   The Braden Scale for predicting pressure sore risk.

Patient_____	Evaluator_____		Date_____	
				Subscore
Sensory Perception Ability to respond to meaningful pressure related discomfort	**1. Completely Limited** Unresponsive to painful stimuli due to diminished level of consciousness or sedation *or* limited ability to feel pain over most of body.	**2. Very limited** Responds only to painful stimuli. Cannot communicate discomfort except by moaning or restlessness *or* has a sensory impairment which limits ability to feel pain or discomfort over ½ of body.	**3. Slightly Limited** Responds to verbal commands, but cannot always communicate discomfort or need to be turned *or* has some sensory impairment, which limits ability to feel pain or discomfort in one or two extremities.	**4. No Impairment** Responds to verbal commands. Has no sensory deficit, which would limit ability to feel or voice pain or discomfort.
Moisture Degree to which skin is exposed to moisture	**1. Constantly Moist** Skin is kept moist almost constantly by perspiration, urine, etc. Dampness is detected every time patient is moved or turned.	**2. Very Moist** Skin is often, but not always, moist. Linen must be changed at least once a shift.	**3. Occasionally Moist** Skin is occasionally moist, requiring an extra linen change approximately once a day.	**4. Rarely Moist** Skin is usually dry; linen only requires changing at routine intervals.
Activity Degree of physical activity	**1. Bedfast** Confined to bed.	**2. Chairfast** Ability to walk severely limited or non-existent. Cannot bear own weight and/or must be assisted into wheelchair.	**3. Walks Occasionally** Walks occasionally during day, but for very short distances, with or without assistance. Spends majority of each shift in bed or chair.	**4. Walks Frequently** Walks outside room at least twice a day and inside room at least once every two hours during waking hours.
Mobility Ability to change and control body position	**1. Completely Immobile** Does not make even slight changes in body or extremity position without assistance.	**2. Very Limited** Makes occasional slight changes in body or extremity position but unable to make frequent or significant changes independently.	**3. Slightly Limited** Makes frequent though slight changes in body or extremity position independently.	**4. No Limitations** Makes major and frequent changes in position without assistance.

(continued)

The lower the total score, the higher the risk of developing a pressure ulcer.
(Used with permission, copyright Barbara Braden and Nancy Bergstrom, 1988.)

TABLE 1.1   Continued

Nutrition Usual food intake pattern	**1. Very Poor** Never eats a complete meal. Rarely eats more than $\frac{1}{3}$ of any food offered. Eats two servings or less of protein per day. Takes fluids poorly. Does not take a liquid dietary supplement *or* is NPO and/or maintained on clear liquids or IVs for more than five days.	**2. Probably Inadequate** Rarely eats a complete meal and generally eats only about ½ of any food offered. Protein intake includes only three servings per day. Occasionally will take a dietary supplement, *or* receives less than optimum amount of liquid diet or tube feeding.	**3. Adequate** Eats over half of most meals. Eats a total of four servings of protein. Occasionally will refuse a meal, but will usually take a supplement when offered *or* is on tube feeding or Total Parenteral Nutrition (TPN) regimen which probably meets most of nutritional needs.	**4. Excellent** Eats most of every meal. Never refuses a meal. Usually eats a total of four or more servings of meat and dairy products. Occasionally eats between meals. Does not require supplementation.
Friction and Shear	**1. Problem** Requires moderate to maximum assistance in moving. Complete lifting without sliding against sheets is impossible. Frequently slides down in bed or chair, requires frequent repositioning with maximum assistance. Spasticity, contractures or agitation leads to almost constant friction.	**2. Potential Problem** Moves feebly or requires minimum assistance. During a move skin probably slides to some extent against sheets, chair, restraints, or other devices. Maintains relatively good position in chair or bed most of the time but occasionally slides down.	**3. No Apparent Problem** Moves in bed and in chair independently and has sufficient muscle strength to lift up completely during move. Maintains good position in bed or chair.	
			Total Score	

TABLE 1.2   Secondary conditions commonly affecting clients with disabilities that must be taken into account when developing a health care plan

Osteoporosis

Osteoarthritis

Decreased balance

Decreased strength

Decreased endurance

Decreased fitness

Decreased joint flexibility

Decreased musculotendinous extensibility

Increased spasticity

Weight problems

Depression

> ## Key Point:
> Prior to the development of the Nagi model, level of health was based on the disease or pathologic state, not on how the disease or pathologic state affected the client's life.

expected, and personally desired societal roles.[102] Jette[103] stated that disablement is a global term reflecting all of the diverse consequences that disease, injury, or congenital abnormalities may have on human function at many different levels. Disablement also provides a useful framework for identifying important clinical treatment outcomes. According to Jette[103] the purpose for the development of disability models is essentially twofold: 1) to help theorize the potential effects of disease, injury, or congenital abnormalities on the functioning of specific organs or body systems on fundamental physical and mental actions, and on individual behavior or roles in daily life, and 2) to provide a construct for the description of various personal and environmental factors that can accelerate (such as predisposing risk factors) or retard (such as therapeutic exercise intervention) the disablement process. Developed in 1965, the Nagi model[104] (**Figure 1.12**) was the first disability model that examined a client's health status in relation to their disease state. Prior to this, a client's level of health was primarily based directly on the manifestation of a disease or pathologic state, rather than on the magnitude with which the disease or pathologic state affected the client's life.

The *Nagi model* consists of four concepts: pathology, impairment, functional limitation, and disability.[104] Pathology has many potential etiologies including infec-

tion, trauma, degenerative conditions, and disease. *Impairments* occur at the organ level (e.g., knee joint flexion contracture, rotator cuff muscle group weakness). *Functional limitations* are only visible at the level of the whole organism (e.g., dressing, bathing, eating, stair climbing, throwing a ball). Nagi's definition of *disability* refers to a client's inability or limitation in performing socially defined roles. In Virgil's case these include, but are not limited to, his involvement as a husband and father in addition to being a cattle rancher.

The World Health Organization (WHO) developed the *International Classification of Impairment, Disabilities, and Handicaps (ICIDH) model* in the mid-1970s (**Figure 1.13**).[105] Today, treatment of pathology is more likely than ever to result in manageable conditions that are chronic or disabling. Within these conditions, the interaction between impairments and disabilities becomes important. The ICIDH disablement model has four components related to the health state: disease, impairment, disability, and handicap. In this model, the term "disease" refers to changes that occur at the level of the organ (e.g., infection, inflammation, or, as in Virgil's case, a fractured bone). This is quite similar to Nagi's definition for pathology, but not exactly. The ICIDH concept of disease refers specifically to changes in body structure or function. The term impairment is synonymous in both the Nagi and

> ## Key Point:
> The term impairment is the same for both the Nagi and ICIDH models. Examples include pain, swelling, effusion, instability, reduced joint range of motion, muscle weakness, joint laxity, and loss of proprioception or balance.

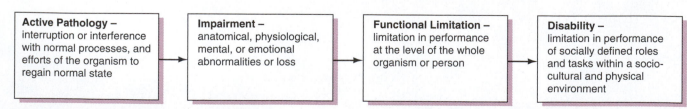

Active Pathology – interruption or interference with normal processes, and efforts of the organism to regain normal state

Impairment – anatomical, physiological, mental, or emotional abnormalities or loss

Functional Limitation – limitation in performance at the level of the whole organism or person

Disability – limitation in performance of socially defined roles and tasks within a sociocultural and physical environment

Figure 1.12   Nagi Disablement Model.[104]

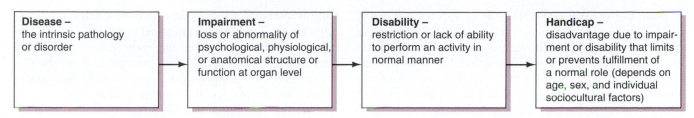

Figure 1.13   International Classification of Impairment, Disabilities, and Handicaps (ICIDH) Model.[105]

ICIDH models. Examples of impairments include pain, swelling, effusion and instability, range of motion restrictions, muscle weakness or fatigue, joint laxity, and loss of proprioception or balance.

In the WHO model disability occurs at the client level, representing a restriction in or lack of ability to perform common activities in a "normal" manner. The definition of disability in the ICIDH model is similar to what the Nagi model describes as functional limitations. Functional limitations include restrictions in the ability to perform activities of daily living, instrumental activities of daily living, and sporting activities.

> ## Key Point:
> According to the Nagi model, functional limitations include any restriction in the ability to perform activities of daily living, instrumental activities of daily living and/or sporting activities.

The term functional limitation is synonymous with activity restriction.[102] The inability to walk up and down stairs, move from sitting to standing or roll over in bed would all be termed disabilities according to the ICIDH model. Any movement limitations that result from impairments would also be categorized as disabilities in the ICIDH model. Disability refers to restrictions in performance of a client's roles in society such as the ability to care for self or others, to work, and to participate in recreational or sporting activities. Disability can be considered synonymous with participation restrictions.

> ## Key Point:
> Disability refers to any restrictions that limit a client's ability to carry out his or her role or to otherwise participate in society. Examples of disabilities include the ability to care for self or others, to work, or to participate in recreational or sporting activities.

The use of the term "handicap" in the ICIDH model refers to societal or social role limitations. Therefore, the ICIDH definition of handicap is comparable to Nagi's concept of disability in that both address limitations imposed by the physical environment, society, or both. In contrast to Nagi's model, handicap, disability, and impairment on the ICIDH model should be considered concurrent interactive concepts, not a hierarchical progression. Recently, the National Center for Medical Rehabilitation Research (NCMRR) proposed a *modified disablement model* that expanded Nagi's model by introducing the concept of *societal limitation* as a separate characteristic of the functional problems associated with disability. According to the NCMRR, societal limitations are restrictions attributable to social policy or barriers (structural or attitudinal) that limit fulfillment of roles or deny access to services and opportunities associated with full participation in society. Societal limitations as described by the NCMRR are similar to the concept of handicap discussed in the ICIDH. No consensus currently exists on any of the conceptual models of disablement described.

Health related quality of life refers to total well being, encompassing physical, social, and psychological domains of health.[106] Health related quality of life is largely based on the client's perception of their health including emotional well being, energy and vitality, sleep and rest, behavioral competence, and general life satisfaction.

> ## Key Point:
> Health related quality of life encompasses physical, social, and psychological domains of health. It includes the client's perception of his or her own health, including emotional well being, energy and vitality, sleep and rest, behavioral competence, and general life satisfaction.

The ability of the client to function without limitation in their role performance (e.g., husband, father, farmer) is an essential component of quality of life. Rehabilitation clinicians must consider whether the client's physical condition or the treatment provided causes dependency on the clinician or depression related to the disability. Either of these factors may limit their role performance. Quality of life is an important consideration in the development of treatment plans and goals. Since quality of life depends on physical, emotional and social functional abilities and interaction with the environment, then these areas must be addressed in rehabilitation. The client's perception of quality of life can have a tremendous influence on motivation and compliance with a therapeutic exercise program. Jette[106] related quality of life directly to the client's ability to relate to his or her environment (**Figure 1.14**); therefore, functional limitations and handicaps or disabilities would have the most influence on quality of life. Continued modification and elaboration of disablement models and health related quality of life measurements are likely to occur, particularly with the recent increases in research support. This continued dialogue has potential for improving interdisciplinary communication and research hypothesis development to further help minimize disability.

The rehabilitation clinician who works with Virgil will become familiar with his pathology from his medical records and while taking his history. Essential to the history-taking interview is the clinician's ability to develop a positive rapport with the client in an effort to develop a comprehensive and accurate understanding of his disabilities, essentially the functional consequences of the pathology. Concurrently from a prevention and wellness perspective, how can a positive health behavior be promoted for Virgil? Considerations need to be given to helping him achieve and restore his optimal level of function, minimizing functional ramifications of his existing impairments, functional limitations, and disabilities, helping prevent further condition deterioration or future illness, and creating appropriate environmental adaptations to enhance independent function.

Prevention of Disability

Prevention should consider three components (primary, secondary and tertiary).[107] *Primary prevention* attempts to deter disease, illness, or pathology in a susceptible or potentially susceptible individual through general health pro-

motion intervention. *Secondary prevention* refers to deterring disease, illness, or pathological condition severity, duration and their sequelae by early identification and intervention. *Tertiary prevention* attempts to limit the disability level and promote the restoration of function in clients with chronic and irreversible disease.

Virgil has sustained two traumatic injuries to his musculoskeletal system, a pubic rami fracture of his pelvis, and a non-displaced tibia fracture. We presently have limited information about Virgil. However, we know that prolonged bed rest, and limited weight bearing may have negative effects on multiple bodily systems. From a primary prevention standpoint, we need to design our therapeutic exercise intervention to decrease Virgil's risk for developing muscle weakness, decreased bone mineral density, depression, a deep vein thrombosis, and so on. From a secondary prevention standpoint, our intervention must also attempt to facilitate the functional recovery of his injured musculoskeletal system. Tertiary prevention does not appear to be an obvious consideration with Virgil; however, if he had degenerative osteoarthritis of his knee on the opposite side of his tibial shaft fracture, we would need to be sure that our therapeutic exercise program design does not promote excessive compensatory weight bearing on the opposite lower extremity, thereby exacerbating his osteoarthritis condition.

THERAPEUTIC EXERCISE AND ITS CONTRAINDICATIONS

Exercise training can provoke myriad beneficial physiologic adaptations.[108] Regular exercise induces physiologic changes that constitute what is termed "the exercise response" representing biochemical alterations in the body's control of metabolism.[109] Even modern intensive care units cannot match the body's extraordinary and sophisticated system for delivery of biochemical compounds during exercise, despite the fact that some natural compounds (including hormones) are often used as prescription drugs.[108]

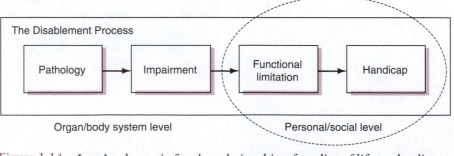

Figure 1.14   Jette's schematic for the relationship of quality of life to the disablement concept. (From Jette AM. Using health related quality of life measures in physical therapy outcomes research. *Phys Ther* 1993;73:528–537.)

From this perspective, exercise itself is "medicine."[108] However, determining the appropriate therapeutic exercise volume, or dosage to reap these positive changes while minimizing exacerbation of an existing medical condition remains a challenge, particularly among older clients.[110]

Although a well designed therapeutic exercise program can benefit numerous body systems, several conditions that either contraindicate therapeutic exercise or more likely warrant program modifications deserve discussion. Specifically, diseases or conditions that affect the cardiovascular or cardiopulmonary system such as coronary artery disease, hypertension, diabetes, obesity, peripheral vascular disease, or conditions that promote heat intolerance, hypernea-dyspnea or increased stress levels warrant careful screening by a cardiologist or similarly prepared physician prior to program initiation. Additionally, clients with a family history of these diseases or conditions or those who undergo pharmaceutical intevention for their control should obtain clearance from a qualified physician prior to initiating a therapeutic exercise program. Disease states that affect connective tissues such as rheumatoid arthritis or lupus erythematosus may require limiting joint range of motion and limiting resistance training to a load that facilitates dynamic joint stability without injuring capsuloligamentous static joint stabilizers, particularly when "flare-ups" periodically appear. Osteoarthritis or degenerative joint disease and osteoporosis may require limited performance of weight bearing activities, particularly tasks that use bounding or plyometric-type training activities. Weight bearing reductions might be easily achieved by changing the therapeutic exercise setting from the clinic to an aquatic therapy environment. Clients with impaired balance or proprioception may benefit from progressive weight bearing activities that require postural control during weight shifting activities in an upright sitting or standing posture, eventually progressing to single leg standing tasks. Many alternative forms of therapeutic exercise provide useful strategies for achieving this end. Blending integrated trunk and lower extremity strength training

with postural control and balance training should enhance the functional relevance of the therapeutic exercise program. Clients with impaired coordination or agility may benefit from therapeutic exercise interventions that incorporate progressively more challenging upper and/or lower extremity movements, first with manual tactile cueing prior to using progressive resistance in the form of free weights or resistive bands.

While the rehabilitation clinician may attempt to bias the therapeutic exercise program focus more toward anerobic or aerobic energy system requirements, it is essential that he or she understand that no single system ever functions completely in isolation and the maintenance of at least baseline function in both systems is necessary for the client to perform all activity of daily living, recreational, and vocational functions. The client who has never participated in an organized therapeutic exercise program before may need additional instruction and evaluation of understanding, proactive strategies to enhance program compliance or adherence, more frequent re-evaluation, and multi-media examples of appropriate performance of a limited number of therapeutic exercises. Consideration of the high "learning curve" associated with the selection of particular therapeutic exercise movements given their potential injury risk-to-benefit ratio also warrants consideration by the rehabilitation clinician. Foundational to the client reaping any benefits from regular therapeutic exercise program participation is an understanding of adequate nutrition and hydration and recovery time between sessions based on intensity level and program focus. Appreciation of the client's level of understanding (particularly regarding attaining their fully informed consent to participate in the program), support system, health locus of control, and real and/or perceived barriers will help the rehabilitation clinician design a therapeutic exercise program that adequately matches the client's individuality as well as functional needs (see Chapter 11). The rehabilitation clinician should also become familiar with both the prescribed (including hormone replacement therapy) and over-the-counter medications and supplements (including herbal preparations) that the client may be taking for musculoskeletal pain-inflammation or neuromuscular contractility and their possible influence on cognition, bone mineral density, tissue healing characteristics, and fatigue. A current copy of the *Physician's Desk Reference*[111] in addition to Internet access to appropriate Web sites and databases provides the rehabilitation clinician with straightforward access to new advances in this area. Consideration of the status of the client's exteroceptive system function (vision, hearing, taste, smell) and use of or need for assistive or adaptive devices will also increase the likelihood of the client achieving his or her goals. Last, preparing the client for an eventual return to full activity and deciding on the appropriate timing of this release are also critical therapeutic exercise program decisions.

Key Point:

Several conditions either contraindicate therapeutic exercise or more likely warrant program modification. Specifically, diseases or conditions that affect the cardiovascular or cardiopulmonary system such as coronary artery disease, hypertension, diabetes, obesity, peripheral vascular disease, or conditions that promote heat intolerance, hypernea-dyspnea or increased stress levels warrant careful screening by a cardiologist or similarly prepared physician prior to program initiation.

Summary

This chapter has provided a comprehensive discussion of ways that the bed rest, immobilization, and relative disuse or inactivity may complicate client recovery (**Figure 1.15**). You are advised to consider the possible ramifications of these complications while progressing through Chapter 2, "The Physiology of Muscle Activation," and Chapter 3, "Stretching for Musculotendinous Extensibility and Joint Flexibility," and begin to consider the essential components of cardiopulmonary and strength training therapeutic exercise program designs covered in Chapters 4 and 5. Following this, you should begin to integrate concepts of training for joint stability (Chapter 6), proprioception-kinesthesia (Chapter 7), coordination and neuromuscular re-education (Chapter 8), and agility and balance (Chapter 9) into your concept of how to optimize a given client's level of function. In Chapter 10, you will be introduced to some alternative and complimentary exercise therapies. In Chapter 11, you will be asked to synthesize this information with greater consideration of developing the appropriate interface with each individual client, designing plan of care algorithms, finalizing particular therapeutic exercise program selections, improving therapeutic exercise program compliance, making sound decisions regarding return to activity, and measuring progress and functional outcomes.

In Section II, you will have the opportunity to use this knowledge to design therapeutic exercise programs for ten "real" clients with varying medical diagnoses, impairments, functional limitations, and disabilities. The authors of each case will provide guidance as you make critical client care decisions. [Specific therapeutic exercises that the case authors have selected are included on a supplemental CD to provide a moving three-dimensional depiction of the therapeutic exercise movement.] Discussions focusing on considerations of the client are also encouraged and you are encouraged to contribute your personal experiences regarding similar client cases to class discussions. You may find that your answers differ somewhat from those proposed by the case author. This is fine, provided you can support your decisions with sound scientific evidence that is relevant to the situation presented by your client.

With appropriate health care team intervention, it should not be long before Virgil is back to doing the things that matter to him, things that he finds to be both rewarding and fun (**Figure 1.16**). As you proceed through the book, please think about Virgil and how you might apply your new knowledge to his situation. As class discussions and laboratory experiences progress through internships and early professional practice, it is our hope that this text will serve you well as a valuable desk reference.

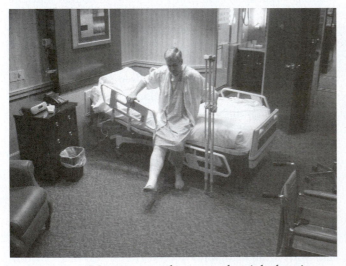

Figure 1.15   Movement and protected weight bearing are instrumental as Virgil begins the recovery process.

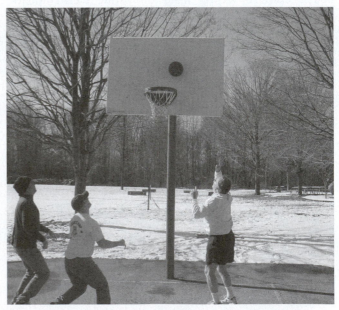

Figure 1.16   Virgil back playing basketball with his son and friend.

References

1. Hippocrates. *The genuine works of Hippocrates*. London: The Sydenham Society, 1849.

2. Serpell MG, Haldane GJ, Jamieson DRS, Carson D. Prevention of headache after lumbar puncture: Questionnaire survey of neurologists and neurosurgeons in United Kingdom. *BMJ*. 1998;316:1709–1710.

3. Carbaat PA, van Crevel H. Lumbar puncture headache: Controlled study on the preventive effect of 24 hours' bed rest. *Lancet*. 1981;ii:1133–1135.

4. Allen C, Glasziou P, Del Mar C. Bed rest: a potentially harmful treatment needing more careful evaluation. *Lancet*. 1999;354:1229–1233.

5. Miles MP, Clarkson PM, Bean M, et al. Muscle function at the wrist following 9 d of immobilization and suspension. *Med Sci Sports Exerc*. 1994;26:615–623.

6. Tesch PA, Berg HE, Haggmark T, et al. Muscle strength and endurance following lower limb suspension in man. *Physiologist*. 1991;34:S104–S106.

7. Veldhuizen JW, Verstappen FTJ, Vroemen JPAM, et al. Functional and morphological adaptations following four weeks of knee immobilization. *Int J Sports Med*. 1993;14:283–287.

8. Vandenborne K, Elliott MA, Walter GA, et al. Longitudinal study of skeletal muscle adaptations during immobilization and rehabilitation. *Muscle Nerve*. 1998;21:1006–1012.

9. Kitahara A, Hamaoka T, Murase N, et al. Deterioration of muscle function after 21-day forearm immobilization. *Med Sci Sports Exerc*. 2003;35(10):1697–1702.

10. Deitrick JE, Whedon GD, Shorr E. Effects of immobilization upon various metabolic and physiologic functions of normal men. *Am J Med*. 1948;4:3–36.

11. LeBlanc A, Rowe R, Evans H, et al. Muscle atrophy during long duration bed rest. *Int J Sports Med*. 1997:18:S283–S285.

12. LeBlanc A, Gogia P, Schneider V, et al. Calf muscle area and strength changes after five weeks of horizontal bed rest. *Am J Sports Med*. 1988;16:624–629.

13. Hikida RS, Gollnick PD, Dudley GA, et al. Structural and metabolic characteristics of human skeletal muscle following 30 days of simulated microgravity. *Aviat Space Environ Med*. 1989;60:664–670.

14. Dudley GA, Duvoisin MR, Convertino VA, Buchanan P. Alterations of the in vivo torque-velocity relationship of human skeletal muscle following 30 days exposure to simulated microgravity. *Aviat Space Environ Med*. 1989;60:659–663.

15. Sale DG, McComas AJ, MacDougall JD, Upton AR. Neuromuscular adaptation in human thenar muscles following strength training and immobilization. *J Appl Physiol*. 1982:53(2):419–424.

16. Bloomfield SA. Changes in musculoskeletal structure and function with prolonged bed rest. *Med Sci Sports Exerc*. 1997;29(2):197–206.

17. LeBlanc A, Schneider V, Spector E, et al. Calcium absorption, endogenous excretion, and endocrine changes during and after long-term bed rest. *Bone*. 1995;6(4, Suppl):301S–304S.

18. Nishimura Y, Fukuoka H, Kiriyama M, et al. Bone turnover and calcium metabolism during 20 days bed rest in young healthy males and females. *Acta Physiol Scand*. 1994;150 (Suppl):616:27–35.

19. Schneider VS, Hulley SB, Donaldson CL, et al. Prevention of bone mineral changes induced by bed rest: modification by static compression, simulated weight bearing, combined supplementation of oral calcium and phosphate, calcitonin injections, oscillating compression, the oral diphosphonate disodium etidronate, and lower body negative pressure (Final Report). NASA CR-141453, Public Health Service Hospital, San Francisco, CA. NTIS No. N75-13331/1st, 1974.

20. Bergmann P, Heilporn A, Schoutens A, et al. Longitudinal study of calcium and bone metabolism in paraplegic patients. *Paraplegia*. 1977–1978;15:147–159.

21. Morukov BV, Orlov OI, Grigoriev. Calcium homeostasis in prolonged hypokinesia. *Physiologist*. 1989;32:S37–S40.

22. Ruml LA, Dubois SK, Roberts ML, Pak CYC. Prevention of hypercalciuria and stone-forming propensity during prolonged bed rest by alendronate. *J Bone Min Res*. 1995;10:655–662.

23. Mack PB, Lachance PL. Effects of recumbency and space flight on bone density. *Am J Clin Nutr*. 1967;20:1194–1205.

24. Krolner B, Toft B. Vertebral bone loss: an unheeded side effect of therapeutic bed rest. *Clin Sci*. 1983;64:537–540.

25. LeBlanc AD, Schneider VS, Evans HJ, et al. Bone mineral loss and recovery after 17 weeks of bed rest. *J Bone Miner Res*. 1990;5:843–850.

26. Vogel JM, Whittle MW. Bone mineral changes: the second manned Skylab mission. *Aviat Space Environ Med*. 1976;47:396–400.

27. Vico L, Chappard D, Alexandre C, et al. Effects of a 120-day period of bed-rest on bone mass and bone cell activities in man: attempts at countermeasure. *Bone Miner*. 1987;2:383–394.

28. Minaire P, Meunier P, Edouard C, et al. Quantitative histological data on disuse osteoporosis: comparison with biological data. *Calcif Tissue Res.* 1974; 17:57–73.

29. Young DR, Niklowitz WJ, Brown RJ, Jee WSS. Immobilization-associated osteoporosis in primates. *Bone.* 1986;7:109–117.

30. Young DR, Niklowitz WJ, Steele CR. Tibial changes in experimental disuse osteoporosis in the monkey. *Calcif Tissue Int.* 1983;35:304–308.

31. Lueken SA, Arnaud SB, Taylor AK, Baylink DJ. Changes in markers of bone formation and resorption in a bed rest model of weightlessness. *J Bone Miner Res.* 1993;8:1433–1438.

32. Pfeilschifter F, Diel I, Pilz K, et al. Mitogenic responsiveness of human bone cells in vitro to hormones and growth factors decreases with age. *J Bone Miner Res.* 1993;8:707–717.

33. Ross RD, Wasnich RD, Vogel JM. Detection of prefracture spinal osteoporosis using bone mineral absorptiometry. *J Bone Miner Res.* 1988;3:1–11.

34. Convertino V, Bloomfield S, Greenleaf J. An overview of the issues: Physiological effects of bed rest and restricted physical activity. *Med Sci Sports Exerc.* 1997;29:187–190.

35. Kannus P. Immobilization or early mobilization after an acute soft-tissue injury. *Physician Sportsmed.* 2000;28(3):55–56;59–60;62–63.

36. Wren TA, Beaupre GS, Carter DR. Tendon and ligament adaptation to exercise, immobilization, and remobilization. *J Rehabil Res Dev.* 2000;37(2): 217–224.

37. Yasuda K, Hayashi K. Changes in biomechanical properties of tendons and ligaments from joint disuse. *Osteoarthritis Cartilage.* 1999;7:122–129.

38. Akeson WH, Amiel D, Mechanic GL, et al. Collagen cross-linking alterations in joint contractures: changes in the reducible cross-links in periarticular connective tissue collagen after nine weeks of immobilization. *Connect Tissue Res.* 1977;5(1): 15–19.

39. Amiel D, Akeson WH, Harwood FL, Frank CB. Stress deprivation effect on metabolic turnover of the medial collateral ligament collagen. *Clin Orthop.* 1983;172:265–270.

40. Kannus P, Jozsa L, Natri A, Jarvinen M. Effects of training, immobilization and remobilization on tendons. *Scand J Med Sci Sports.* 1997;7(2):67–71.

41. Montgomery JB, Steadman JR. Rehabilitation of the injured knee. *Clin Sports Med.* 1985;4(2): 333–343.

42. Tipton CM, Matthes RD, Maynard JA, Carey RA. The influence of physical activity on ligaments and tendons. *Med Sci Sports.* 1975;7(3):165–175.

43. Gelberman RH, Woo SL, Lothringer K, et al. Effects of early intermittent passive mobilization on healing canine flexor tendons. *J Hand Surg.* 1982; 7(2):170–175.

44. Gelberman RH, Manske PR, Akeson WH, et al. Flexor tendon repair. *J Orthop Res.* 1986;4(1): 119–128.

45. Takai S, Woo SL, Horibe S, et al. The effects of frequency and duration of controlled passive mobilization on tendon healing. *J Orthop Res.* 1991;9(5): 705–713.

46. Loitz BJ, Zernicke RF, Vailas AC, et al. Effects of short-term immobilization versus continuous passive motion on the biomechanical and biochemical properties of the rabbit tendon. *Clin Orthop.* 1989;244: 265–271.

47. Buckwalter J. Effects of early motion on healing of musculoskeletal tissues. *Hand Clinics.* 1996:12:13–19.

48. Stehno-Bittel L, Reddy GK, Gum S, et al. Biochemistry and biomechanics of healing tendon: Part I. Effects of rigid plaster casts and functional casts. *Med Sci Sports Exerc.* 1998;30(6):788–793.

49. Pneumaticos SG, Noble PC, McGarvey WC, et al. The effects of early mobilization in the healing of Achilles tendon repair. *Foot Ankle Int.* 2000;21(7): 551–557.

50. Salter R. History of rest and motion and the scientific basis for early continuous passive motion. *Hand Clinics.* 1996:12:1–11.

51. Buckwalter J. Osteoarthritis and articular cartilage use, disuse, and abuse: Experimental studies. *J Rheumatol.* 1995;22(Suppl 43):13–15.

52. Cohen NP, Foster RJ, VC Mow. Composition and dynamics of articular cartilage: Structure, function, and maintaining healthy state. *J Orthop Sports Phys Ther.* 1998;28(4):203–215.

53. Walker JM. Pathomechanics and classification of cartilage lesions, facilitation of repair. *J Orthop Sports Phys Ther.* 1998;28(4):216–231.

54. Praemer AP, Furner S, Rise DP, eds. *Musculoskeletal Conditions in the United States.* Park Ridge: American Academy of Orthopaedic Surgeons, 1992.

55. Wakabayashi S, Akizuki S, Takizawa T, Yasukawa Y. A comparison of the healing potential of fibrillated cartilage versus eburnated bone in osteoarthritic knees after high tibial osteotomy: An arthroscopic study with 1-year follow-up. *Arthroscopy.* 2002; 18(3):272–278.

56. Behrens F, Kraft E, Oegema T. Biochemical changes in articular cartilage after joint immobilization by casting or external fixation. *J Orthop Res.* 1989;7:335–343.

57. Jurvelin J, Kiviranta I, Saamanen A, et al. Partial restoration of immobilization-induced softening of canine articular cartilage after remobilization of the knee (stifle) joint. *J Orthop Res.* 1989;7:352–358.

58. Olah E, Kostenszky K. Effects of altered functional demand on the glysaminoglycan content of the ar-

ticular cartilage of dogs. *Acta Biol Hung.* 1972; 23:195–200.

59. Palmoski M, Brandt K. Immobilization of the knee prevents osteoarthritis after anterior cruciate ligament resection. *Arthritis Rheum.* 1982;25:1201–1208.

60. Stockwell RA. Structure and function of the chondrocyte under mechanical stress. In: Helminen HJ, Kiviranta I, Saamanen A-M, Tammi M, Paukkonen K, Jurvelin J (eds.), *Joint Loading,* pp. 126–148. Bristol: Wright, 1987.

61. Finsterbush A, Friedman B. Reversibility of joint changes produced by immobilization in rabbits. *Clin Orthop.* 1975;236:279–285.

62. Suh J, Aroen A, Muzzonigro T, et al. Injury and repair of articular cartilage: Related scientific issues. *Oper Tech Orthop.* 1997;7(4):270–278.

63. Eberhardt AW. An analytical model of joint contact. *J Biomech Eng.* 1990;112:407–413.

64. Shimizu T, Videman T, Shimazaki K. Experimental study on the repair of full thickness articular cartilage defects: Effects of varying periods of continuous passive range of motion, cage activity and immobilization. *J Orthop Res.* 1987;5:187–197.

65. Salter RB. The biological concept of continuous passive motion of synovial joints. The first 18 years of basic research and its clinical application. *Clin Orthop.* 1989;242:12–25.

66. Kozlovskaya IB, Grigoryeva LS, Gevlich GI. Comparative analysis of effects of weightlessness and its models on velocity and strength properties and tone of human skeletal muscles. *Kosm Biol Aviakosm Med.* 1984;18:22–26.

67. Sale DG, McComas AJ, MacDougall JD, Upton ARM. Neuromuscular adaptation in human thenar muscles following strength training and immobilization. *J Appl Physiol.* 1982;53:419–424.

68. Duchateau J, Hainaut K. Electrical and mechanical changes in the immobilized human muscle. *J Appl Physiol.* 1987;62:2168–2173.

69. Seki K, Taniguchi Y, Narusawa M. Effects of joint immobilization on firing rate modulation of human motor units. *J Physiol.* 2001;530. 3:507–519.

70. White MJ, Davies CT. The effects of immobilization, after lower leg fracture, on the contractile properties of human triceps surae. *Clin Sci.* 1984; 66(3):277–282.

71. Booth FW. Effect of limb immobilization on skeletal muscle. *J Appl Physiol.* 1982;52:1113–1118.

72. MacDougall JD, Elder GC, Sale DG, et al. Effects of strength training and immobilization on human muscle fibres. *Eur J Appl Physiol Occup Physiol.* 1980; 43(1):25–34.

73. Yue GH, Bilodeau M, Hardy PA, Enoka RM. Task-dependent effect of limb immobilization on the fatiguability of the elbow flexor muscles in humans. *Exp Physiol.* 1997;82(3):567–592.

74. Duchateau J, Hainut K. Effects of immobilization on contractile properties, recruitment and firing rates of human motor units. *J Physiol.* 1990;422: 55–65.

75. Convertino V. Cardiovascular consequences of bed rest: effect on maximal oxygen uptake. *Med Sci Sports Exerc.* 1997;29:191–196.

76. Levine B, Zuckerman J, Pawelczyk J. Cardiac atrophy after bed-rest deconditioning. *Circulation.* 1997; 96:517–525.

77. Takenaka K, Suzuki Y, Kawakubo K, et al. Cardiovascular effects of 20 days bed rest in healthy subjects. *Acta Physiol Scand.* 1994:150:Supp 616:59–63.

78. McGuire DK, Levine BD, Williamson JW, et al. A 30-year follow-up of the Dallas Bedrest and Training Study: I. Effect of age on cardiovascular response to exercise. *Circulation.* 2001;104(12): 1350–1357.

79. Faria SH. Assessment of immobility hazards. *Home Care Provid.* 1998;3(4):189–191.

80. Totten VY, Sugarman DB. Respiratory effects of spinal immobilization. *Prehosp Emerg Care.* 1999; 3(4): 347–352.

81. Krohler B, Toft B. Vertebral bone loss: an unheeded side effect of therapeutic bed rest. *Clin Sci.* 1983; 64(5):537–540.

82. Mahoney JE. Immobility and falls. *Clin Geriatric Med.* 1998;14(4):699–726.

83. Convertino V, Bloomfield S, Greenleaf J. An overview of the issues: physiological effects of bed rest and restricted physical activity. *Med Sci Sports Exerc.* 1997;29:187–190.

84. Guyton AC, Hall JE. *Textbook of Medical Physiology,* 10th ed. Philadelphia, PA: Elsevier Science, 2000.

85. Slipman C, Lipetz J, Jackson H, Vresilovic E. Deep venous thrombosis and pulmonary embolism as a complication of bed rest for low back pain. *Arch Phys Med Rehabil.* 2000;81:127–129.

86. Patterson J, Bennett R. Prevention and treatment of pressure sores. *J Am Geriatr Soc.* 1995;43:919–927.

87. Versluysen M. How elderly patients with femoral fractures develop pressure sores in hospital. *Br Med J.* 1986;292(6531):1311–1313.

88. Versluysen M. Pressure sores in elderly patients. The epidemiology related to hip operations. *J Bone Joint Surgery Br.* 1985;67(1):10–13.

89. Jensen TT, Juncker Y. Pressure sores common after hip operations. *Acta Orthop Scand.* 1987;58(3): 209–11.

90. Clarke M, Kadhom HM. The nursing prevention of pressure sores in hospital and community patients. *J Adv Nurs.* 1988;13(3):365–73.

91. Smith D. Pressure ulcers in the nursing home. *Ann Int Med.* 1995;123:433–442.

92. Allman RM, Goode PS, Patrick MM, et al. Pressure ulcer risk factors among hospitalized patients with activity limitation. *JAMA.* 1995;273:865–870.

93. Agency for Health Care Policy and Research. Pressure ulcer in adults: Prediction and prevention. *Clinical Practice Guideline*, Number 3. AHCPR Pub. No. 92-0047. Rockville, MD: Public Health Service, U.S. Department of Health and Human Services; May, 1992.

94. Sussman C, Bates-Jensen B. *Wound Care: A Collaborative Practice Manual for Physical Therapists and Nurses. 2nd edition*, Austin, TX: Pro-Ed, 2001.

95. Bergstrom N, Braden BJ, Laguzza A, Holman V. The Braden Scale for predicting pressure sore risk. *Nurs Res.* 1987;36:205–210.

96. Rybuck RS, Trimble RW, Lewis DF, Jennings CL. Psychological effects of prolonged weightlessness "bed rest" in young healthy volunteer. *Aerospace Med.* 1971;42(4):408–415.

97. Buschbacher RM, Porter CD. Deconditioning, conditioning, and the benefits of exercise. *In* RL Braddom (ed.), *Physical Medicine and Rehabilitation*, 2nd ed. Philadelphia: WB Saunders, 2000, p. 704.

98. Haruna Y, Suzuki Y, Kawakubo K, et al. Decremental reset in basal metabolism during 20-days bed rest. *Acta Physiol Scand.* 1994;150:Supp 616:43–49.

99. Going S, Davis R. Body composition. In JL Roitman (ed.), *ACSM's Resource Manual for Guidelines for Exercise Testing and Prescription*, 3rd ed. Baltimore: Williams & Wilkins, 1998, pp. 378–386.

100. Rimmer J. Health promotion for people with disabilities: the emerging paradigm shift from disability prevention to prevention of secondary conditions. *Phys Ther.* 1999;79:495–502.

101. National Blueprint, Increasing Physical Activity Among Adults Age 50 and Older. The Robert Wood Johnson Foundation, Princeton, NJ, 2001.

102. Irrgang J. Outcomes management for orthopaedic surgery. *Orthopaedic Grand Rounds*, University of Louisville, Louisville, KY, October 16, 2002.

103. Jette AM. Physical disablement concepts for physical therapy research and practice. *Phys Ther.* 1994; 74(5):380–386.

104. Nagi SA. Disability concepts revisited. In A. Pope and A. Tarlov (eds.), *Disability in America: Toward a national agenda for prevention*. Washington, DC: National Academy Press.

105. World Health Organization. *International Classification of Impairments, Disabilities and Handicaps: A manual of classification relating to the consequences of disease*. Geneva, Switzerland, 1980.

106. Jette AM. Using health related quality of life measures in physical therapy outcomes research. *Phys Ther.* 1993;8:528–537.

107. American Physical Therapy Association, *Guide to Physical Therapist Practice*. Alexandria, VA, 1999.

108. Moore GE, Durstine JL. Framework Chapter 2. In JL Durstine, ed., *ACSM's Exercise Management for Persons with Chronic Diseases and Disabilities*. Champaign, IL: Human Kinetics, 1997, pp. 6–16.

109. Woodard CM, Berry MJ. Enhancing adherence to prescribed exercise: Structured behavioral interventions in clinical exercise programs. *J Cardiopulm Rehabil.* 2001;21:201–209.

110. Thompson LV. Skeletal muscle adaptations with age, inactivity, and therapeutic exercise. *J Orthop Sports Phys Ther.* 2002;32(2):44–57.

111. *2004 Physicians' Desk Reference*, 58th ed. Montvale, NJ: Thomson Healthcare, 2003.

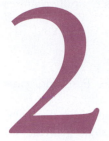

The Physiology of Muscle Activation

J. TIMOTHY NOTEBOOM

Objectives
The reader will be able to:

- Describe the energy systems associated with physical activity.
- Explain how nutrition can affect the neuromuscular system.
- List foundational principles of muscle physiology and function.
- Discuss how pharmacological agents can influence physiological responses to exercise

- Describe the role of motor unit neurophysiology on production and modulation of muscle force.
- Summarize principles of sensory feedback and its effects on motor performance.

Outline

INTRODUCTION

Human activity is highly dependent on a properly functioning neuromuscular system. From the maintenance of stable postures, where there is a balance of competing forces, to the production of finely graded forces resulting in body motions, the neuromuscular system is constantly transferring chemical energy into kinetic energy. Muscle function is dependent on several components of cellular metabolism, especially that of adenosine triphosphate (ATP), the source of energy for many enzymatic reactions in the muscle fiber, including the contractile process itself. Therefore, if rehabilitation clinicians wish to modify and optimize human function, it is critical to understand these bioenergetics mechanisms.

This chapter provides an overview of some of the basic physiological adaptations that occur with exercise training, with special emphasis on muscle metabolism. However, because muscle is an effector organ, responding to output from the central nervous system, portions of the chapter will also focus on the neurophysiological mechanisms underlying the human motion. As the final common pathway of the central nervous system, the motor unit, consisting of the motor neuron and the muscle fibers that the neuron innervates, will be discussed in detail. Factors that alter motor unit function, including physical training and detraining, fatigue, aging, and various disease processes, will also be discussed. The contents of this chapter should allow a greater understanding of the kinesiological principles of movement and exercise training that are introduced in later chapters.

MUSCLE METABOLISM

On average, muscle contributes over 50 percent of the total body mass. In addition, muscle metabolism can vary dramatically, with a tenfold increase in range of activity. Therefore, meeting the energy demands of this type of system is critical not only for the intrinsic function, but also for the production of motion. Metabolic activity is based on the production and use of energy in biological systems. Energy can be defined as the ability to perform work. The various forms of energy, such as chemical, mechanical, and heat, can be transformed from one type to another. *Bioenergetics*, which is the flow of energy in a biological system, is concerned with the conversion of food into biologically usable forms of energy. The breakdown of various bonds in these food molecules—large carbohydrate, protein, and fat molecules containing chemical energy—releases the energy necessary to perform work.[1] Because processes that result in energy production also cost energy, the total of all energy processes is termed metabolism. *Adenosine triphosphate (ATP)* is the intermediary molecule that is released during the breakdown of larger molecules (catabolic reactions), whereas the synthesis of larger molecules from smaller molecules typically requires additional energy (anabolic reactions).

$$ATP \Leftrightarrow ADP + P_i + e$$

(where ADP is adenosine diphosphate; P_i is inorganic phosphate; and *e* is energy).

The composition of ATP includes adenine, a nitrogen-containing base; ribose, a five-carbon sugar (collectively called adenosine); and three phosphate groups. The removal by hydrolysis of a phosphate group yields adenosine diphosphate (ADP). The high-energy bonds linking the two outermost phosphates represent considerable stored energy within the ATP molecule. Within muscle cells, the released energy is used to power several cellular functions. Most of the ATP is used to activate the contractile elements, since ATP is required to detach the myosin cross-bridges from the actin filaments, thereby allowing the bridges to move to new positions on the filaments.[2] In addition, ATP is also necessary to power two important metabolic pumps. The Na^+-K^+ pump maintains the muscle fiber sarcolemma in an excitable state during muscle activity, whereas the other pump returns Ca^{2+} to the sarcoplasmic reticulum at the end of the excitation-contraction coupling of the muscle.

Key Point:

ATP is used to activate the contractile elements and to power the sodium (Na^+)-potassium (K^+) and calcium (Ca^{2+}) pumps.

Despite the ongoing expenditure of energy, the muscle cell stores only small quantities of ATP. McArdle et al.[3] state that at any one time the body stores only about 80–100 g of ATP, providing enough energy for several seconds of explosive, maximal exercise. In addition, it is estimated that a sedentary individual uses an amount of ATP approximately equal to 75 percent of body mass.[3] Obviously, muscle energy stores are not adequate to meet the needs of our daily activities. Therefore, to maintain adequate energy stores within the muscle, several systems are responsible for replenishing ATP supplies. To accommodate situations requiring the immediate need for substantial energy, such as sprinting or heavy lifting, the splitting of an ATP molecule can take place immediately and without oxygen.

ATP-PC system

Some energy for ATP resynthesis comes directly from the splitting (hydrolysis) of a phosphate from another intracellular high-energy compound, phosphocreatine (PCr).

Unlike other cells, the muscle fiber has substantial energy reserves in the form of PCr. As ATP is expended, it is instantly replenished from PCr by the action of the enzyme creatine kinase:

$$ADP + PCr \Leftrightarrow ATP + Cr$$

(where Cr is creatine).

PCr is so effective at maintaining ATP levels that when a muscle is exercised to fatigue, substantial amounts of ATP remain, even though the supply of PCr is exhausted.[2] Resting stores of PCr in the muscle are three to four times greater than that of ATP; however, with the onset of intense exercise, the hydrolysis of PCr reaches a maximum in about 10 sec. Thus, PCr can be considered a "reservoir" of high-energy phosphate bonds that can be accessed without the use of oxygen.

> ## Key Point:
> With 3–4 times greater resting stores, phosphocreatine helps to preserve ATP levels when a muscle is exercised to fatigue.

Generally, type II (fast twitch) muscle fibers contain greater concentrations of phosphogens compared with type I (slow twitch) fibers.[4] (Muscle fiber types will be discussed in more detail in later sections of this chapter.) Furthermore, increasing sarcoplasmic concentration of ADP stimulates the activity level of creatine kinase, the enzymatic catalyst facilitating PCr breakdown, thus providing a crucial feedback mechanism for rapidly forming ATP from the available high-energy phosphates.[3] Creatine kinase activity remains elevated if exercise continues at a high intensity. If exercise is discontinued or continues at an intensity low enough to allow glycolysis or the oxidative system to supply an adequate amount of ATP to meet energy demands, the sarcoplasmic concentrations of ATP will likely increase, thereby inhibiting creatine kinase activity.[1]

The potential for phosphocreatine to enhance athletic performance has contributed to increased dietary supplementation of creatine. In fact, in a survey of Division I college athletes, over 25 percent of respondents were users of creatine.[5] In a recent review, Mesa and colleagues[6] conclude that the use of creatine supplements to increase muscle creatine content above the approximately 20 mmol/kg dry muscle mass leads to improvements in high intensity, intermittent high intensity, and even endurance exercise. However, other authors have stated that limited data is available on the pharmacokinetics of creatine, and that further studies are needed to define absorption char-

acteristics, clearance kinetics, its impact on adequate hydration levels, and the effect of multiple doses.

> ## Key Point:
> Despite its popularity, limited data is available on the pharmacokinetics of creatine, and further studies are needed to define absorption characteristics, clearance kinetics, its impact on adequate hydration levels, and the effect of multiple doses.

Therefore, although creatine does not appear to have obvious adverse effects,[6] athletes should be cautioned in the prolonged usage of oral creatine supplementation.

Finally, ATP can be synthesized from ADP in another way. The enzyme myoadenylate kinase can convert two molecules of ADP to one of ATP and one of adenosine monophosphate (AMP).

$$2\ ADP \Leftrightarrow ATP + AMP$$

However, McComas[2] states that this pathway for the production of ATP probably plays a relatively minor role.

Glycolysis

As muscles continue to contract, the production of ATP from PCr becomes inadequate. At this point, the fibers become completely dependent on the oxidation of other energy sources, fat and glucose, the latter being largely derived from the storage polysaccaride, glycogen.[2] *Glycolysis* is the breakdown of carbohydrates, either glycogen stored in the muscle or glucose delivered via the circulatory system, to produce ATP, thus supplementing the phosphagen system for high-intensity muscular activity. The process of glycolysis can proceed in one of two pathways, fast (anaerobic) glycolysis and slow (aerobic) glycolysis. (It should be noted that use of the terms anaerobic and aerobic incorrectly implies that oxygen involvement differentiates the two pathways. See Brooks et al. for further discussion.[7]) During fast glycolysis, pyruvate is converted to lactic acid, providing ATP at a fast rate compared with slow glycolysis, which results in pyruvate transported to the mitochondria for use in the oxidative system. The fate of the end products is controlled by the energy demands within the muscle cell. For example, if energy must be supplied at a high rate (e.g., during weight training), fast glycolysis is used primarily, whereas lower demands, in the presence of adequate quantities of oxygen, can activate slow glycolysis.[1]

Fast glycolysis occurs during periods of reduced oxygen availability in the muscle cells and results in the formation of the organic end product lactic acid (commonly used interchangeably with the term lactate, its corresponding salt). Prolonged, high intensity exercise is typically associated with corresponding high tissue levels of *lactic acid*, resulting from an imbalance between production and utilization.

Key Point:

Long term, high intensity exercise is associated with corresponding high tissue levels of lactic acid.

Lactic acid accumulation, with corresponding elevation of hydrogen ion concentrations, is believed to inhibit glycolytic reactions and directly interfere with muscle excitation-contraction coupling, possibly by inhibiting calcium binding to troponin, interfering with cross-bridge formation, or the general reduction of cellular enzymatic activity.[8] In humans, the cell's limited capacity for glycolysis assumes a crucial role during physical activities that require maximal effort for up to 90 seconds.[3]

The Oxidative System (Fat and Protein)

The oxidative system is the primary source of ATP at rest and during low-intensity activities using primarily carbohydrates and fats as substrates.[9] Protein is normally not metabolized in significant amounts, except during long-term starvation and long bouts (> 90 min) of exercise. At rest, approximately 70 percent of the ATP produced is derived from fats and 30 percent from carbohydrates. Following the onset of activity, as the intensity of the exercise increases, there is a shift in substrate preferences from fats to carbohydrates.

Key Point:

At rest about 70 percent of the ATP produced comes from fats and 30 percent comes from carbohydrates. Following activity onset and as exercise intensity increases, the substrate preference shifts from fats to carbohydrates.

During high intensity aerobic exercise, almost 100 percent of the energy is derived from carbohydrates, if an adequate supply is available. However, during prolonged, submaximal, steady-state work, there is a gradual shift from carbohydrates back to fats and protein as energy substrates.

The oxidative metabolism of blood glucose and muscle glycogen begins with glycolysis. If oxygen is present in sufficient quantities, the end product of glycolysis, pyruvate, is not converted to lactic acid but is transported to the mitochondria, where it is taken up and enters the *Krebs cycle*, or citric acid cycle. The Krebs cycle consists of a series of reactions that continues the oxidation of the substrate begun in glycolysis and produces two ATPs indirectly from guanine triphosphate (GTP) for each molecule of glucose. Also produced from one molecule of glucose are six molecules of reduced nicotinamide adenine dinucleotide (NADH) and two molecules of reduced flavin adenine dinucleotide ($FADH^2$). These molecules transport hydrogen atoms to the electron transport chain (ETC) to be used to produce ATP from ADP. The ETC uses the NADH and $FADH^2$ molecules to rephosphorylate ADP to ATP. The hydrogen atoms are passed down the chain by a series of electron carriers known as cytochromes, to form a proton concentration gradient, which provides energy for ATP production, with oxygen serving as the final electron acceptor.

Because NADH and $FADH^2$ enter the ETC at different sites, they differ in their ability to produce ATP. One molecule of NADH can produce three molecules of ATP, whereas one molecule of $FADH^2$ can produce only two molecules of ATP. The production of ATP during this process is referred to as oxidative phosphorylation. The oxidative system, beginning with glycolysis, results in the production of approximately 38 ATPs from the degradation of one glucose molecule (**Table 2.1**).[1]

Fat Oxidation

Fats can also be used by the oxidative energy system. An enzyme, hormone-sensitive lipase, can break down triglycerides stored in fat cells, which releases free fatty acids from the fat cells into the blood, where they can be transported to skeletal muscle fibers. Limited quantities of triglycerides, stored within the muscle along with a form of lipase, produce an intramuscular source of free fatty acids. Free fatty acids enter the mitochondria, and undergo beta-oxidation, a series of reactions in which the free fatty acids are broken down, resulting in the formation of acetyl CoA and hydrogen atoms. The acetyl CoA enters the Krebs cycle directly, and hydrogen atoms are carried by NADH and $FADH^2$ to the ETC.

Unlike carbohydrate metabolism, which is closely geared to the energy requirements of the working muscle, fat utilization is not as tightly regulated. No mechanisms exist for matching the availability and metabolism of fatty acids to the prevailing rate of energy expenditure.[10,11] Therefore, the rate of fat oxidation during exercise is principally determined by the rate of carbohydrate utilization and the availability of circulating fatty acids.

Key Point:

The rate of fat oxidation during exercise is primarily determined by the rate of carbohydrate utilization and the availability of circulating fatty acids.

TABLE 2.1   Total energy yield from the oxidation of one glucose molecule.

Process	ATP production
Total Energy Yield from the Oxidation of One Glucose Molecule	
Slow Glycolysis	
Substrate level phosphorylation	4
Oxidative phosphorylation: 2 NADH (3 ATP each)	6
Krebs Cycle (two rotations through the Krebs cycle per glucose)	
Substrate level phosophorylation: 8 NADH (3 ATP each)	2
Oxidative phosphorylation: 8 NADH (3 ATP each)	24
Via guanine triphosphate (GTP): 2 FADH (2 ATP each)	4
	Total = 40*
Total Energy Yield from the Oxidation of One (18-carbon) Triglyceride Molecule	
1 molecule of glycerol	22
18-carbon fatty acid metabolism:**	
147 ATP per fatty acid × 3 fatty acids/triglyceride molecule	441
	Total = 463

Glycolysis consumes 2 ATP (if starting with glucose), so net ATP production is 40 − 2 = 38. This figure can also be reported as 36 ATP depending on which shuttle system is used to transport the NADH to the mitochondria.

**Other triglycerides that contain a different amount of carbons will yield more or less ATP.*

(Reprinted with permission from Conley M. Bioenergetics of Exercise and Training. In TR Baechle, RW Earle (eds), *Essentials of Strength Training and Conditioning*. Champaign, IL: Human Kinetics, 2000, p. 81.)

During rest, fat-based fuels may be the predominant energy source. As the relative exercise intensity increases, there is a shift from fat-based to carbohydrate-based fuels, although if the exercise is maintained for longer durations (> one hour), the greater contribution is from fat to the total energy metabolism. It should be noted, however, that strategies used to increase the availability of fatty acids (such as caffeine ingestion, L-carnitine supplementation, and infusion of intralipid emulsions), have not resulted in improved exercise capacity, despite greater availability of circulating free fatty acids.[11]

Protein Oxidation

Although not a significant source of energy for most activities, protein can be broken down into its constituent amino acids by various metabolic processes. These amino acids can then be converted into glucose (via gluconeogenesis), pyruvate, or various Krebs cycle intermediates to produce ATP. The contribution of amino acids to the production of ATP has been estimated to be minimal during short-term exercise, but may contribute 3–18 percent of the energy requirements during prolonged activity.[12,13] The major amino acids that are oxidized in skeletal muscle are believed to be the branched-chain amino acids (leucine, isolucine, and valine), although alanin, aspartate, and glutamate may also be used. The nitrogenous waste products of amino acid degradation are eliminated through the formation of urea and small amounts of ammonia. The elimination of ammonia is significant because ammonia is toxic and the build-up of ammonia is associated with fatigue.[1]

Oxidative System Regulation

Although there are many significant steps in the Krebs cycle cascade, the key rate-limiting step is the conversion of isocitrate to ∝-ketoglutarate, a reaction catalyzed by the enzyme isocitrate dehydrogenase. Isocitrate dehydrogenase is stimulated by ADP and normally inhibited by ATP. Similarly, the reactions that produce NADH or FADH[2] also influence the regulation of the Krebs cycle. If NAD+ and FAD[2]+ are not available in sufficient quantities to accept hydrogen, the rate of the Krebs cycle is reduced. Also, when GTP accumulates, the concentration of succinyl CoA increases, inhibiting the initial reaction (oxaloacetate + acetyl CoA → citrate + CoA) of the Krebs cycle. The electron transport chain is inhibited by ATP and stimulated by ADP.[7]

Energy Production and Capacity

The phosphagen, glycolytic, and oxidative energy systems differ in their ability to supply energy for activities of various intensities and durations (**Table 2.2 and Table 2.3**). *Exercise intensity* is defined as a level of muscular activity that can be quantified in terms of power (work performed

TABLE 2.2   Effect of event duration on energy systems.

Duration	Intensity	Primary energy systems
0–6 s	Very intense	Phosphagen
6–30 s	Intense	Phosphagen and fast glycolysis
30 s–2 min	Heavy	Fast glycolysis
2–3 min	Moderate	Fast glycolysis and oxidative system
More than 3 min	Light	Oxidative system

(Reprinted with permission from Conley M. Bioenergetics of Exercise and Training. In TR Baechle, RW Earle (eds.), *Essentials of Strength Training and Conditioning*. Champaign, IL: Human Kinetics, 2000, p. 83.)

per unit of time) output.[14] It has been shown that power at maximal oxygen uptake is approximately 20–30 percent of peak power on a cycle ergometer.[15] Therefore, exercise primarily supported by aerobic mechanisms, even at 100 percent of maximal oxygen uptake, should not be classified as high intensity exercise. Activities such as resistance training that are high intensity and thus have a high power output require a rapid rate of energy supplied; they rely almost entirely on the energy supplied by the phosphagen system. Activities that are of low intensity but long duration (e.g., marathon running) require a large energy supply, primarily supplied by the oxidative energy system. The predominant source of energy for activities ranging

TABLE 2.3   Rankings of rate capacity of ATP production.

System	Rate of ATP production	Capacity of ATP production
Phosphagen	1	5
Fast glycolysis	2	4
Slow glycolysis	3	3
Oxidation of carbohydrates	4	2
Oxidation of fats/proteins	5	1

1 = fastest or greatest; 5 = slowest or least

(Reprinted with permission from Conley M. Bioenergetics of Exercise and Training. In TR Baechle, RW Earle (eds.), *Essentials of Strength Training and Conditioning*. Champaign, IL: Human Kinetics, 2000, p. 83.)

between these two extremes shifts depends on the intensity and duration of the event.

Key Point:

The main energy source during activity depends on activity intensity and duration. As activity intensity decreases and the duration increases, the emphasis gradually shifts to slow glycolysis and oxidative energy systems.

In general, short, high intensity activities rely on the phosphagen energy system and fast glycolysis. As the intensity decreases and the duration increases, the emphasis gradually shifts to slow glycolysis and oxidative energy systems.[10,12,16]

Activity duration also influences which energy system is used. Athletic events range in duration from one to three seconds to more than four hours. The extent to which each of the three energy systems contributes to ATP production depends primarily on the intensity of muscular activity and secondarily on the duration. At no time, during either exercise or rest, does any single energy system provide the complete supply of energy.[1]

Key Point:

At no time during either exercise or rest does any single energy system provide the complete energy supply.

Intensity and Duration of Exercise

The body's energy transfer system should be viewed along a continuum of exercise bioenergetics. Anaerobic sources supply most of the energy for fast movements, or during increased resistance to movement at a given speed. Also, when movement begins at a fast or slow speed (from performing a front handspring to starting a marathon run), the intramuscular phosphagens provide immediate anaerobic energy for the required muscle actions.

At the short duration extreme of maximum effort, the intramuscular phosphagens ATP and PCr supply the major energy for the entire exercise. The ATP-PCr and lactic acid systems provide about one-half of the energy required for "best-effort" exercise lasting up to two minutes, whereas aerobic reactions provide the remainder. For top performance in all-out, two-minute exercise, a person must possess a well developed capacity for both aerobic and anaerobic metabolism. Intense exercise for intermediate duration performed for 5 to 10 minutes, such as middle-distance running and swimming or stop-and-go sports such as basketball and soccer, demands greater aerobic energy transfer. Longer-duration exercise, such as marathon running, distance swimming and cycling, recreational jogging, cross-country skiing, and hiking and backpacking, requires a continual energy supply derived aerobically without reliance on lactate formation. Proper training can enhance the performance of these endurance activities without the deleterious effects of increased lactate build-up. Conversely, other factors, such as performing endurance tasks at altitude, can result in greater lactate formation given similar workloads.

Intensity and duration determine which energy system and metabolic mixture predominate during exercise. The aerobic system predominates in low intensity exercise with fatty acids serving as the primary fuel source. The liver markedly increases its release of glucose to active muscle as exercise progresses from low to high intensity. Simultaneously, glycogen stored within muscle serves as the predominant carbohydrate source during the early stages of exercise, and when exercise intensity increases. During high intensity aerobic exercise, the advantage of selective dependence on carbohydrate metabolism lies in its two times more rapid energy transfer capacity compared with fatty acid and protein fuels. Compared with fat, carbohydrate also generates about 6 percent greater energy per unit of oxygen consumed.[3] As exercise continues and muscle glycogen depletes, progressively more fat (intramuscular triglycerides and circulating free fatty acids) enters the metabolic mixture for ATP production. In maximal anaerobic effort (reactions of glycolysis), carbohydrate becomes the sole contributor to ATP production.

> ## Key Point:
> The liver markedly increases glucose release to active muscles as exercise progresses from low to high intensity.

A sound approach to exercise training analyzes an activity for its specific energy components and then establishes a training regimen to ensure the optimal physiologic and metabolic adaptations. An improved capacity for energy transfer usually improves exercise performance.

> ## Key Point:
> Effective exercise programs are based on an analysis of the activity for its specific energy components to ensure the development of optimal physiologic and metabolic adaptations.

Nutrient Related Fatigue

Severe depletion of liver and muscle glycogen during exercise induces fatigue (i.e., "hitting the wall"), despite sufficient oxygen availability to muscle and unlimited potential energy from stored fat. Skeletal muscles do not contain the phosphatase enzyme (present in liver) that releases glucose from cells; thus, relatively inactive muscles retain all of their glycogen. Controversy exists as to why liver and muscle glycogen depletion during prolonged exercise reduces exercise capacity.[3] Part of the answer relates to:

- Central nervous system's use of blood glucose for energy.
- Muscle glycogen's role as a "primer" in fat catabolism.
- Significantly slower rate of energy release from fat compared with carbohydrate breakdown.

Oxygen Uptake During Recovery: The So-Called "Oxygen Debt"

Bodily processes do not immediately return to resting levels after exercise ceases. In light exercises (e.g., golf, archery, bowling), recovery to resting condition takes place rapidly and often progresses unnoticed. With particularly intense physical activity (running full speed for 800m or trying to swim 200 m at maximal effort), however, it takes considerable time for the body to return to resting levels. The difference in recovery from light and strenuous exercise relates largely to the specific metabolic and physiologic processes in each exercise mode.

A.V. Hill (1886–1977), the British Nobel physiologist, referred to *oxygen debt*. Contemporary theory no longer uses this term.[1] Instead, *recovery oxygen uptake* or *excess post-exercise oxygen consumption (EPOC)*, refers to the total oxygen consumed after exercise in excess of a pre-exercise baseline level.

Figure 2.1(a) shows that light exercise rapidly attains steady rate and a small oxygen deficit. Rapid recovery ensues from such exercise with an accompanying small EPOC. In moderate to heavy aerobic exercise (**Figure 2.1(b)**), it takes longer to reach steady rate, and the oxygen deficit becomes considerably larger compared with light exercise. Oxygen uptake in recovery from this relatively strenuous aerobic exercise returns more slowly to the pre-exercise resting level. Recovery oxygen deficit and EPOC uses the steady-rate oxygen uptake to represent the exercise oxygen (energy) requirement. During exhausting exercise, a steady rate of aerobic metabolism cannot be attained. This produces large amounts of lactate. Blood lactate then accumulates and it takes oxygen uptake considerable time to return to the pre-exercise level. It becomes nearly impossible to determine the true oxygen deficit in such exercise because no steady rate exists, and

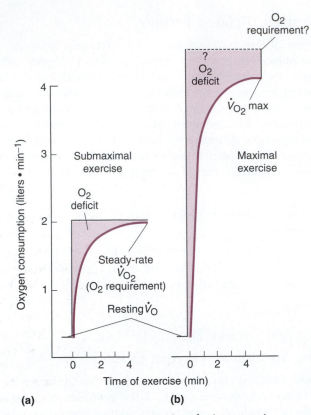

(a)   **(b)**

Figure 2.1   Oxygen consumption during exercise. Oxygen consumption before and during continuous bouts of steady-rate submaximal and maximal exercise. In submaximal exercise (a), the oxygen deficit can be estimated as the difference between the steady-rate VO$_2$ and actual VO$_2$ prior to attainment of the steady-rate VO$_2$. In maximal exercise (b), the oxygen deficit cannot be estimated with certainty for lack of a precise value of the oxygen required. For this reason, scientists have attempted to utilize the "O$_2$ debt" as a measure of anaerobic metabolism during exercise. (Reprinted with permission from GA Brooks, TD Fahey, TP White. *Exercise Physiology: Human Bioenergetics and Its Applications*, 3rd ed. Mountain View, CA: Mayfield Publishing Company, 2000, p. 202 (Figure 10-5)).

the energy requirement exceeds the individual's maximal oxygen uptake.

No matter how intense the exercise or functional task, an oxygen uptake in excess of the resting value always exists when exercise stops. The shaded area under the recovery curve in **Figure 2.1** indicates this quantity of oxygen; it equals the total oxygen consumed in recovery (until attaining the baseline level) minus the total oxygen that would normally be consumed at rest for an equivalent duration.

The recovery curves in **Figure 2.2** illustrate two fundamentals of oxygen uptake during recovery:

1. **Fast component:** In low intensity, primarily aerobic exercise (with little increase in body temperature), about one-half the total EPOC takes place in 30 seconds; complete recovery requires several minutes.
2. **Slow component:** A second slower phase occurs in recovery from more strenuous exercise (often accompanied by considerable increases in blood lactate and body temperature). The slower phase of recovery, depending on exercise intensity and duration, may require 24 hours or more before re-establishing the pre-exercise oxygen uptake.[7]

Updated Theory to Explain EPOC

No doubt exists that the elevated aerobic metabolism in recovery helps restore the body's processes to pre-exercise conditions. Oxygen uptake after light and moderate exercise replenishes high energy phosphates depleted in the preceding exercise and sustains the cost of a somewhat elevated overall level of physiologic function. In recovery from strenuous exercise, some oxygen resynthesizes a portion of lactate to glucose. However, a significant portion of recovery oxygen uptake supports physiologic functions actually taking place during recovery. The considerably larger recovery oxygen uptake compared with oxygen deficit in high intensity, exhaustive exercise results partly from factors such as elevated body temperature. Core temperature frequently increases about 3°C during vigorous exercise and can remain elevated for several hours into recovery. This thermogenic "boost" directly stimulates metabolism and increases EPOC.

In essence, all of the physiologic systems activated to meet the demands of muscular activity increase their need for oxygen during recovery. The recovery oxygen uptake reflects:

■ Anaerobic metabolism of prior exercise.
■ Respiratory, circulatory, hormonal, ionic, and thermal disequilibriums caused by prior exercise.[1]

Implications of EPOC for Exercise and Recovery

Oxygen uptake provides a basis for structuring exercise intervals during training and optimizing recovery from strenuous physical activity. Blood lactate does not accumulate considerably, with either steady rate aerobic exercise or

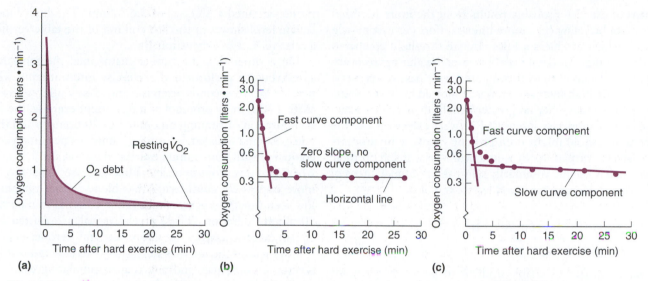

Figure 2.2   Oxygen consumption post-exercise. Oxygen consumption after a period of exercise requiring a constant work output. (a) Plotted on linear coordinates, the O_2 debt is the area under the postexercise VO_2 curve above the resting VO_2 baseline. (b) and (c) VO_2 after easy and hard exercise bouts, plotted on semilogarithmic coordinates. Note one postexercise VO_2 curve component after easy exercise (b) and two components after hard exercise (c). (Reprinted with permission from GA Brooks, TD Fahey, TP White, *Exercise Physiology: Human Bioenergetics and Its Applications,* 3rd ed. Mountain View, CA: Mayfield Publishing Company, 2000, p. 202 (Figure 10-6)).

brief 5- to 10-second bouts of all-out effort powered by the intramuscular high energy phosphates. Recovery proceeds rapidly (fast component), and exercise can begin again within a brief time. In contrast, anaerobic exercise powered mainly by glycolysis causes lactate buildup and significant disruption in physiologic processes. This requires considerably more time for complete recovery (slow component). It poses a problem in sports such as basketball, hockey, soccer, tennis, and badminton because a performer pushed to a high level of anaerobic metabolism may not fully recover during brief rest periods or times out, between points, or even during half-time breaks.

Procedures for speeding recovery from exercise can occur as active or passive. *Active recovery* (often called cooling down or tapering off) involves submaximal aerobic exercise performed immediately post exercise. Many practitioners believe that continued movement prevents muscle cramps and stiffness and facilitates the recovery process. In contrast, in *passive recovery*, a person usually lies down, assuming that complete inactivity reduces the resting energy requirements and "frees" oxygen for the recovery process. Modification of active and passive recovery have included cold showers, massages, specific body positions, ice application, and ingesting cold fluids. Research findings have been equivocal about these recovery procedures.[7]

Optimal Recovery from Exercise

Most people can perform exercise below 55 to 60 percent of VO_{2max} (maximum amount of oxygen in millimeters one can use in one minute per kilogram of body weight) in steady

rate with little blood lactate accumulation.[7] Recovery from such exercise resynthesizes high energy phosphate, replenishes oxygen in the blood, body fluids, and muscle myoglobin, and supports the small energy cost to sustain circulation and ventilation. Passive procedures produce the most rapid recovery in such cases because exercise elevates total metabolism and delays recovery.[3]

Lactate formation exceeds its rate of removal and blood lactate accumulates when exercise intensity exceeds the maximum steady rate level. As work intensity increases the level of lactate increases sharply, and the exerciser soon becomes exhausted. The precise mechanisms of fatigue during intense anaerobic exercise are not fully understood, but the blood lactate level indicates the relative strenuousness of exercise and reflects the adequacy of the recovery.

> ## Key Point:
>
> Although the precise mechanisms of fatigue during intense anaerobic exercise are not fully understood, blood lactate level increases generally indicate the relative strenuousness of exercise and reflect the adequacy of recovery.

Active aerobic exercise in recovery accelerates lactate removal. The optimal level of exercise in recovery ranges between 30 and 45 percent of VO_{2max} for bicycle exercise and between 55 and 60 percent of VO_{2max} when recovery involves treadmill running. The variation between these two forms of exercise probably results from the more localized nature of bicycling (i.e., more intense effort per unit muscle mass), which produces a lower lactate threshold compared with running. Moderate aerobic exercise during recovery facilitates lactate removal compared with passive recovery. Combining high intensity exercise followed by lower intensity exercise may offer no greater benefit than a single exercise bout of moderate intensity. Recovery exercise above the lactate threshold might even prolong recovery by promoting lactate formation. In a practical sense, if left to their own choice, people voluntarily select their optimal intensity of recovery exercise for blood lactate removal.

Intermittent Exercise: The Interval Training Approach

Several approaches enable a client to perform significant amounts of normally exhaustive exercise, while simultaneously reducing the deleterious effects of anaerobic energy transfer through glycolysis. One approach requires training to improve a client's capability of sustaining exercise at a high rate of aerobic energy transfer. A high steady rate capability exists for elite marathon runners, distance swimmers, and cross country skiers who compete at close to 90% VO_{2max} without significant blood lactate accumulation.

One can also exercise at an intensity that would normally prove exhausting within three to five minutes using pre-established spacing of exercise and rest intervals. Adjusting exercise and rest intervals forms the basis of an interval training program. With this approach, the exerciser applies various work-to-rest intervals using "super maximum" effort to overload the specific systems of energy transfer. For example, with all-out exercise of up to 8 seconds duration, intramuscular phosphates provide the major portion of energy, with little demand on the glycolytic pathway. Rapid recovery ensues (fast component), and exercise can begin again after only a brief recovery.

Table 2.4 summarizes the results from experiments using combinations of exercise and rest intervals during intermittent exercise. On one day, the subject ran at a speed that would normally exhaust him within five minutes. This continuous run covered about 0.8 mile, and the

runner attained a VO_{2max} of 5.6 L/min. The high blood lactate level shown in the last column of the table verified a relative state of exhaustion.[14]

On another day, the runner maintained the same fast speed, but he performed the exercise intermittently with periods of 10-seconds exercise and 5-seconds recovery. With a 30-minute protocol of intermittent exercise, the actual duration of running amounted to 20 minutes and distance covered equaled 4.0 miles (5 minutes per mile pace) compared with four-minute exercise duration and 0.8 miles when running continuously. This exercise capability is more impressive considering that blood lactate remained low even though oxygen uptake averaged 5.1 L/min for the 30-minute duration. Thus, a relative balance existed between exercise energy requirements and aerobic energy transfer within the muscles during the exercise and rest intervals.[14] These data indicate that manipulating exercise-to-rest intervals can isolate and overload a specific energy transfer system. Extending the rest interval after a 10-second exercise bout from 5 to 10 seconds decreased the average oxygen uptake 4.4 L/min; with 15-second exercise and 30-second recovery intervals, only a 3.6 L/min oxygen uptake occurred. In each case of 30-minute intermittent exercise, the runner achieved a longer distance and a lower blood lactate compared with the same exercise performed continuously. Rehabilitation clinicians need to consider both exercise and rest intervals in optimizing workouts geared to train specific energy transfer systems.

> ## *Key Point:*
> To optimize therapeutic exercise sessions, rehabilitation clinicians need to consider both exercise and rest intervals to train specific energy transfer systems.

One can also apply the *exercise-to-rest interval* (the E-to-R method) to improve muscular endurance. For example, two basic training approaches can improve sit-up capacity. In one method, the client performs as many sit-ups as possible for a specific time period. Suppose a client completed 40

TABLE 2.4   Exercise: Rest intervals, total distance average oxygen uptake, and blood lactate levels during continuous and intermittent exercise.

Exercise: Rest intervals	Total distance run (yd)	Average oxygen uptake ($L \cdot min^{-1}$)	Blood lactate level ($mg \cdot 100 \ mL \ blood^{-1}$)
4 minutes continuous	1422	5.6	150
Exercise 10 seconds, rest 5 seconds	7294	5.1	44
Exercise 10 seconds, rest 10 seconds	5468	4.4	20
Exercise 15 seconds, rest 30 seconds	3642	3.6	16

(From Christenson EH, Hedman R, Saltin B. Intermittent and continuous running. Acta Physiol. Scand., 1960:50:269–286, as reported in P.O. Astrand, and K. Rodahl, *Textbook of Work Physiology.* New York: McGraw-Hill, 1970, p. 384.)

consecutive sit-ups in 2 minutes. In each subsequent training session, the client would attempt to perform additional sit-ups. With the E-to-R method, sit-ups would be sequenced within intervals. Six sit-ups might be done within 10 seconds, followed by a 20-second rest interval. The sequence of sit-ups and rest would repeat 10 times, resulting in a total of 60 sit-ups. Performing 20, 10-second bouts of sit-ups would obviously double sit-up performance. Although the rest intervals add to the duration of training, the total number of completed sit-ups increases significantly beyond that performed in a single continuous exercise bout. The same E-to-R method can be applied to other types of performances such as push-ups, various flexibility exercises, and workouts with resistance equipment.[14]

NUTRITION

For a person to maintain proper metabolic function at rest, and especially when involved in prolonged exercise, the intake of energy stores has to balance energy expenditures. However, not only does the quantity of the caloric intake affect metabolic function, but the dietary composition of the calories can also influence exercise performance as well as general health status. Therefore, proper nutrition is an important consideration in general health promotion. *Macronutrients* form the cornerstone of optimal caloric intake. A macronutrient is a nutrient that is required in significant amounts in the diet. Three important classes of macronutrients are protein, carbohydrate, and lipids (fats and related compounds).

Protein

Although protein intake has always been of interest to athletes wishing to enhance muscle development, more recently several dietary programs such as the Atkins diet have emphasized the importance of protein intake in a healthy diet. This section reviews the function of *protein* in the body, the effects of exercise on protein metabolism, and dietary requirements for athletes.

Similar to carbohydrates and fats, proteins are composed of carbon, hydrogen, and oxygen atoms. Unlike carbohydrates and fats, proteins also contain nitrogen. Amino acids are the molecules that are critical building blocks for thousands of proteins occurring in nature. Proteins in the body are composed of 20 amino acids, with more than half of these synthesized by the human body and commonly called nonessential amino acids because they do not need to be consumed in the diet.[17] Nine of the amino acids are essential because the body cannot manufacture them: histine, isoleucine, leucine, lysine, methionine, phenylalanine, threonine, tryptophan, and valine. Therefore, the essential amino acids must be consumed through the diet.

Amino acids are joined together through peptide bonds. Two amino acids together are referred to as dipeptide, and several amino acids together are referred to as polypeptide. Polypeptide chains bond together to form a multitude of proteins with various structures and functions. Muscle tissue constitutes the body's highest concentration of proteins, and the majority of the body's protein exists in skeletal muscle, organs, and bone tissue. Although sometimes perceived to be all protein, tissues are mostly water and contain various amounts of protein. For example, protein makes up 20 percent of the weight of the heart, skeletal muscles, liver, and glands and 10 percent of brain tissue.[17] Nonstructural or plasma proteins, such as enzymes, antibodies, lipoproteins, hormones, hemoglobin, albumin, and transferin, constitute only a small proportion of the body's protein, but they are profoundly powerful and are negatively affected by poor nutritional status.

Dietary Protein

The amino acid content of a dietary protein affects how the protein will be used in the body. Whether the protein supplies the amino acids in amounts proportional to the body's needs determines the protein quality. High quality protein, high biological value, and complete protein are synonymous terms used to describe the amino acid pattern of protein that is similar to the body's needs. High quality proteins include proteins of animal origin (those in eggs, meat, fish, poultry, and dairy products). Proteins that are deficient in one or more of the essential amino acids (grains, beans, vegetables, and gelatin) are referred to as incomplete proteins, low quality proteins, or proteins of low biological value. Plant proteins tend to be low in lysine (grains) or methionine and cysteine (beans).[17] Of the plant proteins, soy is the highest quality. Protein quality is one of the issues vegans (those who consume only plant proteins—no meat, fish, poultry, eggs, or milk) must consider. When relying on low quality proteins, it is important to consume a variety of plant foods that provide different amino acids, often referred to as complementary proteins, so that all essential amino acids are consumed over the course of a day.[17,18] Common examples of complementary proteins are beans and rice, corn tortillas and refried beans, or peanut butter and bread. As a general rule of thumb, combining beans or legumes with grain provides the essential amino acids in appropriate ratios. It was believed for some time that complementary proteins had to be consumed at the same meal, however, this is now known to be untrue.

Protein Requirements

Although dietary recommendations are stated as protein requirements, the actual requirement is for amino acids. The need for dietary proteins/amino acids in sedentary, healthy adults results from the constant turnover of cells. During *cell turnover*, which is the constant breakdown and regeneration of cells, the immediate supplier of amino acids is the *amino acid pool*. The pool is replenished from dietary protein digestion, as well as the amino acids released from tissue turnover. Substantially more protein gets broken down daily than is ordinarily consumed, indicating that amino acids are recycled. This process is not completely efficient, however, so dietary amino acid intake is required to replace losses.

When estimating the protein requirements for individuals, two key factors, caloric intake and biological value of the protein should be considered. Protein can be metabolized as a source of energy in a state of negative caloric balance, in which fewer calories are consumed than are expended. In this case, the protein cannot be used for the intended purpose of replacing the amino acid pool; therefore, an inverse relationship exists between caloric intake and protein requirement. When caloric intake goes down, protein requirement goes up. Dietary protein requirements were derived from research on subjects who were consuming adequate calories. Requirements for individuals who are not consuming adequate calories are higher than stated requirements.

Key Point:

Dietary protein requirements were derived from research on subjects who were consuming adequate calories. Dietary protein requirements are higher for individuals who are not consuming adequate calories.

Additionally, approximately 65 to 75 percent of the proteins in those studies were from food of animal origin (meat, fish, poultry, dairy products and eggs), protein of high biological value.[17] The higher the biological value of the protein, the lower the protein requirement. Assuming the adequate caloric intake and two-thirds or more of the protein from animal sources, the recommended dietary allowance (RDA) for protein for adults is 0.8 g/kg of body weight for both adult men and women.[19] Requirements for individuals in a negative calorie balance or who consume lower quality proteins are higher, although they have not been quantified to date.

Beyond the maintenance requirement of protein previously described, training increases athletes' protein requirements. Both aerobic endurance training and strength training can increase protein need, although the exact mechanisms are unclear and may be different for the different types of training. For aerobic endurance athletes, the underlying mechanisms could include tissue repair and the use of the branched-chain amino acids for auxiliary fuel, whereas for strength and power athletes, the mechanisms are probably tissue repair and the maintenance of a positive nitrogen balance so that the hypertrophic stimulus is maximized.[20]

Research indicates that the protein requirement of aerobic endurance athletes is slightly over 0.8 g/kg of body weight and can reach 1.4g/kg of body weight, due in part to the increased use of protein as a fuel source during ex-

ercise.[20] Research has shown that strength training can increase requirements as high as 1.7 g/kg of body weight. Because most athletes do not fall neatly into one category (aerobic endurance or strength training athletes), a general recommendation of 1.5 to 2.0 g/kg of body weight ensures adequate protein intake and a diet with at least 65 percent of the protein of high biological value. Athletes consuming a vegan diet or restricting calories may require more than 2.0 g/kg of body weight.

Concerns regarding potential negative effects of protein intakes greater than 0.8 g/kg of body weight have often been expressed. These concerns are unfounded for the most part, especially in healthy individuals. Proteins consumed in excess of amounts needed for the synthesis of tissue are broken down. The nitrogen is excreted as urea in urine, and the remaining ketoacids are either used directly as sources of energy or converted to carbohydrate (gluconeogenesis) or body fat. Rehabilitation clinicians should be aware that excessively high protein intakes, greater than 4 g/kg of body weight per day, are not indicated for athletes with impaired renal function, or low calcium intake, or who are restricting fluid intake.[17] Finally, data from several recent systematic reviews have provided additional detail on how dietary protein intake can effect general health status. Liu et al.[21] conclude that a convincing cross sectional inverse association between dietary protein intake and blood pressure was demonstrated, indicating that higher levels of protein intake may be associated with lower blood pressure levels. Similarly, conclusions from a recent Cochrane systematic review indicate that supplementation appears to produce a small but consistent weight gain in frail, elderly individuals who are at risk for malnutrition, with a significant beneficial effect on mortality and a shortened length of hospital stay.[22]

Carbohydrates

The primary role of *carbohydrate* in human physiology is energy provision. The importance of carbohydrates in the diets of athletes and physical laborers was recognized very early in the 20th century. Diets high in carbohydrate content were found to enhance the performance of prolonged, heavy physical activity. Numerous studies have documented an ergogenic effect of carbohydrate intake and elevated muscle glycogen concentration on aerobic endurance performance, work output, and high intensity, intermittent activity.

Key Point:

Carbohydrate intake and elevated muscle glycogen concentrations enhance aerobic endurance, work output and the performance of high intensity, intermittent activities.

Additionally, glycogen concentration may be beneficial to high intensity exercise of short duration.[23] Carbohydrates are composed of carbon, hydrogen, and oxygen. Carbohydrates can be classified into three groups according to the number of sugar (saccharide) units they contain: monosaccharides, disaccharides, and polysaccharides.

Monosaccharides (glucose, fructose, and galactose) are single-sugar molecules. Glucose is the most common monosaccharide and is considered the building block of larger sugars. Glucose is present in the body as circulating sugar in the blood, is the primary energy substitute for cells, and is composed of *glycogen*, a polysaccharide stored in muscle and liver cells. In food sources, it is usually combined with other monosaccharides to form, for example, sucrose. Isolated glucose is used in intravenous fluids and is sometimes used in sports drinks as dextrose. Fructose has the same chemical formula as glucose, but because the atoms are arranged differently, it tastes much sweeter and has different properties. Fructose accounts for the sweet taste of honey, and occurs naturally in fruits and vegetables, and is also found in many sweetened beverages (e.g., carbonated soft drinks) as high-fructose corn syrup. In the body, fructose causes less insulin secretion than other sugars, which has made it a focus of much research in the area of aerobic endurance performance. However, large doses of fructose have been shown to increase the risk of gastric cramping and diarrhea, so applications of fructose as the primary source of carbohydrate during exercise are limited.[24] Galactose, the third monosaccharide, combines with glucose to form lactose, also known as milk sugar.

Disaccharides (sucrose, lactose, and maltose) are composed of two simple sugar units joined together. Sucrose (or table sugar), the most common disaccharide, is a combination of glucose and fructose. Its sweetness is derived from fructose. Sucrose occurs naturally in most fruits and is crystallized from the syrup of sugar cane and sugar beets to make brown, powdered, and white sugar. Although lactose (glucose + galactose) is found only in mammalian milk, maltose (glucose + glucose) occurs primarily when polysaccharides are broken down during digestion. It also occurs in the fermentation process of alcohol and is the primary carbohydrate of beer.

Polysaccharides, also known as complex carbohydrates, can contain thousands of glucose units. Some of the most common polysaccharides of nutritional importance are starch, fiber, and glycogen. Starch is the storage form of glucose in plants. Grains, nuts, legumes, and vegetables are good sources of starch. Before starch can be used as a source of energy, it first must be broken down into glucose components. *Dietary fiber*, a constituent of the plant cell wall, is also a form of carbohydrate. Fibers such as cellulose and noncarbohydrate fibrous materials (lignins) are generally resistant to human digestive enzymes and therefore increase bulk and water content and decrease transit time of feces.

Glycogen is found in small amounts of human and animal tissue as a temporary source of stored energy. It is not present to any large extent in the food we eat. When glucose enters the muscles and liver, if it is not metabolized for energy, it is synthesized to form glycogen. Two-thirds of the glycogen in the body is stored in skeletal muscle; the remaining third is stored in the liver.[17] The process of converting glucose to glycogen is called *glycogenesis*. The liver has the highest glycogen content of all the tissues in the body and, in fact, can convert many of the end products of digestion into glycogen—a process called *gluconeogenesis*.

Dietary Carbohydrates

Traditionally, breads, cereals, pasta, fruit, and starchy vegetables have been promoted to athletes as ideal sources of carbohydrate, and indeed they are. It should be understood, however, that all types of dietary carbohydrate, sugars as well as starches, are effective in supplying the athlete with glucose and glycogen. Consumption of a mix of sugars and starches is desirable.[17]

In real life, athletes typically consume a variety of carbohydrates in their normal diets, but occasionally seasoned athletes reach a point in their training when fine-tuning such details as the metabolic response to carbohydrates and the subsequent effect on performance becomes pertinent. Researchers and clinicians are interested in how altering carbohydrate ingestion may impact the glycemic response to foods. Originally used as a food marker for individuals with diabetes mellitus, only recently has the *glycemic index (GI)* been applied to the general population. The GI provides a qualitative indicator of how well ingested carbohydrate raises blood glucose levels.[3] The reference food is glucose, or white bread, which is given a rating of 100.[25] Foods that are digested quickly and rapidly raise blood glucose have a high GI. For example, carrots have a GI of 101, whereas lentils, which take longer to digest and therefore slowly increase blood glucose, have a GI of 41. However, McArdle and colleagues caution that although the GI is of interest and can be used for a general understanding of how foods behave when consumed, it appears that significant variability exists.[3] Although there is growing interest in low carbohydrate diets (e.g., Atkins and South Beach diets), there is growing evidence supporting diets that incorporate high levels of fiber rich carbohydrates, moderate to high levels of protein, and low levels of fat to prevent weight gain in a normal weight population and to help reduce bodyweight in an overweight population, and these diets may have the most beneficial effect on blood lipids and blood pressure levels.[26]

Lipids

Although the terms fat and lipid are often used interchangeably, lipid is a broader term. *Lipids* include triglycerides (fats and oils) as well as related fatty compounds, such as sterols and phospholipids.[17] Triglycerides, fatty acids, phospholipids, and cholesterol are the primary lipids of interest. Like carbohydrate, fat contains carbon, oxygen, and hydrogen atoms, but because the fatty acid chains have more carbon and hydrogen relative to oxygen, fats provide more energy per gram (9 kcal/g vs. 4 kcal/g for carbohydrates and proteins).[17]

A feature that differentiates the various fats is the degree of saturation of the fatty acids. Whereas saturated fats have maximized their hydrogen carrying capacity, some of the potential hydrogen bonding positions are unused in unsaturated fats. In addition, fatty acids containing no double bonds are saturated, whereas fatty acids containing one double bond are called monounsaturated, and fatty acids with two or more bonds are termed polyunsaturated. Although athletes and health care practitioners frequently perceive fatty acids negatively, fats serve several physiological functions. In addition to the insulative and protective function that fats, in the stored form of adipose tissue, can have, several fat soluble vitamins, such as A, D, E and K, rely on fatty acids as carriers.

> ### Key Point:
> Fats serve several important physiological functions including insulation and protection of internal organs, the formation of cell membranes, as carriers of vitamins A, D, E, and K, and in the production of several hormones.

The formation of cell membranes is also a function of several essential fatty acids, as is the production of several hormones.[17]

Similar to fat, cholesterol in the body has a negative reputation, despite its important function as a structural and functional component of cell membranes. Cholesterol is also necessary for the production of vitamin D and several hormones. However, high levels of cholesterol or unfavorable ratios of lipoproteins are associated with obesity and increased risk of heart disease.

PHARMACOLOGICAL AGENTS AND EXERCISE

As we have already seen, the physiological response to exercise is complex, involves multiple systems, and varies depending on the type, intensity, and duration of the activity. Increases in cardiac output and myocardial oxygen consumption, along with significant increases in blood flow to exercising muscles, are just a few of the general changes. It is known that many common medications can affect how the body responds to the physiological demands of exercise. Therefore, rehabilitation clinicians and other health care practitioners should be aware of the interaction of exercise and commonly prescribed pharmacological agents.

Drugs that directly affect the heart by altering either myocardial contractility or the initiation and conduction of the cardiac action potential can influence cardiac output.[27] Digitalis, an inotropic agent, can increase contractility, whereas various beta-adrenergic receptor antagonists (Beta-Blockers) will have opposite effects. Similarly, decreasing the rate of depolarization of the sinoatrial node can decrease heart rate through the use of beta-receptor antagonists. Medications can also affect exercise responses by altering factors that determine myocardial oxygen demands or oxygen delivery.[27] Primary factors that increase oxygen demand include an increase in heart rate, aortic pressure, and stroke volume. Increases in blood flow and oxygen delivery via vasodilation of coronary arteries can match the increased oxygen demands. However, if coronary artery stenosis inhibits the sufficient increase in blood flow, then decreasing oxygen demands by depressing heart rate, myocardial contractility, and/or total peripheral vascular resistance can be used. Accordingly, some medications used to treat angina are effective because they decrease myocardial oxygen requirements via these same mechanisms.[28]

> ### Key Point:
> Medications can also affect exercise responses by altering factors that determine myocardial oxygen demands or delivery.

Peripheral blood flow changes during exercise can also be affected by common medications. If the normal increase in skeletal muscle blood flow is impaired, then exercise duration may be decreased because of an accumulation of metabolites associated with anaerobic metabolism. For example, a nonspecific beta-receptor antagonist could prevent relaxation of the vascular smooth muscle in the exercising muscle by blocking beta-2 receptors. As a result, decreased oxygen delivery could occur due to a decrease in beta receptor–mediated vasodilation. This effect, however, is most likely offset by the vasodilation that occurs in response to the buildup of local metabolites.

Medications can also affect the metabolic response to exercise by interfering with *glycogenolysis* or fatty acid mobilization and subsequent oxidation.[29] Inadequate glycogen may limit endurance time, along with the ability to perform moderate- to high-intensity activities. Inadequate mobilization and oxidation of fatty acids limits the ability to perform exercise for prolonged time periods. The class of medications that has been most thoroughly studied in terms of effects on the metabolic response to exercise is the group of beta-adrenergic receptor antagonists because of the important role played by the sympathetic nervous system and catecholamines in maintaining metabolic homeostasis during strenuous work. By blocking beta-2 receptors in the liver, these medications can impair glycogenolysis. Similarly, studies have shown that there is less reliance on fatty acid oxidation during exercise when a person is taking beta receptor antagonists.[30,31] Additionally, there is no increase in the rate of muscle glycogen breakdown. The lack of compensatory increase in glycogen breakdown probably contributes to the reduction in endurance time.[27]

MOTOR UNITS AND MUSCLE FIBERS

The previous sections of this chapter have focused on the physiological mechanisms that convert food sources into useable forms of energy that not only maintain basal metabolism, but also ultimately produce purposeful movement. Muscle is the effector organ, driven by the electrical signals carried by motor neurons, that is responsible for developing the forces needed for movement. Therefore, it is necessary to understand how motor units function. The dynamic range of forces generated from this motor unit complex is impressive, from the precision grip tasks performed by the hand to the maximal exertion seen in power lifting. The following sections will more closely examine properties of the muscle cell and motor neuron, and how they relate to force production.

Muscle Physiology: a Historical Perspective

McComas provides an excellent historical perspective of the various experiments that contributed to our current understanding of how skeletal muscle fibers contract to produce purposeful movement.[2] In the 1950s, Andrew Huxley and Hugh Huxley (no relation) determined that the myofilaments within the muscle fibers, composed of actin and myosin filaments, moved systematically to produce the changes in muscle length and tension.

With the electron microscope, it was seen that each myofibril within a muscle fiber was composed of many myofilaments and that the latter were of two types, thick and thin.[32] In cross sections of muscle fibers, each thick filament is surrounded by a hexagonal array of thin filaments; in longitudinal sections the thick filaments of myofibril were found to be in alignment with each other. For a long time it had been known that the contractile proteins of muscles were myosin and actin, and next it was shown that these proteins corresponded to the thick and thin filaments, respectively.[32]

At the same time Hugh Huxley was undertaking these important studies, Andrew Huxley was using the interference microscope to examine the muscle striations of living frog muscle fibers during contraction and relaxation. He observed that during contraction the light I-band became shorter while the dark A-band remained the same length;

within the A-band, however the pale H-zone narrowed and might disappear completely.[33] Quite independently, the Huxleys proposed that their respective findings could be explained by sliding movement actin and myosin filaments past each other. This *sliding filament hypothesis* is now accepted.[2]

Figure 2.3 shows that the I-band is the region of the fiber where only actin filaments are present; the A-band corresponds to the position of the myosin filaments.[2] In the relaxed state, although there is some overlap between the actin and myosin filaments, opposing actin filaments are separated from each other along the myosin filament. The gap between the actin filaments is responsible for a pale region (H-zone) at the center of the A-band.

When the muscle contracts, the opposing actin filaments are propelled toward each other and slide along the intervening myosin filament. As they near each other, they cause the H-zone to become narrower; similarly, as more of each actin filament is drawn into the space between the myosin filaments, the I-band becomes shorter. Since the myosin filaments do not alter their shape, the length of the A-band stays unchanged.

The function of the Z-line, or Z-disc, is to tether the actin filaments together, while the M-line in the center of the A-band corresponds to link between the myosin filaments; both types of structure maintain the orderly geometrical relationship of the filaments to one another. The sliding filament mechanism consists of small projections from myosin filaments. These projections were termed cross-bridges, and it was proposed that they could momentarily attach themselves to the actin filaments and propel the latter into new positions. The cross-bridges are approximately 13 nm long and lie in six rows along the myosin filament; each row can engage one of the actin filaments in the hexagonal array surrounding the myosin filament. In a single "working stroke," a cross-bridge moves an actin filament through 10 nm in the space of 2 ms, while hydrolyzing one molecule of ATP.[34]

One of the predictions of the sliding filament hypothesis was that each cross-bridge would act as an independent force generator, and that the force developed in a contraction would then depend on the number of simultaneous interactions between the cross-bridges and the actin filaments. Experimentally, stretching the muscle fiber and so altering the amount of overlap between the actin and myosin filaments can vary the number of cross-bridge-actin interactions. Clinically, this can be done by contracting the calf muscles while placing the ankle in varying degrees of dorsiflexion. It can be seen that the force increases, with muscle lengthening, up to a maximum and then, with further stretching, starts to decline. Similarly, the tension developed is proportional to the degree of overlap between the actin and myosin filaments and thereby to the number of active cross-bridges on the latter. If further shortening is allowed, such that opposing actin filaments now overlap each other as well as the

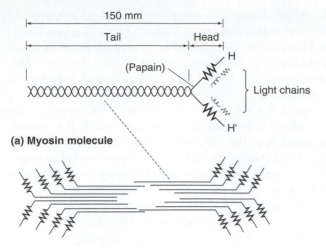

(a) Myosin molecule

(b) Myosin aggregate

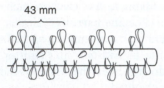

(c) Myosin filament

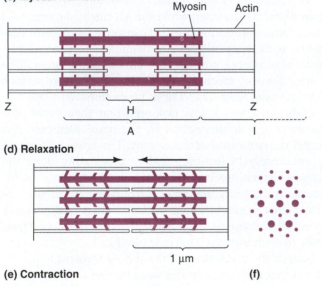

(d) Relaxation

(e) Contraction   **(f)**

Figure 2.3 Actin-myosin. The myosin molecule and its arrangement in the thick filaments of the myofibrils. (a) A single molecule, consisting of a double-helical rod terminating in two globular heads, each of which has two light chains attached. The site of enzymatic cleavage, with papain, is shown. (b) In solution, myosin molecules spontaneously aggregate to form filaments with heads at both ends. (c) In a thick filament, the two globular heads of a myosin molecule project to form a cross-bridge. The next bridge is separated by 14.3 nm and 60 degrees. (d) The overlap of actin and myosin filaments in a relaxed myofibril and the various refractive bands that are created. (e) Contraction is produced by actin filaments sliding over the myosin filament, causing approximation of the Z-lines (discs) and narrowing of the H-region. (f) A cross section through a myofibril to display the hexagonal disposition of the actin filaments around the myosin filaments. (Reprinted with permission from AJ McComas, *Skeletal Muscle: Form and Function*. Champaign, IL: Human Kinetics, 1996, p. 164 (Figure 11.2)).

underlying myosin filament, the isometric tension declines. It is probable that in some way overlapping actin filaments interfere with the cross-bridge mechanism at these short sarcomere lengths.

Key Point:

The tension a muscle can develop is proportional to the amount of overlap between the actin and myosin filaments.

When stretching the muscle fiber so far that there was no overlap between the myosin and the actin filaments, no tension could be developed because the myosin cross-bridges were unable to reach the actin filaments.[35,36] This is exactly the situation that is thought to occur in the cardiac failure associated with ventricular distension. Whether extensive lengthening can ever take place in normal skeletal muscles is doubtful, because the permissible ranges of joint movement are possibly too small. In diseased muscles, however, the possibility of hyperextension seems more likely, since the partial replacement of muscle fibers by relatively inelastic fibrous tissue could well allow surviving segments of fibers to be stretched excessively.[2]

A complete cross-bridge cycle lasts approximately 50 ms; of this time, the myosin head is attached to the actin filament for only 2 ms, and the power stroke is therefore a very brief event. As noted previously, each myosin head contains two *light chains* attached to the neck region of the myosin head and are termed *regulatory* and *essential*, respectively. In some ways the light chains are thought to effect the actions of the myosin heads, possibly by modifying the movement in each power stroke. Phosphorylation of the light chain has been proposed as the mechanism responsible for potentiating isometric twitch tension.[2]

Actin Filaments

Actin filaments, through their attachment to the cross-bridges, can be viewed as one half of the contractile mechanism. In the present section we will learn a little more about their structure and about the special proteins, troponin and tropomyosin, which are associated with them in the thin filaments of the muscle fiber.

With the electron microscope, an actin filament is seen as a thread about 1 μm long and 8 nm wide. The filament contains between 300 and 400 actin molecules, and each of these, in turn, is made up of 375 amino acids.[2] Although the actin molecules are spherical, they have a distinct polarity, and they line up facing the same direction, giving the appearance of a double-helical strand twisted about its own axis. This union of actin molecules is brought about by polymerization, a process that requires the presence of a nucleotide. An actin filament can be "decorated" by exposing it to myosin heads, which then appear as arrowhead-like structures along the filament. Since the actin molecules in each filament face the same way, the arrowheads behave similarly, pointing to the minus end of the filament.

Tropomyosin can be considered the tail of the myosin molecule (**Figure 2.4**). It consists of a double helix that lies on the surface of the actin filament and stiffens it; each tropomyosin molecule spans about seven of the actin mol-

ecules.[2] *Troponin* is a complex of three polypeptides, one of which (troponin T) attaches to tropomyosin. *Troponin I*, in contrast, binds to actin and indirectly prevents the latter from interacting with the myosin head. During a muscle contraction, this inhibitory effect of troponin I is overcome by a sudden rise in cytosolic calcium; each *troponin C* molecule captures four cytosolic calcium ions and, as it does so, undergoes a conformational change that lifts the tropomyosin molecule away from the actin filament. This movement of tropomyosin exposes sites on the actin filament to which the myosin heads can become attached, allowing the contraction to proceed.

Excitation-Contraction Coupling

As previously noted, the signal for a contraction to begin is a sudden rise in the concentration of calcium ions in the vicinity of the myosin and actin filaments. In this way calcium ions act as a second messenger, or an intermediary between the action potential and the contractile apparatus. The cellular mechanism by which the calcium concentration is increased is called excitation-contraction coupling and takes place in two steps: 1) depolarization of the T-tubules and 2) diffusion of calcium ions from the sarcoplasmic reticulum to the myofilaments. The excitation-contraction coupling can also be described as the processes that convert the motor neuron command, or action potential, into a muscle fiber force.

This process, involving seven steps, can be summarized as follows: 1) propagation of the sarcolemmal action potential; 2) propagation of the action potential down the transverse (T) tubule; 3) coupling of the action potential to the change in calcium conductance of the sarcoplasmic reticulum; 4) release of the calcium from the sarcoplasmic reticulum; 5) re-uptake of the calcium by the sarcoplasmic reticulum; 6) calcium binding to the troponin; and 7) interaction of the cross-bridge (myosin) and actin.[2] It should be noted that only step 7 actually represents the interaction between actin and myosin, whereas steps 1–6 are in preparation for this interaction.

Muscle Fiber Type

Human skeletal muscle is composed of a heterogeneous collection of muscle fiber types,[37,38] which allows varied functional activities to be performed efficiently. In addition, muscle fibers can adapt to changing demands by altering the size and fiber type composition of muscle. Because of this plasticity, a variety of intervention strategies have been developed to capitalize on this feature. In this section, an overview of muscle fiber type classifications will be discussed, which will provide a basis for more advanced muscle function. In contrast to the use of direct physiological measurements to distinguish motor units types, some classification schemes are based on histochemical, biochemical, and molecular properties of the muscle fibers. The histochemical and biochemical

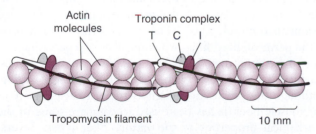

Figure 2.4   Actin. Schematic drawing of part of an actin filament showing the relationship between successive pairs of actin molecules, thin filaments of tropomyosin, and the three types of troponin. (Reprinted with permission from AJ McComas, *Skeletal Muscle: Form and Function.* Champaign, IL: Human Kinetics, 1996, p. 171 (Figure 11.9)).

techniques involve determining the enzyme content of the muscle fibers. Because enzymes are the catalysts for chemical reactions, measuring the amount of enzyme provides an index of the speed and quantity of the reaction. Similarly, molecular techniques can be used to determine the distribution of different isoforms of key molecules involved in a contraction. Thus, the aim of histochemical, biochemical, and molecular techniques is to measure mechanisms responsible for the various physiological properties. Once a correlation can be determined between a chemical reaction or the abundance of a molecule and a physiological response, the quantity of enzyme or molecule can be interpreted as a correlate of the physiological response.[39] Typically, three types of enzymes are measured: one type indicates contractile speed, whereas the other two represent the metabolic basis on which the muscle fiber produces its energy from contraction. Commonly assayed enzymes for aerobic metabolism are succinic dehydrogenase (SDH) and nicotinamide adenine dinucleotide-tetrazolium reductase (NADH-TR); for anaerobic capabilities, the enzymes are phosphorylase and alpha-glycerophosphate dehydrogenase (α-GPD).[39]

On the basis of these enzyme assays of muscle fibers, it is possible to classify muscle fibers into three groups. Two schemes can be used to make these classifications. One scheme, which classifies fibers solely on the basis of myosin ATPase, uses the names *types I, IIa,* and *IIb.* The distinction between *type I* and *type II* muscle fibers is based on the amount of ATPase activity remaining in the muscle fibers after preincubation in a solution with pH of 9.4. Type I represents the slow twitch and type II the fast twitch muscle fibers. Type II muscle fibers can be further separated into two groups (IIa and IIb) after preincubation in solution with pHs of 4.3 (IIa) and 4.6 (IIb). The distinction between muscle fiber types is shown in **Figure 2.5**, with myosin ATPase stain of a thin cross section of a cat hindlimb muscle. The other scheme, which uses enzymes for contraction speed (myosin ATPase), aerobic capacity (SDH or NADH-TR), and anaerobic capacity (phosphorylase and α-GPD), employs the term slow twitch, oxidative *(type SO);* fast twitch, oxidative-glycolytic *(type FG).*

One molecular technique that has been used to identify muscle fiber types assesses the distribution of the genetically defined isoforms of the myosin heavy chain.[40] With this technique, the molecular components of the muscle fiber specimen can be separated by gel electrophoresis and the quantity of each element measured by densitometry. Based on myosin heavy chain (MHC) isoforms, three types of muscle fibers can be identified with this technique in human skeletal muscle: MHC-I, MHC-IIa, and MHC-IId. Although the human MHC-IIb gene and transcript have been identified, type IIb fibers contain the MHC-IId or (MHC-IIx) isoform and not the MHC-IIb isoform. There is a high correspondence between the histochemically determined I, IIa, and IIb fiber types and the MHC-I, MHC-IIa, and the MHC-IId types identified by electrophoresis.

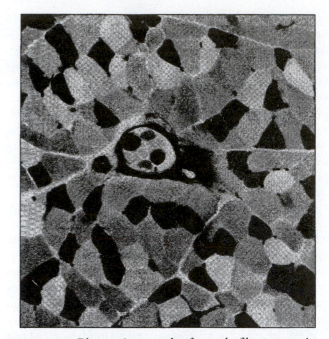

Figure 2.5 Photomicrograph of muscle fibers types in the cat tibialis posterior muscle after staining with myosin adenosine triphosphatase. Type I muscle fibers are the darkest, type IIa are the lightest, and type IIb appear gray. The structure in the middle of the figure is a muscle spindle with its capsule and intrafusal muscle fibers. Photo used with permission of RJ Callister. (Reprinted with permission from RM Enoka. *Neuromechanics of Human Movement.* Champaign, IL: Human Kinetics, 2002, p. 287 (Figure 6.45)).

A significant advantage of the molecular analysis is the possibility of identifying hybrid muscle fibers, that is, those compromising combinations of the MHC isoforms.

While many of the single-fiber characteristics described earlier in the chapter were determined with intact fibers from the frog, technical developments have made it possible to compare some of the properties of type-identified mammalian muscle fibers. The most common preparation is the permeabilized fiber, which involves the permeabilization of the outer membrane by the application of chemicals, the mechanical removal of the membrane, or freeze-drying. Although the preparation disrupts the normal integrity of the muscle fiber, it has been used to compare some of the mechanical properties of the various fiber types. Several studies have shown, for example, that the contractile speed, as indicated by shortening velocity, varies with fiber type. Because permeabilized fibers swell during performance of these measurements, fiber diameter cannot be measured accurately, and so the estimated values for specific tension differ from the values obtained with intact fibers.

The measurement of motor unit properties in human muscle results in a less discrete classification scheme than that of muscle fibers. There are at least four explanations for this discrepancy. First, it is possible that the measured biochemical and molecular characteristics are strongly related to contractile function, but this seems unlikely. Second, the muscle fibers of a motor unit may compromise a range of contractile properties, and we can measure only the net effect. There is evidence that the molecular composition of a muscle fiber can vary along its length, so it seems possible that the contractile function varies among the muscle fibers of the motor unit. Third, the forces exerted by the single muscle fibers might be modified in the transmission pathway from the fiber to the skeleton. The force generated by contractile proteins, for example, is transmitted through the cytoskeleton and connective tissues before it is registered externally. This process might make the contractile properties of muscle fibers appear more similar than they in fact are. Fourth, experiments on humans have largely focused on low threshold motor units; this could mask associations that exist across an entire population of motor units. Because of these possibilities, the classification scheme that should be used for human motor units is unclear.[39]

> ## Key Point:
> Experiments on human subjects have largely studied low threshold motor units; therefore the classification scheme that should be used for all types of human motor units is presently unclear.

Nonetheless, there does appear to be some association between muscle fiber typing and muscle function. When Monster, Chan, and O'Connor[41] examined the extent of usage for 15 muscles during a normal 8 hour working day, they found that muscles with higher proportion of type I fibers were used more frequently. Presumably, muscles with a higher proportion of type I fibers have a greater oxidative capacity and are less likely to fatigue due to metabolic factors. Similarly, there appears to be a positive correlation between the proportion of fast twitch fibers in biceps brachii and the maximum elbow flexor force, and the proportion of type I fibers and peak oxygen consumption.

To explore this issue systematically, Harridge et al.[42] obtained biopsy samples from three different muscles of human volunteers and measured the fiber type distribution and physiological properties of segments from single muscle fibers. The muscles examined in this study were soleus (MHC-I = 70 percent), vastus lateralis (MHC-I = 47 percent), and triceps brachii (MHC-I = 33 percent). Across these three muscles, whole muscle measurements of twitch contraction time, the rate of increase in tetanic force when the muscle was activated by electrical stimulation, and the fatigability after 2 min of intermittent electrical stimulation

were all associated with the proportion of the MHC-II fibers in the muscles (**Figure 2.6**). Although the MHC isoforms determine such physiological properties as the maximum shortening velocity and the maximum rate of tetanic force in single fibers, the associations suggest that the biochemical and molecular determinants of these other properties may co-vary with the MHC-determined fiber types. An important feature of these data, however, is the absence of significant associations within each muscle. It seems that when we are comparing the fiber-type proportions for a

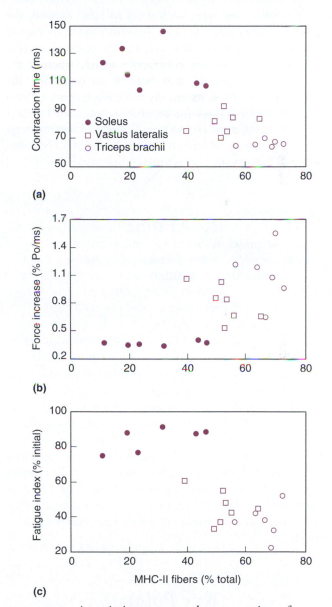

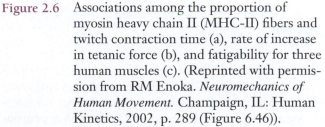

Figure 2.6 Associations among the proportion of myosin heavy chain II (MHC-II) fibers and twitch contraction time (a), rate of increase in tetanic force (b), and fatigability for three human muscles (c). (Reprinted with permission from RM Enoka. *Neuromechanics of Human Movement.* Champaign, IL: Human Kinetics, 2002, p. 289 (Figure 6.46)).

specific muscle across subjects, fiber-type differences can only partially explain the physiological differences.

Although motor unit and muscle fiber activity is often discussed in terms of the slow twitch (S), fast twitch fatigue resistant (FR), and fast twitch fast fatigable (FF) motor unit scheme, this does not appear to be appropriate for human muscles. Additionally the *size principle of motor unit recruitment*, which states motor unit recruitment follows an orderly process from smaller, slow twitch motor units to larger, fast twitch motor units, may not be accurate. First, investigators have been unable to identify comparable motor unit types in human muscle. Second, the first motor units activated in a voluntary contraction can be either slow twitch or fast twitch. Third, the cross sectional area of human muscle fibers often does not increase from type I to type IIb, as it does in many non-human muscles. The relative size of different fiber types appears to vary among muscles and between men and women; type I fibers can be the same size as type II fibers. These findings suggest that much remains to be learned about the functional organization of motor units in humans.[39]

> ## Key Point:
> The size principle of motor unit recruitment may not be accurate. Much remains to be learned about the functional organization of motor units in humans.

Motor Units

Muscle force is graded through activation for the individual components of the neuromuscular system, which are known as motor units. A *motor unit* is defined as the cell body and dendrites of a motor neuron, the multiple branches of its axon, and the muscle fibers that it innervates. Most skeletal muscles comprise a few hundred motor units.[2,43] Because each motor neuron innervates many muscle fibers, ranging from about 5 to 2,000 in various muscles, a few hundred motor neurons are able to activate the thousands of fibers that compose each muscle.

> ## Key Point:
> One motor neuron can innervate 5 to 2,000 individual muscle fibers.

The motor unit has been referred to as the final common pathway, through which the commands from the nervous system are sent to the muscle.[39,44] The motor neurons innervating skeletal muscle are located in the spinal cord and brainstem, and each motor neuron sends its axon via a peripheral nerve to the muscle fibers that it innervates.

The features of the motor neuron that vary within a population include its morphology, excitability, and distribution of input. The morphological feature of the neural component that has received the greatest attention is the motor neuron size. This feature is thought to be important because of its role in the activation of motor neurons. The size of the neuron can be indicated by the diameter of the soma, the surface area of the cell body, the number of dendrites arising from the soma, the diameter of the axon, and the cell capacitance.[39] As indicated by Henneman et al.,[45] there is a strong correlation between the size of a motor neuron and order of activation. For example, small motor neurons have a lower level of excitability, defined by the amount of current that must be injected into the motor neuron for it to generate an action potential, compared to motor neurons of larger size. Other motor neuron properties appear to differ based on size, including the after-hyperpolarization, conduction velocity, and the type of input (number and type of synapses) received.[39]

Although a muscle fiber is innervated by a single motor neuron, each motor neuron innervates more than one muscle fiber. The number of muscle fibers innervated by a single motor unit is referred to as the *innervation ratio* and varies from about 1:1,900 in the lower leg muscles to 1:6 in some ocular muscles. For example, the first dorsal interosseus muscle (a hand muscle) contains about 41,000 muscle fibers and 120 motor units, with an innervation ratio of about 1:342 (**Table 2.5**). In contrast, medial gastrocnemius has about 1,120,000 muscle fibers and 580 motor units, which yields an average innervation ratio of 1:1,934. However, as Enoka and Fuglevand[46] have reported, the range of innervation ratios in a given muscle is unknown. Each time a motor neuron is activated in the central nervous system, it elicits one or more action potentials in all of its muscle fibers; hence, the lower the innervation ratio, the lower the number of muscle fibers that are activated. The innervation ratio is also indicative of the number of times that an axon must branch in order to contact all of its muscle fibers.

Another important concept is that of the distribution of muscle fibers innervated by a single motor unit. Data from cat medial gastrocnemius indicate that muscle fibers belonging to the unit were confined to a sub-volume of the muscle. This territory can extend to up to 15 percent of the volume of the muscle, with a density of two to five muscle fibers per 100 belonging to the motor unit.[47] This means that a given region of a muscle contains muscle fibers from 20 to 50 different motor units.

Not only is the territory of a single motor unit limited to a specific part of a muscle, but it also appears that different parts of a muscle can contain distinct populations of motor units. This observation has given rise to the concept of a *neuromuscular compartment*.[48]

TABLE 2.5 Anatomical estimates of the number of motor axons and muscle fibers in human skeletal muscles.

Muscle	Specimen	Motor axon	Number of muscle fibers	Innervation ratio
Biceps brachii	Stillborn infants	774	580,000	750
First dorsal interosseus	Male 22 yr	119	40,500	340
First lumbrical	Male 54 yr	93	10,038	108
	Female 29 yr	98	10,500	107
Medial gastrocnemius	Male 28 yr	579	1,247,000	1934
Rectus lateralis	Two cadavers	4150	22,000	5
Tibialis anterior	Male 40 yr	445	250,200	562

(Modified and reprinted with permission from RM Enoka, *Neuromechanics of Human Movement.* Champaign, IL: Human Kinetics, 2000, p. 83.)

Key Point:

Neuromuscular compartmentalization refers to a specific portion of a whole muscle having a distinct population of motor units.

Enoka defines a compartment as the volume of muscle supplied by a primary branch of the muscle nerve.[39] A compartment contains a unique population of motor units, and the muscle fibers belonging to one motor unit are confined to a single neuromuscular compartment. The proportion of muscle fiber types can differ between the compartments of a single muscle. Neuromuscular compartments have been found in some, but not all, muscles. Because compartments can be activated independently, a single muscle, which is an anatomical entity, can consist of several distinct regions that each serves a different physiological function.[49] Also, the existence of compartments suggests that it can be misleading to infer the function of a muscle based solely on the location of its attachments. The analysis of muscle function must consider both the architecture and innervation pattern of the muscle.[39]

The biceps brachii muscle is often cited as an example of a muscle with distinct neuromuscular compartments. Three to six primary branches of the musculocutaneous nerve innervate it, and functionally, the motor units in biceps brachii appear to comprise two distinct populations. One population, which is located in the lateral aspect of the long head, is active when a flexion torque is exerted about the elbow joint. The other population is active when the torque about the elbow joint includes flexion and supination components.[39]

Contractile Properties

Motor units can be compared with one another based on a number of physiological properties, including the discharge characteristics of the motor neuron, the speed of contraction, the magnitude of force, and the resistance to fatigue. Most comparisons are based on the contractile properties of the motor unit. Two methodologies are commonly used for evaluating these parameters, one direct and the other indirect. A *direct evaluation* refers to the physiological measurement of the motor unit properties. An *indirect evaluation* is based on the histochemical, biochemical, and molecular measurement of characteristics that are related to contractile function. The direct physiological characterization of a motor unit is based on the discharge pattern of its action potentials and on its contractile properties.

Contractile Speed

A *muscle twitch* is the summative force-time response to a single input (**Figure 2.7**). Under normal conditions, the input is an action potential in response to an activation signal from the nervous system. In some experiments, however, the input is an electric shock that artificially generates an action potential. A *twitch response* is usually characterized by three measurements: the time from force onset to peak force (contraction time), the magnitude of the peak force, and the time it takes for the force to decline to one-half of its peak value (half-relaxation time). Contraction time is used as a measure of the speed of the contractile machinery, although it primarily depends on the rate at which calcium is released from the sarcoplasmic reticulum. If contraction time is long, the motor unit is described as a slow twitch motor unit, whereas a brief contraction time indicates a fast twitch unit.[39]

Motor Unit Force

Motor units are rarely activated to produce individual twitches. Rather, the input typically comprises several action potentials, resulting in a series of twitch responses that overlap and produce a force that is greater than the twitch force. The force-time profile that consists of overlapping twitch responses is known as a *tetanus.* As the frequency of the action potentials increases, the tetanus

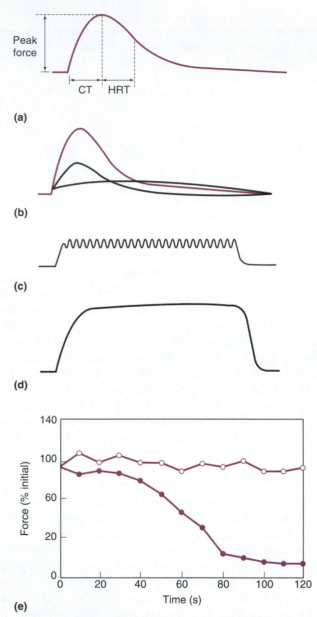

(a)

(b)

(c)

(d)

(e)

Figure 2.7   Twitch and tetanic responses of motor units in a cat hindlimb muscle. (a) Motor unit twitch (contraction time [CT] = 24 ms; half-relaxation time [HRT] = 21 ms; peak force = 0.03N); (b) twitch responses for fast- and slow-twitch motor units; (c) an unfused tetanus (stimulated at 28 Hz) for a fast-twitch unit (peak force = 0.42 N); (d) a fused tetanus (stimulated at 200 Hz) for the motor unit in c (peak force = 1.30 N); (e) fatigue test for fatigue-resistant and fatigable motor units. (Reprinted with permission from RM Enoka. *Neuromechanics of Human Movement.* Champaign, IL: Human Kinetics, 2002, p. 282 (Figure 6.42)).

muscle fibers determines both the magnitude and the smoothness of the motor unit force.

The relation between activation rate and average tetanic force is known as the *force–frequency relation.* To determine the force–frequency relation for a motor unit, the unit must be activated with electric shocks at various rates and the evoked force measured. The resulting graph indicates the force–frequency relation for the motor units. This relation indicates the rate at which the motor units must be activated to achieve maximal force. Therefore, by recording the discharge rate of action potentials during voluntary contractions, the proportion of the maximum force that the motor units exert can be assessed.[39]

The capability of the motor unit to exert force is not measured from the twitch; it is assessed from the peak force of a single fused tetanus. The difference between the peak twitch force and the maximum force in a fused tetanus, known as the *twitch–tetanus ratio,* generally varies from 1:1.5 to 1:10. Thus, in a fused tetanus the force may be 1.5 to 10 times greater than the twitch force. Peak tetanic force for human motor units does not vary as a function of twitch contraction time. Instead, the maximum force from a fused contraction can vary over a substantial range for the same twitch contraction time, and conversely twitch contraction time can double with a systematic change in the maximum force levels. These data indicate that the peak force exerted by motor units in the human thenar muscle is not related to the twitch contraction time, that is, some fast twitch motor units exert relatively low forces.[50]

Fatigability

The force achieved in a single tetanus declines over time if the motor unit is required to produce a series of tetani. The ability of a motor unit to prevent such a decline indicates its resistance to fatigue. The time between the onset of activation and the beginning of the decline in force differs markedly among motor units, and can be assessed by various fatigue tests. Burke and colleagues[51] developed a standard fatigue test used initially in the cat hindlimb, which involves eliciting tetani for two to six minutes at a rate of one tetanus each second—each tetanus lasts for 330 ms and includes 13 stimuli. A ratio between these forces and that exerted during the initial tetanus is used as an *index of fatigue.* This fatigue test seems to stress the connection between the electrical signal from the nervous system and the contraction of the muscle, and thereby distinguishes motor units that are fatigue resistant and those that are not. Fatigue resistant motor units (types S and FR) have a fatigue index greater than or equal to 0.75 compared with an index of less than 0.25 for fatigable motor units (type FF). An index of 0.25 indicates that after 2 min the force exerted by the unit will be only 25 percent of that measured at the beginning of the test. These data suggest that activation of the type S and FR motor units is more appropriate for sustained contractions because they are resistant to fatigue.

changes from an irregular force profile (unfused) to a smooth plateau (fused tetanus). The rate at which the action potentials are sent from the motor neuron to the

Motor Unit Types

Based on the distributions of these contractile properties, it is often possible to identify different groups of motor units. Such classification schemes are based on the physiological properties of the motor units. However, classification systems established from animal data may not accurately represent the function of human motor units.[52] Human motor units can be distinguished based on differences in tetanic force and fatigability, but not contraction time. For example, Enoka[39] and others[53] have analyzed data that indicate the most fatigue-resistant motor units in the human thenar muscle tend to produce a lesser tetanic force. The first motor units activated during a voluntary contraction performed by a human subject are weak and fatigue resistant, but they may be slow or fast contracting. Enoka[39] emphasizes that it is not correct to say that low force contractions performed by humans are sustained solely by slow twitch muscle fibers.

Key Point:

Low force human muscle contractions are not sustained solely by slow twitch muscle fibers.

Although there is not a strong association between force and contraction speed for human motor units, there do appear to be both fast and slow twitch motor units in human muscles. Twitch contraction times of human motor units have been reported to extend along a continuum from 20 to 72 ms (mean = 35 ms) for masseter muscle, 43 to 91 ms (mean = 57 ms) for long finger flexors and hand muscles, and 40 to 110 ms (mean = 76 ms) for medial gastrocnemius.[39] Several factors influence differences in contraction speed, including variations in enzyme myosin ATPase, the rate at which calcium is released from and taken up by the sarcoplasmic reticulum, and the architecture of the muscle.

One feature of contraction speed that may distinguish among human motor units is the activation rate required to achieve half the maximum force. Fuglevand et al.[53] identified two groups of motor units when assessing force–frequency relation of motor units in the long finger flexors and hand muscles. One group of motor units required an activation rate of 9 Hz, whereas the other group needed 16 Hz to achieve half maximum force. The average contraction times for the two groups of motor units were 66 ms and 46 ms, respectively. However, there was no difference in the fatigability of these two groups of motor units.

Motor Unit Activation Patterns

The force that a muscle can exert is varied through alteration in the amount of motor unit activity.[54] This is accomplished by changing either the number of motor units that are active (*motor unit recruitment*) or the rate at which motor neurons discharge action potentials (*discharge rate modulation*). It has long been known that the performance of a particular movement always appears to be accomplished by the activation of motor units in a set sequence.[55] Because the sequence of motor unit activation remains relatively fixed, it has been called *orderly recruitment*. As the force exerted by a muscle increases, additional motor units are activated, or recruited. Once recruited, a motor unit remains active until the force declines (**Figure 2.8**). A motor unit that initially responds to force demands is recruited first and remains active as long as the force does not decrease. The increase in force occurs because of continuing recruitment of motor units and an increase in the activation rate of the recruited motor units. As the force is reduced, motor units are sequentially inactivated, or derecruited, in the reverse order. This means that the last motor unit recruited is typically the first derecruited.[39]

The relative contribution of motor unit recruitment to muscle force varies among muscles. In some hand muscles, for example, all motor units are recruited when force reaches about 50 percent of maximum. In other muscles, such as biceps brachii, deltoid, and tibialis anterior, motor unit recruitment continues up to 85 percent of maximum force.[39,50,56] The increase in muscle force beyond the upper limit of motor unit recruitment is accomplished entirely

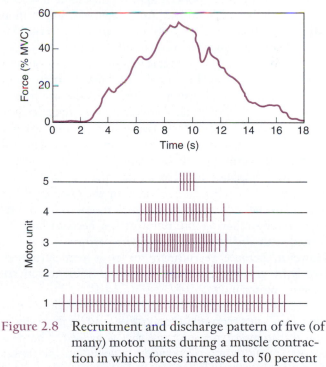

Figure 2.8   Recruitment and discharge pattern of five (of many) motor units during a muscle contraction in which forces increased to 50 percent of maximum (MVC = maximal voluntary contraction). (Reprinted with permission from RM Enoka. *Neuromechanics of Human Movement*. Champaign, IL: Human Kinetics, 2002, p. 289 (Figure 6.47)).

through variation in the discharge rate of action potentials.

Motor Unit Recruitment Order

Orderly recruitment has been demonstrated in a wide variety of muscle groups and animal species for many different tasks. It appears to be the result of several physiological processes rather than a single mechanism.[39] One factor underlying orderly recruitment is motor neuron size, which is indicated by the surface area of the soma and dendrites. This effect is commonly known as the *size principle*, which states that the recruitment order of motor units is determined by differences in motor unit size. According to the size principle, the motor unit with the smallest motor neuron is recruited first and the motor unit with the largest motor neuron is recruited last.[57]

The recruitment of motor units, however, does not depend solely on motor neuron size; it is also influenced by other motor neuron characteristics and by the organization of synaptic inputs on the dendrites and soma of the motor neurons in the pool. It appears that some morphological (number of dendrites, axon diameter, innervation ratio), membrane (input resistance, after-hyperpolarization, rheobase), and synaptic input characteristics vary with motor unit size such that smallest motor neurons can be excited most easily. Because the peak force a motor unit can exert covaries with size, recruitment by the size principle means that muscle force can be graded systematically.

One advantage of orderly recruitment is that when a muscle is commanded to exert a force, the sequence of motor unit recruitment is determined by spinal mechanisms and does not have to be specified by the brain. Therefore, the command generated by the brain does not have to include information on which motor units to activate thereby relieving the brain of the need to be concerned with this level of movement performance detail. However, because recruitment order is predetermined, largely by spinal mechanisms, it is not possible to activate selective motor units.

The consequence of this predetermined order is that the motor units recruited for a task depend on the proportion of the motor neuron pool that is needed. The proportion of motor units recruited depends on the power demands of the task. For example, jogging at a slow speed represents an activity in which the muscle power requirements are minimal, therefore, only low threshold motor units may need to be recruited. Because recruitment order is fixed, the gradual increase in the power demands of a

task involves the progressive recruitment of higher threshold motor units. When power demands of the task are high, as for a vertical jump, both low and high threshold motor units may be recruited in a prescribed order.

Discharge Rate

The force exerted by muscle is due to variable combinations of the number of active motor units and the rate at which the motor neurons discharge action potentials (firing rate). When a motor unit is recruited and the force exerted by the muscle continues to increase, the rate at which the motor neuron discharges usually increases. Although each motor unit action potential results in a motor unit twitch, when the action potentials occur close to one another, the twitches add together and exert a force that is greater than the twitch. The degree to which the twitches summate depends on the rate at which the action potentials are discharged, producing the force–frequency relation (**Figure 2.9**). The increase in the force when action potential rate goes from 5 to 10 Hz is not the same as that due to increasing firing rate from 20 to 25 Hz, even though there is a difference of 5 Hz in each case. The greatest increase in force (steepest slope) occurs at the intermediate discharge rates (9 to 12 Hz).

On the basis of the force–frequency relation, we can measure the rate at which a motor neuron discharges action potentials and infer the relative force that the motor unit exerts. For most tasks that have been examined, discharge rate is well below that necessary to evoke the maximum force for a motor unit. Because of technical limitations, most is known about motor unit discharge during low force, isometric conditions. For such tasks, there is a concurrent increase in motor unit recruitment and discharge rate as the muscle force is recruited.[58] **Figure 2.10** illustrates this scheme by showing that a gradual increase and subsequent decrease in force were accomplished by the recruitment and derecruitment of motor units and a parallel variation in the discharge rate for the earliest recruited motor units.[58] Each thin line in the figure represents the activity of a single motor unit located in rectus femoris muscle, with recruitment occurring at the leftmost dot on each thin line. Motor unit 1, for example, was recruited at a force of about 28 percent of maximum with an initial discharge rate of 9 Hz, which increased to 15 Hz at the peak force. If the force–frequency relation for this motor unit was similar to that shown in **Figure 2.9** then the motor unit would have exerted a peak force that was about 60 percent of maximum. However, it should be

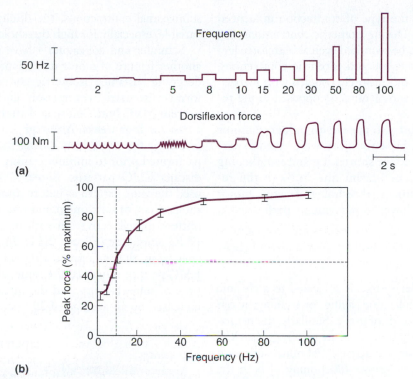

(a)

(b)

Figure 2.9 The force–frequency relation for motor units in human toe extensor muscles. (a) Motor units activated by intraneural stimulation (upper trace) evoked a force in the dorsiflexor muscles (lower trace); (b) force was normalized to the maximum value for each motor unit to produce the force-frequency relation for 13 motor units. (Reprinted with permission from RM Enoka. *Neuromechanics of Human Movement.* Champaign, IL: Human Kinetics, 2002, p. 284 (Figure 6.43)).

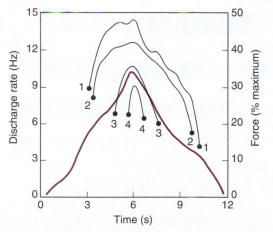

Figure 2.10 Modulation of discharge rate by four motor units during a gradual increase and then decrease in the force (thick line) exerted by the knee extensor muscles. (Reprinted with permission from RM Enoka. *Neuromechanics of Human Movement.* Champaign, IL: Human Kinetics, 2002, p. 292 (Figure 6.50)).

noted that motor neuron discharge rates can vary significantly over the course of a given task.

The minimum rate at which motor neurons discharge action potentials repetitively during voluntary contractions is about 5 to 7 Hz.[50,59,60] Discharge rate is measured while a muscle exerts moderate forces (35 percent of maximum); the maximal discharge rates are greater for low threshold motor units. At high forces, some studies have shown that the high threshold motor units have greater maximum discharge rates, while others have shown that the maximal discharge rate is greater for low threshold units. Maximum discharge rates, however, vary across muscles. The mean rates of 35 to 40 Hz have been recorded for first dorsal interosseus, 29 Hz for deltoid, 20 to 25 Hz for biceps brachii, and 11 Hz for soleus. Linnamo and colleagues[61] recently compared motor unit activation patterns at various force levels during concentric and eccentric muscle contractions. Intramuscular and surface electromyographic (EMG) recordings in the biceps brachii muscle indicated that motor unit recruitment threshold might be lower in dynamic compared to isometric activations. In addition, the type of contraction influenced the recruitment pattern. During isometric contractions, fast motor units continued to be recruited even at high force levels, whereas during concentric and eccentric contractions, higher force levels were more closely coupled with increasing firing rates of active motor units, as opposed to the recruitment of new units.

The rate of movement also appears to influence motor unit activation patterns. When subjects were asked to perform constant velocity, active shortening and lengthening contractions of the biceps brachii muscle, both the recruitment and derecruitment thresholds of active motor units were found to be lower in movements performed at higher velocities.[62]

Fatigue

When the neuromuscular system is subjected to a chronic stimulus, such as immobilization, aging, or training, it can adapt to the altered demands of usage. Similarly, the neuromuscular system can adapt to more acute challenges, such as those associated with sustained activity. Volitional activation of skeletal muscle requires proper functioning of both the central nervous system and peripheral neuromuscular pathways. Failure anywhere along the central or peripheral pathways can result in fatigue. *Fatigue* is defined as any reduction in the force-generating capacity of a muscle due to recent activation and can be attributed to peripheral or central nervous system failure.[63–65] Although many studies have been undertaken in an attempt to identify a single factor, there seems to be little doubt that the concept of fatigue refers to a class of acute effects that can impair motor performance. These observations have led to the notion that the mechanisms underlying fatigue are task dependent.[66]

Key Point:

Fatigue refers to a class of acute effects than can impair motor performance. The mechanisms underlying fatigue are task dependent.

The activity of motor units during a fatiguing contraction depends on the intensity and the type of contraction being performed. The average discharge rates of motor units in many muscles decline during a sustained Maximal Voluntary Contraction (MVC).[67,68] In addition, the average discharge rate of motor units during submaximal isometric contractions does not change substantially, although the change in discharge rate appears to differ for isometric and anisometric contractions.[69] Enoka concludes that the increase in EMG during a fatiguing contraction held at a submaximal force is largely due to the recruitment of additional motor units.[39] The activation history of the muscle also provides flexibility to motor unit recruitment. For example, when a muscle that is in a fatigued state performs

submaximal contractions, the discharge rate can be more variable, especially for high threshold motor units.[70,71]

Semmler and colleagues[72] have recently demonstrated another feature of motor unit adaptability for subjects undergoing sustained isometric contractions. Subjects performed isometric contraction at a target force of 15 percent MVC both before and after the arm was placed in a cast for four weeks. Although the EMG increased progressively for all subjects during the fatiguing contraction performed prior to immobilization, subjects exhibited two distinct EMG patterns. Some subjects (five of six men) used the same pattern as before immobilization. The other subjects (six of six women and one of six men) used intermittent muscle activation with no progressive increase in EMG amplitude (**Figure 2.11**). In addition, there was no change in the endurance time of those subjects whose EMG pattern remained the same, although the endurance time of subjects who used the intermittent EMG pattern increased by an average of 207 percent. The intermittent

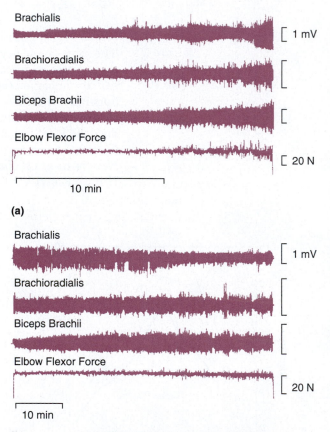

Figure 2.11   EMG activity for the brachialis, brachioradialis, and biceps brachii muscles during a submaximal fatiguing contraction (a) before and (b) after four weeks of casting. (Reprinted with permission from RM Enoka. *Neuromechanics of Human Movement.* Champaign, IL: Human Kinetics, 2002, p. 382 (Figure 8.20)).

EMG pattern was accompanied by an apparent rotation of activity among a selected group of motor units.[72]

Aging

Although men and women can maintain full and active lives as they age, several important changes in the motor system accompany the aging process, including muscles becoming thinner, strength decreasing, and movements becoming slower and less precise.[2,73] In addition, these neuromuscular changes result in a reduction in the magnitude of reflex responses, a slowing of rapid reactions, and increased postural instability, decreased control of submaximal forces, and difficulty with precision movements.[74] The loss of strength and muscular coordination affects men and women similarly and appears to affect most, if not all, muscle groups. As expected, the decline is greatest in the oldest subjects, in whom some muscles can only develop half their former force.[75] However, the extent of age-related declines in performance is gradual, and can be mitigated by training and lifestyle changes.

Key Point:

The effect of aging on muscle performance can be mitigated by a healthy lifestyle and by performing regular exercise activities.

Vandervoort and McComas[76] reported that ankle dorsiflexor and plantar flexor muscles lose approximately 1.3 percent of their former strength each year beyond the age of 50, and conclude that similar rates of strength loss occur in other muscle groups.

One of the most prominent effects of age on the motor system is the unavoidable decline in muscle mass and strength, a condition known as *sarcopenia*.[75,77] The decrease in strength, however, is usually greater than the loss of muscle mass. Frontera et al.[78] reported that cross sectional area of muscle in a longitudinal study declined by 16 percent for the knee extensor muscle group and 15 percent for the knee flexor group compared with the average strength reductions of 20 to 30 percent. One explanation for this dissociation between muscle cross sectional area and strength may be that typical cross sectional area techniques do not account for the fact that contractile elements are frequently replaced by adipose and connective tissue in aging muscle.[76] In addition to the loss of muscle mass and strength with age, the contractile speed of many muscles is also reduced in older individuals,[79] as indicated by an increase in contraction and relaxation time of the twitch response, a decline in the speed of rapid contractions, and a reduction in the power that muscles can produce.

Muscle biopsies taken from aging muscles indicate that individual muscle fibers maintain their sizes into the seventh

decade of life, although beyond that time there is progressive shrinkage of type II fibers, and less changes occurring in the type I fibers.[2] Therefore, age-related changes to the muscle fibers do not account for the all the neuromuscular adaptations associated with declines in performance. Modification in the structure and function of motor units is another factor associated with reduction in motor performance with aging. Until the age of 60, the number of functioning motor units shows little change; beyond the age of 60, there is a progressive fall in the number of functioning units, and by 70 years of age, the population of units is reduced to less than half its original size (**Figure 2.12**). Fortunately, the loss of motor units with advancing age does not imply that all the muscle fibers innervated by a dying motor unit will also become nonfunctional. The development of collateral axonal sprouts will reinnervate some of the abandoned muscle fibers, thereby preserving their function.

Key Point:

Collateral axonal sprouting helps to preserve muscle function with advancing age.

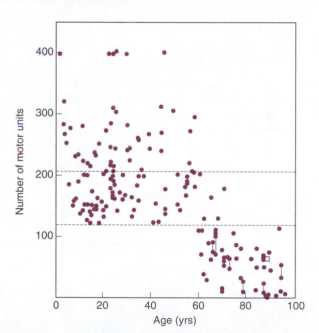

Figure 2.12 Loss of functioning motor units with age. The results were obtained from the extensor digitorum brevis muscles of 207 healthy subjects aged 7 months to 97 years. The upper and lower horizontal lines show respectively the mean value (210 units) and the lower limit of the range for subjects below 60 years (120 units). Linked values are bilateral. (Reprinted with permission from AJ McComas. *Skeletal Muscle: Form and Function*. Champaign, IL: Human Kinetics, 1996, p. 332 (Figure 22.5)).

The re-innervation of denervated muscle fibers by surviving motor units increases the innervation ratio of these units. Because of the increases in innervation ratio, the force exerted by single motor units increases as a function of age.[39,80] This influences the ability of an individual to smoothly grade muscle force in two ways. First, there are fewer low force motor units. Typically a motor unit pool consists of many low force units with an exponentially declining number of high force units. The low force units are important for finely controlled movements that involve submaximal forces. Second, the smoothness (as indicated by absence of fluctuations) of the force exerted by a muscle depends on the force contributed by the most recently recruited motor unit. Because motor units are recruited at low discharge rates that produce unfused tetani, the recruitment of a motor unit contributes to net force fluctuations. Furthermore, the increase in motor unit force with age results in larger fluctuations with each motor unit recruited. As the average force increases, however, the relative contribution of the most recently recruited motor unit to the net force decreases, which suggests that the effect of enlarged motor units on the force fluctuation is greatest at low forces. This is consistent with the observation that old adults are less steady, compared with young adults, when exerting low forces and lifting light loads.[30,81–83]

Spinal Reflexes

Although much is known about the organization of motor units and motor neuron pools, it is less clear how this organization influences motor behavior. Spinal reflexes are a form of sensorimotor integration because they involve connections between the afferent and efferent neurons. Spinal reflexes are mediated at the spinal level, in contrast to others mediated at the brainstem and higher centers. Spinal reflexes serve three important functions in motor control: 1) to adjust for unexpected perturbations; 2) to organize patterns of coordination, such as reciprocal inhibition; and 3) to allow for rapid protection from painful and damaging stimuli.

Key Point:
Spinal reflexes help adjust for unexpected perturbations, organize patterns of coordination such as reciprocal inhibition, and allow for protection from painful and injurious stimuli.

Spinal reflexes that are nonpathologic provide efficiency in motor planning and effectiveness of movement without the need for conscious thought or continuous supraspinal modulation (see Chapter 8). For example, higher centers may provide a goal directed plan for skipping rope, but the details of this plan, such as the reciprocal activation of flexors and extensors, is enabled by the spinal cord reflex circuitry rather than by direct supraspinal control.

Another example can be illustrated by this scenario: I hand you a box that is small but unexpectedly heavy for its size. Without too much effort, you are able to compensate for this unexpected weight automatically. The adequate stimulus for load compensation is muscle stretch; thus the reflex is called the *stretch reflex*, also known as the *myotatic reflex*. The stretch reflex is present even after total destruction of the cerebral cortex. Even though the cortex is involved in the myotatic reflex, the remainder of the central nervous system makes its own contribution.

Several different neural circuits are responsible for increasing muscle activation in response to the increased load (**Figure 2.13**). Much of the circuitry for the stretch reflex appears to be wired into the spinal cord. Returning to the example, when you received the box, the very first change in your muscle activity occurred quickly. Type Ia spindle afferents were excited by the stretch on the muscle due to the weight of the box. These afferents enter the spinal cord through the dorsal root and synapse directly on the motor neurons of the same muscle. If enough type Ia afferents release enough transmitter on the motor neurons, the motor neurons generate action potentials that travel back out of the ventral root of the cord and activate the muscle. We can measure the *reaction time* or time for action potentials to travel from the muscle spindles to the spinal cord, plus the time for action potentials induced in

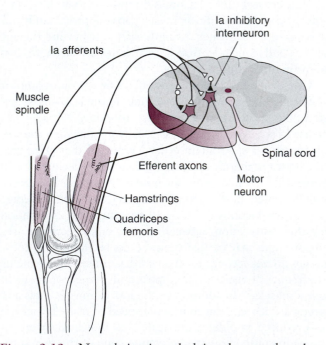

Figure 2.13   Neural circuit underlying the stretch and reciprocal-inhibition reflexes. (Adapted from RM Enoka. *Neuromechanics of Human Movement.* Champaign, IL: Human Kinetics, 2002, p. 299 (Figure 6.59)).

the motor neurons to travel back to the muscle. In humans, the stretch reflex has a reaction time of 19 to 25 milliseconds. Based on the very first reaction potentials in the muscles, action potentials from the stretch reflex spend approximately 0.5 millisecond in the spinal cord, which is just long enough to send transmitter across one synapse. This time period is called the *central delay*. The fastest component of the stretch reflex required only one synapse, which must be formed by a type Ia afferent connected directly to an α motor neuron. The pathway for the earliest component of the stretch reflex, as opposed to other components that take many milliseconds longer to begin, is called the *monosynaptic pathway*. It consists of the shortest possible neuronal circuit, one synapse.

It should be noted, however, that a monosynaptic circuit could still be affected by other inputs, either from supraspinal centers or other afferent inputs from the periphery. Because axonal inputs can be distributed at many locations on the dendritic tree of the linking α motor neuron, the input of a type Ia afferent can be affected by other inputs onto the same dendrite. Therefore, even in the monosynaptic pathway, the input/output relation of the circuit may not be stereotypical.

The traditional definition of a spinal reflex is one in which an adequate stimulus leads to a stereotypic motor response that is graded with the stimulus. A reflex has 1) a sensor, 2) a processor, and 3) an effector. The sensor, or "afferent limb," consists of the receptor and its primary sensory afferent. For example, the muscle spindle and the type Ia afferent are considered the sensor in the stretch reflex. The processor is the integration center in the spinal cord, such as the synapse in the ventral horn in the case of the monosynaptic stretch reflex. Finally, the effector is the "efferent limb," including the α motor neuron and muscle fibers it innervates (i.e., motor unit) in the muscle.

Key Point:
Reflexes have a sensor, a processor, and an effector.

Spinal reflexes can be localized in the spinal cord so that sensor, processor, and effector are all associated with the same spinal segment. Alternatively, *intersegmental spinal reflexes* that involve several spinal segments use interneurons to transmit afferent limb signals to higher or lower spinal segments. Intersegmental reflexes underlie synergistic effector responses, such as the *flexor withdrawal reflex*, discussed later.

More recent advances in neurophysiology indicate that spinal reflexes may not be as "hard-wired" as previously thought. Although nociceptive and protective reflexes (e.g., flexor withdrawal reflex) operating at the spinal and brainstem levels are relatively hard wired, other lower threshold proprioceptive reflexes may become phase and context dependent, as a particular task demands. In other words, whereas the input–output relation for protective reflex pathways may not be fundamentally altered by changes in spinal state, such a change can elicit a reflex reversal of output to the same sensory input.[84] This concept of alternative spinal reflex pathways has been promoted for several decades; however, it is frequently omitted from textbooks describing spinal reflexes.

Stretch Reflex

The stretch reflex is mediated by the muscle spindle with its intrafusal fibers and type Ia and II afferents. When a muscle is stretched, axons from type Ia afferents from that muscle enter the spinal cord through the dorsal root. Branches of these axons cross through the gray matter of the spinal cord to the ventral horn and then synapse directly on the motor neurons projecting to the same muscle. Therefore, any external force stretching the muscle excites the type Ia axons, which excite the motor neuron pool, which oppose the external force by activating the muscle. This process is termed *autogenic facilitation*; the stretch stimulus originated in the same muscle that was activated by the reflex. In addition, through an inhibitory interneuron, the antagonistic muscle is inhibited.

Each type Ia afferent projects to nearly all of the motor neurons in the homonymous motor neuron pool. The recruitment of motor neurons by the stretch reflex follows the size principle: Small, slow motor units are recruited first, and only rarely are large, fast units recruited during a stretch reflex. The size principle also applies to the inhibitory action of type Ia-INs (inhibitory interneurons): The antagonist muscle slow motor units are inhibited more easily than the antagonist fast motor units.

In contrast to the monosynaptic pathway of the type Ia afferent, the type II afferents make polysynaptic connections with the same motor neuron pool. In addition, the average excitatory effect from the type II afferent on the postsynaptic cell is about half the size of that from a type Ia afferent. Thus, the recruitment capability of the type II afferent is less effective than that of the type Ia. Because the monosynaptic pathway is driven by type Ia sensory fibers, a very rapid stretch should be more effective at activating this pathway than a slow stretch. It should be noted that the monosynaptic pathway is only one part of the stretch reflex; other pathways are better suited to deal with slow stretches.

The easiest way to demonstrate a rapid stretch is with the knee-jerk response, elicited by striking the tendon distal to the patella. The muscle is stretched very rapidly, over a short distance. The characteristic knee kick results from maximal stimulation of the monosynaptic pathway. Remember, Type Ia fibers are exquisitely sensitive to rapid stretch, owing to their dynamic sensitivity. Thus, the *knee-jerk reflex*, more generally termed the *deep tendon reflex (DTR)*, is simply a special case of the stretch reflex. The signal is almost a pure signal of the rate of the length change (velocity), and the response is dominated by the type Ia synapse on motor neurons of the same muscle.

This description of a DTR does not address an important problem. When the knee kicks because of the reflex activation of the knee extensor muscles, a rapid stretch of the knee flexors is produced. What prevents the knee flexors from responding with their own jerk reflex? This action, of course, would cause another stretch reflex response. When the sensory axons from the extensors excite the extensor α motor neurons, they simultaneously inhibit the flexor motor neurons through the type Ia-IN described earlier. This two-synapse path ensures that the antagonist muscles do not interfere with the DTR or, more generally, with the stretch reflex. Whenever antagonist muscles are inhibited during the activation of agonist muscles, the process is called *reciprocal inhibition*.

Recurrent inhibition has effects opposite to reciprocal inhibition: inhibition of agonists and synergists, with disinhibition of antagonists. Renshaw cells, interneurons that produce recurrent inhibition, are stimulated by a recurrent collateral branch from the α motor neuron. A recurrent collateral branch is a side branch of an axon that turns back toward its own cell body. Renshaw cells inhibit the same α motor neuron that gives rise to the collateral branch and also inhibit motor neurons of synergists. Renshaw cells focus motor activity, thus isolating desired motor activity from gross activation.[85] Loss of descending influence on Renshaw cell activity may cause difficulty in achieving fine motor control.

> ## *Key Point:*
> Renshaw cells help to isolate desired motor activity from gross activation.

The sensitivity of the muscle spindle can be regulated by the γ motor neurons by the way of the intrafusal fibers—that is, the γ motor neurons help to set the gain of the stretch reflex. If the γ dynamic motor neurons are highly activated, the reflex is even more responsive to rapid stretch. Less γ dynamic activity results in less velocity sensitivity to the type Ia axons and greater difficulty in producing a reflex response. Therefore, if the gain is low, a greater stretch is required to produce a similar change in muscle force.[39]

Golgi Tendon Organs

Another sensory receptor that is important in the reflex regulation of motor activity is the Golgi tendon organ. *Golgi tendon organs* are encapsulated afferent nerve endings located at the junction of the muscle and tendon (**Figure 2.14**) (see Chapters 7 and 8). Each tendon organ is related

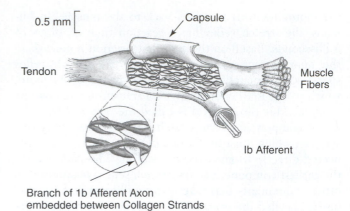

Figure 2.14   Golgi tendon organ. (Adapted from RM Enoka. *Neuromechanics of Human Movement*. Champaign, IL: Human Kinetics, 2002, p. 237 (Figure 5.22)).

to a single group Ib sensory axon (the Ib axons being slightly smaller than the Ia axons that innervate the muscle spindles). In contrast to the parallel arrangement of extrafusal muscle fibers and spindles, Golgi tendon organs are in series with the extrafusal fibers. When a muscle is passively stretched, most of the change in length occurs in the muscle fibers, since they are more elastic than the fibers of the tendon. When a muscle actively contracts, however, the force acts directly on the tendon, leading to an increase in the tension of the collagen fibrils in the tendon organ and compression of the intertwined sensory receptors. As a result, Golgi tendon organs are exquisitely sensitive to increases in muscle tension that arise from muscle contraction but, unlike spindles, are relatively insensitive to passive stretch.[39]

The Ib axons from Golgi tendon organs contact inhibitory local circuit neurons in the spinal cord (Ib inhibitory interneurons) that synapse, in turn, with the α motor neurons that innervate the same muscle. The Golgi tendon circuit is thus a negative feedback system that regulates muscle tension; it decreases the activation of a muscle when exceptionally large forces are generated and thus protects musculotendinous integrity. The reflex circuit also operates at reduced levels of muscle force, counteracting small changes in muscle tension by increasing or decreasing the inhibition of α motor neurons. Under these conditions, the Golgi tendon system tends to maintain a steady force level, counteracting effects that diminish muscle force (such as fatigue). In short, if the *muscle spindle system* is considered a feedback system that monitors and maintains muscle length, then the Golgi tendon system is a feedback system that monitors and maintains muscle force. Similar to the muscle spindle system, the Golgi tendon organ system is not a closed loop. The Ib inhibitory interneurons also receive synaptic inputs from a variety of other sources, including cutaneous receptors, joint receptors, muscle spindles, and descending upper motor neuron pathways. Acting in concert, these inputs regulate the responsiveness of Ib interneurons to activity arising in the Golgi tendon organs.[39,86]

Withdrawal Reflex

Thus far, the focus has been on reflexes driven by sensory receptors located within the muscle or tendons. Other reflex circuitry, however, mediates the withdrawal of a limb from noxious stimuli, such as stepping on a sharp object. Despite the rapid movement associated with the withdrawal response, this reflex involves several synaptic links (**Figure 2.15**). As a result of activity in this circuitry, stimulation of nociceptive sensory fibers leads to excitation of ipsilateral flexor muscles and reciprocal inhibition of ipsilateral extensor muscles. Flexion of the stimulated limb is also accompanied by an opposite reaction in the contralateral limb, e.g., the contralateral extensor muscles are excited while flexor muscles are inhibited. This *crossed extension reflex* serves to enhance postural support during withdrawal of the affected limb from the painful stimulus.

Like other reflex pathways, local circuit neurons in the *withdrawal reflex pathway* receive converging inputs from several different sources, including cutaneous receptors, other spinal cord interneurons, and upper motor neuron pathways. Although the functional significance of this com-

plex pattern of connectivity is unclear, changes in the character of the reflex following damage to descending pathways provides some insight. Under normal conditions, a noxious stimulus is required to evoke the withdrawal reflex; following damage to the descending pathways, however, other types of stimulation, such as squeezing a limb, can sometimes produce the same response. This observation suggests that the descending projections to the spinal cord modulate the responsiveness of the local circuitry of a variety of sensory inputs.[39]

Automatic Responses

Feedback from sensory receptors is also important for a class of behaviors known as *automatic responses.*[39] These behaviors are produced by neural circuits that are more complex than those associated with reflexes.[87] Automatic responses do have similarities with spinal reflexes, such as being evoked by sensory feedback in a rapid time frame. Postural adjustments that precede complex movements are one example of an automatic response. Recently, Hodges and colleagues performed a series of studies investigating how the trunk muscles become active prior to rapid movements of the peripheral joints.[88–93] Using surface EMG to monitor the onset of muscle activity, a comparison was made between the anterior shoulder muscles producing a sudden forward flexing motion and the abdominal and low back muscles responsible for producing an extensor moment of the spine. Three-dimensional trunk motion, trunk muscle electromyography, and intra-abdominal pressure were evaluated to investigate the preparatory control of the trunk associated with voluntary unilateral upper limb movement. Preparatory motion of the trunk occurred in three dimensions in the directions opposite to the reactive moments. Electromyographic recordings from the superficial trunk muscles were consistent with preparatory trunk motion. However, activation of transversus abdominis was inconsistent with control of direction-specific moments acting on the trunk. The results provide evidence that anticipatory postural adjustments result in movements and not simple rigidification of the trunk.[89] Although there appears to be a robust aspect to automatic responses, it appears that several factors can influence the input–output relation of these responses. For example, in subjects with a history of low back pain, the automatic response of the trunk muscles is altered compared with the response from subjects without low back pain.[90] In addition, training appears to normalize these altered responses. However, it is unclear if the alteration in the automatic responses was the cause or the result of the low back pain. Taken together, these data indicate that the central nervous system uses a complex interaction of sensory feedback and motor responses to generate automatic responses to changes in postural demands, even though these responses may be altered by training and other external influences.

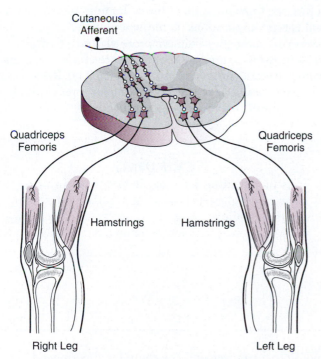

Figure 2.15   Neural circuit for the withdrawal and crossed-extensor reflexes. (Redrawn from RM Enoka. *Neuromechanics of Human Movement.* Champaign, IL: Human Kinetics, 2002, p. 300 (Figure 6.60)).

> ## Key Point:
> The central nervous system uses a complex interaction of sensory feedback and motor responses to generate automatic responses to postural demand changes.

The Effects of Arousal on Motor Performance

Sensory feedback can activate neural mechanisms responsible for physiological functions other than those related to the musculoskeletal system. For example, behaviors such as the *fight-or-flight response* evoked by sensory feedback can result in elevated arousal levels, which may have additional indirect effects on movement. *Arousal* is described as an internal state of alertness, composed of several emotional responses, including fear and anxiety, mediated by the neuroendocrine system.[39] Its physiological manifestations commonly include increases in blood pressure and heart rate; sweating; dryness of the mouth; hyperventilation; and musculoskeletal disturbances such as restlessness, tremor, and feelings of weakness.[94-97] The level of arousal exhibited by an individual varies along a continuum from deep sleep to the fight-or-flight response. It can have a substantial effect on an individual's movements.[39] The neurotransmitters and hormones that elicit the physiological manifestations of arousal, however, can potentially modulate the function of spinal circuits underlying motor performance. Because of this interaction, elevated neuroendocrine activity during heightened arousal has been implicated as a factor that can alter motor performance.[98]

In a series of studies using an electrical shock as a laboratory stressor, Noteboom and colleagues[99] found that subjects experiencing either the threat of shock or the actual delivery of noxious levels of shock had a significant elevation in physiological and cognitive markers of arousal. In addition, the greater levels of arousal were associated with parallel reductions in steadiness, which was quantified as the change in the standard deviation of the force fluctuations around the average force. Interestingly, the effect of arousal on motor performance was more pronounced for the women compared with the men in the shock conditions.[98,100] Electrical shock also appears to impair the performance of maximal contractions. Peak force during a MVC trial was significantly less for trials immediately preceded by an electrical shock compared with trials without shock.

Increased levels of arousal also enhance the amount of muscle activation used to perform a task.[39] For example, Weinburg and Hunt[100] found that subjects with high levels of anxiety (an index of arousability), as compared with less anxious subjects, responded to negative feedback on performance by increasing the amount of muscle EMG during a throwing task. The change in EMG activity caused a decline in performance for the highly anxious subjects but an improvement in the performance of the less anxious subjects.

Activation of the arousal response results in elevated autonomic output, which is primarily represented by the release of neurotransmitters. Although the primary role of the neurotransmitters is rapid neuronal communication, recent evidence suggests that neuroendocrine substrates, such as the neurotransmitters serotonin and norepinephrine, have significant neuromodulatory effects on the spinal circuits underlying motor output.[101-103] Therefore, in addition to elevating cognitive and physiological measures of arousal, stressful situations may also impair motor performance through the activation of neuroendocrine substrates. Obviously, these recent findings may have several clinical implications. Incorporating psychological and behavioral strategies that minimize the effect of potentially stressful events may result in more efficacious therapeutic exercise programs (see Chapter 11). Regardless, clinicians should be cognizant of complex interactions between emotion and physical performance.

> ## Key Point:
> Stressful situations may impair motor performance. Incorporating psychological and behavioral strategies that minimize the effect of stress into therapeutic exercises may increase program effectiveness.

Summary

The neuromuscular system is the primary system responsible for complex human movement. The metabolic energy systems are designed to provide the energy necessary to drive a range of activities, from those classified as low intensity, long duration to very high intensity, short duration tasks. Although muscle is the end effector organ responsible for movement, the central and peripheral nervous systems integrate the sensory and motor actions to drive the function of skeletal muscle. By understanding the musculoskeletal system, from the cellular to the behavioral levels, rehabilitation clinicians will be better able to manage clients who have movement-related dysfunction.

References

1. Conley M. Bioenergetics of exercise and training. In TR Baechle, RW Earle (eds.), *Essentials of Strength Training and Conditioning*. Champaign, IL: Human Kinetics; 2000;73–90.

2. McComas AJ. *Skeletal Muscle: Form and Function.* Champaign, IL: Human Kinetics, 1996.

3. McArdle WD, Katch FI, Katch VL. *Essentials of Exercise Physiology*, 2nd ed. Philadelphia: Lippincott Williams & Wilkins, 2000.

4. Jansson E, Sylven C, Nordevang E. Myoglobin in the quadriceps femoris muscle of competitive cyclists and untrained men. *Acta Physiol Scand.* 1982; 114(4):627–629.

5. LaBotz M, Smith BW. Creatine supplement use in an NCAA Division I athletic program. *Clin J Sport Med.* 1999;9(3):167–169.

6. Mesa JL, Ruiz JR, Gonzalez-Gross MM, et al. Oral creatine supplementation and skeletal muscle metabolism in physical exercise. *Sports Med.* 2002;32 (14):903–944.

7. Brooks GA, Fahey TD, White TP. *Exercise Physiology: Human Bioenergetics and Its Applications.* 3rd ed. Mountain View, CA: Mayfield Publishing Company, 2000.

8. Mader A. Glycolysis and oxidative phosphorylation as a function of cytosolic phosphorylation state and power output of the muscle cell. *Eur J Appl Physiol.* 2003;88(4–5):317–338.

9. Stone MH, O'Bryant HS. *Weight Training: A Scientific Approach.* Minneapolis, MN: Burgess International, 1987.

10. Holloszy JO, Kohrt WM, Hansen PA. The regulation of carbohydrate and fat metabolism during and after exercise. *Front Biosci.* 1998;3:D1011–1027.

11. Hawley JA. Effect of increased fat availability on metabolism and exercise capacity. *Med Sci Sports Exerc.* 2002;34(9):1485–1491.

12. Brooks GA. Amino acid and protein metabolism during exercise and recovery. *Med Sci Sports Exerc.* 1987;19(5 Suppl):S150–S156.

13. Smith SA, Montain SJ, Matott RP, et al. Creatine supplementation and age influence muscle metabolism during exercise. *J Appl Physiol.* 1998;85(4): 1349–1356.

14. Astrand PO, Rodahl K. *Textbook of Work Physiology*, 2nd ed. New York: McGraw-Hill, 1970.

15. Conley MS, Stone M, O'Bryant HS, et al. Peak power versus power at maximal oxygen uptake (abstract). *J Strength Cond Res.* 1993;7(4):253.

16. Hawley JA. Adaptations of skeletal muscle to prolonged, intense endurance training. *Clin Exp Pharmacol Physiol.* 2002;29(3):218–222.

17. Reimers K, Ruud J. Nutritional factors in health and performance. *In* TR Baechle, RW Earle (eds.) *Essentials of Strength Training and Conditioning.* Champaign, IL: Human Kinetics, 2000; pp. 229–257.

18. Young VR, Pellett PL. Plant proteins in relation to human protein and amino acid nutrition. *Am J Clin Nutr.* 1994;59:1203S–1212S.

19. Council NR. *Recommended Dietary Allowances.* Washington, DC: National Academy Press; 1989.

20. Lemon PW. Effects of exercise on dietary protein requirements. *Int J Sports Nutr.* 1998;8:426–447.

21. Liu L, Ikeda K, Sullivan DH, et al. Epidemiological evidence of the association between dietary protein intake and blood pressue: A meta-analysis of published data. *Hypertens Res.* 2002;25(5):689–695.

22. Milne AC, Potter J, Avenell A. Protein and energy supplementation in elderly people at risk from malnutrition. *Cochrane Database Syst Rev.* 2002;3:CD003288.

23. Maughan RJ, Greenhaff PL, Leiper JB, et al. Diet composition and the performance of high-intensity exercise. *J Sports Sci.* 1997;15:265–275.

24. Fujisawa T, Mulligan K, Wada L, et al. The effect of exercise on fructose absorption. *Am J Clin Nutr.* 1993;58:75–79.

25. Jenkins DJ, Wolever TM, Taylor RH, et al. Glycemic index of foods: a physiological basis for carbohydrate exchange. *Am J Clin Nutr.* 1981;34 (3):362–366.

26. Astrup A, Ryan L, Grunwald GK, et al. The role of dietary fat in body fatness: Evidence from a preliminary meta-analysis of ad libitum low-fat dietary intervention studies. *Br J Nutr.* 2000;83 (Suppl 1):S25–32.

27. Ciccone CD. Current trends in cardiovascular pharmacology. *Phys Ther.* 1996;76(5):481–497.

28. Ciccone CD. *Pharmacology in Rehabilitation.* Philadelphia: F.A. Davis; 2002.

29. Peel C, Mossberg KA. Effects of cardiovascular medications on exercise responses. *Phys Ther.* 1995; 75(5):387–396.

30. Frisk-Holmberg M, Jorfeldt L, Juhlin-Dannfelt A. Metabolic effects in muscle during antihypertensive therapy with beta 1- and beta 1/beta 2-adrenoceptor blockers. *Clin Pharmacol Ther.* 1981;30(5): 611–618.

31. Cleroux J, Van Nguyen P, Taylor AW, Leenen FH. Effects of beta 1- vs. beta 1 + beta 2-blockade on exercise endurance and muscle metabolism in humans. *J Appl Physiol.* 1989;66(2):548–554.

32. Huxley H. Changes in the cross-striations of muscle during contraction and stretch and their structural interpretations. *Nature.* 1954;173:973–976.

33. Huxley AF, Niedergerke R. Structural changes in muscle during contraction. Interference microscopy of living muscle fibres. *Nature*. 1954;173:971–973.

34. Huxley HE. Sliding filaments and molecular motile systems. *J Biol Chem*. 1990;265(15):8347–8350.

35. Gordon AM, Huxley AF, Julian FJ. The variation in isometric tension with sarcomere length in vertebrate muscle fibres. *J Physiol*. 1966;184(1):170–192.

36. Gordon AM, Huxley AF, Julian FJ. Tension development in highly stretched vertebrate muscle fibres. *J Physiol*. 1966;184(1):143–169.

37. Staron RS. Human skeletal muscle fiber types: Delineation, development, and distribution. *Can J Appl Physiol*. 1997;22(4):307–327.

38. Pette D, Staron RS. Mammalian skeletal muscle fiber type transitions. *Int Rev Cytol*. 1997;170:143–223.

39. Enoka RM. *Neuromechanics of Human Movement*. Champaign, IL: Human Kinetics, 2002.

40. Pette D. The adaptive potential of skeletal muscle fibers. *Can J Appl Physiol*. 2002;27(4):423–448.

41. Monster AW, Chan H, O'Connor D. Activity patterns of human skeletal muscles: Relation to muscle fiber type composition. *Science*. 1978;200(4339):314–317.

42. Harridge SD, Magnusson G, Gordon A. Skeletal muscle contractile characteristics and fatigue resistance in patients with chronic heart failure. *Eur Heart J*. 1996;17(6):896–901.

43. McComas AJ. Motor unit estimation: Methods, results, and present status. *Muscle Nerve*. 1991;14:585–597.

44. Liddell EGT, Sherrington CS. Recruitment and some other factors of reflex inhibition. *Proc Royal Soc London Biol Sci*. 1925;B97:488–518.

45. Henneman E, Somjen G, Carpenter DO. Excitability and inhibitability of motoneurons of different sizes. *J Neurophysiol*. 1965;28(3):599–620.

46. Enoka RM, Fuglevand AJ. Motor unit physiology: Some unresolved issues. *Muscle Nerve*. 2001;24(1):4–17.

47. Burke RE, Tsairis P. Anatomy and innervation ratios in motor units of cat gastrocnemius. *J Physiol*. 1973;234(3):749–765.

48. Peters SE. Structure and function in vertebrate skeletal muscle. *Am Zool*. 1989;29:221–234.

49. English AW, Wolf SL, Segal RL. Compartmentalization of muscles and their motor nuclei: The partitioning hypothesis. *Phys Ther*. 1993;73(12):857–867.

50. Van Cutsem M, Feiereisen P, Duchateau J, Hainaut K. Mechanical properties and behaviour of motor units in the tibialis anterior during voluntary contractions. *Can J Appl Physiol*. 1997;22(6):585–597.

51. Burke RE, Levine DN, Tsairis P, Zajac FE III. Physiological types and histochemical profiles in motor units of the cat gastrocnemius. *J Physiol*. 1973;234(3):723–748.

52. Bigland-Richie B, Fuglevand RJ, Thomas CK. Contractile properties of human motor units: Is man a cat? *Neuroscientist*. 1998;4:240–249.

53. Fuglevand AJ, Macefield VG, Bigland-Ritchie B. Force–frequency and fatigue properties of motor units in muscles that control digits of the human hand. *J Neurophysiol*. 1999;81(4):1718–1729.

54. Kernell D. Organized variability in the neuromuscular system: A survey of task-related adaptations. *Arch Ital Biol*. 1992;130(1):19–66.

55. Denny-Brown D, Pennybacker JB. Fibrillation and fasciculation in voluntary muscle. *Brain*. 1938;61:311–334.

56. Kukulka CG, Clamann HP. Comparison of the recruitment and discharge properties of motor units in human brachial biceps and adductor pollicis during isometric contractions. *Brain Res*. 1981;219(1):45–55.

57. Henneman E. Relation between the size of neurons and their susceptibility to discharge. *Science*. 1957;126:1345–1347.

58. Person RS, Kudina LP. Discharge frequency and discharge pattern of human motor units during voluntary contraction of muscle. *Electroencephalogr Clin Neurophysiol*. 1972;32(5):471–483.

59. Spiegel KM, Stratton J, Burke JR, et al. The influence of age on the assessment of motor unit activation in a human hand muscle. *Exp Physiol*. 1996;81(5):805–819.

60. Kudina LP, Alexeeva NL. After-potentials and control of repetitive firing in human motoneurones. *Electroencephalogr Clin Neurophysiol*. 1992;85(5):345–353.

61. Linnamo V, Moritani T, Nicol C, Komi PV. Motor unit activation patterns during isometric, concentric and eccentric actions at different force levels. *J Electromyogr Kinesiol*. 2003;13(1):93–101.

62. Christova P, Kossev A. Human motor unit activity during concentric and eccentric movements. *Electromyogr Clin Neurophysiol*. 2000;40(6):331–338.

63. Bigland-Ritchie B, Woods JJ. Changes in muscle contractile properties and neural control during human muscular fatigue. *Muscle Nerve*. 1984;7(9):691–699.

64. Bigland-Ritchie B, Furbush F, Woods JJ. Fatigue of intermittent submaximal voluntary contractions: Central and peripheral factors. *J Appl Physiol*. 1986;61(2):421–429.

65. Gandevia SC, Allen GM, Butler JE, Taylor JL. Supraspinal factors in human muscle fatigue: Evidence for suboptimal output from the motor cortex. *J Physiol*. 1996;490(2):529–536.

66. Enoka RM, Stuart DG. Neurobiology of muscle fatigue. *J Appl Physiol.* 1992;72(5):1631–1648.

67. Bigland-Ritchie B, Johansson R, Lippold OC, et al. Changes in motoneurone firing rates during sustained maximal voluntary contractions. *J Physiol.* 1983;340:335–346.

68. Peters EJ, Fuglevand AJ. Cessation of human motor unit discharge during sustained maximal voluntary contraction. *Neurosci Lett.* 1999;274(1):66–70.

69. Griffin L, Ivanova T, Garland SJ. Role of limb movement in the modulation of motor unit discharge rate during fatiguing contractions. *Exp Brain Res.* 2000;130(3):392–400.

70. Carpentier A, Duchateau J, Hainaut K. Motor unit behaviour and contractile changes during fatigue in the human first dorsal interosseus. *J Physiol.* 2001;534 (Pt 3):903–912.

71. Duchateau J, Balestra C, Carpentier A, Hainaut K. Reflex regulation during sustained and intermittent submaximal contractions in humans. *J Physiol.* 2002; 541 (Pt 3):959–967.

72. Semmler JG, Kutzscher DV, Enoka RM. Limb immobilization alters muscle activation patterns during a fatiguing isometric contraction. *Muscle Nerve.* 2000;23(9):1381–1392.

73. Enoka RM, Burnett RA, Graves AE, et al. Task- and age-dependent variations in steadiness. *Prog Brain Res.* 1999;123:389–395.

74. Grabiner MD, Enoka RM. Changes in movement capabilities with aging. *Exerc Sport Sci Rev.* 1995; 23:65–104.

75. Hurley BF. Strength training in the elderly: Effects on risk factors for age-related diseases. *Sports Med.* 2000;30(4):249–268.

76. Vandervoort AA, McComas AJ. Contractile changes in opposing muscles of the human ankle joint with aging. *J Appl Physiol.* 1986;61(1):361–367.

77. Vandervoort AA. Aging of the human neuromuscular system. *Muscle Nerve.* 2002;25(1):17–25.

78. Frontera WR, Hughes VA, Fielding RA, et al. Aging of skeletal muscle: A 12-yr longitudinal study. *J Appl Physiol.* 2000;88(4):1321–1326.

79. Hunter SK, White M, Thompson M. Techniques to evaluate elderly human muscle function: A physiological basis. *J Gerontol.* 1998;53A:B204–B216.

80. Galganski ME, Fuglevand AJ, Enoka RM. Reduced control of motor output in a human hand muscle of elderly subjects during submaximal contractions. *J Neurophysiol.* 1993;69(6):2108–2115.

81. Graves AE, Kornatz KW, Enoka RM. Older adults use a unique strategy to lift inertial loads with the elbow flexor muscles. *J Neurophysiol.* 2000;83(4):2030–2039.

82. Laidlaw DH, Bilodeau M, Enoka RM. Steadiness is reduced and motor unit discharge is more variable in old adults. *Muscle Nerve.* 2000;23(4): 600–612.

83. Fuglevand AJ, Zackowski KM, Huey KA, Enoka RM. Impairment of neuromuscular propagation during human fatiguing contractions at submaximal forces. *J Physiol.* 1993;460:549–572.

84. Stuart DG. Reflections on spinal reflexes. *Adv Exp Med Biol.* 2002;508:249–257.

85. Thach WT. Fundamentals of motor systems. *In* MJ Zigmond (ed.), *Fundamental Neuroscience.* San Diego: Academic Press; 1999, 855–863.

86. Nichols TR. The contributions of muscles and reflexes to the regulation of joint and limb mechanics. *Clin Orthop.* 2002;403 (Suppl):S43–50.

87. Prochazka A, Clarac F, Loeb GE, et al. What do reflex and voluntary mean? Modern views on an ancient debate. *Exp Brain Res.* 2000;130(4):417–432.

88. Hodges PW, Cresswell AG, Thorstensson A. Perturbed upper limb movements cause short-latency postural responses in trunk muscles. *Exp Brain Res.* 2001;138(2):243–250.

89. Hodges PW, Cresswell AG, Daggfeldt K, Thorstensson A. Three dimensional preparatory trunk motion precedes asymmetrical upper limb movement. *Gait Posture.* 2000;11(2):92–101.

90. Hodges PW, Richardson CA. Altered trunk muscle recruitment in people with low back pain with upper limb movement at different speeds. *Arch Phys Med Rehabil.* 1999;80(9):1005–1012.

91. Hodges PW, Butler JE, McKenzie DK, Gandevia SC. Contraction of the human diaphragm during rapid postural adjustments. *J Physiol.* 1997;505 (Pt 2):539–548.

92. Hodges PW, Richardson CA. Relationship between limb movement speed and associated contraction of the trunk muscles. *Ergonomics.* 1997;40:1220–1230.

93. Hodges PW, Richardson CA. Contraction of the abdominal muscles associated with movement of the lower limb. *Phys Ther.* 1997;77(2):132–142.

94. Bonnet M, Bradley MM, Lang PJ, Requin J. Modulation of spinal reflexes: Arousal, pleasure, action. *Psychophysiology.* 1995;32:367–372.

95. Hoehn-Saric R, Hazlett RL, Pourmotabbed T, McLeod DR. Does muscle tension reflect arousal? Relationship between EMG and EEG recordings. *Psychiatry Res.* 1997;71:49–55.

96. Spielberger CD, Rickman RL. Assessment of state and trait anxiety. *In* N Sartorius (ed.), *Anxiety: Psychobiological and Clinical Perspectives.* New York: Hemisphere Publishing, 1990, 69–83.

97. Noteboom JT, Fleshner M, Enoka RM. Activation of the arousal response can impair performance of a simple motor task. *J Appl Physiol.* 2001;91(2):821–831.

98. Marder E. From biophysics to models of network function. *Ann Rev Neurosci.* 1998; 21:25–45.

99. Noteboom JT, Barnholt KR, Enoka RM. Activation of the arousal response and impairment of performance increase with anxiety and stressor intensity. *J Appl Physiol.* 2001;91(5):2093–2101.

100. Weinberg R, Hunt V. The interrelationships between anxiety, motor performance and electromyography. *J Mot Behav.* 1976;8(3):219–224.

101. Katz PS. Intrinsic and extrinsic neuromodulation of motor circuits. *Curr Opin Neurobiol.* 1995;5:799–808.

102. Dickinson PS. Interactions among neural networks for behavior. *Curr Opin. Neurobiol.* 1995;5:792–798.

103. Marder E. From biophysics to models of network function. *Ann Rev Neurosci.* 1998;21:25–45.

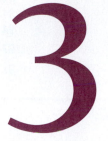

3

Stretching for Musculotendinous Extensibility and Joint Flexibility

HARVEY WALLMANN

J. TIMOTHY NOTEBOOM

Objectives

The reader will be able to:

- Diagram a stress-strain curve and discuss factors that influence curve changes.
- Describe the structural and biomechanical properties of connective tissue and the effects that outside factors can impose on their mechanical characteristics.
- Define viscoelastic properties and discuss their ability to alter connective tissue properties.

- Discuss clinical techniques and strategies related to flexibility and extensibility and critical components that influence their design.
- Discuss the performance benefits of musculotendinous stretching techniques.
- Summarize precautions and essential components of stretching program development.

Outline

(continued)

INTRODUCTION

Along with cardiopulmonary system endurance and muscular strength, stretching to enhance flexibility has long been recognized as an important component of a total fitness program. Many rehabilitation clinicians would agree that stretching is useful for generating and maintaining overall flexibility, not only for sport-specific events but for activities of daily living (ADLs) as well. The need for stretching becomes even more important after sustaining an injury, particularly if mobility has been impaired, resulting in compromised joint range of motion (ROM) and flexibility. Changes in joint positions associated with shortened musculotendinous structures may potentially create faulty postural alignment that may lead to injury and joint dysfunction. Since restoring ROM is crucial to any rehabilitation program, understanding and incorporating stretching exercises to restore normal ROM and flexibility becomes a primary goal to help facilitate non-impaired function.

Conventional wisdom would dictate that the main goal of stretching is to enhance overall flexibility. However, many experts argue that stretching also helps prevent injury, allows quicker recovery from workouts, reduces post exercise soreness, facilitates relaxation, and improves performance.[1] They further emphasize that a flexible body is more efficient, is more easily able to undergo strength and endurance training, maintains balanced musculotendinous length between opposing muscle groups, and improves posture.

> ## Key Point:
> Flexibility is essential to undergo safe strength and endurance training and to maintain balanced musculotendinous lengths between opposing muscle groups, thereby improving posture.

The previously ascribed benefits have resulted in a variety of perceived notions that have become popular in the lay literature. Research indicates, however, that limited scientific evidence exists to support some of these popular notions. In fact, research is currently ongoing in an attempt to determine the effects of stretching on the body.

As a result, some of the long-held beliefs about stretching, especially prior to exercise, are being challenged.

In this chapter, intrinsic and extrinsic factors impacting joint flexibility and musculotendinous extensibility will be discussed. Additionally, evidence concerning the different types of stretching, the purported benefits of stretching and flexibility, and the effects of stretching on performance will be addressed, culminating in the discussion of criteria necessary for development of a stretching and flexibility program.

VISCOELASTIC TISSUE PROPERTIES

Before discussing the biological and mechanical properties of specific tissues, we will review several general biomechanical concepts that form a foundation for later material. Specifically, concepts of stress and strain, along with associated variables of tensile load, deformation, loading rates, and viscosity will be discussed.

Stress and Strain

Although the terms stress and strain have commonly been used to describe emotional or behavioral qualities, they have specific mechanical meaning that must be understood. *Stress* or *load* is given in units of force per area, such as used to describe pressure, where the units may be pounds per square inch or Newtons per square centimeter. Therefore, stress, which is directly related to the magnitude of force and inversely related to the unit area, is independent of the amount of a material.[2]

An example of a mechanical stress is applying an external load to a structure, such as that applied by the foot when standing on a wooden box. The weight of the body is the external load, whereas the surface contact between the foot and box is the unit area. In this situation, intuition tells us that the wooden box will support the weight placed on it and the box will maintain its structural integrity. However, if the wooden box was replaced by a similar sized piece of foam rubber, the question would be whether the piece of foam could support a weight with its structure intact. Although the same stress is applied in each situation, different responses are expected. In other words, the response to a given stress is dependent on other variables. The complementary measure related to stress is *strain* or *deformation*.

Therefore, strain (e) is defined as the change in length of a material divided by the original length:

$$e = \frac{\Delta L}{L_0} = \frac{L - L_0}{L_0}$$

where L is the length at the time of measurement, L_0 is the original length, and ΔL is the calculated change in length. Although strain is dimensionless (units of measure cancel each other out), units are often provided (e.g., inches/inch) to give a perspective of scale applied to the loads.

Returning to the example of stepping on a wooden box or a piece of foam, the strain is very different for these two materials, although the stresses applied are identical. Obviously, the materials of wood and rubber are very different, which differentiates the two strain values. Some materials, such as wood, may have a high threshold, or resistance to strain, but once that level of stress is reached, the materials may strain only a small amount before they break. In contrast, other materials, such as foam rubber, may have a low threshold for stresses that will produce significant strains, but the magnitude of strain may be significant before the material breaks down. The mechanical stress of stepping on the foam may cause significant strain,

but the structure can deform by a much larger magnitude (compared with the wood material) before breaking. In this case, the load of the body weight causes a compression of the foam material, which is the material's response to the applied load. Other loads could be applied that produce different responses to the material, depending on how the load is applied. For example, a stretching load could be applied by having a client pull the foot into dorsiflexion using elastic tubing or a rolled up towel, resulting in a tensile load to the triceps surae muscle group and Achilles tendon. Other types of loads include bending, shear, torsion, and various loading combinations.

From the above discussion it can be seen that the relation of stress and strain is dependent on several factors, including the properties of the material in question, the magnitude of the stresses, and the rate at which the stresses are applied. Therefore, the graphic representation of the relation between stress and strain will be different for each material type. This representation is known as the *stress-strain* or *load-deformation* curve.[3] **Figure 3.1** demonstrates several regions of the stress-strain relation for ligamentous tissue where the slope of the line defining the relationships is fundamentally different.

Each region demonstrates a biomechanical property of the tissue. In Zone A, called the *toe region*, the slightly stretched tissue (i.e., a ligament) produces only a small amount of tension within the tissue, resulting in the slack of the tissue being taken up. This minimally elevating slope indicates that the collagen fibers within the tissue must first be pulled tight prior to any significant tension being recorded. However, if the tissue were continued to be pulled at higher stress levels, there would be a linear change in strain, represented by Zone B. The linear rela-

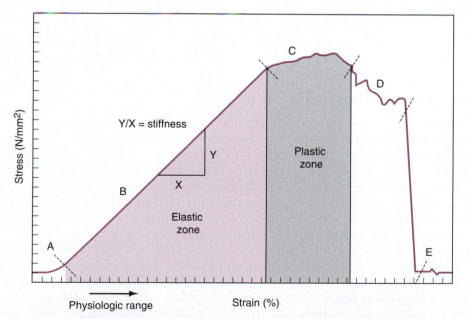

Figure 3.1   Stress-strain curve. (Modified from DA Neumann: Arthrokinesiologic considerations for the aged adult. In AA Guccione (ed.): *Geriatric Physical Therapy*, 2nd ed. Chicago: Mosby-Yearbook, 2000.)

tion between stress and strain in Zone B is similar to the common model of a stretched rubber band. The greater the load stress on the rubber band, the more the band stretches. Similarly, as the tension placed on the rubber band is removed, the band shortens closer to its original length. Because of this, Zone B is referred to as the *elastic zone* of the stress-strain relation or the Hookean Region. The amount of stretch (strain) applied to the tissue in this zone is significant and likely experienced during many natural movements of the body. Within this zone, the tissue returns to its original length or shape once the deforming force is removed. It should be noted that the slope of the stress-strain relation in this zone is indicative of the relative *stiffness* of the tissue, where stiffness is defined as the change in force per unit change in length.[4] Therefore, the stiffer the tissue, the steeper the slope. In other words, tissues such as tendon will only change length at higher levels of stress compared with tissues of less stiffness, such as loose connective tissue or ligament.

A finite point at the upper level of Zone B marks a transition from the linear relation of stress and strain to one where the slope begins to flatten. Therefore, there is a point where an increasing level of stress on the tissue results in proportionately increased changes in tissue length. At this extreme and abnormally large stretch, the tissue undergoes increased elongation, presumably due to microscopic failure of the tissue. Because this tissue damage results in permanent deformation, this Zone C is termed the *plastic zone*. Unlike the elastic zone (Zone B), the plastic energy is not recoverable in its entirety when the deforming load is removed, and there is a change in its resting length. If the tissue underwent continued stretch, additional deformation of the tissue would occur until it reached its *initial point of failure* in Zone D and *complete failure* in Zone E. Although the strain values associated with the various zones are dependent on many factors, especially tissue type, for tendon, Zone A can include strains up to 3 percent, Zone B from 6 to 10 percent, and Zone C and D from 10 to 15 percent.[4,5]

Viscoelasticity and Tissue Function

Although connective tissue appears in many forms throughout the body, all connective tissue exhibits the common property of *viscoelasticity*. The behavior of viscoelastic materials is a combination of the properties of elasticity and viscosity.[6,7] As stated in the previous section, *elasticity* refers to a material's ability to return to its original state following deformation (change in dimensions, i.e., length or shape) after the removal of the deforming load. *Viscosity* refers to a material's ability to dampen shearing forces. When forces are applied to viscous materials, the tissues exhibit time-dependent and rate-dependent properties.

Viscoelastic materials are capable of undergoing deformation under either a tensile (distractive) force or a compressive force before returning to their original state after the removal of the force. However, under normal conditions viscoelastic materials do not return to their original state immediately. Viscoelastic materials, unlike pure elastic materials, have time-dependent mechanical properties. In other words, viscoelastic materials are sensitive to the duration of the force application. When a viscoelastic material is subjected to either a constant compressive or tensile load, the material initially responds by rapidly deforming and then continues to deform over a finite length of time (hours, days, and months) even if the load remains constant. Deformation of the tissue continues until a state of equilibrium is reached when the load is balanced. This phenomenon is called *creep* and is attributed to different mechanisms in different materials.[6] Creep is simply the gradual increase in tissue length that is necessary to maintain a constant stress. In bone, at the microscopic level, compressive forces resulting in creep have been attributed to the slip of lamellae within the osteons (Haversian system) and the flow of the interstitial fluid. Similarly, in hyaline articular cartilage subjected to a compressive force, creep is attributed to the gradual loss of fluid from the tissue. In tendons and ligaments, creep is due to motion of long glycosaminoglycan (GAG) chains in the solid matrix. Generally, the longer the duration of the applied force, the greater the deformation. Similarly, increases in the magnitude of the applied load tend to increase the rate of creep. In some tissues, an acceleration of the rate of creep occurs after a prolonged rate of time. Changes in temperature also affect the rate of creep. High temperatures increase the rate of creep and low temperatures decrease the rate. Theoretically, if one wishes to stretch out (elongate) a connective tissue structure, one should heat it and use a large load over a long period of time to produce creep. A clinical example of creep deformation as a transient biomechanical phenomenon can be illustrated using the hamstring muscles. If one uses a constant force against the muscle when slowly and passively stretching it, the muscle will eventually elongate. However, when unloaded, the tissue does not return to its original prestretched length immediately. This imperfect recovery is believed to be due to the collagen's viscous property.[7]

Stress-relaxation or *force-relaxation*, unlike creep, occurs when a viscoelastic material experiences a constant deformation. It responds initially with a high initial stress that decreases over time until equilibrium is reached and the stress equals zero, hence the label "relaxation." As a result, no change in length is produced. Using the previous scenario, if the hamstring muscle is held at a certain length over time, the stress would diminish, but there would be no change in length (no stretch occurs). Viscoelastic properties of biological tissue also influence the loading and unloading phases of the tissue. The difference between the stress-strain relation for loading and unloading can be quantified by measuring the *hysteresis* area (**Figure 3.2**). When a load is applied to a tissue and then released, the stress and strain are measured during the loading (up arrow on **Figure 3.2**) and unloading (down arrow) phases.

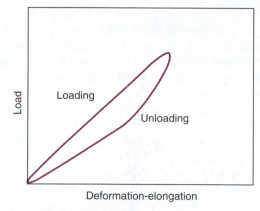

Figure 3.2   Hysteresis loop.

For biological material, the line for the unloading phase lies below that for the loading phase. The area between the two lines is known as the hysteresis area, which represents the amount of energy dissipated in the loading and unloading process.[4,7]

> ## Key Point:
> Understanding the viscoelastic properties of creep, stress relaxation, and hysteresis are critical to the rehabilitation clinician who desires to alter connective tissue length via flexibility and extensibility training.

ADAPTATIONS IN CONNECTIVE TISSUE

The material properties of tendon and ligaments tend to decline with such conditions as reduced use (immobilization, prolonged bed rest, sedentary lifestyle, etc.), age, and steroid use, but increase with regular exercise.[5,8,9] For example, when humans reach the fifth and sixth decades of life, the connections between ligaments and tendons with bone are weaker, and there are more cross-links in tendon and ligament, making these tissues less compliant.[5,10] Furthermore, exercise appears to increase the strength and stiffness of ligaments, but probably only by about 10–20 percent.[11] Conversely, joint immobilization appears to decrease ligament strength and stiffness.[8,10] Determination of the optimal exercise stimulus to attain the desired "mechano-biologic" effect in specific bodily tissues is a growing area of research.

STRUCTURE, VISCOELASTIC PROPERTIES, AND FUNCTION OF TISSUE

Tendons and Ligaments

Although tendons (attaching muscle to bone) and ligaments (attaching bone to bone) vary considerably in their function, like all dense connective tissues, they are composed of two major components, cells and extracellular matrix. Comprising only 20 percent of the total tissue volume, cells such as the fibrocyte, also known as fibroblast, manufacture and secrete the components of the extracellular matrix that makes up the remaining 80 percent. Approximately 86 percent of the dry weight of tendon and ligament consists of type I collagen, which is a fibrous protein that has considerable mechanical stability.[4,12] Collagen fibers are made of short subunits (fibrils), which are the typical load-bearing units of both tendon and ligament. The structure of the fibrils, from the alpha chains of the triple helix to the packing of the tropocollagen molecules in the microfibril, is the same for tendon and ligament (**Figures 3.3–3.4**).

Type I collagen fibers are thick, rugged fibers that are gathered into bundles and elongate very little when placed under tension. In contrast, type II collagen fibers are thinner and possess slightly less tensile strength. These fibers provide a flexible woven framework for maintaining the general shape and consistency of more complex structures, such as articular cartilage. Still, type II collagen provides internal strength to all connective tissues. One structural

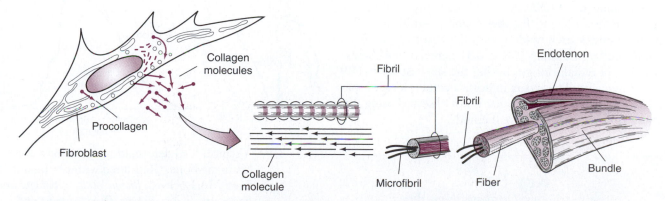

Figure 3.3   Schematic representation of collagen fibrils, fibers, and bundles of tendons and collagenous ligaments. (Reprinted with permission from M Nordin, VH Frankel. *Basic Biomechanics of the Musculoskeletal System*, 3rd ed. Philadelphia: Lippincott Williams and Wilkins, 2001, Figure 4.1).

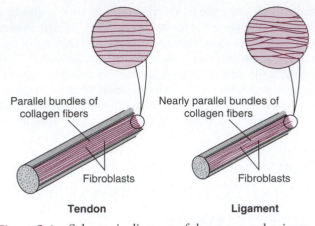

Parallel bundles of
collagen fibers

Nearly parallel bundles of
collagen fibers

Fibroblasts

Fibroblasts

Tendon   **Ligament**

Figure 3.4   Schematic diagram of the structural orientation of the fibers of tendon and ligament. (Reprinted with permission from M Nordin, VH Frankel. *Basic Biomechanics of the Musculoskeletal System*, 3rd ed. Philadelphia: Lippincott Williams and Wilkins, 2001, Figure 4.4).

difference between the collagen types that directly impacts tissue strength is the number and state of the cross-linkages between the collagen molecules. These cross-links occur both within and between the rows of collagen molecules in the microfibril.

Direct measurement of tendon strain in animals during passive loading of a muscle-tendon unit[13,14] and during muscle contraction[15] indicate that tendons strain approximately 3 percent at muscle maximum tetanic tension. However, it is less clear if human tendon properties under difficult to measure physiological conditions are similar to values obtained from less physiological conditions in animals. Lieber suggested that in order for tendon properties to be determined under loads to which they would normally be exposed, the relationship between muscle physiological cross-sectional area (PCSA) and maximum tetanic tension (P_o) must be overcome.[13] Using the prime movers of the wrist as a model, Loren and Lieber[16] first analyzed the architecture of the muscle-tendon complex in cadavers to determine the PCSA. After subsequently loading the muscle-tendon units to P_o, they found a significantly different strain for each tendon, with the flexor carpi ulnaris having the largest strain (3.8 ± 0.31 percent) and the extensor carpi radialis longus having the smallest strain (1.9 ± 0.14 percent). These data indicate a certain level of specialization between tendons that is not observed using traditional elongation-to-failure methods.

Key Point:

In contrast to tendons, ligaments insert directly into bone or periosteum, and thereby assume full time responsibility for maintaining joint stability.

The major protein present in ligament is collagen, which exists in fibrillar form and enables ligaments to resist tensile forces. Collagen comprises about 75 percent of the dry weight of a ligament.[4] Although the strength of the collagen fibers depends on its diameter, the load-deformation characteristics of whole ligament depend on the number of adjacent collagen fibers and the length of those fibers.[5,8] Tipton et al.[11] and Viidik[17] have demonstrated, using animal models, that ligaments responded to repetitive strength training loads with increases in tensile load.

The concepts related to the stress-strain curve were introduced in earlier sections. **Figure 3.5** demonstrates a typical curve for ligament. In the toe region there is very little increase in the stress, allowing tissue elongation and resultant strains of 1.2-1.5 percent.[18] The stresses that produce these types of strains are similar to those applied by clinicians during an examination of knee joint ligamentous laxity. In contrast, the steeper slope associated with the linear, or elastic region of the curve indicates that the applied loads result in greater elongation of the tissue. It is believed that structural microfailure begins in this region due to stretching of the straightened collagen fibers. In this region, the ligament returns to its pre-stressed length when the tensile load is removed. Therefore, the linear portion of the curve is associated with the stress and strain that are part of normal physiological motion.

The third region of the curve is associated with progressive failure, also known as the plastic range. In this range tensile loads disrupt sufficient collagen fibers to decrease the slope of the curve. Therefore, the ligament is not able to completely return to pre-stretched levels when the deforming load is removed, which is consistent with the clini-

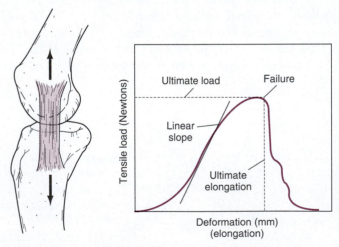

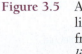

Figure 3.5   A typical load deformation curve for a bone-ligament-bone. (Reprinted with permission from MA Lockard. *Biomechanics of tendons and ligaments. In Kinesiology: The mechanics and pathomechanics of human movement*, CA Oatis (ed). Philadelphia: Lippincott Williams & Wilkins, 2002, pp. 80–95 (Figure 6.3)).

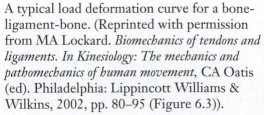

cal pathology of a sprain. If deformation loads were to exceed those experienced in the plastic range, then major failure can occur. Although the ligament may still be intact, ultrastructure damage occurs, which may be visualized as a narrowing of the tissue. The final stage is that of complete failure, which can occur when deformation loads produce strains of 8 percent or more.[19] It should be noted that wide variability may exist across different ligaments and tendons, and may be influenced by the rate and magnitude of deformation, age, sex hormone levels, and activity level.[18]

Muscle

The predominant collagen in skelatal, cardiac, and smooth muscle is type I and III. Since the initial proposal of the sliding filament theory of muscle contraction, it has become obvious that there must exist additional structures that facilitate the force-generating function of the myofilaments.[20,21] These structures, which are termed the cytoskeleton, align the thin and thick filaments and transmit force from the sarcomeres to the skeleton. Furthermore, this same cytoskeleton structure is involved when motion is imposed on the skeleton, such as that occurring during passive stretching of a limb. The cytoskeleton has been described as consisting of two lattices; the endosarcomeric cytoskeleton maintains the orientation of the thin and thick myofilaments within the sarcomeres and the exosarcomeric cytoskeleton maintains the lateral (side by side) alignment of the myofibrils.

As described in the classic length–tension relation, when muscle is stretched beyond resting length, the sarcomeres generate passive tension. However, it remains unclear as to exactly where this passive tension originates. A seminal study by Magid and Law[22] demonstrated that the origin of the passive muscle tension is within the myofibrils themselves, rather than the presumed extracellular connective tissue in striated muscle, and is most likely due to the large structural protein titin. As pointed out by Lieber,[13] the discovery of titin has tremendous clinical significance. During the traditional physical examination, it is the passive properties of skeletal muscles that are the most readily appreciated and quantified, forming the basis for clinical decision making. Because passive properties are dominated by titin, it is probably the titin molecule that most strongly influences such an examination.[13] In addition, titin may serve as a sensor for altered muscle mechanical conditions such as chronic length changes produced by stretching regimes discussed later in this chapter. (For a more detailed discussion on titin and other structural proteins, see Lieber[13].)

Although extracellular connective tissue may not have as expanded a role in passive tissue tension generation as once thought, the exosarcomeric cytoskeleton does provide connections that transmit the force generated by the actin and myosin to intramuscular connective tissue and to the skeleton. The exosarcomeric proteins, including the intermediate filaments and costameres (also known as focal adhesions), are especially involved in the lateral transmission of force.[23] It is possible that as much as 80 percent of the force generated by a single muscle fiber is transmitted laterally rather than longitudinally.[24] Costameres are made up of a number of structural proteins: desmin, integrins, dystrophin, and ankyrin, among others. These groups of molecules have the capability of binding both intracellular and extracellular molecules and thus provide a link between the basement membrane and the cytoskeleton.[24] The presence of these molecules at both the myotendinous junction and costameres suggests they have a role in the force transmission mechanism at both sites, although much remains to be learned about the functional interactions of these molecules.

Key Point:

Improving our understanding of the effects of active forces produced by, and passive forces, imposed on a muscle will enhance our ability to develop more effective strength and flexibility training interventions.

Articular Cartilage

Articular cartilage is a specialized type of hyaline cartilage the forms the load bearing surface of joints. Articular cartilage, which is avascular and aneural, covers the ends of bones with thicknesses ranging from 1 to 4 mm in areas of low compression forces to 5–7 mm in areas of high compression.[25,26] Composed of a relatively small number of cells known as chondrocytes, articular cartilage is a composite of materials with a wide variability in mechanical properties. Although small in number, the chondrocytes vary in shape and location, residing at different layers within the ground substance. The cells, bathed in the nutrient-rich synovial fluid, benefit from the milking action of articular surface deformation during intermittent joint loading (**Figure 3.6**).[3]

The remainder of the tissue is composed primarily of proteoglycans and collagen. Proteoglycans, which make up about 30 percent of the dry weight of articular cartilage, consist of a protein core and glycosaminoglycans GAGs (e.g., chondroitin sulfate, and keratin sulfate) attachments that, when bound to a backbone of hyaluronic acid, form a macromolecule. Proteoglycan concentration and water content vary inversely to each other. At the articular surface, proteoglycan concentration is relatively low, whereas water content is greater compared to other levels. Similarly, in the deeper regions of the cartilage, such as the area near subchondral bone, the proteoglycan concentration is greatest, and the water content is lowest. In contrast to proteoglycans, collagen is a fibrous protein that makes up 60 percent to 70 percent of the dry weight of articular cartilage. Primarily type II collagen is typically

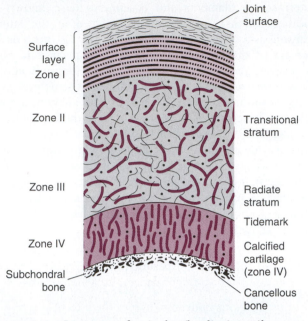

Figure 3.6   Structure of articular (hyaline) cartilage.

arranged to form a restraining network that adds structural stability to the tissue. The deepest fibers in the calcified zone are firmly anchored to the subchondral bone. These fibers are linked to the vertically oriented fibers in the adjacent deep zone (IV) which, in turn, are linked to the obliquely oriented fibers of the middle zone (II, III), and finally to the transversely oriented fibers of the superficial tangential zone (I). The series of chemically interlinked fibers form a netlike fibrous structure that entraps the large GAG molecules beneath the articular surface. The GAGs, in turn, attract water that provides a unique element of rigidity to articular cartilage. The rigidity increases the ability of cartilage to adequately withstand loads.[3] The main function of articular cartilage is to protect the bone from high stresses. Articular cartilage stiffness is about 1/20 that of the subchondral cancellous bone and about 1/65 that of cortical bone. Therefore it deforms more than bone under the same applied loads. Like a waterbed, articular cartilage fills in incongruities and spreads the load over the articulating surface in order to increase contact area and therefore decrease contact stress.

Bone

Bone gives rigid support to the body and provides the muscles with a system of levers, thereby transferring muscular activations into movement. Similarly, the rehabilitation clinician imposing passive movements that produce deformation loads at a client's connective tissues can use these same bony levers. Although bone is more resistant to mechanical loads, it is still a very dynamic structure that can be influenced by intrinsic and extrinsic factors. The mechanical properties of bone are determined primarily by its structural components. Like other forms of connective tissue,

bone consists of a cellular component and an extracellular matrix. Collagen and *hydroxyapatite* (HA) are the primary organic and inorganic materials, respectively, making up bone. Collagen is responsible for approximately 90 percent of the organic material in bone, with organic material making up 40 percent of bone's dry weight. The collagen in bone is primarily type I collagen, although other cartilage-specific collagens are present.[27] The remaining 60 percent of the dry weight of bone is from inorganic materials, with the calcium phosphate–based mineral HA being the primary one. The HA crystals, which have ceramic properties, are found primarily between collagen fibers.

The structural subunit of bone is the *osteon* or *Haversian* system, which organizes the collagen fibers into a series of concentric spirals that form *lamellae*. The cells of bone are confined with narrow *lacunae*, or spaces, positioned between the lamellae of the osteon.[3] Because bone deforms very little, the vascular supply can be routed within bone structure between the outer periosteal and the inner endosteal surfaces. The connective tissue of the periosteum and endosteum are richly vascularized and innervated with sensory receptors for pressure and pain.[3,28]

The cellular components of bone consist of fibroblasts, fibrocytes, osteoblasts, osteocytes, and osteoprogenitor cells. These cells are responsible for the ongoing remodeling that occurs in response to forces generated during physical activities and to other regulatory mechanisms, such as the hormonal regulation of systemic calcium stores. The *fibroblasts* and *fibrocytes* are essential for the production of collagen, whereas *osteoblasts* not only synthesize bone, but also regulate the deposition and mineralization of bone. When osteoblasts stop their bone-making activity, they turn into *osteocytes*, becoming another component in the bone lattice. In contrast, *osteoclasts*, which are large polymorphous cells, are responsible for bone resorption.

Perhaps, mature bone is heterogeneous so that it can better withstand varying structural demands. Whereas cortical bone is dense and hard, cancellous bone, also called spongy bone, is less dense and tends to fill inner spaces of the whole bone. For example, cortical bone is found in the mid-shaft (*diaphysis*) of the femur, with cancellous bone occupying the interior portion of the femoral head and the flared areas at each end (*metaphysis*). In the immature animal, each metaphysis is covered by an *epiphysis*, which is united to its metaphysis by a cartilaginous growth plate (*epiphyseal plate*). The growth plate is the region where calcification of articular cartilage takes place. At the cessation of growth, the epiphyses (composed of cancellous bone) become fused with the adjacent metaphyses. A thin layer of cortical bone continuous with the cortical bone of the diaphysis covers the epiphyses and metaphyses like a shell. In cancellous bone, the calcified tissue forms thin plates called *trabeculae*, which are laid down in response to stresses placed on the bone, thereby undergoing self-regulated modeling.[28] Compact bone is strongest under compressive loads, displays intermediate strength under tension loads, and is weakest under shear or torsion loads.

> ### Key Point:
> The structure and function of cancellous and cortical bone is very likely influenced by the dynamic loads placed on the developing and mature bone.

Nigg and Grimston, in a restatement of Wolff's Law, point out that physical laws are a major factor influencing bone modeling and remodeling.[29]

INFLUENCE OF TRAINING, DISUSE, AGING, AND GENDER ON TISSUES OF THE MUSCULOSKELETAL SYSTEM

At this point, the reader should realize that connective tissue is a vital component of all tissues in the musculoskeletal system. The structural and biomechanical properties of these tissues have been described. This section will go into more depth on several factors that can influence tissue, namely training or therapeutic exercise intensity, disuse (or immobilization), aging, and gender.

Bone

As previously mentioned, bone is a very dynamic tissue. Of tissues involved with joints, bone has a markedly better capacity for tissue remodeling, repair, and regeneration.[3] The physiological response of trabecular bone to an increasing load is to hypertrophy, whereas with decreased or absent loads, the trabeculae become smaller and thus are less able to provide support.[6] Reduced physical activity displays a direct relationship to decreased bone mass.[30]

> ### Key Point:
> Reduced physical activity is directly related to decreased bone mass.

Although a recent review estimated that on average 1–2 percent of site specific bone mineral density is lost per month during exposure to microgravity, the range of individual responses may be substantially larger.[31] Similarly, the rate, frequency, duration, and type of loading affect bone, in that repeated loadings, whether high repetition coupled with low load or low repetition with high load, can cause permanent strain and lead to bone failure. Bone loses stiffness and strength with repetitive loading as a result of creep strain, which occurs when a tissue is loaded repetitively during the time the material is undergoing creep.

At advancing ages, metabolism of bone contributes to the slow healing of fractures. The altered metabolism also con-

tributes to *osteoporosis*, particularly type II osteoporosis—a type that thins both trabecular and cortical bone in both males and females.[32] Osteoporosis is a de-ossification or decrease of overall bone mass that decreases the structural integrity of bony tissue. Zioupos and Currey[33] studied bones from people between 35 and 92 years of age and found that several mechanical properties decreased with age. The primary changes were 1) a 2.3 percent decrease in *Young's Modulus of Elasticity* for every 10 years after age 35; 2) a decreased resistance to bone fracture, as measured by bone toughness, at a rate of 4 percent per 10 years; and 3) decreased bending strength by about 3.7 percent per 10 years. Young's Modulus of Elasticity is the ratio of tissue stress to strain at any point in the elastic zone or Hookean Region of a load-deformation curve, yielding a value for stiffness. Human models of disuse osteoporosis, namely bed rest, spinal cord injury, and exposure to microgravity demonstrate that negative calcium balance, alterations in biochemical markers of bone turnover, and resultant loss of bone mineral density in the lower limbs occur with reduced weight bearing loading[34] mechanisms that may also be related to bone aging.

Ligaments/Joint Capsule

Ligaments have a lower percentage and more random organization of collagen, and a higher percentage of ground substance than tendons. Skeletal maturity and aging have significant effects on the biomechanical properties of ligaments.[18] The geometric and material properties of ligaments and other connective tissues change during growth and development. While some of the changes occur in the absence of mechanical loading, normal development requires the mechanical stimulus provided by normal physical activity.[35] Generally, tensile strength, load to failure, and elastic modulus all improve rapidly during maturation until skeletal maturity, as defined by the closure of epiphyses. Similarly, stress relaxation and creep in response to both static and cyclic loads are also greater in very young animals and improve with maturation.[18] Using empirical data from a series of animal studies, Woo et al.[36,37] concluded that maximal tissue strength is achieved around the time of skeletal maturity and gradually declines during adulthood and into old age. Injury patterns are subsequently affected, as young animals with open epiphyses may be more prone to avulsion fractures, whereas similar tensile loads applied to mature animals result in mid-substance ligamentous ruptures.[36]

The rate and process by which tissue ages are individual-specific. However, general changes associated with aging include slowing of the rate of collagen fiber and GAG replacement and repair.[38,39] The GAG molecules produced by aging cells are fewer in number and smaller in size than those produced by young cells. Similarly, GAG-related reductions in water binding capacity result in connective tissues that do not slide across each other as easily. Consequently, bundles of fibers in ligaments do not align in parallel with imposed forces, thereby hindering the resistance to rapidly applied forces. For example, the stiffness, ultimate load, and elastic modulus of human anterior cruciate ligament specimens from young adults (age 22–35 years) are about threefold greater compared with those from older adults.[40,41]

Although there can be a tendency to think of the synovial joint capsule as a homogenous structure, several studies have identified regional differences in mechanical properties of joint capsules of the glenohumeral joint,[42–44] hip,[45] and cervical spine.[46,47] For example, Tonetti et al.[46] reported regional differences in the joint capsules of the lower cervical spine that closely matched the descriptive anatomy of the capsule, where ligamentous reinforcement of capsule resulted in increased mechanical properties such as stiffness. These data indicate that the mechanical properties of the joint capsule are similar to those of connective tissue in general, with differences being related primarily to the cross-sectional area of the structure. This view would be consistent with the view that two capsule structures with the same cross sectional area would have similar stiffness. Therefore, generally the mechanical properties of joint capsule will vary by the cross sectional area and length of the tissue, and in this way have properties similar to ligamentous structures.

The rate of decline in strength of connective tissue is somewhat dependent on the normal metabolic activity of the specific tissue. For example, immobilization produces a marked decrease in tensile strength of the ligaments of the knee within a few weeks.[9,48]

Tendon

As a component of the musculotendinous complex that can produce dynamic motion and stability to any joints that it crosses, tendon is integral to normal movement. Primarily because of their collagen fiber composition and orientation, tendons have the highest tensile strength of any soft tissue. Tendon, which has connective tissue properties similar to those for ligaments, can be influenced by a wide variety of intrinsic and extrinsic factors. As stated previously, tendon strain has been reported to be approximately 3 percent, although tendon type, muscular interaction, and measurement technique can influence this value. Tendon and ligaments are not equally affected by strain rate.

Tendons are more strain rate sensitive compared with ligaments.[18] For example, as the rate of force application increases, stiffness and ultimate load also increase; thus, failure is more likely to occur by rupture. Conversely, at slow speeds, failure occurs predominately by avulsion at the tendon–bone interface. Under normal conditions, the tendon is most vulnerable at either of its ends (both the site of bone attachment, and the histological "gray-zone" between muscle–tendon transition) rather than in its midsubstance, and in fact rarely ruptures under typical loading conditions.

> ## *Key Point:*
> Tendons are more sensitive to strain rate than ligaments. At higher loading rates failure is more likely to occur by rupture. Conversely, at slower rates failure occurs predominantly by avulsion at the tendon–bone interface.

As stated in the previous section on ligaments, biochemical and histological alterations occur during maturation and aging. Collagen fibril size increases, along with collagen concentration and synthesis, are greater for mature adults compared with adolescents. In addition, the cross links between collagen fibers are also greater in adults. Beyond the fifth and sixth decades, however, collagen concentrations are reduced, and the number of small-diameter collagen fibrils increases resulting in reduced levels of maximal tissue strength[49]. Although changes in mechanical properties of aged tendon may alter the muscle–tendon interaction, this has not been adequately studied in vivo for humans.

Prolonged joint immobilization can have profound deleterious effects on the biochemical, histological, and mechanical properties of connective tissue in general, and it particularly affects tendons. Prolonged immobilization (a period as short as several weeks) can reduce the biomechanical properties of load at failure and stiffness of connective tissues.[50] The underlying biochemical and histological changes associated with these mechanical changes include collagen synthesis and degradation increases, resulting in collagen turnover. Similarly, collagen cross linking, which is also affected by immobilization, increases, although much of the newly synthesized collagen is immature and may not result in improved tensile strength. The cross links, along with water content and total GAGs, may be associated with the development of connective tissue contractures or adhesions in immobilized dense connective tissue structures.[51] It should be noted, however, that immobilizing limbs to place the tendon under greater tension can improve the collagen fiber organization.

Muscle

Non-contractile or passive elements of muscle, including the fascicles, sarcolemma, epimysium, perimysium, and endomysium are four orders of magnitude more compliant than is tendon.[24] Therefore, these structures are likely to receive most of the mechanical stress that is generated by passive stretching. Williams and Goldspink[52,53] demonstrated, using mouse muscle, that when a muscle was immobilized with a constant stretch, for 4 weeks the muscle responded with an approximately 20 percent increase in sarcomere number. Therefore, the muscle, sensing the passive stretch, synthesized new sarcomeres to return individual sarcomeres back to their normal length. In contrast, muscle immobilized in a shortened position for four weeks (i.e., the antagonists to the lengthened muscles) were shown to be much stiffer, or more resistant to passive stretch, with a decrease in sarcomere number by 40 percent.[52,53] Lieber[13] suggested that the adaptive tendencies of muscle to length changes may differ between anti-gravity postural muscles and those without such a role.

Using a model that more closely mimicked clinical conditions, Williams et al.[54] used an intermittent immobilization model, where mouse soleus muscle was taken out of a cast and mobilized by performing passive range of motion (ROM) daily. When the joint was passively stretched throughout the range in a relatively slow rate for as little as 30 min/day, the intervention was sufficient to prevent loss of motion and decrease in sarcomere number.[54] The close correlation between sarcomere number and ROM suggested that the contractile elements of muscle were responsible for length changes, rather than changes in the non-contractile connective tissue elements.[13] De Deyne,[24] in an excellent review on the consequences of passive stretch to muscle fibers, concurs with this view of muscle being the prominent component of extensibility changes. Increased ROM immediately following passive stretching can be explained by the viscoelastic behavior of muscle and short term changes in muscle extensibility. However, it is not clear if the mobility gained by stretch based exercise protocols is due to the hysteresis process as depicted by the stress–strain curve, or if the changes in the sarcomeres in series are the primary mechanism. To explain how myofibrillogenesis could contribute to muscle extensibility, De Deyne proposed three potential mechanisms: 1) the phosphorylation of integral membrane proteins (integrins, dystroglycan complex) and associated cytoskeletal molecules; 2) the secretion of selective growth factors, regulated by the autocrine (mode of hormone action affecting the cell type that produced it) or paracrine (mode of hormone action affecting cells other than the type that produced it) mechanisms; or 3) changes in the intracellular ion flux through stretch activated ion channels.[24] Regardless of the specific mechanisms, it may be that traditional stretching techniques used to gain ROM may be found primarily in the cellular and molecular adaptive mechanism of the muscle fiber.

Key Point:

Similar to other connective tissues, muscle is affected by immobilization, aging, and other chronic factors that can alter its mechanical properties and function. Unlike ligaments and tendons, however, muscle has a contractile component that also is affected by these same factors.

As discussed in previous chapters, immobilization, or disuse, can result in atrophy of the muscle secondary to a reduction in protein synthesis and a loss of muscle fibers.[55,56] In addition, short term immobilization can re-
sult in a decline in electrical activity of the muscle, loss of muscle mass, reduced cross sectional area, and impaired performance. Another commonly reported observation from limb immobilization studies is the slow-to-fast conversion of muscle fiber types, with the proportion of slow twitch, oxidative muscle fibers decreasing and that of fast twitch, oxidative-glycolytic muscle fibers increasing.[4]

Although the relative importance of this conversion is unclear and has been debated, impaired neuromuscular performance has been consistently demonstrated following immobilization. For example, the effect of immobilization on the fatigability of muscle appears to differ for high and low force contractions. The endurance time of elbow flexor muscles immobilized for four weeks was similar to pre-immobilization levels for high force contractions of 65 percent maximal volitional contraction (MVC), whereas endurance time for the contractions of 20 percent MVC was increased by approximately 60 percent. In addition, endurance times for women were greater compared than those for men when the subjects performed contractions at 15 percent MVC force levels.[57] Another consequence appears to be the altered motor drive to the immobilized muscle. Six to eight weeks of immobilization affects both the properties and the behavior of motor units.[58] Although there was an increase in the number of high threshold motor units, the average force exerted by the units was less and the peak-to-peak amplitude of the motor unit action potentials was reduced. These findings indicate that immobilization changes the activation strategy used to grade muscle force.[4]

With aging, muscle becomes weaker for several reasons. First, muscle fiber size decreases, which results in a muscle that has a smaller cross sectional area. Second, the number of fast twitch muscle fibers decreases, which itself implies a strength loss. In addition, there is evidence that the ability to activate motor units decreases with age so that even the fibers that remain in the muscle are not fully used. It is less clear, however, to what extent these changes are due strictly to the aging process and what effects are due to the low level of use experienced by muscles as an individual ages. More recent evidence indicates that reduced activity level has at least some effect. Therefore, the quality of life experienced by older adults depends on the lifestyle that one chooses. Strength and flexibility training is associated with improvements in strength, improved postural stability maintenance, reduced levels of muscle atrophy, and improvements in mobility.[4] See Enoka[4] for a more in depth discussion on the effects of aging and reduced activity on the neuromuscular system.

INFLUENCE OF SENSORY AND MOTOR SYSTEMS ON FLEXIBILITY

Before clinical techniques and strategies related to flexibility are discussed, it is important to remember that creating short term or long term changes in biological tissues depends on more than just the biomechanical properties of tissue. Many of the flexibility strategies discussed later in this chapter are influenced by the contractile component of muscle. For example, a clinical technique designed to improve hamstring flexibility may have very different results depending on the level of relaxation of the hamstring muscles (along with their antagonists, the knee extensors) during the stretching technique. Therefore, the sensory and motor components of the nervous system can significantly impact the efficacy of flexibility programs. Because of this, readers are encouraged to review Chapters 2, 7 and 8 for more detail on muscle spindles and other receptors, along with sensory motor reflexes responsive to receptor input.

Key Point:

The relative state of muscle activation or relaxation is a critical component of many flexibility programs.

The muscle spindle and golgi tendon organs (GTOs) are the two sensory receptors that monitor muscle activity and, via afferent pathways, can activate both spinal reflexes and long-loop pathways involving supraspinal centers. The muscle spindle, whose mechanoreceptor sensitivity can be adjusted, has two types of intrafusal muscle fibers that can be made to contract and relax. Therefore, the muscle spindle is ideally positioned within the extrafusal muscle to monitor not only overall muscle length, but also, more important, the rate of change in muscle length. When the sensory nerve endings in the intrafusal fibers are stimulated by changes in length, the sensory input is transmitted to the spinal cord via Ia and II sensory axons. If sufficiently large, these axons may activate homonymous motor neurons that will activate the stretched muscle, resulting in a muscle contraction that can thereby reduce the stretch of the muscle.

In contrast to the muscle spindle, the GTO is a relatively simple sensory receptor, as it has a single afferent and no efferent connections. Despite its name, few tendon organs are located in the tendon proper. Most organs are grouped around a few extrafusal muscle fibers near the aponeurosis of the attachment.[4] When a muscle and its connective tissue attachments are stretched, either through passive stretch or active contraction of the muscle, the organs excite the Group Ib afferent nerve. Therefore, the tendon organ is a monitor of muscle force, whose threshold for activation can be task and state dependent.[4,59]

STRETCHING AND MUSCULOTENDINOUS FLEXIBILITY

What Is Stretching?

Stretching involves the elongation or increased extensibility of the muscles and tendons by moving parts of the body, generally to the end of the available ROM. When a muscle is subjected to a tensile (pulling) force, transient deformation occurs, thereby elongating the musculotendinous unit, resulting in a stretch.[1,60] The amount of stretching that takes place is dependent on the physiology of the muscles and connective tissue (i.e., skin, fascia, ligaments, tendons, joint capsules, and muscle fascia). Collagen levels primarily dictate the viscoelastic behavior of connective tissues.[7,61]

Stretching also affects different sensory organs in the muscle and tendon, resulting in important neurophysiological phenomena. Although the resultant muscle and tendon lengthening serve to gradually increase flexibility, other types of adaptations may occur from a regular stretching program. Research has demonstrated that adaptive plasticity is possible in the central nervous system.[62,63] As a result of training, the stretch reflex may be reset to a different level. In animal studies, increased stretching has resulted in an increased number of sarcomeres.[52,64] Several types of stretching exercises have been detailed in the literature and will be described in a later section.

What Is Flexibility?

Maintaining a reasonable amount of flexibility is necessary for efficient movement. Decreased joint mobility and ROM may lead to incorrect postural alignment, which could potentially result in chronically tight muscles, faulty compensation patterns, inefficient body mechanics, and possibly increased risk of injury. Flexibility has been defined as the ability to move muscles and joints through a full ROM[1] and refers to the amount of extensibility of muscles and connective tissue in order to allow adequate ROM in joints. Whereas stretching refers to the process of elongation of muscles and other connective tissues, flexibility generally refers to the amount of normal motion available.

Key Point:

Flexibility refers to the capacity to move muscles and joints through a full range of motion. Whereas stretching refers to the process of elongation of muscles and other connective tissues, flexibility generally refers to the amount of normal motion available.

Flexibility can be classified into different categories, depending on the type of stretching that is performed. For example, static flexibility refers to the ROM about a joint as a result of *static stretching* (no velocity involved), whereas *dynamic flexibility* relates to the ability to move through a ROM with normal or rapid velocity.[1] However, based on the available literature, there is no evidence to assume that flexibility exists as a single general characteristic of the body; rather, it is specific to particular joints, joint actions, or movements.[65–67] Flexibility is highly variable among different individuals, as are muscle and joint stiffness, resulting in different levels of flexibility in various movements. Many studies have identified a functional ROM for specific joints, which occurs during the performance of certain functional tasks.[68–71] For example, approximately 105° of knee flexion is necessary to ascend and descend stairs (depending on the height of the step).

Of course, the flexibility needed for athletic endeavors usually differs from activities of daily living. Just as flexibility is joint specific, it is also sport or activity specific. For example, a baseball pitcher exhibits increased shoulder ROM with external rotation and decreased internal rotation in the throwing arm as compared to the non-throwing arm (**Figure 3.7**).[72,73] A swimmer would require more bilateral shoulder flexibility than would a track and field sprinter.

Many people consider good flexibility essential for successful athletic performance and injury prevention. Although it may seem intuitive that increased flexibility could improve athletic performance, there is virtually no research to substantiate this claim. Common sense suggests that including stretching activities in most therapeutic exercise or fitness programs is a good idea. Decreased flexibility in a hurdler, for example, could potentially hinder his or her ability to get over the hurdle efficiently. Flexibility is an important part of any training program, since it dictates movement ability during sports activities. However, with notable exceptions, maximal flexibility is not vital in all sports because most sport skills require an effective balance between joint flexibility and stability (e.g., shooting a basketball, playing golf).

Flexibility is maintained through regular and proper stretching regimens and will diminish over time if tissues are not stretched or exercised.[1] Therefore, a loss of flexibility would result in a decreased ROM about a joint secondary to a decreased ability of the muscle to deform.[74] It stands to reason then that the goal of any flexibility pro-

gram would be to improve ROM at all joints by enhancing musculotendinous extensibility around those joints, rather than isolating capsuloligamentous structures. Based on evidence from numerous studies, the American College of Sports Medicine (ACSM) has developed guidelines for flexibility training, as follows[75]:

- **Type:** A general stretching routine that exercises the major muscle and/or tendon groups using static stretching or proprioceptive neuromuscular facilitation techniques (PNF)
- **Frequency:** A minimum of 2–3 days per week
- **Intensity:** To a position of mild discomfort
- **Duration:** 10–30 seconds for static; 6-second contraction followed by 10–30 seconds assisted stretch for PNF
- **Repetitions:** 3–4 for each stretch

FLEXIBILITY AND ASSOCIATED TOPICS

Limitations to Flexibility

Although muscles, tendons, and their surrounding fascia are most likely to be responsible for limiting ROM, other factors, such as bony structures, fat, connective tissue lesions, skin, and postural problems, may all lead to flexibility and joint ROM limitations. During the assessment, the rehabilitation clinician must determine if ROM restrictions or limitations are contributing to functional movement limitations. Additionally, given joint specificity, the clinician must identify what is causing the restriction and then select the appropriate exercise techniques to improve flexibility. Other factors that may affect flexibility are age and gender.

Aging and Flexibility

Early research indicates that children appear to have greatest flexibility during their elementary school years. With adolescence, flexibility seems to level off and then begins to decrease throughout adulthood.[76,77] Some authors have suggested that a muscle-tendon unit may experience an increased *preload* if the bone grows faster than the muscle-tendon unit.[78] A preload is simply the amount of force sustained by a tissue in the body's normal relaxed state and can be assessed via flexibility measurement. This increase in tissue preload may result in decreased flexibility and an increase in tissue stiffness, which may explain the loss of back and leg flexibility in boys between the ages of 8 and 13 years.[78] The physiological changes that occur with aging beyond adolescence can also lead to a decrease in overall musculoskeletal flexibility. This is particularly true in the elderly. Alongside the loss of muscle function, an increase in intramuscular connective tissue stiffness occurs, resulting in decreased ROM and a gradual decline in the efficiency of activities of daily living (ADL) performance. Certain physical and biochemical changes occur to collagen with aging that result in decreased extensibility.

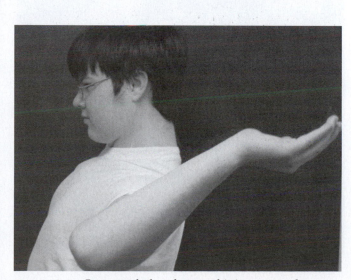

Figure 3.7   Increased glenohumeral joint external rotation.

It appears that an increased number of intra- and inter-molecular cross links form, which, coupled with a concomitant decline in tissue hydration, restrict the ability of the collagen fibers to move past each other.[79]

Evidence suggests that elderly people who regularly participate in flexibility training programs display improved joint ROM.[80–87] It should be noted that increased ROM did not relate directly to improved functional capacity in some of these studies. Time is also an important consideration when dealing with decreased flexibility in the elderly. This is mainly because collagen is less mobile and responds more slowly to stretching in the elderly than in their younger counterparts.[88] However, given some compensation for time, the older person is also capable of improving his or her flexibility.[89] Further study is suggested regarding optimal stretching intervention parameters for older subjects.

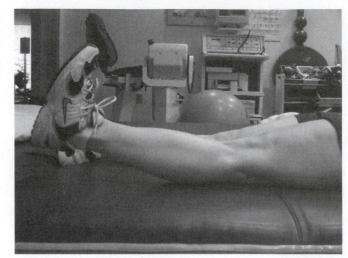

Figure 3.8   Knee hyperextension.

Gender Differences

Evidence suggests that women are generally more flexible than men.[1] This level of increased flexibility may be in some part due to the physiological and anatomical differences. One study, examining the differences between men and women over an 18-year period, revealed that men had less flexibility than women only in their hamstring muscles.[90] Flexibility in women is also affected by pregnancy, during which time the pelvic joints and capsuloligamentous tissues are relaxed and are capable of greater movement. Additionally, some of the differences in flexibility may be due to the nature of different regular and social activities performed by people of each gender.[76] Although no firm conclusions can be drawn, hormonal fluctuations may play a role in ligamentous laxity of certain joints, thus potentially predisposing women to greater ROM differences than their male counterparts.

Pathology and Joint Laxity

The goal of any flexibility program is to improve joint ROM by improving the muscle extensibility. However, it should be kept in mind that some individuals exhibit skeletal malalignment, which alters soft tissue loading of joints and may affect musculoskeletal extensibility. Subsequently, this can lead to compensatory postures resulting in pathological conditions, along with abnormal joint load distribution and contact pressures, which can lead to articular cartilage degeneration.[91]

Although not necessarily a limitation of flexibility, joint laxity may affect the way flexibility is assessed. Many people have greater joint laxity than average but poor musculotendinous extensibility. Some researchers have suggested that hypermobile individuals avoid strenuous physical activity because of their potentially increased risk for in-

jury.[92] The hypermobility screening method developed by Carter and Wilkinson[93] and later modified by Beighton et al.,[94] has been used extensively to examine specific joint flexibility. This method examines the ability to hyperextend the knees (**Figure 3.8**) and elbows (**Figure 3.9**) beyond 10°, to passively extend the fingers so they are parallel to the forearm (**Figure 3.10**), to passively abduct the thumb so that it touches the forearm (**Figure 3.11**), and to forward flex the trunk so that the palms easily touch the floor (**Figure 3.12**). Therefore, when demonstrating a stretching program with these individuals, it is necessary to isolate the muscle to be stretched, focusing on stretching the muscle only and not the joint capsule.

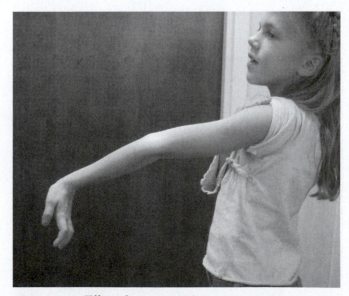

Figure 3.9   Elbow hyperextension.

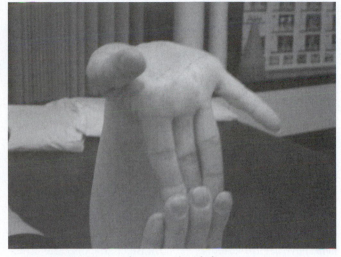

Figure 3.10   Finger hyperextensibility.

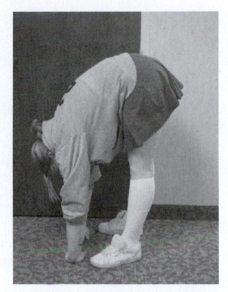

Figure 3.12   Trunk hypermobility.

This produces a more effective stretch than simply performing a component stretch across two or three joints.

Flexibility Assessment

Although many people speak in terms of overall flexibility, no one composite test can provide a satisfactory index of an individual's flexibility characteristics.[65] Assessment of flexibility usually involves ROM measurement about a specific joint, since flexibility is specific to individual joint movements. Therefore, some measurements of overall flexibility may prove to be difficult, as it may involve a complexity of movements over several joints (i.e., sit and reach test) (**Figure 3.13**). Although a variety of instruments are used to measure joint motion, the measuring device most commonly used to measure ROM, which is fairly accurate, is the universal goniometer (**Figure 3.14**).

A goniometer is simply a protractor with degree measurements. The arms of the goniometer are placed along the proximal and distal components around a joint with the axis centered over the joint. Moving the goniometer's distal component toward the proximal component results in a measurement of an arc of motion about that specific joint. Due to its versatility, it can be used to measure joint position and ROM at almost all joints of the body. Other types of goniometers used in the clinical setting, albeit less frequently, are the inclinometer, the pendulum goniometer, and the fluid goniometer. Electrogoniometers are also available but are used primarily for research purposes to obtain dynamic joint measurements. The Leighton

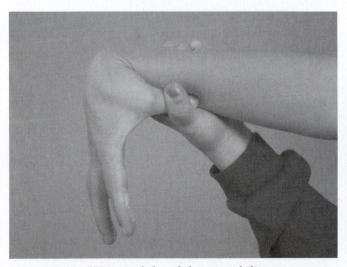

Figure 3.11   Wrist and thumb hypermobility.

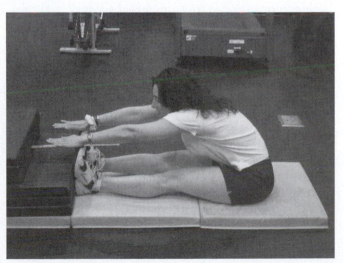

Figure 3.13   Sit and reach test.

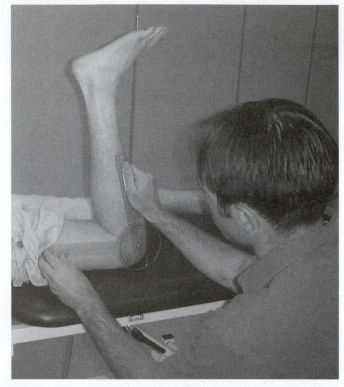

Figure 3.14   Goniometric measurement.

GENERAL EFFECTS OF STRETCHING

Although difficult to believe, a limited knowledge of stretching of the muscle–tendon unit with respect to its mechanisms and efficacy exists, despite its widespread use. Stretching effectiveness is attributed to its *mechanical* and *neurophysiological* effects.[61,123] Biomechanically, the muscle–tendon unit has been shown to respond viscoelastically during stretching. Alternatively, some stretching exercises are based on the neural inhibition of the muscle undergoing stretch. In other words, decreased reflex activity results in reduced resistance to stretch, resulting in further gains of joint ROM. Although there appears to be a dichotomy presented in the literature, most likely both mechanisms are responsible for stretching of the human muscle–tendon unit in vivo. It should be noted that, in the discussion of stretching, interest lies primarily in increasing end range joint flexibility. Arguably, therefore, the issue deals more with the connective tissue component, since many authors contend that the primary resistance to flexibility is not likely to be the contractile elements of the muscle.[61,124] Muscle relaxation during stretch may have little or no direct effect on the ROM achieved,[99,125] which would argue against the basis for proprioceptive neuromuscular facilitation (PNF) techniques.

Connective tissue is composed of both collagen (viscous component) and elastin fibers (elastic component), which gives it the property of viscoelasticity. As described earlier, viscoelasticity describes the ability to exhibit both viscous and elastic properties. Viscous properties allow *plastic* or permanent deformation, while elastic properties permit recoverable deformation.[126] When under tensile stress, connective tissue behaves in a viscoelastic manner.[127] In this case, collagen gives the tissue its strength and stiffness to resist mechanical deformation, while the elastin gives the tissue its spring-like properties, allowing it to recover from deformation.[128] Being time dependent, the time required to stretch collagen varies inversely with the force used.[129] So high force, short duration favors primarily elastic tissue deformation, whereas low force, long duration favors plastic deformation.[130,131]

Stiffness is a tissue's ability to resist stretch and indicates the amount of deformation proportional to the load applied[124] and is a measure of the rate of increase of *passive tension* as a muscle is stretched. Therefore, the stiffer the tissue, the less likely it is to stretch and the less *compliance* it has; less stiffness means greater compliance.

Flexometer, a device that contains a rotating circular dial marked off in degrees, has also been used for measuring flexibility.[95]

Consistency is crucial when using a specific type of goniometer for a specific client. Since different goniometer types may provide differing results, they should not be used interchangeably in the clinical setting. For example, if an inclinometer is selected as the measurement device for a particular client, it should be used with that client for all future re-assessments. Although visual estimates are also used in a clinical setting, most authorities recommend using goniometry due to its increased accuracy and reliability of measurement.[96,97]

PRINCIPLES OF STRETCHING

Many people perform stretching exercises without a clear understanding of why, how, and when they should stretch. Most of the research performed on stretching includes the various types of stretching,[98–101] its effects on flexibility and strength,[102–108] how it should be performed,[109–111] and when stretching should be implemented in the exercise regime.[112,113] Other research reveals the effects of stretching on the occurrence of injury,[105,106,113–118] while also alluding to enhancement of athletic performance.[119–122] While the aforementioned research concludes that stretching may indeed increase flexibility, decrease the chance of injury, and reduce strength, it also provides data to the contrary.

Flexibility training is designed to decrease the stiffness of the muscle–tendon unit.[61,123]

Key Point:

Flexibility training is designed to decrease the stiffness of the muscle–tendon unit.

Moreover, the more rapidly a stretch is applied to a viscoelastic tissue, the greater the resistance to stretch. It has been reported that slow twitch muscle has greater stiffness than fast twitch muscle, suggesting that long term use influences the mechanical properties of muscle.[132] Although muscular flexibility has both mechanical and neurophysiological components,[61,98,133–136] the ability of stretching to produce greater flexibility appears to be primarily a result of the viscoelastic nature of muscle and connective tissue.[61,137] The greatest resistance to stretching comes from the connective tissue framework and sheathing from within and around the muscle and not the muscle itself (since the muscle itself can be stretched to 150 percent of its resting length); this is known as the parallel elastic component and includes the epimysium, perimysium, endomysium, and may even include the sarcolemma.[23,126,138–140] The collagenous make-up of these tissues is what is responsible for its inherent viscoelastic properties. Taylor et al.[61] suggested that static stretching as well as PNF stretching results in stress relaxation of connective tissue.

Whereas many researchers contend that the muscle–tendon units are the limiting structures preventing increases in ROM,[61,102,124,141,142] others suggest that the immediate result of stretching may be attributed to neurophysiological phenomena.[123] These phenomena can be categorized as either a *stretch tolerance* or active contractile responses. A stretch tolerance is simply an accommodation to the discomfort of stretching over time and may be associated with free nerve endings. Muscle spindles and GTOs constitute the mechanoreceptors responsible for the contractile responses. The limiting factor during stretching, in this line of thinking, would be the muscular resistance secondary to reflex activity.[123] The aim of stretching would therefore be to inhibit the reflex activity, thereby decreasing the resistance and improving ROM. Several researchers have recommended certain types of stretching because of reductions in reflex activity.[98,133–136,143,144] Others, however, have reported that certain types of stretching actually heighten stretch reflex activation, making the stretch more difficult to perform.[145] Despite this evidence, many have reported that a significant decline in resistance to stretch occurs in the absence of any meaningful electromyographic (EMG) activity during a static stretch,[124,146] suggesting that the effect may be more mechanical in nature; others[137,147] have also demonstrated

viscoelastic stress relaxation in human skeletal muscle with stretching, concluding that it was independent of detectable EMG activity. They reported that slow, passive muscle stretching through the ROM produced no electrical activity in normal relaxed subjects. Thus, it appears from the existing literature that a resistance to stretch may be possible, despite the lack of EMG activity.

TYPES OF STRETCHING

Research on stretching has focused on the comparisons of the different stretching techniques and their effectiveness at increasing ROM, as well as what the optimal times of stretching are for maximizing increases in ROM. Although several different types of stretching techniques are used to enhance musculotendinous and connective tissue extensibility; they usually fall into four main categories: static (active and passive), ballistic, PNF, and dynamic. All four techniques have been shown to increase flexibility.[98,100,103,148–150] The proper execution of the selected mode of stretching is the most important element of any flexibility program.

Static Stretching

Static stretching is the most common form of stretching and is a technique used to safely increase the ROM in a joint by sustaining a controlled muscle stretch (**Figure 3.15a–b**).[110] In order to obtain optimal passive stretching, all voluntary and reflex muscular resistance should be eliminated. There is abundant evidence to support that slow passive stretching through the ROM will not produce muscle activity in normal relaxed subjects.[126,147] So, for the static stretch, the muscle is slowly and passively stretched to a new length where further motion is limited by its own tension, thereby not eliciting the stretch reflex of the stretched muscle. The stretch should be tolerable and should not elicit pain or discomfort.[98,143] It is then maintained for an extended period of time, during which time the tension is reduced, before being returned to its starting position. As a result, a relaxation and concurrent elongation of the muscle is accomplished. It is recommended that the muscle be stretched slowly and with a low force, either externally or internally, so as to avoid the chance of injury to muscles and tendons.[7] A *passive static stretch* implies that the force is applied externally with a partner or using gravity (**Figure 3.16**). If the force is produced by an opposing muscle action, then the stretch is called an *active static stretch*. Passive and active muscle stretching are not comparable processes. Active stretching involves the muscle (series elastic) components and is ineffective at stretching non-muscular structures such as ligaments and joint capsules. Passive stretching, on the other hand, involves the non-muscular (parallel elastic)

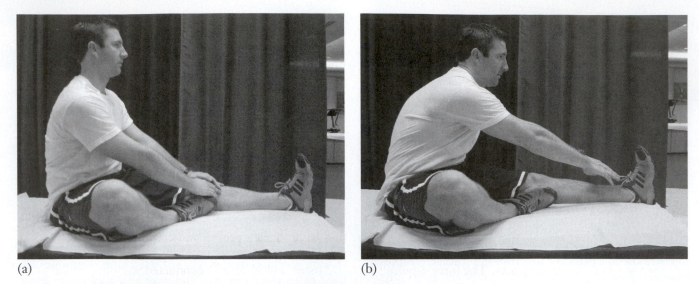

(a)   (b)

Figure 3.15   Static hamstring stretching. (a) start position; (b) finish position.

components (myofascial, ligaments, and joint capsules) as well as the series elastic components (**Figure 3.17**).[7]

The type of static stretch used is one of choice, or may depend upon the availability of a partner. For example, in the sit and reach toe touch, the individual sits with the legs extended and the trunk and hips flexed forward; with the arms straight and the hands reaching toward the toes, as the individual flexes forward. If this were performed as an active static stretch, the subject would lean forward while actively using the hip and trunk flexors until the end ROM is reached. This would result in a stretch of the lower back and hamstrings and would be held for several seconds. If the same technique was performed as a passive static stretch, then the subject would relax and have a partner press against the back until the end ROM was reached, holding that position for several seconds.[151] In most warm-up programs, static stretches are primarily active static stretches, using gravity to assist the stretch.

Ballistic Stretching

The second technique is ballistic stretching. For many people, this is the least desirable and most controversial technique, as it involves the use of jerking or bouncing movements to stretch the muscles, potentially placing the tissue at risk.[152] Ciullo and Zarins[120] warn that if bouncing occurs while the muscle is contracting, the musculotendinous unit must absorb the added energy eccentrically while concentrically contracting, which could result in tissue rupture. The muscle is stretched by momentum created from the movement of the body segments, supplying the tensile force used for the stretch. When the end ROM is reached, the person quickly relaxes the muscle. This is done in a cyclical bouncing motion, repeated several

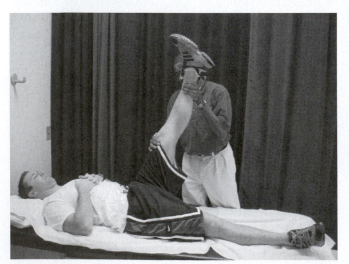

Figure 3.16   Passive hamstring stretch.

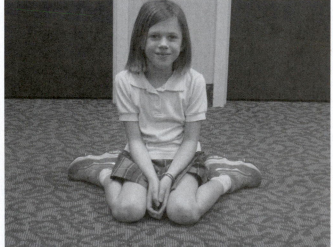

Figure 3.17   The "W" sit position, a not so desirable form of passive stretching because of the plastic deformation it creates at the capsuloligamentous structures of the medial knee joint.

times, thus engaging the neurological component called active resistance. This resistance results from the contraction of skeletal muscles that resist elongation in the form of muscle reflex activity.[153] When a muscle is rapidly stretched, the muscle spindles are activated, sending a signal to the central nervous system (CNS), which responds by causing motor units to contract and overcome the stretch.[60,98] Ballistic stretches are considered undesirable because they stimulate the muscle spindles during the stretch, resulting in a continuous resistance to further stretch and thereby causing a high rate of tension strong enough to potentially injure the musculotendinous unit.[110,126,154]

For example, one would perform a toe touch stretch from a standing position with the feet close together, the knees extended, the trunk and hips flexed, and the arms extended reaching toward the toes. The force required to move the body would vary, depending on the speed of the stretch. This would be done several times with hopes that each bounce would increase the ROM.

In contrast, static stretches move the musculotendinous unit to its end ROM slowly where it is held for several seconds, bypassing muscle reflex activity. Studies using EMG techniques have shown that there is low muscle activity with static stretch.[99,155,156] These findings are also dependent on the subject voluntarily relaxing and being comfortable with the stretch.

Proprioceptive Neuromuscular Facilitation (PNF)

The third technique to facilitate ROM increases is proprioceptive neuromuscular facilitation (PNF). PNF is actually an entire system of therapy comprising a broad spectrum of techniques designed to promote neuromuscular responses through proprioceptive stimulation.[144] PNF may be recognized as classical or modified. "Classical" refers to the clinical approach described by Knott and Voss, and the modified approach adapts certain PNF techniques and principles for use in physical conditioning. Stretching is only one of the many aspects attributed to this modified PNF approach. These stretching techniques use volitional contractions in an attempt to increase ROM by minimizing the resistance attributed to the spinal reflex pathways.[125] Currently, it is used to strengthen and increase flexibility of the muscle and has been used in sports, neuromuscular rehabilitation, and orthopaedic clinical settings for over 50 years.[134] Key components of PNF stretching are the execution of movement in diagonal patterns and the use of an isometric contraction prior to the stretch in order to achieve greater gains than stretching alone. (See Chapter 6) Many clinicians have modified the PNF patterns considerably, deviating significantly from the proposed diagonal patterns originally described by Knott and Voss to straight plane patterns. Subsequently, it

is difficult to ascertain if the effects of PNF treatment are consistent among practitioners.

Theoretically, PNF techniques increase ROM through the stimulation of the proprioceptors.[1] Taylor et al.[61] explained that voluntary isometric contraction of the stretched muscle group leads to self-inhibition of that muscle (autogenic inhibition) through the GTO reflexes. Voluntary isometric contraction of the antagonistic muscle group results in a subsequent reflex inhibition on the muscle groups being stretched (reciprocal inhibition). So, at the same time the agonist muscle (e.g., hamstrings) is facilitated, the antagonistic (e.g., quadriceps) muscle is inhibited or relaxed (**Figure 3.18**). This reciprocal inhibition of the antagonistic muscle combines with GTO facilitation to produce a greater muscle relaxation by inhibiting reflex activity.

Moore and Hutton[99] conducted a study to determine the relative muscle relaxation during PNF and static stretching. Despite producing greater increases in ROM, they reported that the PNF contract-relax with agonist contraction produced increased muscle activity with stretching than did static stretching. Their findings contradicted the theory that increased EMG activity levels in the stretched muscle would inhibit ROM increases. They additionally explained that the voluntary discomfort felt in the antagonistic muscle (in this case the hamstrings) might have been masked during the agonist muscle contraction (quadriceps), which may have attributed to increased ROM by increasing the tolerance of stretching discomfort. Therefore, factors other than muscle relaxation are important in attaining increased ROM.[99,157] However, Etnyre and Abraham[135] dismissed this line of reasoning for greater muscle activity during stretching, stating that the appearance of co-contraction between antagonist muscles were actually cross talk between the electrodes. Many different PNF techniques are employed, but some of the more commonly used techniques are contract-relax, contract-relax with agonist contraction, hold-relax, and slow-reversal-hold relax. These will be discussed in more detail in Chapter 6.

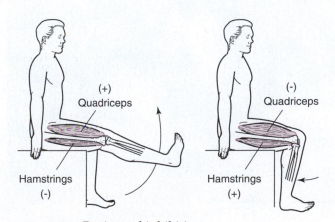

Figure 3.18   Reciprocal inhibition.

The *contract-relax* technique involves a dynamic contraction of the antagonist against maximal resistance of the clinician, followed by relaxation of the muscle. It begins by the rehabilitation clinician moving the limb to the end ROM until the subject feels a stretch. The subject then contracts the muscle against the clinician's resistance for 5–10 seconds with subsequent relaxation. The limb is then passively moved into its new limit; the subject is instructed to relax and the clinician holds the stretch for 10 seconds (**Figure 3.19a–b**). This process is repeated until the required number of repetitions are performed, each time starting and continuing from the point where the limb is moved to its new limit of pain-free motion. For example, the subject contracts the hamstring muscle (extends it) against the clinician's resistance and then relaxes the leg, allowing the clinician to further stretch the hamstring and move the leg toward hip flexion. This position is held for 10 seconds before starting the next repetition.

In the *contract-relax with agonist contraction* technique, the limb is initially taken to the point of stretch and the rehabilitation clinician applies resistance against the muscle being stretched for 5 seconds (as in the contract-relax method). The muscle is then relaxed while the agonist concentrically contracts; this helps to facilitate the stretch utilizing the principle of reciprocal inhibition. The rehabilitation clinician again takes up any slack and holds the new position for 10 seconds.

Using the previous example, after the contract-relax portion has been performed, the subject would then concentrically contract the quadriceps to help move the limb toward further hip flexion (with the clinician taking up the slack), thereby enhancing the stretch and increasing ROM. The new position would be held for 10 seconds before starting the next repetition.

The *hold-relax* technique is similar to the contract-relax, except that isometric, rather than dynamic contraction against maximal resistance, is applied prior to the relaxation of the limb. So, in our example, the subject would contract the hamstrings isometrically before relaxing and being stretched further.

The *slow reversal hold-relax* movement comprises primarily the same movements as the contract-relax with agonist contraction. With this technique, the limb is stretched by the rehabilitation clinician as before to the point of stretch. The subject then isometrically contracts the muscle (in this case the hamstrings) against the clinician. The subject then concentrically contracts the opposing muscle (in this case the quadriceps) as the rehabilitation clinician takes up the slack, stretching the limb further into the ROM. The subject then relaxes and the position is held for 10 seconds. All of the techniques listed may be repeated three to five times.

Dynamic Stretching

The fourth type of stretching is dynamic stretching. In this type of stretching, a muscle is stretched by a muscular contraction, thereby increasing or decreasing the joint angle where the muscle crosses, and elongating the musculotendinous unit as the end ROM is obtained.[158,159] Dynamic stretching uses activity specific movements, making it a specific warm-up because it prepares the muscles by taking them through the movements used in a particular sport. For example, a sprinter would walk using long strides, which emphasizes hip flexion and extension, subsequently actively contracting and stretching the muscles used by the sprinter, namely the hip flexors and extensors.[151] Dynamic stretching does not incorporate end

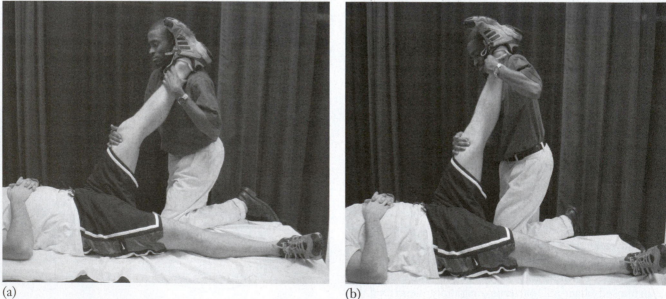

(a)   (b)

Figure 3.19   (a). Hamstring contract-relax (starting position). (b). Hamstring contract-relax (finish position).

range ballistic movements that are bouncy or jerky in nature. Rather, all movements are under control (**Figure 3.20**).

STRETCHING COMPARISONS

It has been well documented that static stretching, ballistic stretching, dynamic stretching, and PNF techniques all facilitate flexibility and therefore ROM increases.[160–163] However, evidence suggests that further research is still needed to determine the appropriate stretching frequency and duration for lasting changes in flexibility.[164] Although comparative studies have been conducted in an attempt to elucidate the efficacy of the different techniques, it is not clearly evident which stretching technique increases flexibility most effectively. Early research comparing ballistic stretching with static stretching did not report differences between the two techniques.[98,100,148,160,162] Little research has been compiled on dynamic stretching, but the existing research indicates that it may produce equal or less flexibility gains than static and ballistic stretching.[148,159,162]

Many studies have provided support for PNF as the preferred method for increasing flexibility over static and ballistic stretching.[98–101,133,148,159,162,163,165,166] However, direct comparison between methods is virtually impossible to determine secondary to differences in experimental de-sign, measurement instrumentation, the lack of control groups or use of inadequate control groups, and inconsistent application of stretching techniques. In several studies, significant differences were not observed between stretching techniques;[99,148,162,167] therefore, it could not be concluded that PNF methods produced more favorable results than did the static stretching. Some authors have reviewed stretching studies and reported conflicting evidence as to the efficacy of these methods[134,166] and stated that most of the differences between studies could be explained by variations in training methods, measuring instruments, and confounding variables. Other researchers, citing the linear relationship between EMG activity and isometric force development, have hypothesized that the ROM gains obtained in previous studies reporting the superiority of PNF compared with static stretching may have been due to the viscoelastic effects of greater forces within the musculotendinous unit rather than autogenic or reciprocal inhibition.[168]

Although PNF may be the preferred method for many practitioners to increase ROM, it may not be the most practical method to use. PNF requires a partner during the early stages of instruction to ensure that the client follows the appropriate movement pattern(s). Once the appropriate patterns have been established, many PNF exercises can use other forms of resistance (elastic bands or tubing) in place of the exercise partner, albeit without the partner's guidance or feedback. Partners are not always available, and clients may not possess the knowledge required to perform PNF. PNF exercises are not widely used as components of a fitness plan for healthy adults. Static stretching is the most popular form of stretching because it does not require the use of a partner and it can be performed in large groups where resources and time are limited. Additionally, static stretching offers a couple of advantages: (1) there is less of a danger in exceeding the tissue's limits of extensibility, (2) the energy requirements are lower, and (3) it may help to decrease muscle soreness, though this has yet to be definitively shown.[103,169] Although ballistic stretching may be equivalent to static stretching at increasing flexibility, ballistic stretches are often not used because of the potential muscle injury from abrupt stretching.[1,134] For the above reasons, static stretching has been recommended and widely implemented in most flexibility programs.

PROPOSED STRETCHING BENEFITS

Enhanced Flexibility

Stretching can promote greater tissue compliance of the muscle–tendon unit, resulting in enhanced flexibility. Research has shown that prolonged or routine stretching can produce long term improvements in flexibility, whereas acute stretching does not.[170–172] Wiktorsson-Moller et al.[104] in studying eight male subjects reported that a four

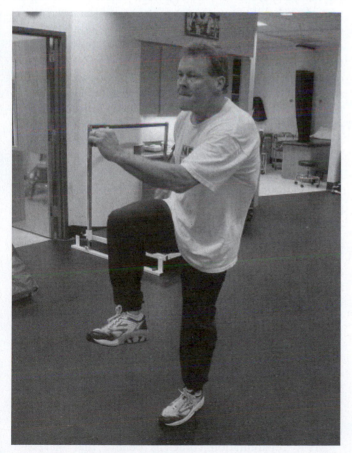

Figure 3.20 Dynamic stretching.

to six second isometric contraction followed by two seconds of relaxation, followed by eight seconds of passive stretching significantly increased range of motion for hip flexion/extension, hip abduction, knee flexion, and ankle dorsiflexion compared to that achieved via massage and warming up separately or in combination. The entire stretching program took 15 minutes. Other studies have had similar results. From this, an assumption can be made that if a warm-up specific to the joint is used along with a stretch, greater benefit in flexibility will be shown. As a part of health, flexibility training may help keep good posture and joint mobility.[173] It should be kept in mind, however, that although clinical investigations of flexibility in humans have used maximal joint ROM as the dependent variable,[98,99,135,136,140,157,163,165] maximal joint ROM provides limited information about the behavior of the muscle–tendon unit to stretch.[124]

Relief of Muscular Soreness

Early research suggests that slow stretching exercises may be able to reduce post-exercise muscular soreness. Utilizing EMG, de Vries[160,174] demonstrated that static stretching relieved muscle soreness and decreased muscle activity. Another study examining the effect of static stretching on soreness, however, revealed that when compared with a control group, static stretching significantly reduced EMG muscle activity but had no significant effect on perceived pain.[175] This was confirmed in a later study that showed that stretching had no effects on decreasing exercise soreness over the post-exercise period or immediately after an acute bout of stretching.[169,176]

Interestingly enough, research has demonstrated that stretching may also cause muscle soreness. Findings from a study conducted to determine if static and ballistic stretching would induce significant amounts of delayed onset muscle soreness (DOMS) indicated that similar bouts of static and ballistic stretching induced significant increases in DOMS in subjects unaccustomed to such exercise. Furthermore, static stretching induced significantly more DOMS than did ballistic stretching.[177] In an attempt to determine the extent to which pre-exercise static stretching affected pain associated with DOMS, High et al.,[178] reported that stretching did not aid in its prevention among 62 healthy male and female volunteers.

Muscle Relaxation

Many individuals use various forms of stretching as a way to facilitate relaxation. This type of flexibility training is used in yoga,[1] where the belief is that muscles under chronic tension become less strong, less supple, and not as capable of absorbing the shock and stress of various types of movements (see Chapter 10). Research has shown that undesirably high levels of muscular tension can result in negative side effects such as high blood pressure, headaches, ulcers, and muscle and joint pain. Consequently, undue muscular tension may result in muscular tightness. Research has shown that stretching, as part of a total fitness program, can therefore be implemented to facilitate muscular relaxation, thereby promoting the release of stress and muscular tension.[179] Plausible explanations may involve either neurophysiological or mechanical phenomena. For example, with stretching, the muscle spindles may become desensitized and adapt to the stretch or, while held at a constant length, force relaxation may occur, which would decrease the tension on the muscle itself. Using EMG to measure muscle activity, Mohr et al.[155] reported that 30 seconds or perhaps less for a static stretch was sufficient to attain muscle relaxation (low or no EMG activity) among 16 healthy volunteers between 23 and 36 years of age.

Injury Prevention

The literature is conflicting on whether stretching prior to or after exercise actually decreases or increases the chance of injury; for many advocates, it is an empirical clinical observation. Some studies have reported that stretching may decrease the rate of injury.[105,106,115,180] When stretching was performed three times a day,[105] or a static stretching program was incorporated immediately before strenuous activity,[106] it was associated with a decrease in the incidences of musculotendinous strains of the lower extremity. Other studies reported that stretching before exercise, as part of a warm-up, or stretching as part of a rehabilitation program, decreased the percentage or recurrence of injuries.[142,180] Conversely, other research has shown that stretching is not effective in preventing injury. According to van Mechelen et al.,[116] an intervention of warm-up and stretching performed prior to each running session, and cool-down after, was not effective in reducing the number of running injuries. Furthermore, a randomized trial of male military recruits by Pope et al.[114] showed that stretching had little influence on injuries associated with weight-bearing physical training such as running, marching, and walking. In their study, they tested 1538 male army recruits in a 12-week training program to observe the effects of static stretching on injury prevention. Army recruits were randomly divided into two groups (stretching and no stretching). Both groups performed aerobic warm-ups; however, the stretch group included 20-second duration static stretching of all major leg muscle groups. In 12 weeks, 333 lower limb injuries were observed, but there were no significant differences between the stretching and no stretching groups. Fitness level (measured by a 20 meter shuttle run), weight, age, and date of enlistment were also recorded and were reported to be a stronger predictors of injury risk. The least fit subjects were 14 times more likely to sustain an injury than the fittest. Recruits who were older and who had enlisted later in the exercise program were also more likely to be injured when compared to the younger recruits.

Many rehabilitation clinicians believe that increased joint flexibility will prevent injury, especially in those activities that require maximum musculotendinous extensibility (i.e., gymnastics). Even though some rehabilitation clinicians state that clinical data exist to show the need for flexibility training to prevent injuries,[76] available data do not support that a lack of flexibility predisposes one to injury or if a minimal amount of flexibility is necessary to prevent injury. In reviews of the literature involving flexibility, stretching, and injury prevention,[117,181] the reviewers state that one of the most accepted reasons for adding stretching to warm-up is based on the concept that stretching will reduce the risk of muscular injury; however, they reported that the studies were often retrospective in nature. They concluded that the literature supports the epidemiological evidence that stretching before exercise does not decrease the risk of injury.

Key Point:

Stretching alone as a means of reducing injury risk is not well supported in the literature.

PERFORMANCE ENHANCEMENT

Long Term Effects

Few researchers have examined the effect that flexibility programs have on strength and performance. Wilson et al.[121] studied the effects of an eight-week progressive static stretching program (six to nine sets, 8 to 30 seconds per set for chest stretch) on the chest musculotendinous stiffness and bench press performance of 16 male power lifters. The stretch group showed significant decreases in musculotendinous stiffness, increases in glenohumeral joint ROM, and better performance in the rebound bench press than the no stretch group. The authors concluded that a compliant musculotendinous unit (less stiff) was able to produce significantly more work due to the increased loading and release of energy in the series elastic component of the muscle.

Klinge et al.[156] examined whether isometric strength training or isometric strength training combined with flexibility training of the hamstring muscles changed the viscoelastic response during stretch. Twelve male subjects performed isometric training (strength) on one side and isometric and flexibility training (strength and flexibility) on the other side for 13 weeks; 10 other subjects served as controls. After 13 weeks of training, isometric strength increased in both training groups by 43 percent; musculotendinous stiffness and passive torque also increased in both training groups, whereas EMG activity remained low. There was no significant difference between the training groups in strength, stiffness, or passive torque. The authors suggested that strength training was a stronger stimulus than stretching because the material properties of the

muscle were not altered by the addition of stretching. In a comparative study involving 6 week old baby chicks with hereditary muscular dystrophy, Ashmore[182] reported that when the wing muscle was stretched for 1 week, the effects on muscle growth and on muscle pathology were variable. However, when the muscle of 1 week old chicks was stretched for 6 weeks, muscle weight and cross sectional area were dramatically increased.

Short Term Effects

Those who propose that athletic performance is enhanced by pre-activity stretching point to sports that require attaining ROM extremes at particular joints, such as gymnastics and baseball pitching. However, no conclusive data have been found to support a correlation between flexibility and performance. For many athletes, coaches, and rehabilitation clinicians, stretching is widely accepted as an important part of the warm-up, and they view flexibility as an important factor in skilled performance.[172] Furthermore, stretching performed immediately prior to physical activity has traditionally been accepted as a way to improve performance.[117,183] It is plausible that increased flexibility may enhance the potential for improved performance in many activities where measured ROM is necessary to perform certain skills, such as in gymnastics, diving, and figure skating. However, whether pre-performance stretching can actually improve performance or not has been questioned by many researchers.[172,173] Some studies have concluded that pre-performance stretching neither helps nor inhibits performance.[161,184] Conversely, several pre-performance stretching studies have revealed negative performance effects.[107,108,183,185–188] It appears that the muscle–tendon unit may become weaker and less able to produce high intensity force immediately after acute stretching, resulting in a period of time during which the muscle–tendon unit stays stretched. If this is the case, there may be a lag period after stretching in which the muscle–tendon unit may need to "take up the slack" before peak tension is reached. Therefore, stretching immediately prior to a task may cause a strength deficit, thereby impeding performance. As a result, it has been suggested that low intensity muscle contractions should probably be performed immediately prior to sport performance (i.e., dynamic stretching).[189]

Few studies have provided evidence that pre-performance stretching enhances performance. Godges et al.[161] studied the effects of PNF and static stretching on the hip range of motion and gait economy (the amount of O_2 consumed at a given speed) of 25 healthy male college students. Hip flexors and hip extensors were stretched for two minutes using each technique. Both techniques resulted in significant increases in hip range of motion. Improvements in ROM were related to gait economy at running speeds of 40 percent, 60 percent, and 80 percent VO_{2max}. Post-stretching running economy with static stretching significantly decreased VO_{2max} when compared to baseline running speeds. PNF stretching significantly improved gait economy, but only at 60 percent VO_{2max} running speed. Other research demonstrates an inverse relationship between the ROM of selected joint movements (flexibility) and running economy. Craib et al.,[190] in testing 19 well-trained male subelite distance runners, reported that runners who were less flexible in the trunk and lower limbs were more economical. Their conclusions suggested that inflexibility in the trunk and lower limbs increased the storage and return of elastic energy from the musculotendinous unit, thereby decreasing the need for muscular activity and increasing running economy. When investigating a long term stretching program on 16 female and 16 male physically active college students, Nelson et al.[191] concluded that a chronic stretching program does not necessarily negatively influence running economy, since neither the stretching group nor the control group exhibited a significant change in the O_2 cost for a submaximal run.

The majority of studies indicate that pre-performance stretching does not improve immediate post-stretching performance. Several authors studied the effects of passive stretching on maximal voluntary contraction (i.e., plantar flexor torque) and muscle activity (EMG). They showed that both twitch torque and motor unit activation were all significantly decreased after passive stretching and, in some cases, remained depressed for up to one hour.[107,183,192] Behm et al.[193] investigated the factors underlying the force loss occurring after 20 minutes of prolonged, static, passive stretching among nonimpaired adult male subjects (20–43 years of age). Their data analysis suggested that post-stretch force decrements were more affected by muscle inactivation than changes in muscle elasticity.

Other researchers have also investigated the effects of pre-performance stretching on maximal strength performance. It was suggested that pre-exercise stretching could have a negative impact on the performance of skills in which success is related to maximal force output. Kokkonen et al.[108] examined the effects of static stretching on maximal strength performance in knee flexion and extension among 15 male and 15 female college physical education class students (22 ± 5 years of age) and reported significant decreases in both. Sit and reach scores showed that flexibility significantly increased due to the stretching regime, which negatively correlated with the strength deficits. The authors suggested that the stretching decreased musculotendinous stiffness (increased muscle compliance), rather than decreased muscle activation (they discounted the likelihood of autogenic inhibition secondary to the increased rest time after the stretch). This can be construed as shifting the contractile properties of the muscle to a less optimal range on the length-tension curve. Nelson et al.[188] measured the effects of four sets of static stretches (one active and three passive) on the quadriceps muscle group for five different maximal torque velocities among 10 men and 5 women between 22 and 28 years of age. Compared to the baseline torque measurements, torque significantly decreased only in the two

slowest velocities. They concluded that static stretching might concentrate primarily upon slow-twitch muscle fibers. Other research has shown that the effects of stretching are not only velocity specific but are also joint angle specific, citing that the average maximal voluntary contraction for each joint angle was reported to be significantly less than pre-stretch values.[187]

In attempting to determine the relationship between hamstring flexibility and hamstring muscle performance, Worrell et al.[194] examined the effects of PNF and static stretching on isokinetic peak torque among 19 subjects. They reported no difference in flexibility between the different stretches. However, they reported that significant increases in knee flexor eccentric force production occurred at 60°/sec and 120°/sec, while improvements in peak concentric force occurred only at 120°/sec. The increases in eccentric force production were attributed to the significant increases in flexibility and musculotendinous compliance (decreased stiffness), which allowed the musculotendinous unit to store more elastic energy for force production.

Nelson et al.[195] investigated the effect of pre-performance stretching on the musculotendinous stiffness of 10 untrained college age male subjects and the amount of stored elastic energy to determine if it enhanced vertical jump performance. After stretching, both squat jump and countermovement vertical jump heights were significantly reduced. The authors concluded that net force production for the vertical jump was reduced due to stretching, but the performance decrease did not appear to be from changes in the elastic properties of the muscle. In an effort to determine the mechanism responsible for the decreased performance, Cornwell et al.[185] examined if either musculotendinous stiffness or decreased muscle activity was the cause. They investigated the effect of passive stretching on the neuromechanical properties of the plantar flexors using squat jumps and countermovement jumps among 10 male subjects. Following the stretch, a significant difference in musculotendinous stiffness was noted. Countermovement jump height decreased significantly, but no decrease in muscle activity (EMG) was noted. However, squat jump height did not change, but a significant decrease in muscle activity (EMG) was observed. The performance decrease was concluded to be due to a change in plantar flexor musculotendinous stiffness rather than from changes in motor activation because countermovement jumps, which rely on musculotendinous stiffness, were significantly decreased in height, while there was no significant changes in squat jump heights.

Rationale for Stretching Affecting Performance

There have been two main theories proposed to explain the subsequent decrease in performance secondary to stretching. The first proposed theory is based upon research performed by Wilson et al.,[122] who concluded that the stiffness of the musculotendinous system, which maximizes isometric and concentric performance, appears to be skewed toward stiffness on the elasticity continuum. A stiff musculotendinous unit appears to enhance the force production capacity of the contractile component through a combination of an improved contractile component length and rate of shortening. In addition, Wilson et al.[122] did not find a correlation between eccentric contractions and musculotendinous stiffness among the 13 trained subjects who participated in their study. Also supporting the theory of musculotendinous stiffness, in their review paper, Gleim et al.[117] concluded that increased flexibility is important for performance in some sports that rely on extremes of motion for movement, but decreases in flexibility may actually increase economy of movement in sports, which use only the mid-portion of ROM. This was shown by static flexibility measurements that correlated with musculoskeletal tightness and concentric strength in professional American football players. This supports the idea that a stiffer muscle provides a more efficient transmission of contractile force production. Furthermore, according to Fowles et al.,[107] reduced muscle stiffness can affect evoked muscle twitch amplitude and shape because of greater time needed to "take up slack" in compliant in-series elements. In addition, increased muscle length may alter the fine balance of muscle properties and joint kinematics that combine to produce force at a given joint angle.

The second theory states that stretching of the muscle produces autogenic inhibition. Muscle or joint proprioceptors (e.g., Golgi tendon organs and low threshold pain receptors) respond to a sustained stretch by producing a reflexive inhibition (autogenic inhibition) of both the muscle being stretched and its synergists. Furthermore, when a person stretches to their pain threshold repeatedly, the pain receptors located in the muscles, tendons, and joint capsule can also inhibit the neural pathways responsible for activation of the muscle. This diminishes the available number of motor units, thus limiting force production. Also supporting the principle of autogenic inhibition, Fowles et al.[107] reported that after a two minute, sustained stretch of the plantar flexors, a 25 percent loss of MVC resulted for 30 min post-stretching among the 10 young adults who participated in the study (six men, four women). Sixty percent of this loss was due to lack of muscle fiber activation and the other 40 percent was due to other factors affecting force generation (e.g., musculotendinous stiffness and force–tension relationships). There remained an average MVC loss of 10 percent up to one hour. One percent of the (10 percent) MVC loss was due to muscle fiber activation; the remaining 99 percent was due to force generating factors. It should again be emphasized that voluntary strength was impaired for up to one hour following a prolonged two minute stretch.

> **Key Point:**
> From the research reviewed, it appears that stretching can decrease strength due both to factors of autogenic inhibition and musculotendinous stiffness changes. When these changes occur, the force production can be compromised, thereby directly affecting performance.

STRETCHING PRECAUTIONS

Although some speculate that stretching can lead to joint "over flexibility" or laxity, this view has not been supported in the literature. It would appear that most laxity is an anatomical characteristic and not a result of stretching. Stretching is an activity in which almost anyone can participate. Remember, stretching is a slow and adaptive process. So, when considering a stretching program or performing rehabilitation using stretching, some crucial guidelines and precautions should be followed or considered:[173]

1. Warm up the tissue prior to stretching.
2. The stretch should be comfortable and not to the point of pain (overstretch).
3. Flexibility is specific to each joint, so a stretching program should consider all the joints that will be involved in the exercises (whether stretching before or after the activity).
4. Use pain as a guide and exercise caution when stretching areas around known pathologies or disorders (e.g., fracture, inflammation, infection, osteoporosis, sprains and strains, hypermobility, skin diseases).
5. Be specific about proper stretching technique and positioning.
6. Stretch agonists as well as antagonists to avoid muscular imbalance.
7. Adhere to the individual guidelines for the different types of stretching to ensure safety and effectiveness.

STRETCHING AIDS

In addition to the various techniques shown for stretching, specifically designed stretching aids are available for use to enhance ROM (i.e., the incline board) (**Figure 3.21**). Many of these devices are used in therapeutic exercise programs and vary in cost and sophistication. Factors to be considered include safety, effectiveness, and durability of the product. Rehabilitation clinicians should research the different types of stretching aids and be able to evaluate their safety and effectiveness prior to prescribing them for clients.

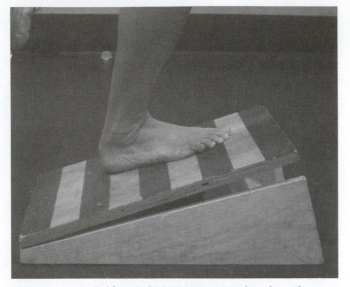

Figure 3.21   Calf stretching using an incline board.

ESSENTIALS OF A STRETCHING PROGRAM

When to Stretch

Limited scientific literature is available to discern the role of and appropriate place for stretching in an exercise program. First of all, it should be noted that stretching and warm-up are not the same. Warm-up is an activity that raises total body and muscle temperatures to prepare the body for vigorous exercise,[143] although some would argue that stretching may also be sufficient to increase muscle temperature.[102] Many believe that stretching should be an integral part of the warm-up regimen to enhance musculotendinous extensibility, but should not constitute a complete warm-up.[196] Depending upon the type of stretching performed, the literature seems to bear this latter idea out. Wiktorsson-Moller et al.[104] reported that warm-up prior to stretching resulted in significant changes in joint ROM, although they questioned whether the warm-up actually affected the musculotendinous extensibility attained from stretching. Some believe stretching should probably not be performed at the beginning of a warm-up routine, because the tissue temperatures are too low for optimal muscle-tendon function, leading to a less compliant tissue, which may ultimately make the tissue less prepared for activity. Many authors recommend that at least five minutes of light, but progressively more intense exercise be performed before stretching,[126,196] while others discourage exercise before stretching altogether, stating that warmed up muscle tissue does not necessarily stretch better nor is it less likely to be injured. Additionally, the demands on ROM from exercise are generally not great.

The reason that many authors promote stretching before the actual event or workout is to give the individual protection against injury. Some advocate stretching after an exercise session, citing that the increased musculotendinous extensibility leads to the potential for improved joint flexibility. However, Cornelius et al.[112] reported that including stretching in a six-week workout program did not make a significant difference in increasing ROM. In their study, static stretching was done before, after, and both before and after each workout. All produced significant increases in ROM.

Program

Warm-up.   The purpose of warm-up exercises is to prepare the body for the stresses it will encounter during an activity or sport. Warm-up exercises increase the core body temperature and disrupt transient connective tissue bonds. As muscle contracts, heat is produced, which increases the intramuscular temperature.[120] The effect of increased muscle temperature will (1) increase dissociation of oxygen from hemoglobin and myoglobin, (2) increase conduction velocities of action potentials, (3) increase metabolic rate, (4) increase blood flow to the muscles, (5) decrease viscosity of the muscles, and (6) increase connective tissue compliance.[60] As a result, ROM should be increased.[126] A warmed muscle has the ability to contract more forcefully and relax more quickly[197,198] thereby potentially enhancing performance and work production for those muscles used.[199,200] Davies and Young[201] who studied the effect of temperature on contractile properties of the triceps surae among five healthy male subjects, reported that when muscle temperature increased 3.1° C above normal, the contractile elements of the muscle significantly increased the velocity of contraction (by 7 percent) and relaxation time (by 22 percent). In a study examining the effects of warm-up without stretch on the behavior of muscle–tendon units, Safran et al.[115] reported that a greater force and increase in length were needed to tear warmed tissue. However, this was not the case with the cold tissue, which was more inelastic at each increase in length.

> # *Key Point:*
> A warmed muscle can contract more forcefully and relax more quickly.

Widely accepted warm-up protocols include two components: *general*, which consists of 5 to 10 minutes of aerobic work, and *specific*, which includes sport or activity specific movements. Specific warm-ups usually last 8 to 15 minutes and include dynamic activities as well as specific stretches.[151] Of course, these warm-up times may vary somewhat, depending on the nature of the activity or event. Whatever type of warm-up is chosen, it should be intense enough to cause an increase in body temperature, but not so intense as to cause fatigue. One should taper the warm-up 5 to 10 minutes prior to the actual exercise event.[143] Traditionally, stretching has been included in specific warm-up because it was thought to enhance performance and prevent injury.

It is agreed that to most effectively stretch a muscle–tendon unit, intramuscular temperature should be increased. The clinical assumption, of course, is that a more compliant muscle can be stretched further and is therefore less susceptible to injury.[117] However, many think that the warm-up period is not the best time to stretch for increasing ROM, primarily because of increased tissue stiffness. The likelihood of enhancing performance and injury prevention has come under question, and the perceived benefits of stretching prior to activity may be incorrect. Light to moderate muscle actions of gradually increasing intensity (dynamic stretching) may be more appropriate than static stretching as a warm-up activity. Studies examining the combination of stretching and active warm-up have revealed that the decrease in stiffness is mainly a result of increased muscle temperature and not the effect of stretching.[202,203] The inclusion of stretching would increase the time spent in the warm-up portion.

Increasing intramuscular temperature can also be achieved through external means, which also may have an effect on ROM.[113] In a randomized study of the effects of heat alone, stretching alone, or combined heat and stretching on hip joint ROM among 15 adult males and 15 adult females (30 ± 6 years of age), Henricson et al.[204] reported that, although heat alone (electric heating pad at 43° C for 20 minutes) did not improve hip ROM, stretching without heat did increase hip ROM, and stretching combined with heat gave the greatest increase in ROM, maintaining it for 30 minutes. These results are in accordance with the findings of other investigators,[205,206] who reported that heat increases collagen extensibility and decreases musculotendinous stiffness. However, most recommend using exercise as the primary way of increasing intramuscular temperature.

Stewart and Sleivert[207] studied the effect of warm-up intensity on the ROM and anaerobic performance of nine male subjects. Subjects performed 15 minutes of treadmill running at 60, 70, and 80 percent VO_{2max}. Following the warm-up, PNF (contract-relax) stretching was performed. Results showed that ankle dorsiflexion ROM significantly increased in all warm-ups. However, intensity of the warm-up did not change the ROM obtained except for hip flexion, which significantly increased only after the 80 percent VO_{2max} warm-up. Aerobic warm-ups at 60–70 percent VO_{2max} were also shown to increase anaerobic performance (observed in a maximal treadmill run); the warm-up done at 80 percent VO_{2max} did not improve performance. The 15-minute warm-up at an intensity of 60–70 percent VO_{2max} was therefore recommended to improve ROM and enhance subsequent anaerobic performance.

Wiemann and Hahn[208] studied the effects of resistance training, static and ballistic stretching, and stationary cycling on ROM and stretch-induced EMG activity of the hamstrings among 69 nonimpaired adult male subjects (20–34 years of age). They reported that static stretching, ballistic stretching, and aerobic cycling all increased ROM in the knee flexors. Pre- and post-testing of the knee flexors revealed a decrease in EMG activity from static stretching, ballistic stretching, and cycling. They suggested that the subjects' tolerance to higher stretching strain brings about increased ROM after short term stretching exercises. However, they found no decreases in musculotendinous stiffness, which agreed with Magnusson et al.,[209] who also reported no significant decreases in musculotendinous stiffness in the knee flexors of 12 recreational athletes after 10 minutes of static and ballistic stretching.

Taylor et al.[210] studied changes in the viscoelastic characteristics of rabbit muscle using passive static stretching versus isometric muscular contractions. They concluded that stretching and contracting both resulted in stress relaxation of the muscle-tendon unit. This finding may have been a result of changes in the viscous elements of the connective tissue secondary to the forces generated by either stretches or contractions, since both isometric contractions and passive stretching result in connective tissue elongation. This study suggested that isometric muscular contractions might be responsible for decreased passive tension in a muscle at neutral length, a finding that is normally associated with passive stretching. Rosenbaum and Hennig[203] also reported that the force characteristics observed after stretching indicate improved muscle compliance; however, the changes brought about after an additional warm-up had a more pronounced effect with regard to improved force development and decreased EMG activity among 50 male subjects. Moller et al.[111] studied the effects of warm-up, massage, and stretching on the ROM of eight male volunteers. In contrast to other reports, their results showed that stretching alone was greater at increasing flexibility than massage, warm-up, or stretching combined with massage and warm-up.

Duration and Frequency. The specific duration, frequency, and number of stretching repetitions is varied among differing research reports. The duration of each stretch will depend upon the joint targeted, the flexibility goal, and the type of stretching technique used. Evidence to date has shown that stretches can be held anywhere from 10 to 60 seconds. Most research has prompted recommendations that stretches be held between 15 and 30 seconds.[109,124,170,211] Researchers have varied the duration of stretch to determine what effect holding the stretch has on increased ROM. However, very little research has been conducted on the number of repetitions of a stretch in an exercise session. When the muscle–tendon unit is cyclically stretched to a fixed tension or length, the properties of creep and stress relaxation occurs with each cycle. Using rabbit muscle–tendon units, Taylor et al.[61] reported that 80 percent of the length changes occurred in the first four stretches of 30 seconds each. Decreases in passive tension and stiffness in the hamstrings have also been shown with cyclical stretching.[124] McNair et al.[212] pointed out when stretching the ankle joint the greatest change in tension was found in the first 20 seconds among 15 adult males and 8 adult females. It should be noted that because of the structural and morphological diversity of tissue, it is very difficult to predict the duration of stretching for each tissue.[7] Current ACSM guidelines recommend three to five repetitions for each stretching exercise.[213]

Madding et al.[149] compared one repetition of 15 seconds, 45 seconds, or 120 seconds of passive stretches on hip abduction ROM among 72 adult males (27.1 ± 4.4 years of age), assessing ROM immediately following each stretch. Results showed that hip abduction ROM was significantly increased after each of the three stretches. However, there was no significant difference between the three stretches. They concluded there was no difference between holding a stretch for 15, 45, or 120 seconds. In a six week study of 57 non-impaired adult subjects, Bandy and Irion[109] attempted to show which stretch duration was most beneficial at increasing knee ROM for three groups who performed stretching five days a week. The lengths of time used for stretching were 15, 30, and 60 seconds. Data analysis showed significant increases in knee ROM in all groups, but reported that between the treatments, 30 and 60 seconds were found to be significantly more effective than 15 seconds. However, 60 seconds did not significantly differ from 30 seconds.

In a later study of 93 non-impaired adult subjects, Bandy et al.[170] questioned the length of time and frequency of stretching at increasing knee ROM. As in their previous study, the stretching programs were implemented five days a week for six weeks. Stretching treatments consisted of three one minute stretches, three 30 second stretches, a single one minute stretch, and a single 30 second stretch. They reported that increasing the frequency of the stretching did not significantly increase the ROM. The three repetition stretch group did not have significantly greater gains in ROM than the one repetition group. Additionally, the one minute stretch group produced no greater results than the 30 second stretch group. The authors concluded that one repetition of 30 seconds was optimal for increasing flexibility. Roberts and Wilson[211] compared 5 seconds of passive stretching for nine repetitions to 15 seconds of passive stretching for three repetitions among 19 adult men and 5 adult women. They reported no difference between the groups for passive ROM, but reported a significant difference in active ROM for the 15 second stretch. These findings suggest that holding stretches for 15 seconds, as opposed to five seconds, may result in greater improvements in active ROM.

Sustaining a stretch may not significantly affect the improvements gained in passive ROM, however. Borms et al.[214] studied the effects of different durations of static stretching exercises on hip flexibility among sedentary adult women. Three subgroups were formed (group 1, 10 seconds; group 2, 20 seconds; group 3, 30 seconds), each following the same program, except that the duration of the static stretch differed. Data analysis revealed that the hip flexibility had improved significantly in the treatment groups after 10 weeks (two 50 minute sessions/week). However, no differences were noted between the subgroups. This finding suggested that a duration of 10 seconds static stretching is sufficient for improving hip flexibility.

Intensity.   The intensity of stretch can significantly affect the increase in ROM and should be carefully considered, especially as it relates to tissue repair.[126,215] Controlled stresses will favorably affect the different repair phases contributing to improvement in the tissue's mechanical properties and length.[7] Stretching with increased levels of force may create structural damage and result in acute structural weakening of the muscle-tendon unit, thus increasing the risk of injury.[216,217] For static stretching, the appropriate intensity is to stretch slowly and hold the elongated position at low force levels. This is most often communicated to the individual as "pain free" stretching only to the point of tension or mild discomfort. Whatever the technique employed, bear in mind the viscoelastic properties of muscle and connective tissue.

Cool Down.   The cool down phase incorporates light exercises post activity and is a valuable part of the overall activity, as it is a time to help maintain or increase flexibility. Many practitioners recommend this time period as the optimal time to stretch, when the tissue temperatures are the highest.[126,172] It has been shown that elevated temperature has a significant influence on the mechanical behavior of connective tissue under tensile stress. Maintaining a tensile force during cooling on tissue that has been previously heated has been shown to significantly increase plastic deformation of the tissue.[205]

How Long Does It Last?   Little is reported on how long the effects of stretching last. If stretching is important in a warm-up, it would certainly behoove one to know if a single session of stretching persists over the specified period involved during exercise or an athletic event or if the response is modified or muted by activity. This could be important information, especially for athletes who are suddenly required to play after 30 minutes of sitting. Furthermore, it becomes an important clinical issue, because limitations with certain joint movements can bring about compensatory movement patterns resulting in future pathologies or disorders. Therefore, if stretching does not have a lasting affect, then clinicians must seriously question the use of this treatment for rehabilitation purposes.

Starring et al.,[218] in studying groups of nonimpaired men and women, reported that techniques utilizing cyclic and sustained stretching for 15 minutes on five consecutive days increased hamstring muscle length and that a significant percentage of the increased length was retained one week post-treatment. Using four consecutive knee flexor static stretches of 30 seconds among 30 male cadets (19.8 ± 5.1 years of age), DePino et al.[219] reported that the new knee ROM was maintained for three minutes, but had returned to pre-stretched levels in six minutes. Kirsch et al.,[220] using a 60 second stretch, concluded that plantar flexor passive torque returned to baseline within five minutes among non-impaired adult subjects. Zito et al.[221] stretched the ankle for two repetitions of 15 seconds and reported no significant change in dorsiflexion ROM among 19 non-impaired volunteers. Magnusson et al.[222] observed a 18–20 percent decrease in plantar flexor musculotendinous stiffness with a 45 second stretch, but noted a return to baseline after a 30 second rest period among non-impaired subjects.

Others have reported that increased ROM from stretching remained for up to 90 minutes.[107,111] Zito et al.[221] stated that these differences could be explained by variations in warm-up, stretching position, stretching force, and stretching duration. Whereas Moller et al.[111] used an extensive warm-up, which included a low intensity (50 Watt) 15 minute bicycle ergometer aerobic exercise followed by one maximal isometric contraction of the muscle to prepare for stretch, DePino et al.[219] and Magnusson et al.[222] used no warm-up prior to stretching.

Willy et al.[223] tested the effects of cessation and resumption of a hamstring muscle stretching protocol on the knee ROM of college students (12 men, 6 women). They reported that there was no retention of the knee ROM gains made over the initial six week duration stretching protocol when measured at four weeks following the intervention. Additionally, following the completion of another six week duration stretching protocol, knee ROM did not improve above the gains observed following the initial six week session. In other words, the gains in flexibility in the second six week period were no different from the gains in the first six weeks. The significance of this finding could be applied to exercise programs where greater flexibility gains are desired but due to long intervals between seasons, any gained flexibility may most likely be lost. In studying the effect of stretching among 47 adult men who were assigned to one of four stretching frequency groups, Wallin et al.[154] reported that stretching at least once a week after a 30 day training program helped subjects maintain the flexibility gains they had made during the training program.

Summary

Human movement is a carefully orchestrated process that involves the driving force of the neuromuscular system and the structural apparatus of the skeletal system. One factor impacting movement is the ability of tissues to be responsible for both the generation of joint motion and limitation of excessive and potentially injurious motions. For example, the same process that can produce purposeful motion at the knee joint can also result in forces that exceed the normal physiological ranges tolerated by muscle, tendon, ligament, articular cartilage, articular cartilage or bone. Therefore, it is critical to understand the biomechanical and physiological properties of tissues supporting human movement. Knowing these properties allows the rehabilitation clinician to modulate appropriate variables such that client specific recommendations can be made regarding therapeutic exercise programs impacting strength, coordination, endurance, and flexibility.

References

1. Alter MJ. *Science of Flexibility*, 2nd ed. Champaign, IL: Human Kinetics; 1996.
2. Topoleski LD. Mechanical properties of materials. *In* C.A. Oatis (ed.), *Kinesiology: The mechanics and pathomechanics of human movement.* Philadelphia: Lippincott Williams & Wilkins, 2004, pp. 21–35.
3. Threlkeld AJ. Basic structure and function of the joints. *In* D.A. Neumann (ed.): *Kinesiology of the Musculoskeletal System.* St. Louis: Mosby, 2002, pp. 25–40.
4. Enoka RM. (ed.) *Neuromechanics of Human Movement.* Champaign: Human Kinetics, 2002.
5. Woo SL-Y, An K-N, Arnoczky SP, et al. Anatomy, biology, and biomechanics of tendon, ligament, and meniscus. *In* S.R. Simon (ed.), *Orthopaedic Basic Science.* Park Ridge, IL: American Academy of Orthopaedic Surgeons, 1994, pp. 45–87.
6. Levangie PK, Norkin CC. *Joint Structure and Function: A comprehensive analysis,* 3rd ed. Philadelphia: F.A. Davis, 2001.
7. Lederman E. (ed.) *Fundamentals of Manual Therapy: Physiology, Neurology, and Psychology.* New York: Churchill Livingstone, 1997.

8. Butler DL, Grood ES, Noyes FR, et al. Biomechanics of ligaments and tendons. *Exerc Sport Sci Rev.* 1978;6:125–181.

9. Noyes FR. Functional properties of knee ligaments and alterations induced by immobilization: A correlative biomechanical and histological study in primates. *Clin Orthop.* 1977;(123):210–242.

10. Frank CB. Ligament injuries: Pathophysiology and healing. *In* J.E. Zachazewski, D.J. Magee, W.S. Quillen (eds.), *Athletic Injuries and Rehabilitation.* Philadelphia: Saunders, 1996, pp. 9–26.

11. Tipton CM, Matthes RD, Maynard JA, et al. The influence of physical activity on ligaments and tendons. *Med Sci Sports.* 1975;7(3):165–175.

12. Burgeson RE, Nimni ME. Collagen types. Molecular structure and tissue distribution. *Clin Orthop.* 1992;(282):250–272.

13. Lieber RL. *Skeletal Muscle Structure, Function and Plasticity: The physiological basis of rehabilitation.* Philadelphia: Lippincott Williams & Wilkins; 2002.

14. Lieber RL, Leonard ME, Brown CG, et al. Frog semitendinosis tendon load-strain and stress-strain properties during passive loading. *Am J Physiol.* 1991;261(1 Pt 1):C86–92.

15. Lieber RL, Leonard ME, Brown-Maupin CG. Effects of muscle contraction on the load-strain properties of frog aponeurosis and tendon. *Cells Tissues Organs.* 2000;166(1):48–54.

16. Loren GJ, Lieber RL. Tendon biomechanical properties enhance human wrist muscle specialization. *J Biomech.* 1995;28(7):791–799.

17. Viidik A. Elasticity and tensile strength of the anterior cruciate ligament in rabbits as influenced by training. *Acta Physiol Scand.* 1968;74(3):372–380.

18. Lockard MA. Biomechanics of tendons and ligaments. *In* C.A. Oatis (ed.), *Kinesiology: The mechanics & pathomechanics of human movement.* Philadelphia: Lippincott Williams & Wilkins, 2004, pp. 80–95.

19. Kannus P. Structure of the tendon connective tissue. *Scand J Med Sci Sports.* 2000;10(6):312–320.

20. Roy RR, Talmadge RJ, Hodgson JA, et al. Differential response of fast hindlimb extensor and flexor muscles to exercise in adult spinalized cats. *Muscle Nerve.* 1999;22(2):230–241.

21. Sheard PW. Tension delivery from short fibers in long muscles. *Exerc Sport Sci Rev.* 2000;28(2):51–56.

22. Magid A, Law DJ. Myofibrils bear most of the resting tension in frog skeletal muscle. *Science.* 1985;230(4731):1280–1282.

23. Street SF. Lateral transmission of tension in frog myofibers: A myofibrillar network and transverse cytoskeletal connections are possible transmitters. *J Cell Physiol.* 1983;114(3):346–364.

24. De Deyne PG. Application of passive stretch and its implications for muscle fibers. *Phys Ther.* 2001;81(2):819–827.

25. Kurrat HJ, Oberlander W. The thickness of the cartilage in the hip joint. *J Anat.* 1978;126(1):145–155.

26. Stockwell RA. The interrelationship of cell density and cartilage thickness in mammalian articular cartilage. *J Anat.* 1971;109(3):411–421.

27. Topoleski LD. Biomechanics of bone. *In* C.A. Oatis (ed.), *Kinesiology: The mechanics and pathomechanics of human movement.* Philadelphia: Lippincott Williams & Wilkins, 2004, pp. 36–43.

28. Turner CH, Robling AG. Designing exercise regimens to increase bone strength. *Exerc Sport Sci Rev.* 2003;31(1):45–50.

29. Nigg BM, Grimston SK (ed.). *Biomechanics of the Musculoskeletal System.* Chichester: John Wiley & Sons, 1994.

30. Bikle DD, Halloran BP. The response of bone to unloading. *J Bone Miner Metab.* 1999;17(4):233–244.

31. Holick MF. Perspective on the impact of weightlessness on calcium and bone metabolism. *Bone.* 1998;22 (5 Suppl):105S–111S.

32. Glaser DL, Kaplan FS. Osteoporosis. Definition and clinical presentation. *Spine.* 1997;22 (24 Suppl): 12S–16S.

33. Zioupos P, Currey JD. Changes in the stiffness, strength, and toughness of human cortical bone with age. *Bone.* 1998;22(1):57–66.

34. Giangregorio L, Blimkie CJ. Skeletal adaptations to alterations in weight-bearing activity: A comparison of models of disuse osteoporosis. *Sports Med.* 2002;32(7):459–476.

35. Wren TA, Beaupre GS, Carter DR. A model for loading-dependent growth, development, and adaptation of tendons and ligaments. *J Biomech.* 1998; 31(2):107–114.

36. Woo SL, Orlando CA, Gomez MA, et al. Tensile properties of the medial collateral ligament as a function of age. *J Orthop Res.* 1986;4(2):133–141.

37. Woo SL, Peterson RH, Ohland KJ, et al. The effects of strain rate on the properties of the medial collateral ligament in skeletally immature and mature rabbits: A biomechanical and histological study. *J Orthop Res.* 1990;8(5):712–721.

38. Hamerman D. Aging and the musculoskeletal system. *Ann Rheum Dis.* 1997;56(10):578–585.

39. Buckwalter JA, Woo SL, Goldberg VM, et al. Soft-tissue aging and musculoskeletal function. *J Bone Joint Surg Am.* 1993;75(10):1533–1548.

40. Noyes FR, Grood ES. The strength of the anterior cruciate ligament in humans and Rhesus monkeys. *J Bone Joint Surg Am.* 1976;58(8):1074–1082.

41. Woo SL, Hollis JM, Adams DJ, et al. Tensile properties of the human femur-anterior cruciate ligament-tibia complex. The effects of specimen age and orientation. *Am J Sports Med.* 1991;19(3):217–225.

42. Bigliani LU, Kelkar R, Flatow EL, et al. Glenohumeral stability. Biomechanical properties of pas-

sive and active stabilizers. *Clin Orthop.* 1996;(330): 13–30.

43. Debski RE, Sakone M, Woo SL, et al. Contribution of the passive properties of the rotator cuff to glenohumeral stability during anterior-posterior loading. *J Shoulder Elbow Surg.* 1999;8(4):324–329.

44. Debski RE, Wong EK, Woo SL, et al. In situ force distribution in the glenohumeral joint capsule during anterior-posterior loading. *J Orthop Res.* 1999; 17(5):769–776.

45. Hewitt JD, Glisson RR, Guilak F, et al. The mechanical properties of the human hip capsule ligaments. *J Arthroplasty.* 2002;17(1):82–89.

46. Tonetti J, Peoc'h M, Merloz P, et al. Elastic reinforcement and thickness of the joint capsules of the lower cervical spine. *Surg Radiol Anat.* 1999;21(1): 35–39.

47. Yoganandan N, Kumaresan S, Pintar FA. Geometric and mechanical properties of human cervical spine ligaments. *J Biomech Eng.* 2000;122(6):623–629.

48. Woo SL, Gomez MA, Sites TJ, et al. The biomechanical and morphological changes in the medial collateral ligament of the rabbit after immobilization and remobilization. *J Bone Joint Surg Am.* 1987;69(8):1200–1211.

49. Strocchi R, De Pasquale V, Facchini A, et al. Age-related changes in human anterior cruciate ligament (ACL) collagen fibrils. *Ital J Anat Embryol.* 1996;101(4):213–220.

50. Kannus P, Jozsa L, Renstrom P, et al. The effects of training, immobilization and remobilization on musculoskeletal tissue. I. Training and immobilization. *Scand J Med Sci Sports.* 1992;2:100–118.

51. Amiel D, Frey C, Woo SL, et al. Value of hyaluronic acid in the prevention of contracture formation. *Clin Orthop.* 1985;(196):306–311.

52. Williams PE, Goldspink G. Longitudinal growth of striated muscle fibres. *J Cell Sci.* 1971;9(3):751–767.

53. Williams PE, Goldspink G. The effect of immobilization on the longitudinal growth of striated muscle fibres. *J Anat.* 1973;116(1):45–55.

54. Williams PE, Catanese T, Lucey EG, et al. The importance of stretch and contractile activity in the prevention of connective tissue accumulation in muscle. *J Anat.* 1988;158:109–114.

55. Gibson JN, Halliday D, Morrison WL, et al. Decrease in human quadriceps muscle protein turnover consequent upon leg immobilization. *Clin Sci (Lond).* 1987;72(4):503–509.

56. Oishi Y, Ishihara A, Katsuta S. Muscle fibre number following hindlimb immobilization. *Acta Physiol Scand.* 1992;146(2):281–282.

57. Yue GH, Bilodeau M, Hardy PA, et al. Task-dependent effect of limb immobilization on the fatigability of the elbow flexor muscles in humans. *Exp Physiol.* 1997;82(3):567–592.

58. Duchateau J, Hainaut K. Effects of immobilization on contractile properties, recruitment and firing rates of human motor units. *J Physiol.* 1990;422: 55–65.

59. Binder MD, Kroin JS, Moore GP, et al. The response of Golgi tendon organs to single motor unit contractions. *J Physiol.* 1977;271(2):337–349.

60. Enoka R. *Neuromechanical Basis of Kinesiology,* 2nd ed. Champaign, IL: Human Kinetics, 1994.

61. Taylor DC, Dalton JD, Seaber AV, et al. Viscoelastic properties of muscle-tendon units. The biomechanical effects of stretching. *Am J Sports Med.* 1990; 18(3):300–309.

62. Wolpaw JR, Carp JS. Memory traces in spinal cord. *Trends Neurosci.* 1990;13(4):137–142.

63. Wolpaw JR. Acquisition and maintenance of the simplest motor skill: Investigation of CNS mechanisms. *Med Sci Sports Exerc.* 1994;26(12):1475–1479.

64. Goldspink G. Sarcomere length during post-natal growth of mammalian muscle fibres. *J Cell Sci.* 1968;3(4):539–548.

65. Harris M. A factor analytic study of flexibility. *Res Q Exerc Sport.* 1969;40:62–70.

66. Merni F, Balboni M, Bargellini S, et al. Differences in males and females in joint movement range during growth. *Med Sport.* 1981;15:168–175.

67. Hupprich FL, Sigerseth PO. The specificity of flexibility in girls. *Res Q.* 1950;21:25–33.

68. Livingston LA, Stevenson JM, Olney SJ. Stair-climbing kinematics on stairs of differing dimensions. *Arch Phys Med Rehabil.* 1991;72(6):398–402.

69. Jevsevar DS, Riley PO, Hodge WA, et al. Knee kinematics and kinetics during locomotor activities of daily living in subjects with knee arthroplasty and in healthy control subjects. *Phys Ther.* 1993;73(4): 229–239.

70. Safaee-Rad R, Shwedyk E, Quanbury AO, et al. Normal functional range of motion of upper limb joints during performance of three feeding activities. *Arch Phys Med Rehabil.* 1990;71(7):505–509.

71. Ostrosky KM, VanSwearingen JM, Burdett RG, et al. A comparison of gait characteristics in young and old subjects. *Phys Ther.* 1994;74(7):637–644.

72. Magnusson SP, Gleim GW, Nicholas JA. Shoulder weakness in professional baseball pitchers. *Med Sci Sports Exerc.* 1994;26(1):5–9.

73. Donatelli R, Ellenbecker TS, Ekedahl SR, et al. Assessment of shoulder strength in professional baseball pitchers. *J Orthop Sports Phys Ther.* 2000;30(9): 544–551.

74. Zachazewski JE, Magee DJ, Quillen WS (eds.). *Athletic Injuries and Rehabilitation.* Philadelphia: Saunders, 1996.

75. American College of Sports Medicine Position Stand. The recommended quantity and quality of exercise for developing and maintaining cardiorespiratory and

muscular fitness, and flexibility in healthy adults. *Med Sci Sports Exerc.* 1998;30(6): 975–991.

76. Corbin CB, Noble L. Flexibility: A major component of physical fitness. *J Phys Educ Rec.* 1980;51 (6):23–24.

77. Sermeev BV. Development of mobility in the hip joint in sportsmen. *Yessis Rev.* 1966;2(1):16–17.

78. Hawkins D, Metheny J. Overuse injuries in youth sports: Biomechanical considerations. *Med Sci Sports Exerc.* 2001;33(10):1701–1707.

79. Elliott DH. Structure and function of mammalian tendon. *Bio Rev.* 1965;40(3):392–421.

80. Brown M, Holloszy JO. Effects of a low intensity exercise program on selected physical performance characteristics of 60- to 71-year-olds. *Aging (Milano).* 1991;3(2):129–139.

81. Mills EM. The effect of low-intensity aerobic exercise on muscle strength, flexibility, and balance among sedentary elderly persons. *Nurs Res.* 1994;43 (4):207–211.

82. Pendergast DR, Fisher NM, Calkins E. Cardiovascular, neuromuscular, and metabolic alterations with age leading to frailty. *J Gerontol.* 1993;48:61–67.

83. Raab DM, Agre JC, McAdam M, et al. Light resistance and stretching exercise in elderly women: Effect upon flexibility. *Arch Phys Med Rehabil.* 1988; 69(4):268–272.

84. Skelton DA, Greig CA, Davies JM, et al. Strength, power and related functional ability of healthy people aged 65–89 years. *Age Ageing.* 1994;23(5):371–377.

85. Germain NW, Blair SN. Variability of shoulder flexion with age, activity and sex. *Am Correct Ther J.* 1983;37(6):156–160.

86. Drummer GM, Vaccardo P, Clarke DH. Muscular strength and flexibility of two female master swimmers in the eighth decade of life. *J Orthop Sports Phys Ther.* 1985;6(4):235–237.

87. Bell RD, Hoshizaki TB. Relationships of age and sex with range of motion of seventeen joint actions in humans. *Can J Appl Sport Sci.* 1981;6(4):202–206.

88. Lewis CB. *Aging: The Health-care Challenge: An Interdisciplinary Approach to Assessment and Rehabilitative Management of the Elderly,* 4th ed. Philadelphia: F.A. Davis Co., 2002.

89. Frekany GA, Leslie DK. Effects of an exercise program on selected flexibility measurements of senior citizens. *Gerontol.* 1975;15(2):182–183.

90. Barnekow-Bergkvist M, Hedberg G, Janlert U, et al. Development of muscular endurance and strength from adolescence to adulthood and level of physical capacity in men and women at the age of 34 years. *Scand J Med Sci Sports.* 1996;6(3):145–155.

91. Riegger-Krugh C, Keysor JJ. Skeletal malalignments of the lower quarter: Correlated and compensatory motions and postures. *J Orthop Sports Phys Ther.* 1996;23(2):164–170.

92. Decoster LC, Vailas JC, Lindsay RH, et al. Prevalence and features of joint hypermobility among adolescent athletes. *Arch Pediatr Adolesc Med.* 1997; 151(10):989–992.

93. Carter CO, Wilkinson JA. Genetic and environmental factors in the etiology of congenital dislocation of the hip. *Clin Orthop.* 1964;33:119–128.

94. Beighton P, Solomon L, Soskolne CL. Articular mobility in an African population. *Ann Rheum Dis.* 1973;32(5):413–418.

95. Leighton JR. The Leighton flexometer and flexibility test. *J Assoc Phys Ment Rehabil.* 1966;20(3):86–93.

96. Salter N. Methods of measurement of muscle and joint function. *J Bone Joint Surg Br.* 1955;34:474.

97. Watkins MA, Riddle DL, Lamb RL, et al. Reliability of goniometric measurements and visual estimates of knee range of motion obtained in a clinical setting. *Phys Ther.* 1991;71(2):90–96.

98. Sady SP, Wortman M, Blanke D. Flexibility training: Ballistic, static or proprioceptive neuromuscular facilitation? *Arch Phys Med Rehabil.* 1982;63(6): 261–263.

99. Moore MA, Hutton RS. Electromyographic investigation of muscle stretching techniques. *Med Sci Sports Exerc.* 1980;12(5):322–329.

100. Holt LE, Travis TM, Okita T. Comparative study of three stretching techniques. *Percept Mot Skills.* 1970;31(2):611–616.

101. Etnyre BR, Abraham LD. H-reflex changes during static stretching and two variations of proprioceptive neuromuscular facilitation techniques. *Electroencephalogr Clin Neurophysiol.* 1986;63(2):174–179.

102. Hubley CL, Kozey JW, Stanish WD. The effects of static stretching exercises and stationary cycling on range of motion at the hip joint. *J Orthop Sports Phys Ther.* 1984;6(2):104–109.

103. de Vries HA. Evaluation of static stretching procedures for improvement of flexibility. *Res Q.* 1962; 33(2):222–229.

104. Wiktorsson-Moller M, Oberg B, Ekstrand J, et al. Effects of warming up, massage, and stretching on range of motion and muscle strength in the lower extremity. *Am J Sports Med.* 1983;11(4):249–252.

105. Hartig DE, Henderson JM. Increasing hamstring flexibility decreases lower extremity overuse injuries in military basic trainees. *Am J Sports Med.* 1999; 27(2):173–176.

106. Cross KM, Worrell TW. Effects of a static stretching program on the incidence of lower extremity musculotendinous strains. *J Athl Train.* 1999;34(1): 11–14.

107. Fowles JR, Sale DG, MacDougall JD. Reduced strength after passive stretch of the human plantarflexors. *J Appl Physiol.* 2000;89(3):1179–1188.

108. Kokkonen J, Nelson AG, Cornwell A, Kokkonen J. Acute muscle stretching inhibits maximal strength

performance. *Res Q Exerc Sport.* 1998;69(4): 411–415.

109. Bandy WD, Irion JM. The effect of time on static stretch on the flexibility of the hamstring muscles. *Phys Ther.* 1994;74(9):845–850; discussion, 850–882.

110. Knudson D. Stretching: From science to practice. *J Phys Ed Rec Dance.* 1998;69(3):38–45.

111. Moller M, Ekstrand J, Oberg B, et al. Duration of stretching effect on range of motion in lower extremities. *Arch Phys Med Rehabil.* 1985;66(3): 171–173.

112. Cornelius WL, Hagemann RW, Jr., Jackson AW. A study on placement of stretching within a workout. *J Sports Med Phys Fitness.* 1988;28(3):234–236.

113. Shellock FG, Prentice WE. Warming-up and stretching for improved physical performance and prevention of sports-related injuries. *Sports Med.* 1985;2(4):267–278.

114. Pope RP, Herbert RD, Kirwan JD, et al. A randomized trial of preexercise stretching for prevention of lower-limb injury. *Med Sci Sports Exerc.* 2000;32(2): 271–277.

115. Safran MR, Garrett WE, Jr., Seaber AV, et al. The role of warmup in muscular injury prevention. *Am J Sports Med.* 1988;16(2):123–129.

116. van Mechelen W, Hlobil H, Kemper HC, et al. Prevention of running injuries by warm-up, cool-down, and stretching exercises. *Am J Sports Med.* 1993;21(5):711–719.

117. Gleim GW, McHugh MP. Flexibility and its effects on sports injury and performance. *Sports Med.* 1997;24(5):289–299.

118. Strickler T, Malone T, Garrett WE. The effects of passive warming on muscle injury. *Am J Sports Med.* 1990;18(2):141–145.

119. Kubo K, Kawakami Y, Fukunaga T. Influence of elastic properties of tendon structures on jump performance in humans. *J Appl Physiol.* 1999;87(6): 2090–2096.

120. Ciullo JV, Zarins B. Biomechanics of the musculotendinous unit: Relation to athletic performance and injury. *Clin Sports Med.* 1983;2(1):71–86.

121. Wilson GJ, Elliott BC, Wood GA. Stretch shorten cycle performance enhancement through flexibility training. *Med Sci Sports Exerc.* 1992;24(1):116–123.

122. Wilson GJ, Murphy AJ, Pryor JF. Musculotendinous stiffness: Its relationship to eccentric, isometric, and concentric performance. *J Appl Physiol.* 1994;76(6):2714–2719.

123. Hutton RS. Neuromuscular basis of stretching exercise. *In* P. V. Komi (ed.), *Strength and Power in Sports.* Oxford: Blackwell Science Publications, 1993, pp. 29–38.

124. Magnusson SP, Simonsen EB, Aagaard P, et al. Mechanical and physical responses to stretching with and without preisometric contraction in human skeletal muscle. *Arch Phys Med Rehabil.* 1996;77(4):373–378.

125. Condon SM, Hutton RS. Soleus muscle electromyographic activity and ankle dorsiflexion range of motion during four stretching procedures. *Phys Ther.* 1987;67(1):24–30.

126. Sapega AA, Quedenfeld RA, Moyer RA, et al. Biophysical factors in range of motion exercise. *Physician Sportsmed.* 1981;9(12):57–65.

127. Stromberg DD, Wiederhielm CA. Viscoelastic description of a collagenous tissue in simple elongation. *J Appl Physiol.* 1969;26(6):857–862.

128. Hukins DW, Kirby MC, Sikoryn TA, et al. Comparison of structure, mechanical properties, and functions of lumbar spinal ligaments. *Spine.* 1990; 15(8):787–795.

129. Warren CG, Lehmann JF, Koblanski JN. Heat and stretch procedures: an evaluation using rat tail tendon. *Arch Phys Med Rehabil.* 1976;57(3):122–126.

130. Kottke FJ, Pauley DL, Ptak RA. The rationale for prolonged stretching for correction of shortening of connective tissue. *Arch Phys Med Rehabil.* 1966; 47(6):345–352.

131. Laban MM. Collagen tissue: Implications of its response to stress in vitro. *Arch Phys Med Rehabil.* 1962;43:461–466.

132. Kovanen V, Suominen H, Heikkinen E. Collagen of slow twitch and fast twitch muscle fibres in different types of rat skeletal muscle. *Eur J Appl Physiol Occup Physiol.* 1984;52(2):235–242.

133. Tanigawa MC. Comparison of the hold-relax procedure and passive mobilization on increasing muscle length. *Phys Ther.* 1972;52(7):725–735.

134. Etnyre BR, Lee EJ. Comments on proprioceptive neuromuscular facilitation techniques. *Res Q Exerc Sport.* 1987;58:184–188.

135. Etnyre BR, Abraham LD. Antagonist muscle activity during stretching: a paradox re-assessed. *Med Sci Sports Exerc.* 1988;20(3):285–9.

136. Guissard N, Duchateau J, Hainaut K. Muscle stretching and motoneuron excitability. *Eur J Appl Physiol Occup Physiol.* 1988;58(1–2):47–52.

137. McHugh MP, Magnusson SP, Gleim GW, et al. Viscoelastic stress relaxation in human skeletal muscle. *Med Sci Sports Exerc.* 1992;24(12):1375–1382.

138. Stolov WC, Weilepp TG, Jr. Passive length-tension relationship of intact muscle, epimysium, and tendon in normal and denervated gastrocnemius of the rat. *Arch Phys Med Rehabil.* 1966;47(9):612–620.

139. Nordin M, Frankel VH. *Basic Biomechanics of the Musculoskeletal System,* 2nd ed. Philadelphia: Lea & Febiger, 1989.

140. Cornelius WL, Hands MR. The effects of a warm-up on acute hip joint range of motion using modified PNF stretching techniques. *J Athl Train.* 1992;27:112–114.

141. Johns RJ, Wright V. Relative importance of various tissues in joint stiffness. *J Appl Physiol.* 1962;17: 824–828.

142. Ekstrand J, Gillquist J. The avoidability of soccer injuries. *Int J Sports Med.* 1983;4(2):124–128.

143. Anderson B, Burke ER. Scientific, medical, and practical aspects of stretching. *Clin Sports Med.* 1991;10(1):63–86.

144. Voss DE, Ionta MK, Myers BJ, et al. *Proprioceptive Neuromuscular Facilitation: Patterns and Techniques,* 3rd ed. Philadelphia: Harper & Row, 1985.

145. Edin BB, Vallbo AB. Stretch sensitization of human muscle spindles. *J Physiol.* 1988;400:101–111.

146. Magnusson SP, Simonsen EB, Aagaard P, et al. Viscoelastic response to repeated static stretching in the human hamstring muscle. *Scand J Med Sci Sports.* 1995;5(6):342–347.

147. Becker RO. The electrical response of human skeletal muscle to passive stretch. *Surg Forum.* 1960;10: 828–831.

148. Hartley-O'Brien SJ. Six mobilization exercises for active range of hip flexion. *Res Q Exerc Sport.* 1980; 51:625–635.

149. Madding S, Wong J, Medeiros J. Effect of duration of passive stretch on hip abduction range of motion. *J Orthop Sports Phys Ther.* 1987;8:409–416.

150. Markos PD. Ipsilateral and contralateral effects of proprioceptive neuromuscular facilitation techniques on hip motion and electromyographic activity. *Phys Ther.* 1979;59(11):1366–1373.

151. Holcomb W. Stretching and warm-up. *In* T. Baechle, R. Earle (eds.): *Essentials of Strength Training and Conditioning,* 2nd ed. Champaign, IL: Human Kinetics, 2000, pp. 321–342.

152. Lamontagne A, Malouin F, Richards CL. Viscoelastic behavior of plantar flexor muscle-tendon unit at rest. *J Orthop Sports Phys Ther.* 1997;26(5):244–252.

153. Muir IW, Chesworth BM, Vandervoort AA. Effect of a static calf-stretching exercise on the resistive torque during passive ankle dorsiflexion in healthy subjects. *J Orthop Sports Phys Ther.* 1999;29(2): 106–113.

154. Wallin D, Ekblom B, Grahn R, et al. Improvement of muscle flexibility. A comparison between two techniques. *Am J Sports Med.* 1985;13(4):263–268.

155. Mohr KJ, Pink MM, Elsner C, Kvitne RS. Electromyographic investigation of stretching: The effect of warm-up. *Clin J Sport Med.* 1998;8(3): 215–220.

156. Klinge K, Magnusson SP, Simonsen EB, et al. The effect of strength and flexibility training on skeletal muscle electromyographic activity, stiffness, and viscoelastic stress relaxation response. *Am J Sports Med.* 1997;25(5):710–716.

157. Osternig LR, Robertson R, Troxel R, et al. Muscle activation during proprioceptive neuromuscular facilitation (PNF) stretching techniques. *Am J Phys Med.* 1987;66(5):298–307.

158. Hardy L, Jones D. Dynamic flexibility and proprioceptive neuromuscular facilitation. *Res Q Exerc Sport.* 1986;57(2):150–153.

159. Bandy WD, Irion JM, Briggler M. The effect of static stretch and dynamic range of motion training on the flexibility of the hamstring muscles. *J Orthop Sports Phys Ther.* 1998;27(4):295–300.

160. de Vries HA. Electromyographic observations of the effects of static stretching upon muscular distress. *Res Q. Exerc Sport* 1961;32(4):468–479.

161. Godges JJ, MacRae H, Longdon C, et al. The effects of two stretching procedures on hip range of motion and gait economy. *J Orthop Sports Phys Ther.* 1989;7:350–357.

162. Lucas RC, Koslow R. Comparative study of static, dynamic, and proprioceptive neuromuscular facilitation stretching techniques on flexibility. *Percept Mot Skills.* 1984;58(2):615–618.

163. Prentice WE. A comparison of static stretching and PNF stretching for improving hip joint flexibility. *Athl Train.* 1983;18(1):56–59.

164. Pratt K, Bohannon R. Effects of a 3-minute standing stretch on ankle-dorsiflexion range of motion. *J Sport Rehabil.* 2003;12(2):162–173.

165. Cornelius WL, Hinson MM. The relationship between isometric contractions of hip extensors and subsequent flexibility in males. *J Sports Med Phys Fitness.* 1980;20(1):75–80.

166. Hardy L. Improving active range of hip flexion. *Res Q Exerc Sport.* 1985;56(2):111–114.

167. Medeiros JM, Smidt GL, Burmeister LF, et al. The influence of isometric exercise and passive stretch on hip joint motion. *Phys Ther.* 1977;57(5): 518–523.

168. Sullivan MK, Dejulia JJ, Worrell TW. Effect of pelvic position and stretching method on hamstring muscle flexibility. *Med Sci Sports Exerc.* 1992;24(12): 1383–1389.

169. Buroker K, Schwane J. Does postexercise static stretching alleviate delayed muscle soreness? *Physician Sportsmed* 1989;17(6):65–83.

170. Bandy WD, Irion JM, Briggler M. The effect of time and frequency of static stretching on flexibility of the hamstring muscles. *Phys Ther.* 1997;77(10): 1090–1096.

171. Bohannon RW. Effect of repeated eight-minute muscle loading on the angle of straight-leg raising. *Phys Ther.* 1984;64(4):491–497.

172. Knudson D. Stretching during warm-up: Do we have enough evidence? *J Phys Educ Rec Dance.* 1999;70(7):24–32.

173. Smith CA. The warm-up procedure: To stretch or not to stretch. A brief review. *J Orthop Sports Phys Ther.* 1994;19(1):12–17.

174. de Vries HA. Quantitative electromyographic investigation of the spasm theory of muscle pain. *Am J Phys Med.* 1966;45(3):119–134.

175. McGlynn GH, Laughlin NT, Rowe V. Effect of electromyographic feedback and static stretching on artificially induced muscle soreness. *Am J Phys Med.* 1979;58(3):139–148.

176. Gulick DT, Kimura IF, Sitler M, et al. Various treatment techniques on signs and symptoms of delayed onset muscle soreness. *J Athl Train.* 1996;31(2):145–152.

177. Smith LL, Brunetz MH, Chenier TC, et al. The effects of static and ballistic stretching on delayed onset muscle soreness and creatine kinase. *Res Q Exerc Sport.* 1993;64(1):103–107.

178. High DM, Howley ET, Franks BD. The effects of static stretching and warm-up on prevention of delayed-onset muscle soreness. *Res Q Exerc Sport.* 1989;60(4):357–361.

179. de Vries HA, Wiswell RA, Bulbulian R, et al. Tranquilizer effect of exercise. Acute effects of moderate aerobic exercise on spinal reflex activation level. *Am J Phys Med.* 1981;60(2):57–66.

180. Millar AP. An early stretching routine for calf muscle strains. *Med Sci Sports.* 1976;8(1):39–42.

181. Shrier I. Stretching before exercise does not reduce the risk of local muscle injury: A critical review of the clinical and basic science literature. *Clin J Sport Med.* 1999;9(4):221–227.

182. Lieber RL, Woodburn TM, Friden J. Muscle damage induced by eccentric contractions of 25% strain. *J Appl Physiol.* 1991;70(6):2498–2507.

183. Knudson D, Bennett K, Corn R, et al. Acute effects of stretching are not evident in the kinematics of the vertical jump. *J Strength Cond Res.* 2001;15(1):98–101.

184. Cornwell A, Nelson A, Sidaway B. Acute effects of passive stretching on the neuromechanical behavior of the triceps surae muscle complex [abstract]. *Med Sci Sports Exerc.* 1999;31(5):S221.

185. Nelson AG, Kokkonen J. Acute ballistic muscle stretching inhibits maximal strength performance. *Res Q Exerc Sport.* 2001;72(4):415–419.

186. Nelson AG, Allen JD, Cornwell A, et al. Inhibition of maximal voluntary isometric torque production by acute stretching is joint-angle specific. *Res Q Exerc Sport.* 2001;72(1):68–70.

187. Nelson AG, Guillory IK, Cornwell C, et al. Inhibition of maximal voluntary isokinetic torque production following stretching is velocity-specific. *J Strength Cond Res.* 2001;15(2):241–246.

188. Bracko MR. Can stretching prior to exercise and sports improve performance and prevent injury? *ACSM's Health & Fitness Journal.* 2002;6(5):17–22.

189. Craib MW, Mitchell VA, Fields KB, et al. The association between flexibility and running economy in sub-elite male distance runners. *Med Sci Sports Exerc.* 1996;28(6):737–743.

190. Nelson AG, Kokkonen J, Eldredge C, et al. Chronic stretching and running economy. *Scand J Med Sci Sports.* 2001;11(5):260–265.

191. Avela J, Kyrolainen H, Komi PV. Altered reflex sensitivity after repeated and prolonged passive muscle stretching. *J Appl Physiol.* 1999;86(4):1283–1291.

192. Behm DG, Button DC, Butt JC. Factors affecting force loss with prolonged stretching. *Can J Appl Physiol.* 2001;26(3):261–272.

193. Worrell TW, Smith TL, Winegardner J. Effect of hamstring stretching on hamstring muscle performance. *J Orthop Sports Phys Ther.* 1994;20(3):154–159.

194. Nelson AG, Cornwell A, Heise G. Acute stretching exercises and vertical jump stored elastic energy. *Med Sci Sports Exerc.* 1996;28(5)Suppl:156 [abstract].

195. Kulund DN, Tottossy M. Warm-up, strength, and power. *Orthop Clin North Am.* 1983;14(2):427–448.

196. Martin BJ, Robinson S, Wiegman DL, et al. Effect of warm-up on metabolic responses to strenuous exercise. *Med Sci Sports.* 1975;7(2):146–149.

197. Bergh U. Human power at subnormal body temperatures. *Acta Physiol Scand Suppl.* 1980;478:1–39.

198. Bergh U, Ekblom B. Influence of muscle temperature on maximal muscle strength and power output in human skeletal muscles. *Acta Physiol Scand.* 1979;107(1):33–37.

199. Bergh U, Ekblom B. Physical performance and peak aerobic power at different body temperatures. *J Appl Physiol.* 1979;46(5):885–889.

200. Davies CT, Young K. Effect of temperature on the contractile properties and muscle power of triceps surae in humans. *J Appl Physiol.* 1983;55(1, Pt 1):191–195.

201. McNair PJ, Stanley SN. Effect of passive stretching and jogging on the series elastic muscle stiffness and range of motion of the ankle joint. *Br J Sports Med.* 1996;30(4):313–317.

202. Rosenbaum D, Hennig EM. The influence of stretching and warm-up exercises on Achilles tendon reflex activity. *J Sports Sci.* 1995;13(6):481–490.

203. Henricson A, Fredriksson K, Persson I, et al. The effect of heat and stretching on range of hip motion. *J Orthop Sports Phys Ther.* 1984;6(2):110–115.

204. Hunter SK, Enoka RM. Sex differences in the fatigability of arm muscles depends on absolute force during isometric contractions. *J Appl Physiol.* 2001;91(6):2686–2694.

205. Lehmann JF, Masock AJ, Warren CG, et al. Effect of therapeutic temperatures on tendon extensibility. *Arch Phys Med Rehabil.* 1970;51(8):481–487.

206. Stewart IB, Sleivert GG. The effect of warm-up intensity on range of motion and anaerobic performance. *J Orthop Sports Phys Ther.* 1998;27(2):154–161.

207. Wiemann K, Hahn K. Influences of strength, stretching and circulatory exercises on flexibility parameters of the human hamstrings. *Int J Sports Med.* 1997;18(5):340–346.

208. Magnusson SP, Aagard P, Simonsen E, et al. A biomechanical evaluation of cyclic and static stretch in human skeletal muscle. *Int J Sports Med.* 1998;19(5): 310–316.

209. Taylor DC, Brooks DE, Ryan JB. Viscoelastic characteristics of muscle: passive stretching versus muscular contractions. *Med Sci Sports Exerc.* 1997;29 (12):1619–1624.

210. Roberts JM, Wilson K. Effect of stretching duration on active and passive range of motion in the lower extremity. *Br J Sports Med.* 1999;33(4):259–263.

211. McNair PJ, Dombroski EW, Hewson DJ, et al. Stretching at the ankle joint: Viscoelastic responses to holds and continuous passive motion. *Med Sci Sports Exerc.* 2001;33(3):354–358.

212. Pollock ML, Gaesser GA, Butcher JD, et al. American College of Sports Medicine Position Stand. The recommended quantity and quality of exercise for developing and maintaining cardiorespiratory and muscular fitness, and flexibility in healthy adults. *Med Sci Sports Exerc.* 1998;30(6):975–991.

213. Borms J, Van Roy P, Santens JP, et al. Optimal duration of static stretching exercises for improvement of coxo-femoral flexibility. *J Sports Sci.* 1987;5(1): 39–47.

214. Walter J, Figoni SF, Andres FF, et al. Training intensity and duration in flexibility. *Clin Kinesiol.* 1996;50(2):40–45.

215. Taylor DC, Dalton JD, Jr., Seaber AV, et al. Experimental muscle strain injury. Early functional and structural deficits and the increased risk for reinjury. *Am J Sports Med.* 1993;21(2):190–194.

216. Noonan TJ, Best TM, Seaber AV, et al. Identification of a threshold for skeletal muscle injury. *Am J Sports Med.* 1994;22(2):257–261.

217. Starring DT, Gossman MR, Nicholson GG, Jr., et al. Comparison of cyclic and sustained passive stretching using a mechanical device to increase resting length of hamstring muscles. *Phys Ther.* 1988;68(3):314–320.

218. DePino G, Webright W, Arnold B. Duration of maintained hamstring flexibility after cessation of an acute static stretching protocol. *J Athl Train.* 2000;35(1):56–59.

219. Kirsch RF, Weiss PL, Dannenbaum RM, et al. Effect of maintained stretch on the range of motion of the human ankle joint. *Clin Biomech.* 1995;10(3): 166–168.

220. Zito M, Driver D, Parker C, et al. Lasting effects of one bout of two 15-second passive stretches on ankle dorsiflexion range of motion. *J Orthop Sports Phys Ther.* 1997;26(4):214–221.

221. Magnusson SP, Aagaard P, Nielson JJ. Passive energy return after repeated stretches of the hamstring muscle-tendon unit. *Med Sci Sports Exerc.* 2000;32(6):1160–1164.

222. Willy RW, Kyle BA, Moore SA, et al. Effect of cessation and resumption of static hamstring muscle stretching on joint range of motion. *J Orthop Sports Phys Ther.* 2001;31(3):138–144.

223. Ashmore CR. Stretch-induced growth in chicken wing muscles: effects on hereditary muscular dystrophy. *Am J Physiol.* 1982;242(3):178–183.

4

Training for Cardiopulmonary and Cardiovascular Fitness

MARK F. REINKING

HARVEY WALLMANN

Objectives

The reader will be able to:

- Describe the physiological responses of the cardiovascular system and pulmonary system to aerobic exercise.

- Define maximal oxygen uptake and describe the factors influencing this physiological characteristic.

- Compare maximal and submaximal graded exercise testing, their common modes, and discuss the advantages and disadvantages of each mode.

- Identify the primary variables used in prescribing exercise to improve aerobic power.

- Identify appropriate aerobic exercise training volume levels (intensity, duration, frequency).

- Discuss the benefits of cross training.

- Compare and contrast various modes of aerobic exercise with regard to cardiovascular and pulmonary response, equipment requirements, and injury risk.

- Discuss exercise-related cardiac events and discuss strategies to minimize such events.

- Describe necessary modifications to aerobic exercise prescription in certain conditions including pregnancy, diabetes, and other disease conditions.

- List the changes that occur in the cardiovascular and pulmonary systems with aging, and relate these changes to aerobic exercise in these populations.

Outline

INTRODUCTION TO TRAINING FOR CARDIOPULMONARY AND CARDIOVASCULAR FITNESS

The benefits of physical activity on health are well established, with evidence of decreased mortality rates from cardiorespiratory disease and cancer for those with greater levels of fitness.[1,2] The Healthy People 2010 project identified 10 health indicators reflecting the major public health concerns in the United States. Two of those indicators—being overweight or obese—have a direct relationship to physical fitness and physical activity.[3] The most recent National Health and Nutrition Examination Survey indicated that 35 percent of U.S. adults are overweight, with a Body Mass Index (BMI) of 25.0–29.9 and 26 percent are obese (BMI > 30.0).[4] As compared to the previous published survey in 1994, this is an increase from 55 percent of Americans who are overweight or obese to 61 percent. A particularly alarming statistic is that the percentage of children who are overweight increased from 11 percent in 1994 to 14 percent in 1999.[5] These data reflect the overall decline in physical activity by Americans.

In 1995, the Center for Disease Control and Prevention and the American College of Sports Medicine (ACSM) developed a consensus statement regarding the recommended amount of physical activity for adults. The recommendation stated, "every American adult should accumulate 30 minutes or more of moderate-intensity physical activity on most, preferably all, days of the week."[2] However, the reality is that over 60 percent of adults and 50 percent of children in the United States are not regularly physically active.[6] Those persons who do not have physically active lifestyles are at higher risk of coronary artery disease, hypertension, cerebrovascular disease, obesity, adult onset diabetes, osteoarthritis, osteoporosis, depression, and colon cancer.

Cardiopulmonary training, or training for aerobic power, is an underutilized form of training in rehabilitation settings. Most patients seeking rehabilitative services have integumentary, musculoskeletal or neuromuscular impairments and the interventions are focused on these problems. Unfortunately, the cardiovascular and pulmonary systems are often not evaluated by clinicians. Many of the clients that we encounter daily have risk factors for cardiopulmonary disease and may have significant existing impairments of these systems. In order to comprehensively address health care needs, a screening examination should be completed for all clients seeking rehabilitation services. This screening examination may reveal risk factors for cardiovascular or cardiopulmonary disease that should be considered when developing a therapeutic exercise program. A brief and limited screening examination should include client and family history and an assessment of blood pressure, heart rate, respiratory rate, and edema.[7] If risk factors or system impairments are identified, the clinician should communicate these to the client's physician. Based on the examination findings, appropriate therapeutic exercise intervention is provided that will prevent or delay the development of cardiopulmonary disease, and contribute to the restoration of the client's functional status.

The focus on health promotion in Healthy People 2010[3] is reflected in the development of primary prevention patterns in the Guide to Physical Therapist Practice.[7] One of the preferred practice patterns in the guide is primary prevention/risk reduction for cardiovascular/pulmonary disorders. This pattern identifies cardiovascular and cardiopulmonary system risk factors for disease, including family history of heart disease, sedentary lifestyle, obesity, smoking, diabetes, hypercholesterolemia, and hypertension. The addition of therapeutic exercise focused on improving aerobic power can contribute to a client's improved fitness, increased sense of well being, weight management, tolerance of exertion, and lower mortality rates.[1,8–10] Pate et al.[2] reported that lifestyle modifications which ensured a total of 30 minutes of moderate intensity activity daily was sufficient to stimulate weight loss and improve cardiopulmonary fitness, even in the absence of a structured aerobic exercise program.

Training the cardiopulmonary system results in physiological adaptations that affect the entire body. The specific training effects are determined by the training mode as well as the intensity, duration, and frequency of training. The physiological training effects as well as the ability to coordinate muscular activity ultimately determine performance and may differ as a result of individual differences in the ability to train aerobically.

The type of therapeutic exercise performed is the most important determinant of pulmonary and cardiovascular response to exercise.[11] However, the training level and current aerobic fitness level should also be considered when determining the type of exercise stimulus. An individual's genetic potential dictates the magnitude of training adaptation possible. As an individual approaches the upper limit of this training adaptation, smaller physiological gains will be observed, thereby prompting the individual to carefully monitor and fine-tune the therapeutic exercise program design in order to further enhance performance capability. The complex integration of the cardiovascular and cardiopulmonary systems allows for optimal endurance training and performance.

METABOLIC PATHWAYS

As mentioned in Chapter 2, three pathways are responsible for supplying energy to the body during skeletal muscle contraction: the adenosine triphosphate-creatine phosphate (ATP-CP) (phosphagen) system, the glycolytic (glycolysis or glycogen-lactic acid) system, and the oxidative (aerobic) system. The latter two pathways are metabolic pathways, since they involve a sequence of reactions. In contrast, the ATP-CP system is not considered a metabolic pathway because it consists of only a single reaction (**Figure 4.1**). The relative contribution of each system to ATP production varies and depends upon exercise parameters such as intensity, duration, and rest intervals. Anaero-

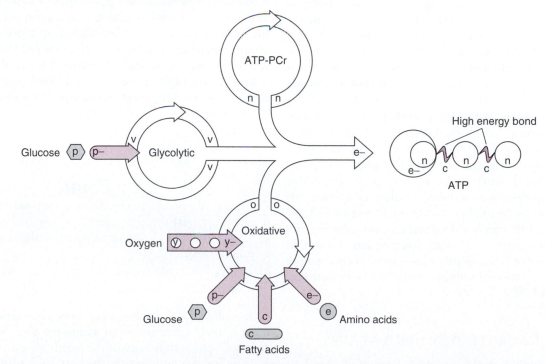

Figure 4.1   Energy systems. (Reprinted with permission from Axen K, Vermitsky Axen K. *Illustrated Principles of Exercise Physiology.* Upper Saddle River, NJ: Prentice Hall, 2002.)

bic metabolism primarily involves the phosphagen system and glycolysis (or anaerobic glycolysis), whereas aerobic energy production stems from the oxidative system.

Muscle cell CP concentrations are about four to six times greater than concentrations of ATP, making it the high energy phosphate reservoir. The energy supplied for high intensity exercise is primarily limited, however, not by the unavailability of fuel sources, but by the inability of the body to tolerate lactate buildup. If exercise is continued in the absence of oxygen, lactate levels begin to accumulate in the muscles, affecting muscle contraction and causing fatigue. However, lactate can be used as a fuel during aerobic metabolism. Anaerobic training can develop physical tolerance for intense exercise.[12,13]

Key Point:

Aerobic energy production occurs with submaximal exercise where carbohydrates and fat are used as fuel sources to produce ATP. If more than adequate oxygen is present with increased exercise intensity, more free fatty acids will be used for energy production. As intensity increases, more carbohydrates are used for fuel. With maximal exercise intensity, carbohydrates provide a greater proportion of the fuel, while fat use decreases.

Aerobic energy production occurs with submaximal exercise in which carbohydrates and fat are used as fuel sources to produce ATP. If more than adequate oxygen is present with decreased intensity or workload, more fat (free fatty acids rather than carbohydrates) is used for energy production. As intensity increases, more carbohydrates are used to supply energy. So, with maximal exercise intensity, the proportion of carbohydrates used as a fuel source increases dramatically, while the proportion of fat as a fuel decreases.

Peak performance gains are typically related to changes to more than one physiological system, making total conditioning necessary. Additionally, one has to be careful not to train one system at the expense of another. For example, if aerobic training is the desired primary exercise stimulus, then resistance training should play a lesser role in the training program, but should still be performed. Although resistance training does not enhance aerobic metabolism when performed alone, research has shown that when a resistance training program is used in conjunction with aerobic endurance training, aerobic metabolism may be improved.[14–18]

Blood Lactate Accumulation

Pyruvate formation in the muscle as a result of glycolysis can result in the production of both carbon dioxide and water (oxidized aerobically) or lactate (oxidized anaerobi-

cally). Lactate production occurs when the rate of production of pyruvate and hydrogen atoms by glycolysis exceeds their rate of removal by the Krebs cycle and electron transport chain. Reduced activity of the electron transport chain decreases the rate at which pyruvate is oxidized to carbon dioxide by the Krebs cycle as well as decreases the rate at which hydrogen atoms are removed from the cytoplasm. Ultimately, this results in increased lactate concentrations. Blood lactate levels remain nearly constant from states of rest to moderate exercise. However, lactate is formed continuously at all levels of exercise. In fact, fivefold levels of lactate production can occur without a concomitant increase in blood lactate levels. In other words, the nearly constant levels of blood lactate observed during rest and up to moderate levels of exercise occur as a result of an equilibrium between lactate production and lactate removal.[19] During light to moderate exercise, any lactate formed is rapidly oxidized by the heart and other muscle fibers with high oxidative capacities (remember, lactate can be used as a fuel). So, during aerobic activity, lactate formation is matched by its rate of removal by other tissues. This allows the blood lactate levels to be relatively stable, despite the increase in oxygen uptake. It is only when removal does not match production that blood lactate levels accumulate. The most rapidly accumulating and highest lactate levels are produced during sustained maximal exercise (up to 180 seconds duration).

Since increased blood lactate levels can be a result of either an increase in the rate of lactate production or a decrease in the rate of lactate removal, or a combination of the two, it stands to reason that the concentration of blood lactate is not a very good indicator of lactate production. Still, blood lactate concentration does indicate the amount of lactate accumulation at a point in time. Many researchers and exercise scientists call this point the *lactate threshold* or *anaerobic threshold*. Lactate threshold is defined as the highest exercise level that is not associated with an elevation in blood lactate concentration above the pre-exercise level.

Key Point:

Lactate threshold is the highest exercise level the client can perform that is not associated with an elevation in blood lactate concentration above the pre-exercise level.

Essentially, it is a transitional stage representing a shift from a solely oxidative to an additional glycolytic energy supply.[20] The significance of the lactate threshold is that it is an index representing the highest level of exercise intensity that can be indefinitely sustained. This becomes extremely important for the trained athlete, since accumulated lactate leads to fatigue in skeletal muscle. Training above the lactate threshold level improves the body's ability to process lactate, thereby allowing the lactate threshold level to increase without compromising the ability to sustain a high submaximal exercise intensity.[21,22]

Another term used to describe a systematic increase in blood lactate level is the *onset of blood lactate accumulation.* The terms lactate threshold and onset of blood lactate accumulation are often used interchangeably. However, the onset of blood lactate accumulation refers to an increase in blood lactate level equal to some predetermined amount, usually equal to or above a 4-mMol baseline.

RESPONSE TO EXERCISE

In order to appreciate the effects of aerobic training, it is necessary to have a basic understanding of the acute physiological responses to exercise. Pursuant to this, however, is the need to understand the importance of cardiopulmonary function. The cardiopulmonary system is responsible for delivery of oxygen to the working muscles, in addition to removing the byproducts of exercise. This is particularly crucial for maintenance of homeostasis during exercise as it relates to exchange of oxygen and carbon dioxide. Two major components are considered responsible for oxygen transportation during aerobic exercise. The first is the *central* component, which refers to the ability of the cardiopulmonary system to oxygenate blood and deliver it to the exercising muscles. The second component is referred to as the *peripheral* component, which deals with the ability of the exercising muscles to use oxygen aerobically to convert fuel to energy for muscular contractions.[23] Several factors come into play for each component. The effectiveness of the central component to deliver oxygen to the muscles is dependent upon pulmonary diffusion, cardiac output, and hemoglobin affinity. Important factors affecting the peripheral component are the degree of vascularization of the exercising muscles; glycogen stores in the muscles; the number, size, and distribution of the mitochondria; myoglobin content; and the status of the oxidative enzymes.[23,24] These factors all dictate how much oxygen can be consumed in a given amount of time. In summary, the central component delivers the oxygen and the peripheral component uses it to the best of its ability.

> ## *Key Point:*
> Both central and peripheral components influence oxygen use during exercise.

In any case, the major characteristic of the acute response associated with an increase in exercise intensity is an increase in oxygen consumption (VO_2). The annota-

tion V is the scientific shorthand for the rate of volume flow. The equation that expresses the determinants of VO_2 is known as the *Fick equation:*

$$VO_2 = \text{cardiac output} \times (A - vO_2)$$

In this equation, a–v O_2 is the arteriovenous oxygen difference.[11] Cardiac output refers to the amount of blood pumped by the heart (usually during a one minute period) and increases during progressive aerobic exercise, showing a linear relationship to VO_2 (**Figure 4.2**). Normal cardiac output at rest is five liters/min for males and 4.5 liters/min for females. The maximal value for cardiac output reflects the functional capacity of the circulation to meet the demands of exercise. Cardiac output depends on heart rate and the quantity of blood ejected with each stroke or stroke volume, represented by the equation

$$\text{cardiac output} = \text{heart rate} \times \text{stroke volume}$$

(**Figures 4.3–4.4**). Increases in cardiac ouput during exercise are largely determined by an increase in heart rate.[25] Stroke volume also contributes to an increase in the cardiac output, especially early in exercise, primarily as a result of the increase in venous return due to the pumping action of the exercising muscles.

At rest, the tissues of the body normally deplete arterial blood of about one-quarter of the oxygen it carries and results in a difference of 5 ml oxygen per 100 ml of blood between the oxygen content of arterial blood and that of

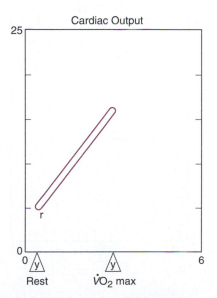

Figure 4.2   Relationship of cardiac output to oxygen uptake during exercise. (Reprinted with permission from Axen K, Vermitsky Axen K. *Illustrated Principles of Exercise Physiology.* Upper Saddle River, NJ: Prentice Hall, 2002.)

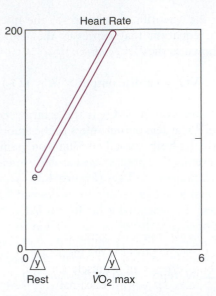

Figure 4.3 Relationship of heart rate to oxygen uptake during exercise. (Reprinted with permission from Axen K, Vermitsky Axen K. *Illustrated Principles of Exercise Physiology.* Upper Saddle River, NJ: Prentice Hall, 2002.)

mixed venous blood, the a−v O_2 difference. During exercise, muscle tissues extract more oxygen from arterial blood, thereby widening the a−v O_2 difference.[11] This is considered the "peripheral" extraction of the delivered oxygen. Central oxygen delivery is determined by cardiac output and initial arterial oxygen content, with maximal

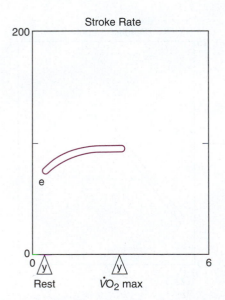

Figure 4.4 Relationship of stroke volume to oxygen uptake during exercise. (Reprinted with permission from Axen K, Vermitsky Axen K. *Illustrated Principles of Exercise Physiology.* Upper Saddle River, NJ: Prentice Hall, 2002.)

limits imposed by heart rate and stroke volume limits, as well as maximal arterial oxygen content. Thus, the physiologic response to exercise results in changes in all of these parameters, thereby ultimately increasing VO_2. In other words, VO_2 can increase by either increasing cardiac output, a−v O_2, or both, and cardiac output can increase by increasing heart rate, stroke volume, or both. The Fick equation shows that training induced increases in VO_2 can be attributed to higher levels of cardiac output coupled with increased oxygen extraction by the tissues, as evidenced by a wider a−v O_2 difference.

Resting heart rate is determined largely by parasympathetic control via the vagus nerve. However, once exercise is initiated, this vagal control is subsumed by central nervous system mechanisms, resulting in an initial rapid increase in heart rate.[11] Progression of exercise intensity results in subsequent increases in heart rate, which are mediated by increases in the sympathetic nervous system as well as increases in circulating catecholamines (epinephrine and norepinephrine).

AEROBIC CAPACITY AND ENDURANCE

An ideal system would be if the central component could deliver as much oxygen to the body as was needed and if the peripheral component could use as much oxygen as was delivered. However, anyone who has ever trained for an endurance event knows this is not the case. There is a limit to how much oxygen can be used by the muscles. The increased muscle activity during exercise requires increased oxygen delivery to the active muscles to support the demands of aerobic metabolism. *Aerobic capacity* refers to the greatest amount of oxygen an individual can consume during exercise. Oxygen delivery can increase virtually instantaneously during activity by as much as twenty fold, whereas the demand on the inactive muscles may remain essentially unchanged.

> ## *Key Point:*
> Aerobic capacity refers to the greatest amount of oxygen an individual can consume during exercise.

Endurance is the capacity for an individual to maintain a certain level of exercise over a certain time frame. In other words, endurance can be defined as the capacity to sustain a given velocity or *power output* for the longest possible time.[26] Whereas aerobic capacity is an absolute factor, endurance is more likely a relative one. An improvement in endurance may refer to either being able to endure a particular exercise intensity for a longer period or being able to endure an increased intensity for a shorter period. However, it is generally described as the ability to maintain a certain fraction of aerobic capacity for a specific period.

Having at least a minimal level of cardiopulmonary and cardiovascular fitness is generally considered a prerequisite for all sports and is recommended for anyone participating in endurance activities. This minimal aerobic fitness level is referred to as an *aerobic base*. Of course, the extent to which someone trains is dependent upon the level of participation. Some sports and activities have greater reliance on aerobic energy sources than others do (e.g., endurance running vs. sprinting). Programs for cardiopulmonary and cardiovascular system training may include interval training or continuous training, described later in this chapter. The determination of which program to follow depends upon the specific nature of the sport performed. It is well accepted that enhancement of the cardiopulmonary and cardiovascular systems increase the overall physiological function and well being of an individual. Cardiopulmonary and cardiovascular conditioning is typically measured by O_2 consumption or the efficiency of O_2 use during exercise (exercise economy).

MAXIMAL OXYGEN UPTAKE (VO$_{2MAX}$)

Hill and Lupton[27] were among the first to describe a linear relationship between O_2 consumption and workload (running speed). They postulated that shortly before maximum work capacity was reached, the rate of O_2 consumption plateaued and did not increase further, even though the individual was able to exercise a little harder beyond that point. They termed this the point of maximum oxygen consumption or VO$_{2max}$ (**Figure 4.5**).

Key Point:

Maximum oxygen consumption refers to the instant at which maximal oxygen consumption does not increase further.

Another term used in the literature describing VO$_{2max}$ is *maximal aerobic power*. A commonly accepted definition of maximal aerobic power is the maximal rate at which energy can be produced in a muscle through oxidative metabolism.[28] In other words, maximal aerobic power is the ability to take up, transport, and utilize O_2 by the working muscle and is usually expressed as VO$_{2max}$.[23] It is in this context that VO$_{2max}$ is taken as a measure of cardiopulmonary fitness. Research has revealed a high correlation between VO$_{2max}$ and performance in aerobic endurance events.[29,30] It has long been associated with success in endurance sports and is usually expressed relative to body weight to adjust for body size (i.e., ml/kg/min).[29,31] It is also highly reproducible from day to day in a given individual when he or she is tested with the same protocol and on the same piece of equipment. Many researchers and rehabilitation clinicians use a VO$_{2max}$ measure of aerobic

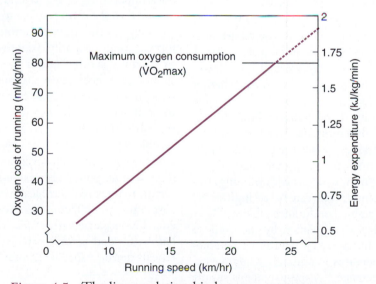

Figure 4.5   The linear relationship between oxygen consumption and running speed, showing the point at which maximum oxygen consumption (VO$_{2max}$) is believed to occur. (Reprinted with permission from T. Noakes. *Lore of Running*, 3rd ed. Figure 22, Champaign, IL: Leisure Press; 1991, p. 19.)

power because it measures exercise performance capabilities and can be used across different exercise modes.

Research performed during the past few decades has fueled a debate concerning VO_{2max}. The most critical issue involves the question that has been most widely researched: What limits maximal oxygen uptake? Of particular interest is the fact that VO_{2max} is not only a measure of aerobic energy exchange, but also a precise measurement of the capacity to transport and utilize oxygen (i.e., central and peripheral components). Many researchers have concluded that the limiting factor is the muscle mitochondria, whereas others have suggested that oxygen transport in the muscle is the limiting factor.[32,33] Although there is a widely accepted notion that VO_{2max} is limited by the rate at which oxygen can be supplied to the muscles and not by the muscle's ability to extract O_2 from the blood,[34] no consensus exists and current views continue to be far apart. An in-depth discussion of the physiology of these factors is beyond the scope of this chapter. Nonetheless, the question of what limits VO_{2max} is unlikely to be definitively answered in the near future.

FACTORS AFFECTING VO₂MAX

As previously mentioned, the ability to perform prolonged exercise depends on aerobic metabolism. It follows that the magnitude of increase in exercise capacity following training depends on the magnitude of increase in VO_{2max}. However, healthy individuals embarking on a running program can expect a VO_{2max} increase of only about 5 percent to 15 percent,[35] suggesting that major VO_{2max} differences between individuals (greater than 15 percent) likely result from factors other than training (e.g., heredity). The VO_{2max} values of healthy young men and women are usually between 45 and 55 ml/kg/min, about 60 percent lower than that of elite athletes. Women typically have lower VO_{2max} values than men, due in part to a woman's higher body fat content and smaller muscle mass. Resting oxygen uptake is very similar in trained and untrained individuals, but there is a substantial difference (as much as twofold higher) in VO_{2max} in the trained versus the untrained individual.[24] For example, in normal young men, the VO_{2max} is approximately 45 ml/kg/min, whereas with training, this can increase to 60 ml/kg/min, and can be as high as 80 ml/kg/min in world class, trained endurance athletes.[36]

Increases in VO_{2max} are accompanied by increases in maximum cardiac output and a−v O_2. The a−v O_2 values increase because of the increases in systemic oxidative capacity and vascular conductance.[37] Conductance is simply the measure of the blood flow through a vessel for a given pressure difference and is the reciprocal of resistance. Cardiac output increases largely by an increase in stroke volume, because maximum heart rate in trained individuals does not differ from that of untrained individuals. In other words, increased heart rate alone cannot explain the increased cardiac output response of the trained athlete.[11]

Therefore, the ability to increase stroke volume is the prime cardiovascular system response to training.[38] During maximal exercise, increases in cardiac output and a−v O_2 by the exercising muscle result in a greater VO_{2max}.[39]

Since most endurance training studies show some increase in VO_{2max} with time, the optimal exercise volume and intensity for increasing VO_{2max} is not known. However, the increase probably depends on several factors, most notably the initial fitness level of the individual, training program duration and intensity, and the frequency of the training sessions.[26] There is some evidence in the literature to suggest that a high intensity of training may be necessary for improvement in VO_{2max}. Several studies have shown increases ranging anywhere from 5 percent to 10 percent in VO_{2max} with short term endurance training programs,[40,–46] while other researchers have reported as high as a 23 percent increase in VO_{2max} with over nine weeks of endurance training.[47] There is also evidence that during longer term training programs, VO_{2max} will eventually stabilize, with subsequent performance improvements resulting from increased exercise economy and lactate threshold.[48,49]

TRAINING FOR MAXIMAL AEROBIC CAPACITY

Aerobic endurance training programs should be designed to increase VO_{2max}. Since during endurance sports the athlete relies heavily on aerobic capacity (also called *aerobic power*), it should be apparent that a high aerobic capacity is of tremendous importance in events that require prolonged exercise. *Maximal aerobic capacity* refers to this aspect of aerobic fitness and involves the maximal amount of work that can be performed using primarily oxidative metabolism.[23] The ability to produce aerobic power is crucial in competition and should be a goal during training, as this allows repeated bouts of exercise to occur. For example, it is common for a track athlete or swimmer to race in more than one event; therefore, the enhanced recovery rate associated with a high aerobic capacity could play a significant role in how well the athlete deals with multi-event competitions. The benefits of high aerobic power also extend to anaerobic sports. Since lactate is removed aerobically, good aerobic capability will have a positive effect on recovery from high intensity exercise. This is particularly crucial during training, since an athlete with good aerobic capacity can perform more quality repeats during a specific amount of practice time.

EXERCISE ECONOMY AND AEROBIC CAPACITY

Exercise economy can be defined as the oxygen uptake required at a given absolute exercise intensity.[26] Increased exercise economy simply means that less oxygen is consumed when performing the same activity. For example, athletes with high aerobic capacity, but with poor exercise economy, may not match the performance of those with less aerobic capacity but who use oxygen more efficiently. Individual variability in the oxygen cost of submaximal exercise exists, even in individuals having similar levels of aerobic fitness (VO_{2max}). Researchers have reported that, regardless of VO_{2max} values, elite runners run at very similar intensities during competition.[50,51] Other researchers have reported that there are marked differences in the oxygen requirement for different athletes running at the same racing speeds. They suggest that differences in exercise economy on the efficiency of oxygen utilization could be a major factor in explaining the running performance differences between athletes with similar VO_{2max} values.[52] Some differences were as much as 30 percent, even in trained athletes.[53] Horowitz et al.[54] demonstrated that elite cyclists exercising at the same power output required different rates of oxygen uptake. The more efficient cyclists had a greater percentage of type I (slow twitch) muscles fibers in the vastus lateralis, suggesting that a motor unit recruitment pattern during exercise may affect exercise economy.

> **Key Point:**
> Greater exercise economy means that less oxygen is needed to perform an activity at the same performance level during aerobic energy system function.

Research has shown that the best athletes usually display high exercise efficiency.[55] Conley and Krahenbuhl[56] reported that 10 km race performance was closely related to running economy in a group of 12 male runners with similar high VO_{2max} values. Although they were unable to predict their 10 km time, they reported excellent correlations between the amount of oxygen used and their best times for the race. The runners who used the least oxygen and were the most efficient had the fastest 10 km time. In other words, running efficiency and not VO_{2max} was the factor determining success in the 10 km race. It appears that better exercise economy (i.e., lower VO_{2max} values for a given absolute running speed or power output) is advantageous to endurance performance because of the utilization of a lower percentage of VO_{2max} at a particular exercise intensity.[26] Lower VO_{2max} values reported for some elite endurance athletes may be compensated for by enhanced exercise economy.[57,58] Runners with very high VO_{2max} values may have less impressive running performances because they are simply less efficient and require more oxygen than average to run at any speed. Gender has no effect on running efficiency; trained men and women appear to be equally efficient.[30,50]

Children may be less efficient in running economy than adults. Davies[59] reported improved running efficiencies when child runners ran with weights. He concluded that because of their lesser bodyweight, children are normally less able to transfer energy in the horizontal plane. He attributed the increase in efficiency with the weights to a depressed vertical movement, allowing his subjects to better transfer this energy forward. Similar results were noted with slower runners of similar heights, weights, and VO_{2max} values. The slower runners ran with a more upright stance, covered less ground and used up twice as much energy in the vertical axis as the faster runners.[60]

Using extra weight added to the legs or feet may also greatly affect exercise economy during rehabilitation. In research involving runners, Martin[61] reported that the addition of 0.5 kg to each thigh or to each foot increased the O_2 cost of running by 3.5 percent and 7.2 percent, respectively. Other studies corroborated these results, showing that an addition of 1 kg to the feet increased the O_2 cost of walking and running by about 6 percent to 10 percent, with the increase being the same for men and women.[62,63] The increased weight of in-shoe orthotics has been shown to adversely affect exercise economy as well. Researchers have reported that the addition of an orthotic to each running shoe increased the O_2 cost of running anywhere from 0.4 percent to 1.4 percent.[64,65]

The concept of exercise economy is important with any activity, whether it is athletic, recreational, or occupational in nature. An individual with high exercise economy will burn less fuel than will an inefficient person during the performance of the same task. This becomes particularly important for endurance activities, because depleted body fuel stores create an earlier fatigue onset.

EFFECTS OF ENDURANCE TRAINING

Oxygen Uptake Adaptations

One of the most commonly measured endurance training adaptations is an increase in VO_{2max}. Aerobic training increases the oxidative capacity of the trained muscle, resulting in the trained muscle's ability to consume O_2 at a higher rate than the untrained muscle, thereby increasing VO_{2max}. Depending on the initial fitness level, aerobic endurance training can increase aerobic power by 5 percent to 30 percent. Individuals with lower starting fitness levels can expect greater improvement with training. Since most VO_{2max} adaptations occur within a 6 to 12 month period, subsequent performance improvements are more likely related to improved exercise economy, increases in the aerobic capacity of skeletal muscle (i.e., fast and slow twitch muscle fibers), and changes in anaerobic metabolism (i.e., increased lactate threshold level). Additionally, there is an increase in muscle myoglobin content, which enhances the transport of oxygen from the cell membrane to the mitochondria. This may help to explain why training helps individuals attain aerobic steady state in a shorter period of time, thus reducing the oxygen deficit during the initial period of exercise.

Cardiovascular Adaptations

Cardiovascular system adaptations to endurance exercise training include a larger cardiac muscle mass, a higher maximum cardiac output, and a lower heart rate for any given level of submaximal exercise. During exercise, an elevated heart rate results in less time spent in diastole (the relaxation phase of the cardiac cycle). Training enhances the weight and volume of the heart and left ventricular thickness and chamber size. This allows for an increased stroke volume, alongside a more forceful contraction, by facilitating a more complete filling of the left ventricle during diastole. As a result, stroke volume increases during submaximal and maximal exercise as well as during rest.

Trained individuals display a lower heart rate at rest and at submaximal exercise levels, but have a correspondingly higher stroke volume than the untrained individual at any given cardiac output level or VO_2. This results in performing the same amount of work with less effort. Subsequently, heart rate at a given intensity can be regarded as an index of cardiovascular fitness, whereas a reduced heart rate at the same exercise intensity is evidence of a cardiovascular training effect. No change occurs in cardiac output at rest or during submaximal exercise as a result of training because heart rate decreases and stroke volume increases (remember, cardiac output = heart rate $\times$ stroke volume). However, the trained individual exhibits significantly higher VO_{2max} values and maximum cardiac output values (due to an increase in stroke volume during maximum exercise) than the untrained individual. During exercise, cardiac output increases up to 18 to 34 liters/min, with initial increases due to increases in both heart rate and stroke volume.[66]

Vascular system adaptations to endurance training result in increases in overall blood volume by expanding plasma volume and by increasing the number of red blood cells. The increase in blood plasma is due both to changes in hormone levels that increase water reabsorption in the kidneys (antidiuretic hormone from the posterior pituitary gland and aldosterone from the adrenal cortex) and an increase in plasma proteins (i.e., albumin). Plasma proteins serve to increase plasma volume through their effect on plasma osmotic pressure, thus causing more water to be retained in the blood vessels. Training also stimulates red blood cell production in bone marrow, which may contribute to the increase in blood volume. An increase in blood volume improves cardiovascular function primarily through increased ventricular preload (the stretch of the left ventricle just before the onset of contraction), which increases stroke volume. This helps the endurance athlete to produce a larger stroke volume than a sedentary person.

Respiratory or Pulmonary Adaptations

The maximum rate at which oxygen can be transported to the alveoli of the lungs does not appear to limit maximum oxygen transport, indicating that the pulmonary or respiratory component of performance is not a limiting factor during endurance training. The reason for this is that more air can be moved into and out of the lungs than is required during exercise. In other words, the capacity of the pulmonary system to deliver oxygen to the body surpasses the ability of the body to use oxygen.

> ## *Key Point:*
> In the healthy individual, the pulmonary system's ability to deliver oxygen to the body far surpasses the ability of the body to use oxygen as a fuel source.

Despite this, adaptations do occur during aerobic training. These adaptations include an improved economy of ventilation and a higher maximum voluntary ventilation due primarily to improvements in respiratory muscle endurance and economy. An improved *economy of ventilation* refers to the respiratory muscles consuming less oxygen at any given level of ventilation, which improves the exercise economy because a greater proportion of the oxygen uptake is consumed by the working muscles. *Maximum voluntary ventilation* is the highest level of ventilation that a seated person can voluntarily achieve over a 15 sec period. The fact that observed values are higher (usually by about 25 percent) than the actual values attained during maximal exercise supports the notion that ventilation is not stressed maximally in exercise and is therefore not a limiting factor.

Gas exchange is unchanged at rest and at submaximal levels of exercise, but increases during maximal exercise, thus resulting in increased O_2 perfusion. Additionally, a−v O_2 difference increases during maximal exercise as a result of training occur secondary to enhanced O_2 extraction by the tissues.

Metabolic Adaptations

Metabolic adaptations to endurance training include increases in the number and size of mitochondria compared to less active muscle tissue. A nearly twofold increase in the level of aerobic system enzymes is also noted. These adaptations greatly increase the capacity to generate ATP via oxidative phosphorylation. Training also results in an increased ability to store glycogen and a slower depletion of muscle and liver glycogen stores, thus allowing exercise to continue for a longer period of time. The lower rate of carbohydrate utilization as an energy source results in a glycogen sparing effect and allows a higher rate of fatty acid utilization by the body during submaximal exercise. However, endurance training does not increase the activity of the ATP-CP or glycolytic system enzymes. This is consistent with the view that muscle strength is not affected by endurance training.

Blood Lactate Adaptations

Aerobic training improves the oxidative capacity of skeletal muscle, delays the onset of blood lactate accumulation, and delays the point at which anaerobic metabolism needs to assist for high intensity exercise to continue. As a result, the onset of blood lactate accumulation occurs at a higher percentage (80 percent to 90 percent) of the trained individual's aerobic capacity.[66,67] Training above the lactate threshold level (anaerobically) serves to improve the body's ability to process lactate, allowing lactate threshold levels to increase.[15,16,21,22] Since accumulated muscle lactate is associated with fatigue, being able to increase the lactate threshold level results in the ability to sustain a higher intensity of continuous submaximal exercise and in a lowering of the muscle and blood levels of lactate during any given level of submaximal exercise.[66,67] In other words, blood lactate accumulation is lower at standard workloads for trained individuals compared to untrained individuals. A low blood lactate level in a trained individual probably reflects both increased lactate production in active skeletal muscle and increased lactate clearance.

*E*XERCISE AND *O*XYGEN *D*ELIVERY

At rest, the primary muscles of inspiration are the diaphragm, the scalene muscles, and the parasternal muscles. Collectively these muscles expand the thorax by producing lower rib cage expansion (diaphragm), rib cage elevation (scalene muscles), and an increase in the anterior-posterior dimension of the rib cage (parasternal muscles). During activity, additional muscles are recruited, including the sternocleidomastoid and external intercostal muscles. The abdominal muscles indirectly assist in inspi-

ration by pushing the diaphragm upward during expiration, increasing its length prior to inspiration. The internal intercostal muscles also assist with expiration during intense exercise. Once air enters the lungs, gas exchange between the alveoli and pulmonary capillary blood occurs. Commonly measured normal lung volume or capacity measurements are displayed in **Figure 4.6.** For this to occur, the alveoli that receive fresh air must be perfused with blood. The blood must have an adequate transit time in the pulmonary capillary to allow time for diffusion of gases. The time needed for CO_2 to move into the alveoli and for O_2 to move into capillary blood is approximately 0.25 seconds.[67,68]

Another important factor for an adequate O_2 delivery system is the O_2 carrying capacity of the blood. The O_2 content of the blood is determined by the amount of hemoglobin in the blood and by the partial pressure of oxygen (PO_2) in the blood. A shift in the oxyhemoglobin curve to the left impairs the amount of O_2 extracted by muscle, whereas a shift to the right facilitates the unloading of O_2 from hemoglobin. An increased concentration of carboxyhemoglobin that occurs with smoking produces a leftward shift of the curve, impairing O_2 delivery. Acidosis and increased body temperature that occur with exercise facilitate the unloading of O_2 from hemoglobin and the diffusion of O_2 from the capillaries to the muscle cells.[67,68]

A final critical factor is the need for a method of regulation that prevents large fluctuations in arterial blood gases and pH. Changes in the partial pressure of O_2 in arterial blood (PaO_2), the partial pressure of CO_2 in arterial blood ($PaCO_2$), and hydrogen ion concentration stimulate the respiratory system and produce changes in ventilation that serve to return the blood gases to normal. The increase in metabolism with exercise results in an increase in

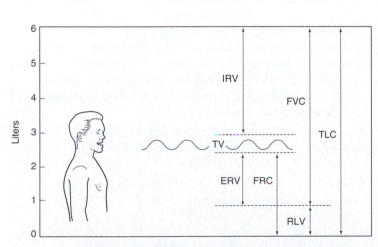

Lung Volume/ Capacity	Definition	Average Values (mL)	
		Men	Women
TV (tidal volume)	Volume inhaled and exhaled with each breath	600	500
IRV (inspiratory reserve volume)	Maximum inhalation at end of tidal inhalation	3000	1900
ERV (expiratory reserve volume)	Maximum exhalation at end of tidal exhalation	1200	800
FRC (functional residual capacity)	Volume in lungs after tidal exhalation	2400	1800
FVC (forced vital capacity)	Maximum volume exhaled after maximum inhalation	4800	3200
RLV (residual lung volume)	Volume in lungs after maximum exhalation	1200	1000
TLC (total lung capacity)	Volume in lungs after maximum inhalation	6000	4200

Figure 4.6   Normal lung volume or capacity measurements. (From WD McArdle, FI Katch, VL Katch. *Exercise Physiology Energy, Nutrition, and Human Performance,* 4th ed. Philadelphia: Lippincott Williams & Wilkins, 1996, Figure 12.7, Chapter 12, p. 223.)

CO_2 production so that arterial blood gases and pH remain close to baseline during mild to moderate exercise. The exact mechanism of control is unknown and may involve the rate of CO_2 flow to the lungs or the central nervous system.[67,68] Because of the multiple steps that are involved in the transfer of O_2 from the atmosphere to the skeletal muscles, there are a variety of problems that can contribute to cardiovascular and pulmonary system dysfunction (**Table 4.1**) and their various signs and symptoms (**Table 4.2**).

TABLE 4.1   Components that contribute to cardiovascular and pulmonary system dysfunction[67]

Problem	Mechanism	Examples
Respiratory muscle dysfunction and chest wall deformities	Limits the ability of the thorax to expand, compromising pulmonary ventilation	• Partial or complete paralysis of the respiratory muscles as with some cervical spine disorders, Guillain-Barré syndrome. Progressive muscular diseases such as muscular dystrophy and amyotrophic lateral sclerosis. • Chest wall deformities associated with anklylosing spondylitis, kyphosis, and scoliosis. A less compliant or rigid chest as occurs with normal aging may also limit thoracic expansion.
Ventilation-perfusion mismatching	An imbalance between areas of ventilation and perfusion	• Occurs with obstructive lung diseases such as emphysema and chronic bronchitis.
Diffusion abnormalities	Abnormalities in the alveolar-capillary membrane due to an accumulation of fluid in the alveoli or interstitial space	• Caused by pulmonary diseases that thicken the capillary membrane causing impaired diffusion. This occurs with idiopathic pulmonary fibrosis. In pulmonary edema or congestive heart failure, fluid fills the space between the capillaries and alveoli. Both of these conditions result in impaired O_2 diffusion from the alveoli to the capillary blood. This condition worsens with activity as the blood moves faster through the pulmonary capillaries and there is less time for diffusion.
Inadequate cardiac output	Caused by cardiac abnormalities	• Common causes include myocardial ischemia, heart failure, valvular abnormalities, and cardiac dysrhythmias. Coronary artery vasospasm and atherosclerosis can create myocardial ischemia. Chronic heart failure refers to impaired cardiac muscle contractile properties occurring as a result of many causes including coronary artery disease, myocarditis, hypertension, and some systemic diseases. If any of these conditions is severe the cardiac output may not be sufficient to serve the needs of the body. With less severe conditions cardiac output may be sufficient at rest; however, it becomes inadequate with activity. When this occurs increased demands are placed on the anaerobic metabolic pathways resulting in increased blood lactate levels producing metabolic acidosis.
Limitations in peripheral blood flow	Caused by impaired vasodilation or vasoconstriction capability	• Atherosclerosis of the peripheral arteries decreases blood flow directly because of the lesion or by decreasing the ability of the artery to vasodilate.
Low oxygen-carrying capacity	Caused by anemia	• Lower hemoglobin levels carry less O_2. As the blood reaches the skeletal muscle, the lower PO_2 levels may not provide a sufficient gradient for O_2 diffusion from the blood to the skeletal muscle. Lactic acid then increases, and metabolic acidosis and fatigue result. Tachycardia (rapid heart rate) is a common compensatory mechanism that attempts to increase cardiac output.

TABLE 4.2   Signs and symptoms of cardiovascular and pulmonary system dysfunction

Condition	Signs/symptoms
Respiratory distress	• Difficult breathing, shortness of breath, increased respiration rate, increased use of accessory respiratory muscles, flared nostrils • Chronic coughing • Skin color changes (pallor or cyanosis)
Cardiac dysfunction	• Abnormal responses to activity such as an excessively high or low heart rate, decreasing systolic blood pressure, increased diastolic blood pressure, changes in electrocardiogram (ECG) activity or heart sounds, excessive fatigue • Chest pain • Dyspnea
Peripheral vascular disease	• Intermittent claudication • Decreased or absent peripheral pulses • Changes in the appearance of the involved extremities, which may include dry or cool skin, hair loss, or muscular atrophy

From C Peel. The cardiopulmonary system and movement dysfunction. *Phys Ther*. 1996;76:448–455.

THERMOREGULATION

Humans have the ability to regulate body temperature. This is especially important during exercise, since excess heat is produced by muscle contraction. At rest approximately 70 percent of the body's heat is generated by the internal organs, while during exercise skeletal muscle can account for as much as 90 percent of heat production.[69] Due to the inefficiency of the conversion of chemical energy to mechanical energy, as much as 70 percent of the chemical energy used during muscular contraction is released as heat. However, only a small amount of the heat produced in active skeletal muscle is lost from the skin. Most of the heat is transferred to the body core through venous return to the heart. These increases in body core temperature are sensed by thermoreceptors located in the hypothalamus, which also receives sensory input from the skin.[68,70]

> ## Key Point:
> As much as 70 percent of the chemical energy used during muscular contractions is released as heat.

The body's core temperature must be maintained by neural and hormonal mechanisms at a fairly constant level (37 ± 1°C) despite fluctuations in environmental temperatures. These mechanisms act as a negative feedback control system that causes the body to gain heat when the environmental temperature decreases (when the core temperature falls below 37°C) and to lose heat when the temperature increases (core temperature rises above 37°C). Heat gain is due to an increased rate of heat production associated with a decreased rate of heat removal, whereas heat loss is due to an increased rate of heat removal.

Body temperature during exercise reflects a balance between the rate of added body heat and the rate of removal of body heat. During high intensity exercise (especially in the heat), the rate of heat production surpasses the rate of heat loss, resulting in the rising of core temperature. For example, when a fit individual is exercising at about 80 percent to 90 percent VO_{2max}, heat production could potentially cause body temperature to increase by 1°C every five to eight minutes, if there was no ability of the body to dissipate the heat. Given this scenario, the body temperature could approach dangerous levels, thus forcing the individual to quit exercising.[68,70] When the heat gain exceeds heat loss, the resulting condition is known as *hyperthermia*. Conversely, when heat loss exceeds heat gain, a condition referred to as *hypothermia* may result. To help prevent these conditions from occurring, the body must be able to call upon different heat-losing or heat-conserving mechanisms.

Temperature Regulatory Control

Body temperature is regulated via two types of thermoreceptors: *central* and *peripheral thermoreceptors*. The central thermoreceptors (which reside in the hypothalamus) detect core temperature, while the peripheral thermoreceptors (free nerve endings) detect skin temperature. The hypothalamus serves as the body's temperature servomechanism. The anterior hypothalamus helps to control heat loss, whereas the posterior hypothalamus helps to serve as a heat production and conservation center.

Hyperthermia

Blood flow to the muscles increases with exercise onset and is preferentially diverted away from the non-working muscles, toward the working muscles and skin. As the core temperature increases, afferent signals from the central and peripheral thermoreceptors stimulate the hypothalamus to increase the rate of heat loss by increasing sweating and vasodilation. During vigorous exercise in hot weather, blood flow is diverted to the skin in an effort to dissipate heat. This presents a conflict with the blood flow to the exercising muscles, thus interfering with the body's need to receive fuel and oxygen to continue exercise. However, when faced with conflicting demands, the body will opt to increase blood flow to the muscles so less heat is dissipated through the skin. This causes the body to overheat and explains the decline in exercise performance during hot and humid conditions.

Several adaptive responses take place with regular exercise in a hot, humid environment, especially for individuals accustomed to training in cool weather conditions. These adaptive responses are referred to as *heat acclimatization*. The best way to achieve heat acclimatization is to train daily in the heat for 2–4 hours. Heat acclimatization is fully developed within 7–10 days after initial exposure to exercise in the heat. Once attained, heat acclimatization is usually retained for about two weeks. Adapted responses include (1) an expanded blood volume, (2) an earlier onset

of sweating and a higher sweat rate, and (3) lower concentrations of sodium and chloride in the sweat. Because evaporation of sweat is the primary mechanism of heat dissipation in the exercising client, anything that interferes with this will contribute to the pathophysiology of heat illness. Factors that affect evaporative heat loss include sweat gland acclimatization, the state of hydration, and relative humidity. Normal sweat rates during exercise in an untrained individual may be up to 1.5 L/hour, while a trained individual may lose 2-3 L/hour. Total sweat loss is generally held to be a maximum of 10–15 L/day, and the increase in sweating parallels increases in core temperature.[69] Initially sweat rate is increased by recruiting more sweat glands and subsequently by increasing the sweating rate of each gland. *Relative humidity* (the ratio of water in ambient air to total quantity of water that could be carried in the air) is a vital factor in determining evaporative heat loss effectiveness (**Figure 4.7**). The greater the air temperature and relative humidity, the greater the risk of heat illness.

Hypothermia

Since lower body core temperatures caused by exposure to severe cold causes many biochemical reactions and pathways to become distorted or slowed, it negatively affects athletic performance via all organ systems and especially

Air temperature, °F

Relative humidity	70°	75°	80°	85°	90°	95°	100°	105°	110°	115°	120°
	Heat Sensation										
0%	64°	89°	73°	78°	83°	87°	91°	95°	99°	103°	107°
10%	65°	70°	75°	80°	85°	90°	95°	100°	105°	111°	116°
20%	66°	72°	77°	82°	87°	93°	99°	105°	112°	120°	130°
30%	67°	73°	78°	84°	90°	96°	104°	113°	123°	135°	148°
40%	68°	74°	79°	86°	93°	101°	110°	123°	137°	151°	
50%	69°	75°	81°	88°	96°	107°	120°	135°	150°		
60%	70°	76°	82°	90°	100°	114°	132°	149°			
70%	70°	77°	85°	93°	106°	124°	144°				
80%	72°	78°	88°	97°	113°	136°					
90%	71°	79°	88°	102°	122°						
100%	72°	80°	91°	108°							

Heat sensation	Risk of heat injury
90° – 105°	Possibility of heat cramps
105° – 130°	Heat cramps or heat exhaustion likely Heat stroke possible
130°+	Heat stroke a definite risk

Figure 4.7 Relative humidity (Reprinted with permission from WD McArdle, FI Katch, VL Katch. *Exercise Physiology Energy, Nutrition, and Human Performance*, 4th ed. Baltimore: Lippincott Williams & Wilkins, 1996, Chapter 25, p. 518, Figure 25.10.)

the central nervous and cardiovascular systems. Low body shell temperature can also interfere with athletic performance by weakening and slowing muscle activations, by delaying nerve conduction time, and by facilitating both local and systemic cold induced injuries.[70,71]

Cooling causes the body to shiver. As the core temperature decreases, afferent signals from the central and peripheral thermoreceptors stimulate the hypothalamus to increase the rate of heat production to the body and to decrease the amount of heat loss to the environment. This is accomplished by increasing sympathetic activity to increase the metabolic rate (i.e., shivering, and thermogenic hormones) and by increasing cutaneous vasoconstriction.

The human body remains thermoneutral at ambient temperatures ranging from 82° to 93°F (28°–34°C) and can survive in temperatures as low as −58°F (−50°C).[72] However, the temperature of the body core, internal organs such as the brain, heart, and lungs, must remain within a range of 75° to 105°F (24–40.5°C),[73] remaining more or less constant at 99°F (37.2°C), with some changes resulting from circadian rhythm, altitude, hydration status, and sleep deprivation.[74] When core body temperature is less than 95°F (< 35°C), many biochemical pathways become altered or slowed. Other organ system changes resulting from low core temperature may include decreased insulin activity, increased lactate production resulting in tissue acidosis, and diuresis resulting from increased renal filtration of core blood.[74] Severe cold affects all organ systems, especially the central nervous system and cardiovascular system (**Table 4.3**).

In contrast to core temperature, the body's shell temperature (skin, muscles and extremities) fluctuates widely because of its close contact with environmental stresses.

Cooling of the shell can interfere with athletic ability by weakening and slowing muscle activation and by delaying nerve conduction time.[74]

Outdoor sports performed in cold weather have gained increasing popularity, and the most at risk are clients who engage in cross country sports like skiing (cross country and downhill), backpacking, mountaineering, snowmobiling, and hunting. Almost all cold induced injuries result from an inability to protect oneself from the environment. The physiologic changes of exercise are affected in direct proportion to the intensity of cold stimulation, and cold induced injury may be local (frostbite) or systemic (hypothermia), depending on outdoor temperature and the length of exposure to it.

Hypothermia is defined as core temperature of less than 95°F (< 35°C).[72,75] Primary or accidental hypothermia occurs when normal heat conservation mechanisms cannot overcome low environmental temperature.[72] Secondary hypothermia occurs when heat conservation mechanisms are disturbed by underlying diseases that potentially affect hypothalamic temperature regulation, shivering, redistribution of blood, or ability to leave a cold environment.[76] Infants, because of their large body surface area, which predisposes them to rapid heat loss, and the elderly, because of impaired ability to either sense decreasing temperature[77] or to limit heat loss by peripheral vasoconstriction or shivering, are at greater risk for succumbing to hypothermia than non-impaired young adults.

Drugs that alter the sensory system or that otherwise act on the central nervous system (i.e., barbiturates, phenothiazines) may inhibit the body's response to cold and thus increase susceptibility to cold. Risk of hypothermia is increased by hypothyroidism, hypopituitarism, hypoadrenalism, diabetes, sepsis, and head injury.[77]

TABLE 4.3   Organ system effects observed with decreasing core body temperature measured rectally

Core body temperature		
°F	(°C)	Observed organ system effect
98.6	(37)	Normal functioning
95	(35)	Distorted/slowed biochemical reactions
90	(32)	Decreased cerebral blood flow
90	(32)	Myocardial irritability, atrial fibrillation
82	(28)	Ventricular fibrillation
77	(25)	Changes in cardiovascular autoregulation, decreased heart rate
65	(18)	Asystole
61	(16)	Lowest reported adult hypothermia survival
59	(15)	Lowest reported infant hypothermia survival

From R Sallis, CM Chassay. Recognizing and treating common-cold induced injury in outdoor sports. *Med Sci Sports Exerc* 1999;31(10):1367–1373.

Mild hypothermia occurs when core temperature is 90°–95°F (32°–35°C). During mild hypothermia clients will appear to be pale, cool, and will have maximally vasoconstricted blood flow to the skin. Clients may shiver uncontrollably, and have varying degrees of confusion, disorientation, incoherence, ataxic gait, and be unable to perform fine movements of the hand. These clients have tachycardia, tachypnea, and cold diuresis induced by increased cardiac output and resultantly increased renal perfusion.[76]

Moderate hypothermia occurs when core temperature is 82°–90°F (28°–32°C), with more severe symptoms including severely impaired judgment, muscle rigidity with areflexia, and dilated pupils. In moderate hypothermia the shivering reflex is lost and blood pressure, heart rate, and respiration rate decrease. At this point with no ability to generate heat, the client cools to the ambient temperature and dies if warming is not accomplished.[71]

During *severe hypothermia* core temperature is less than 82°F (< 28°C). In severe hypothermia the client will appear to be dead with undiscernible blood pressure, extremely slow respiration, and in a coma with pupils dilated and rigid and areflexic muscles. Atrial arrhythmia may be present and verticular fibrillations are easily induced even by moving the client slightly.[71]

Out in the field the degree of hypothermia can be estimated by noting the client's level of consciousness and whether they are shivering. A shivering client probably has a core temperature of more than 90°F (32°C) and less severe hypothermia, while clients who are not shivering or who have impaired consciousness generally have a core temperature of less than 90° F (32°C) and more severe hypothermia.[71]

CLINICAL EXERCISE TESTING

Screening

Before embarking on any aerobic endurance training exercise program, it is essential that the rehabilitation clinician examine the client to determine his or her general health status and physiological responses to exercise. This helps to assure the safety of exercise testing and training. Although such an examination is routinely performed with athletes, it is particularly important when attempting to assess functional deficits that may be present in high risk populations. Pre-program clinical exercise testing is useful because it documents the physiologic and subjective responses of the client to exercise. Clients' symptoms generally develop or become most marked during exercise. Important clinical uses of exercise testing include the assessment of exercise capability, to aid in the diagnosis of the cause of exercise limitations/symptoms, to assess factors that might contribute to exercise limitation, to select the components and parameters of a prescriptive exercise training program, to assess the need for specific therapy to

improve exercise performance (oxygen therapy during exercise), and to assess the clients' probable response to a therapeutic exercise program.[78] Common cardiovascular and pulmonary system responses for clients with differing medical conditions are presented in **Table 4.4.** These deficits may be reflected in abnormal responses to exercise and/or reduced exercise capacities. Guidelines for health and evaluation have been established to help delineate symptomatic and asymptomatic individuals through exercise testing.

Graded Exercise Testing

Appropriate development of a therapeutic exercise prescription for cardiopulmonary endurance involves accurate testing of VO_{2max}. This is known as a *graded exercise test*, knowledge of which provides feedback about an individual's aerobic capacity to perform endurance exercise. However, although establishing training intensity from measures of oxygen uptake is fairly accurate, testing of oxygen consumption is not feasible for many clinicians, because of the limited availability of facilities and access to laboratory equipment to directly measure these levels. As a result, effective alternative methods that incorporate a variety of submaximal and maximal tests have been devised to regulate exercise for relative intensity and thereby help to establish training protocols.

Maximal Graded Exercise Testing

A maximal graded exercise test requires that the individual exercise to the point of fatigue. Direct measurement via the use of open-circuit spirometry is used to assess VO_{2max}. Although many accepted protocols can be used to administer a maximal graded exercise test, all protocols employ regular progressive increments of work intensity.[70] It should be noted that, for the average individual, VO_{2max} and HR_{max} values vary when they are measured on different pieces of equipment (e.g., VO_{2max} values are generally higher during testing on a treadmill than on a cycle ergometer). However, when exercise intensity is expressed as a percentage of their respective maximal values, the relationship is nearly identical. Because a maximal graded exercise test is costly and often not a feasible method of assessment for most rehabilitation clinicians to perform, it is primarily reserved for testing specific client populations, for research, and for testing athletes. However, VO_{2max} can be estimated from prediction equations and submaximal tests. Subsequently, submaximal tests are commonly used to assess cardiopulmonary system endurance.

Submaximal Graded Exercise Testing

The equations used during submaximal exercise testing make assumptions that tend to increase their error (**Table 4.5**). Although not as precise as maximal exercise testing,

TABLE 4.4   Cardiovascular and pulmonary system responses for common medical conditions

	Chronic Obstructive Pulmonary Disease (COPD)	Restrictive lung disease	Congestive heart failure	Mitral valve disease	Pulmonary vascular disease	Poor fitness level
VO_{2Max}	Decreased	Decreased	Decreased	Decreased	Decreased	Decreased
Heart rate during submaximal work	Increased	Increased or no change	Increased	Increased	Increased	Increased
Maximal heart rate	Decreased, rarely no change	Decreased	Decreased or no change	No change	Decreased	No change
Minute ventilation during submaximal work	Increased or no change	Increased	Increased	Increased	Increased	Increased above anaerobic threshold
Peak minute ventilation/ maximal voluntary ventilation	Both components are increased	Increased	No change	No change	No change	No change / decreased
Peak tidal volume/ vital capacity	No change or decreased	No change	No change	No change	No change or questionable effects	No change
Arterial O_2 desaturation	$+$ or $-$ O_2 desaturation with exercise	$+$ O_2 desaturation with exercise	$-$ O_2 desaturation with exercise	$-$ O_2 desaturation with exercise	$+$ O_2 desaturation with exercise	$-$ O_2 desaturation with exercise

(From CG Gallagher. Exercise and chronic obstructive pulmonary disease. *Med Clin N Am.* 1990;74(3):619–641.)

submaximal exercise testing is commonly used to predict VO_{2max}. Nevertheless, submaximal graded exercise testing provides a useful estimate of an individual's aerobic fitness level. Procedures involved in the submaximal graded exercise testing require that the individual exercise at a progressively increasing work rate to cause the heart rate to gradually increase in a systematic manner. When the heart rate equals 85 percent of the age adjusted maximal heart rate, the test is terminated. Plotting the points on a graph allows the VO_{2max} (work rate) to be estimated.

TABLE 4.5   Assumptions made during submaximal exercise tests

- A steady-state heart rate is obtained for each exercise work rate.
- A linear relationship exists between heart rate and work rate.
- The maximal heart rate for a given age is uniform.
- Mechanical efficiency (i.e., VO_2 at a given work rate) is the same for everyone.

(Reprinted with permission from *American College of Sports Medicine's Guidelines for Exercise Testing and Prescription*, 6th ed. Baltimore: Lippincott Williams & Wilkins, 2000, p. 69.)

The supervision of a physician is recommended during maximal or submaximal graded exercise testing for individuals who are symptomatic or who are experiencing coronary artery disease. The ACSM also recommends physician supervision during graded exercise testing for men over 40 years of age or women over 50 years of age who have two or more risk factors for coronary artery disease, but who are asymptomatic. However, physician supervision is generally not required for testing of men and women under the age of 40 and 50, respectively, who are asymptomatic. In these cases, rehabilitation clinicians who are familiar with the specific graded exercise testing protocols can safely administer testing. For further information, refer to the *ACSM's Guidelines for Exercise Testing and Prescription*[70] and the comprehensive work of Noonan and Dean on clinical application and interpretation of submaximal exercise testing.[79]

LABORATORY TESTING

Laboratory exercise tests such as the treadmill, cycle ergometer, and step tests are commonly used to predict VO_{2max}. Test selection should be based on several criteria: safety, knowledge of testing protocol, equipment availability, and client's limitations.

Treadmill

Submaximal treadmill tests have been developed for low-fit to high-fit individuals. The goal of the test is to raise the steady-state heart rate of the subject to 85 percent of the age predicted maximal heart rate (HR_{max}) for at least two consecutive stages. A single stage submaximal treadmill test has been developed for testing low risk individuals. However, according to the ACSM, the stages of the test should be three minutes or longer; this limitation is placed in an effort to ensure a steady state heart rate response for each stage.[70] Common testing protocols are presented in **Figure 4.8.** Normative values for maximal aerobic power are given in **Table 4.6.** Using a modified Balke test, research by Blair et al.[1] suggested that an increased risk of death from all causes is associated with a VO_{2max} below the 20th percentile.

Cycle Ergometer

The Astrand-Rhyming test[80] is a six minute single stage test with the work rate based on gender and activity status. In this test, heart rate is measured during the fifth and sixth minute of work. A nomogram is then used to estimate VO_{2max} from the average of the two heart rates, which is then adjusted for age (since heart rate decreases with age) according to a correction factor (**Figure 4.9; Table 4.7**).[70] The YMCA cycle test is another commonly used graded exercise test.[81]

Step

A wide variety of step tests have been developed to categorize cardiopulmonary and cardiovascular fitness and can be used to test large numbers of individuals. For example, Astrand and Rhyming[80] used a single-step height of 33 cm for women and 40 cm for men at a rate of 22.5 steps/min to estimate VO_{2max}. The work rate can be varied by increasing the step rate and keeping the step height the same, or by increasing the step height and varying the cadence. This allows testing of low fit as well as active individuals. The ACSM recommends that these tests be modified to suit the population being tested.[70]

FIELD TESTING

Field tests are submaximal in nature, are used for testing large groups of people, and are fairly easy to administer. The two most commonly used field tests are the Cooper 12 minute test and the 1.5 mile test for time. The goal of the Cooper 12 minute test is for the individual to cover the greatest amount of distance possible during the 12 minute time period. The objective of the 1.5 mile test is to run the distance in the shortest amount of time possible. VO_{2max} can then be estimated from the 1.5 mile test using the equation, $VO_{2max} = 3.5 + 483/(\text{time in minutes})$.[70] A potential risk exists in that individuals are encouraged to

Functional class	Clinical status	O₂ cost mL·kg⁻¹·min⁻¹	Mets	Bicycle ergometer	Bruce 3 Min stages MPH/GR	Kattus MPH/GR	Balke-Ware /Grade at 3.3 mph 1-min stages	Ellestad 3/2/3 min stages MPH/GR	USAFSAM MPH/GR	"Slow" USAFSAM MPH/GR	McHenry MPH/GR	Stanford /Grade at 3 mph	Stanford /Grade at 2 mph
Normal and I (Healthy, dependent on age, activity)				1 watt = 5 kpm/min	5.5 / 20		26						
		56.0	16	For 70 kg body weight kpm/min 1500	5.0 / 18		25, 24	6 / 15					
		52.5	15				23		3.3 / 25				
		49.0	14			4 / 22	22, 21	5 / 15					
		45.5	13	1350	4.2 / 16		20, 19		3.3 / 20				
		42.0	12	1200		4 / 18	18				3.3 / 21	22.5	
		38.5	11	1050			17	5 / 10		2 / 25	3.3 / 18	20.0	
		35.0	10	900		4 / 14	16, 15		3.3 / 15		3.3 / 15	17.5	
	(Sedentary healthy)	31.5	9	750	3.4 / 14		14, 13	4 / 10		2 / 20		15.0	
		28.0	8			4 / 10	12		3.3 / 10	2 / 15	3.3 / 12	12.5	
		24.5	7	600	2.5 / 12	3 / 10	11, 10	3 / 10				10.0	17.5
II (Limited)		21.0	6	450		2 / 10	9, 8		3.3 / 5	2 / 10	3.3 / 9	7.5	14
		17.5	5	300	1.7 / 10		7	1.7 / 10			3.3 / 6	5.0	10.5
III (Symptomatic)		14.0	4		1.7 / 5		6, 5		3.3 / 0	2 / 5		2.5	7
		10.5	3	150			4, 3				2.0 / 3	0.0	3.5
		7.0	2		1.7 / 0		2			2.0 / 0			
IV		3.5	1				1						

Figure 4.8   Common exercise protocols. Stage I of the conventional Bruce treadmill protocol starts at 1.7 mph, 10 percent grade. The modified Bruce protocol may start at 1.7 mph, 0 percent grade, or at 1.7 mph, 5 percent grade, shown here. (Reprinted with permission from *American College of Sports Medicine's Guidelines for Exercise Testing and Prescription*, 6th ed. Baltimore: Lippincott Williams & Wilkins, 2000, p. 98.)

TABLE 4.6   Percentile values for maximal aerobic power $(mL \cdot kg^{-1} \cdot min^{-1})$*

Percentile	Age				
	20–29	30–39	40–49	50–59	60+
Men					
90	51.4	50.4	48.2	45.3	42.5
80	48.2	46.8	44.1	41.0	38.1
70	46.8	44.6	41.8	38.5	35.3
60	44.2	42.4	39.9	36.7	33.6
50	42.5	41.0	38.1	35.2	31.8
40	41.0	38.9	36.7	33.8	30.2
30	39.5	37.4	35.1	32.3	28.7
20	37.1	35.4	33.0	30.2	26.5
10	34.5	32.5	30.9	28.0	23.1
Women					
90	44.2	41.0	39.5	35.2	35.2
80	41.0	38.6	36.3	32.3	31.2
70	38.1	36.7	33.8	30.9	29.4
60	36.7	34.6	32.3	29.4	27.2
50	35.2	33.8	30.9	28.2	25.8
40	33.8	32.3	29.5	26.9	24.5
30	32.3	30.5	28.3	25.5	23.8
20	30.6	28.7	26.5	24.3	22.8
10	28.4	26.5	25.1	22.3	20.8

Data provided by Institute for Aerobics Research, Dallas, TX (1994). The study population for the data set was predominantly white and college educated. A modified Balke treadmill test was used with VO_{2max} estimated from the last grade/speed achieved. The following may be used as descriptors for the percentile rankings: well above average (90), above average (70), average (50), below average (30), and well below average (10).

(Reprinted with permission from *American College of Sports Medicine's Guidelines for Exercise Testing and Prescription*, 6th ed. Baltimore: Lippincott Williams & Wilkins, 2000, p. 77.)

put forth a maximal effort, which may be inappropriate for sedentary and symptomatic individuals.

LIFESPAN CHANGES

The primary component for the age related decline in VO_{2max} is the decline in maximum cardiac output.[82,83] After 25 years of age, individuals experience gradual decreases in VO_{2max} of about 5 percent to 9 percent per decade, depending on the level of exercise maintained by

the individual.[83] A potential cause for the decrease in VO_{2max} with age may be the age related decrease in maximum heart rate and therefore maximum cardiac output. It also may reflect a progressive decrease in muscle contractility or a loss of muscle mass with age. Interestingly, research has suggested that changes in aerobic capacity associated with increasing age may not be entirely age related. Age therefore may not influence the degree to which VO_{2max} increases with training, with similar increases observed in the elderly as in younger individuals.[84,85]

There is evidence to support that an inactive lifestyle contributes to the decline in cardiac function and, therefore, VO_{2max}. In examining endurance trained men, Meredith et al.[86] reported that maximal aerobic capacity was not related to age but rather to the total number of hours spent exercising per week. Studies have shown that a decline in VO_{2max} can be slowed down with endurance training and that sufficient exercise training in older sedentary adults could increase VO_{2max} to the same level as it did in younger people.[87,88]

Other research has revealed that the absolute gains in aerobic capacity were similar between initially sedentary 20–30 year old subjects and subjects who were 60–70 years of age.[84] In this study, the researchers reported that the mechanism for adaptation to regular submaximal exercise appeared to differ between the two groups. A more than twofold increase in the oxidative capacity of the muscles in the older subjects over the younger subjects was identified via muscle biopsies taken after training.

It has also been shown that the mechanisms involved in training-induced VO_{2max} increases differ between older men and women. Spina et al.[89] reported that older men increased VO_{2max} primarily via an increase in stroke volume (66 percent). In contrast, older women demonstrated no change in stroke volume; the entire increase in VO_{2max} was accounted for by a greater a-v O_2 difference during maximal exercise. In summary, maintenance of regular exercise is associated with greater cardiopulmonary and cardiovascular system benefits among older adults.

INTRODUCTION TO AEROBIC EXERCISE PRESCRIPTION

Considerations in Aerobic Exercise Prescription

Rehabilitation clinicians face a significant challenge designing therapeutic exercise programs that both elicit the desired physiological response and accommodate the lifestyle and motivation of each individual client. Appropriate therapeutic exercise prescription requires careful consideration of factors that may influence program effectiveness, efficiency, and safety. Addressing these issues

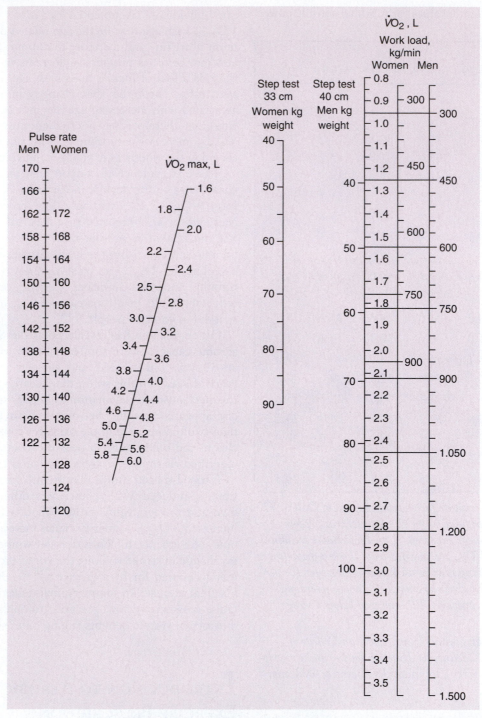

Figure 4.9   The Modified Astrand-Ryhming nomogram. (Reprinted with permission from PO Astrand, I Ryhming. A nomogram for calculation of aerobic capacity [physical fitness] from pulse rate during submaximal work. *J Appl Physiol* 1954;7:218–221.)

requires knowledge of physiology, anatomy, biomechanics, neuroscience, and psychology and application of these basic sciences to the clinical decision making process. When prescribing therapeutic exercises specifically aimed at improving aerobic power, answers to certain key questions are critical. The question list below is not meant to be comprehensive but to stimulate consideration of issues that impact therapeutic exercise program development.

- What is the person's general health status?
- Are there personal or family health history findings that indicate risk factors for pulmonary or cardiovascular disease?

TABLE 4.7   Age correction factors

Age	Correction factor
15	1.10
25	1.00
35	0.87
40	0.83
45	0.78
50	0.75
55	0.71
60	0.68
65	0.65

(Reprinted with permission from *American College of Sports Medicine's Guidelines for Exercise Testing and Prescription*, 6th ed. Baltimore: Lippincott Williams & Wilkins, 2000, p. 74.)

- Is the person taking any medications and if so, how do those medicines affect exercise?
- Does the person have pathology and subsequent impairments that affect exercise?
- What are the physiological and biomechanical demands of the person's work or recreational activities?
- What is the person's exercise history? What is their attitude towards exercise?
- How much time does the person have in their schedule for exercise? Do they have access to exercise facilities?
- What is the person's social support system?
- What is the person's preferred learning style?
- What are the person's specific goals?

Exercise Program Adherence

An understanding of the behavioral influences that affect therapeutic exercise adherence is critical for the rehabilitation clinician. Approximately 50 percent of people who start exercise programs will discontinue the program during the first year. Exercise program adherence is influenced by personal factors, including behavioral and attitudinal characteristics, social factors, and program factors.[90,91] Research has shown that major personal factors negatively influencing exercise program adherence include cigarette smoking, inactivity in occupation and leisure, and blue collar employment.[92,93] Social factors affecting compliance include spousal support, exercise companions, and the presence of positive feedback. Program variables which effect exercise adherence include time and location, exercise variety, exercise intensity, and program leadership.[92] In an effort to maximize the client's commitment to health and wellness, rehabilitation clinicians should consider implementing strategies that will encour-

TABLE 4.8   Strategies to encourage therapeutic exercise program adherence

- Patient/client participation in goal setting
- Appropriate selection and variety of exercises based on the patient/client's needs and goals
- Appropriate exercise program progression. Pushing a client too hard or not providing sufficient progression will discourage adherence
- Use of some form of positive reinforcement for achievement
- Use of visual charts or logs to document exercise progress
- Education on how to prevent musculoskeletal injury
- Well trained and enthusiastic leadership
- Create social support systems for clients through group programs and/or spousal support
- Focus on fun
- Creation of exercise habits: time of day, days of the week, etc.

age exercise program adherence. A list of possible strategies is provided in **Table 4.8.** Further information regarding methods of improving therapeutic exercise program compliance is reported in Chapter 11.

COMPONENTS OF AEROBIC POWER EXERCISE PRESCRIPTION

Following clinical exercise testing, an appropriate therapeutic exercise program can be designed. Cardiopulmonary rehabilitation programs should focus on reducing the work of breathing, improving pulmonary function, normalizing arterial blood gases, alleviating dyspnea, increasing the efficiency of energy utilization, correcting nutritional habits, improving exercise and activities of daily living performance, restoring a positive emotional outlook in the client, decreasing health care costs, improving the quality of life, and improving survival time.[95] Components of a comprehensive cardiopulmonary rehabilitation program should include both client and family education, dyspnea assessment, a comprehensive therapeutic exercise program, nutritional assessment and support, breathing retraining and expectoration techniques, and psychosocial support.[96] Troosters et al.[97] evaluated the effects of a therapeutic exercise program on clients with severe COPD. In their randomized study, 50 clients received a program consisting of stationary cycling, walking and strength training, and 50 clients received only the usual medical care. At six months after program intervention, the therapeutic exercise group displayed greater significant and clinically relevant improvements in 6 min walking distance, maximal exercise performance, peripheral and respiratory muscle strength, and quality of life compared to the control group. Most of these positive training effects were still evident at 18 months after program initiation. Cardiopulmonary training programs vary greatly in their level of complexity and expense. There is little evidence that supports the superiority of more complex, comprehensive programs in achieving improved subjective and objective outcome parameters compared to simple therapeutic exercise programs supervised by knowledgeable rehabilitation clinicians.[98] O'Donnell et al.[98] proposed a pulmonary training program with primary goals of reducing breathlessness and improving exercise capacity. Their program consisted of a multimodality endurance training program with an education component, which was conducted by two physical therapists in consultation with a pulmonologist. Their program was individualized for each client based on preliminary testing results. Aerobic training of as large a muscle mass as possible was achieved using walking, stair climbing, treadmill exercise, cycle ergometry, and arm ergometry. Their program regulated training intensity primarily on the basis of symptom tolerance. They abandoned conventional heart rate training targets because they are considered to be less reliable for clients who have COPD compared with non-impaired clients.[99] Training intensity was guided by targeted Borg perceived exertion ratings for breathlessness relative to levels observed during pre-program evaluation. Using a graduated, step-wise approach, clients were encouraged to train at progressively higher intensity levels until achieving their highest attainable work level for the longest tolerable duration. Their eight-week program consisted of three, two- to three-hour sessions per week and bi-weekly educational sessions aimed at increasing clients' knowledge about their disease and the rationale for effective management. For clients with incapacitating breathlessness, they also employed breathing re-training techniques including pursed-lips breathing.[98]

The primary variables in prescribing exercise for improving aerobic power are intensity, duration, frequency, and mode. However, these variables must be considered in the context of client-specific factors such as medical history, health status, exercise history, functional needs, motivation, client goals, and psychosocial issues to insure that the therapeutic exercise program will be both safe and effective. Therapeutic exercise prescription requires an effective integration of exercise science with behavioral techniques (see Chapter 11). When these components are effectively integrated, the result is long-term program compliance and the attainment of the individual's goals.

Overload Principle

As the body adapts to a given level of exercise stimulus, manipulation of the primary exercise variables must occur in order to improve performance. In other words, for a training adaptation to occur, the individual must exercise at a level beyond that which is typically performed; this is known as the overload principle. The concept of overload applies to sedentary people and disabled individuals as well as athletes. Applied appropriately, overload enables the body to function more efficiently at a higher level. How much one improves performance depends on factors such as age, gender, genetics, and current level of fitness.

Reversibility Principle

In order to maintain a high level of conditioning, it is important to adhere to a regular training program. When training stops, training-induced gains in physical performance disappear very quickly. This concept is referred to as the *reversibility principle* or detraining, and it encompasses the notion that substantial decreases in exercise capacity may occur in as little as one to two weeks of inactivity. Regardless of how many prior years of exercise or training an individual has undergone, the beneficial effects of exercise can be reversed. Therefore, it is important to maintain current levels of conditioning during rehabilitation and to initiate a reconditioning program if needed to offset exercise capacity decreases.

Aerobic Exercise Intensity

Intensity is a critical issue in appropriately prescribing therapeutic exercise to improve aerobic power. This variable will most strongly influence the client's perception of how "hard" the exercise is to perform. Several clinical measures of exercise intensity are described in the literature, including percentage of VO_{2max} or *oxygen uptake reserve* (VO_2R), percentage of HR_{max} or *heart rate reserve* (HRR), *rating of perceived exertion* (RPE), multiples of metabolic equivalents (METs), and exercising below, at, or above the lactate threshold. The VO_2R is the difference between $VO_{2\ max}$ and resting oxygen uptake, and the HRR is the difference between maximal and resting heart rates. Swain et al.[100] have shown that the percentage of heart rate reserve is equivalent to the percentage of VO_2R. Ideally, exercise intensity should be based on maximum heart rate or VO_{2max} as determined through mode specific clinical exercise testing as described earlier in the chapter. If these data are available, then calculations using HR_{max}, HRR, VO_{2max} or VO_2R can be used, provided they are used to set standards on the same exercise device as that used during testing.

If exercise-testing data are not available, HR_{max} can be predicted based on age (predicted maximum heart rate = 220 − age). However, this prediction model has potential inaccuracies.[101,102] The "220 − age" equation may overestimate HR_{max} for younger individuals and underestimate HR_{max} for older individuals. A recent meta-analysis confirmed that this method underestimates the HR_{max} for older adults, and the authors recommended revising the equation for predicted HR_{max} to $208 - (0.7 \times age)$.[103] This revised formula slightly lowers the predicted HR_{max} for the young adult but significantly raises the predicted HR_{max} for older adults.

A meta-analysis conducted by Londeree and Moeschberger[104] confirmed that age was the most important predictor of HR_{max} and that there was considerable variability in its estimate. Others have reported that estimated HR_{max} values are too variable to be relied upon for precisely guiding exercise intensity during cycling or running. O'Toole et al.[105] recommended that formal maximal exercise tests be performed to determine true HR_{max} values in each exercise mode. Given the error involved in estimating HR_{max}, it is important to remember to use it only as a guideline.

According to the ACSM,[70] exercise intensity should range between 55 percent and 90 percent of HR_{max}, or 40 percent and 85 percent of VO_2R or HRR. The individual's fitness level and goals will determine what specific percentage of maximum heart rate, VO_2R or HRR are used. For highly deconditioned clients, 55 percent of HR_{max} or 40 percent of VO_2R or HRR is appropriate to begin improving their aerobic fitness.[106] Swain and Franklin[107] reported that training studies support the use of 45 percent VO_2R as a minimal effective training intensity for higher fit subjects, and 30 percent VO_2R for lower fit subjects. However aerobic power training of highly conditioned athletes requires intensities of 85 percent to 90 percent of HR_{max} or 80 percent to 85 percent of VO_2R or HRR. For most individuals without cardiopulmonary or cardiovascular system pathology, training in the 70 percent to 85 percent of HR_{max} or 60 percent to 80 percent VO_2R or HRR is appropriate to stimulate improvement in their aerobic function as measured by VO_{2max} or lactate threshold.[106]

Establishing exercise intensity based on lactate threshold has been shown to be an effective method of improving aerobic power.[108] As previously described, lactate threshold can be quantified by the onset of blood lactate accumulation defined as a 4.0 mM blood lactate value. Training at the lactate threshold is essential for stimulating the body to work at elevated intensities, serves to improve the body's ability to process lactate, and increases VO_{2max} as well as the percentage of VO_{2max} that can effectively be used before the onset of blood lactate accumulation.[20] The disadvantage of this method is that it requires periodic drawing of blood samples during exercise to plot the blood lactate concentration in relation to exercise intensity. Exercising at or slightly above the onset of blood lactate accumulation ensures that the individual is training at an intensity that will stimulate an improvement in aerobic power. As aerobic fitness improves, the lactate threshold will change. Therefore, periodic lactate threshold re-evaluation should be performed to know when the exercise intensity should be increased.

Another measure used to establish exercise intensity is metabolic equivalents or *METs*. One MET describes the energy expenditure of an individual at rest (resting metabolic rate) and is equal to about 3.5 ml/kg/min. The MET is also equivalent to one Kcal/kg/hr. This measure allows rehabilitation clinicians and researchers to describe the energy requirements of an activity or exercise session as multiples of the resting metabolic rate. Ainsworth[109] presented a summary of the metabolic costs of over 500 physical activities (**Table 4.9**). This compendium was obtained primarily from previously published physical activity energy expenditure lists. A "T" followed by a code numbr identifies activity energy expenditures taken from the Minnesota Leisure Time Physical Activity Questionnaire. For example, the energy requirement of walking three miles per hour on a level, firm surface is approximately 3.5 METs.[109] Maximal aerobic capacity for men and women usually range from 8 to 12 METs, with older adults generally averaging a maximal capacity of five to eight METs. Highly trained adults, however, have been shown to attain 15 to 20 METs or more capacity.[110] The range for exercise intensity prescribed corresponds to the percentage of VO_{2max} desired (i.e., 60 percent to 80 percent of VO_{2max} would equal 60 percent to 80 percent of the total METs). The exercise prescription in terms of METs requires knowledge of maximal MET values based on graded exercise test results. If this value is known, the target MET level can be calculated and then used in the formula below:

$$\text{Target MET} = (\text{desired exercise intensity})(\text{maximal MET} - \text{resting MET}) + \text{resting MET}$$

In this equation, the VO_{2rest} is expressed as 1 MET, or 3.5 ml/kg · min. In an example in which a client had a maximal VO_{2max} of 14 METs, or 49 ml/kg · min, and the desired exercise intensity was 65 percent, the target MET level would be 9.45 METs or 33 ml/kg · min. Using **Table 4.9**, an appropriate physical activity would be chosen based on that desired MET level. In this example, jogging at an 11 minute per mile pace would be appropriate to achieve the targeted MET level. This method of determining exercise is quite simple, but has its limitations. The MET values listed in **Table 4.9** are estimates of energy expenditure; the actual values vary based on metabolic rate, skill, and environmental conditions. While this method of setting exercise intensity does not require heart rate or oxygen consumption monitoring, it should be used with caution, and physiological monitoring of clients is encouraged. It has been shown that a regular exercise program can increase the maximal MET level by $20 \pm 10\%$ in three months.[106]

Ratings of perceived exertion can also be used to regulate training intensity during aerobic endurance training, as this measure correlates well with other indices of exercise intensity such as heart rate and oxygen consumption

TABLE 4.9   Compendium of physical activities (code, METS)

01009	8.5	Bicycling	Bicycling, BMX or mountain
01010	4.0	Bicycling	Bicycling, < 10 mph, general, leisure, to work or for pleasure (T115)
01020	6.0	Bicycling	Bicycling, 10–11.9 mph, leisure, slow, light effort
01030	8.0	Bicycling	Bicycling, 12–13.9 mph, leisure, moderate effort
01040	10.0	Bicycling	Bicycling, 14–15.9 mph, racing or leisure, fast, vigorous effort
01050	12.0	Bicycling	Bicycling, 16–19 mph, racing/not drafting or >19 mph drafting, very fast, racing general
01060	16.0	Bicycling	Bicycling, >20 mph, racing, not drafting
01070	5.0	Bicycling	Unicycling
02010	5.0	Conditioning exercise	Bicycling, stationary, general
02011	3.0	Conditioning exercise	Bicycling, stationary, 50 W, very light effort
02012	5.5	Conditioning exercise	Bicycling, stationary, 100 W, light effort
02013	7.0	Conditioning exercise	Bicycling, stationary, 150 W, moderate effort
02014	10.5	Conditioning exercise	Bicycling, stationary, 200 W, vigorous effort
02015	12.5	Conditioning exercise	Bicycling, stationary, 250 W, very vigorous effort
02020	8.0	Conditioning exercise	Calisthenics (e.g., pushups, pullups, situps), heavy, vigorous effort
02030	4.5	Conditioning exercise	Calisthenics, home exercise, light or moderate effort, general (T 150) (example: back exercises), going up & down from floor
02040	8.0	Conditioning exercise	Circuit training, general
02050	6.0	Conditioning exercise	Weight lifting (free weight, nautilus or universal-type), power lifting or body building, vigorous effort (T 210)
02060	5.5	Conditioning exercise	Health club exercise, general (T 160)
02065	6.0	Conditioning exercise	Stair-treadmill ergometer, general
02070	9.5	Conditioning exercise	Rowing, stationary ergometer, general
02071	3.5	Conditioning exercise	Rowing, stationary, 50 W, light effort
02072	7.0	Conditioning exercise	Rowing, stationary, 100 W, moderate effort
02073	8.5	Conditioning exercise	Rowing, stationary, 150 W, vigorous effort
02074	12.0	Conditioning exercise	Rowing, stationary, 200 W, very vigorous effort
02080	9.5	Conditioning exercise	Ski machine, general
02090	6.0	Conditioning exercise	Slimnastics
02100	4.0	Conditioning exercise	Stretching, hatha yoga
02110	6.0	Conditioning exercise	Teaching aerobic exercise class
02120	4.0	Conditioning exercise	Water aerobics, water calisthenics
02130	3.0	Conditioning exercise	Weight lifting (free, nautilus or universal-type), light or moderate effort, light workout, general
02135	1.0	Conditioning exercise	Whirlpool, sitting
03010	6.0	Dancing	Aerobic, ballet or modern, twist
03015	6.0	Dancing	Aerobic, general
03020	5.0	Dancing	Aerobic, low impact
03021	7.0	Dancing	Aerobic, high impact
03025	4.5	Dancing	General
03030	5.5	Dancing	Ballroom, fast (disco, folk, square) (T 125)
03040	3.0	Dancing	Ballroom, slow (e.g., waltz, foxtrot, slow dancing)
04001	4.0	Fishing and hunting	Fishing, general

TABLE 4.9   Compendium of physical activities (code, METS) (continued)

04010	4.0	Fishing and hunting	Digging worms, with shovel
04020	5.0	Fishing and hunting	Fishing from river bank and walking
04030	2.5	Fishing and hunting	Fishing from boat, sitting
04040	3.5	Fishing and hunting	Fishing from river bank, standing (T 660)
04050	6.0	Fishing and hunting	Fishing in stream, in waders (T 670)
04060	2.0	Fishing and hunting	Fishing, ice, sitting
04070	2.5	Fishing and hunting	Hunting, bow and arrow or crossbow
04080	6.0	Fishing and hunting	Hunting, deer, elk, large game (T 710)
04090	2.5	Fishing and hunting	Hunting, duck, wading
04100	5.0	Fishing and hunting	Hunting, general
04110	6.0	Fishing and hunting	Hunting, pheasants or grouse (T 680)
04120	5.0	Fishing and hunting	Hunting, rabbit, squirrel, prairie chick, raccoon, small game (T 690)
04130	2.5	Fishing and hunting	Pistol shooting or trap shooting, standing
05010	2.5	Home activities	Carpet sweeping, sweeping floors
05020	4.5	Home activities	Cleaning, heavy or major (e.g., wash car, wash windows, mop, clean garage), vigorous effort
05030	3.5	Home activities	Cleaning, house or cabin, general
05040	2.5	Home activities	Cleaning, light (dusting, straightening up, vacuuming, changing linen, carrying out trash), moderate effort
05041	2.3	Home activities	Wash dishes-standing or in general (not broken into stand/walk components)
	2.3	Home activities	Wash dishes; cleaning dishes from table-walking
05050	2.5	Home activities	Cooking or food preparation-standing or sitting or in general (not broken into stand/walk components)
05051	2.5	Home activities	Serving food, setting table-implied walking or standing
05052	2.5	Home activities	Cooking or food preparation-walking
05055	2.5	Home activities	Putting away groceries (e.g., carrying groceries, shopping without a grocery cart)
05056	8.0	Home activities	Carrying groceries upstairs
05060	3.5	Home activities	Food shopping, with grocery cart
05065	2.0	Home activities	Standing-shopping (non-grocery shopping)
05066	2.3	Home activities	Walking-shopping (non-grocery shopping)
05070	2.3	Home activities	Ironing
05080	1.5	Home activities	Sitting, knitting, sewing, light wrapping (presents)
05090	2.0	Home activities	Implied standing-laundry, fold or hang clothes, put clothes in washer or dryer, packing suitcase
05095	2.3	Home activities	Implied walking-putting away clothes, gathering clothes to pack, putting away laundry
05100	2.0	Home activities	Making bed
05110	5.0	Home activities	Maple syruping/sugar bushing (including carrying buckets, carrying wood)
05120	6.0	Home activities	Moving furniture, household
05130	5.5	Home activities	Scrubbing floors, on hands and knees
05140	4.0	Home activities	Sweeping garage, sidewalk or outside of house
05145	7.0	Home activities	Moving household items, carrying boxes

TABLE 4.9   Compendium of physical activities (code, METS) (continued)

05146	3.5	Home activities	Standing-packing/unpacking boxes, occasional lifting of household items light-moderate effort
05147	3.0	Home activities	Implied walking-putting away household items-moderate effort
05150	9.0	Home activities	Move household items upstairs, carrying boxes or furniture
05160	2.5	Home activities	Standing-light (pump gas, change light bulb, etc.)
05165	3.0	Home activities	Walking-light, noncleaning (ready to leave, shut/lock doors, close windows, etc.)
05170	2.5	Home activities	Sitting-playing with child(ren)-light
05171	2.8	Home activities	Standing-playing with child(ren)-light
05175	4.0	Home activities	Walk/run-playing with child(ren)-moderate
05180	5.0	Home activities	Walk/run-playing with child(ren)-vigorous
05185	3.0	Home activities	Child care: sitting/kneeling-dressing, bathing, grooming, feeding, occasional lifting of child-light effort
05186	3.5	Home activities	Child care: standing-dressing, bathing, feeding, occasional lifting of child-light effort
06010	3.0	Home repair	Airplane repair
06020	4.5	Home repair	Automobile body work
06030	3.0	Home repair	Automobile repair
06040	3.0	Home repair	Carpentry, general, workshop (T 620)
06050	6.0	Home repair	Carpentry, outside house (T 640) installing rain gutters
06060	4.5	Home repair	Carpentry, finishing or refinishing cabinets or furniture
06070	7.5	Home repair	Carpentry, sawing hardwood
06080	5.0	Home repair	Caulking, chinking log cabin
06090	4.5	Home repair	Caulking, except log cabin
06100	5.0	Home repair	Cleaning gutters
06110	5.0	Home repair	Excavating garage
06120	5.0	Home repair	Hanging storm windows
06130	4.5	Home repair	Laying or removing carpet
06140	4.5	Home repair	Laying tile or linoleum
06150	5.0	Home repair	Painting, outside house (T 650)
06160	4.5	Home repair	Painting, papering, plastering, scraping, inside house, hanging sheet rock, remodeling (T 630)
06170	3.0	Home repair	Put on and removal of tarp-sailboat
06180	6.0	Home repair	Roofing
06190	4.5	Home repair	Sanding floors with a power sander
06200	4.5	Home repair	Scrape and paint sailboat or powerboat
06210	5.0	Home repair	Spreading dirt with a shovel
06220	4.5	Home repair	Wash and wax hull of sailboat, car, powerboat, airplane
06230	4.5	Home repair	Washing fence
06240	3.0	Home repair	Wiring, plumbing
07010	0.9	Inactivity, quiet	Lying quietly, reclining (watch television), lying quietly in bed-awake
07020	1.0	Inactivity, quiet	Sitting quietly (riding in a car, listening to a lecture or music, watch television or movie)
07030	0.9	Inactivity, quiet	Sleeping

TABLE 4.9   Compendium of physical activities (code, METS) (continued)

07040	1.2	Inactivity, quiet	Standing quietly (standing in a line)
07050	1.0	Inactivity, light	Recline-writing
07060	1.0	Inactivity, light	Recline-talking or talking on phone
07070	1.0	Inactivity, light	Recline-reading
08010	5.0	Lawn and garden	Carrying, loading or stacking wood, loading/unloading or carrying lumber
08020	6.0	Lawn and garden	Chopping wood, splitting logs
08030	5.0	Lawn and garden	Clearing land, hauling branches
08040	5.0	Lawn and garden	Digging, sandbox
08050	5.0	Lawn and garden	Digging, spading, filling garden (T 590)
08060	6.0	Lawn and garden	Gardening with heavy power tools, tilling a garden (see occupation, shoveling)
08080	5.0	Lawn and garden	Laying crushed rock
08090	5.0	Lawn and garden	Laying sod
08095	5.5	Lawn and garden	Mowing lawn, general
08100	2.5	Lawn and garden	Mowing lawn, riding mower (T 550)
08110	6.0	Lawn and garden	Mowing lawn, walk, hand mower (T 570)
08120	4.5	Lawn and garden	Mowing lawn, walk, power mower (T 590)
08130	4.5	Lawn and garden	Operating snow blower, walking
08140	4.0	Lawn and garden	Planting seedlings, shrubs
08150	4.5	Lawn and garden	Planting trees
08160	4.0	Lawn and garden	Raking lawn (T 600)
08170	4.0	Lawn and garden	Raking roof with snow rake
08180	3.0	Lawn and garden	Riding snow blower
08190	4.0	Lawn and garden	Sacking grass, leaves
08200	6.0	Lawn and garden	Shoveling, snow, by hand (T 610)
08210	4.5	Lawn and garden	Trimming shrubs or trees, manual cutter
08215	3.5	Lawn and garden	Trimming shrubs or trees, power cutter
08220	2.5	Lawn and garden	Walking, applying fertilizer or seeding a lawn
08230	1.5	Lawn and garden	Watering lawn or garden, standing or walking
08240	4.5	Lawn and garden	Weeding, cultivating garden (T 580)
08245	5.0	Lawn and garden	Gardening, general
08250	3.0	Lawn and garden	Implied walking/standing-picking up yard, light
09010	1.5	Miscellaneous	Sitting, card playing, playing board games
09020	2.0	Miscellaneous	Standing-drawing (writing), casino gambling
09030	1.3	Miscellaneous	Sitting-reading, book, newspaper, etc.
09040	1.8	Miscellaneous	Sitting-writing, desk work
09050	1.8	Miscellaneous	Standing-talking or talking on the phone
09055	1.5	Miscellaneous	Sitting-talking or talking on the phone
09060	1.8	Miscellaneous	Sitting-studying, general, including reading and/or writing
09065	1.8	Miscellaneous	Sitting-in class, general, including note-taking or class discussion
09070	1.8	Miscellaneous	Standing-reading
10010	1.8	Music playing	Accordion
10020	2.0	Music playing	Cello

TABLE 4.9   Compendium of physical activities (code, METS) (continued)

10030	2.5	Music playing	Conducting
10040	4.0	Music playing	Drums
10050	2.0	Music playing	Flute (sitting)
10060	2.0	Music playing	Horn
10070	2.5	Music playing	Piano or organ
10080	3.5	Music playing	Trombone
10090	2.5	Music playing	Trumpet
10100	2.5	Music playing	Violin
10110	2.0	Music playing	Woodwind
10120	2.0	Music playing	Guitar, classical, folk (sitting)
10125	3.0	Music playing	Guitar, rock and roll band (standing)
10130	4.0	Music playing	Marching band, playing an instrument, baton twirling (walking)
10135	3.5	Music playing	Marching band, drum major (walking)
11010	4.0	Occupation	Bakery, general
11020	2.3	Occupation	Bookbinding
11030	6.0	Occupation	Building road (including hauling debris, driving heavy machinery)
11035	2.0	Occupation	Building road, directing traffic (standing)
11040	3.5	Occupation	Carpentry, general
11050	8.0	Occupation	Carrying heavy loads, such as bricks
11060	8.0	Occupation	Carrying moderate loads up stairs, moving boxes (16–40 pounds)
11070	2.5	Occupation	Chambermaid
11080	6.5	Occupation	Coal mining, drilling coal, rock
11090	6.5	Occupation	Coal mining, erecting supports
11100	6.0	Occupation	Coal mining, general
11110	7.0	Occupation	Coal mining, shovelling coal
11120	5.5	Occupation	Construction, outside, remodeling
11130	3.5	Occupation	Electrical work, plumbing
11140	8.0	Occupation	Farming, baling hay, cleaning barn, poultry work
11150	3.5	Occupation	Farming, chasing cattle, nonstrenuous
11160	2.5	Occupation	Farming, driving harvester
11170	2.5	Occupation	Farming, driving tractor
11180	4.0	Occupation	Farming, feeding small animals
11190	4.5	Occupation	Farming, feeding cattle
11200	8.0	Occupation	Farming, forking straw bales
11210	3.0	Occupation	Farming, milking by hand
11220	1.5	Occupation	Farming, milking by machine
11230	5.5	Occupation	Farming, shoveling grain
11240	12.0	Occupation	Fire fighter, general
11245	11.0	Occupation	Fire fighter, climbing ladder with full gear
11246	8.0	Occupation	Fire fighter, hauling hoses on ground
11250	17.0	Occupation	Forestry, ax chopping, fast
11260	5.0	Occupation	Forestry, ax chopping, slow

TABLE 4.9   Compendium of physical activities (code, METS) (continued)

11270	7.0	Occupation	Forestry, barking trees
11280	11.0	Occupation	Forestry, carrying logs
11290	8.0	Occupation	Forestry, felling trees
11300	8.0	Occupation	Forestry, general
11310	5.0	Occupation	Forestry, hoeing
11320	6.0	Occupation	Forestry, planting by hand
11330	7.0	Occupation	Forestry, sawing by hand
11340	4.5	Occupation	Forestry, sawing, power
11350	9.0	Occupation	Forestry, trimming trees
11360	4.0	Occupation	Forestry, weeding
11370	4.5	Occupation	Furriery
11380	6.0	Occupation	Horse grooming
11390	8.0	Occupation	Horse racing, galloping
11400	6.5	Occupation	Horse racing, trotting
11410	2.6	Occupation	Horse racing, walking
11420	3.5	Occupation	Locksmith
11430	2.5	Occupation	Machine tooling, machining, working sheet metal
11440	3.0	Occupation	Machine tooling, operating lathe
11450	5.0	Occupation	Machine tooling, operating punch press
11460	4.0	Occupation	Machine tooling, tapping and drilling
11470	3.0	Occupation	Machine tooling, welding
11480	7.0	Occupation	Masonry, concrete
11485	4.0	Occupation	Masseur, masseuse (standing)
11490	7.0	Occupation	Moving, pushing heavy objects, 75 lbs or more (desks, moving van work)
11500	2.5	Occupation	Operating heavy duty equipment/automated, not driving
11510	4.5	Occupation	Orange grove work
11520	2.3	Occupation	Printing (standing)
11525	2.5	Occupation	Police, directing traffic (standing)
11526	2.0	Occupation	Police, driving a squad car (sitting)
11527	1.3	Occupation	Police, riding in a squad car (sitting)
11528	8.0	Occupation	Police, making an arrest (standing)
11530	2.5	Occupation	Shoe repair, general
11540	8.5	Occupation	Shoveling, digging ditches
11550	9.0	Occupation	Shoveling, heavy (more than 16 lbs. min^{-1})
11560	6.0	Occupation	Shoveling, light (less than 10 lbs. min^{-1})
11570	7.0	Occupation	Shoveling, moderate (10–15 lbs. min^{-1})
11580	1.5	Occupation	Sitting-light office work, in general (chemistry lab work, light use of hand-tools, watch repair or micro-assembly, light assembly/repair)
11585	1.5	Occupation	Sitting-meetings, general, and/or with talking involved
11590	2.5	Occupation	Sitting; moderate (heavy levers, riding mower/forklift, crane operation)
11600	2.5	Occupation	Standing; light (bartending, store clerk, assembling, filing, xeroxing, put up Christmas tree)

TABLE 4.9   Compendium of physical activities (code, METS) (continued)

11610	3.0	Occupation	Standing; light/moderate (assemble/repair heavy parts, welding, stocking, auto repair, pack boxes for moving, etc.), patient care (as in nursing)
11620	3.5	Occupation	Standing; moderate (assembling at fast rate, lifting 50 lbs, hitch/twisting ropes)
11630	4.0	Occupation	Standing; moderate/heavy (lifting more than 50 lb, masonry, painting, paper hanging)
11640	5.0	Occupation	Steel mill, fetting
11650	5.5	Occupation	Steel mill, forging
11660	8.0	Occupation	Steel mill, hand rolling
11670	8.0	Occupation	Steel mill, merchant mill rolling
11680	11.0	Occupation	Steel mill, removing slag
11690	7.5	Occupation	Steel mill, tending furnace
11700	5.5	Occupation	Steel mill, tipping molds
11710	8.0	Occupation	Steel mill, working in general
11720	2.5	Occupation	Tailoring, cutting
11730	2.5	Occupation	Tailoring, general
11740	2.0	Occupation	Tailoring, hand sewing
11750	2.5	Occupation	Tailoring, machine sewing
11760	4.0	Occupation	Tailoring, pressing
11766	6.5	Occupation	Truck driving, loading and unloading truck (standing)
11770	1.5	Occupation	Typing, electric, manual or computer
11780	6.0	Occupation	Using heavy power tools such pneumatic tools (jackhammers, drills, etc.)
11790	8.0	Occupation	Using heavy tools (not power) such as shovel, pick, tunnel bar, spade
11791	2.0	Occupation	Walking on job, less than 2.0 mph (in office or lab area), very slow
11792	3.5	Occupation	Walking on job, 3.0 mph, in office, moderate speed, not carrying anything
11793	4.0	Occupation	Walking on job, 3.5 mph, in office, brisk speed, not carrying anything
11795	3.0	Occupation	Walking, 2.5 mph, slowly and carrying light objects less than 25 lbs
11800	4.0	Occupation	Walking, 3.0 mph, moderately and carrying light objects less than 25 lbs
11810	4.5	Occupation	Walking, 3.5 mph, briskly and carrying objects less than 25 lbs
11820	5.0	Occupation	Walking or walk downstairs or standing, carrying objects about 25–49 lbs
11830	6.5	Occupation	Walking or walk downstairs or standing, carrying objects about 50–74 lbs
11840	7.5	Occupation	Walking or walk downstairs or standing, carrying objects about 75–99 lbs
11850	8.5	Occupation	Walking or walk downstairs or standing, carrying objects about 100 lbs and over
11870	3.0	Occupation	Working in scene shop, theater actor, backstage, employee
12010	6.0	Running	Job/walk combination (jobbing component of less than 10 min) (T 180)
12020	7.0	Running	Jogging, general
12030	8.0	Running	Running, 5 mph (12 min $\cdot$ mile^{-1})
12040	9.0	Running	Running, 5.2 mph (11.5 min $\cdot$ mile^{-1})
12050	10.0	Running	Running, 6 mph (10 min $\cdot$ mile^{-1})
12060	11.0	Running	Running, 6.7 mph (9 min $\cdot$ mile^{-1})
12070	11.5	Running	Running, 7 mph (8.5 min $\cdot$ mile^{-1})
12080	12.5	Running	Running, 7.5 mph (8 min $\cdot$ mile^{-1})
12090	13.5	Running	Running, 8 mph (7.5 min $\cdot$ mile^{-1})

TABLE 4.9   Compendium of physical activities (code, METS) (continued)

Code	METS	Category	Activity
12100	14.0	Running	Running, 8.6 mph (7 min · mile^{-1})
12110	15.0	Running	Running, 9 mph (6.5 min · mile^{-1})
12120	16.0	Running	Running, 10 mph (6 min · mile^{-1})
12130	18.0	Running	Running, 10.9 mph (5.5 min · mile^{-1})
12140	9.0	Running	Running, cross-country
12150	8.0	Running	Running, general (T 200)
12160	8.0	Running	Running, in place
12170	15.0	Running	Running, stairs, up
12180	10.0	Running	Running, on a track, team practice
12190	8.0	Running	Running, training, pushing wheelchair, marathon wheeling
12195	3.0	Running	Running, wheeling, general
13000	2.5	Self-care	Standing-getting ready for bed, in general
13009	1.0	Self-care	Sitting on toilet
13010	2.0	Self-care	Bathing (sitting)
13020	2.5	Self-care	Dressing, undressing (standing or sitting)
13030	1.5	Self-care	Eating (sitting)
13035	2.0	Self-care	Talking and eating or eating only (standing)
13040	2.5	Self-care	Sitting or standing-grooming (washing, shaving, brushing teeth, urinating, washing hands, put on make-up)
13050	4.0	Self-care	Showering, toweling off (standing)
14010	1.5	Sexual activity	Active, vigorous effort
14020	1.3	Sexual activity	General, moderate effort
14030	1.0	Sexual activity	Passive, light effort, kissing, hugging
15010	3.5	Sports	Archery (nonhunting)
15020	7.0	Sports	Badminton, competitive (T 450)
15030	4.5	Sports	Badminton, social singles and doubles, general
15040	8.0	Sports	Basketball, game (T 490)
15050	6.0	Sports	Basketball, nongame, general (T 480)
15060	7.0	Sports	Basketball, officiating (T 500)
15070	4.5	Sports	Basketball, shooting baskets
15075	6.5	Sports	Basketball, wheelchair
15080	2.5	Sports	Billiards
15090	3.0	Sports	Bowling (T 390)
15100	12.0	Sports	Boxing, in ring, general
15110	6.0	Sports	Boxing, punching bag
15120	9.0	Sports	Boxing, sparring
15130	7.0	Sports	Broomball
15135	5.0	Sports	Children's games (hopscotch, 4-square, dodgeball, playground apparatus, t-ball, tetherball, marbles, jacks, arcade games)
15140	4.0	Sports	Coaching: football, soccer, basketball, baseball, swimming, etc.
15150	5.0	Sports	Cricket (batting, bowling)
15160	2.5	Sports	Croquet
15170	4.0	Sports	Curling

TABLE 4.9   Compendium of physical activities (code, METS) (continued)

15180	2.5	Sports	Darts, wall or lawn
15190	6.0	Sports	Drag racing, pushing or driving a car
15200	6.0	Sports	Fencing
15210	9.0	Sports	Football, competitive
15230	8.0	Sports	Football, touch, flag, general (T 510)
15235	2.5	Sports	Football or baseball, playing catch
15240	3.0	Sports	Frisbee playing, general
15250	3.5	Sports	Frisbee, ultimate
15255	4.5	Sports	Golf, general
15260	5.5	Sports	Golf, carrying clubs (T 090)
15270	3.0	Sports	Golf, miniature, driving range
15280	5.0	Sports	Golf, pulling clubs (T 080)
15290	3.5	Sports	Golf, using power cart (T 070)
15300	4.0	Sports	Gymnastics, general
15310	4.0	Sports	Hacky sack
15320	12.0	Sports	Handball, general (T 520)
15330	8.0	Sports	Handball, team
15340	3.5	Sports	Hang gliding
15350	8.0	Sports	Hockey, field
15360	8.0	Sports	Hockey, ice
15370	4.0	Sports	Horseback riding, general
15380	3.5	Sports	Horseback riding, saddling horse
15390	6.5	Sports	Horseback riding, trotting
15400	2.5	Sports	Horseback riding, walking
15410	3.0	Sports	Horseshoe pitching, quoits
15420	12.0	Sports	Jai alai
15430	10.0	Sports	Judo, jujitsu, karate, kick boxing, tae kwan do
15440	4.0	Sports	Juggling
15450	7.0	Sports	Kickball
15460	8.0	Sports	Lacrosse
15470	4.0	Sports	Moto-cross
15480	9.0	Sports	Orienteering
15490	10.0	Sports	Paddleball, competitive
15500	6.0	Sports	Paddleball, casual, general (T 460)
15510	8.0	Sports	Polo
15520	10.0	Sports	Racketball, competitive
15530	7.0	Sports	Racketball, casual, general (T 470)
15535	11.0	Sports	Rock climbing, ascending rock
15540	8.0	Sports	Rock climbing, rapelling
15550	12.0	Sports	Rope jumping, fast
15551	10.0	Sports	Rope jumping, moderate, general
15552	8.0	Sports	Rope jumping, slow
15560	10.0	Sports	Rugby

TABLE 4.9   Compendium of physical activities (code, METS) (continued)

15570	3.0	Sports	Shuffleboard, lawn bowling
15580	5.0	Sports	Skateboarding
15590	7.0	Sports	Skating, roller (T 360)
15600	3.5	Sports	Sky diving
15605	10.0	Sports	Soccer, competitive
15610	7.0	Sports	Soccer, casual, general (T 540)
15620	5.0	Sports	Softball or baseball, fast or slow pitch, general (T 440)
15630	4.0	Sports	Softball, officiating
15640	6.0	Sports	Softball, pitching
15650	12.0	Sports	Squash (T 530)
15660	4.0	Sports	Table tennis, ping pong (T 410)
15670	4.0	Sports	Tai chi
15675	7.0	Sports	Tennis, general
15680	6.0	Sports	Tennis, doubles (T 430)
15690	8.0	Sports	Tennis, singles (T 420)
15700	3.5	Sports	Trampoline
15710	4.0	Sports	Volleyball, competitive, in gymnasium (T 400)
15720	3.0	Sports	Volleyball, noncompetitive; 6–9 member team, general
15725	8.0	Sports	Volleyball, beach
15730	6.0	Sports	Wrestling (one match = 5 min)
15731	7.0	Sports	Wallyball, general
16010	2.0	Transportation	Automobile or light truck (not a semi) driving
16020	2.0	Transportation	Flying airplane
16030	2.5	Transportation	Motor scooter, motor cycle
16040	6.0	Transportation	Pushing plane in and out of hangar
16050	3.0	Transportation	Driving heavy truck, tractor, bus
17010	7.0	Walking	Backpacking, general (T 050)
17020	3.5	Walking	Carrying infant or 15-lb load (e.g., suitcase), level ground or downstairs
17025	9.0	Walking	Carrying load upstairs, general
17026	5.0	Walking	Carrying 1- to 15-lb load, upstairs
17027	6.0	Walking	Carrying 16- to 24-lb load, upstairs
17028	8.0	Walking	Carrying 25- to 49-lb load, upstairs
17029	10.0	Walking	Carrying 50- to 74-lb load, upstairs
17030	12.0	Walking	Carrying 74+-lb load, upstairs
17035	7.0	Walking	Climbing hills with 0- to 9-lb load
17040	7.5	Walking	Climbing hills with 10- to 20-lb load
17050	8.0	Walking	Climbing hills with 21- to 42-lb load
17060	9.0	Walking	Climbing hills with 42+-lb load
17070	3.0	Walking	Downstairs
17080	6.0	Walking	Hiking, cross country (T 040)
17090	6.5	Walking	Marching, rapidly, military
17100	2.5	Walking	Pushing or pulling stroller with child

TABLE 4.9   Compendium of physical activities (code, METS) (continued)

17110	6.5	Walking	Race walking
17120	8.0	Walking	Rock or mountain climbing (T 060)
17130	8.0	Walking	Up stairs, using or climbing up ladder (T 030)
17140	4.0	Walking	Using crutches
17150	2.0	Walking	Walking, less than 2.0 mph, level ground, strolling, household walking, very slow
17160	2.5	Walking	Walking, 2.0 mph, level, slow pace, firm surface
17170	3.0	Walking	Walking, 2.5 mph, firm surface
17180	3.0	Walking	Walking, 2.5 mph, downhill
17190	3.5	Walking	Walking, 3.0 mph, level, moderate pace, firm surface
17200	4.0	Walking	Walking, 3.5 mph, level, brisk, firm surface
17210	6.0	Walking	Walking, 3.5 mph, uphill
17220	4.0	Walking	Walking, 4.0 mph, level, firm surface, very brisk pace
17230	4.5	Walking	Walking, 4.5 mph, level, firm surface, very, very brisk
17250	3.5	Walking	Walking, for pleasure, work break, walking the dog
17260	5.0	Walking	Walking, grass track
17270	4.0	Walking	Walking, to work or class (T 015)
18010	2.5	Water activities	Boating, power
18020	4.0	Water activities	Canoeing, on camping trip (T 270)
18030	7.0	Water activities	Canoeing, portaging
18040	3.0	Water activities	Canoeing, rowing, 2.0-3.9 mph, light effort
18050	7.0	Water activities	Canoeing, rowing, 4.0-5.9 mph, moderate effort
18060	12.0	Water activities	Canoeing, rowing, 6 mph, vigorous effort
18070	3.5	Water activities	Canoeing, rowing, for pleasure, general (T 250)
18080	12.0	Water activities	Canoeing, rowing, in competition, or crew or sculling (T 260)
18090	3.0	Water activities	Diving, springboard or platform
18100	5.0	Water activities	Kayaking
18110	4.0	Water activities	Paddleboat
18120	3.0	Water activities	Sailing, boat and board sailing, windsurfing, ice sailing, general (T 235)
18130	5.0	Water activities	Sailing, in competition
18140	3.0	Water activities	Sailing, Sunfish/Laser/Hobby Cat, keel boats, ocean sailing, yachting
18150	6.0	Water activities	Sking, water (T 220)
18160	7.0	Water activities	Skimobiling
18170	12.0	Water activities	Skindiving or scuba diving as frogman
18180	16.0	Water activities	Skindiving, fast
18190	12.5	Water activities	Skindiving, moderate
18200	7.0	Water activities	Skindiving, scuba diving, general (T 310)
18210	5.0	Water activities	Snorkeling (T 320)
18220	3.0	Water activities	Surfing, body or board
18230	10.0	Water activities	Swimming laps, freestyle, fast, vigorous effort
18240	8.0	Water activities	Swimming laps, freestyle, slow, moderate or light effort
18250	8.0	Water activities	Swimming, backstroke, general
18260	10.0	Water activities	Swimming, breaststroke, general

TABLE 4.9   Compendium of physical activities (code, METS) (continued)

18270	11.0	Water activities	Swimming, butterfly, general
18280	11.0	Water activities	Swimming, crawl, fast (75 yards $\bullet$ min^{-1}), vigorous effort
18290	8.0	Water activities	Swimming, crawl, slow (50 yards $\bullet$ min^{-1}), moderate or light effort
18300	6.0	Water activities	Swimming, lake, ocean, river (T 280, T 295)
18310	6.0	Water activities	Swimming, leisurely, not lap swimming, general
18320	8.0	Water activities	Swimming, sidestroke, general
18330	8.0	Water activities	Swimming, synchronized
18340	10.0	Water activities	Swimming, treading water, fast vigorous effort
18350	4.0	Water activities	Swimming, treading water, moderate effort, general
18360	10.0	Water activities	Water polo
18365	3.0	Water activities	Water volleyball
18370	5.0	Water activities	Whitewater rafting, kayaking, or canoeing
19010	6.0	Winter activities	Moving ice house (set up/drill holes, etc.)
19020	5.5	Winter activities	Skating, ice, 9 mph or less
19030	7.0	Winter activities	Skating, ice, general (T 360)
19040	9.0	Winter activities	Skating, ice, rapidly, more than 9 mph
19050	15.0	Winter activities	Skating, speed, competitive
19060	7.0	Winter activities	Ski jumping (climb up carrying skis)
19075	7.0	Winter activities	Skiing general
19080	7.0	Winter activities	Skiing, cross-country, 2.5 mph, slow or light effort, ski walking
19090	8.0	Winter activities	Skiing, cross-country, 4.0–4.9 mph, moderate speed and effort, general
19100	9.0	Winter activities	Skiing, cross-country, 5.0–7.9 mph, brisk speed, vigorous effort
19110	14.0	Winter activities	Skiing, cross-country, > 8.0 mph, racing
19130	16.5	Winter activities	Skiing, cross-country, hard snow, uphill, maximum
19150	5.0	Winter activities	Skiing, downhill, light effort
19160	6.0	Winter activities	Skiing, downhill, moderate effort, general
19170	8.0	Winter activities	Skiing, downhill, vigorous effort, racing
19180	7.0	Winter activities	Sledding, tobogganing, bobsledding, luge (T 370)
19190	8.0	Winter activities	Snow shoeing
19200	3.5	Winter activities	Snowmobling

(Reprinted with permission from (Appendix I) BE Ainsworth et al. Compendium of physical activities: Classification of energy costs of human physical activities. *Med Sci Sports Exerc.* 1993;25(1):71–80.)

(**Table 4.10**). This method is recommended if physiological measurements are not possible, or if heart rate measurements are inappropriate to judge intensity because of a client's medication use or disease status. Ratings of perceived exertion has been shown to be valid for monitoring exercise intensity.[111–115]

Perceived effort can be rated numerically using the 15-point Borg scale (**Figure 4.10**).[116,117] The client rates their level of perceived exertion on the numeric scale ranging from 6 to 20 based on descriptors provided, ranging from "very, very light" to "very, very hard." The higher the levels of energy expenditure and physiologic strain, the higher the perceived exertion rating. Although heart rate values generally coincide with perceived exertion ratings, at the same perceived exertion ratings some individuals will display lower heart rates while others will display higher heart rates. To establish the accuracy of the perceived exertion rating, a graded exercise test should be used to correlate the rating of perceived exertion with physiological measures over a wide range of exercise

TABLE 4.10 Classification of physical activity intensity based on physical activity lasting up to 60 minutes

	Relative intensity		
Intensity	%HRR or %VO_2R	%HR_{max}	RPE
Very light	<20	<35	<10
Light	20–39	35–54	10–11
Moderate	40–59	55–69	12–13
Hard	60–84	70–89	14–16
Very hard	≥ 85	≥ 90	17–19
Maximal	100	100	20

(Reprinted with permission from *American College of Sports Medicine's Guidelines for Exercise Testing and Prescription*, 6th ed. Baltimore: Lippincott Williams & Wilkins; 2000, p. 150.)

intensities. Using this method enables therapeutic exercise to be performed at a rating of perceived exertion that corresponds with the desired heart rate or VO_2. One advantage of the perceived exertion rating method of setting therapeutic exercise intensity is that it truly encourages individuals to "listen to their bodies." A therapeutic exercise intensity that feels "too hard" may well be beyond the individual's safe exercise intensity level.

Aerobic Exercise Duration

Duration is the length of time spent exercising in one session. The combination of exercise intensity and exercise duration establishes the energy expenditure in an exercise session. The determination of an optimal duration is dependent on the exercise goals of the client and his or her fitness level. The ACSM recommends a duration of 20–60 minutes of aerobic exercise.[106] If the exercise is intermittent rather than continuous, the ACSM suggests that each bout of exercise be at least 10 minutes, and that bouts be repeated to reach the 20–60 minute recommendation.[106] At present, there is no conclusive evidence of an optimal combination of duration and intensity for training for aerobic power. The range of duration recommended by the ACSM allows the client to choose between a lower intensity exercise for a longer duration and a higher intensity exercise for a shorter duration. The research findings of Pollock, Ward, and Ayres[118] supported the equivalence of lower intensity, higher duration exercise to higher intensity, lower duration exercise if the total energy expenditure is equal. As higher intensity exercise is associated with a greater risk of musculoskeletal and cardiovascular injury and greater attrition,[119] low to moderate intensity aerobic exercise for 30–40 minutes is desirable for a general training program not focused on athletic preparation. This is consistent with the 1995 consensus statement of the Center for Disease Control and the ACSM that "Every Amer-

Category scale		Category-ratio scale		
6		0	Nothing at all	"No I"
7	Very, very light	0.3		
8		0.5	Extremely weak	Just noticeable
9	Very light	0.7		
10		1	Very weak	
11	Fairly light	1.5		
12		2	Weak	Light
13	Somewhat hard	2.5		
14		3	Moderate	
15	Hard	4		
16		5	Strong	Heavy
17	Very hard	6		
18		7	Very strong	
19	Very, very hard	8		
20		9		
		10	Extremely strong	"Strongest I"
		11		
		•	Absolute maximum	Highest possible

Figure 4.10 Category and category-ratio scales for ratings of perceived exertion (RPE). On the category-ratio scale "I" represents intensity. For correct usage of the Borg scales, it is necessary to follow the administration and instructions given in Borg's Perceived Exertion and Pain Scales. (Champaign, IL: Human Kinetics; 1998.) (Reprinted with permission from *American College of Sports Medicine's Guidelines for Exercise Testing and Prescription*, 6th ed. Baltimore: Lippincott Williams & Wilkins, 2000, p. 79.)

ican adult should accumulate 30 minutes or more of moderate-intensity physical activity on most, preferably all, days of the week."[2]

Aerobic Exercise Frequency

The number of exercise sessions per week is referred to as the frequency of exercise. The ACSM recommends a frequency of three to five days/week for cardiopulmonary fitness.[106] For those individuals who are limited to low intensity activities (less than three METs), multiple bouts of activity per day are desirable to reach the energy expenditure for weight control and general fitness. For an individual exercising at a high level of intensity, three days/week is sufficient to maintain or improve VO_{2max} whereas for those exercising at moderate intensities, four to five days/week is desirable. Once again, the specific therapeutic exercise prescription should be crafted based on the client's pre-exercise fitness as well as their preferences and fitness goals.

The sum total of aerobic exercise intensity, duration, and frequency is referred to as training volume. Is the "more is better" philosophy accurate with regard to the effect of increased training volume on fitness? Currently, the literature does not support this philosophy with regard to cardiopulmonary fitness measures. In a study of collegiate male swimmers, Costill et al.[120] found that swimmers who completed two, 1.5-hour training sessions daily for six weeks exhibited a decrease in sprint velocity as compared to an increase in sprint velocity in those swimmers who trained only one, 1.5-hour session daily. Pollock et al.[119] found that although there was a greater improvement in VO_{2max} with higher intensity running, there was a greater incidence of injury and attrition with training at this level as compared to lower intensity training. In an earlier study by Fox et al.,[121] there was no difference in improvement in VO_{2max} between groups that trained two or four days/week. A study of NCAA Division I cross-country runners found that running twice daily during the precompetition phase of training was associated with decreased performance.[122]

While increased training volume does not necessarily result in improved cardiopulmonary fitness measures, it does increase the total caloric expenditure as compared to lower volume training. Depending on the specific aerobic fitness goals of the exercise, a greater volume may be desirable for weight loss goals. However, this decision must be made cautiously as the injury risks associated with high training volume may not justify the benefit of increased caloric expenditure.

Aerobic Exercise Preparation

As a part of the aerobic exercise prescription, the client should be educated about preparation for exercise activities, such as the concept of "warming-up." These activities should precede the actual exercise session and serve as a physiologic and mental preparation for exercise. Warm-up can be achieved via active or passive means. Active warm-up consists of low intensity exercise, whereas passive warm-up involves the use of external means to increase body temperature. Although both methods have been shown to improve performance times, active warm-up appears to result in better performances.[123] Active warm-up helps to increase the metabolic rate from the resting level of one MET to that of the aerobic requirements for that exercise.

Physiologically, the primary benefit of a pre-exercise warm-up is an increase in tissue temperature. The effects of the thermal response include increased blood flow to muscle, improved oxygen dissociation from myoglobin, an increase in nerve conduction velocity, and increased elasticity of the muscle–tendon units.[124] Taken together, these mechanisms seem to prepare muscles well for exercise, leading to the common belief that a warm-up period serves to reduce the likelihood of injury. This belief may have a strong influence on the psychology of the warm-up. As the person prepares for the exercise session, the warm-up helps to get them "in the mood" as well as providing a sense of confidence that injury is unlikely because of this activity. Although evidence for the effectiveness of the warm-up in preventing musculoskeletal injury is lacking, there is also no evidence to refute this belief. Consequently, a gradual warm-up period to increase core and muscle temperature continues to be recommended by exercise specialists.

> ### *Key Point:*
> Although evidence for the role of warming up to prevent musculoskeletal injury is lacking, there is no evidence to refute this belief. Therefore a gradual warm-up period to increase core body and intramuscular temperature continues to be recommended.

Another significant consideration in prescribing exercise to improve aerobic power is the potential negative cardiac effects of sudden onset moderate to high intensity exercise. Studies have shown that sudden strenuous exercise without warm-up may cause acute myocardial ischemia, resulting in electrocardiogram (ECG) abnormalities, as well as significant increases in systolic blood pressure.[125] These studies demonstrated that a two-minute warm-up significantly improved the myocardial and blood pressure response to exercise. This is crucial in maximizing the safety of aerobic exercise programs.

The inclusion of a stretching program prior to aerobic exercise is another common recommendation by rehabilitation clinicians. Historically, stretching has been incorporated into warm-up activities as a method of injury prevention. Using a rabbit tendon model, Safran et al.[124] provided evidence that warming up a muscle prior to exertion resulted in greater elasticity and a higher strain to failure value. Gleim et al.[126] found that musculotendinous tightness resulted in poorer running economy. However, the literature is mixed on the evidence to support stretching as an injury prevention strategy. This is covered in greater detail in Chapter 3. In a review of the basic science evidence regarding stretching, Shrier[127] concluded that stretching prior to exercise might be more likely to cause injury than to prevent it. They reported that studies that have shown beneficial pre-exercise stretching effects used multiple interventions, and the specific effect of stretching alone was unknown.[127] In a randomized clinical trial of stretching to prevent injury in military recruits, Pope et al.[128] reported that stretching did not significantly reduce the risk of injury. Consequently, there is not a preponderance of evidence at present to support the inclusion of stretching in the warm-up prior to aerobic exercise.

A gradual cool-down following endurance activity is as important as the warm-up. The cool-down helps to keep the blood from pooling in the lower extremities and facilitates venous return to the heart, thereby preventing dizziness. It also encourages removal of metabolic waste products from the tissues. By not cooling down, individuals run the risk of slowing the recovery and adaptation necessary for continued improvements in performance. Failure to perform a cool-down immediately after exercise may also increase cardiovascular complications. The cool-down should last about 5 to 10 minutes and include light aerobic and/or stretching activities.

Aerobic Exercise Mode

The mode of aerobic exercise describes the specific activity that the client engages in to increase aerobic power. The effect of cardiopulmonary training is dependent on training volume—the combination of intensity, duration, and frequency—rather than the specific exercise mode.

> ## Key Point:
> Aerobic training effectiveness is more dependent on training volume than on the specific exercise mode used.

Therapeutic exercises used to improve aerobic power should involve rhythmic contractions of major muscle groups (particularly the larger lower extremity muscle groups). For a client who is not preparing for athletic competition, personal preferences, fitness goals, and available equipment influence the choice of aerobic exercise mode as well as issues related to the neuromuscular and musculoskeletal stresses of that activity. For example,

treadmill running involves significant ground reaction forces during impact-weight acceptance (three to four $\times$ body weight), which are transmitted through the skeletal and joint elements of the lower extremities. In addition, running on a treadmill requires adequate balance and spatial perception. This mode of exercise may be appropriate for a healthy non-obese adult but may be inappropriate for a person who is obese or has neurological impairments that affect kinesthesia (see Chapter 7) or balance (see Chapter 9). To facilitate aerobic exercise program adherence, the mode or modes of exercise selected should be enjoyable to the client while meeting his or her fitness goals. This is another major consideration in the art of therapeutic exercise prescription.

For an athlete, the aerobic exercise mode choice is driven by the demands of the sport. The specificity of training principle indicates that the effects of training are specific to the muscles used and energy systems required in a training activity. Accordingly, to design an aerobic training program specific to a sport requires a thorough knowledge of the physiologic and biomechanical demands of the sport.

> ## Key Point:
> To design an aerobic training program that addresses the energy system demands of a specific sport, a thorough knowledge of the physiologic and biomechanical demands of the sport is required.

Helgerud et al.[129] investigated the effect of an aerobic training program on the performance of soccer players. Using previous studies that examined the physiological demands of soccer, they designed a training program to closely simulate the demands of soccer. Players from two teams were randomly assigned to a training group or a control group. All groups completed routine technical, tactical, strength, and speed training. The training group did an additional interval-training program consisting of running for four bouts of four minutes at 90 percent to 95 percent of HR_{max}, followed by three minutes of jogging at 50 percent to 60 percent HR_{max}. Dependent variables of vertical jump, one repetition-maximum (RM) bench press, one RM squat, 40 m sprint speed, kicking velocity, kicking precision, VO_{2max}, and lactate threshold were measured before and after the eight week training period. The authors reported improved VO_{2max} in the training group but no change in jump height, sprint speed, or kicking measures. Video analysis of two games showed that players in the training group ran a greater distance, performed more sprints, and had a greater number of "involvements with the ball" during a match as compared to players in the control group. The authors concluded that enhanced aerobic performance improved soccer performance.[129]

Published articles regarding the physiological demands are available for many sports, including swimming,[130,131] field hockey,[132] volleyball,[133,134] American football,[135] Nordic skiing,[136–139] alpine skiing,[140] cross-country running,[141,142] basketball,[143–145] softball,[146] gymnastics,[147] ice hockey,[148–150] and wrestling.[151–154] It is beyond the scope of this chapter to discuss the details of the physiological demands of individual sports. However, it is incumbent on the rehabilitation clinician who designs an aerobic power conditioning program for athletes in a specific sport to understand the physiologic requirements of that sport and to design the program accordingly.

Cross-Training

Cross training is a method of training that involves the supplemental use of more than one mode of exercise. In an athletic population, cross training is pursued for several reasons. Cross training may be obligatory in an elite athlete because of the likelihood of overtraining or injury associated with the use of a single exercise mode. After injury, the individual's therapeutic exercise program is generally designed to enhance cardiopulmonary, cardiovascular, and musculoskeletal system function within the constraints of tissue healing.[20] For example, a female cross country athlete who develops a tibial stress fracture may need to cross train to allow for healing of this bony pathology. The cross training in this example would initially require activities that did not apply load to the tibia. Such activities might include aquatic therapy activities such as pool running and swimming, or dry land activities such as arm cycling and stationary biking. As the bone healing proceeds, the athlete would progress to weight bearing activities that do not involve impact loading, such as stair stepping machines or elliptical trainers. In the terminal phase of her rehabilitation, she would progress to lower extremity impact loading exercise, starting with fast walking on the treadmill and advancing to jogging and running as tolerated.

Non-injured athletes can cross train in two different ways. First, they may switch from their normal mode of exercise to an alternative mode in an attempt to improve performance or to minimize injury risk. Secondly, some athletes add an alternative training mode to their primary mode to increase overall training volume. In a comprehensive literature review on cross training, Loy et al.[155] concluded that cross training using a dissimilar exercise mode to the primary exercise mode can positively affect performance and cardiorespiratory fitness in novice athletes or those with lower aerobic capacity. Overall, however, the greater the aerobic capacity of an athlete, the less performance and fitness benefit from cross-training. For an elite athlete whose primary goal is to improve performance, similar modes of cross training are more effective than dissimilar modes. Research by Foster et al.[156] found that adding swimming to the training program of a group of runners resulted in some increase in running perform-

ance, but not to the degree of the group that added additional run training to their workouts. In a study comparing the effect of stair climbing training on run performance, Loy et al.[157] found stair climbing was an effective cross training method for runners, resulting in improved running performance. They concluded that the similar demands of stair climbing and running enabled the training benefits of stair climbing to be transferred effectively to running performance. Generally, however, there is no evidence that cross training using similar or dissimilar aerobic exercise modes has a greater positive effect on performance than one would obtain from training in the primary activity mode. In fact, the time in cross training may be detrimental to an athlete's performance in his or her primary activity. Simply put, to improve running, one should run, to improve swimming, one should swim, to improve cycling, one needs to get on the bike.

> ## Key Point:
> Although cross training may help with injury prevention, to improve as a runner, swimmer or cyclist, one should perform running, swimming or cycling.

Because adaptations are specific to the muscles involved in training, activities that incorporate different muscle groups may not result in the desired improvements. This becomes particularly important when the client trains for strength and endurance concurrently. Adaptations to one type of exercise may interfere with the training effects of another type of exercise. Investigations into combined strength and endurance training reveal that combining resistance and aerobic endurance activities may be important for enhancing endurance performance[14] but may interfere with strength and power performances.[158–160]

> ## Key Point:
> Combined resistance training for strength and aerobic training to enhance endurance may hinder anaerobic strength and power development.

Although there are frequent anecdotal references to the use of cross training to prevent injury, there is little evidence in the literature. In following a group of NCAA Division I female swimmers over a seven year period, McFarland and Wasik[161,162] reported that 44 percent of injuries were a result of swimming, and 44 percent of injuries were a result of cross training. The swimming injuries were typically upper extremity, and the cross training injuries primarily involved the lower extremities. These data do not support the hypothesis of cross training as a method of overall injury prevention in elite athletes.

In clients who are not involved in competitive sport, cross training may be desirable as a technique to encourage therapeutic exercise program compliance. Rather than engaging in only one mode of exercise, the client selects multiple modes for mental, visual, and physiological variety. Not only does this encourage therapeutic exercise program compliance, but it also minimizes overuse injury risk by limiting the repetitive loading of any one activity over time. Cross training may also be seasonally driven; cross country skiing in the winter may be replaced by cycling in the summer for those living in northern climates.

Continuous vs. Interval Training

Within each exercise mode, there is potential of training at a consistent intensity throughout the workout, referred to as continuous training, or varying the intensity, also known as interval training. For continuous training, the intensity is selected based on the client's health and fitness as well as personal goals and preferences. This type of training is appropriate for a client who is beginning a therapeutic exercise program or for a person with specific weight loss goals. Continuous training can be accomplished at a moderate intensity level for long periods of time, resulting in significant caloric expenditure. For competitive athletes involved in long distance running, swimming, or cycling, continuous training is appropriate according to the specificity of training principle. As their competitive event requires continuous performance over time, the physiologic demand of continuous training develops specific motor unit recruitment and metabolic pathways.

One advantage of interval training is the incorporation of high-intensity exercise that cannot be performed continuously because of energy demands. For example, running a four minute mile is an athletic feat that only a few persons have achieved. Even running 400 meters in less than one minute is a challenge for most runners. It is possible, however, to run at a four minute mile pace for a few seconds. If provided with some recovery time, a person may be able to repeat several bouts of this pace. As such, interval training involves bouts of high intensity exercise followed by a rest period of no or lower intensity exercise. Critical to this training method is prescription of the level of intensity of the exercise bouts, the duration of the high intensity interval and the rest period, as well as the number of cycles to be performed. For competitive athletes in sports requiring interval performance, this prescription is based on knowledge of sport energy system demands as previously described. In this case, interval training is consistent with the specificity of training principle. The ratio of exercise to rest depends on the desired energy system to be trained, as summarized in **Table 4.11.**

Which mode of exercise—continuous or interval—is more effective in improving aerobic power? Smith and Wengner[162] compared the effect of cycle ergometer continuous training and interval training at low and high aerobic power on groups of non-impaired male subjects over a 10 day period. They concluded that high power continuous training was most effective for improving aerobic power over a 10 day period. Using the aerobic dance mode of exercise, Perry et al.[163] compared interval and continuous training among non-impaired subjects. Their results showed that the interval dance method was more effective in improving VO_{2max} than the continuous method. Overend et al.[164] compared continuous cycle ergometer training with low power and high power interval training among untrained male subjects. After a 10 week training period, all three groups showed improvement in aerobic parameters but no group was superior. In a study of patient groups who were 24–26 days status post coronary artery bypass surgery, Meyer et al.[165] found that interval training on a cycle ergometer was superior to continuous training in terms of improvement in both aerobic and anaerobic measures of cardiopulmonary fitness. At present, there is not a preponderance of evidence to support one training method over the other in terms of improving aerobic power. However, this variable is an important consideration in the art and science of therapeutic exercise prescription as it may influence a client's perception of effort and enjoyment, ultimately affecting program compliance.

> ## *Key Point:*
> There is not a preponderance of evidence to support the superiority of either continuous or interval training for improving aerobic power.

TABLE 4.11   Interval Training Guidelines

Energy system	Exercise interval (exercise duration:rest duration)
Immediate energy system (< 10 seconds)	1:3
Short term energy system (> 10 seconds, < 1.5 minutes)	1:2
Long term energy system (> 1.5 minutes)	1:1 to 1.5

EXERCISE MODES TO IMPROVE AEROBIC FITNESS

Walking

One of the simplest forms of aerobic exercise is walking. This exercise mode is safe, is appropriate across the lifespan, requires only appropriate footwear, and can be done individually or in groups, indoors or outdoors, and on a treadmill (**Figure 4.11**) or overground (**Figure 4.12**). Rippe et al.[166] reviewed several research studies on the fitness effect of walking and concluded that walking decreases anxiety, improves mood, and can result in weight loss and improved aerobic performance. The primary variable influencing the effect of walking on aerobic power is walking intensity, determined by walking pace and surface grade. The addition of hand held weights or walking poles increase the energy expenditure of walking,[167,168] but there is also an associated increase in systolic blood pressure[168] which may contraindicate this practice in clients who have a history of cardiac pathology.

In a randomized clinical trial, Duncan et al.[169] studied the walking intensity required to improve cardiopulmonary fitness in non-impaired, premenopausal women. Subjects were assigned to one of four groups: no walking, aerobic walkers, brisk walkers, and strollers. Walkers began training at 70 percent of the assigned intensity (8.0 km/h for aerobic walkers, 6.4 km/h for brisk walkers, and 4.8 km/h for strollers) and increased to 100 percent of intensity by the 14th week of training. The results showed that greater walking intensity resulted in greater improvement in aerobic capacity. However, all subject groups showed an improvement in lipoprotein profile regardless of exercise intensity. The authors concluded that walking even at a low intensity that did not have a major effect on cardiopulmonary fitness might nonetheless produce equally favorable changes in the cardiovascular risk profile.[169]

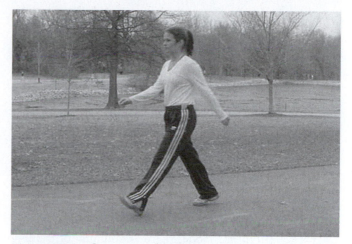

Figure 4.12   Overground walking.

A recent study by Kukkonen-Harjula, et al.[170] supported the results of Duncan et al.[169] These researchers found that non-impaired, middle-aged subjects who performed a moderate intensity walking program over a 15 week training period had improved VO_{2max} and improved lipoprotein profiles.[170] Manson et al.[171] investigated the association of physical activity and coronary events among 72,000 nurses over the 1986–1994 period. A questionnaire was used to assess details regarding modes and intensity of exercise. Overall, the researchers found a strong negative correlation between physical activity and the risk of coronary events. Vigorous activity, defined as greater than six METs, had a similar risk reduction as brisk walking (4.0–4.5 METs). A study of the effects of a six month walking program on 38 non-impaired, elderly (79–91 years of age) females showed improvement in morale, cardiorespiratory fitness, and activity level.[172] These studies substantiate the recommendations of Pate et al.[2] that clients meet the current physical activity standard by briskly walking two miles daily.

The injury risk of walking is quite low; estimates have ranged from 1.4%[173] to 14%,[174] with increased injury rate from increased walking pace.[174] The most common walking injuries affect the leg and foot.[174,175] Walking has been reported to be beneficial as an aerobic exercise for individuals with lower extremity arthritis.[175] Hootman et al.[176] examined the relationship between mode and duration of physical activity and musculoskeletal injury rates among 4,034 men and 967 women. They concluded that walking was a safe form of physical activity for most adults and was associated with a lower risk of injury than running or sport participation.[176]

Running

Running has similar advantages to walking, requiring only appropriate footwear as equipment, and can also be performed individually or in groups, indoors or outdoors, and on a treadmill (**Figure 4.13**) or over ground (**Figure 4.14**).

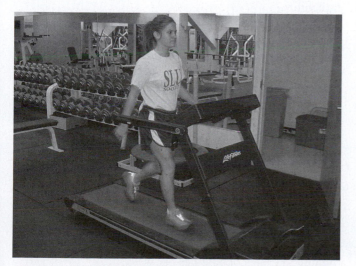

Figure 4.11   Walking on a treadmill.

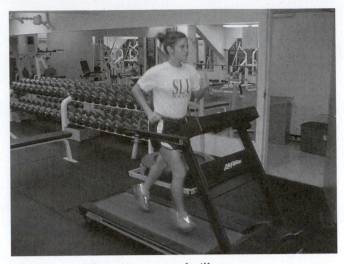

Figure 4.13   Running on treadmill.

However, running significantly differs from walking in terms of greater joint range of motion requirements at the hip, knee, and ankle, higher ground reaction forces, and increased intensity and caloric expenditure.[177,178] Variables that influence running intensity include pace and surface grade. Research has shown that the caloric expenditure of running is relatively constant (1 kcal/km · kg) regardless of running pace. Accordingly, a 80 kg adult running for five km burns approximately 400 kcal, whether the five km is run in 15 minutes or 30 minutes. The client who runs at a slower pace burns fewer calories per minute, but runs more minutes than the client who runs at a faster pace.

Running and jogging have been shown to improve cardiopulmonary fitness in both novice and experienced per-

sons. Research has demonstrated improvements in VO_{2max}[157,179–182] decreased blood pressure,[183] and improved blood lipoprotein profiles.[181, 183,184] Marti[184] described additional benefits of running including weight control and improved bone mineral density. Zeni et al.[185,186] compared energy expenditure at a given RPE level across different pieces of equipment used for aerobic exercise. Treadmill walking/jogging/running was identified as the "optimal" aerobic exercise machine for cardiorespiratory training and caloric expenditure at RPE levels ranging from 11 to 15. Moyna et al.[187] reported similar findings in a comparison across different exercise machines including a treadmill, stair stepper, cross country ski simulator, stationary cycle, rowing ergometer, and rider.

Is there a difference between running overground and running on a treadmill? McMiken and Daniels[188] studied eight runners and compared VO_{2max} for track running in calm air and treadmill running. They found no differences between the two conditions at three different speeds. Other research has shown a difference in the kinematics of running on treadmill and overground. Nigg[189] reported that non-impaired subjects who usually ran on the treadmill had a "flatter" foot plant on the treadmill than overground. Subjects also displayed other changes in lower extremity kinematic variables, but these changes were not consistent between subjects. Schache et al.[190] studied the difference in lumbo-pelvic-hip complex motion between overground running and treadmill running, reporting that a high powered treadmill with a minimal belt speed fluctuation and similar surface stiffness to the relevant ground surface condition produced a close representation of the typical three dimensional kinematic pattern of the lumbo-pelvic-hip complex that occurs during overground running. In summary, there may be minor kinematic differences between treadmill and overground running, but both are appropriate modes of exercise for improving aerobic power. The decision to recommend one mode over the other should be based primarily by the client's preference and equipment availability.

One disadvantage of running as an exercise mode to increase aerobic power is an increased risk of musculoskeletal injury as compared to other exercise modes.[191] Walter et al.[192] followed 1680 runners over a 12 month period and reported that 48 percent of the runners experienced at least one injury, with 54 percent of those injuries being first-time injuries. Van Mechelen[193] reviewed running epidemiology literature and reported an injury rate ranging from 37 percent to 56 percent. Running injuries are predominately caused by accumulated microtrauma (overuse), with injuries to the feet, legs, and knees as the most commonly affected regions. Greater training mileage is commonly associated with an increased risk of musculoskeletal injury;[184, 192,194–196] Wexler[196] is very specific in identifying a threshold of increased musculoskeletal risk as running in excess of 40 miles per week.

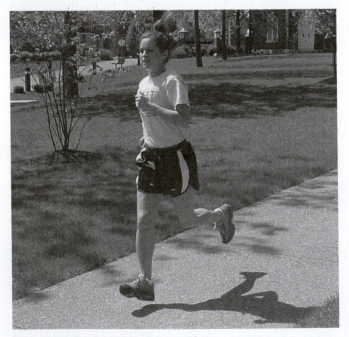

Figure 4.14   Overground running.

In-line Skating

In-line skating, or roller blading (**Figure 4.15**) has become a popular mode of aerobic exercise over the past two decades. This exercise mode requires in-line skates that have three to five wheels arranged in line with each other, attached to a rigid boot. Originally, in-line skating developed as a dry land training technique for ice skaters and ice hockey players. However, it is now the fastest growing recreational sport in the United States,[197] attracting participants of all ages. In-line skating enthusiasts claim that a significant advantage of this exercise mode is decreased impact loading as compared to running. Mahar et al.[198] compared the impact characteristics of in-line skating and running, reporting significantly lower impact during in-line skating. They concluded that in-line skating might be a useful exercise alternative to running for those who wish to reduce impact shock during aerobic training.[198]

Stimulated by an increase in the popularity of in-line skating, several researchers have investigated the physiological demands and training effects of this exercise mode. Snyder et al.[199] and Wallick et al.[200] examined the physiologic responses to in-line skating compared with conventional modes of aerobic exercise, running and cycling. Snyder et al.[199] found oxygen utilization for in-line skating was lower than running or cycling using heart rate as a determinant for exercise intensity, but was sufficient to enable aerobic power training. They suggested that fit individuals need to train uphill or at greater velocities to achieve significant cardiopulmonary benefits. Wallick et al.[200] reported that skating at a pace of 17.7–20.9 km/h resulted in an aerobic exercise intensity of 60 percent to 75 percent VO_{2max}, or 75 percent to 90 percent HR_{max}. These values correspond to the recommended ACSM training ranges earlier described. The researchers concluded from these data that "in-line skating elicits physiological responses comparable to treadmill running and thus would be another exercise alternative for improving aerobic capacity or maintaining body weight."[200]

Two studies by Melanson et al.[180,201] provide further support for the effectiveness of in-line skating in improving aerobic power. In the first study, Melanson et al.[201] reported a significantly higher VO_{2max} with running but no differences in heart rate, rating of perceived exertion, or ventilation between running and in-line skating. In a follow-up study, Melanson et al.[180] compared the changes in VO_{2max} after nine weeks of treadmill training and in-line skating, reporting similar VO_{2max} improvements with both training modes that were equivalent to their training volumes.

A significant issue pertaining to in-line skating is the risk of injury. Concurrent with the rise in popularity is the number of emergency room visits because of injuries sustained while in-line skating. Schieber et al.[202,203] reported that 100,000 (4 percent) of the estimated 22.5 million in-line skating participants were seen for emergency room visits in 1995. The most common in-line skating injuries are wrist, forearm, and elbow fractures.[197,202] Approximately 20 percent of all injuries involve the lower extremities, including contusions, lacerations, and fractures, and head injuries, accounted for 5 percent of all injuries.[197] Most injuries occur in novice skaters and the most common cause of injury was a loss of control. Behavioral patterns that increased the risk of injury were non-use of protective equipment and excessive speed.[197,202] Most in-line skating injuries are preventable by 1) using elbow pads, knee pads, wrist guards, and helmets, and 2) skating in control. If these practices are implemented, in-line skating can be an effective and safe means of improving aerobic power.

> ## *Key Point:*
> Since loss of control is the primary reason for in-line skating injuries among novices, appropriate helmet and pad use must be advised in addition to a training speed that enables consistently controlled movements.

Step Aerobics

Step, or bench, aerobics (**Figure 4.16**) is an exercise mode performed using a platform 4 inches to 10 inches in height. The participant follows the guidance of an instructor who combines body movements with stepping onto and off of the platform. Each participant works in an area around the step platform; there is not a significant amount of transitional movement during a workout. Exercise intensity is controlled by such variables as stepping rate, upper extremity activity, and step height. Sutherland et al.[203] examined the physiological responses and perceived

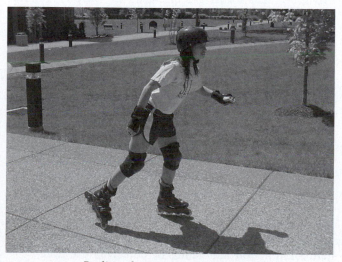

Figure 4.15   In-line skating.

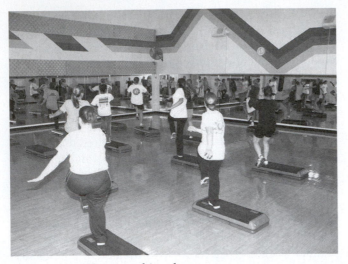

Figure 4.16   Step aerobics class.

exertion in a step aerobics session using three different step heights. In the study, 10 regularly exercising female participants performed a 40 minute step routine at three step heights (6 inches, 8 inches, 10 inches) presented in random order. All of the participants followed the same workout choreography and the dependent variables of oxygen uptake, heart rate, and ratings of perceived exertion were collected. The authors reported that the 8 inch step height and 10 inch step height workouts were of sufficient intensity to improve or maintain cardiopulmonary fitness as established by the ACSM. They concluded that the six inch platform routine was less than adequate in terms of rating of perceived exertion and aerobic training measurements in improving aerobic power, suggesting it be used only for participants who were at lower fitness levels.[203] The investigators also found that heart rate may overestimate the intensity of exercise in a step aerobics session, and ratings of perceived exertion had low correlation to oxygen uptake and therefore, may not be useful in judging the intensity of this particular exercise mode.

Anderson et al.[10] compared the effect of a 16 week program of structured lifestyle activity modification versus step aerobics on cardiovascular risk factors in obese women. Both groups showed weight loss over the 16 weeks, although the step aerobics group maintained more of their muscle mass, or lean body mass, than the lifestyle modification group. In addition, both groups showed significant reduction in total cholesterol and triglycerides. The authors concluded that both modes of activity offered health benefits, including weight loss and improved lipid profiles. Kraemer et al.[204] investigated the physiological effects of a step aerobics program as compared to a step aerobics program with additional resistance training. Thirty-five healthy female participants were randomly assigned to one of the training groups: 25 minute step aerobics session, 25 minute step-aerobics session plus resistance training, 40 minute step aerobics session, and a control group. Their results showed that all three training groups significantly improved VO_{2max}, had a decrease in resting heart rate, and decreased body fat percentage. Williford et al.[182] compared bench stepping and running among healthy young women, concluding that aerobic bench stepping exercise produced similar changes in VO_{2max} as running, confirming the efficacy of step aerobics as an exercise mode to improve aerobic power.

There is little research regarding injury rates in persons undertaking step aerobics. Anecdotal reports identify the common injuries from step aerobics as exercise-related leg pain, foot pain, and patellofemoral pain. Maybury and Waterfield[205] examined the relationship between step height and ground reaction forces. According to their results, the 8 inch and 10 inch steps resulted in significantly higher ground reaction force than the 6 inch step, causing the authors to recommend use of the lower platforms to avoid injury to the lower extremities. A higher stepping rate produces higher ground reaction forces during step aerobics.[207] Ground reaction forces of 1.5–1.87 × body weight have been reported during step aerobics, which are lower than the ground reaction forces of running, but higher than those of walking.[206,207] Consequently, this exercise mode appears to be relatively safe with moderate impact forces and minimal risk for traumatic injuries.

Aerobic Dance

Aerobic dance is similar to step aerobics but does not typically involve the use of a platform. This mode of aerobic exercise is typically performed in a group format with an instructor but can also be performed at home with video instruction. The instructor leads participants though choreographed dance movements to music; the genre of music is variable, depending on the preferences of the instructor and the participants. Dance movements involve a combination of upper and lower extremity motions and may include steps from jazz, ballet, hip-hop, disco, Latin, or funk styles of dance. Dance therapy and other alternative movement forms are discussed in Chapter 10. Recently, a blend of aerobic dance and martial arts or boxing-type movements has been popularized, such as kickboxing and Tae Bo. Generally, there are two levels of aerobic dance, low impact and high impact. The low impact classes require that at least one foot is in contact with the floor at all times and is designed for individuals with impact limitations secondary to age, pregnancy, or weight. High impact activities may include hopping or jumping where both feet are momentarily not in contact with the floor. In their comparison of high impact and low impact aerobic dance, Grant et al.[208] concluded that fit individuals may not gain a training benefit from low impact aerobic dance, as this mode of exercise is most appropriate for poorly conditioned or overweight individuals.

Increased cadence and impact level cause increased oxygen consumption and rating of perceived exertion;[208,209] addition of arm movements had the greatest effect on increasing heart rate during aerobic dance.[209] Schaeffer et al.[210] found that perceived exertion ratings displayed poor correlations with heart rate and VO_{2max} of instructors during an aerobics dance session and concluded that perceived exertion ratings should not be used as a singular measure of exercise intensity in this training mode. In a follow-up study, Schaeffer-Gerschutz et al.[211] recommended that both heart rate and rating of perceived exertion be used to judge exercise intensity during an aerobics dance session. Bell and Bassey[212] reported that pulse palpation by healthy adult females who participated in an aerobics dance class consistently underestimated exercise heart rate as measured by a telemetry system. Accordingly, the rehabilitation clinician must be cautious in relying on participant-measured heart rate alone as an exercise intensity measure.

Multiple studies have shown that aerobic dance is an effective mode for increasing aerobic power. Milburn and Butts[213] compared the effect of aerobic dance and jogging on the cardiopulmonary fitness of college-aged women, reporting that the exercise modes were equally effective in improving cardiopulmonary endurance over a seven week training program. Research by McCord et al.[214] examined the effect of a 12 week program of low impact aerobic dance on VO_{2max} and body composition in college-aged women. These researchers concluded that low impact aerobic dance was as effective as other modes of aerobic exercise both in improving aerobic power and in decreasing body fat. Perry et al.[163] compared the training effect of continuous and interval aerobic dance. The continuous group performed a 30–35 minute continuous dance workout with a warm up and cool down period three times/week. The interval group trained for the same period of time but performed alternating bouts of three to five minutes of aerobic dance and three minutes of brisk walking or mild jogging. Both groups showed improvement in body composition and anaerobic threshold over the 12 week training program. The interval group demonstrated significantly greater VO_{2max} improvements compared to the control group and to the continuous group. The continuous group did not show a significant improvement in VO_{2max} compared to the control group. These researchers concluded that interval dance training can be successfully applied to aerobic dance and should be considered an effective training alternative to conventional aerobic dance programs that use continuous training.[163]

Injuries in persons engaged in aerobic dance are typically of the overuse type and most commonly involve the ankle, leg, knee, and back.[215] In their research on injury rate during fitness activities, Requa[191] reported that the injury rate in aerobic dance was in the intermediate category, along with running. The reported injury rate among aerobic dance participants varies in the literature from 24 percent[216] to 77 percent,[217] with fewer injuries occurring in low impact classes than high impact.[191, 216] These data are consistent with the research of Michaud et al.[218] which demonstrated significantly higher ground reaction forces in high impact aerobic dance than in low impact activities. Garrick et al.[219] found that risk factors for injury in aero-

bic dance included a history of musculoskeletal problems, lack of involvement in other fitness activities, and the type of aerobic dance program. Two studies have shown a greater incidence of injury in aerobics dance instructors;[216,217] this is likely a consequence of overuse by the instructors as a result of teaching multiple classes.

Stair Stepping

Step ergometers (**Figure 4.17**) have become very popular in fitness centers and rehabilitation clinics over the past 15 years. The two most commonly used types of stair stepping or climbing machines are one in which steps revolve on a track with the step height consistent and the step speed variable, and one in which there are two steps that move independently of each other and the exerciser can vary step height and step cadence. In the latter category, step movement can be driven by an electric motor or mechanically, through hydraulic pistons. As it is often inconvenient and unsafe to perform aerobic exercise on actual stairs, these units provide the opportunity for the client to perform repeated stair ascent without encountering the top of the stairs.

Aerobic exercise intensity is typically adjusted on stair climbers using step height, step cadence, and upper body support. Howley et al.[220] found that the use of arms and

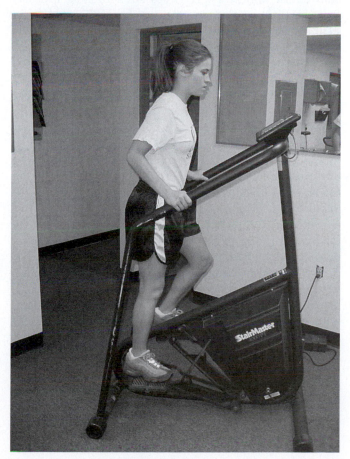

Figure 4.17   Stepping device.

hands significantly lowered the heart rate and the VO_{2max} at the 10 MET level, but not at the four and seven MET level. They found that step rate had no effect on heart rate at any of the MET level workouts. Anecdotal observations suggest that as clients increase step cadence on these machines, they typically decrease their step height. This combination of increased cadence and decreased step height may result in minimal changes in overall work, therefore not significantly changing the VO_{2max}. The rehabilitation clinician needs to cue the client who uses these devices about appropriate posture and the physiologic importance of movement quality.

Stair stepping has been shown to be an effective exercise mode to improve aerobic power. Ben-Ezra and Verstraete[221] examined the task specific training response of healthy men who were assigned to either a stair stepper or treadmill training group. Both groups were tested on both machines before and after the 10-week training period. Their results showed that step ergometry was effective in improving VO_{2max} and the training effect was not specific to stair stepping but transferred to running on the treadmill. Loy et al.[157] compared the training effect of stair climbing and running on physically active college age women over a nine week period. Both groups showed improvement in VO_{2max} and in 2414 m run time. In a follow-up study, Loy et al.[222] showed stair climbing to be an effective exercise for middle-aged women both as an aerobic exercise and as a quadriceps strengthening exercise. Ryan et al.[223] studied the effect of forward or backward stepping on heart rate, perceived exertion rating, blood pressure, and caloric expenditure among healthy college age male subjects during a stair climber exercise session. Their results suggested greater physiologic responses during the retrograde movement at higher intensity levels; however, they did not consider the differences to be practically meaningful.[223]

Very little has been published regarding injury rates in stair stepper devices. In the training study by Loy et al.,[222] they reported an injury rate of 16 percent, similar to that reported for walking programs. In a survey study of 212 members of seven health clubs, Vereschagin et al.[224] reported that 39 percent reported transient paresthesia in the plantar aspect of the feet and toes as a result of overtraining on a stair stepper machine. Based on the patellofemoral reaction forces in stair climbing, it is plausible that this exercise mode may potentially irritate the patellofemoral joint (particularly the articular cartilaginous surface) of clients who are predisposed to this problem.[225] The personal experience of the authors suggests a tendency for clients to demonstrate undesirable postural changes during a workout with increased trunk flexion and dependency on upper extremity support when using this exercise mode. Clients for whom the use of these devices is deemed appropriate should be educated about maintaining an appropriate upright posture and good balance with minimal arm support during a workout.

Elliptical Trainers

Elliptical trainers (**Figure 4.18**) are one of the newest additions to the growing list of devices targeting the development of aerobic power. These machines have footplates that move through reciprocal elliptical motions, simulating the kinematics of running gait. However, the client's feet are always in contact with the footplates, thus reducing impact forces. Some elliptical machines combine arm and leg movement similar to a cross country ski machine to increase the overall muscle mass involved in the exercise. Intensity is manipulated by resistance and speed variables, as well as the addition of upper extremity exercise.

We could find only one report from a peer reviewed source regarding the effects of this aerobic exercise mode. Mercer et al.[226] compared physiological responses of VO_{2max} and heart rate during elliptical trainer and treadmill exercise among physically active college students. They reported no significant differences in VO_{2max}, heart rate, and ratings of perceived exertion during maximal exercise between these two aerobic exercise modes and concluded that the elliptical trainer is a "suitable alternative"[226] to running on the treadmill. Given the very recent development of and interest in this device, there is not yet any information regarding injury rates. However, based on the decrease in impact forces, it is expected that injury patterns would be similar to those of the stair steppers rather than the pattern seen in runners. If this is shown true in future research, the elliptical trainer would be a very attractive form of training with minimal injury risk and significant aerobic training benefits.

Cross-Country skiing

Cross-country skiing is a total body exercise mode that involves the major muscle groups of the lower extremity in the skiing action and the upper extremity muscle groups in

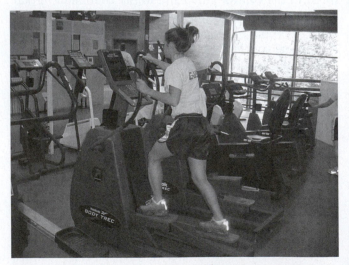

Figure 4.18   Elliptical training with upper extremity contributions.

the pole action. True cross-country skiing (**Figure 4.19**) requires cross-country skis, boots, and poles, as well as the most important prerequisite, snow. Unquestionably, outdoor cross-country skiing is an excellent mode of exercise for maintaining or improving aerobic power. World class cross-country skiers have some of the highest recorded VO_{2max} values of all athletes.[31,227] The simultaneous use of arms and legs for propulsion during this exercise mode demands concurrent activity in upper and lower extremity muscle groups, resulting in significant energy expenditure and oxygen demand. Exercise intensity in cross-country skiing is determined by speed, skiing technique, topography, and snow characteristics, such as packed or powder, temperature, and water content. Oja et al.[228] conducted a training study on untrained middle-aged Finnish men, comparing running and cross-country skiing with both groups training at a prescribed intensity for 40 minutes, three times per week over a 9–10 week duration. Their results indicated that both cross-country skiing and running are equally effective in improving cardiopulmonary fitness.

Although cross-country skiing is a good choice for improving aerobic power, the equipment and climate requirements limit widespread access to and interest in this aerobic exercise mode. Consequently, cross-country ski simulators have been developed to provide this mode of aerobic training without special equipment or snow. As with true cross-country skiing, these simulators are designed to provide resistance to both upper and lower extremity motions. However, a disadvantage of these machines is the client must display appropriate balance and normal motor control to coordinate arm and leg movements. Goss et al.[229] studied the physiological requirements of aerobic exercise during ski simulator exercise among five male subjects reporting high VO_{2max} demands which increased with increased pace on the machine. They concluded that simulated cross-country skiing was an effective mode to improve aerobic power and was a useful alternative to conventional cardiovascular exercise.[229] Research by Zeni et al.[185] demonstrated that healthy women who exercised on a cross-country ski simulator at perceived exertion ratings of 13–16 displayed oxygen uptake increases that were within the range prescribed by the ACSM for improving cardiopulmonary fitness. Moyna et al.[187] reported that persons using the ski simulator and treadmill displayed consistently higher energy expenditures at a given rating of perceived exertion than persons using stair stepper, stationary cycle, rowing, and rider devices.

In true cross-country skiing, the injury rate is between 0.49–5.63 per 1,000 skier days.[230] The most common traumatic injuries are medial collateral ligament sprains of the knee and ulnar collateral ligaments injury to the thumb. Overuse injuries are common, occurring in the foot, lower leg, knee, and low back.[231] No data are published regarding injuries during simulated cross-country skiing.

Bicycling

Bicycling, using a stationary cycle ergometer (**Figure 4.20**) or a road or trail bicycle (**Figure 4.21**) is a very popular mode of aerobic exercise. A primary advantage of cycling is minimization of weight bearing and impact forces

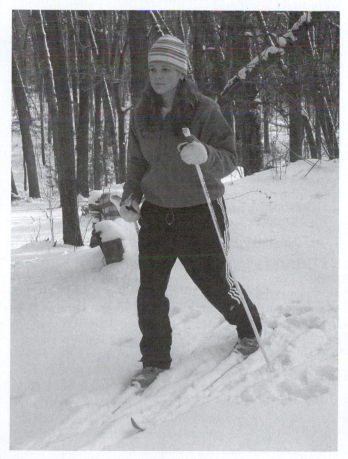

Figure 4.19   Cross-country skiing.

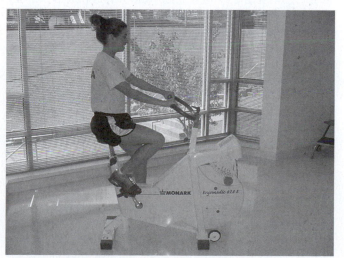

Figure 4.20   Standard stationary cycling.

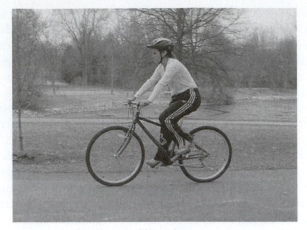

Figure 4.21   Overground bicycling.

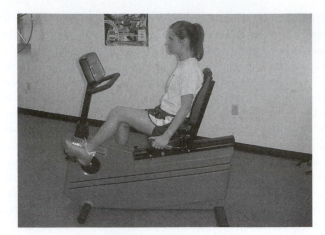

Figure 4.22   Recumbent stationary cycling.

on the hips, knees, and ankles. It does, however, involve rhythmic contractions of large mass muscle groups of the lower extremity, including the quadriceps, hamstrings, iliopsoas, gluteus maximus, and gastrocnemius-soleus complex. Contraction of these muscles creates a significant oxygen demand during cycling, stimulating training of the cardiopulmonary systems.

Multiple variables affect the energy requirements and comfort of cycling. Variables common to stationary and overground cycling include the rider's position, pedal cadence, and linkage of the pedal and the rider's shoe. Seat height should be adjusted so that at the bottom of the stroke, the knee is slightly flexed (10°–20°) with the metatarsal heads located over the pedal axles.[175,232] Nordeen-Snyder[233] compared the effect of three seat height positions on recorded VO_2 values during cycling and found if the seat is too high or too low, it will negatively affect energy efficiency. The seat, or saddle, should be either level or the nose tilted slightly downward. This seat position will prevent excessive pressure on the perineal region in men and women, and will also help prevent pudendal neuropathy and impotence in men.[232] To achieve aerobic exercise benefits, pedal speed should be kept relatively high (70–90 RPM) to maximize exercise efficiency while minimizing joint compressive forces.[175,234] The use of toe clips, forefoot strap, or cleats may improve mechanical efficiency and VO_{2max} in elite cyclists[235] but has no effect on metabolic and cardiopulmonary responses in untrained cyclists.[236]

Stationary cycles come in two basic types: upright (**Figure 4.20**) and recumbent (**Figure 4.22**). Two studies on the effect of rider position have shown no difference in oxygen consumption between these two types of exercise cycles.[237,238] The upright position more closely simulates body position on a bicycle, with weightbearing primarily through the ischial tuberosities on the saddle. Some individuals prefer the recumbent cycle because they can sit on a much larger, bucket-style seat with back support. This

exercise cycle type may be a more desirable choice for individuals who are overweight or pregnant. Regardless of body position, energy expenditure on a stationary cycle is primarily determined by the combination of pedal cadence and pedal resistance. Depending on the exercise cycle design, the resistance may be created by a fan, magnet, friction belt, friction pad, or hydraulic mechanism. The resistance should be set at a level that enables the client to maintain a cadence of 70–90 RPM and provides sufficient load to reach the intensity goal for the aerobic exercise session.

A relatively new form of stationary cycle exercise is "spinning." This exercise mode requires a specialized stationary bike that allows the rider different hand positions and movement on and off of the saddle. Spinning is done in a class setting with an instructor leading the participants through an interval-type workout. The intensity of the exercise program is based on heart rate response to the exercise, and participants are encouraged to follow their own body response to exercise and are discouraged from competing with other class participants. At present, there is no published literature regarding the effectiveness of spinning as a method of training for aerobic power.

In related investigations on the effectiveness of aerobic exercise equipment, Zeni et al.[185, 186] found stationary cycling to produce a lower heart rate at a given perceived exertion rating than simulated cross country skiing, rowing ergometry, stair stepping, and treadmill running. Furthermore, Zeni et al.[186] reported that at a perceived exertion rating of 11 or 13, the cycle ergometer training did not meet the ACSM guidelines for enhancing cardiopulmonary fitness regarding oxygen consumption values. Moyna et al.[187] published similar results in a study comparing energy expenditure using different modes of aerobic exercise. They reported that cycle ergometry had the lowest energy expenditure and heart rate response at a given perceived exertion rating of the six devices examined. Consequently, for a given exercise time period, continuous stationary cycling is not as effective in burning calories as treadmill running or simulated cross country skiing. It is, however, a very safe mode of exercise; Requa et al.[191] reported that stationary cycling had a lower injury rate than any other adult fitness activity, including walking. Given the low impact nature of stationary cycling, it is a good choice for persons with arthritic conditions in their lower extremity joints.[175]

> ## *Key Point:*
> Since stationary cycling is a low impact activity, it is a good aerobic exercise device for clients who have arthritic conditions at their lower extremities.

Overground bicycles also come in three basic types: road (touring) bicycles, trail (mountain) bicycles, and hybrid (comfort) bicycles. There are numerous books available to assist a person in making the decision as to which bicycle to buy. A major part of the decision is where one intends to ride and how comfortable one is on the bicycle. Regardless of the type of bicycle chosen, however, outdoor cycling can be an excellent form of aerobic training. Additional variables affecting energy expenditure in overground cycling include rolling resistance, air resistance, and terrain. *Rolling resistance* is the resistance between the tires and the riding surface. In touring bicycles, the tires are very narrow and are filled with air at a high pressure. Consequently, very little tire surface is in contact with the road, which minimizes the rolling resistance. On the contrary, mountain bikes have wide, knobby tires to maximize traction on off road surfaces. These tires have a greater rolling resistance on a flat hard surface but are better designed for rough, irregular surfaces. *Air resistance* increases with the speed of the bicycle and with the frontal area of the rider. To minimize this resistance, touring bicycle design includes down turned handlebars and aerodynamic frame and wheel construction. By minimizing frontal area in the drop bar position and by wearing smooth riding apparel, the rider can further contribute to less air resistance. When a rider is on flat terrain, the mass of the rider is supported by the bicycle and contributes to the rolling resistance. However, when a rider encounters an incline, the effect of gravity results in a force opposing the uphill motion. Consequently, the rider has to increase power to overcome this force, and oxygen consumption will increase. It is no surprise that elite cyclists have very low body fat percentages, as this plus lightweight bicycle design minimize the challenge of uphill cycling.[234]

One challenge to using outdoor cycling as an exercise mode to increase aerobic power is maintaining consistent exercise intensity during a ride. Depending on terrain, traffic, and pedal speed, it may be difficult for an outdoor cyclist to maintain the requisite intensity to meet fitness

goals. For some, outdoor cycling is a recreational activity to enjoy the company of others and local scenery. Innovative communities have begun to appreciate the development of bike paths to provide a safe exercise outlet for their citizens.

Another consideration in prescribing overground cycling for improving aerobic power is injury risk. Wilber et al.[239] reported that 85 percent of more than 500 recreational bicyclists reported one or more overuse injuries that required medical attention. The areas most commonly affected were the neck, knees, groin, and hand. Positioning on a bicycle is a primary factor in the development of overuse injuries. Improper spinal positioning, seat height, saddle angle, and hand position can cause abnormal loads on body tissues, resulting in musculotendinous or nerve pathology. It is crucial that the outdoor cyclist be counseled regarding bicycle set-up, use of appropriate protective equipment, and proper body positioning to avoid such injuries.

Accidents on bicycles have resulted in the largest number of emergency room visits of all recreational activities.[240] Factors contributing to traumatic bicycle accidents include intoxication,[241] inexperience,[242] rider carelessness, bicycle malfunction, and environmental conditions.[240] A major concern regarding outdoor bicycling is the risk of brain injury. Traumatic brain injury is the cause of 67 percent of bicycle-related fatalities, and 5 percent of all bicycle accidents involve some degree of head injury.[243] Multiple investigations have shown that brain injuries in bicycling are preventable with the use of helmets.[243–246] Unfortunately, bicycle helmet use is still not universal, with estimates in the literature ranging from 13 percent to 69 percent of riders using a helmet regularly. This is one area that health care providers must be active in, advocating and modeling helmet use for all bicyclists.

Rowing

Rowing machines (**Figure 4.23a–b**), like the cross country ski simulators, utilize contractions of the upper extremity, lower extremity, and trunk muscle groups simultaneously. For this reason, rowing advocates promote this mode of exercise for attaining total body fitness. In the exercise mode comparison study by Moyna et al.,[187] the rowing ergometer produced greater energy expenditure than the cycle ergometer and the rider in men, but less than the treadmill, stair stepper, and ski simulator. In women, rowing ergometry was equal to the treadmill and ski simulator and greater than the rider, stair stepper, and cycle ergometer.[187] Zeni et al.[186] reported that exercise on a rowing ergometer by untrained volunteers at RPE values of 11–15 resulted in oxygen uptake values within the ACSM recommended range for enhancing cardiopulmonary fitness.

Marriott and Lamb[247] examined the accuracy of using perceived exertion ratings during rowing ergometry to

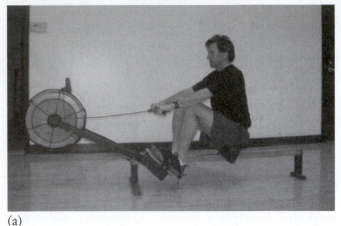

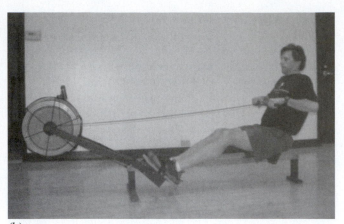

(a)   (b)

Figure 4.23   Indoor rowing. (a) start, (b) finish.

determine aerobic exercise intensity. Using nine competitive male rowers, these authors found a strong relationship between perceived exertion ratings, work output, and heart rate and concluded that perceived exertion rating was a valid estimate of aerobic exercise intensity among this subject group. Cardiopulmonary responses during cycle and rowing ergometry were compared by Hagerman et al.[248] using a sample of untrained men and women. Keeping the power outputs constant, the investigators reported that the energy cost for rowing was significantly higher than for stationary cycling. They concluded that rowing, if performed with a sliding seat that emphasizes large lower extremity muscle use, places a greater demand on the aerobic energy system than some of the more traditional aerobic exercises and therefore has a definite place in the spectrum of prescribed exercises in contemporary physical fitness and cardiac rehabilitation programs.[248]

Little information is published regarding injury in rowing exercise. Requa[191] reported a low injury rate for rowing in his review of injuries in fitness activities. The overuse injury most commonly mentioned in the literature as associated with rowing is rib stress fractures.[249,250] Another region of potential injury in rowing is the spine; Soler[251] reported a 16.9 percent incidence of spondylolysis in competitive rowers.

Arm Ergometry

Some aerobic exercise modes such as rowing, cross country skiing, some elliptical trainers, and some stationary bicycles incorporate simultaneous upper and lower extremity muscle activation. However, lower extremity injury or disease may prevent some clients from using these devices. Upper body ergometry (**Figure 4.24**) may be the best clinically accessible option for some clients to maintain or improve their cardiopulmonary fitness. Additionally, individuals without lower extremity problems might

use arm exercise for cross training or exercise variety reasons. Based on specificity of training, arm exercise may be desirable for persons who engage in work or sport activities that are highly arm dominant. Other advantages of arm ergometry are safety, comfortable positioning, and ease of use.

A major consideration in the application of arm exercise for training is the difference in the cardiovascular response to arm exercise as compared to leg exercise. This difference in physiologic response is a result of the decreased muscle mass that is engaged in upper body exercise as compared to lower body exercise. The VO_{2max} is 20 percent to 30 percent lower in persons engaging in arm exercise than in those engaging in lower extremity exercise.[252] Similarly, HR_{max} and stroke volume are also lower during arm ergometry.[252,253] During arm ergometry there is a greater physiological strain at any given power output as compared to leg ergometry, as evidenced by higher

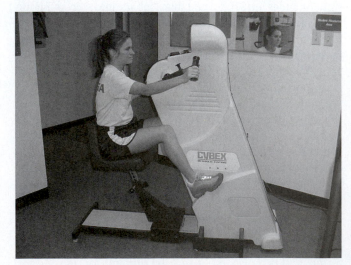

Figure 4.24   Upper body ergometry.

heart rate, oxygen uptake, ventilatory rate, diastolic and systolic blood pressure, and perceived exertion rating.[254]

When prescribing aerobic exercise intensity for arm ergometry, the rehabilitation clinician must consider the unique physiological stresses of this exercise mode. Heart rate intensity prescriptions for arm ergometer training should ideally be based on graded arm ergometer testing. Prescriptive use of arm ergometry as a therapeutic exercise mode based on graded exercise testing performed on a treadmill or cycle ergometer will be inappropriately high. Franklin[253] recommends that therapeutic exercise heart rate levels based on lower extremity graded exercise tests be lowered by 10 beats/minute for training on an arm ergometer. Perceived exertion ratings during use of an arm ergometer have been shown to be effective and valid for regulating the intensity in arm ergometry and are a useful tool for confirming intensity levels set by heart rate.[254]

Arm ergometry training has been shown to improve the VO_{2max} of healthy subjects over a 10 week training period.[255] This exercise mode has also been used successfully in aerobic training for cardiac patients.[256,257] No reports of injury as a result of arm ergometer training were found in the literature. Obviously, there is no concern regarding lower extremity injury with this exercise mode. As there is no impact loading of the upper extremity joints in arm ergometry, there appears to be little risk of injury if the client is properly positioned on the arm ergometer and vital signs and perceived exertion are monitored.

Aquatic Exercise

Exercise to improve aerobic power can be performed in an aquatic environment using swimming (**Figure 4.25a–b**) or pool running (**Figure 4.26**). These exercise modes are particularly desirable for persons with musculoskeletal impairments that limit weight bearing exercise. However, disadvantages of aquatic exercise include the need for regular accessibility to a pool or appropriate body of water, the need for a lifeguard or swim partner, fear or anxiety about water exercise, and for swimming, a requisite level of skill.

Similar to arm ergometer training, the physiological responses in swimming are different than land based, lower extremity exercise. These responses are consequent to the combination of the aquatic medium, joint motion and muscle action, resistive forces, thermal conditions, and body position in swimming. The human body encounters drag when moving through water. Drag is dependent on body position, the swimmer's shape and size, water turbulence, and the interface between the water and the skin.[258] A swimmer has to exert power to overcome these drag forces and these forces increase exponentially as swimming velocity increases.[259] As these drag forces are much greater in water than in air, the energy cost of swimming a distance is approximately four times that of running an equal distance. As the average woman is smaller and has a greater body fat percentage than the average man, women have greater buoyancy, less drag, and, thus, a 30 percent lower energy cost of swimming as compared to men.

Swim training to improve aerobic power can be done with any of the basic four strokes: front crawl, backstroke, breaststroke, and butterfly. The energy costs of these strokes are not the same; breaststroke and butterfly have almost twice the energy demand as the front crawl and backstroke.[259,260] Energy costs of swimming are also affected by training; competitive swimmers exhibit greater energy efficiency in swimming than recreational swimmers.[261] Swim velocity is determined by the product of stroke frequency and stroke length. Novice swimmers will attempt to swim faster by increasing their stroke frequency rather than the stroke length. The greater efficiency of trained swimmers reflects their greater stroke length.

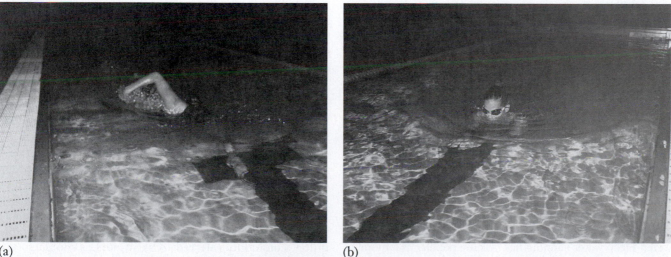

(a)   (b)

Figure 4.25   Swimming. (a) freestyle or crawl stroke, (b) breaststroke.

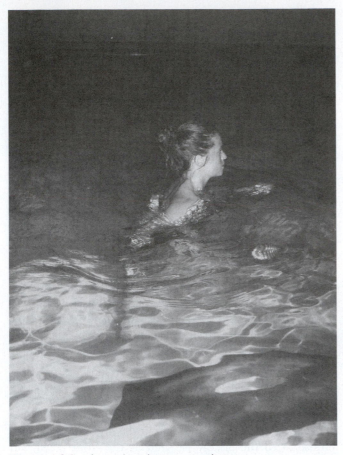

Figure 4.26   Aqua-jogging or running.

Cardiac output and HR_{max} in swimming is lower than in land based, lower extremity exercise. This is a result of body position, smaller muscle mass engaged in propulsion, cooling of the periphery, and the phenomenon described as the diving reflex. The diving reflex elicits a bradycardiac effect when the face is immersed in water. When prescribing intensity for swimming, the age-adjusted HR_{max} should be decreased by 10–15 beats/minute. Research by Tanaka[262] and Magel et al.[263] has shown that VO_{2max} improvements from swim training are specific to swimming with minimal transfer to treadmill running or cycling. These data may reflect the unique cardiopulmonary responses to swim training as compared to land exercise.

If swimming is not feasible, deep water jogging or running is another mode of aquatic exercise for cardiopulmonary and cardiovascular conditioning. In deep water running the participant performs the running motion but without foot contact on the pool bottom. Consequently, there are no impact forces as are encountered in dry land running. The exercise is typically performed with a flotation belt or vest to help keep the person in a vertical position with the head out of the water. Deep water running has become popular as a mode of exercise for persons who have weightbearing limitations and for non-injured persons as a mode of cross training.[264–266]

Wilber et al.[266] studied the effectiveness of deep water running as compared to treadmill running in the maintenance of aerobic conditioning for a group of trained male distance runners. The results of this study showed a six week training period of deep water running was an effective alternative to treadmill running, as there were no significant differences between the two groups in VO_{2max}. Other research has shown that deep water running does not negatively affect running performance in competitive runners.[265,267] Burns and Lauder[264] specifically examined the implementation of a deep water running program for military personnel who were injured and given a non-weightbearing status. Over a 22 month period, 181 military personnel participated in the program, during which they trained in the pool for one hour, three times per week. The researchers reported that deep water running was an ideal exercise for maintaining conditioning and land running performance in military personnel who were on a temporary non-weightbearing status.[264] In a related study, Gehring et al.[268] examined the difference between deep water running with and without a flotation vest in recreational and competitive runners, reporting that competitive runners were able to reach intensities equal to land-based training with or without flotation belt use. In contrast, recreational runners were not able to achieve a level of training intensity during deep water running with flotation vest use that would stimulate effective cardiopulmonary training.

D'Acquisito et al.[269] assessed the metabolic and cardiovascular response to shallow-water exercise in a group of older women (60–80 years). The exercise program was completed in chest deep water and included a 10 minute warm-up period of water walking and stretching followed by a 25 minute primary workout of pool calisthenics, jogging variations, and various multiplanar functional movements. The program finished with a five minute cool down period of water walking and stretching. The researchers concluded that the exercise intensity during this program met the ACSM guidelines for aerobic exercise as measured by both percentage of predicted HR_{max} and MET. An advantage of shallow water exercise is a significant decrease in weightbearing stress to the lower extremity joints. In a depth of water up to the xiphoid process level of the sternum, an individual has approximately 40 percent of their dry land body weight transmitted through their lower extremities when standing still.[175]

There are no reports in the literature about exercise injuries sustained in deep water running or shallow water exercise. Swimming, however, can lead to upper extremity overuse injury, particularly at the shoulder. Repetitive freestyle, back, or butterfly stroke can lead to accumulative microtraumatic damage to the rotator cuff. This condition, commonly referred to as swimmer's shoulder, is a type of shoulder impingement syndrome that primarily involves the subacromial region. Joint instability, improper technique, and overtraining can lead to this condition.[270] Other potential negative consequences of swimming include overexposure to the sun in outdoor swimming and severe injury to the head or neck when diving into a pool. It is of prime importance that a swimmer never swim alone, given the risk of drowning should they encounter any unforeseen adverse events.

Aerobic Exercise Progression

Aerobic Exercise Initiation (Phase I)

The initial phase of an aerobic exercise program is critical in setting the stage for success in achieving the client's exercise goals and encouraging adherence. When prescribing an exercise program to improve aerobic power, the rehabilitation clinician must be cognizant of avoiding being too aggressive in the initial phase of the program. An inappropriate exercise prescription regarding any of the exercise variables—intensity, frequency, duration, or mode—may result in injury or cessation of the program. The ACSM recommends that the initial stage of a conditioning program include easy muscular endurance exercises and moderate level aerobic activities (40–60 percent of HRR). Swain and Franklin[107] reported that a training intensity of 45 percent VO_2R in fit individuals and 30 percent VO_2R in less fit individuals is the minimum training intensity for aerobic fitness. This stage may last four to six weeks, depending on the client's response to exercise. By the end of this stage, the client should be able to exercise three to five times per week for 30 minutes each session without undue muscle soreness, fatigue, or injury.

Aerobic Exercise Advancement (Phase II)

While the focus of phase I was to gradually acclimate the client to the physical and psychological demands of the aerobic exercise program, the goal of phase II is to increase the exercise load and to stimulate improvement in the client's cardiopulmonary and cardiovascular fitness. As reviewed in the introductory information on exercise prescription, the ACSM recommends that aerobic exercise intensity should range between 55 percent and 90 percent of HR_{max}, or 40 percent and 85 percent of VO_2R or HRR.

> ## Key Point:
> Aerobic exercise intensity should range between 55 percent and 90 percent of maximum heart rate, or 40 percent and 85 percent of VO_2 reserve or heart rate reserve.

Accordingly, the participant should be advanced to higher percentages of their HR_{max}, VO_2R, or MET level, depending on what measure was used to set the initial intensity level. Determination of how quickly and how much the intensity has increased is based on the client's previous exercise history, age, and tolerance of and response to the exercise. Duration may or may not be adjusted during this period; this decision is based on the time the individual has available for exercise program participation and caloric expenditure goals. The rehabilitation clinician has to consider the total training volume (intensity × duration × frequency) and monitor the client for muscle soreness, fatigue, injury, or decreased adherence during this period as a barometer of the exercise challenge. A rule of thumb is to increase the training volume no more than 10 percent per week, although this may be too conservative for more highly conditioned individuals. This period of training lasts four to six months and should result in improvement in the physiological response to exercise and achievement of weight loss goals.

> ## Key Point:
> A rule of thumb is to increase training volume by no more than 10 percent per week, but this may be too conservative for more highly conditioned clients.

Aerobic Exercise Maintenance (Phase III)

As implied by the title, the focus of this final phase of exercise is maintenance of the level of aerobic fitness achieved in the first two phases of the exercise program. This phase begins when the client has achieved his or her fitness goals set at the initiation of the aerobic exercise program. By this time, aerobic exercise should be part of the client's weekly routine, and they should be enjoying the benefits of improved fitness.

One potential problem during this phase is development of exercise boredom. Ideally, this maintenance phase should extend from the second phase throughout the client's life. However, as the client ages, interests or fitness goals may change, and changes in health status may affect therapeutic exercise program compliance. A strategy to prevent therapeutic exercise program boredom and maximize compliance is to diversify the client's modes of performing aerobic exercise. Introducing the client to a new aerobic exercise mode during this stage may be just the stimulus they need to invigorate interest in therapeutic exercise program participation.

It is also important that the rehabilitation clinician help the client recognize the value of physical activity in daily life, including walking, stair climbing, lawn work, and house cleaning. Rather than envisioning "exercise" as a separate part of life that requires time away from other activities, the person should come to recognize the incorporation of physical activity into daily life as a healthy lifestyle choice. Combining regular physical activity with proper nutrition, restful sleep, moderation in alcohol use, and no smoking results in maximizing one's health potential.

Key Point:

Ultimately the client should begin to recognize the importance of incorporating physical activities into their daily life as a healthy lifestyle choice.

SPECIAL CONSIDERATIONS IN AEROBIC EXERCISE

Exercise-Related Cardiac Events

The risk of sudden cardiac death, acute myocardial infarction, and cardiac arrhythmias is greater during exercise than non-exercise and is also greater with more vigorous exercise.[271] The risk for sudden death during jogging in men 30–65 years of age is one death for every 15,240–18,000 joggers. In persons over 30 years old, the most common cause of sudden cardiac death or acute myocardial infarction is coronary artery disease.[272,273] In those under the age of 30, the most common cause of sudden cardiac death is congenital abnormalities or hypertrophic cardiomyopathy.[272] In a study by Giri et al.,[274] the authors showed that those most likely to have a cardiac event related to exertion were habitually inactive persons with multiple cardiac risk factors. Thompson[273] described two strategies to reduce the number of adverse cardiac events during exercise: recognizing prodromal symptoms and stress testing of clients in the high risk category. Several authors agree that large scale cardiac screening of asymptomatic individuals without multiple risk factors is cost prohibitive.[271–273]

Key Point:

Two strategies for reducing the number of adverse cardiac events during exercise include the early recognition of their signs and symptoms (chest discomfort, shortness of breath, discomfort in the neck, back, arms, jaw or stomach areas, nausea, lightheadedness, diaphoresis) and pre-activity stress testing for high risk clients.

Firor and Faulkner[272] described the issue of exercise-related cardiac death as a "paradox" because the risk of an adverse cardiac event increases with exercise, but exercise reduces the overall risk of an adverse cardiac event. Their conclusion was the overall protective effect of exercise outweighs the transient increase in risk during exercise, supported by several other authors.[271, 273,275]

Pregnancy

Before initiating, progressing, or maintaining an aerobic exercise program, a pregnant woman must consult her physician to rule out any possible conditions that would contraindicate exercise. These contraindications include pregnancy-induced hypertension, incompetent cervix, placenta previa, pre-term membrane rupture, pre-term labor during present or prior pregnancy, persistent second or third trimester bleeding, or intrauterine growth retardation. In 2002, the American College of Obstetricians and Gynecologists (ACOG) released new recommendations regarding exercise and pregnancy. The ACOG suggests that in the absence of medical or obstetric complications, 30 minutes or more of moderate exercise a day on most, if not all, days of the week is recommended for pregnant women.[276] These recommendations are consistent with the 1995 consensus statement of the Center for Disease Control and ACSM.[2] Although some research data suggest that regular weight bearing aerobic exercise may lead to lower birth weight, this has not had any unfavorable affect on infant health.

When prescribing aerobic exercise for a pregnant woman, consideration should be given to issues of exercise intensity and mode. The ACOG recommends using ratings of perceived exertion rather than heart rate to set and monitor intensity given the effect of pregnancy on heart rate.[276] Regarding mode, the safest forms of aerobic exercise during pregnancy are low impact activities without the risk of abdominal trauma, including swimming, stationary cycling, low impact aerobics, and walking. The ACOG recommends against collision sports, activities that have an increased risk of falling, and scuba diving.[276] Women exercising during pregnancy should be educated regarding appropriate caloric intake, proper hydration, avoiding exercise in hot and humid conditions, and listening closely to their body's response to exercise. A woman should stop exercise and seek care from her physician if any of the following symptoms are experienced: vaginal bleeding, persistent uterine contractions (> 30 minutes), weight loss or insufficient weight gain (< one kg/month), elevated pulse or blood pressure after exercise, or abdominal pain.[277]

Diabetes Mellitus

Aerobic exercise is an important part of the total health management program of persons with types 1 and 2 diabetes. In fact, inactivity is one of the major risk factors in the development of type 2 diabetes.[278–280] Uncontrolled diabetes results in hyperglycemia, and this state can lead to damage and dysfunction of the eyes, heart, vasculature, peripheral nerves, and kidneys. In type 1 diabetes, glycemic control is accomplished by taking exogenous insulin on a specified dose schedule as prescribed by a physician. Type 2 diabetes may be controlled by weight management and exercise in some individuals; others may need an oral hypoglycemic agent. The primary challenge in prescribing aerobic exercise for a person with diabetes is addressing the risk of a hypoglycemic event. Exercise and insulin have similar effects of decreasing blood glucose levels. Consequently, the exerciser needs to recognize symptoms of hypoglycemia and know appropriate treatment and, more importantly, understand strategies to minimize the risk of a hypoglycemic event.

In the exercise initiation phase, clients with diabetes should be advised to start at a lower intensity level and to frequently monitor their blood sugar levels to understand their body's response to the exercise activity. During this phase, they will need to work closely with their physician in determining the appropriate glycemic control strategies. Progress during this stage may be very gradual based on the client's glycemic response to exercise. For clients using exogenous insulin, the dosage should be decreased before and after exercise; dosage reduction will vary dependent on the training volume. It is crucial that the client has appropriate nutrition, because inadequate carbohydrate levels combined with an insulin dose and exercise can quickly lead to a hypoglycemic state. Symptoms of hypoglycemia include tachycardia, palpitations, restlessness, trembling, hunger, sweating, headache, moodiness, and confusion. If untreated, this can progress to drowsiness, impaired mental state, unconsciousness, and convulsions.

To minimize the risk of an adverse hypoglycemic event, the client with diabetes should wear a medical alert piece of jewelry, should not exercise alone, and should have a readily accessible source of carbohydrate available while exercising. If any of the hypoglycemic symptoms are noted, the client should immediately stop exercise and ingest the carbohydrate. This carbohydrate supplementation should be in a source that has no or low fat, as fat will interfere with rapid absorption; good choices include a sport drink, sugar cube, juice, or fruit. After resting for 10–15 minutes, blood glucose levels should be above 100 mg/dL. If the glucose level is still below 100 mg/dL, the client should ingest more carbohydrate. Exercise should not be restarted on that day, and blood sugar levels should be monitored for the rest of the day. Complex carbohydrates should be consumed following an exercise session to avoid a late onset hypoglycemic event. If the client with diabetes follows these basic strategies, exercise to improve aerobic power should be successful and rewarding, and should positively contribute to the management of the diabetic condition.

Age: Children and Elderly

Exercise prescription for an individual must take into consideration the metabolic, anatomic, physiological, and psychological changes across the lifespan. Accordingly, one should not use standards developed for young to middle-aged adults to prescribe aerobic exercise for children or elderly clients. If a rehabilitation clinician fails to recognize the unique demands of exercise for the young or old, it may result in poor exercise program compliance, or worse, adverse effects on the individual participant.

Children exhibit a higher resting heart rate and a lower stroke volume, with a lower cardiac output at a given work level as compared to adults.[282] They also show a lower absolute VO_{2max}, but when expressed in relation to body weight, values are equal to or greater than in adults.[281] Children are less mechanically efficient than adults, losing more energy to heat in metabolic processes. Although children have the ability to thermoregulate under normal conditions, they do not respond as well under high thermal stress conditions. In hot and humid environments, children and parents should be advised to allow for appropriate acclimatization, ensure proper hydration, and minimize training volume. In cold environments, children become hypothermic more quickly than adults, as they have a higher surface area to body mass ratio. Consequently, attention should be given to proper clothing, hydration, and exposure time.

A significant public health problem in the United States is the increased incidence of obesity in children. A major factor contributing to this trend is decreased levels of physical activity among children.[282] Children should be encouraged to get away from the television and computer and participate in active play. The ACSM does not promote specific intensity guidelines for training healthy children, as they will self-select appropriate levels of activity during play. Children should be encouraged to engage in a variety of physical activities for at least 30 minutes daily, most, if not all, days of the week. A troubling recent trend is increases in the number of overuse injuries in active children, primarily attributable to early sports specialization.[283] The American Academy of Pediatrics recently published a recommendation that children not specialize in one sport year round before adolescence.[283]

> ## *Key Point:*
> Because of the high number of overuse injuries experienced by active children, the American Academy of Pediatrics has recommended that children not specialize in one sport year round prior to adolescence.

Unlike children, it is imperative that older adults (men ≥ 45 years of age and women ≥55 years of age) have a complete physical examination by a physician before initiating an exercise program. The ACSM recommends that this testing include an exercise stress test if the person intends to engage in vigorous exercise (> six MET) or if the person intends to engage in moderate exercise but has additional risk factors or cardiopulmonary signs or symptoms. Age-related changes in cardiopulmonary measures of older adults include decreased HR_{max} and cardiac output, decreased VO_{2max}, and decreased vital capacity. An unanswered question at present is whether those changes are truly age related, or if they reflect a general decrease in the physical activity of older adults.

Unquestionably, aerobic exercise to improve cardiopulmonary fitness has numerous health benefits in the older population that can significantly affect quality of life. These benefits include improvement in cardiopulmonary physiologic performance measurements, decreased coronary artery disease risk, improvement in blood lipid profiles, decreased incidence of type 2 diabetes, increased bone mineral density, and an improvement in overall sense of well being.[284] However, appropriate therapeutic exercise prescription is essential to encourage compliance. The general guidelines for therapeutic exercise prescription presented earlier in the chapter can be used, but the initial intensity should be set carefully and the client should be monitored closely for response to exercise. Swain and Franklin[107] have shown that for poorly conditioned individuals, cardiopulmonary system improvement can occur at exercise levels as low as 30 percent VO_2R. Intensity can be monitored using heart rate, perceived exertion rating, or MET level depending on the equipment and personnel available. If using heart rate, it is advised to set training levels based on peak heart rate measured during a graded exercise test than on an age predicted heart rate given the variability of the measurement among the elderly. Another important consideration in setting intensity using heart rate as a training intensity guide is the effect of some prescription medicines. If the client is taking a β blocker, nitrates, calcium channel blockers, diuretics, ACE inhibitors, antiarrythmic agents, bronchodilators, or similar medicines, heart rate should not be used as a measure of exercise intensity. In these cases, perceived exertion ratings are more appropriate indicators of exercise intensity.

Key Point:

Perceived exertion ratings rather than heart rate should be used as an exercise intensity measurement among older clients who use a β blocker, nitrates, calcium channel blockers, diuretics, ACE inhibitors, antiarrythmic agents, bronchodilators, or similar medicines.

The Center for Disease Control–ACSM consensus statement on physical activity—30 minutes of moderate intensity exercise on most, if not all, days of the week—applies to the population of older adults. Older adult clients should be advised that the physical activity that they participate in need not be continuous to have a positive effect; 30 minutes of accumulated activity in a day is beneficial. The choice of mode of exercise is made based on the client's interests, general health, and availability of facilities. Pool walking, swimming, and cycling are desirable for those who have weight bearing limitations. If possible, weight bearing exercises are desirable for bone health and walking is an ideal choice for the older adult. As is true with children, a variety of activities are desirable to encourage compliance, minimize burnout, and avoid overuse injuries.

Summary

Therapeutic exercise focused on improving aerobic power contributes to a person's overall health and wellness, encourages a sense of well being, and lowers the risk of heart disease and type II diabetes. Research has shown positive effects of aerobic exercise on cardiac muscle mass, cardiac output, resting heart rate, blood pressure, and ventilatory capacity. Therapeutic exercise programs following injury or disease should always include a component of training for aerobic power. However, before aerobic exercise is prescribed, a physician should clear the client, and appropriate exercise testing should be performed.

Training-induced changes in cardiovascular and respiratory parameters are dependent on training volume—the combination of training intensity, duration, and frequency. The key to a safe and effective aerobic exercise prescription is the appropriate selection of these variables based on the individual's health history, fitness, functional activities, exercise goals, and motivation. Careful consideration should be given to the selection of the exercise mode to minimize injury risk, maximize exercise efficiency, and encourage exercise adherence. Special consideration in therapeutic exercise prescription are made for individuals who have health conditions, including heart or lung disease, pregnancy, diabetes, degenerative joint disease, and for children and older adults. To maximize aerobic exercise adherence and training effects, the cardiopulmonary or cardiovascular exercise program should be conceptualized as an integral part of a healthy lifestyle, along with strengthening and flexibility exercises, good nutrition, restful sleep, avoidance or cessation of tobacco use, and moderation of alcohol use.

References

1. Blair SN, Kohl HW, III, Paffenbarger RS, Jr., et al. Physical fitness and all-cause mortality: A prospective study of healthy men and women. *JAMA*. 1989;262(17):2395–2401.

2. Pate RR, Pratt M, Blair SN, et al. Physical activity and public health: A recommendation from the Centers for Disease Control and Prevention and the American College of Sports Medicine. *JAMA*. 1995;273(5):402–407.

3. U.S. Department of Health and Human Services. Healthy People 2010: Understanding and Improving Health, 2nd ed. Washington, DC: U.S. Government Printing Office, 2000.

4. National Center for Health Statistics. Prevalence of overweight and obesity among adults: United States, 1999. Hyattsville, MD: U.S. Department of Health and Human Services, 2000.

5. National Center for Health Statistics. Prevalence of overweight among children and adolescents: United States, 1999. Hyattsville, MD: U.S. Department of Health and Human Services; 2000.

6. U.S. Department of Health and Human Services. Physical Activity and Health: A Report of the Surgeon General. Atlanta: U.S. Department of Health and Human Services, Centers for Disease Control and Prevention, National Center for Chronic Disease Prevention and Health Promotion, 1996.

7. American Physical Therapy Association. Guide to Physical Therapist Practice. *Phys Ther*. 2001;81(1):9–744.

8. Norris R, Carroll D, Cochrane R. The effects of aerobic and anaerobic training on fitness, blood pressure, and psychological stress and well-being. *J Psychosomatic Res*. 1990;34(4):367–375.

9. McMurdo ME, Burnett L. Randomised controlled trial of exercise in the elderly. *J Epidemiol Com Health*. 1992;46(3):222–226.

10. Andersen RE, Wadden TA, Bartlett SJ, et al. Effects of lifestyle activity vs. structured aerobic exercise in obese women: A randomized trial. *JAMA*. 1999;281 (4):335–340.

11. Charlton GA, Crawford MH. Physiologic consequences of training. *Cardiol Clin*. 1997;15(3):345-354.

12. Kraemer WJ, Noble BJ, Clark MJ, Culver BW. Physiologic responses to heavy-resistance exercise with very short rest periods. *Int J Sports Med*. 1987; 8(4):247–252.

13. Kraemer WJ, Fleck SJ, Callister R, et al. Training responses of plasma beta-endorphin, adrenocorticotropin, and cortisol. *Med Sci Sports Exerc*. 1989; 21(2):146–153.

14. Hickson RC, Dvorak BA, Gorostiaga EM, et al. Potential for strength and endurance training to amplify endurance performance. *J Appl Physiol*. 1988; 65(5):2285–2290.

15. Dudley GA, Fleck SJ. Strength and endurance training. Are they mutually exclusive? *Sports Med*. 1987;4(2):79–85.

16. Fleck SJ. Cardiovascular adaptations to resistance training. *Med Sci Sports Exerc*. 1988;20(5 Suppl): S146–51.

17. Kraemer WJ, Volek JS, Clark KL, et al. Physiological adaptations to a weight-loss dietary regimen and exercise programs in women. *J Appl Physiol*. 1997; 83(1):270–279.

18. Kraemer WJ, Duncan ND, Volek JS. Resistance training and elite athletes: Adaptations and program considerations. *J Orthop Sports Phys Ther*. 1998;28 (2):110–119.

19. Brooks GA. Anaerobic threshold: Review of the concept and directions for future research. *Med Sci Sports Exerc*. 1985;17(1):22–34.

20. Wallmann H, Rosania J. An introduction to periodization training for the triathlete. *Strength Cond J*. 2001;23(6):55–64.

21. Weltman A, Seip RL, Snead D, et al. Exercise training at and above the lactate threshold in previously untrained women. *Int J Sports Med*. 1992;13 (3):257–263.

22. Belman MJ, Gaesser GA. Exercise training below and above the lactate threshold in the elderly. *Med Sci Sports Exerc*. 1991;23(5):562–568.

23. Docherty D, Sporer B. A proposed model for examining the interference phenomenon between concurrent aerobic and strength training. *Sports Med*. 2000;30(6):385–394.

24. Sutton JR. VO$_{2max}$—new concepts on an old theme. *Med Sci Sports Exerc*. 1992;24(1):26–29.

25. Stone HL, Liang IY. Cardiovascular response and control during exercise. *Am Rev Respir Dis*. 1984; 129(2, Pt 2):S13–16.

26. Jones AM, Carter H. The effect of endurance training on parameters of aerobic fitness. *Sports Med*. 2000;29(6):373–386.

27. Hill AV, Lupton H. Muscular exercise, lactic acid and the supply and utilization of oxygen. *Quarterly Med J*. 1923;16:135–171.

28. Thoden J. Testing aerobic power. *In* J. MacDougall, H. Wenger, H. Green, (eds.). *Physiological Testing of the High-Performance Athlete*. Champaign, IL: Human Kinetics, 1991, pp. 107–173.

29. Costill DL, Thomason H, Roberts E. Fractional utilization of the aerobic capacity during distance running. *Med Sci Sports*. 1973;5(4):248–252.

30. Maughan RJ, Leiper JB. Aerobic capacity and fractional utilisation of aerobic capacity in elite and

non-elite male and female marathon runners. *Eur J Appl Physiol.* 1983;52(1):80–87.

31. Saltin B, Astrand PO. Maximal oxygen uptake in athletes. *J Appl Physiol.* 1967;23(3):353–358.

32. Taylor CR. Structural and functional limits to oxidative metabolism: Insights from scaling. *Ann Rev Physiol.* 1987;49:135–146.

33. Wagner PD, Reeves JT, Sutton JR. Possible limitations of maximal O_2 uptake by peripheral tissue diffusion. *Ann Rev Resp Dis.* 1986;133:A202.

34. Saltin B, Strange S. Maximal oxygen uptake: "Old" and "new" arguments for a cardiovascular limitation. *Med Sci Sports Exerc.* 1992;24(1):30–37.

35. Daniels JT, Yarbrough RA, Foster C. Changes in VO_{2max} and running performance with training. *Eur J Appl Physiol.* 1978;39(4):249–254.

36. Mitchell JH, Blomqvist G. Maximal oxygen uptake. *N Engl J Med.* 1971;284(18):1018–1022.

37. Rowell LB. Muscle blood flow in humans: How high can it go? *Med Sci Sports Exerc.* 1988;20(5 Suppl):S97–103.

38. Blomqvist CG, Saltin B. Cardiovascular adaptations to physical training. *Ann Rev Physiol.* 1983;45:169–189.

39. Spina RJ. Cardiovascular adaptations to endurance exercise training in older men and women. *Exerc Sport Sci Rev.* 1999;27:317–332.

40. Weston AR, Myburgh KH, Lindsay FH, et al. Skeletal muscle buffering capacity and endurance performance after high-intensity interval training by well-trained cyclists. *Eur J Appl Physiol.* 1997;75(1):7–13.

41. Billat VL, Flechet B, Petit B, et al. Interval training at VO_{2max}: Effects on aerobic performance and overtraining markers. *Med Sci Sports Exerc.* 1999;31(1):156–163.

42. Franch J, Madsen K, Djurhuus MS, Pedersen PK. Improved running economy following intensified training correlates with reduced ventilatory demands. *Med Sci Sports Exerc.* 1998;30(8):1250–1256.

43. Mier CM, Turner MJ, Ehsani AA, Spina RJ. Cardiovascular adaptations to 10 days of cycle exercise. *J Appl Physiol.* 1997;83(6):1900–1906.

44. Gibbons ES, Jessup GT, Wells TD, Werthmann DA. Effects of various training intensity levels on anaerobic threshold and aerobic capacity in females. *J Sports Med Phys Fitness.* 1983;23(3):315–318.

45. Carter H, Jones AM, Doust JH. Effect of 6 weeks of endurance training on the lactate minimum speed. *J Sports Sci.* 1999;17(12):957–967.

46. Spina RJ, Chi MM, Hopkins MG, et al. Mitochondrial enzymes increase in muscle in response to 7-10 days of cycle exercise. *J Appl Physiol.* 1996;80(6):2250–2254.

47. Hickson RC, Hagberg JM, Ehsani AA, Holloszy JO. Time course of the adaptive responses of aerobic power and heart rate to training. *Med Sci Sports Exerc.* 1981;13(1):17–20.

48. Pierce EF, Weltman A, Seip RL, Snead D. Effects of training specificity on the lactate threshold and VO_2 peak. *Int J Sports Med.* 1990;11(4):267–272.

49. Rusko HK. Development of aerobic power in relation to age and training in cross-country skiers. *Med Sci Sports Exerc.* 1992;24(9):1040–1047.

50. Davies CT, Thompson MW. Aerobic performance of female marathon and male ultramarathon athletes. *Eur J Appl Physiol.* 1979;41(4): 233–245.

51. Scrimgeour AG, Noakes TD, Adams B, Myburgh K. The influence of weekly training distance on fractional utilization of maximum aerobic capacity in marathon and ultramarathon runners. *Eur J Appl Physiol.* 1986;55(2):202–209.

52. Daniels J. Physiological characteristics of champion male athletes. *Res Quart Exerc Sport.* 1974;45:342–348.

53. Svedenhag J, Sjodin B. Physiological characteristics of elite male runners in and off-season. *Can J Appl Sport Sci.* 1985;10(3):127–133.

54. Horowitz JF, Sidossis LS, Coyle EF. High efficiency of type I muscle fibers improves performance. *Int J Sports Med.* 1994;15(3):152–157.

55. Noakes TD. Implications of exercise testing for prediction of athletic performance: A contemporary perspective. *Med Sci Sports Exerc.* 1988;20(4):319–330.

56. Conley DL, Krahenbuhl GS. Running economy and distance running performance of highly trained athletes. *Med Sci Sports Exerc.* 1980;12(5):357–360.

57. Londeree BR. The use of laboratory test results with long distance runners. *Sports Med.* 1986;3(3):201–213.

58. Morgan DW, Bransford DR, Costill DL, et al. Variation in the aerobic demand of running among trained and untrained subjects. *Med Sci Sports Exerc.* 1995;27(3):404–409.

59. Davies CT. Metabolic cost of exercise and physical performance in children with some observations on external loading. *Eur J Appl Physiol.* 1980;45(2-3):95–102.

60. Miyashita M, Miura M, Murase Y, Yamaji K. Running performance from the viewpoint of aerobic power. In L. J. Folinsbee, J. A. Wagner, J. F. Borgia, B. L. Drinkwater, J. A. Gliner, J. F. Bedi (eds.). *Environmental Stress: Individual Human Adaptations.* New York: Academic Press, 1978, pp. 183–194.

61. Martin PE. Mechanical and physiological responses to lower extremity loading during running. *Med Sci Sports Exerc.* 1985;17(4):427–433.

62. Jones BH, Toner MM, Daniels WL, Knapik JJ. The energy cost and heart-rate response of trained and

untrained subjects walking and running in shoes and boots. *Ergonomics.* 1984;27(8):895–902.

63. Jones BH, Knapik JJ, Daniels WL, Toner MM. The energy cost of women walking and running in shoes and boots. *Ergonomics.* 1986;29(3):439–443.

64. Berg K, Sady S. Oxygen cost of running at submaximal speeds while wearing shoe inserts. *Res Q Exerc Sport.* 1985;56:86–89.

65. Burkett LN, Kohrt WM, Buchbinder R. Effects of shoes and foot orthotics on VO_2 and selected frontal plane knee kinematics. *Med Sci Sports Exerc.* 1985;17(1):158–163.

66. Williams CA, Armstrong N, Powell J. Aerobic responses of prepubertal boys to two modes of training. *Br J Sports Med.* 2000;34(3):168–173.

67. Peel C. The cardiopulmonary system and movement dysfunction. *Phys Ther.* 1996;76:448–455.

68. Gleeson M. Temperature regulation during exercise. *Int J Sports Med.* 1998;19 Suppl 2:S96–99.

69. Wenger CB. Human heat acclimatization. In K.B. Pandolf, M.N. Sawka, R.R. Gonzalez (eds). *Human Performance Physiology and Environmental Medicine at Terrestrial Extremes.* Indianapolis, IN: Benchmark Press, 1988, pp. 153–199.

70. American College of Sports Medicine. *ACSM's Guidelines for Exercise Testing and Prescription,* 6th ed. Baltimore: Lippincott Williams & Wilkins, 2000.

71. Sallis R, Chassay CM. Recognizing and treating common cold-induced injury in outdoor sports. *Med Sci Sports Exerc.* 1999;31(10):1367–1373.

72. Hixson EG. Cold injury. *In* JC DeLee, D. Drez Jr (eds). *Orthopaedic Sports Medicine: Principles and Practice.* Philadelphia: Saunders, 1994, pp. 385–396.

73. Bowman WD Jr. Safe exercise in the cold and cold injuries. In M.B. Mellion, W.M. Walsh, GL Shelton (eds). *The Team Physician's Handbook.* St Louis: Mosby-Yearbook, 1990, pp. 70–77.

74. Lloyd EL. ABC of sports medicine: temperature and performance. I. Cold. *Br Med J.* 1994;309:531–534.

75. Danzl DF, Pozos RS. Accidental hypothermia. *N Engl J Med.* 1994;331:1756–1760.

76. Varon J, Sadovnikoff N, Sternbach GL. Hypothermia: saving patients from the big chill. *Postgrad Med.* 1992;92:47–54,59.

77. Weinberg AD. Hypothermia. *Ann Emerg Med.* 1993;22:370–377.

78. Gallagher CG. Exercise and chronic obstructive pulmonary disease. *Med Clin N Am.* 1990;74(3):619–641.

79. Noonan V, Dean E. Submaximal exercise testing: Clinical application and interpretation. *Phys Ther.* 2000;80(8):783–807.

80. Astrand P O, Rhyming I. A nomogram for calculation of aerobic capacity (physical fitness) from pulse rate during submaximal work. *J Appl Physiol.* 1954;7:218–221.

81. Golding LA, Myers CR, Sinning WE (eds.). *Y's Way to Physical Fitness,* 3rd ed. Champaign, IL: Human Kinetics Publishers, 1989.

82. Stratton JR, Levy WC, Schwartz RS, et al. Beta-adrenergic effects on left ventricular filling: Influence of aging and exercise training. *J Appl Physiol.* 1994;77(6):2522–2529.

83. Pollock ML, Foster C, Knapp D, et al. Effect of age and training on aerobic capacity and body composition of master athletes. *J Appl Physiol.* 1987;62(2):725–731.

84. Meredith CN, Frontera WR, Fisher EC, et al. Peripheral effects of endurance training in young and old subjects. *J Appl Physiol.* 1989;66(6):2844–2849.

85. Hagberg JM, Graves JE, Limacher M, et al. Cardiovascular responses of 70- to 79-yr-old men and women to exercise training. *J Appl Physiol.* 1989;66(6):2589–2594.

86. Meredith CN, Zackin MJ, Frontera WR, Evans WJ. Body composition and aerobic capacity in young and middle-aged endurance-trained men. *Med Sci Sports Exerc.* 1987;19(6):557–563.

87. Pickering GP, Fellmann N, Morio B, et al. Effects of endurance training on the cardiovascular system and water compartments in elderly subjects. *J Appl Physiol.* 1997;83(4):1300–1306.

88. Kohrt WM, Malley MT, Coggan AR, et al. Effects of gender, age, and fitness level on response of VO_{2max} to training in 60-71 yr olds. *J Appl Physiol.* 1991;71(5):2004–2011.

89. Spina RJ, Ogawa T, Kohrt WM, et al. Differences in cardiovascular adaptations to endurance exercise training between older men and women. *J Appl Physiol.* 1993;75(2):849–855.

90. Robinson JI, Rogers MA. Adherence to exercise programmes. Recommendations. *Sports Med.* 1994;17(1):39–52.

91. Rhodes RE, Martin AD, Taunton JE, et al. Factors associated with exercise adherence among older adults. An individual perspective. *Sports Med.* 1999;28(6):397–411.

92. Franklin BA. Program factors that influence exercise adherence: Practical adherence skills for clinical staff. In R.K. Dishman (ed.,). *Exercise Adherence: Its Impact on Public Health.* Champaign, IL: Human Kinetics, 1988, pp. 237–258.

93. Oldridge NB, Jones NL. Preventive use of exercise rehabilitation after myocardial infarction. *Acta Med Scand - Supplementum.* 1986;711:123–129.

94. Swain DP, Leutholtz BC. Heart rate reserve is equivalent to $\%VO_2$ reserve, not to $\% VO_{2max}$. *Med Sci Sports Exerc.* 1997;29(3):410–414.

95. Celli BR. Pulmonary rehabilitation for patients with advanced lung disease. *Clin Chest Med.* 1997;18:521–534.

96. Lacasse Y, Guyatt GH, Goldstein RS. The components of a respiratory rehabilitation program: A systematic overview. *Chest.* 1997;111:1077–1088.

97. Troosters T, Gosselink R, Decramer M. Short- and long-term effects of outpatient rehabilitation in patients with chronic obstructive pulmonary disease: A randomized trial. *Am J Med.* 2000;109(3):207–212.

98. O'Donnell DE, Webb KA, McGuire MA. Older patients with COPD: Benefits of exercise training. *Geriatrics.* 1993;48:59–66.

99. Belman MJ. Exercise in chronic obstructive pulmonary disease. *Clin Chest Med.* 1986;7:585–597.

100. Swain DP, Leutholtz BC, King ME, et al. Relationship between % heart rate reserve and % VO$_2$ reserve in treadmill exercise. *Med Sci Sports Exerc.* 1998;30(2):318–321.

101. Engels H-J, Zhu W, Moffatt RJ. An empirical evaluation of the prediction of maximal heart rate. *Res Q Exerc Sport.* 1998;69(1):94–98.

102. Whaley MH, Kaminsky LA, Dwyer GB., et al Predictors of over- and underachievement of age-predicted maximal heart rate. *Med Sci Sports Exerc.* 1992;24(10):1173–1179.

103. Tanaka H, Monahan KD, Seals DR. Age-predicted maximal heart rate revisited. *J Am Col Cardiol.* 2001;37(1):153–156.

104. Londeree BR, Moeschberger ML. Effect of age and other factors on maximal heart rate. *Res Q Exerc Sport.* 1982;53(4):297–304.

105. O'Toole ML, Douglas PS, Hiller WD. Use of heart rate monitors by endurance athletes: Lessons from triathletes. *J Sports Med Phys Fitness.* 1998;38(3):181–187.

106. Pollock ML, Gaesser GA, Butcher JD, et al. American College of Sports Medicine Position Stand. The recommended quantity and quality of exercise for developing and maintaining cardiorespiratory and muscular fitness, and flexibility in healthy adults. *Med Sci Sports Exerc.* 1998;30(6):975–991.

107. Swain DP, Franklin BA. VO$_2$ reserve and the minimal intensity for improving cardiorespiratory fitness. *Med Sci Sports Exerc.* 2002;34(1):152–157.

108. Londeree BR. Effect of training on lactate/ventilatory thresholds: A meta-analysis. *Med Sci Sports Exerc.* 1997;29(6):837–843.

109. Ainsworth BE, Haskell WL, Leon AS, et al. Compendium of physical activities: classification of energy costs of human physical activities. *Med Sci Sports Exerc.* 1993;25(1):71–80.

110. Franklin BA, Fletcher GF, Gordon NF, et al. Cardiovascular evaluation of the athlete. Issues regarding performance, screening and sudden cardiac death. *Sports Med.* 1997;24(2):97–119.

111. Okura T, Tanaka K. A unique method for predicting cardiorespiratory fitness using rating of perceived exertion. *J Physiol Anthropol Appl Hum Sci.* 2001;20(5):255–261.

112. Dishman RK. Prescribing exercise intensity for healthy adults using perceived exertion. *Med Sci Sports Exerc.* 1994;26(9):1087–1094.

113. Dunbar CC, Glickman-Weiss EL, Edwards WW, et al. Three-point method of prescribing exercise with ratings of perceived exertion is valid for cardiac patients. *Percept Mot Skills.* 1996;83(2): 384–386.

114. Dunbar CC, Robertson RJ, Baun R, et al. The validity of regulating exercise intensity by ratings of perceived exertion. *Med Sci Sports Exerc.* 1992;24(1):94–99.

115. Dunbar CC, Bursztyn DA. The slope method for prescribing exercise with ratings of perceived exertion (RPE). *Percept Mot Skills.* 1996;83(1):91–97.

116. Borg G. Perceived exertion as an indicator of somatic stress. *Scand J Rehabil Med.* 1970;2(2):92–98.

117. Borg GA. Psychophysical bases of perceived exertion. *Med Sci Sports Exerc.* 1982;14(5):377–381.

118. Pollock ML, Ward A, Ayres JJ. Cardiorespiratory fitness: Response to differing intensities and durations of training. *Arch Phys Med Rehabil.* 1977;58(11):467–473.

119. Pollock ML, Gettman LR, Milesis CA, et al. Effects of frequency and duration of training on attrition and incidence of injury. *Med Sci Sports.* 1977;9(1):31–36.

120. Costill DL, Thomas R, Robergs RA, et al. Adaptations to swimming training: influence of training volume. *Med Sci Sports Exerc.* 1991;23(3):371–377.

121. Fox EL, Bartels RL, Billings CE, et al. Frequency and duration of interval training programs and changes in aerobic power. *J Appl Physiol.* 1975;38(3):481–484.

122. Kurz MJ, Berg K, Latin R, DeGraw W. The relationship of training methods in NCAA Division I cross-country runners and 10,000-meter performance. *J Strength Cond Res.* 2000;14(2):196–201.

123. deVries HA. Effects of various warm up procedures on 100-yard times of competitive swimmers. *Res Q Exerc Sport.* 1959;30:11–20.

124. Safran MR, Garrett WE, Jr., Seaber AV, et al. The role of warmup in muscular injury prevention. *Am J Sports Med.* 1988;16(2):123–129.

125. Barnard RJ, Gardner GW, Diaco NV, et al. Cardiovascular responses to sudden strenuous exercise—heart rate, blood pressure, and ECG. *J Applied Physiol.* 1973;34(6):833–837.

126. Gleim GW, Stachenfeld NS, Nicholas JA. The influence of flexibility on the economy of walking and jogging. *J Orthop Res.* 1990;8(6):814–823.

127. Shrier I. Stretching before exercise does not reduce the risk of local muscle injury: A critical review of the clinical and basic science literature. *Clin J Sport Med.* 1999;9(4):221–227.

128. Pope RP, Herbert RD, Kirwan JD, Graham BJ. A randomized trial of preexercise stretching for prevention of lower-limb injury. *Med Sci Sports Exerc.* 2000;32(2):271–277.

129. Helgerud J, Engen LC, Wisloff W, Hoff J. Aerobic endurance training improves soccer performance. *Ann Neurol.* 2001;50(2):133–141.

130. Holmer I. Swimming physiology. *Ann Physiol Anthropol.* 1992;11(3):269–276.

131. Lavoie JM, Montpetit RR. Applied physiology of swimming. *Sports Med.* 1986;3(3):165–189.

132. Reilly T, Borrie A. Physiology applied to field hockey. *Sports Med.* 1992;14(1):10–26.

133. Fleck SJ, Case S, Puhl J, Van Handle P. Physical and physiological characteristics of elite women volleyball players. *Can J Appl Sport Sci.* 1985;10(3):122–126.

134. Smith DJ, Roberts D, Watson B. Physical, physiological and performance differences between Canadian national team and universiade volleyball players. *J Sports Sci.* 1992;10(2):131–138.

135. Pincivero DM, Bompa TO. A physiological review of American football. *Sports Med.* 1997;23(4):247–260.

136. Mahood NV, Kenefick RW, Kertzer R, Quinn TJ. Physiological determinants of cross-country ski racing performance. *Med Sci Sports Exerc.* 2001;33(8):1379–1384.

137. Hoffman MD. Physiological comparisons of cross-country skiing techniques. *Med Sci Sports Exerc.* 1992;24(9):1023–1032.

138. Hoffman MD, Clifford PS. Physiological aspects of competitive cross-country skiing. *J Sports Sci.* 1992;10(1):3–27.

139. Eisenman PA, Johnson SC, Bainbridge CN, Zupan MF. Applied physiology of cross-country skiing. *Sports Med.* 1989;8(2):67–79.

140. Andersen RE, Montgomery DL. Physiology of alpine skiing. *Sports Med.* 1988;6(4):210–221.

141. Mayers N, Gutin B. Physiological characteristics of elite prepubertal cross-country runners. *Med Sci Sports.* 1979;11(2):172–176.

142. Butts NK. Physiological profiles of high school female cross country runners. *Res Q Exerc Sport.* 1982;53(1):8–14.

143. Vaccaro P, Clarke DH, Wrenn JP. Physiological profiles of elite women basketball players. *J Sports Med Phys Fitness.* 1979;19(1):45–54.

144. Smith HK, Thomas SG. Physiological characteristics of elite female basketball players. *Can J Sport Sci.* 1991;16(4):289–295.

145. McInnes SE, Carlson JS, Jones CJ, McKenna MJ. The physiological load imposed on basketball players during competition. *J Sports Sci.* 1995;13(5):387–397.

146. Withers RT, Roberts RG. Physiological profiles of representative women softball, hockey and netball players. *Ergonomics.* 1981;24(8):583–591.

147. Kirkendall DT. Physiologic aspects of gymnastics. *Clin Sports Med.* 1985;4(1):17–22.

148. Agre JC, Casal DC, Leon AS, et al. Professional ice hockey players: physiologic, anthropometric, and musculoskeletal characteristics. *Arch Phys Med Rehabil.* 1988;69(3, Pt 1):188–192.

149. Montgomery DL. Physiology of ice hockey. *Sports Med.* 1988;5(2):99–126.

150. Cox MH, Miles DS, Verde TJ, Rhodes EC. Applied physiology of ice hockey. *Sports Med.* 1995;19(3):184–201.

151. Horswill CA. Applied physiology of amateur wrestling. *Sports Med.* 1992;14(2):114–143.

152. Kraemer WJ, Fry AC, Rubin MR, et al. Physiological and performance responses to tournament wrestling. *Med Sci Sports Exerc.* 2001;33(8):1367–1378.

153. Shaver LG. Effects of a season of varsity wrestling on selected physiological parameters. *J Sports Med Phys Fitness.* 1974;14(2):139–145.

154. Taylor AW. Physiological effects of wrestling in adolescents and teenagers. *J Sports Med.* 1975;3(2):76–84.

155. Loy SF, Hoffmann JJ, Holland GJ. Benefits and practical use of cross-training in sports. *Sports Med.* 1995;19(1):1–8.

156. Foster C, Hector LL, Welsh R, et al. Effects of specific versus cross-training on running performance. *Eur J Appl Physiol.* 1995;70(4):367–372.

157. Loy SF, Holland GJ, Mutton DL, et al. Effects of stair-climbing vs. run training on treadmill and track running performance. *Med Sci Sports Exerc.* 1993;25(11):1275–1278.

158. Hickson RC. Interference of strength development by simultaneously training for strength and endurance. *Eur J Appl Physiol.* 1980;45(2-3):255–263.

159. Kraemer WJ, Patton JF, Gordon SE, et al. Compatibility of high-intensity strength and endurance training on hormonal and skeletal muscle adaptations. *J Appl Physiol.* 1995;78(3):976–989.

160. Dudley GA, Djamil R. Incompatibility of endurance- and strength-training modes of exercise. *J Appl Physiol.* 1985;59(5):1446–1451.

161. McFarland EG, Wasik M. Injuries in female collegiate swimmers due to swimming and cross training. *Clin J Sports Med.* 1996;6(3):178–182.

162. Smith DJ, Wengner HA. The 10 day aerobic minicycle: the effects of interval or continuous training at two different intensities. *J Sports Med Phys Fitness.* 1981;21(4):390–394.

163. Perry A, Mosher P, La Perriere A, et al. A comparison of training responses to interval versus continuous aerobic dance. *J Sports Med Phys Fitness.* 1988;28(3):274–279.

164. Overend TJ, Paterson DH, Cunningham DA. The effect of interval and continuous training on the

aerobic parameters. *Can J Sport Sci.* 1992;17(2): 129–134.

165. Meyer K, Lehmann M, Sunder G, et al. Interval versus continuous exercise training after coronary bypass surgery: a comparison of training-induced acute reactions with respect to the effectiveness of the exercise methods. *Clin Cardiol.* 1990;13(12): 851–861.

166. Rippe JM, Ward A, Porcari JP, Freedson PS. Walking for health and fitness. *JAMA.* 1988;259(18): 2720–2724.

167. Rodgers CD, VanHeest JL, Schachter CL. Energy expenditure during submaximal walking with Exerstriders. *Med Sci Sports Exerc.* 1995;27(4):607–611.

168. Evans BW, Potteiger JA, Bray MC, Tuttle JL. Metabolic and hemodynamic responses to walking with hand weights in older individuals. *Med Sci Sports Exerc.* 1994;26(8):1047–1052.

169. Duncan JJ. Women walking for health and fitness. How much is enough? *J Am Geriatrics Soc.* 1991;39 (12):1155–1159.

170. Kukkonen-Harjula K, Laukkanen R, Vuori I, et al. Effects of walking training on health-related fitness in healthy middle-aged adults—a randomized controlled study. *Scand J Med Sci Sports.* 1998;8 (4):236–242.

171. Manson JE, Hu FB, Rich-Edwards JW, et al. A prospective study of walking as compared with vigorous exercise in the prevention of coronary heart disease in women. *New Engl J Med.* 1999;341(9): 650–658.

172. Hamdorf PA, Penhall RK. Walking with its training effects on the fitness and activity patterns of 79-91 year old females. *Aust New Zeal J Med.* 1999;29(1): 22–28.

173. Powell KE, Heath GW, Kresnow MJ, et al. Injury rates from walking, gardening, weightlifting, outdoor bicycling, and aerobics. *Med Sci Sports Exerc.* 1998;30(8):1246–1249.

174. Carroll JF, Pollock ML, Graves JE, et al. Incidence of injury during moderate- and high-intensity walking training in the elderly. *J Gerontol.* 1992;47(3): M61–66.

175. Westby MD. A health professional's guide to exercise prescription for people with arthritis: A review of aerobic fitness activities. *Arthritis Rheum.* 2001;45(6):501–511.

176. Hootman JM, Macera CA, Ainsworth BE, et al. Association among physical activity level, cardiorespiratory fitness, and risk of musculoskeletal injury. *Am J Epidemiol.* 2001;154(3):251–258.

177. Ounpuu S. The biomechanics of walking and running. *Clin Sports Med.* 1994;13(4):843–863.

178. Pink M, Perry J, Houglum PA, Devine DJ. Lower extremity range of motion in the recreational sport runner. *Am J Sports Med.* 1994;22(4):541–549.

179. Mutton DL, Loy SF, Rogers DM, et al. Effect of run vs. combined cycle/run training on VO$_{2max}$ and running performance. *Med Sci Sports Exerc.* 1993;25 (12):1393–1397.

180. Melanson EL, Freedson PS, Jungbluth S. Changes in VO$_{2max}$ and maximal treadmill time after 9 wk of running or in-line skate training. *Med Sci Sports Exerc.* 1996;28(11):1422–1426.

181. Suter E, Marti B, Gutzwiller F. Jogging or walking—comparison of health effects. *Ann Epidemiol.* 1994;4(5):375–381.

182. Williford HN, Richards LA, Scharff-Olson M, et al. Bench stepping and running in women. Changes in fitness and injury status. *J Sports Med Phys Fitness.* 1998; 38(3):221–226.

183. Suter E, Marti B, Tschopp A, et al. Effects of self-monitored jogging on physical fitness, blood pressure and serum lipids: A controlled study in sedentary middle-aged men. *Int J Sports Med.* 1990; 11(6):425–432.

184. Marti B. Health effects of recreational running in women. Some epidemiological and preventive aspects. *Sports Med.* 1991;11(1):20–51.

185. Zeni AI, Hoffman MD, Clifford PS. Relationships among heart rate, lactate concentration, and perceived effort for different types of rhythmic exercise in women. *Arch Phys Med Rehabil.* 1996;77 (3):237–241.

186. Zeni AI, Hoffman MD, Clifford PS. Energy expenditure with indoor exercise machines. *JAMA.* 1996;275(8):1424–1427.

187. Moyna NM, Robertson RJ, Meckes CL, et al. Intermodal comparison of energy expenditure at exercise intensities corresponding to the perceptual preference range. *Med Sci Sports Exerc.* 2001;33(8): 1404–1410.

188. McMiken DF, Daniels JT. Aerobic requirements and maximum aerobic power in treadmill and track running. *Med Sci Sports.* 1976;8(1):14–17.

189. Nigg BM, De Boer RW, Fisher V. A kinematic comparison of overground and treadmill running. *Med Sci Sports Exerc.* 1995;27(1):98–105.

190. Schache AG, Blanch PD, Rath DA, et al. A comparison of overground and treadmill running for measuring the three-dimensional kinematics of the lumbo-pelvic-hip complex. *Clin Biomech.* 2001; 16(8):667–680.

191. Requa RK, DeAvilla LN, Garrick JG. Injuries in recreational adult fitness activities. *Am J Sports Med.* 1993;21(3):461–467.

192. Walter SD, Hart LE, McIntosh JM, Sutton JR. The Ontario cohort study of running-related injuries. *Arch Int Med.* 1989;149(11):2561–2564.

193. van Mechelen W. Running injuries. A review of the epidemiological literature. *Sports Med.* 1992;14(5): 320–335.

194. Koplan JP, Rothenberg RB, Jones EL. The natural history of exercise: a 10-yr follow-up of a cohort of runners. *Med Sci Sports Exerc.* 1995;27(8):1180–1184.

195. Hootman JM, Macera CA, Ainsworth BE, et al. Predictors of lower extremity injury among recreationally active adults. *Clin J Sport Med.* 2002;12(2): 99–106.

196. Wexler RK. Lower extremity injuries in runners. Helping athletic patients return to form. *Postgrad Med.* 1995;98(4):185–187.

197. Frankovich RJ, Petrella RJ, Lattanzio CN. In-line skating injuries: patterns and protective equipment use. *Physician Sportsmed.* 2001;29(4):57–64.

198. Mahar AT, Derrick TR, Hamill J, Caldwell GE. Impact shock and attenuation during in-line skating. *Med Sci Sports Exerc.* 1997;29(8):1069–1075.

199. Snyder AC, O'Hagan KP, Clifford PS, et al. Exercise responses to in-line skating: comparisons to running and cycling. *Int J Sports Med.* 1993;14(1): 38–42.

200. Wallick ME, Porcari JP, Wallick SB, et al. Physiological responses to in-line skating compared to treadmill running. *Med Sci Sports Exerc.* 1995;27(2): 242–248.

201. Melanson EL, Freedson PS, Webb R, et al. Exercise responses to running and in-line skating at self-selected paces. *Med Sci Sports Exerc.* 1996;28(2): 247–250.

202. Schieber RA, Branche-Dorsey CM, Ryan GW, et al. Risk factors for injuries from in-line skating and the effectiveness of safety gear. *N Engl J Med.* 1996;335 (22):1680–1685.

203. Sutherland R, Wilson J, Aitchison T, Grant S. Physiological responses and perceptions of exertion in a step aerobics session. *J Sports Sci.* 1999;17(6): 495–503.

204. Kraemer WJ, Keuning M, Ratamess NA, et al. Resistance training combined with bench-step aerobics enhances women's health profile. *Med Sci Sports Exerc.* 2001;33(2):259–269.

205. Maybury MC, Waterfield J. An investigation into the relation between step height and ground reaction forces in step exercise: A pilot study. *Br J Sports Med.* 1997;31(2):109–113.

206. Scharff-Olson M, Williford HN, Blessing DL, et al. Vertical impact forces during bench-step aerobics: Exercise rate and experience. *Percep Mot Skills.* 1997;84(1):267–274.

207. Scharff-Olson M, Williford HN, Blessing DL, Brown JA. The physiological effects of bench/step exercise. *Sports Med.* 1996;21(3):164–175.

208. Grant S, Davidson W, Aitchison T, Wilson J. A comparison of physiological responses and rating of perceived exertion between high-impact and low-impact aerobic dance sessions. *Eur J Appl Physiol.* 1998;78(4):324–332.

209. Darby LA, Browder KD, Reeves BD. The effects of cadence, impact, and step on physiological responses to aerobic dance exercise. *Res Q Exerc Sports.* 1995;66(3):231–238.

210. Schaeffer SA, Darby LA, Browder KD, Reeves BD. Perceived exertion and metabolic responses of women during aerobic dance exercise. *Percep Mot Skills.* 1995;81(2):691–700.

211. Schaeffer-Gerschutz SA, Darby LA, Browder KD. Differentiated ratings of perceived exertion and physiological responses during aerobic dance steps by impact/type of arm movement. *Percep Mot Skills.* 2000;90(2):457–471.

212. Bell JM, Bassey EJ. Postexercise heart rates and pulse palpation as a means of determining exercising intensity in an aerobic dance class. *Br J Sports Med.* 1996;30(1):48–52.

213. Milburn, Butts NK. A comparison of the training responses to aerobic dance and jogging in college females. *Med Sci Sports Exerc.* 1983;15(6):510–513.

214. McCord P, Nichols J, Patterson P. The effect of low impact dance training on aerobic capacity, submaximal heart rates and body composition of college-aged females. *J Sports Med Phys Fitness.* 1989;29(2): 184–188.

215. Rothenberger LA, Chang JI, Cable TA. Prevalence and types of injuries in aerobic dancers. *Am J Sports Med.* 1988;16(4):403–407.

216. Janis LR. Aerobic dance survey. A study of high-impact versus low-impact injuries. *J Am Pod Med Assoc.* 1990;80(8):419–423.

217. du Toit V, Smith R. Survey of the effects of aerobic dance on the lower extremity in aerobic instructors. *J Am Pod Med Assoc.* 2001;91(10):528–532.

218. Michaud TJ, Rodriguez-Zayas J, Armstrong C, Hartnig M. Ground reaction forces in high-impact and low-impact aerobic dance. *J Sports Med Phys Fitness.* 1993;33(4):359–366.

219. Garrick JG, Gillien DM, Whiteside P. The epidemiology of aerobic dance injuries. *Am J Sports Med.* 1986;14(1):67–72.

220. Howley ET, Colacino DL, Swensen TC. Factors affecting the oxygen cost of stepping on an electronic stepping ergometer. *Med Sci Sports Exerc.* 1992; 24(9):1055–1058.

221. Ben-Ezra V, Verstraete R. Step ergometry: Is it task-specific training? *Eur J Appl Physiol.* 1991;63 (3–4):261–264.

222. Loy SF, Conley LM, Sacco ER, et al. Effects of stairclimbing on VO$_{2max}$ and quadriceps strength in middle-aged females. *Med Sci Sports Exerc.* 1994; 26(2):241–247.

223. Ryan PT, Plowman SA, Ball TE, Looney MA. Physiologic responses to forward and retrograde simulated stair stepping. *Arch Phys Med Rehabil.* 1994;75(7):798–802.

224. Vereschagin KS, Firtch WL, Caputo LJ, Hoffman MA. Transient paresthesia in stair-climbers' feet. *Physician Sportsmed.* 1993;21(2):63–69.

225. Powers CM. Rehabilitation of patellofemoral joint disorders: A critical review. *J Orthop Sports Phys Ther.* 1998;28(5):345–354.

226. Mercer JA, Dufek JS, Bates BT. Analysis of peak oxygen consumption and heart rate during elliptical and treadmill exercise. *J Sports Rehabil.* 2001;10: 48–56.

227. Rusko H, Havu M, Karvinen E. Aerobic performance capacity in athletes. *Eur J Appl Physiol.* 1978; 38(2):151–159.

228. Oja P, Kukkonen-Harjula K, Nieminen R, et al. Cardiorespiratory strain of middle-aged men in mass events of long-distance cycling, rowing, jogging, and skiing. *Int J Sports Med.* 1988;9(1):45–51.

229. Goss FL, Robertson RJ, Spina RJ, et al. Aerobic metabolic requirements of simulated cross-country skiing. *Ergonomics.* 1989;32(12):1573–1579.

230. Smith M, Matheson GO, Meeuwisse WH. Injuries in cross-country skiing: A critical appraisal of the literature. *Sports Med.* 1996;21(3):239–250.

231. Renstrom P, Johnson RJ. Cross-country skiing injuries and biomechanics. *Sports Med.* 1989;8(6): 346–370.

232. Weiss BD. Clinical syndromes associated with bicycle seats. *Clin Sports Med.* 1994;13(1):175–186.

233. Nordeen-Snyder KS. The effect of bicycle seat height variation upon oxygen consumption and lower limb kinematics. *Med Sci Sports.* 1977;9(2): 113–117.

234. Ryschon TW. Physiologic aspects of bicycling. *Clin Sports Med.* 1994;13(1):15–38.

235. Brodowicz GR, King DS, Ribisl PM. Effect of toe-clip use during cycle ergometry on ventilatory threshold and VO_2 max in trained cyclists and runners. *Ergonomics.* 1991;34(1):49–56.

236. Wilde SW, Knowlton RG, Miles DS, et al. Effects of toeclip use on metabolic and cardiopulmonary responses to bicycle ergometer exercise. *J Hum Ergol.* 1980;9(1):47–54.

237. Welbergen E, Clijsen LP. The influence of body position on maximal performance in cycling. *Eur J Appl Physiol.* 1990;61(1-2):138–142.

238. Begemann-Meijer MJ, Binkhorst RA. The effect of posture on the responses to cycle ergometer exercise. *Ergonomics.* 1989;32(6):639–643.

239. Wilber CA, Holland GJ, Madison RE, Loy SF. An epidemiological analysis of overuse injuries among recreational cyclists. *Int J Sports Med.* 1995;16(3): 201–206.

240. Kiburz D, Jacobs R, Reckling F, Mason J. Bicycle accidents and injuries among adult cyclists. *Am J Sports Med.* 1986;14(5):416–419.

241. Yelon JA, Harrigan N, Evans JT. Bicycle trauma: a five-year experience. *Am Surg.* 1995;61(3):202–205.

242. Dannenberg AL, Needle S, Mullady D, Kolodner KB. Predictors of injury among 1638 riders in a recreational long-distance bicycle tour: Cycle Across Maryland. *Am J Sports Med.* 1996;24(6): 747–753.

243. American Academy of Pediatrics. Committee on Injury and Poison Prevention. Bicycle helmets. *Pediatrics.* 2001;108(4):1030–1032.

244. Goh KY, Zhu XL, Poon WS, Linn S. Epidemiology of bicycle injury, head injury, and helmet use among children in British Columbia: A five year descriptive study. Canadian Hospitals Injury, Reporting and Prevention Program (CHIRPP). *Childs Nerv Sys.* 1996;12(10):611–614.

245. Linn S, Smith D, Sheps S. Epidemiology of bicycle injury, head injury, and helmet use among children in British Columbia: A five year descriptive study. Canadian Hospitals Injury, Reporting and Prevention Program (CHIRPP). *Inj Prevent.* 1998;4(2): 122–125.

246. Attewell RG, Glase K, McFadden M. Bicycle helmet efficacy: A meta-analysis. *Accid Anal Prev.* 2001;33(3):345–352.

247. Marriott HE, Lamb KL. The use of ratings of perceived exertion for regulating exercise levels in rowing ergometry. *Eur J Appl Physiol.* 1996;72(3): 267–271.

248. Hagerman FC, Lawrence RA, Mansfield MC. A comparison of energy expenditure during rowing and cycling ergometry. *Med Sci Sports Exerc.* 1988; 20(5):479–488.

249. Karlson KA. Rib stress fractures in elite rowers. A case series and proposed mechanism. *Am J Sports Med.* 1998;26(4):516–519.

250. Gregory PL, Biswas AC, Batt ME. Musculoskeletal problems of the chest wall in athletes. *Sports Med.* 2002;32(4):235–250.

251. Soler T, Calderon C. The prevalence of spondylolysis in the Spanish elite athlete. *Am J Sports Med.* 2000;28(1):57–62.

252. Miles DS, Cox MH, Bomze JP. Cardiovascular responses to upper body exercise in normals and cardiac patients. *Med Sci Sports Exerc.* 1989;21 (5 Suppl):S126–131.

253. Franklin BA. Aerobic exercise training programs for the upper body. *Med Sci Sports Exerc.* 1989;21 (5 Suppl):S141–48.

254. Kang J, Chaloupka EC, Mastrangelo MA, Angelucci J. Physiological responses to upper body exercise on an arm and a modified leg ergometer. *Med Sci Sports Exerc.* 1999;31(10):1453–1459.

255. Magel JR, McArdle WD, Toner M, Delio DJ. Metabolic and cardiovascular adjustment to arm training. *J Appl Physiol.* 1978;45(1):75–79.

256. Clausen JP, Klausen K, Rasmussen B, Trap-Jensen J. Central and peripheral circulatory changes after training of the arms or legs. *Am J Physiol.* 1973;225 (3):675–682.

257. Ben Ari E, Kellermann JJ. Comparison of cardiocirculatory responses to intensive arm and leg training in patients with angina pectoris. *Heart & Lung.* 1983;12(4):337–341.

258. Troup JP. The physiology and biomechanics of competitive swimming. *Clin Sports Med.* 1999;18(2): 267–285.

259. Sharp RL. Physiology of swimming. *In* W.E. Garrett, Jr., D.T. Kirkendall (ed.). *Exercise and Sports Science.* Philadelphia, PA: Lippincott Williams & Wilkins, 2000.

260. Holmer I. Propulsive efficiency of breaststroke and freestyle swimming. *Eur J Appl Physiol.* 1974;33(2): 95–103.

261. Holmer I. Oxygen uptake during swimming in man. *J Appl Physiol.* 1972;33(4):502–509.

262. Tanaka H. Effects of cross-training. Transfer of training effects on VO_{2max} between cycling, running and swimming. *Sports Med.* 1994;18(5):330–339.

263. Magel JR, Foglia GF, McArdle WD, et al. Specificity of swim training on maximal oxygen uptake. *J Appl Physiol.* 1974;38(1):151–155.

264. Burns AS, Lauder TD. Deep water running: An effective non-weightbearing exercise for the maintenance of land-based running performance. *Mil Med.* 2001;166(3):253–258.

265. Bushman BA, Flynn MG, Andres FF, et al. Effect of 4 wk of deep water run training on running performance. *Med Sci Sports Exerc.* 1997;29(5): 694–699.

266. Wilber RL, Moffatt RJ, Scott BE, et al. Influence of water run training on the maintenance of aerobic performance. *Med Sci Sports Exerc.* 1996;28(8): 1056–1062.

267. Eyestone ED, Fellingham G, George J, Fisher AG. Effect of water running and cycling on maximum oxygen consumption and 2-mile run performance. *Am J Sports Med.* 1993;21(1):41–44.

268. Gehring MM, Keller BA, Brehm BA. Water running with and without a flotation vest in competitive and recreational runners. *Med Sci Sports Exerc.* 1997;29(10):1374–1378.

269. D'Acquisto LJ, D'Acquisto DM, Renne D. Metabolic and cardiovascular responses in older women during shallow-water exercise. *J Strength Cond Res.* 2001;15(1):12–19.

270. Ciullo JV. Swimmer's shoulder. *Clin Sports Med.* 1986;5(1):115–137.

271. Vuori I. The cardiovascular risks of physical activity. *Acta Med Scand Suppl.* 1986;711:205–214.

272. Firor WB, Faulkner RA. Sudden death during exercise: How real a hazard? *Can J Cardiol.* 1988;4(6): 251–254.

273. Thompson PD. Cardiovascular risks of exercise. *Physician Sportsmed.* 2001;29(4):33–42.

274. Giri S, Thompson PD, Kiernan FJ, et al. Clinical and angiographic characteristics of exertion-related acute myocardial infarction. *JAMA.* 1999;282(18): 1731–1736.

275. Kiningham RB. Exercise and primary prevention of cardiovascular disease. *Clin Fam Pract.* 2001;3(4): 707–732.

276. American College of Obstetricians and Gynecologists Committee on Obstetric Practice. ACOG Committee Opinion: Exercise during Pregnancy and the Postpartum Period. Washington, DC: American College of Obstetricians and Gynecologists, 2002, p. 3.

277. Wang TW, Apgar BS. Exercise during pregnancy. *Am Fam Physician.* 1998;57(8):1846–1852, 1857.

278. Narayan KM, Gregg EW, Fagot-Campagna A, et al. Diabetes—A common, growing, serious, costly, and potentially preventable public health problem. *Diabetes Res Clin Pract.* 2000;50(Suppl 2):S77–84.

279. Fletcher B, Gulanick M, Lamendola C. Risk factors for type 2 diabetes mellitus. *J Cardiovasc Nurs.* 2002;16(2):17–23.

280. Pfohl M, Schatz H. Strategies for the prevention of type 2 diabetes. *Exp Clin Endocrinol Diabetes.* 2001;109 (Suppl):S240–S249.

281. Cook PC, Leit ME. Issues in the pediatric athlete. *Orthop Clin North Am.* 1995;26(3):453–464.

282. Luepker RV. How physically active are American children and what can we do about it? *Int J Obes Relat Metab Disord.* 1999;23(Suppl 2):S12–17.

283. Hawkins D, Metheny J. Overuse injuries in youth sports: Biomechanical considerations. *Med Sci Sports Exerc.* 2001;33(10):1701–1707.

284. Nied RJ, Franklin B. Promoting and prescribing exercise for the elderly. *Am Fam Physician.* 2002;65(3): 419–426.

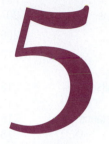

5

Training for Muscular Strength, Power, Endurance and Hypertrophy

JOSEPH A. BROSKY, JR.

GLENN A. WRIGHT

Objectives
The reader will be able to:

- Design a resistance-training program to improve: 1) muscular strength, 2) muscular hypertrophy, 3) muscular endurance, and 4) muscular power.

- Explain the influence of 1) training volume, 2) load, 3) rest time between sets, 4) velocity of movement, 5) training frequency, 6) exercise selection, and 7) order of exercises on the specificity of adaptations to resistance training programs.

- Demonstrate a greater appreciation of the use of a multi-planar approach to facilitate and/or minimize movements when designing specific therapeutic activities for selected conditions.

- Describe the functional significance of the ready position as it relates to dynamic postural stability and musculoskeletal balance.

- Describe the importance and efficiency of the squat exercise and its variations as vital components to lower extremity and trunk therapeutic exercise programs.

- Give examples of an upper and lower limb axial-appendicular musculoskeletal system and discuss why this serves as the foundation for developing core stability.

- Describe the neurophysiological principles behind plyometric training for the development of explosive power.

- List common methods of resistance training and their advantages and disadvantages.

- Discuss the strengths and weaknesses of commonly used functional performance tests.

- Describe characteristics that are common to all to effective anterior cruciate ligament injury prevention programs.

Outline

(continued)

INTRODUCTION

In 1998, the American College of Sports Medicine (ACSM) published their position stand, entitled "The recommended quantity and quality of exercise for developing and maintaining cardiopulmonary and muscular fitness, and flexibility in healthy adults."[1] In 2001, the ACSM published a position stand specific to recommended resistance training progressions for healthy adults.[2] This was one of the first acknowledgements by the scientific community that resistance training was important to health and fitness. The recommendations in this position stand were conservative, at best, but adults of all ages took notice that resistance training was not just for athletes any more. Resistance training is now part of the exercise programs of children, older adults, competitive athletes, and clients interested in general fitness.

Although the primary purpose for resistance training is to increase muscular strength, power, and endurance, other health benefits have also been observed in clients who participate in regular resistance training, including reduction of risk factors for coronary heart disease, non–insulin dependent diabetes, and colon cancer; improved bone health; reduced body fat levels; and prevention of musculoskeletal injuries.[3] Resistance training may also improve dynamic postural stability as related to standing balance and mobility (see Chapter 9), thereby preserving functional independence with aging. Non-impaired, complete active joint range of motion enables resistance training to be applied safely through the ranges of motion needed to perform the majority of activities of daily living (*ADL* = selfcare, mobility, communication), instrumental activities of daily living (*IADL* = other activities vital to the maintenance of independent living, shopping, household chores, etc.), as well as vocational and recreational demands with full functional independence. For these reasons, the attainment of non-impaired joint range of motion is considered prerequisite to the implementation of resistance training programs that rely on a high training volume or resistance level.

RESISTANCE TRAINING CONSIDERATIONS

Existing Health and Fitness Status

Prior to beginning any resistance training program, at risk clients should indergo a complete medical screening by a qualified physician. This becomes more important with advancing age or with a history of medical complications following prior bouts of physical activity, regardless of age.

After receiving medical clearance for the client, an individualized muscular fitness evaluation should also be performed to determine client needs and goals. Initial training status plays an important role in developing realistic goals and objectives for the training program. Untrained clients or those with lower initial strength levels can expect a greater relative muscular fitness increase than clients who have been involved in a resistance training program for the last three to six months or more. Clients who have little or no training experience can expect muscular strength increases of approximately forty percent. Those with more than six months of training can expect 16–20 percent increases in strength, and those with years of resistance training experience who have already attained significant improvements in muscular fitness can expect up to approximately a 10 percent increase in strength at the onset of a new resistance training program.[2]

Key Point:

Clients who have little or no training experience can expect the most dramatic increases in strength following resistance training program intervention.

Client Goals

Once the client's needs have been identified from the muscular fitness evaluation, it is important to develop realistic goals for the resistance training program. Unrealistic goals can lead to adverse outcomes, namely discouragement, poor therapeutic exercise program compliance/adherence (see Chapter 11), and possibly injury or re-injury.[4] An understanding of both expected physiological and behavioral adaptations to a resistance training program are important when helping the client decide on realistic goals that they strive to reach, and the time frame of when to expect these goals to be attained. (see Chapter 11)

Performance vs. Health-Related Fitness and Training

Athletically active clients and individuals with strenuous vocations such as the service professions (e.g., military, fire fighting, postal service) have greater vested interest in *performance-related fitness* (high intensity levels, competitive) than *health-related fitness* (maintaining appropriate health, preventing disease, injury, or negating the deleterious effects of normal aging). Rehabilitation clinicians should be interested in both. Fitness can be thought of as a state of well being that provides an optimal performance or functional level, whereas training is an organized program of exercises designed to stimulate positive long term or chronic adaptations. Therapeutic exercise training as a component of a rehabilitation plan also seeks to stimulate positive long term or chronic adaptations in the client.

Who do you suppose might jump more often during a single "work" session, a college basketball player, or someone who works as an urban parcel delivery employee? Who performs more overhead motions in a single work session, a professional baseball pitcher or a drill press operator? While some of these vocational demands may be similar, the specific motor patterns, muscle activation characteristics, joint movement velocities, postural positioning and changes, and performance techniques may differ, requiring the prescriptive therapeutic exercise interventions to differ with consideration for the *specificity of training principle* (discussed later).

Types of Muscular Actions

Most resistance training programs include dynamic repetitions with both *concentric* (shortening) and *eccentric* (lengthening) muscle actions, whereas *isometric* (tightening

without observable length change) muscle actions play a secondary role.[2] During eccentric actions, a greater force is produced by the active muscle mass as it performs negative work in resisting gravitational forces to decelerate the body. Eccentric muscle actions produce less lactate[5] and seem to be necessary for increasing muscular mass during resistance training; however, eccentric muscle activations result in a greater amount of delayed onset muscle soreness than concentric muscle contractions.[6] It is therefore recommended that both concentric and eccentric muscle actions be included during resistance training for the purpose of increasing muscular strength in a functionally relevant manner.[2]

RESISTANCE TRAINING PRINCIPLES

Overload

The *overload principle* is the basis for all training programs. In simple terminology, the overload principle states that for a muscle or muscle group to increase strength, it must, on a regular basis, be challenged to overcome resistances that are greater than those that are usually encountered. When designing therapeutic exercise programs, the rehabilitation clinician must determine a way to progressively and systematically overload the physiological systems that are the focus of the exercise. Overload can be accomplished in a number of ways:

- Increase load or resistance.
- Increase number of repetitions (one repetition equals one complete exercise movement).
- Increase number of sets (number of consecutive repetitions performed without rest for a given exercise).
- Decrease the rest time between sets or exercises.

Progression

The amount of overload required to bring about positive resistance training adaptations depends on the current level of muscular fitness. Too much overload may result in undue fatigue and soreness, musculoskeletal injury, or overtraining (discussed later). On the other hand, for the human body to continue to make positive adaptations, the magnitude of the physiological demands placed on the targeted system must continually be increased or changed. Since the adaptations to a resistance training program take place quickly, systematically increasing the overload is necessary to continue seeing improvement. A common method of progressive overload involves the modification of both the training load and the number of repetitions. In this method, known as the *double progression method*, a repetition range is prescribed, such as 8 to 12. This means that when the client can complete 12 repetitions at the given load, the load should be increased and the client should use the new load as long as at least 8 repetitions can be successfully performed. If the client cannot perform 8 repetitions, then the load increase was too great. The new load should be used until 12 repetitions again can be successfully performed, and then the load should be increased again and the process started over.

Specificity

There is a high degree of task specificity involved in human movement and adaptation that encompasses both movement patterns and muscle force velocity characteristics.[7] The development of muscular strength and endurance is specific to the muscle groups trained, the energy systems used, and the type of muscle contraction (isometric, concentric, eccentric) used in training.[8] The speed of the therapeutic exercise movement and joint ranges of motion are also specific to the strength improvement. With isometric training, strength is gained at the angles that are used in training with lesser strength gains observed at other joint angles through the full range of motion with approximately a 20° physiologic overlay.[9] Similarly, with isokinetic training, strength gains will be greatest when tested at velocities similar to those used in the training program. The *Specific Adaptations to Imposed Demands (S.A.I.D.) Principle* implies that for training to be effective, the system should be trained in a manner similar to how it will be used. The S.A.I.D. principle has implications to functional anatomy, neuromuscular recruitment, motor skill patterns, cardiovascular function, and muscle energy metabolism. Skeletal muscle metabolism is often the most emphasized component of training specificity. Shorter duration activities place greater demands on glycolytic metabolism and creatine phosphate or adenosine triphosphate (ATP) regeneration, while longer duration activities place greater demands on ATP regeneration from mitochondrial respiration. However, activities never have total reliance on a single metabolic pathway (see Chapter 2). Beyond the blend of metabolic pathways that converge to fuel a given activity, other factors including weight bearing magnitude, range of motion, velocity, postural positioning and the interaction of adjacent joint segments during movement performance are of equal importance to the rehabilitation clinician. There may be a transfer of fitness from one mode of training to another (e.g., cross training), if the training stimulus and muscles are used similarly.[10] Most research on cross-training has been performed on cycling, running, and arm ergometry comparing VO_{2max} (maximal oxygen uptake) indicating that central cardiovascular adaptations do occur between different therapeutic exercise modes if the training stimulus is large enough. Again, it is feasible that the specificity principle is likely the most important training guideline. The concept of specificity has other applications when applied to resistance training. When designing resistance training programs, the specific movement patterns that take place in sports and vocations need to be taken into consideration. Muscles are activated in a sequential order specific to the movement performed, and central and peripheral nervous system adaptations with training occur with similar specificity. Therefore, training athletically active clients for sports specific movements and other clients for specific work, ADL, or IADL related movement tasks is essential.

Key Point:

To prepare clients for the demands of daily activities including vocational and athletic activity challenges, it is critical to design resistance training programs in accordance with the S.A.I.D. principle.

Reversibility

Any improvements in muscular fitness (strength, endurance, hypertrophy, power, and extensibility) will be reversed if the overload on the muscles is decreased. The extent of the reversal depends primarily on the extent that the overload decreases. For example, a greater decrease in muscle strength will occur if a client ceases resistance training altogether than if the same client decreases any of the individual factors that can be modified during resistance exercise (decreased number of sets or repetitions, decreased load, or decreased frequency of workouts).

FUNDAMENTALS OF MUSCULAR FITNESS

There are four basic areas of muscular fitness:

- Muscular strength.
- Muscular hypertrophy.
- Muscular endurance.
- Muscular power.

Any resistance training program will help the client achieve some increase in each of these areas, especially if they have not performed resistance training in the recent past. Untrained beginners gain on almost any resistance training program as long as progressive overload is applied. Ultimately, optimal strength, hypertrophy, local muscular endurance and power require the systematic use of various loading strategies.[11]

Training for Muscular Strength

Muscular strength is defined as the maximal force that can be generated in a single effort by a muscle or muscle group. Increasing muscular strength is primarily a function of the nervous system's ability to recruit a great number of motor units to overcome a resistance. Adaptation to repetitive overloads takes places quickly, with neural mechanisms such as more efficient neural recruitment patterns of more and larger motor units, more efficient rate coding of the neural impulse, improved agonist muscle synchrony, decreased antagonist muscle activation, increased central nervous system activation, and a lowering of neural inhibitory reflexes and a raising of Golgi tendon organ activation thresholds (see Chapters 2, 7, 8)[12,13] being noticed within the initial weeks of training. Transformations of fast twitch glycolytic muscle fibers to more fast twitch oxidative, glycolytic muscle fibers, increased number and size of myofibrils, and stronger, more organized connective tissue components also occur as strength increases.[14] The magnitude of strength increases are based on a number of factors, including the load, training volume, rest time between sets, velocity of movement, training frequency, exercise selection, and exercise order.

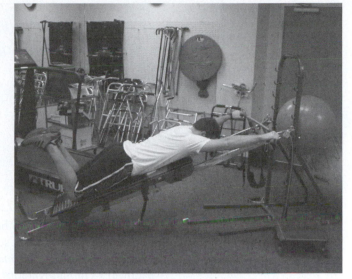

Figure 5.1   Total Gym.™

Load (Resistance) and the Repetition Maximum. There is an inverse relationship between the amount of weight that can be lifted and the number of repetitions that can be performed.[11] The overload principle dictates that a greater than normal physical demand be placed on the muscles for improvement in muscular fitness to be achieved. Altering the training load affects the acute metabolic, hormonal, neural, and cardiovascular responses to resistance exercise.[2]

The *repetition maximum* (RM) is used to establish baseline loads for starting resistance training (based on the number of repetitions that can be correctly performed at a given resistance). Percentages of a client's 10 RM for a given exercise are often used when choosing the resistance to be used during multiple therapeutic exercise sets. When preparing conditioning programs for non-impaired athletic clients, a percentage of the resistance that can be lifted for a five or one RM are commonly used. This is an extremely important concept that some rehabilitation clinicians have avoided in favor of safety concerns, though perhaps their reasoning is ill founded. Clients with acute injuries or debilitating conditions, especially conditions involving surgical reconstructions, should never be subjected to potentially injurious environments or activities. However, it is feasible to impart safe, biomechanically sound, and appropriate stresses to healing tissues in order to stimulate favorable changes through the manipulation of the environment, limiting weight bearing and range of motion with equipment such as the Total Gym™ (EFI, Total Gym,™ San Diego, CA) **(Figure 5.1)**. (● **Section 1, Animation 1**)

A training load of 40–60 percent of the amount the client can maximally use to perform one RM of an exercise is sufficient for the development of muscular strength in most normally active clients. Resistance loads of 80–100 percent of one RM, however, have been shown to produce the most rapid gains in muscular strength.[4,15] Al-

though a percentage of the resistance that can be lifted appropriately for a five or one RM is commonly used to set the appropriate training resistance, a safer, easier, and possibly more precise method is to select a training resistance that allows only a specific number of repetitions to be performed. The effect of load on muscular strength and muscular endurance has been demonstrated by the repetition maximum continuum as depicted in **Figure 5.2.**[16]

Periodization. Periodized training or "periodization" refers to a variation in the training stimulus (i.e., different workouts with different intensities and volumes of exercise) and planned recovery periods to prevent overtraining. Periodization of training allows for changes in the intensity as well as changes in the volume of exercise, which theoretically keeps the exercise stimulus effective for long range resistance training progressions.[11,17] Periodization is a highly structured, sequential development of athletic skill or physiologic capacity brought about by organizing training regimens into blocks of time to focus specifically on particular training goals related to strength, power, endurance, or hypertrophy. These time blocks range from a single training session of several hours to countless sessions spread out over several months up to even a year or more of training. Much has been written about periodization protocols for a variety of purposes. Although usually considered to be something reserved for training the elite athlete, these blocks of time are conceptually similar to what is routinely performed in many therapeutic exercise sessions and appreciation for it's use in the health and fitness arena is growing. *Macrocycles* can be compared to the long term client treatment goals, which may include further subdivisions of shorter time blocks called *mesocycles* and *microcycles*, which are analogous to intermediate and short term client treatment goals, respectively.

RM	3	6	10	12		20	25
	Strength/power	Strength/power		Strength/power		Strength/power	Strength/power
	High-intensity endurance	**High-intensity endurance**		High-intensity endurance		High-intensity endurance	High-intensity endurance
	Low-intensity endurance	Low-intensity endurance		Low-intensity endurance		Low-intensity endurance	**Low-intensity endurance**
	Maximal power output				to		Low power output

RM = repetition maximum

Figure 5.2 Schematic of relationship between repetitions, intensity, strength, power, and endurance. (Used with permission from S Fleck, WJ Kraemer. *Designing Resistance Training Programs*, 2nd ed. Champaign, IL: Human Kinetics, 1997.)

In general, it is recommended that clients who are novice to intermediate weight lifters train with loads corresponding to 8 to 12 RM and advanced clients use loads of one to six RM in a periodized fashion to maximize muscular strength development. For progression in those clients who train at a specific RM load (e.g., 8 to 12 repetitions), it is recommended that a 2–10 percent resistance increase be applied, with greater load increases used for exercises that train larger muscle groups across multiple joints, and smaller increases used for smaller muscles or muscle groups and more isolated muscles. These increases should be applied when the client can perform one to two repetitions over the desired number of training repetitions for two consecutive training sessions.

Training Volume. Training volume is determined by multiplying the number of repetitions by the number of sets by the resistance used for each exercise. Variations in resistance training volume affect the central and peripheral nervous systems, increase muscle size (hypertrophy), and influence hormonal responses, including increased serum testosterone and human growth hormone levels and decreased serum cortisol levels.[12] Cortisol plays several regulatory roles in metabolism and negatively impacts protein metabolism when attempting to conserve glycogen stores. Decreased resting serum cortisol levels may be important for reducing muscle protein catabolism and supporting hypertrophic accretion of protein by reducing protein degradation.[18] The testosterone:cortisol ratio has been used as an indicator of tissue anabolism.[19] Hormonal responses are not only caused by the magnitude of the load or the intensity of the work performed, but also the volume of training.[20]

In general, the greater the cross sectional area of the muscle, the greater its strength. To increase strength, muscle hypertrophy is beneficial. Muscle mass tends to increase with high volume (three to five sets of 10–12 repetitions), moderate intensity (65–75 percent one RM) resistance training. Increasing volume to promote muscle hypertrophy is a matter of increasing the number of repetitions of a given exercise, and/or increasing the number of total exercise sets per training session. High volume training with shorter recovery times between sets (approximately 60 sec; see hypertrophy section) produces an anabolic hormonal environment that promotes a gain in lean muscle mass.

Low volume (three to five sets of two to six repetitions) training with high intensity (80–95 percent one RM) programs tend to improve larger fast twitch muscle fiber motor unit recruitment, which is necessary to increase muscular strength. Considering that the early phase of resistance training is characterized by improvements in neuromuscular activation and coordination, it may be that the overall training volume is not as critical during the first 6–12 weeks of resistance training.[11] Regardless of how the overall training volume is manipulated, it is vital to remember that resistance training goals will not be met without the inclusion of adequate rest between sessions, recovery between sets, and appropriate nutrition between therapeutic exercise sessions.

Key Point:

Adequate rest between sessions, recovery between sets, and nutrition are essential for resistance training goals to be met.

Rest Time Between Sets. The amount of rest between sets and between different exercises affects the metabolic, hormonal, and cardiovascular responses to resistance exercise, as well as the performance of subsequent sets and training adaptations.[2] Short rest periods between sets (60 seconds) may increase the metabolic, cardiovascular, and hormonal responses, but strength increases may be reduced. When the primary resistance training goal is to increase muscular strength, the general guideline is to activate as much total muscle mass as possible (number of muscles, larger muscles), with a greater intensity (load) of exercise, and with longer rest periods between exercise sets. For multi-joint exercises that use heavy loads, a minimum of two to three minutes between sets is recommended. For single joint exercises or exercises with a smaller muscle mass involvement, one to two minute rest periods are usually sufficient.

Movement Velocity. Movement velocity affects the neural, hypertrophic, and metabolic responses to resistance exercise.[1,2] In *isokinetic training* (constant velocity), for example, the greatest strength increases occur at the speed at which training takes place. Therefore, if the client desires to improve his or her strength over a wide range of movement velocities, they should train using a spectrum of fast, moderate, and slow velocities.

Training using constant resistance (*isotonic*) has other variables to consider with movement velocity: whether the slow velocity is *unintentional* or *intentional*. Unintentional slow velocities take place during high load repetitions in which either the load or fatigue is responsible for slowing the movement. For example, the lifter may be attempting to move the load at a fast velocity, but the weight of the load is too great for them to lift quickly. Intentional slow velocity contractions (also referred to as super slow training) involve, as the name implies, purposely moving the load at a slow velocity through the desired range of motion. To be able to move the weight more slowly, the lifter must use a lesser load; because of this, super slow training may not stimulate recruitment of the larger fast twitch motor units to as great an extent as exercise performed at moderate training velocities. Therefore, intentionally slow velocity training may not provide an optimal stimulus for strength enhancement.

It is recommended that beginners initially use slow to moderate resistance training velocities to concentrate more on proper exercise technique. Those with a little experience with resistance training should use moderate velocity movements to enhance muscular strength. For advanced training, exercises should be performed at a variety of velocities: intentionally slow, moderate, and fast. At all movement velocities, proper exercise technique must be used to reduce any risk of injury.

Training Frequency. The optimal resistance training frequency depends on the training status of the client, the intensity and volume of the exercise sessions, the exercises selected, the ability of the client to recover between sessions, and the number of muscle groups trained per session.[1,2]

For most clients, it is recommended that they train each major muscle group no more than two to three times per week to see improvement in muscular strength. For beginning lifters, a total body workout (a workout where all of the major muscle groups are trained in the same exercise session) is recommended two to three times per week. Intermediate lifters are advised to maintain these guidelines of two to three times per week. For those intermediate lifters who are looking to make changes in the design of their resistance training program, changes in training frequency are one way to provide variety and changes in overload. Training frequency might be three to four days per week, with each major muscle group being trained one to two days per week.

As a lifter becomes more experienced, optimal training frequency for improved strength varies. Regardless of whether the client participates in resistance training for general fitness, body building, weight lifting, or for other reasons, training frequency (the volume of work performed by each muscle or muscle group each week) depends on the specific program goals. In some cases, because training volume is high for a particular muscle group per workout, such as during a body builder's resistance training program, frequency may be two training sessions per day, one training session for one muscle group in the morning plus one training session for a separate muscle group later in the day. This type of two-a-day training session (split routine) may lead to 8 to 12 workouts per week. Although this type of training is not rare, to see optimal muscular strength improvements it is recommended that each major muscle group be trained only two to three times per week in those experienced in resistance training. This would typically be accomplished in four to six training sessions using a split routine resistance training program design.

Exercise Selection. Exercise selection is partially determined by the outcome goals of the client for whom the training program is designed. Exercises selected for the client who is interested in increasing greater overall muscular strength to more effectively perform basic ADLs and IADLs should differ from those selected for the athletic client who desires to improve sport specific performance. However, it is also possible that both clients have common resistance training program needs, with the primary difference resting with the magnitude of strength that must be attained for the clients to achieve their goals.

Exercises are classified in a number of different ways. *Whole body exercises* receive contributions from the largest number of muscles, since the entire body contributes to the movement. *Integrated or multiple joint exercise* movements such as the squat, power clean, hang pull, lunge, or bench press use the next largest number of muscles, and *isolated or single joint exercises* such as the seated knee extension or the bicep curl use the least. Many daily movements, such as bending over to pick something up from the floor or reaching high up on a shelf to retrieve a package, are examples of movements requiring whole body strength. Athletes in sports such as football, basketball, wrestling, and track and field have whole body strength or power requirements, since participation in their sport is rarely a matter of using single joints or a few multiple joint movements. Exercises that incorporate the use of the legs, trunk, and shoulder joints within the same movement are considered whole body movements. In recent years, there has been a trend to incorporate more of these types of movements into resistance training and therapeutic exercise programs. Another name for exercises that incorporate whole body movements is *functional training*. These whole body exercises should be used to some extent in the strength training programs of both athletic and non-athletic clients to train muscle groups in the movement patterns that are used in the performance of their sport, job, ADLs or IADLs.

Key Point:

Whole body exercises are becoming more popular therapeutic exercise program components because they can be easily modified to simulate a wide variety of client functions.

The number of joints moving during an exercise allows it to be classified as either a single, or multiple-joint exercise. Both single and multiple joint exercises have been shown to be effective for increasing muscular strength. Multiple joint exercises typically require complex neural activation and coordination that use more muscle mass and allow a greater load to be used for training a specific muscle group. As a result, these exercises, along with whole body exercises, are recommended to make up a high percentage of a resistance training program designed for increasing muscular strength or power. Single joint exercises are usually used to isolate specific muscles or muscle groups. As such, lesser amounts of muscle mass are involved in these movements. Single joint exercises are useful for increasing strength in the target muscles or muscle groups. Therefore, it is recommended that both exercise types be blended into a resistance training program, with emphasis on multiple joint exercises for maximizing muscle strength or power.[1,2]

Resistance training loads can be attained from a variety of sources, including gravity effects on body weight, free weights, exercise machine weight stacks, elastic tubing or bands, springs, water, hydraulic or pneumatic cylinders, and electromagnets. Overall, regardless of the method of resistance training, the important factor for increasing

strength is the overload that is placed on the muscle or groups of muscles that contribute to the movement and the ranges and velocities of the joint movements. Traditional forms of resistance training include the use of free weights and resistance machines. Advantages of free weights include the ability to mimic the intra- and intermuscular coordination and motor patterns needed to effectively perform a specific task. To some extent, resistance training using rubber tubing or using water as resistance in an aquatic environment can also provide resistance, but with a greater focus on concentric muscle activation. While resistance machines are regarded as safer to use and easier to learn to use, and, in some cases, allow resistance to be applied more effectively (e.g., seated knee extension, latissimus dorsi pulldown), they also require stabilization of proximal and distal segments such as the trunk and/or upper or lower extremities to maintain proper positioning within the machine. This could be an advantage or disadvantage depending on the condition and training level of the client and his or her therapeutic exercise program goals. To increase strength in a particular movement specific to ADLs, IADLs, or sports participation, this would be a disadvantage. However, if training a specific muscle or muscle group is a therapeutic exercise program goal, resistance machines could provide a safe and effective means of increasing muscular strength and carefully controlling overload to other connective tissues (ligaments and tendons).

Exercise Order.   The order in which the selected exercises are performed will influence resistance training results. Strength improvement is dependent on the intensity of the work performed by the muscles. Whole body and multiple joint exercises require high amounts of energy, since the muscle mass involvement is great. Therefore, performing these exercises early in the training session when fatigue is minimal will allow higher quality work in the training session. However, isolated, single joint exercises that train muscle groups of larger mass such as the quadriceps femoris and hamstrings may also need to be performed relatively early during a resistance training session.

The order of exercises can also depend on which muscle or muscle group is the focus of the training session. The larger the muscle mass involvement, the greater are the energy requirements. It is recommended to train the larger muscles or muscle groups early in a training session. Many smaller muscle groups are also weaker than the larger muscle groups. Therefore, for optimal results, isolated exercises should not be performed early in a training session using small muscles or muscle groups that may be called upon later in the same training session during the execution of a multiple joint exercise, because the fatigued smaller muscles could limit performance during the multiple joint exercise.

Recommendations for arranging the exercise order for beginning, intermediate, and advanced strength training include the following:

- When training all of the major muscle groups in one session, large muscle group exercise should be performed before small muscle group exercise, and whole body and multiple joint or integrated exercises should be performed before single joint or isolated exercises. A rotation of upper and lower body exercises or opposing muscle groups (agonist-antagonist pairs) during the training session has also been used with success.
- When training upper body muscles on one day and lower body muscles on a separate day, the client should perform the large muscle group exercises before small muscle group exercises and the multiple joint and whole body exercises before the single joint exercises, or should rotate exercises of opposing muscle groups.
- When training individual muscle groups, the client should perform multiple joint exercises before single joint exercises and higher intensity exercises before lower intensity exercises.[1,2]

Training for Muscular Hypertrophy

Many clients begin a resistance training program for the primary purpose of increasing muscle mass. *Muscle hypertrophy* is an increase in muscle cross sectional area caused primarily by increases in the size of the specific muscle fibers that are recruited to work during physical activity. Since fast twitch (type II) muscle fibers tend to achieve hypertrophy to a greater extent than slow twitch (type I) fibers, it is imperative to overload the muscle in a manner that recruits an abundance of fast twitch fibers. Training for musclar hypertrophy (e.g., moderate to heavy loads for 6 to 12 repetitions with moderate to short rest intervals) is supported primarily by energy from the ATP-PC (see Chapters 2 and 4) system and glycolysis, with minor contributions from aerobic metabolism.[11]

Muscle hypertrophy results from an increase in protein accretion, through an increase in protein synthesis, a decrease in protein degradation, or a combination of the two. Protein synthesis peaks at approximately 24 hours following exercise and remains elevated for hours to days after exercise. Muscle hypertrophy is at least partially a function of the hormone response (increased testosterone, increased growth hormone, decreased cortisol, and increased insulin-like growth factors) and the inclusion of eccentric exercises in the training program. It seems the mechanical damage produced with eccentric exercise is a stimulus for hypertrophy, although it is not a requirement for hypertrophy to take place.

Noticeable hypertrophy may take more than two months to develop. Most early adaptations to resistance training are related to central and peripheral nervous system adaptations and increases in voluntary muscular strength. Hypertrophy becomes evident by six to eight weeks of training in relatively untrained clients. Increases in functional muscle mass complements nervous system adaptations to increase voluntary muscular strength. Ultimately, it is the combination of muscular hypertrophy and central and peripheral nervous system adaptations that influence the client's muscle strength increases. Since modifications in resistance training loads and volume influence muscle size increases and nervous system adaptations, specific periods of varying training emphasis are often used to effect the desired systems (see periodization). Program design variables need to be specifically modified to enhance muscle hypertrophy. The following section highlights some of these recommendations.

Load and Volume. Gains in muscle hypertrophy are related to the total work performed during the training sessions. Although traditional strength training (high load, low repetition, longer rest periods) has produced significant hypertrophy, training programs with high volume (multiple sets), and moderate number of repetitions (8 to 12) that are similar to bodybuilding training programs have shown greater results at increasing muscle mass. Moderate to heavy loads, moderate to high repetitions, and multiple sets per exercise are characteristic of hypertrophy training.[11] Since total work seems to be the underlying factor of successful resistance training programs for the purpose of increasing muscle mass, it is not necessary to routinely train using specific repetition maximums. In other words, it may not be necessary to frequently perform sets to the point at which no additional repetitions can be performed (momentary muscular failure) on a regular basis, especially for clients who are new to resistance training. Clients who are more experienced lifters should perform a higher percentage of sets to muscle failure to recruit a greater number of motor units, since muscle fibers that are not active in training will not respond by increasing their size. In addition, clients who are more experienced lifters should also employ a percentage of their training at higher resistances to recruit the larger, stronger motor units that contribute more to muscle hypertrophy. Therefore, the recommendations for beginning and intermediate level clients are to use moderate resistance for 8 to 12 repetitions of one to three sets per exercise to exceed not more than six sets per muscle group. For more advanced training, it is recommended to use loads of one to 12 RM per set for three to six sets per exercise in a periodized manner; however, the majority of training should use 6 to 12 RM resistance rather than one to six RM resistance.[11] Although each RM training zone has it advantages, devoting 100 percent of training to one general RM zone or intensity (e.g., 80 percent of one RM) runs a high risk of the client's progress plateauing or failing to progress efficiently.[11] No more than 10 to 12 sets for large muscle groups (legs, hips, torso) and no more than six to eight sets for smaller muscle groups (upper arms, lower leg) within a given resistance training session should be used, even during advanced training.

Exercise Selection and Order.   The more muscle mass involved in an exercise, the greater the hypertrophy stimulus. Therefore, multiple joint and whole body exercises play an important role in developing a systemic hypertrophy effect. These exercises are complex, and it takes time for the nervous system adaptations from these exercises to take place. Therefore, with these types of exercises, it may take longer before significant hypertrophy is noticed. In the end, however, more hypertrophy will be seen than with single joint exercises. There is ample evidence to show that hypertrophy is promoted with single joint exercises, though usually not to the extent of that seen with multiple joint exercises.

Less is understood concerning the effect of exercise order on muscle hypertrophy. However, it appears that the exercise order recommendations for strength training may also be applied for promoting muscle hypertrophy.[1,2] Therefore, to promote muscle hypertrophy, both single and multiple joint exercises should be included in a resistance training program, with the order similar to that recommended for increasing muscular strength.

Rest Periods.   Rest periods between sets of the same exercise are known to affect muscular strength development, but less is known concerning the effects of rest periods on hypertrophy.[2] The rest period between sets determines the metabolic recovery of the active muscle. Shorter recovery time between sets leads to increases in blood lactate levels, which are thought to be somehow related to an increase in anabolic hormonal responses to acute resistance training. Short rest periods (one to two minutes) coupled with moderate to high resistance training intensity and volume elicit greater acute anabolic hormone responses than programs utilizing very heavy loads with long rest periods (see Chapter 2). Generally speaking, when the client trains at a 90–100 percent maximal power intensity over a 5 to 10 second duration (as with the shotput, 100 yard dash, long jump, < 10 RM weight lifts), the primary dependence on the phosphagen system requires a 12:1 to 20:1 rest-to-work ratio range between sets or bouts of activity for optimal recovery.[11] When they train at a 75–90 percent maximal power intensity over a 15–30 second duration, the primary dependence on the fast glycolysis system requires a 3:1 to 5:1 rest-to-work ratio range between sets or bouts of activity for optimal recovery. When they train at a 30–75 percent maximal power intensity over a one to three minute duration (as with basketball or soccer), the combi-

nation of dependence on the fast glycolysis and oxidative systems requires a 3:1 or 4:1 rest-to-work ratio range between sets or bouts of activity for optimal recovery.[11] When they train at a 20–35 percent maximal power intensity for durations of > three minutes, a 3:1 to 1:1 rest-to-work ratio range is needed between sets or bouts of activity for optimal recovery.[11] Although hormonal response is not an accurate way to judge the effects on hypertrophy, the shorter rest periods seem to create a better physiological environment that is needed for hypertrophy to take place.

In general, based on the anabolic hormone response, it is recommended that one to two minute rest periods be used for beginners and those clients with moderate experience in resistance training. For clients who are more advanced lifters, the length of the rest periods should correspond to the goals of each exercise or the training phase, such that two to three minute rest periods may be used with heavy resistance for the key strength building exercises. One to two minute rest periods may be sufficient for other exercises performed at moderate to high training intensities.[2]

Movement Velocity.   The optimal movement velocity to enhance muscle hypertrophy has not been thoroughly researched. Keeping the force–velocity relationship for muscle force generation during concentric activation in mind (the faster the movement speed, the lower the force produced), recruitment of the larger fast twitch (type II) muscle fibers with a high potential for hypertrophy is not as likely with high speed movement. Higher forces during concentric muscle activations are produced at slower movement speeds. However, "too slow" a speed may necessitate the use of a lighter load, thereby decreasing fast twitch (type II) muscle fiber recruitment. Therefore, the recommendation is to use slow to moderate speed resistance training movements when muscular hypertrophy is the resistance training program goal.

Training Frequency.   Training frequency for muscular hypertrophy depends on the client's capacity for recovery. Training status, age, physical demands outside of training, and nutritional status influence the client's ability to recover after exercise. Resistance training programs could be designed for three to six sessions per week, although training of the same muscle group should occur only two to three times per week. The total training frequency therefore would depend on whether the entire body was trained in one session, three times per week, or whether different muscle groups were trained on alternating days four to six times per week. Clients who increase their resistance training frequency to four to six times per week are at greater risk of *overtraining*—reaching a plateau or experiencing decreased performance due to chronic fatigue (discussed in greater detail later).

Training for Muscular Endurance

Muscular endurance is the ability of a muscle to move a submaximal load repetitiously without a degradation in performance. Training to improve local muscle endurance (e.g., high repetition, short rest intervals) involves a higher contribution of energy from aerobic metabolism.[11] Increasing muscular endurance can be achieved in several ways. The specific training program depends on the type of muscular endurance necessary and may depend on the client's recreational activities, such as long distance cycling or running, or occupational demands, such as for a hospital orderly who routinely transports patients throughout the day. In the case of long term recreational activities, low power muscular endurance (sets of approximately 25 RM intensity over longer duration) is called for, whereas many occupational demands require a higher power muscular endurance (sets of approximately 10–12 RM intensity over shorter duration) (see **Figure 5.2**). Specific adaptations can be fostered by modifying program design, but the basic principle for the development of muscular endurance is to use a moderate to light load for a relatively high number of repetitions with short rest periods between sets and exercises. Minimizing recovery time between sets is an important training stimulus to skeletal muscle, promoting increased numbers of mitochondria, increased capillary number, muscle fiber type transformations, and improved lactate acid buffering capacity. The rest interval between sets and exercises greatly influences the relative contribution of the three metabolic energy pathways, and the metabolic, hormonal, and cardiovascular reponses to an acute exercise bout, in addition to performance during subsequent sets and training adaptations.[11]

Key Point:

Resistance training to improve muscular endurance requires the performance of a relatively high number of repetitions with a light to moderate resistance with short rest periods between sets and exercises.

It should also be mentioned that increasing the strength of a particular muscle group usually coincides with an increase in muscular endurance, when tested with the same absolute load pre- and post-training. Since the relative load is lighter following an increase in strength, the client is typically capable of performing more repetitions at the testing load used prior to training.

Exercise Selection and Order. Designing an appropriate resistance training program for improving muscular endurance needs to include exercises that incorporate the muscles or muscle groups involved in the task that requires muscular endurance. In general, multiple joint exercises will create the greatest metabolic demand. Metabolic demand is an important stimulus to create the desired skeletal muscle adaptations for improving local muscular endurance.[2] Single joint exercises can also be included to increase muscular endurance of specific muscles or muscle groups.

Fatigue within a muscle or muscle group is a necessary aspect of a resistance training program to increase muscular endurance. Therefore, exercise order does not seem to be as important during training to improve muscle endurance as it is when training for muscular strength. One method of increasing muscular endurance is to perform several exercises consecutively that train the same muscle or muscle group. This practice is also known as *pre-exhaustion training* and typically will use a single joint exercise followed by a multiple joint exercise that emphasizes the same muscle or muscle group with minimal rest between exercises. Another method to train muscle endurance is through various types of circuit weight training. Circuit weight training progressions have been developed that alternate upper extremity and lower extremity exercises or that have a "push exercise" such as a bench press followed by a "pull exercise" such as a latissimus dorsi pulldown. Circuit weight training examples for therapeutic exercise program consideration are discussed later in this chapter.

Exercise Resistance and Volume. Light resistance coupled with high volume (two to three sets of 15 to 20 repetitions) has been shown to be most effective for increasing low power muscular endurance. However, moderate to heavy exercise resistance (three to four sets of 10 to 12 repetitions) with short rest periods is more effective for increasing high intensity muscular endurance. In general, the higher the training volume is within a given muscle or muscle group, the greater will be the muscular endurance increase.

Rest-to-Work Intervals. The length of the rest period between sets may be the determining factor in the production of muscular endurance. Again, keep in mind that fatigue is important as a stimulus and is necessary to improve muscle endurance. Therefore, rest periods must be relatively short to produce these effects. It is recommended that rest periods used for low power muscular endurance (15–20 repetitions) use one to two minute rest periods between sets and high intensity muscular endurance (10–12 repetitions) use less than one minute rest periods between sets.[2]

Training Frequency. The recommended frequency for muscular endurance training is similar to that for hypertrophy training.

Training for Muscular Power

There are essentially two ways to increase *muscle power*. Since power is a function of work and time (muscle power = work/time), one can either increase the work performed or decrease the time in which it is performed by increasing neuromuscular reaction time and efficiency. This is contrasted with *muscle strength*, which considers the ability to overcome a resistance, thereby performing work without consideration for the time component. Strength and power training (e.g., heavy loads, one to six repetitions with long rest intervals) predominantly stress the ATP-PC system. A well planned resistance training program should address increasing strength followed by training the responsiveness and efficiency of the neuromuscular system to increase muscle power. Neuromuscular adaptations that may contribute to increased power include increased maximal rate of force production, increased muscular strength at slow and fast repetition velocities, efficient stretch shortening cycle performance (discussed in the plyometric section), and improved movement pattern coordination and skill.[21] Bobbert and Van Soest[22] suggest that maximal power training requires both heavy resistance training and use of rapid muscular activation or "explosive exercise movements." One of the best methods to achieve the development of muscular power is through plyometric training, which will be discussed later in this chapter.

RESISTANCE TRAINING PROGRAM DESIGN

In designing the resistance training component of a therapeutic exercise program, the rehabilitation clinician should have a foundational understanding of the metabolic demands, primary joints and muscle groups involved, and the biomechanical characteristics of each exercise movement that they select. Understanding these variables helps the rehabilitation clinician develop what is referred to as a *demands or needs analysis profile*.[23] In addition to understanding the specifics of the activity demands, this analysis profile includes the client's age, previous exercise and activity experience, past medical history, motivation level (see Chapter 11), and baseline physical characteristics of speed, power, strength, flexibility (see Chapter 3), coordination (see Chapter 8), and work capacity (see Chapter 4). The ACSM recommends that novices who participate in a resistance training program perform one set of 8 to 12 repetitions for 8 to 10 exercises, including one exercise for each of the major muscle groups.[1] For older or more frail clients, 10 to 15 repetitions using a lower resistance is recommended.[1] These guidelines should be used for the initial three to four months of training with a frequency of two to three exercise sessions per week. As the goals of the client change, as for example, for a client who desires to continue past the

novice stage, the resistance training recommendations should also change.

Gambetta[23] has presented several useful philosophical and physiological constructs that may provide some guiding principles to rehabilitation clinicians in designing resistance training programs to develop strength, power, endurance, or hypertrophy.

- Postural alignment and muscle balance are the foundation for all training and rehabilitation.
- Train synergists before prime movers.
- Train entire movements, not individual muscles.
- Develop core (proximal stability) strength before extremity strength.
- The whole is greater than the sum of its parts.

Other Resistance Training Methods

Power Lifting. Power lifting has been reserved for the competitive setting to determine the maximum amount of weight that can be lifted, to develop a clients' overall strength and explosiveness (rapid muscular power development) during specific lifts such as the bench press, squat, and dead lift. Power lifts are traditionally used as a conditioning form for American football. These particular lifts are not generally recommended to be used competitively for young or elderly populations (with greater focus on skill and technique rather than load), or those participating in acute or intermediate stages of rehabilitation. Power lifting is effective but does have some inherent dangers if performed without supervision, by those with limited experience, or with the use of faulty techniques.

Olympic Weight Lifting. Olympic style weight lifting includes two lifts: the snatch, and the clean and jerk. The objective of the snatch is to lift the barbell from the floor to an extended arms position overhead in one continuous motion (**Figure 5.3a–d**). The clean and jerk is actually two separate movements. The first, the clean involves lifting the barbell in one continuous motion from the floor to a position resting on the front of the shoulders. The second, the jerk, involves lifting the barbell to an extended

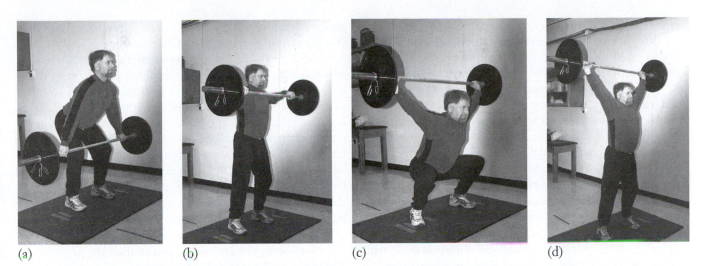

Figure 5.3   Olympic style weight lifting: the snatch. (a) initiation, (b) pull, (c) receiving the bar, (d) finish.

arms overhead position as with the snatch movement (**Figure 5.4a–d**). The major component of both of these lifts is the pull, whose object is to get the weight as high as possible off the floor before the lifter moves underneath it. The lower extremities, shoulders and the entire back are the primary regions of the body involved in the pull. These are highly skilled lifts that require sessions dedicated strictly to perfecting technique rather than increasing load. Foundational lifts used in training to prepare for Olympic weight lifting include the front and back squat. Training volume often varies from session to session based on the principles of periodization.

Body Building.   Body building uses resistance training to optimize muscle hypertrophy, definition and symmetry while reducing body fat to optimize appearance.[11]

THERAPEUTIC EXERCISE PROGRAM APPLICATIONS OF CROSS TRAINING AND CIRCUIT TRAINING

Cross Training and Crossover Effect

Cross training refers to training in different modes, or training in a secondary activity to supplement or augment the metabolic adaptations and training effects of a primary activity (e.g., adding resistance to increase the training intensity of the same muscles involved during an endurance exercise or activity). One important aspect of cross training may be the possibility that it helps prevent overuse (micro-traumatic) injuries, although this is only speculative and not well supported by conclusive research.[10] The

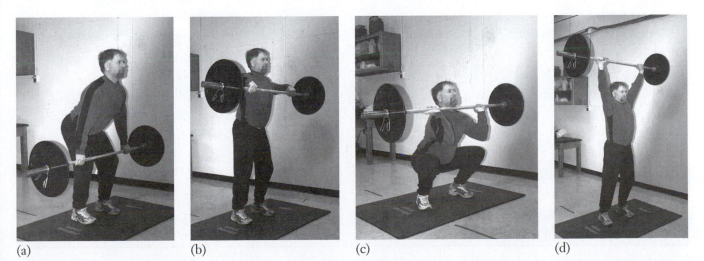

Figure 5.4   Olympic style weight lifting: the clean and jerk. (a) initiation, (b) pull, (c) receiving the bar, (d) finish.

term cross training should not be confused with the physiological phenomenon known as the *crossed education* or *crossover* effect that occurs when training one extremity results in strength gains at the contralateral extremity as has been reported in the homologous muscles of the contralateral extremity during high intensity training.[24–27] Studies that have used neuromuscular stimulation and eccentric quadriceps femoris activations[28] or imagined muscle contractions of the hypothenar muscles of the hand (visual imagery)[29] have also been reported to produce contralateral extremity strength increases. These reports support the use of visual imagery and resistive training exercises of uninvolved extremities during periods of immobilization or convalescence due to an injury, trauma, or surgical procedure and should be administered with greater enthusiasm and regularity than currently exists.

Circuit Training

Morgan and Adamson first reported circuit training as a formal training method at the University of Leeds in England in the 1950s.[30,31] A system was designed that would permit the training of several fitness components (strength, cardiovascular, balance) simultaneously. Circuit training is basically a series of exercise stations performed sequentially in a given time or for a specific number of repetitions, and may be designed to increase muscular strength, endurance, flexibility, balance and cardiopulmonary endurance. Though heart rates can be significantly elevated during circuit training, the magnitude of the cardiopulmonary endurance effects are generally not as great as those achieved through training programs consisting entirely of aerobic activities such as running, swimming, Nordic skiing or cycling (see Chapter 4).

Circuit training can be designed to be highly sports specific, with greater or lesser emphasis on eccentric muscle activation.[32] It provides an excellent method of adding variety to a therapeutic exercise program to prevent boredom, and minimize the likelihood of overuse injuries associated with training. Additionally, with creativity, circuit training can provide an excellent environment for the rehabilitation clinician to group exercise activities that simulate the demands of specific athletic or vocational movement needs. Both anaerobic and aerobic benefits can be achieved but this will depend on the circuit design (exercises, rest-to-work intervals, duration, etc). Sample circuits for the upper and lower extremities are provided in **Table 5.1** and **Table 5.2**, respectively.

PYRAMIDS, SPLIT ROUTINES, SUPER SETS, AND COMPOUND SETS

The *pyramid system* involves continuous sets of an exercise that progresses from light to heavy resistance, with the number of repetitions per set decreasing as the exercise intensity is increased. The *split routine* refers to dividing up exercise sessions by body region. A typical split routine system might involve training upper and lower body antagonistic muscle groups on successive days, for example exercises for the chest, shoulders, and back on Monday, Wednesday, and Friday and exercises for the arms, legs, and abdominals on Tuesday, Thursday, and Saturday. *Super sets* involve training opposing muscle groups in

TABLE 5.1   Example of activities for lower extremity therapeutic exercise circuit

Activity/Exercise Intervention	Comments
Cycling	5–10 minutes as a general warm-up
Single leg stands	Alternating, eyes open/closed
Biomechanical Ankle Platform System (BAPs) or wobble board	Levels 1–5, clockwise/counterclockwise
Standing heel raises	Single or double support
Single leg medicine ball toss	To a partner or inclined trampoline
Heel-to-toe inline walking (forward/retro)	May use handheld dumbbells for overload
Step ups/downs	Variable heights, forward, retro, or lateral
Squats	Partial, quarter, or half
Lateral sliding board	Variable lengths
Carioca/grapevine/braiding	Variable speeds
Lunges	Forward, lateral, or posterior rotational
Hops in place, quadrant drills	Single or double support
Sportcord, elastic tubing resisted walking	Forward, retro, lateral

Example conditions or diagnoses may include ankle sprain, post-arthroscopic knee surgery, musculotendinous lesions of the hip/thigh, etc., and may consist of 40–45 seconds for exercise duration with 15–20 seconds rest between stations.

TABLE 5.2   Example of activities for upper extremity therapeutic exercise circuit

Activity/exercise intervention	Comments
Upper body ergometer	5–10 minute warm-up, moderate intensity
Seated rowing	Machine, elastic tubing
Medicine ball around waist	Facilitate shoulder internal rotation, extension, adduction
Bodyblade™ oscillations	Multiple planes of motion
Wall approximation/push off with ball	Variable positions to facilitate co-contraction
Upper extremity combination movements with dumbbells	Alternate punches (protraction/retraction with trunk rotation)
Medicine ball chest passes	With partner or inclined trampoline
Medicine ball diagonal passes	With partner or inclined trampoline
Wall dribbling with a medicine ball	Multiple positions (overhead, eye level, etc.)
Floor or wall push up with a plus	Facilitate scapular protraction
Pull downs	Machine, elastic tubing

Example conditions or diagnoses may include rotator cuff tendinitis, post-arthroscopic knee surgery, lateral epicondylitis, etc. and may consist of 40–45 seconds for exercise duration with 15–20 seconds rest between stations.

quick succession, one after another, such as hamstring curls followed by seated knee extensions. *Compound sets* entail the sequential performance of two or more sets of different resistance exercises for the same muscle group. Elements of these different intervention systems, methods, or strategies have features and benefits that may enhance any therapeutic exercise program with variety and a means of systematic progression. However, evidence regarding the efficacy or superiority of any of these training approaches is sorely lacking, particularly in the health or fitness arena of resistance training.

Key Point:

Many different methods of grouping resistance training exercises are currently popular. The rehabilitation clinician is encouraged to make strategic use of these methods to add variety to their client's therapeutic exercise program. However, evidence regarding the efficacy of superiority of any of these training approaches is lacking.

EXERCISE, THERAPEUTIC EXERCISE, OR REHABILITATION?

In the previous section, and in the preceding chapters, a great deal has been presented on definitions and principles of exercise, training, and rehabilitation. A unique feature of this textbook is to provide information that serves as the foundation for clinical problem solving and critical thinking required of all rehabilitation clinicians who design therapeutic exercise interventions or programs. An unspoken or unchallenged assumption that prevails, at least conceptually, in the realm of rehabilitation science is that *therapeutic exercise* differs from *regular exercise*. It appears easy to argue that all exercise might be considered therapeutic, in the sense that it is beneficial physiologically, and psychologically. Exercise can be performed through many methods and just about anywhere and is recognized as an important part of healthy living. Increasing emphasis placed on health promotion and disease prevention has intentionally blurred some of the distinctions between regular exercise and therapeutic exercise.[1,2,33,34] Physical therapists, for example, have traditionally been viewed as professionals who are reactive to injury, disease, or pathology, although they are increasingly being seen as important proactive health care professionals involved in the prevention (primary, secondary, and tertiary) of movement related disorders.

Therapeutic exercise may differ in the sense that it is organized in a systematic fashion, with or without apparatus or equipment, used for restoring normal function to diseased or injured tissues, aimed to prevent muscular atrophy, restore joint/muscle function, increase strength, and improve cardiovascular and pulmonary system efficiency.[35] While differentiation of *regular exercise* and *therapeutic exercise* may exist only among the clientele served, for instance apparently healthy versus those with movement or mobility related dysfunctions, the essential principles and guidelines remain the same. Rehabilitation clinicians who provide and design therapeutic exercise interventions and programs for their clients must consider such parameters as the exercise type, mode, frequency, duration, repetitions, sets, and intensity, in the same way a strength and conditioning specialist does for a healthy athlete. Additionally, rehabilitation clinicians must possess an appreciation of how applied resistance training principles interface with biological healing constraints, pathological processes involving connective tissue, cardiopulmonary and cardiovascular system limitations, and neurological system injury. Sufficient knowledge of functional musculoskeletal anatomy and applied kinesiology should not be neglected, and its importance to therapeutic exercise and resistance training is accentuated in a statement by Fernel: "Anatomy is to physiology, as geography is to history; it describes the theatre of events."[36] Furthermore, according to Lieber, the rehabilitation clinicians' understanding of muscle structure, function, and capacity for adaptations with training (strength, power, endurance, hypertrophy) may be the most important consideration involved with therapeutic exercise program design and intervention.[37] It is this understanding of functional anatomy and applied kinesiology that should drive the clinical decision making process regarding the selection of specific exercise interventions, and not those ideas that are trendy or popular for the moment.

The remainder of this chapter discusses therapeutic exercise program design and addresses principles of creating appropriate functional therapeutic exercise environments, multi-planar resistance training considerations, the frequently referred to and sometimes misconstrued conventions of open and closed kinetic chain movements, the basis of trunk or core stability concepts as they relate to upper and lower extremity rehabilitation, and selected modes in which these concepts can be applied.

Key Point:

The differentiation between the terms exercise and therapeutic exercise are based on the clientele who are served. The essential resistance training principles and guidelines are the same.

GENERAL PRINCIPLES OF THERAPEUTIC EXERCISE INTERVENTION

Creating a Functional Therapeutic Exercise Environment

The term functional implies a meaningful manner in which clients perform tasks and roles required for ADLs or IADLs. The capacity for the client to adequately perform his or her chosen role in society should be at the center of therapeutic exercise program design. A large

part of this planning involves the selection of exercise movements that replicate the functional tasks that they value (for example, Virgil in Chapter 1 desires to be able to care for his cattle; therefore, he must be able to lift feedbags, shovel stalls, climb fences, etc.).

Arguably, few rehabilitation clinicians have had a greater influence than Gray[38] on the understanding of biomechanical strategies or approaches to therapeutic exercise program design from a standpoint of function through appreciation of multi-planar analysis, integration of segmental linkages, and consideration of synergistic muscle function. Many of Gray's simple, yet insightful teachings begin with specific guidelines referred to as the *"Rules of Rehabilitation"* (**Table 5.3**).[38] These principles or rules are similar to those proposed by Salter in his *Textbook of Disorders and Injuries of the Musculoskeletal System* (**Table 5.4**).[39] Both offer a useful framework for both novice and experienced rehabilitation clinicians on which to base their client management strategies, timetables, and therapeutic exercise intervention programs.

To create an environment or therapeutic exercise setting that is conducive for optimal healing the rehabilitation clinician needs to have a thorough knowledge of a client's history, and a solid background in functional anatomy or applied kinesiology. An appreciation of the wide variation of what might be considered normal or non-impaired promotes a wide spectrum of therapeutic exercise possibilities. Two omnipresent forces that must always be considered and are easily modified by rehabilitation clinicians are related to body weight and gravity. There are countless means of accomplishing modifications of these forces through creative positional changes and the use of simple basic equipment. Appreciating *fundamental planes of motion* (sagittal, frontal or coronal, and transverse or horizontal) (**Figure 5.5**) and those that are primary and secondary to particular tasks, activities, or sporting events provide the framework for selecting or creating appropriate therapeutic exercises.

By recognizing how adjacent body segments may compensate for impaired mobility or weakness at an injured body region, the rehabilitation clinician can select or create therapeutic exercises that more effectively facilitate desired joint movements from the injured body region. An

TABLE 5.3   Rules of Rehabilitation as suggested by Gray

1. Create an environment for optimal healing.
2. Above all else, do no harm.
3. Be as aggressive as you can without breaking rule number 2.

(Reprinted with permission from Chain Reaction Seminars, Adrian, MI: Wynn Marketing, 1989.)

TABLE 5.4   General principles of musculoskeletal treatment

1. First do no harm (*primum non nocere*).
2. Base treatments on an accurate diagnosis and prognosis.
3. Select treatment with specific aims.
4. Cooperate with the laws of nature.
5. Be realistic and practical in your treatment.
6. Select treatment for your client as an individual.

(Reprinted with permission from RB Salter, General principles and specific methods of musculoskeletal treatment, *pp. 91–93.* In *Textbook of Disorders and Injuries of the Musculoskeletal System*, 3rd ed. Baltimore:Williams & Wilkins, 1999.)

example of this application to the upper extremity can be illustrated in selected interventions designed to improve the range of motion, strength and functional use of the upper extremity through glenohumeral joint external rotation. If this motion is analyzed holistically through tasks such as throwing or reaching, and contributions from the torso are considered, it is observed that glenohumeral joint external rotation is frequently accompanied by the transverse plane dominated motions of ipsilateral scapular retraction and depression, ipsilateral spinal rotation, and

contralateral hip external rotation. If the client initially displays weak or painful glenohumeral joint external rotation, these synergistic motions can be exaggerated to facilitate the desired glenohumeral joint movement pattern. These mass movement patterns reflect a portion of the basic theory behind the hypothetical effectiveness of proprioceptive neuromuscular facilitation (PNF) techniques (as discussed in Chapter 6) and are consistent with Beevor's axiom that "the brain knows nothing of individual muscle action but knows only of movement."[40] This important axiom should provide some guidance to astute rehabilitation clinicians as they blend isolated and integrated therapeutic exercise movements during program planning.

An example in the lower extremity follows: Squatting activities are accompanied by physiologic valgus at the knee and subtalar pronation through the frontal plane and, if excessive and uncontrolled, may lead to injury of the medial stabilizing structures of the knee and ankle. It is not by accident that the medial collateral ligament of the knee and the deltoid ligament complex at the ankle are broader, stronger and more robust than their lateral counterparts. This is an excellent example of how structure and function are related. When these medial structures are compromised through injury, the rehabilitation clinician must find ways to protect the structure and minimize stress in the early phases of therapeutic exercise performance, which may mean limiting frontal (coronal) plane activities. However, in order to obtain a favorable tissue healing response, it will be necessary to gradually introduce increasing frontal plane stresses to these collagenous structures if they are to heal into organized, functionally competent structures. Judging exactly when and how much stress is needed can be challenging, and unfortunately there are no exact time tested protocols for individual clients and conditions. Decisions regarding resistance training loads and volume are largely based on known biological tissue healing constraints and the clinical demonstration of any signs of involved tissue pain and/or inflammation. Specific loading during functionally relevant therapeutic exercise movements, and not necessarily isolated loading (which is often the case on many types of isotonic and isokinetic devices) of all musculoskeletal structures, namely muscle, tendon, and bone, is required to obtain favorable outcomes.

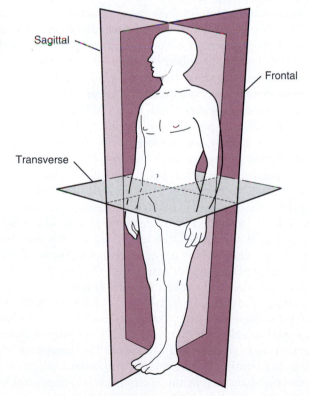

Figure 5.5   Cardinal motion planes.

Key Point:
Appreciating the fundamental planes of motion (sagittal, frontal or coronal, and transverse or horizontal) and those that are primary and secondary to particular movement tasks, activities or sporting events provide the framework for selecting appropriate therapeutic exercises.

The S.A.I.D. principle,[41] which was discussed earlier in this chapter, should be applied whenever possible. Therapeutic exercise programs that consider the functions that the client will need to perform make it easier to achieve training specificity. Expanding on this concept requires somewhat of a paradigm shift in how rehabilitation clinicians view muscle actions and muscle functions, which are often distinctly different. The quadriceps femoris is classified as a knee extensor in most textbooks, and while it is certainly capable of performing this *action* quite well, this is a *function* that it rarely performs. Understanding the gait cycle and muscle activation patterns during its many subdivisions helps to guide rehabilitation clinicians in developing specific interventions for the lower extremities (see Chapter 9). Isokinetic testing has been proven to be useful (see section on isokinetics) for providing a reliable, objective measurement of isolated muscle or muscle group torque producing capability. Additional performance variables of interest can be obtained through isokinetic testing, such as torque, time to peak torque, total work, torque/body weight ratios, agonist:antagonist ratios, and endurance. Evaluating parameters such as torque may be useful for bilateral comparison between limbs, but offers little information regarding integrated muscle group performance.

Using a circular measurement grid, the *Lower Extremity Functional Profile (LEFP)*[42] (**Figure 5.6**), provides an inter-esting approach to quantitatively (distance) and qualitatively (observation of technique) evaluating three-dimensional composite lower extremity function. The LEFP uses a testing grid that consists of eight vectors that are spaced 45° apart radiating from the circle center and serving as a two dimensional measure of three dimensional movement patterns, in which all of the lower extremity joints function in unison throughout all three movement planes under a continuum of concentric, eccentric, and isometric muscle activations. Measurements of multiple joint movements such as forward (**Figure 5.7a–b**), diagonal (**Figure 5.8a–b**), or lateral (**Figure 5.9a–b**) lunges may serve as a useful complement to more isolated single joint evaluation methods (such as manual muscle testing or standard isokinetic testing), potentially having a greater functional significance. Research is needed to better determine the association between composite measurements such as these and commonly performed ADLs and IADLs, including vocational or sporting activities.

Planes of Motion

Planes of motion and *degrees of freedom* (the motion available at a given joint, see Chapters 3, 6 and 8) are important biomechanical concepts used to describe total body as well as segmental movement and function. These parameters provide a means for understanding *osteokinematics* (bony lever movements) and *arthrokinematics* (joint surface movements). Without an understanding of these principles, it would be impossible to measure joint range of motion and mobility and interpret the influence of therapeutic exercise program intervention on these measurements.

The three traditional or cardinal planes of motion (sagittal, frontal or coronal, and transverse or horizontal) are commonly used for body position and movement references. However, these traditional planes and their axes of motion may be inadequate for accurately describing most athletic maneuvers and many ADLs and IADLs. Many activities, especially sport skills such as throwing, hitting and kicking, are performed in diagonal patterns lying outside of the cardinal motion planes, diagonal to the longitudinal axis of the body (the spine). The range of motion available at the hip and shoulder joints essentially describes these diagonal planes of motion. Logan and McKinney[43] described three diagonal planes, which they referred to as the *Logan-McKinney Diagonal Planes of Motion:* 1) high diagonal for upper extremities (**Figure 5.10**), 2) low diagonal for upper extremities (**Figure 5.11**), and 3) low diagonal for lower extremities (**Figure 5.12**). Appreciating the relationship between spinal (*axial*) and extremity (*appendicular*) movements and the synergistic aggregate muscle activity involved with purposeful movement patterns establishes a framework for therapeutic exercise intervention strategies. The importance of this will be discussed further in the section on axio-appendicular relationships.

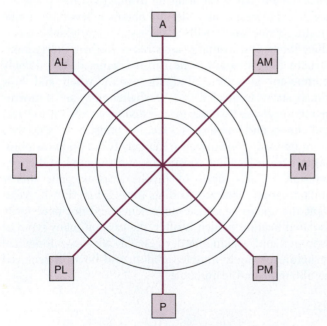

LEFP test vs grid (reference left)

Figure 5.6   Left foot grid vector starting positions using the Lower Extremity Functional Profile. A = anterior, AM = anteromedial, M = medial, PM = posteromedial, P = posterior, PL = posterolateral, L = lateral; AL = anterolateral. (Redrawn from Wynn Marketing, Adrian, MI, 1995.)

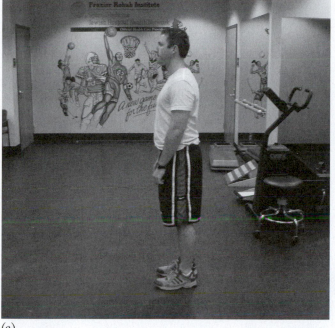
(a)

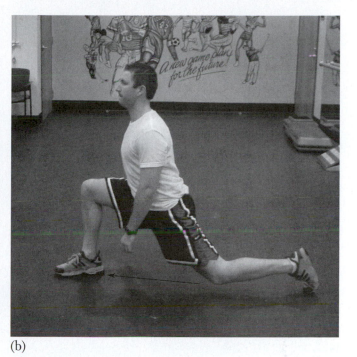
(b)

Figure 5.7   Forward lunge excursion test with the right lower extremity. (a) starting position; (b) completion.

Key Point:

The three traditional planes of motion (sagittal, frontal and transverse) are commonly used for body position and movement references. The three diagonal planes of motion (the high diagonal for the upper extremities, the low diagonal for the upper extremities, and the low diagonal for the lower extremities) are used to refer to activities performed through planes that are diagonal to the longitudinal axis of the body (the spine).

Posture and the "Ready Position"

A client's posture may be the single most influential factor in the design of an appropriate therapeutic exercise environment. Postural alignment and antagonist-agonist musculotendinous strength and length balance are foundational components to all therapeutic exercise programs.[23,44] Sahrmann[44] and Kendall et al.[45] have written extensively in the area of posture, muscle balance and ideal alignment. While ideal postural alignment may not be realistic for all to achieve, understanding a client's resting or baseline posture helps the rehabilitation clinician better appreciate the movement patterns clients assume during activities.

For a therapeutic exercise program to be successful, postural faults and deviations should be addressed and monitored during exercise performance. In addition to using a plumb line, mirror, or posture grid, a quick and easy screening technique for postural faults and deficits is the *vertical compression test* (VCT).[46] To perform the VCT, the rehabilitation clinician stands (on a stool or plinth) above and behind the client, who is assuming a relaxed stance position, and provides a controlled and gradual axial load through the shoulders. This additional force may illustrate abnormal stress points, which can be reported by the client or observed by the rehabilitation clinician as a mild buckling or giving way. Simple positional changes can easily be made, and the VCT reapplied, with both the client and rehabilitation clinician observing changes. Educating clients about postural biomechanics and how simple postural improvements can positively influence their stability and appearance can be empowering and motivating.

The *position of readiness* or *ready position*[43] is one of the most universal and important positions for many types of physical labor and virtually all sporting activities (**Figure 5.13**). Since the ready position is central to the balance and stability required for successful and rapid changes of vertical and lateral directions, it is a common starting point for therapeutic exercises performed in a standing position. It can be described as a partial squat with a forward leaning trunk and slight flexion of the ankles (dorsiflexion), knees, and hips. The primary muscles involved with maintenance and control of this critical position are the large extensors or anti-gravity muscles: the erector spinae, quadriceps, gluteus maximus, and triceps surae. These muscles collectively serve as the foundation for the

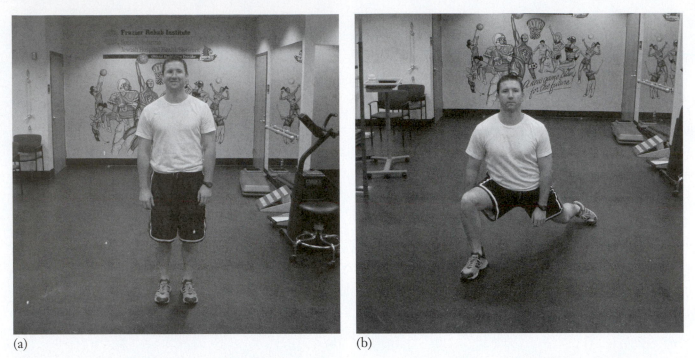

(a)   (b)

Figure 5.8   Diagonal lunge excursion test with the right lower extremity. (a) starting position; (b) completion.

superimposition of most skilled lower extremity movements.

A review of basic musculotendinous biomechanics and length–tension relationships reinforces the importance of this position, as muscles have the potential to develop their greatest tension when they are placed on slight stretch and the articulations are in midrange. The ready position supports the popularity and importance of the many variations of the squat movement as a key therapeutic exercise (see considerations of the squat).

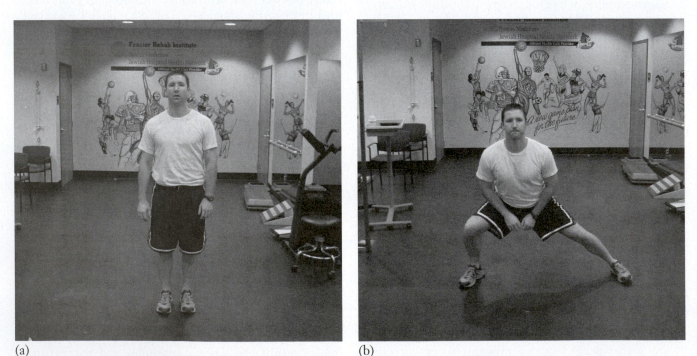

(a)   (b)

Figure 5.9   Lateral lunge excursion test with the right lower extremity. (a) starting position; (b) completion.

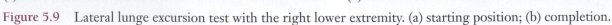

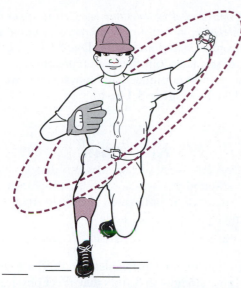

Figure 5.10   High diagonal plane motion used by a left handed pitcher.

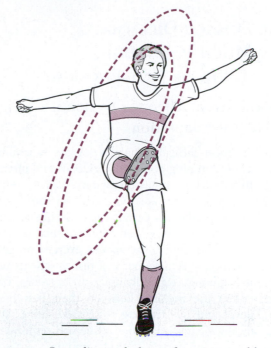

Figure 5.12   Low diagonal plane of motion used by a soccer player.

> ## Key Point:
> A client's posture may be the single most influential factor in the design of an appropriate therapeutic exercise environment. The "ready position", which is central to balance, stability and is required as a starting point for rapid changes in vertical and lateral directions, often serves as a common starting point for therapeutic exercises.

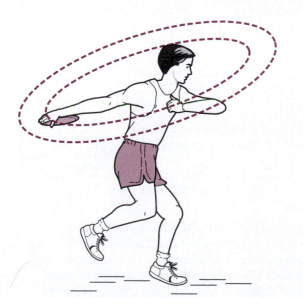

Figure 5.11   Low diagonal plane of motion used by a discus thrower.

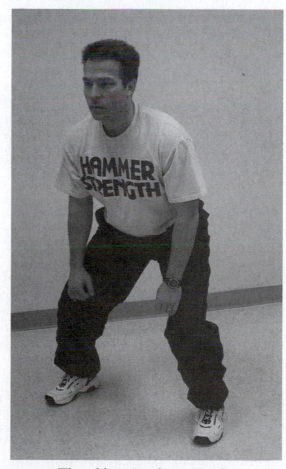

Figure 5.13   The athletic "ready position."

THE DOSAGE DILEMMA: HOW MUCH IS ENOUGH, TOO MUCH, OR NOT ENOUGH?

Physical Stress Theory, Overload, and Neural Adaptation

One of the most difficult struggles for the rehabilitation clinician is determining accurate workloads and intensities in order to obtain a favorable therapeutic exercise response and ultimately a favorable long term outcome for the client. Dosage guidelines pertaining to frequency, intensity, and duration were discussed earlier in this chapter and should assist with planning therapeutic exercise programs.

In an attempt to achieve optimal results, clients undergoing elite training (e.g., Olympic, professional, college athletes) often toe the line between their best possible training level and overtraining (discussed later). Wolff's Law promotes the idea that bone tissue will respond in accordance with the stresses placed upon it.[47] This same concept or theory is easily applied to other collagenous/connective tissue structures such as ligament, tendon, and muscle.[48] Are there benefits in providing isolated stress to target tissues in non-specific, non-functional movement patterns? Mueller and Maluf[49] have presented a *physical stress theory* (PST) suggesting that changes in physical stress levels cause one of five predictable adaptive responses in all (biological) tissues. These five tissue responses to physical stress are *decreased stress tolerance*, as seen in cases of atrophy; *maintenance; increased stress tolerance*, as noted in cases of hypertrophy; *injury;* and *death*. Dye[50] has described an envelope of safe knee joint function representing a range of joint loads that do not induce supraphysiologic overload or structural failure (**Figure 5.14a–b**).

Key Point:
The physical stress theory suggests that biological tissues respond to physical stress by either decreased stress tolerance, maintenance, increased stress tolerance, injury or tissue death.

Twelve fundamental principles for PST are discussed and presented along with factors that affect physical stress, such as movement and alignment factors, extrinsic factors, and psychosocial and physiological factors.[49] This is a challenging area, where the art and science of therapeutic exercise program planning coexist and clinical decision making skills by the rehabilitation clinician are improved only through education, research, and experience.

Many rehabilitation clinicians, especially those involved with cardiovascular and cardiopulmonary therapeutic exercise program development, are familiar with rating of perceived exertion scales used to assess exercise intensity.[51] The original 6–22 scale was devised by Borg to correlate with the average adult heart rate from approxi-

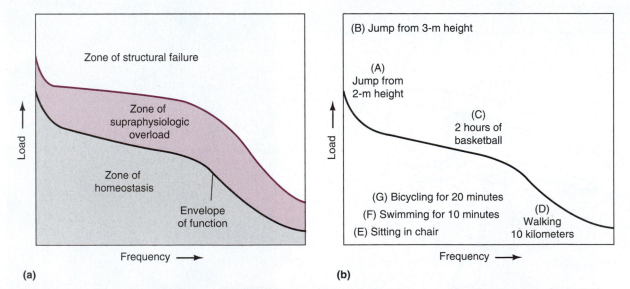

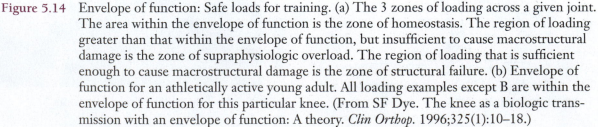

Figure 5.14   Envelope of function: Safe loads for training. (a) The 3 zones of loading across a given joint. The area within the envelope of function is the zone of homeostasis. The region of loading greater than that within the envelope of function, but insufficient to cause macrostructural damage is the zone of supraphysiologic overload. The region of loading that is sufficient enough to cause macrostructural damage is the zone of structural failure. (b) Envelope of function for an athletically active young adult. All loading examples except B are within the envelope of function for this particular knee. (From SF Dye. The knee as a biologic transmission with an envelope of function: A theory. *Clin Orthop.* 1996;325(1):10–18.)

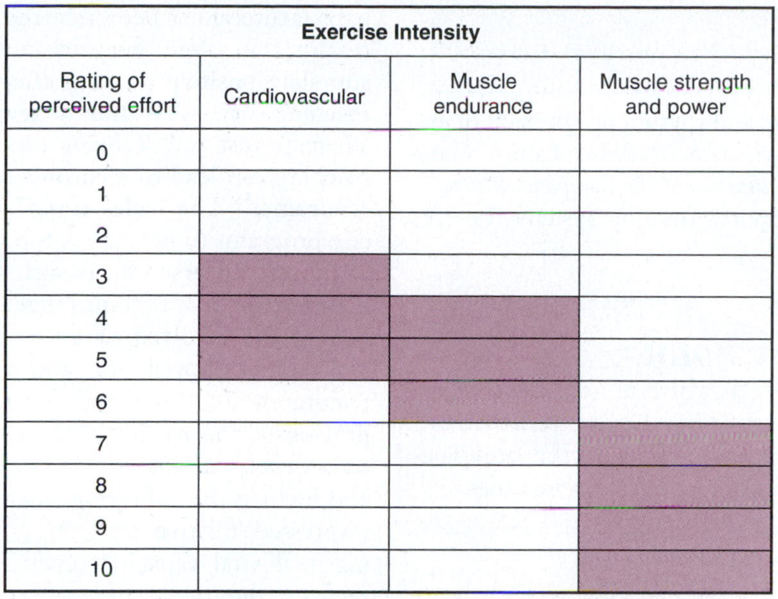

Exercise Intensity			
Rating of perceived effort	Cardiovascular	Muscle endurance	Muscle strength and power
0			
1			
2			
3	▓		
4	▓	▓	
5	▓	▓	
6		▓	
7			▓
8			▓
9			▓
10			▓

Figure 5.15   Rating of perceived effort. The shaded areas indicate the recommended zone to achieve the desired type of conditioning. Redrawn from MC Siff. *Supertraining*, 5th Ed., Denver, CO: Supertraining Institute, 2000.

mately 60 beats/minute at rest to a maximum of 220 beats/minute. The scale was modified, or simplified, to a 0–10 scale, with cardiovascular conditioning taking place in the 3 to 5 range. Siff proposed an adaptation of this scale for use with muscular strength and muscular endurance therapeutic exercise activities (**Figure 5.15**).[30] In Siff's scale, maximal effort is rated at 10, and no effort at 0. Muscle endurance can be developed with loads of 40–60 percent of 1 RM range, and strength and power with loads of 70–100 percent of 1 RM. Research validating this proposal with differing clientele is needed. The use of a rating of perceived exertion scale can help monitor how difficult a particular load feels during any given set during therapeutic exercise sessions, providing an individualized means of adjusting program intensity.

As mentioned earlier, strength and power training may cause early changes within the neurological system that produce better muscle activation coordination in the absence of actual structural adaptations in the muscle itself. Neural adaptations from therapeutic exercise program performance encourage positive short and long term changes in muscular strength and power.[52] The establishment of therapeutic exercise program volume and progressions will largely depend on the program goals. A general guideline regarding the progression of repetitions is found in **Table 5.5.** Another variable that is less frequently addressed in therapeutic exercise program planning is the *exercise rhythm* or *cadence*. The necessity of movement cadence variability is obvious in many ADLs and IADLs and sporting activities. Examples might include stopping, starting, a sudden unplanned movement to avoid stepping on a rambunctious

child or pet running through the kitchen, or in sports, a premeditated hesitation move to elude a defender. The rhythm or cadence of exercise can be as important as the more familiar frequency, intensity and duration variables and can range from very slow to explosive (**Figure 5.16**).[23]

It is important that safety, through controlled therapeutic exercise movements, be emphasized at all times. Verbal cues and feedback can be given instructing clients to move as fast as they can, provided they can control their movements. Speed of movement is an important factor in the development of power that can be achieved through plyometric training (discussed later). The history, physiology, and guidelines for developing power through more advanced training methods utilizing plyometrics is offered by Chu (see plyometric section).[53]

TABLE 5.5   General recommendations of functional goals and repetition number based on set/repetition maximum

Function/goal	Number of repetitions
Absolute strength	1–6
Muscle hypertrophy	6–12 (performed slowly)
"Explosive" strength	6–12 (performed rapidly, plyometrics)
Strength endurance (Commonly used for rehabilitation goals)	15–30

Very slow – Slow – Moderate – Fast – Variable – Explosive

Figure 5.16 Variable rate and rhythm progression of exercise performance. (Redrawn from V Gambetta. *Rehabilitation of the Complete Athlete,* Gambetta Sports Training Systems, 1992.)

> # Key Point:
> The rhythm or cadence at which an exercise is performed (slow to explosive) can be as important to achieving the desired training effects as the more familiar frequency, intensity, and duration variables.

Overload vs. Overtraining

Positive adaptations to therapeutic exercise program intervention do not occur unless the body experiences greater stress than that to which it is accustomed. Proper overload stimulus optimizes training adaptations, while overstressing leads to overtraining. *Overtraining* refers to training with excessive frequency, volume, or intensity leading to fatigue, burnout or staleness, illness, or injury. Overtraining may be associated with increased sympathetic nervous system activity at rest and/or increased parasympathetic nervous system activity at rest or with exercise.[54] Overtraining which occurs over a short term basis (acutely) has been referred to as *overreaching.* Overreaching is often factored into training programs to stimulate positive training effects. Recovery from overreaching occurs within a few days. However, when adequate rest and recovery time are not provided, overreaching can lead to a chronic or long term overtraining syndrome.[55] The "rules of too" apply to therapeutic exercise programs (don't do . . . too much, too soon, too fast), to prevent adverse effects such as increased joint inflammation/pain, loss of joint range of motion, injury or reinjury to the involved or to an adjacent body region, or maladaptive movement patterns that stop or delay the restoration of functional independence. As mentioned previously, the nature of the overload stimulus depends on a variety of factors, which can be altered or modified and include the following: therapeutic exercise intensity (expressed relative to VO_{2max}, maximal heart rate, or maximal vital capacity, repetitions, resistance, cadence, recovery duration), therapeutic exercise duration (length of training, frequency of exercise sessions and duration of recovery, days per week, active or passive recovery), type of therapeutic exercises selected, and initial (baseline) level of fitness. Larger magnitude improvements are expected for clients who begin their training at a lower relative level of specific fitness. Remember that therapeutic exercises provide the stimulus to adapt, and that adaptation occurs during the recovery periods, provided proper nutrition and hydration are also obtained. Guidelines for signs and symptoms of overtraining and overly aggressive therapeutic exercise program intervention are listed in **Table 5.6.**

TABLE 5.6 Signs and symptoms of overtraining or an overly aggressive therapeutic exercise program

Overtraining	Overly aggressive program
Increased resting heart rate	New onset, or persistent swelling/effusion
Loss of body weight	Poor tolerance to previous levels of activity
Suppressed or decreased appetite	Loss or setbacks in range of motion, strength, endurance
Muscle soreness/tenderness >24 hours	Muscle tenderness/joint soreness lasting more than 6–8 hours
Increased serum enzyme activity for creatine kinase and lactate dehydrogenase	
Increased submaximal heart rate	
Increased incidence and risk for colds, flu, infections	
Irregular bowel habits	
Decreased performance, coordination	
Lack of desire in training, practice, or competition	
Easily fatigued, sleep disturbances	

Key Point:

Positive adaptations to therapeutic exercise intervention do not occur unless the client experiences more stress than that to which they are accustomed. However, doing too much, too soon, and/or too fast can lead to adverse effects that stop or delay the restoration of functional independence.

Closed and Open Kinematic or Kinetic Chains

"The animal that moves makes its change of position by pressing against that which is beneath it."[56] The statement credited to Aristotle illustrates the recognition that the interaction between movement, structure, and the environment are inseparable.[57] The application of this important concept can be observed in any appropriately designed functionally relevant therapeutic exercise program. Concepts of closed and open *kinematic* (motion alone) and *kinetic* (motion and force considerations) chain concepts applied to therapeutic exercise performance have intrigued biomechanists, surgeons, rehabilitation clinicians, and researchers for decades. Much of this evolution and interest has paralleled developments with improved understanding of anterior cruciate ligament (ACL) reconstruction, biomechanics, and rehabilitation. Palmitier et al.[58] provides some important historical background of the kinetic chain concept to knee rehabilitation. Investigations by Grood et al.[59] and Henning et al.[60] were instrumental in increasing the awareness of the benefits of weight bearing exercise, and utilizing a closed kinetic chain environment to reduce anterior tibial translation and ACL strain. Another related milestone in this area came from Shelbourne and Nitz,[61] realizing that clients who resumed functional activities (e.g., removed brace, initiated early weight bearing and returned to work) earlier than specified in the post-operative protocol appeared to have as good or better outcomes without detrimental effects than clients who followed a more restrictive protocol, giving us the previously referred to accelerated ACL rehabilitation protocol, which has become widely accepted as the norm.

The origin of the kinetic chain terminology as applied to human movement has been credited to Steindler,[62] who observed muscle recruitment and joint motion differences between limbs during different loading conditions, suggesting that the differences were significant enough to differentially classify the two conditions as open or closed kinetic chains. An *open kinetic chain* (OKC) exists when the distal, or terminal, segment (e.g., hand or foot) can move freely, and a *closed kinetic chain* (CKC) exists whenever the terminal segment meets (considerable) resistance. These distinctions or classifications to human movement appear oversimplified when one considers the multitude and complexity of ADLs, IADLs, and sport movement variability, and may not be well understood, or agreed upon.[63–67] Comparisons and differences between CKC and OKC exercises generally deal with concepts of specificity, especially as related to gravitational effects, biomechanically consistent stress and strain characteristics, proprioceptive feedback, velocity, and stabilization.[38]

Snyder-Mackler,[48] citing the adequacy of training stimulus of selected CKC exercises on quadriceps function,[68–70] cautions rehabilitation clinicians to be aware of accepting all CKC activities as functional, and that judicious use of uni-axial OKC activities may be warranted as part of a complete and balanced therapeutic exercise program. Manual muscle testing procedures are based upon an understanding of the important interactions of musculotendinous attachment sites, fiber direction, muscles that work together in groups (*synergists*) or in relative isolation and other factors such as muscle length, joint angle, position relative to gravity, and leverage.[45] Testing of a muscle or muscle group in a relatively isolated manner remains an important responsibility of the rehabilitation clinician in ascertaining the weakest link as a muscle that performs poorly in isolation will likely perform poorly when subjected to gross, multi-segmental functional demands.

Key Point:

Identification of the weak link through the use of isolated manual muscle testing enables the rehabilitation clinician to select or design functionally relevant therapeutic exercises that require contributions from this region for the movement to be successful.

The concept of OKC and CKC movements alone clearly illustrates the important role of the rehabilitation clinician in understanding possible compensatory movement patterns and selecting or designing therapeutic exercise interventions that restore more natural function. Meanings and definitions change over time as understanding improves and new discoveries are made. While use of the terms OKC and CKC are currently quite common in everyday communication in the world of therapeutic exercise, confusion and inconsistencies exist.[48,71] To illustrate this point, the reader is challenged to categorize accurately the following activities as occurring in either a purely OKC or a purely CKC environment: leg press, cycling, Nordic, downhill, or water skiing, ice or roller skating, rollerblading, surfing, or sliding board activities. Applying the CKC requirement of the "distal segment being fixed," or "meeting some considerable resistance," to the aforementioned activities can produce some classification dilemmas.

An important characteristic of CKC therapeutic exercise related to the concept of training specificity involves what Steindler[62] described as the *concurrent shift*. This concurrent shift illustrates the action of bi-articular muscles acting across two joints simultaneously. For example, flexion at one joint and extension at the second joint by a bi-articular muscle results in a relative situation of constant length, or what has been called a *pseudoisometric* action.[58] In other words, many bi-articular muscles will undergo shortening (concentric) at one joint, and lengthening (eccentric) at an adjacent joint that allows them to exert a greater force throughout the action than if they were shortened at only one end.[43] The gastrocnemius, rectus femoris, semimembranosus, semitendinosus, sartorius, long head of the biceps femoris, and the long heads of the biceps brachii and triceps brachii are examples of biarticular muscles that maintain active sufficiency[72] through constant length changes and adjustments. For example, in running and jumping, the gastrocnemius is an important component that maintains its mechanical advantage by lengthening across the knee as it shortens across the ankle during plantar flexion (propulsion).[43]

The complex ability of a single muscle (or muscle group) to undergo dramatically different actions intrinsically may also be related to *muscle compartmentalization* or the *muscle partitioning hypothesis* (see Chapter 2). The muscle partitioning hypothesis states that individual muscles have complex arrangements of neuromuscular compartments or subunits that are innervated by a distinct muscle nerve branch with unique motor unit territories. These muscle partitions have been demonstrated to have task specific functions that could enhance our understanding of neuromuscular synergies as related to specificity of training.[73]

In controlling the musculoskeletal system, bi-articular muscles offer many advantages related to movement efficiency and velocity, and the redistribution of muscle torque, joint power, joint stability and mechanical energy throughout a limb. Many of the bi-articular muscles, along with their one joint synergists, are activated simultaneously with antagonists to provide joint stability through *coactivation* or *co-contraction*. Co-contraction occurs as a mechanism used for increasing joint stiffness and stability, and appears to be facilitated efficiently through weight bearing activities for the lower extremity, or joint approximation activities for the upper extremities (see Chapter 6). These principles are readily applied in a CKC environment, and rarely if ever to the same degree during OKC or isolated, single joint movement patterns. One of the best examples and most common practical interventions of a CKC exercise used in lower extremity therapeutic exercise programs is the squat and its many variations.

CONSIDERATIONS OF THE SQUAT AND ITS VARIATIONS AS CORNERSTONES OF LOWER EXTREMITY EXERCISE

The ready position, as was discussed earlier, is common to most competitive sports and is essentially nothing more than a partial squat. Additionally, transitioning through the ready position is also applicable to many important ADLs, such as getting up and down from a chair, crouching to pick up an object off the floor or a low shelf, or getting in and out of an automobile. Klein[74] reported that the full or deep squat might be inherently dangerous to knee joint stability, but numerous reports take issue with this finding. Various modifications of the squat exercise have gained recognition as important components of many lower extremity therapeutic exercise protocols. Chandler and Stone[75] provided an excellent literature review of the squat exercise and its effects and offer guidelines for proper performance (**Table 5.7**). One of the nine summary highlights of this position paper is that squats are not only safe (when performed correctly) but may be significant for knee injury prevention. There appears to be an increasing level of understanding and agreement that the squat, and variations or modifications of squat-type movements (limited range of motion, cadence, motion plane), when performed correctly, can contribute favorably to the development of lower extremity strength and stability without compromising safety.[75]

Patellofemoral problems are a commonly encountered lower extremity condition, and clients often report that these symptoms are aggravated by activities like squatting and stair climbing. The visibility and clinical vulnerability of the knee (e.g., easy to see, easy to palpate, and a "that's where the pain is so this must be the problem" attitude) make the patella the apparent culprit of the lower extremity movement dysfunction. In reality, the patellofemoral joint reacts to forces imparted on it by the hip from above through the femur and the ankle from below through the tibia, an idea best summarized by the statement that "knee joint function is somewhat at the mercy of ankle and hip joint function." Gray has emphasized this point by encouraging the rehabilitation clinician to consider both the "train" (patella) and the "track" that it follows (femoral groove).[38] A recent study by Powers et al.[76] using magnetic resonance imaging techniques has supported this claim. The multi-segmental linkages of the lower extremity and the multifactorial etiologies that coexist with patellofemoral syndrome(s) make it a challenging con-

TABLE 5.7   Guidelines and considerations for proper form and performance of the standard squat exercise

Use approximately a shoulder width foot stance.

Descend in a controlled manner.

Proper breathing is important to support the torso.

Avoid bouncing or twisting.

Maintain a normal lordotic posture, with torso as close to vertical as possible.

Generally, descend only until the tops of the thighs are parallel to the floor or slightly below. (This will need to be carefully monitored, modified and progressed systematically according to individual client needs, goals, conditions, and diagnosis.)

Feet should be kept flat on the floor.

Forward leaning can increase shear forces on the knee. Shins should be kept perpendicular with knees no more than just slightly in front of the toes. Knees should move directly over midline of feet, with second and third metatarsals as a guide.

(Reprinted with permission from TJ Chandler and MH Stone. The squat exercise in athletic conditioning: A review of the literature. *NSCA Journal* 1991;13(5):52–68.)

dition to manage. Successful therapeutic exercise interventions will blend progressive quadriceps femoris strengthening and modifications such as foot position (perhaps with orthotic use), altered hip and trunk alignment during squatting type movements, weight bearing modifications, and non-rigid bracing or taping interventions. Powers,[77] in his critical review of effective rehabilitation strategies for patellofemoral joint dysfunction, citing investigations by Steinkamp et al.[78] and Hungerford and Barry,[79] suggests that quadriceps strengthening exercises be performed for OKC (non-weight bearing) through a knee arc of 90–45°, and for CKC or weight bearing from approximately 45–0°. Fitzgerald[80] has provided an excellent review of knee joint forces during OKC and CKC exercises and Beynnon et al.[81] have described how many of these movements affect ACL strain. Escamilla et al.,[82] investigating technique variations (e.g., foot placement), recommended that clients use the foot position most comfortable for them and also recommended training in a functional range with a knee angle between 50° and 0° to minimize joint stress.[82]

THE SPINAL ENGINE

Gracovetsky[83] and others[84] have offered thought-provoking ideas related to the *theory of the spinal engine* concerning the important contributions made by the passive tension generated within the posterior ligamentous system, which includes the zygoapophyseal joints and joint

Key Point:

The squat and variations or modifications of the squat when performed with appropriate technique can contribute favorably to the development of lower extremity strength and stability without risk of injury.

capsules, interspinous, supraspinous, intertransverse ligament, and the thoracolumbar fascia. This tension is controlled through pelvic tilting by the powerful hip extensors, and the *hydraulic amplifier effect*. The hydraulic amplifier effect occurs through passive tightening of the thoracolumbar fascia as it surrounds and invests the paraspinal muscles, possibly enhancing low back muscle strength by up to 30 percent.[84] Although intra-abdominal pressure increases (e.g., the Valsalva maneuver) should be avoided by some clients (e.g., those with hypertension), with client education in proper breathing patterns, safe, intra-abdominal pressure increases needed to control axial spine rotation can occur.

Optimum body movement strategies seem to involve a combination of the hip, pelvic, and spinal musculotendinous and capsuloligamentous contributions previously mentioned. The spine is the primary engine that drives the pelvis and the shoulder girdle, and therapeutic exercise programs which focus on upper and lower extremity function should involve the trunk and lumbopelvic region early and often. The converse of this axio-appendicular relationship is also true in that therapeutic exercise programs that focus on the trunk and lumbopelvic regions should involve the upper extremities and lower extremities to adequately challenge core stability in a functionally relevant manner. However, advocates of core stabilization programs discuss the importance of isolated training of the genuine or deep back muscles, namely the interspinales, intertransversarii, rotatores, and the multifidi. These muscles have been referred to previously by Bergmark[85] as a *local muscular system*, with a *global muscular system* involving the more superficial trunk muscles used to produce greater torques and movements (see the serape effect section). (see Chapter 6)

Key Point:

According to Gracovetsky, the spine is the primary engine that drives the pelvis and the shoulder girdles, therefore therapeutic exercise programs which focus on upper and lower extremity function should also involve the trunk and lumbopelvic regions, early and often.

Axial–Appendicular Relationship and Anatomical Rationale for Core Stability

The term dynamic postural stabilization seems paradoxical, as "dynamic" implies movement and "stabilization" implies movement prevention.[43] The importance of spinal, or core (trunk and lumbopelvic region) stabilization has received considerable attention in the therapeutic exercise literature; however, dynamic postural stabilization via steady and prolonged isometric activation of specific muscles to help maintain posture may rarely, if ever, occur during most ADLs.

Therapeutic exercise creation for the core, as with any body region, warrants a review of anatomical structure prior to analyzing function. Of particular importance to core or spinal stabilization therapeutic exercise program development is having a sound understanding of the functional relationships between the upper extremity, lower extremity, trunk, and lumbopelvic regions. The spiral (diagonal) characteristic movements of proprioceptive neuromuscular facilitation (PNF) patterns (discussed in Chapter 6) and many athletic and vocational activities are integrally related to the spiral or rotatory orientation of musculoskeletal structures, including bones (torsions, versions), joints, ligaments, and muscle fiber direction. The torsional relationships of many of the long bones, especially of the femur, tibia, and humerus, exist for reasons of efficiency and mechanical advantage, while alterations secondary to trauma, injury, or congenital abnormalities can have significant detrimental effects on performance.

The role of trunk muscles for dynamic stability depends upon the instantaneous demands placed upon the spinal column. Generally, muscles that are antagonistic to a task are most effective for increasing dynamic stability. On average, the larger, more global muscles are better able to improve spinal stability than the smaller, intersegmental muscles. Kavic et al.[86] recommended the use of therapeutic exercises that train motor patterns that involve contributions from many of the potentially important lumbar stabilizers.[86] Cholewicki and McGill[87] suggested that no single muscle, local or global, possesses a dominant responsibility for lumbar spine stability and therefore concluded that training efforts should not focus on a single muscle. There is no single abdominal exercise that challenges all of the abdominal muscles. Therefore more than one exercise is needed if the therapeutic exercise program goal is to increase the force capability or endurance of these muscles (**Table 5.8**).[88] Compromised trunk muscle endurance appears to be involved in many spinal injuries that occur during the performance of submaximal effort tasks (such as bending over to pick up a pencil).

Ideally, therapeutic exercises that challenge muscles but impose minimal joint loads are desired unless they produce a considerably higher muscle loading rate than joint loading rate. McGill[89] stated that core exercises that best suit a particular client may depend on a number of variables, including their history of previous spinal injuries, the mechanism of their current injury, fitness level, training goals, and other factors specific to the client. McGill advises that a client who is beginning a post-spinal joint or

TABLE 5.8 Low back moment, muscle activity, and lumbar compressive load during several types of abdominal exercises[a]

	Moment (N-m)	Muscle activation		Compression (N)
		Rectus abdominis muscle (%MVC)	External oblique muscle (%MVC)	
Straight-leg sit-up	148	121	~ 70	3,506
Bent-knee sit-up	154	103	70	3,350
CSTF curl-up, feet anchored	92	87	45	2,009
CSTF curl-up, feet free	81	67	38	1,991
Quarter sit-up	114	78	42	2,392
Straight-leg raise	102	57	35	2,525
Bent-knee raise	82	35	24	1,767
Cross-knee curl-up	112	89	67	2,964
Hanging, straight leg	107	112	90	2,805
Hanging, bent knee	84	78	64	3,313
Isometric side support	72	48	50	2,585

[a] *Maximal voluntary contractions (MVCs) were isometric. Muscle activation values higher than 100 percent are often seen during other types of exercise. CSTF = Canadian Standardized Test of Fitness.*

(From CT Axler, SM McGill. Low back loads over a variety of abdominal exercises: Searching for the safest abdominal challenge. *Med Sci Sports Exerc.* 1997;29:804–811.)

soft tissue injury therapeutic exercise program should be advised to avoid loading the spine throughout the range of motion, whereas a trained athlete may indeed achieve higher performance levels by doing so.[89] With a bias toward safety the key is to minimize spinal loads while presenting the trunk muscles with sufficient loads to create a training stimulus. As a general rule, McGill proposed that the natural low back curve or slight lordosis (as observed during standing) or a slight modification of this posture (more neutral) which creates minimal discomfort should be maintained during therapeutic exercise performance.[89] Successful therapeutic exercise interventions for the trunk with emphasis on this neutral spinal alignment have promoted increasing the mobility of the hips and knees.[89]

Each client's clinical picture should influence the design of his or her therapeutic exercise program. McGill recommends that most therapeutic exercise programs for the low back begin with flexion–extension cycles performed in a quadriped position.[89] Then, hip and knee mobility exercises are recommended to facilitate spine-conserving postures. Finally, McGill recommends training specific muscles or muscle groups beginning with anterior abdominal exercises while maintaining a neutral spine posture, and progressing with lateral muscle exercises for the quadratus lumborum and abdominal wall muscles (**Figure 5.17**), and trunk extensor exercises.[89] Generally, for most tasks of daily living, very modest levels of abdominal wall co-contraction are sufficient.

A critical role of the trunk musculature is to stiffen the spine in all modes of instability (three rotational and three translational modes) at each intervertebral joint. Ideally, on an individualized basis, an optimal balance between stability, mobility, and moment generation occurs. The stiffness provided by noncontractile tissues is decreased with injury, and the stiffness provided by contractile tissues throughout the range of motion may be compromised by disturbed motor patterns following injury. The amount of muscle activation needed to ensure sufficient low back stability depends on the task. Again, depending on the task, co-contraction with the extensors (including quadratus lumborum and latissimus dorsi) and the abdominals (rectus abdominus, the obliques and transverse abdominus) will ensure stability. However if a joint has lost noncontractile stability due to injury, increased muscular co-contraction is needed to compensate for the deficiency.[90]

According to McGill[89] therapeutic exercise that "grooves motor patterns" to ensure a stable trunk (including the lumbopelvic region) through repetition constitutes a core stabilization exercise. Achieving sufficient trunk stability is a "moving target," which continually changes as a function of the three dimensional torques needed to support postures, provide the necessary stiffness needed in anticipation of enduring unexpected loads, or to prepare to move quickly. Motor control fitness is essential to achieving the stability target under all possible conditions for performance and injury avoidance (see Chapter 8). Virtually all trunk muscles work together to create the dynamic stiffness balance needed to ensure sufficient stability in all degrees of freedom (or to maintain the appropriate level of potential energy of the spine). With the evidence supporting the importance of muscle endurance (not strength) and "healthy" motor patterns to assure stability, further basic and applied research in this area is needed.

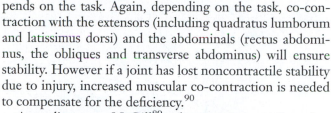

Key Point:
With a bias toward safety, the key to a successful therapeutic exercise program to manage a spinal joint or soft tissue injury is to minimize the spinal load while presenting the trunk muscles with a sufficient load to create a training stimulus.

The Serape Effect

A review of the musculoskeletal system from popular anatomical charts or textbooks reveals unique diagonal patterns of muscle fiber orientation from proximal and distal attachments that frequently extend across the midline of the body from right to left.[91] An example of this arrangement in the torso was described by Logan and McKinney as the *serape effect*.[43] "Serape" is a Spanish word for a colorful woolen blanket used as an outer garment. This garment is worn across the shoulders and is crossed diagonally over the anterior aspect of the trunk, terminating on the contralateral pelvis (**Figure 5.18**). The area covered by the serape closely follows the fiber direction of distinct muscle pairs, including the rhomboids, serratus anterior, external and internal obliques (**Figure 5.19**).[91] The aggregate actions of theses muscles[43] can essentially be thought of as "*synergists at a distance*"[92] and are extremely common in many gross or large scale motor activities, such as throwing and kicking.

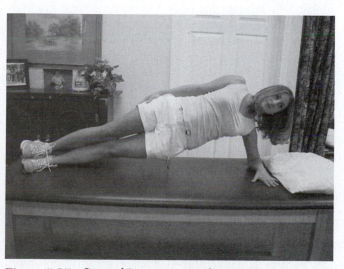

Figure 5.17   Lateral isometric trunk exercise.

Kinesiological Monitors

If one examines the relationship between structure and function, the morphology (small size, small cross sectional area) and considerable mechanical disadvantage of the genuine (deep) back muscles suggest these muscles are likely incapable of providing any appreciable force to the spine. These anatomical descriptions seem contradictory to the development of core stabilization from a strength or force standpoint. Of particular significance, and likely related to the empirical support of the efficacy of core stability exercise training, is that these muscles positioned in parallel combinations with larger and longer trunk muscles may serve more important roles as proprioceptive transducers, or kinesiological monitors.[93] It has been reported that all of the unisegmental muscles of the spine have two to six times the muscle spindle density of the longer paraspinal muscles.[93–95] Similar parallel muscle combinations can be found in the peripheral joints of the upper and lower extremities (triceps:anconeus, quadriceps femoris:articularis genu, gluteus maximus:piriformis, gastrocnemius:plantaris).[93]

Examples of Dynamic Core Stabilization Exercises

Core stabilization exercises can be performed in supine, prone, and sitting positions. These positions may be quite useful or even considered necessary as a starting point for acute conditions, but rehabilitation clinicians should ask, if indeed the deep back muscles do play such an important role in kinesiological monitoring of the spine, what carryover effect can be expected when forces are introduced to the spinal joints as normally occur when standing? It may be fallacious to think that core (trunk) and peripheral (extremity) stability can be achieved independently or in isolation of one another. It becomes obvious that there is still a great deal of clinical research needed in this important area of core stability. Saunders[96] provides some very basic guidelines that emphasize core strength and flexibility testing through simple, functionally relevant methods. He presents some clinically useful therapeutic exercises and evaluation methods that require minimal or no equipment with well defined procedures and scoring criteria (though perhaps arbitrary) that assess both trunk flexibility and strength: 1) shoulder girdle and upper back mobility and strength test (**Figure 5.20**), 2) abdominal muscle strength curl ups (**Figure 5.21**), 3) abdominal muscle strength-double leg lift (**Figure 5.22**), and 4) back strength-prone extension (**Figure 5.23**).

Soncrant[97] and Gambetta et al.[98,99] advocate the use of six core exercises using medicine ball that include the figure 8 (**Figure 5.24**), tight side-to-side rotations in standing position (**Figure 5.25**) (● **Section 1, Animation 2**), wide rotations in standing that combine a lunge with ipsilateral trunk rotations (**Figure 5.26**) (● **Section 1, Animation 3**), stepping and performing an overhead press to the ipsilateral side (**Figure 5.27**) (● **Section 1, Animation 4**), a single leg squat and touch

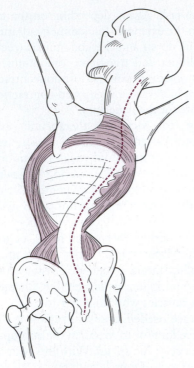

Figure 5.18   "Serape," posterior view.

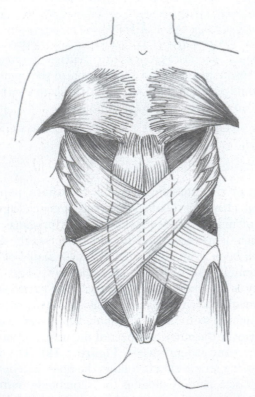

Figure 5.19   The muscular "serape." (Redrawn from GA Logan, WC McKinney. *Kinesiology*, 3rd ed. Wm. C. Brown Company Publishers, Dubuque, Iowa: 1972.)

Purpose

To test the mobility and strength of the shoulder flexors, the shoulder girdle muscles and the upper back.

Rationale

Workers who stand or sit in a forward bent position often adopt the forward bent, rounded shoulder posture. Loss of shoulder girdle and upper back mobility and strength often results. This contributes to a further deterioration of posture, which can make the worker more susceptible to upper back, neck and shoulder injuries.

Procedure

1. Client lies prone with the forehead supported on the floor. The arms are positioned overhead, with the elbows extended. The straight arms are held close to the head.

2. The client grasps stick, hands at shoulder width, elbows straight and raises arms straight up toward the ceiling as far as possible. The forehead should remain on the floor and the trunk should not move. Wrists remain neutral.

Scoring

1. Able to raise stick 9" from floor (flexibility) and hold 30 seconds (strength) = satisfactory.

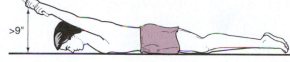

2. Able to raise stick 6" to 9" from floor (flexibility) and hold 30 seconds (strength) = marginal.

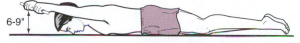

3. Unable to raise stick 6" from floor (flexibility) and hold 30 seconds (strength) = unsatisfactory.

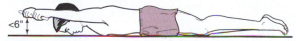

Note: Inability to perform this test can be due to either weakness or stiffness. Therefore, if the client cannot raise the stick, the examiner should assist by helping lift the stick. If the client is able to raise the stick with the examiner's assistance, any deficiency is due to muscle weakness, not inflexibility. Score the test for both strength and flexibility.

Figure 5.20   Shoulder girdle and upper back mobility and strength test. (Redrawn from HD Saunders. *Assessing Flexibility and Strength in Industrial Workers*, 2nd ed. Chaska, MN: The Saunders Group, 1991.)

with forward trunk lean (**Figure 5.28**) (● **Section 1, Animation 5**), and a total body exercise performed as the client moves forward using a quadruped gait pattern (the "Spider-man crawl") (**Figure 5.29**) (● **Section 1, Animation 6**).

Total Gym™

The Total Gym™, as its name implies, is an exercise device that has applications for the entire body, including the upper extremities, lower extremities, and the core.

The Total Gym™ also utilizes body weight resistance through the modification of the effect of gravitational forces on the body by adjustments between 10 different incline angles (10–30°), enabling the client to exercise between approximately 7 percent to 70 percent of body weight. Upper extremity interventions such as chin-ups and pull-ups can be performed easily with the pulleys and other attachments. Several core exercises can be performed with the Total Gym™ and the Backstrong Spinal Rehabilitation Machine™ (BackStrong International, Brea, CA). A few examples of the variability of therapeutic exercises for the core using the Total Gym™ include abdominal crunches, latissimus pulls (**Figure 5.30**), and progressive resistance trunk rotations (**Figure 5.31**) (● **Section 1, Animation 7**).

One important therapeutic exercise consideration frequently encountered during the acute and sub-acute stages following injury or surgical procedure is the need for protected, controlled or limited weight bearing and range of motion. While the Total Gym™ device has countless applications for specific therapeutic exercise interventions (examples include a standard double lower extremity squat, single lower extremity squats through a partial range of knee joint motion, heel raises, prone heel raises with flexed knees (soleus emphasis), diagonal squats, and lunges), it can also be used for evaluation particularly in comparing involved lower extremity to non-involved lower extremity function.

The concept of *bilateral equivalence*[100] is the customary standard used for comparing an injured or involved limb to an uninjured or uninvolved limb. While this construct may have some limitations, for example, in clients who are involved in unilateral dominant activities such as the high jump, where true limb symmetry may not exist, or clients who have bilateral deficits and therefore have no "normal" comparison limb, it is quite traditional and has some clinical practicality. Lower extremity power and endurance tests have been developed and can easily be performed on the Total Gym™ by clients with many different conditions in order to provide a means of comparison between the involved and the uninvolved limb. The lower extremity power test evaluates how many single leg squats can be performed in a pre-determined time (e.g., 20 seconds), while the endurance test evaluates the time it takes for a client to complete a specific number of single leg squats (e.g., 50). Clinical research is needed however to validate the functional significance of these measurements.

Several different testing parameters and variables can be controlled and documented including the range of motion (e.g., 0–90° of knee flexion), start and finish knee joint positions, and the slide board angle used during testing (lowest resistance with horizontal setting, maximal resistance at steepest slide board angle). As a client progresses, intensity can be increased accordingly by advancing to more vertical slide board angles and/or with additional resistance added to the slide board.

Purpose

To test the strength of the upper abdominal muscles.

Rationale

One of the functions of the abdominal muscles is to aid in the support of the lower back. If the abdominal muscles are firm, the strain on the low back muscles and the discs will be decreased and injury will be less likely to occur.

Procedure

1. Client lies supine with knees and hips bent and lest flat on floor.
2. Client reaches toward knees with arms extended, flexing the neck and trunk. The scapulae raise off the floor, and the trunk is flexed until the lower lumbar spine is off the floor. No lumbar fordosis is allowed except in the case where inability to flex the lumbar spine is due to stiffness.
3. Client repeats above test with a slight twist to the right, touching left fingertips to the outside of the left knee.
4. Client holds each position as long as he can, for a maximum of ten seconds.

Scoring

1. Client can hold each of the three positions ten seconds = satisfactory.

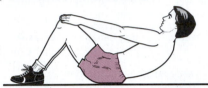

2. Client can assume positions but cannot hold for ten seconds = marginal.

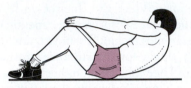 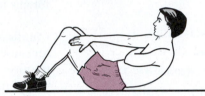

3. Client cannot assume position correctly = unsatisfactory. All drawings shown at right and below are examples of incorrect positioning.

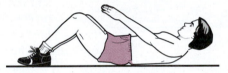

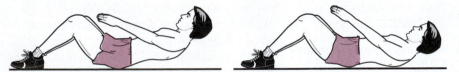

Figure 5.21   Abdominal muscle strength curl-up test. (Redrawn from HD Saunders. *Assessing Flexibility and Strength in Industrial Workers,* 2nd ed. Chaska, MN: The Saunders Group, 1991.)

Key Point:

Bilateral equivalence is the customary standard used for comparing an injured or involved extremity to an uninjured or uninvolved extremity.

PLYOMETRICS: TRAINING FOR POWER

Plyometric training has become a popular and efficient method of developing "explosive" reactive power and has important applications in many therapeutic exercise programs. Fred Wilt, a former Olympic runner and university track and field coach, has been given credit for coining the term plyometrics, which actually means "measurable increases."[53,101] Plyometric training involves exercises that enable a muscle (or muscle group) to reach maximum strength in the shortest time possible, or, stated in another way, uses quick counter-movements to produce a rapid muscle stretch (eccentric activation) followed by a rapid muscle contraction (concentric activation) (known as the *stretch-shortening cycle*) for the purpose of performing specific movements or activities.

The basic concept behind plyometrics is to exploit the muscular lengthening and shortening cycle to increase power via the series of elastic components, which include the musculotendinous units and actin/myosin cross bridges, and the stretch or myotatic reflex (see Chapter 2). The goal of plyometric training is to train the neuromus-

Purpose

To test the strength of the lower abdominal muscles.

Rationale

One of the functions of the abdominal muscles is to aid in the support of the lower back. If the abdominal muscles are firm, the strain on the low back muscles and the discs will be decreased and injury will be less likely to occur.

Procedure

1. Client lies supine with legs held straight up, knees straight.

2. Client flattens lower back against the floor by contracting abdominal muscles and squeezing buttock muscles together.

3. Client bilaterally lowers the legs to within 6" of the floor, keeping the back flat on the floor.

4. Client holds the above position as long as they can, for a maximum of 10 seconds.

Scoring

1. Client can assume and hold position with feet 6" from the floor for 10 seconds = satisfactory

2. Client can assume and hold position with knees bent to 90° and feet 6" from the floor for 10 seconds = marginal

3. Client is unable to hold any correct position = unsatisfactory. All drawings below show examples of failure. Note that the lower back must stay flat on the floor to pass.

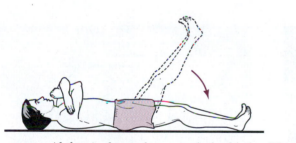

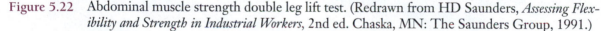

Figure 5.22   Abdominal muscle strength double leg lift test. (Redrawn from HD Saunders, *Assessing Flexibility and Strength in Industrial Workers,* 2nd ed. Chaska, MN: The Saunders Group, 1991.)

culoskeletal system to react quickly to the stretch-shortening cycle by reducing the neuromuscular reaction time to reach maximum tension. Training can also increase the Golgi tendon organ threshold, and increase tolerance to stretch loads. This injury prevention benefit has recently become recognized and applied in jump-training programs designed to reduce ACL injuries.[102,103]

> ## *Key Point:*
> The stretch-shortening cycle involves an eccentric muscle action followed as quickly as possible by a powerful concentric muscle action to maximize the use of stored elastic energy.

To understand the physiological principles behind plyometric training it is important to recall the basic types of muscle actions and their unique characteristics. Isometric muscle action is best thought of as a stabilizing action occurring when there is no visible overall muscle length change, and when the internal muscle force matches the external force or load. Concentric muscle action can be referred to as an accelerating action and involves muscle shortening, or positive work. Eccentric action refers to a decelerating action and involves muscle lengthening, or negative work. Eccentric, or negative training has been advocated for the treatment of tendonitis or tendonosis[32] and is an important aspect of plyometrics training. However, clients undergoing specific eccentric loading exercises must be monitored and educated about the potential

Purpose

To test the overall strength of the back muscles.

Rationale

Studies show that individuals with strong back muscles have fewer back injuries.

Procedure

1. Client lies prone on floor with arms overhead.
2. Client lifts chest, arms and legs off floor.
3. Client holds the above position as long as they can, for a maximum of 60 seconds.

Scoring

1. Client can hold position for 60 seconds = satisfactory.
2. Client can assume position, and hold for 30-60 seconds = marginal.
3. Client cannot hold for 30 seconds = unsatisfactory.

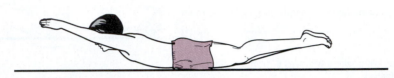

Note: Extreme stiffness of back and hip extension may make this test difficult or impossible for a few clients. The examiner should consider the client's back extension flexibility and use an alternate back strength test when necessary.

Figure 5.23   Back strength test. (Redrawn from HD Saunders. *Assessing Flexibility and Strength in Industrial Workers,* 2nd ed. Chaska, MN: The Saunders Group, 1991.)

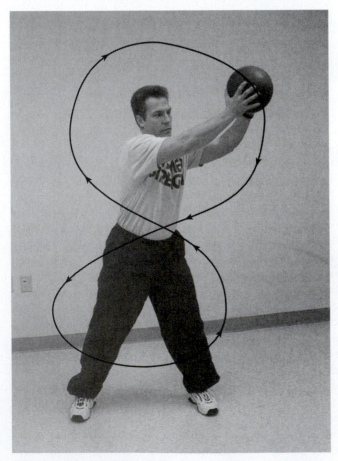
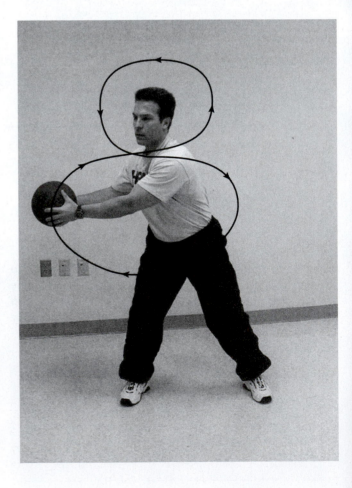

Figure 5.24   Medicine ball exercise: Figure "8" patterns.

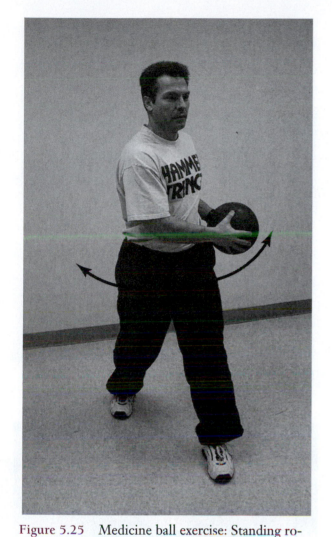

Figure 5.25 Medicine ball exercise: Standing rotations (tight or short arms).

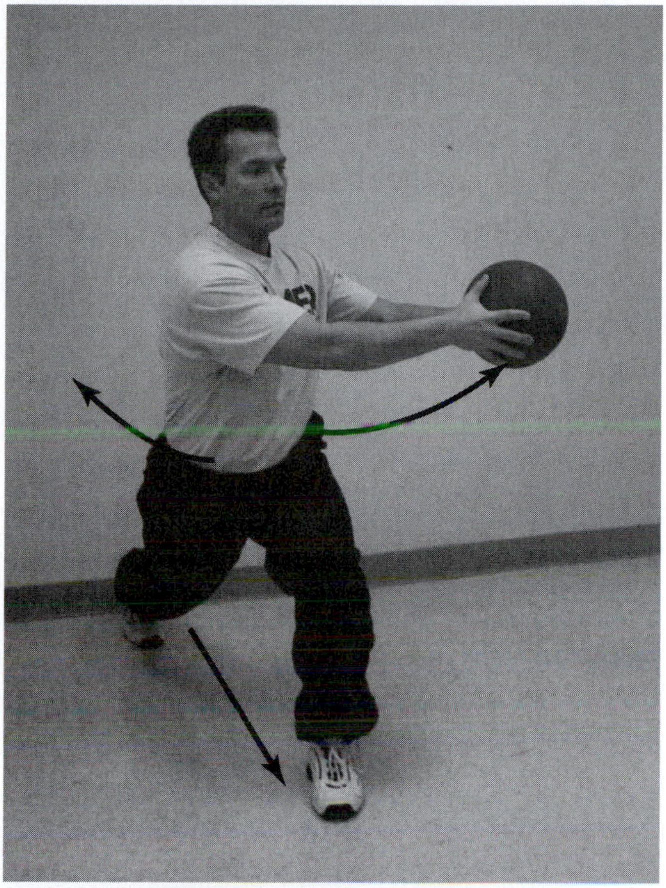

Figure 5.26 Medicine ball exercise: Standing rotations (long arms) with lunge.

of developing delayed onset muscle soreness (DOMS) or post-exercise muscle soreness (PEMS).

> ## Key Point:
> Isometric muscle action serves a joint stabilization function. Concentric muscle action involves muscle shortening or positive work. Eccentric muscle action involves controlled muscle lengthening, producing negative work. Plyometrics train the efficient transfer of energy stored during eccentric muscle activation to powerful concentric muscle activation.

In considering the absolute strength of the different types of muscle activations, the *Elftman principle*[104] describes a hierarchy of muscle force production where eccentric force is greater than isometric force, which in turn is greater than concentric force. It has been estimated that the same muscle or muscle group can typically produce 1.8 times greater force eccentrically than concentrically.[105] Recalling the biomechanical and physiological principles of length-tension (**Figure 5.32**) and force-velocity (**Figure 5.33**) relationships helps in understanding that the speed of muscle activation and muscle length changes are important factors in determining the force of muscle action. A key concept in understanding the development of power relies on the development of either increasing the amount of work performed or, decreasing the amount of time it takes to perform a movement (power = work/time).[106] By decreasing the time it takes to perform a movement, power or "explosiveness," can be improved.

> ## Key Point:
> While strength represents the work performed, power is the work performed within a certain time interval. Therefore power has a greater direct application to most athletic endeavors.

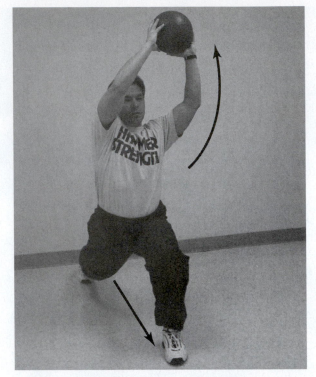

Figure 5.27   Medicine ball exercise: Lunge with ipsilateral overhead reach/press.

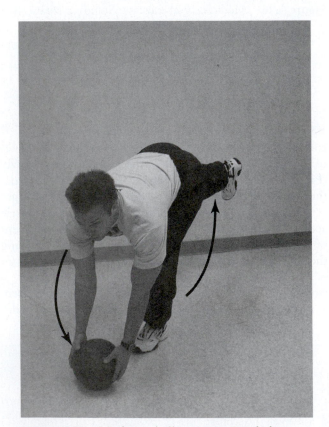

Figure 5.28   Medicine ball exercise: Single leg squat and touch with forward trunk lean.

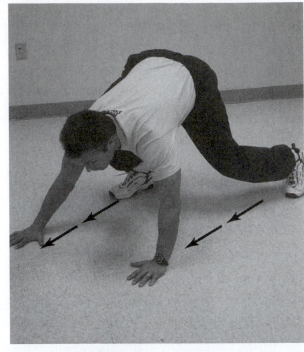

Figure 5.29   "Spiderman crawl."

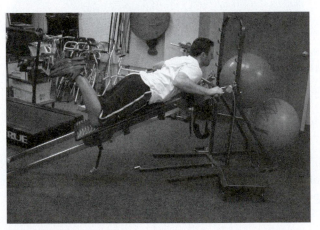

Figure 5.30   Latissimus dorsi pull-ups on the Total Gym.™

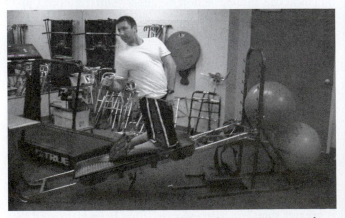

Figure 5.31   Trunk rotation in kneeling position on the Total Gym.™

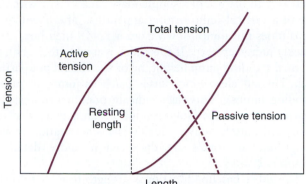

Figure 5.32   The active and passive tension exerted by a whole muscle during a maximal isometric activation is plotted against the muscle's length. Active tension is produced by the contractile muscle components and passive tension by the series and parallel elastic components, which develop stress when the muscle is stretched beyond its resting length. As stretching increases, the larger is the contribution of the elastic components to the total tension. Adapted from M Nordin, Frankel VH. *Basic Biomechanics of the Musculoskeletal System*, 2nd Ed. Lea & Febiger, Philadelphia, 1989 (from Chapter 5, Figure 5-9).

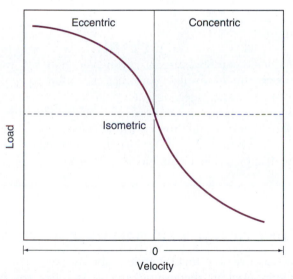

Figure 5.33   Load-velocity curve. With minimal external loads a muscle contracts concentrically with maximal speed. When the external load and the muscle force are equal, the muscle fails to shorten (zero velocity) and is activated isometrically. When the load is increased further, the muscle lengthens eccentrically. This lengthening becomes more rapid with even greater loads. Adapted from M Nordin, Frankel VH. *Basic Biomechanics of the Musculoskeletal System*, 2nd Ed. Lea & Febiger, Philadelphia, 1989 (from Chapter 5, Figure 5-10).

The time it takes to shift from eccentric to concentric action is known as the *amortization phase*.[53] A brief support time is necessary to prevent energy loss through muscle heat dissipation. The coupling of the eccentric–concentric action (stretch– shortening), has been referred to as "*eccentric*"[107] and may more precisely describe the true phenomenon that occurs with many muscle powered movements. The downward movement preceding a vertical jump, the wind-up before a pitch, and the back swing of a golfer's swing are all examples of this countermovement concept.

Plyometrics are often used during the final stages of therapeutic exercise programs, such as functional testing to determine readiness for return to sports (see Chapter 11). Training program variables including intensity, volume, frequency, and recovery just as with other forms of training, should be considered and modified according to individual client needs. Intensity of plyometric drills for the lower extremities range from jumps in place (low intensity) to depth jumps (high intensity), with intermediate jumps including standing jumps, multiple hops and jumps, bounding and box drills.[53] Volume is generally measured by the number of foot contacts, and frequency refers to the number of training sessions per week. Recovery time between sessions has been recommended to be 48–72 hours, with a 1:5 to 1:10 work-to-rest ratio and a progression of no more than 10 percent per week in any of the variables.[53]

Some basic equipment commonly used for lower extremity plyometric training includes boxes, cones (**Figure 5.34**), hurdles, stairs, elastic resistance cords, mini-trampolines. Variable resistance medicine balls are commonly used for both lower and upper extremity training. Plyometric training is generally reserved for higher level athletic clients during the terminal stages of the therapeutic exercise program and should never be used with clients with recent post-operative conditions, in the presence of pain or other inflammatory conditions, or with clients who have gross joint instability and/or weakness. Some important clinical guidelines have been suggested in determining whether a client is appropriate for plyometrics training.[53,101] These include the presence of good relative flexibility of the spine, shoulders, and hips and good baseline eccentric strength of the primary muscle groups involved in the training. Other considerations include the need for supportive footwear (and/or supplemental orthotic use) and cushioned training surface(s), the use of the upper extremities (arm swings, etc.) for normal postural mechanisms, and proper landing techniques which include a respective order of toe-midfoot-heel contacts.

Screening for Plyometric Training Readiness

Radcliffe and Farentinos[101] recommended that some baseline criteria or requirements[53] be exhibited by clients prior to participation in a plyometrics program. Prior to allowing clients to participate in plyometric training, the

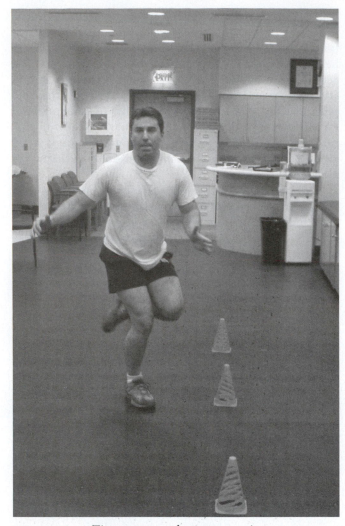

Figure 5.34   Zigzag pattern hop progression.

rehabilitation clinician should evaluate their general readiness by having them perform some progressive-intensity, sports-specific agility maneuvers. Then their squat technique should be evaluated, with particular attention paid to lower extremity posture and joint excursion of the lumbar spine, hips, knees, and ankles.[101]

Limitations in joint range of motion or isolated muscle strength deficits should be addressed through stretching (see Chapter 3) and/or joint mobilization and focused strength training, respectively, prior to any plyometric training. Inadequate range of motion can lead to excessive joint stresses and poor utilization of eccentric muscle actions and the series-parallel elastic components that are crucial to dampening forces and returning energy to the system.

A description of the standing jump and reach test follows: The client's standing overhead reach distance is noted and recorded. The client then performs a standing jump and reach movement, with a countermovement, but without stepping. The maximal standing jump height is then recorded. This can be measured a number of ways

such as with the use of a simple mark on a wall or with the use of a vertical jump testing apparatus. The client then steps (does not jump) down from a 12–18 inch box, then quickly jumps upward. If the client is unable to reach the original standing jump height, he or she should not participate beyond elementary levels (such as jumps in place, standing jumps). This may indicate poor neuromuscular control and perhaps Golgi tendon organ activity that inhibits the muscle activity during the amortization phase. Golgi tendon organs are discussed in more detail in Chapters 2 and 7.

Two other baseline functional strength tests that can be used as evaluative criteria to assist in determining the readiness for plyometric training are parallel squat performance with 75 percent of body weight and the five-repetition/five-second parallel squat at 60 percent body weight.[53]

Upper extremity plyometric testing can be administered through a medicine ball chest pass or medicine ball put, either from a seated position[101] or a standing position.[108] (see also Chapter 8). The seated test is performed with a medicine ball of 9, 12, or 15 pounds and the distance from the chair to the landing point of the ball is measured. Passes under 10–12 feet may indicate the need for training/testing with a lighter medicine ball. The standing test is administered in a similar fashion. These criteria may assist the rehabilitation clinician in determining whether a client has the foundational strength and neuromuscular control required for such training.

> ### *Key Point:*
> Prior to participating in plyometric training, the client should display non-impaired strength with manual muscle testing and pain-free component lower extremity joint range of motion. The client should also be able to perform pain-free squats and moderate intensity sports specific agility maneuvers with appropriate technique.

FUNCTIONAL PERFORMANCE TESTING

The majority of testing for athletic ability, sports skills, and function used in therapeutic exercise settings has been modified or developed largely from the physical education literature.[109] Every rehabilitation clinician involved in therapeutic exercise program planning understands the importance of functional testing as the final component to help determine the safe and timely return to work, recreational activity or athletic competition (see Chapter 11). A battery of clinical outcome measures, subjective reports by the client, and both qualitative (how appropriate the technique) and quantitative (how far, how fast, etc.) data are needed to develop a comprehensive profile and assure that all therapeutic exercise program goals have been achieved. Although physical characteristics like range of motion, girth, isokinetic strength, and tests of capsuloligamentous joint stability provide important objective information about the post-injury and post-operative condition, they do not relate strongly to function.[100,110] Testing that simulates actual performance demands is critical in the assessment of readiness for return to intense functional activities.

Bandy et al.[111] defined functional testing as the performance of one manual effort or a series of activities, in an attempt to quantify function. Many commonly used functional tests have been described and developed for use in assessing upper and lower extremity performance and have been reported to possess good reliability in both non-impaired and impaired client populations when specific testing criteria are followed.[110-113] Some examples of commonly used functional tests for the lower extremity include single leg hops for distance (**Figure 5.35a–c**), the single leg vertical jump test (**Figure 5.36a–b**), the cocontraction test, the carioca test, and the shuttle run test.[114-119] While the majority of these hop or jump tests are typically used in assessing knee functional stability and performance after ACL injury and/or reconstruction, it appears that these same tests could easily be used with other lower extremity conditions (see Chapter 11). The contention exists, however, that jump and hop tests may not be sensitive enough maneuvers to adequately test strength, power, and stability.[120] Previous investigations analyzing ground reaction force, joint moment, and kinematic data have reported that segmental contributions of the ankle, knee, hip, and upper extremities are quite variable between subjects.[121-123] These variable contributions from the ankle (22 percent to 23 percent), knee (4 percent to 56 percent), and hip (10 percent to 46 percent) should caution the rehabilitation clinician to not make

judgments on the results of a single functional test and instead reinforce the need for a battery of clinical, functional and subjective (client reported) outcome measures.

Timm[100] presented an interesting model for functional performance measurement and identified some shortcomings with traditional approaches. His suggested functional drill performance time models[100] incorporating task specificity for sports such as hockey, basketball, and football, potentially address some of the validity and predictability problems that exist with the traditional methods of authority, instrumentation, normative data from performance drills, and bilateral equivalence (**Figure 5.37a–c**). For instance, rehabilitation clinicians commonly compare performance of the involved (e.g., injured) extremity with performance by the non-involved extremity to define a percentage of functional normalcy (bilateral equivalence). While bilateral equivalence has tremendous clinical practicality to the return of a client to ADLs and IADLs, rehabilitation clinicians must consider that many vocational, recreational, and higher level sporting activities involve the presence of unilateral limb dominance and a normal condition of limb *asymmetry*. Common examples are throwing sports like pitching, racquet sports, or jumping

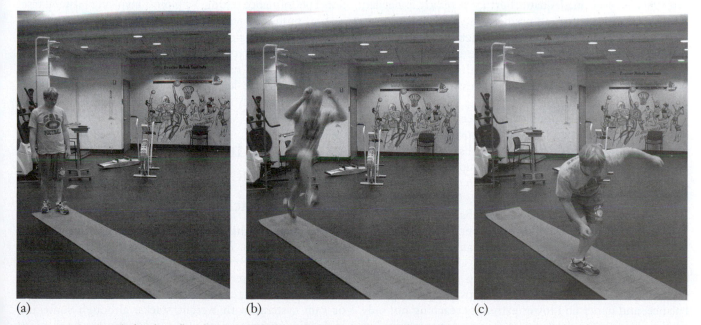

(a) (b) (c)

Figure 5.35 Single leg hop for distance. (a) start; (b), hop; (c) hold the landing.

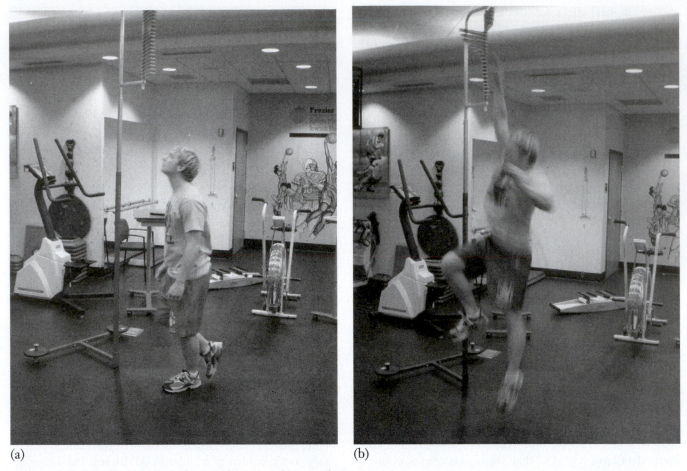

(a)   (b)

Figure 5.36   Single leg vertical jump. (a) start; (b) completion.

activities encountered in track and field. Therefore, simply restoring the strength or functional capacity of a dominant extremity to 100 percent of the uninvolved, non-dominant extremity may be inadequate. Further research is needed to improve the validity and predictability of the previously mentioned traditional methods of functional testing, and the functional drill performance time model provides a means of accomplishing this, perhaps through routine administration during meaningful pre-season or pre-placement physical examinations.

As previously mentioned, the Lower Extremity Functional Profile developed by Gray[124] provides a specific set of rules and guidelines involving a grid system with reference vectors used for evaluating temporal (timed) and spatial (distance) abilities through multiple planes of movement using hops, jumps, steps, lunges, upper or lower extremity reach distances and balance maneuvers. The principles established in the Lower Extremity Functional Profile are simple and safe and can be used to evaluate functional progression from the acute to the final phases of rehabilitation. Functionally specific activities such as multi-directional single leg hops, jumps, stepping, balance, and upper and lower extremity reaching not only have meaningful applications as therapeutic exercises, but

also show promise as reliable and valid lower extremity functional performance tests.

Less information exists regarding upper extremity functional performance testing, with most involving bilateral tests such as push-ups, pull-ups, and the medicine ball put test. Unilateral throwing or functional skill tests can easily be developed with accuracy or distance as the measured variables. Some examples of functional performance tests such as the vertical and single leg hop tests and the Edgren sidestep test[125] to name only a few, can be found in **Table 5.9**.[126]

COMMON METHODS OF RESISTANCE TRAINING

Resistance Machines

There are many different models and types of resistance training machines. Most of these devices have been designed for commercial use and placed in fitness clubs and rehabilitation centers, although home models continue to be popular. Most resistance training machines use pulley or cam systems with weight stacks, although some use hydraulic, pneumatic, or electromagnetic mechanisms to

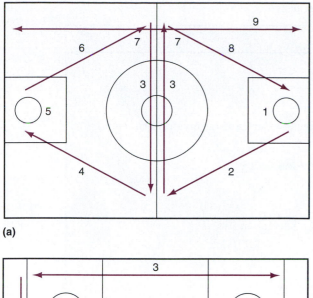

(a)

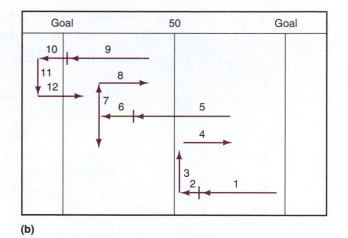

(b)

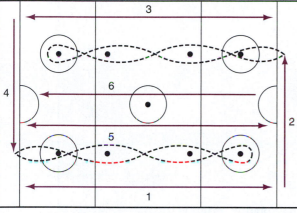

(c)

Figure 5.37   Functional drills. (a) Basketball. 1) Mikan drill; 2) sprint dribble; 3) defensive shuffle; 4) sprint dribble; 5–8) repeat of above four elements; 9) run the lines. (b) Football. 1) 40-yard dash; 2) drive blocking sled 10 yards; 3) Carioca 20 yards; 4) defensive run 20 yards; (5–12) repeat above four elements twice. (c) Ice hockey. 1) Sprint skate the lines; 2) figure 8 the dots; 3) sprint skate the lines; 4) figure 8 the dots; 5) forward/background lines; 6) sprint skate to score. (Redrawn from KE Timm, EA Dobrzykowski. Functional outcomes measurement in sports physical therapy: Determination on return to competition. *J Rehabil Outcomes Meas.* 1997;1(1):35–44.)

apply resistance. Cam systems attempt to alter resistance based on changes in joint moments/leverage and musculotendinous length–tension relationships. Hydraulic and pneumatic devices have been shown to produce strength gains similar to those achieved with free weights; however, they focus on concentric muscle activation.[127] Resistance training machines allow for quick and rather easy independent adjustments to accommodate most average sized clients and may be safer for some clients who are apprehensive or have balance and stability problems. However, this is a relative safety advantage, as some of these machines can be cumbersome and challenging to get on and off because of small seats, raised platforms, and narrow entry/exit points. Some resistance machine manufacturers have developed equipment especially designed for the older adult.[128]

In contrast to this is equipment designed especially for youth that accounts for size differentials between children and adults, using bodyweight resistance that is ultimately safer and provides a means for increased body awareness (International Youth Fitness, Mount Airy, MD) (**Figure 5.38**). Specific guidelines for youth fitness and strength training have been reported by the National Strength and Conditioning Association.[129] Important guidelines are offered and emphasized, including 5–10 minutes of general warm-up, thorough instruction, and complete supervision to ensure safety and performance with proper technique, and careful attention to each child's physical and mental abilities. Sessions should include single and multi-joint exercises, beginning with relatively light loads (12–15 RM), and, depending on the therapeutic exercise program goal(s), one to three sets of 6 to 15 repetitions performed

TABLE 5.9   Sports and some suggested functional tests

Sport	Functional tests
Baseball	T-test
	Medicine ball put test
	300 yard shuttle
	Isokinetic shoulder internal–external rotation strength
Basketball	Edgren sidestep test
	Vertical jump test-single/double leg
	300 yard shuttle
Cross country/track	2 mile run
	Time/distance/height for specific event
	Single leg hop tests
Football	*Lineman:*
	10 yard sprint
	Medicine ball put test
	Vertical jump
	300 yard shuttle
	Backs:
	40 yard sprint
	T-test
	300 yard shuttle
	Quarterbacks:
	Isokinetic shoulder internal rotation–external rotation strength
	Medicine ball put test
Soccer	T-test
	300 yard shuttle
Softball	T-test
	Medicine ball put test
	300 yard shuttle
	Isokinetic shoulder internal–external rotation strength
Swimming	Timed distance swimming preferred stroke
	Isokinetic internal–external rotation strength
Tennis	T-test
	300 yard shuttle
Volleyball	Edgren sidestep test
	Vertical jump test-single/double leg
	300 yard shuttle
Wrestling	Medicine ball put test
	300 yard shuttle

Reprinted with permission of David M. Williams, MPT, ATC, CSCS, University of Iowa.

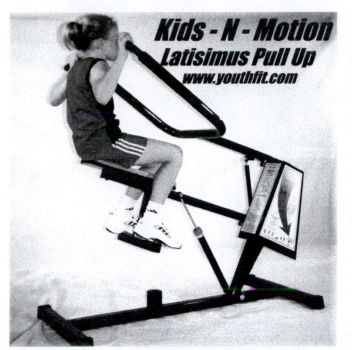

Figure 5.38 Bodyweight resistance machine designed for children. (Kids-N-Motion Latisimus Pull-Up. Reprinted with permission from International Youth Fitness, Mount Airy, MD; www.youthfit.com.)

on two or three non-consecutive days a week, with no more than a 5–10 percent increase in load between successive sessions.[129]

Conceptually, the majority of resistance training machines are designed for training specific muscles or muscle groups, not movements, and this aspect may be viewed as one of the limitations of many isotonic or dynamic constant external resistance devices. Generally, these machines provide a controlled resistance through uniplanar motions, with stabilization at both the proximal and distal segments. Movements are often performed from a seated position in resistance training machines and are sometimes referred to as a *fixed form technique*. Two joint or biarticular muscles or muscle groups naturally function as limb or segment stabilizers (isometric), accelerators (concentric) or decelerators (eccentric). These "isotonic" devices are limited in the sense that they provide loads to only a portion of a muscle acting on only one of the joints. For example, many of the two joint muscles may actually shorten at one attachment site, and lengthen at another (recall the earlier discussion of pseudoisometric action). The overall change in muscle length may be minimal (concurrent shift–pseudoisometric) and has been described previously. This can be observed in many two joint muscles when analyzing common movements or activities such as rising from a chair and squatting. It should be also appreciated that spinal (disc) stresses are increased when a client exercises (such as pushing or pulling a load) from a seated position as compared to equivalent exercises

performed while standing. It has been estimated that exercises performed when seated increase lumbar disk pressure 40 percent more than those performed when standing.[130–133] This must be a consideration for all clients, especially those with existing spinal pathology.

An arguable advantage or disadvantage of many upper extremity resistance machines is their required bilateral movement. This limitation can easily be addressed through the use of free weight dumbbells and medicine balls, sometimes referred to as *free form techniques*, that actually have several therapeutic exercise advantages over many resistance training machines. These advantages might include improved hand-eye coordination, superior integration of trunk and extremity function, trunk and extremity interactions, and enhanced movement pattern specificity. Recent innovations in resistance training machine design and application have effectively corrected many of the aforementioned (**Figure 5.39**).

Key Point:

Following proper instruction, free form techniques using dumbbells or medicine balls as resistance provide a useful method of performing upper extremity resistance exercises in a functionally relevant manner.

Free Weights, Dumbbells and Medicine Balls

Free form techniques of resistance training, such as free weights, dumbbells, and medicine balls have always been popular in the sports performance and fitness/conditioning arenas. These tools are equally important for the rehabilitation clinician and offer unique features over many of the resistance training machines. Free weights (dumbbells) can be used for complete strength training of the trunk and both upper and lower extremities, and often with exercises that can appropriately overload the entire system through combination movement patterns.[107] Apparent advantages of free weights include the requirement of naturally occurring joint stabilization methods with synergistic muscle actions requiring proximal stability, the need for natural proprioceptive feedback and postural neuromuscular responses, (see Chapters 6–8) and the ability to train through multiple movement planes to achieve desired goals. Free weight exercises with dumbbells can also incorporate PNF (proprioceptive neuromuscular facilitation) patterns, which are difficult if not virtually impossible to perform on most isokinetic or resistance machines/devices. Dumbbells can be used in isolation, although combination patterns using multiple joints may be more efficient and provide less risk of injury or overuse when performed correctly. One area where dumbbell interventions can be used effectively is with various shoulder conditions associated with rotator cuff muscle group weakness. There have been several investigations that have

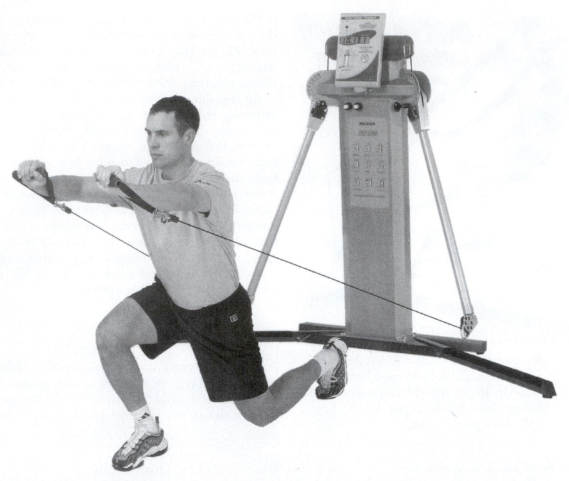

Figure 5.39   Forward lunge (low setting) on Keiser Infinity Series ™ Functional Trainer (Keiser Corp., Fresno, CA).

examined selected shoulder girdle muscles and therapeutic exercises, and some have recommended specific exercises based on peak EMG activity.[134]

Blackburn et al.,[135] with the use of intramuscular EMG, investigated 23 variations of commonly prescribed exercises used in shoulder therapeutic exercise programs noting greater EMG activity throughout the posterior rotator cuff musculature (supraspinatus, infraspinatus, and teres minor) when performed in a prone position as compared to a standing position (**Figures 5.40a–d**). Townsend et al.[136] also conducted EMG investigations on the deltoids, pectoralis major, latissimus dorsi, and the four rotator cuff muscles while performing 17 different shoulder exercises (● **Section 1, Figures 8–24**). Based on the criteria established in their investigation, they recommended that an effective shoulder therapeutic exercise program should include the following exercises: humeral elevation in the scapular plane with thumbs down ("scaption"), shoulder flexion, horizontal abduction with the humerus externally rotated, and the press-up. In a similar investigation, Moseley et al.[137] reported significant activity in the scapular rotators with the performance of the following exercises:

scaption with humeral external rotation ("thumbs up" position), rowing, seated press-ups and "push-ups with a plus" (exaggerated scapular protraction at end range) (**Figure 5.41**). Previous studies that have supported the use of press-ups and "push-ups with a plus" underscore the importance and inter-relationship between trunk and upper extremity musculature in providing strength and stability to the shoulder complex. Many of the aforementioned therapeutic exercises may produce overload to both muscles and tendons, thereby improving the tensile properties of both of these structures. These investigations have provided very useful information regarding the onset and relative degree of EMG activity and have improved our understanding of shoulder muscle actions during movement and exercise.

Rehabilitation clinicians must always consider the client's position during upper extremity therapeutic exercise performance (for example, prone vs. standing), as this can have profound effects on desired therapeutic exercise strategies and interventions. Although higher levels of EMG activation suggest greater shoulder muscle activation when a given therapeutic exercise is performed in a particular position, further research is needed to validate the impact of these re-

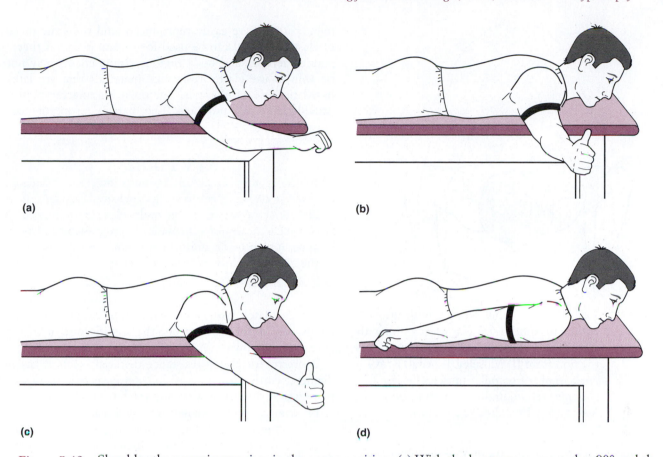

Figure 5.40   Shoulder therapeutic exercises in the prone position. (a) With the humerus supported at 90° and the elbow flexed to 90°, the subject externally rotates the arm. (b) With the arm hanging from the table, the subject lifts the arm into horizontal abduction at 90° and extreme external rotation. (c) With the arm hanging from the table, the subject lifts the arm into horizontal abduction at 100° and extreme external rotation. (d) With the arm hanging from the table, the subject extends and externally rotates the shoulder. (From TA Blackburn, et al. EMG analysis of posterior rotator cuff exercise. *J Athl Train.* 1990;25(1):41–45.)

lationships on client functional outcomes. Is it possible that the supposed benefits of performing certain isolated rotator cuff exercises occur at the cost of disrupting natural interactive motor processes between muscular synergists that normally interact through both the upper extremity and trunk?

Additional therapeutic exercises that combine upper extremity and trunk movement patterns and synergistic muscular activity include punches with protraction and trunk rotation (**Figure 5.42a**), overhead press with lateral trunk flexion (**Figure 5.42b**), trunk/hip flexion-rotation with shoulder external rotation (**Figure 5.42c–d**), and wrist cross forward trunk flexion followed by trunk extension/scapular retraction/external rotation (**Figure 5.42e–f**). The use of weighted boxing gloves and punch blocking mitts can provide a variety of higher speed functional upper extremity movements in standing (**Figure 5.43**).

Dumbbells, often used for upper extremity strength programs, also provide a means for effective training of the lower extremities by way of intrinsic overload with

countless variations of squats, multi-directional lunges, and stepping exercises (**Figures 5.44a–d**).

Medicine balls come in a variety of sizes and weights, and are generally covered by leather (older models), though newer models are rubberized or have polyurethane coverings and offer advantages of indoor and outdoor use as well as possessing improved rebound/return characteristics. Chu[138] classifies plyometric exercises with the medicine ball into arm, trunk, and leg exercises and denotes important differences between tosses and throws. According to Chu, tosses are short passes made from below 90° of shoulder elevation, and throws are longer distance passes made from above 90° of shoulder elevation.[138] Medicine balls provide an excellent tool for rehabilitation clinicians during all stages of upper extremity therapeutic exercise program intervention (acute, sub-acute, return to activity testing, maintenance conditioning). Activities might include variations of scapular protraction-retraction against a wall to facilitate co-contraction with concurrent

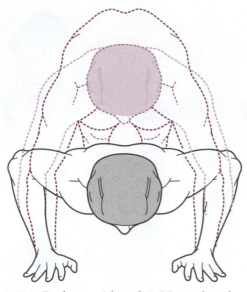

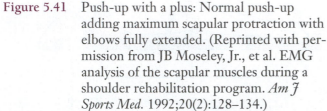

Figure 5.41 Push-up with a plus: Normal push-up adding maximum scapular protraction with elbows fully extended. (Reprinted with permission from JB Moseley, Jr., et al. EMG analysis of the scapular muscles during a shoulder rehabilitation program. *Am J Sports Med.* 1992;20(2):128–134.)

trunk rotation (**Figure 5.45a–b**), or wall dribbling activities to develop midrange functional strength and endurance (**Figure 5.46a–b**). The seated medicine ball chest pass, discussed previously, is a commonly used functional test to determine upper extremity strength and power. The motor control and plyometric aspects of medicine ball training are discussed in Chapter 8.

Elastic Resistance Devices

Elastic or rubber bands or tubing of differing thickness, material properties, or diameters are the fundamental sources of this type of resistance. One of the more popular brands of elastic resistance materials is Theraband™ (The Hygenic Corp, Akron, OH) whose product comes in several different color codes to assist rehabilitation clinicians in determining the appropriate resistance level for a given exercise. The ability to quantify the true force-generating properties of these devices can be difficult based on length, wear, age, and environmental conditions in which it is used, but recent studies that investigated the material properties of Theraband™ have provided information and agreement on force and strain characteristics.[139,140]

Elastic materials provide benefits of being relatively inexpensive, being easy to use just about anywhere, allowing for multi-planar movements, providing a means for a systematic resistance progression (color-coding), and providing uniform resistance regardless of the client's position relative to gravitational forces. Diagonal PNF-type move-

ment patterns are easily reproduced, and the same piece of elastic material can be used for several different therapeutic exercises and body regions. Some clients may not be able to use elastic resistance materials that are latex based because of allergies, but most manufacturers also provide latex-free products. The material properties be-

> ## Key Point:
> Elastic materials used in resistance exercise provide benefits of being relatively inexpensive, easy to use just about anywhere, enable multi-planar movements, provide a means for systematically progressing resistance, and provide uniform resistance regardless of the client's position relative to gravity.

tween the latex based, and non–latex based tubing or bands may differ slightly, but the significance of this is currently unknown.

More robust elastic resistance materials such as larger diameter cords allow for resisted sports specific therapeutic exercises such as forward and retro running, lateral and cross over stepping maneuvers, and various forms of squats, lunges, and resisted jumping or hopping. The Pro Fitter™ (Fitter International Inc., Calgary, Alberta, Canada) provides a unique combination of elastic resistance and balance training during movement patterns that simulate sports activities such as skiing (**Figure 5.47**). When performing these important gross total movement patterns, the rehabilitation clinician must remember to always inspect the attachment sites, handles, cords, belts, or bands for signs of wear to prevent injury caused by failure of the system. Furthermore, the rehabilitation clinician must pay particular attention to and address movement compensations or substitutions as the client performs each therapeutic exercise. Depending on the goal(s), different movements, activities, and primary motion planes can be emphasized, or avoided to maximize desired or minimize undesired stresses (**Figure 5.48(a–g)**).

Manual Resistance and Body Weight Resistance

The use of manual resistance deserves some mention as it serves as the basis for manual muscle testing and PNF techniques, including rhythmic stabilization, hold-relax, and contract-relax movements (see Chapter 6). Manual resistance exercise and training provides a benefit over many other forms of resistance training in that it allows the rehabilitation clinician to continuously monitor force output by the client and provide proprioceptive feedback. It provides a means for rapid changes in applied resistance, which if applied by a skilled rehabilitation clinician, is similar to the accommodating resistance concept touted

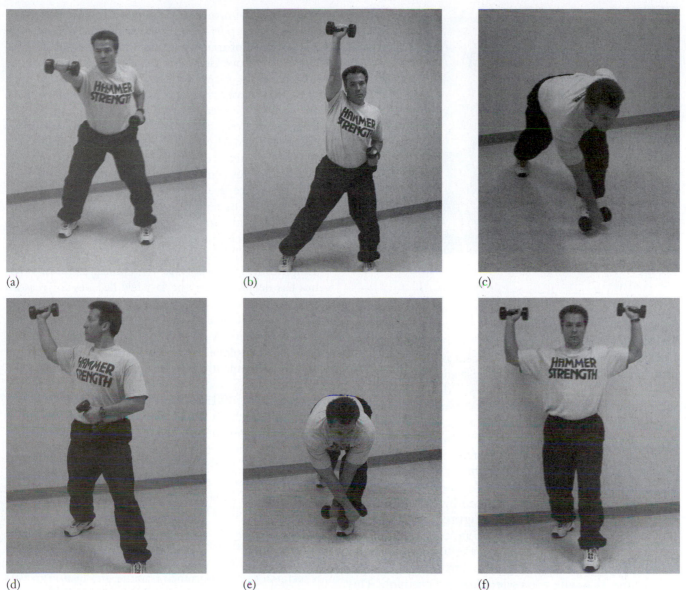

(a)   (b)   (c)

(d)   (e)   (f)

Figure 5.42   Upper extremity combination patterns with dumbbells. (a) shoulder flexion-internal rotation-scapular protraction/elbow extension-forearm pronation; (b) overhead press with lateral trunk flexion; (c), (d) forward trunk flexion to trunk extension with unilateral scapular retraction/external rotation (c, start; d, completion). (e), (f) forward trunk flexion with wrist cross to trunk extension with bilateral scapular retraction/external rotation (e, start; f, completion).

as one of the important features of isokinetics. The "laying on of hands" may be a powerful component to any therapeutic exercise intervention as well and must be considered when discussing the benefits or effects of manual resistance. Manual resistance is also easily taught to clients for self application, as is commonly prescribed during the acute stages of post-operative conditions where isometric exercises may be indicated to reduce the effects of immobilization and disuse and maintain neuromuscular association. Often the uninvolved extremity can be used to apply graded (submaximal to maximal where indicated) resistance, such as with multi-angle isometrics for knee extension/flexion or upper extremity strengthening.

Key Point:

Manual resistance exercises provide a benefit over many other forms of resistance training in that they enable the rehabilitation clinician to continuously monitor force output and provide feedback to the client. They also provide a means of applying rapidly changing resistive forces or sudden perturbations to the client.

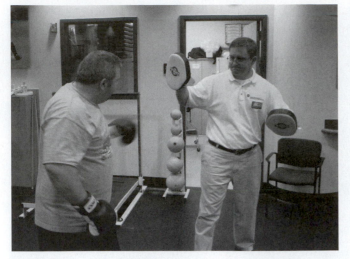

Figure 5.43 Punch blocking.

Isokinetics

In the 1960s, Hislop and Perrine[141] were among the first to describe and investigate the concept of isokinetic exercise. Clinical devices used for exercise and testing became commercially available in the 1970s with limited angular velocities. A detailed history and overview of isokinetics and a compendium of the clinical usage are available for more in depth understanding.[142,143] One of the benefits of isokinetics as a therapeutic exercise is the accommodating resistance, where a dynamometer is able to generate a force or load opposite in direction, but equal in magnitude of that which is produced by a client (muscle torque = dynamometer torque) (**Figure 5.49**). This accommodating resistance provides an environment that automatically adjusts or accommodates to changing leverage, moment arms, and muscle length tension changes (all factors that affect muscle force production). This serves as an advantage over isotonic exercises that are essentially limited by the weakest point in a range of motion a limb segment or joint can produce. Predetermined angular velocities provide operator control (degrees/second) over the speed of movement variable when desired. This predetermined velocity could also be viewed as contradictory to the concept of training specificity as most movements (functional or naturally occurring) seldom involve constant angular velocities, and instead require continual refinements, adjustments, and regulation. The upper range limits for velocity of most commercially available isokinetic devices are 450–500°/second, which does not approach the velocities encountered during running, throwing, and jumping.

There are several parameters from isokinetic testing that may provide useful information for between limb comparisons. Many rehabilitation clinicians use the principle of bilateral equivalence (discussed earlier in this chapter) as the gold standard during clinical examinations, which is the comparison of one extremity (usually involved, injured, or impaired) to the other (uninvolved, un-injured, or non-impaired).[100] Studies of isokinetic resistance training support velocity specificity and demonstrate the importance of training at fast, moderate, and slow velocities to improve isokinetic force production across all testing velocities. Fleck and Kraemer[16] reported that most studies that have examined isokinetic resistance have shown strength increases specific to the training velocity with some carryover above and below the training velocity. Kanehisa and Miyashita[144] reported that training at a moderate velocity (180–240°/sec) produced the greatest strength increases across all testing velocities for the knee extensors. There are several isokinetic parameters reported that may be useful for obtaining information comparing one limb to another regarding deficits and therapeutic exercise program effectiveness (**Tables 5.10–5.12**).[142]

Empirically, it appears that the clinical usage of isokinetics has declined over the last few decades for reasons related to improved understanding and appreciation of applied kinesiology and the importance of therapeutic exercise specificity. A great deal of research has been performed since isokinetic concepts entered into strength testing and therapeutic exercise arenas. It is a reliable and clinically controlled alternative means of strength testing and exercise.[110,142] Like many other forms of strength testing and exercise it has advantages and disadvantages. It seems a bit extreme to discount the use of isokinetics completely, and indeed some manufacturers have recently applied isokinetic methods to weight bearing and CKC environments. Isokinetic evaluations provide an objective measurement of isolated muscle or muscle group torque producing capability. We should appreciate what we have learned from isokinetic research (force velocity, length tension relationships), training, and therapeutic exercise applications and continue to look for better ways to use this technology for resistance training and testing to better assess a client's true functional status.

> ### *Key Point:*
> One of the benefits of isokinetics as a form of therapeutic exercise is the accommodating resistance it produces. By controlling movement velocities, isokinetic dynamometers are able to provide resistances that match that produced by the client (muscle torque = dynamometer torque).

OTHER RESISTANCE TRAINING ENVIRONMENTS

The Aquatic Environment

The unique properties of the aquatic environment offer rehabilitation clinicians and their clients an alternative to land based therapeutic exercise. This environment can

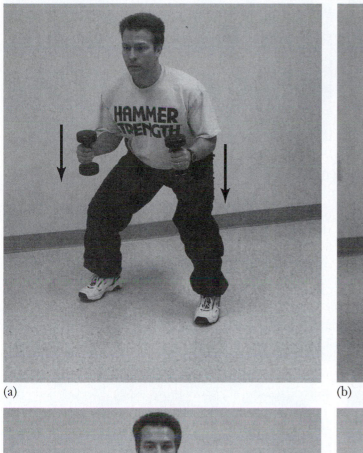

(a)

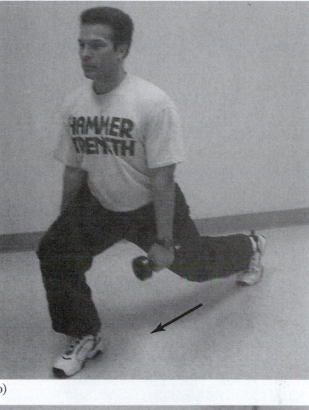

(b)

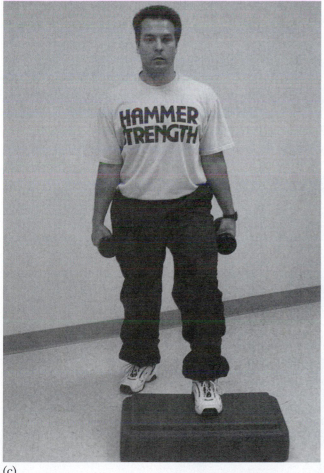

(c)

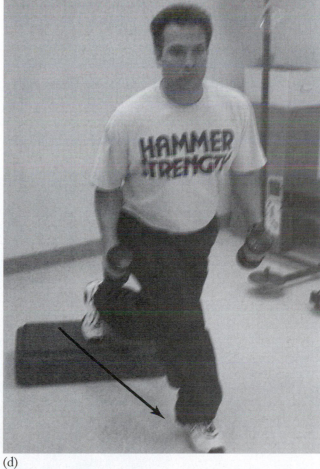

(d)

Figure 5.44   Lower extremity combination patterns with dumbbells. (a) squats; (b) lunges (forward/lateral/diagonal); (c), (d) crossover stepping from a box (c, start; d, completion).

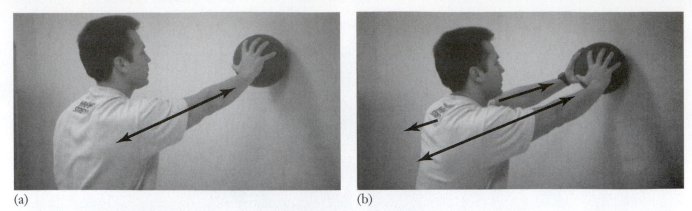

(a)   (b)

Figure 5.45 Scapular protraction/retraction against a wall. (a) unilateral; (b) bilateral.

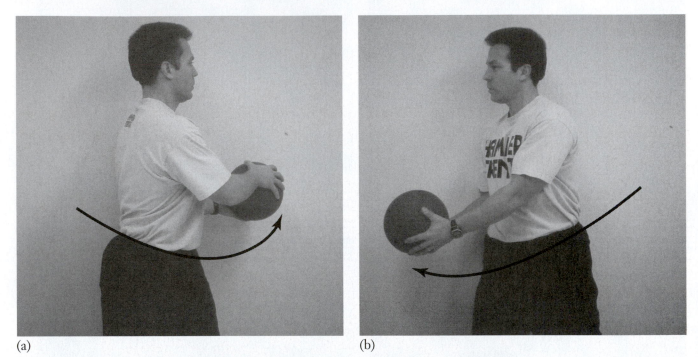

(a)   (b)

Figure 5.46 Wall dribbling activities to develop midrange functional strength and endurance. (a) start; (b) completion.

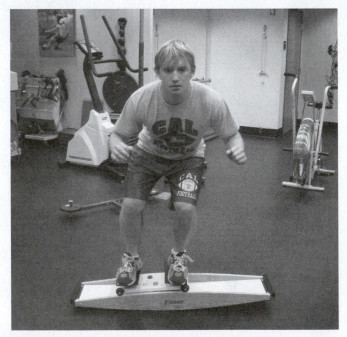

Figure 5.47 Pro-Fitter™ training.

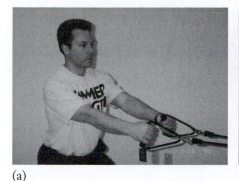
(a)

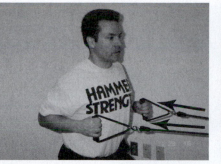
(b)

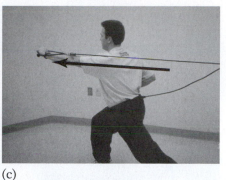
(c)

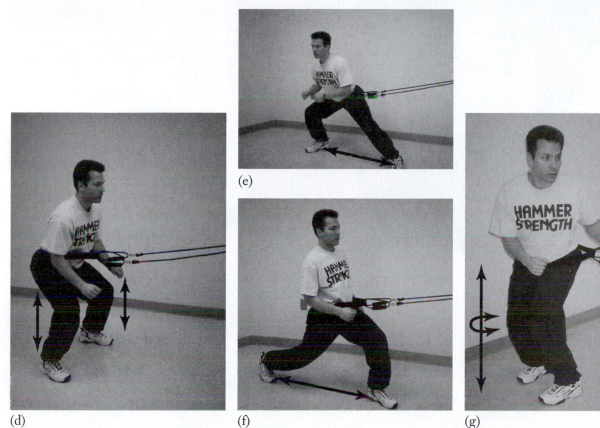
(d)   (e)   (f)   (g)

Figure 5.48   Exercises with elastic resistance. (a) (b) rowing motion (a, start; b, finish); (c) combined upper extremity punch and contralateral lunge; (d) squat with anterior resistance; (e) lateral lunge; (f) retro lunge with anterior resistance; (g) ski squat.

provide benefits especially for clients with weight bearing limitations during fracture healing, status post-open reduction internal fixation of a fracture, total joint replacement, various spinal pathologies, or those with articular cartilage injury (**Figure 5.50**). The physical properties of water include specific gravity, buoyancy, hydrostatic pressure, viscosity, cohesion/adhesion, and surface tension. Each of these properties can be used to achieve certain therapeutic exercise program goals. When considering aquatic program design, Irion reminds rehabilitation clinicians to appreciate body type and swimming skills, as these factors can influence decisions regarding client safety.[145] Clients with a greater lean body mass (less body

fat) percentage will have a higher specific density and a greater tendency to sink, while those with more overall fat mass have a greater tendency to remain afloat. Water temperature is an environmental variable that should be considered just as ambient temperature and humidity are with dry land training and exercise. Thermo-neutral temperatures in the range of 31–34° C (88–93° F) have been recommended.[145]

Buoyancy refers to the upward thrust (opposite gravity) imparted on a body immersed in a fluid and is applied to assist, support, or resist a particular movement pattern. Position, depth of water, length of lever arms used, and aquatic therapy equipment (foam dumbbells, paddles,

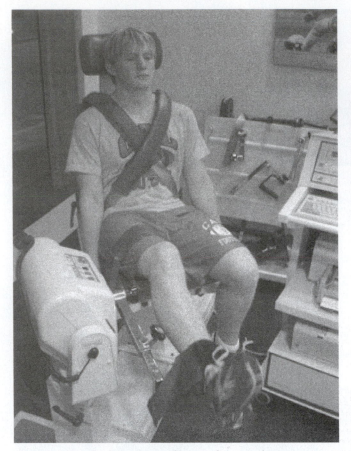

Figure 5.49   Isokinetic quadriceps femoris-hamstring testing.

TABLE 5.10   Isokinetic test parameters

Peak torque to body weight ratio
Bilateral mean peak torque comparison
Torque curve analysis
Bilateral total work comparison
Unilateral peak torque ratio
Average power to body weight ratio
Bilateral peak torque comparison
Time ratio to torque development
Endurance ratio (first repetition to last repetition)

(Reprinted with permission from KE Wilk, Dynamic muscle strength testing. In LR Admundsen (ed.), *Muscle Strength Testing: Instrumented and Non-instrumented Systems.* New York: Churchill Livingstone, 1990.)

TABLE 5.11   Hamstrings/quadriceps unilateral ratios

Dynamometer speed (degrees/sec)	Ratio (percent)
60	60–69
180	70–79
300	80–84
450	95–100

(Reprinted with permission from KE Wilk, Dynamic muscle strength testing. In LR Admundsen (ed.), *Muscle Strength Testing: Instrumented and Non-Instrumented Systems.* New York: Churchill Livingstone, 1990.)

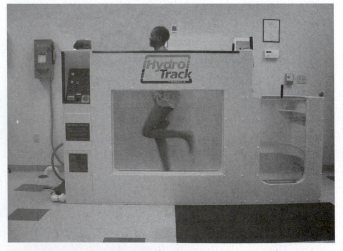

Figure 5.50   Aquatic treadmill.

TABLE 5.12   Isokinetic quadriceps torque to body weight ratios

Dynamometer speed (degrees/sec)	Men (%)	Women (%)
60	100–115	80–95
180	60–75	50–65
300	40–55	30–45
450	30–40	20–29

(Reprinted with permission from KE Wilk, Dynamic muscle strength testing. In LR Admundsen (ed.), *Muscle Strength Testing: Instrumented and Non-Instrumented Systems,* New York: Churchill Livingstone, 1990.)

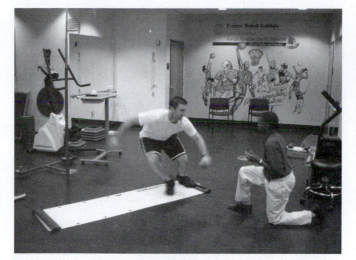

Figure 5.51   Sliding board with simultaneous upper extremity exercise.

cuffs, gloves and belts) are all variables used to modify the effects of buoyancy according to desired therapeutic exercise program strategies.[146] Estimates of the buoyancy effects on weight bearing status in a standing position and during ambulation have been reported by Harrison et al. and are presented in **Table 5.13**.[147,148] Hydrostatic pressure results in additionally important physiologic sequelae that must also be considered. Immersion in water creates changes in peripheral blood flow and edema, blood pressure, heart rate and increases in heart and pulmonary blood volume. Additional information regarding aquatic therapeutic exercise is presented in Chapter 4.

Aquatic therapeutic exercise interventions may provide an excellent transitional environment for clients with many acute and sub-acute conditions, while at the same time providing some program variety. Rehabilitation clinicians should remember to balance the metabolic system demands of the program based on client goals, consider the degree of functional carryover, and emphasize the return to land based environments as soon as they are deemed appropriate.

Friction: Lower Extremity Sliding Boards (Inertial/Isoinertial)

Another therapeutic exercise tool based on the concepts of friction and inertia is the lower extremity sliding board (**Figure 5.50**). Sliding boards involve eccentric and concentric muscle activity incorporating selective loading of the series elastic components through horizontal, submaximal, plyometric principles. Inertia, which is the resistance (of an object) to a change in motion, is another principle of physics that results in this rapid reversal of muscle activation from concentric to eccentric, which is necessary for quick changes in directions. Intensity, volume, and duration can be controlled through the modification of movement speed and distance traveled, repetitions, and time. Sliding board activities are very useful for the development of frontal plane control and stability of the lower extremity, with a particular emphasis on training the hip abductor and adductor muscle groups. Originally developed for office training and conditioning for speed skaters and hockey players, sliding boards have become popular and effective for enhancing lateral movements common in to many sporting activities.

Swiss Ball

The Swiss (Pezzi) ball has been used for the treatment of neurodevelopmental conditions for nearly 45 years in rehabilitation settings throughout Europe.[149,150] Klein-Vogel-

TABLE 5.13   Buoyancy

Quantification of approximate weight bearing percentages in water based on level of immersion.		
	Standing	**Slow Ambulation**
Vertebral Level C7	8–10% BW	25% BW
Xiphoid Process	28–35% BW	25–50% BW
A.S.I.S.	47–54% BW	50–75% BW

BW = body weight, A.S.I.S. = Anterior Superior Iliac Spine, C7 = seventh cervical spinous process.

(Reprinted with permission from Harrison RA, et al. Loading the lower limb when walking partially immersed: Implications for clinical practice. *Physiother.* 1992;78:164–166.)

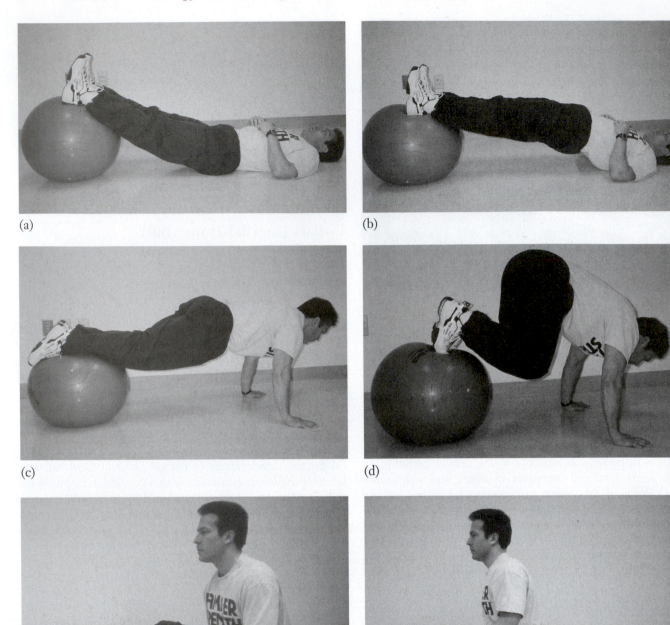

Figure 5.52   Exercises with a Swiss ball. (a), (b) supine hip and trunk extension (a, start; b, completion); (c), (d) Easter bunny exercise (c, start; d, completion); (e), (f) swing exercise (e, start; f, completion).

bach, considered one of the pioneers of Swiss ball training, incorporated its use through her teachings in functional kinetics in Basel, Switzerland.[150,151] Beate Carriere popularized the use of the Swiss ball in the United States and has written one of the most comprehensive texts to date on the theory behind its clinical applications.[150] The Swiss ball can be found in nearly all therapeutic exercise program settings as well as in health and fitness clubs, and in many homes with literally hundreds, if not thousands, of applications including—but not limited to—balance, stability, postural training, stretching, strengthening, endurance, and automobilization techniques. Some common applications used for upper, lower, and torso strengthening include the supine extension (**Figure 5.52a–b**), "Easter bunny" (**Figure 5.52c–d**), and the "Swing" (**Figure 5.52e–f**). Uses for the Swiss ball during dynamic joint stability training are discussed in Chapters 6 and 11.

Common Denominators of Successful Knee Injury Prevention Programs

Recent research has provided support to the notion that specially designed therapeutic exercise programs can help prevent knee injuries (especially the ACL).[102,103,152,153]

Common characteristics associated with each of these programs include an emphasis on weight bearing (see Chapter 1), proprioception-kinesthesia (see Chapter 7), balance (see Chapter 9), coordination (see Chapter 8), effective neuromuscular power, appropriate jump landing techniques (see Chapter 11), and sudden deceleration and running directional change techniques (see Chapter 9) to avoid the pathomechanics associated with knee injury. Each of these programs relies on multi-joint, integrated, and functionally relevant movement patterns with a focus on technique and feedback to facilitate appropriate motor learning for joint preservation (see Chapter 8). Opportunities exist for similar therapeutic exercise program development to prevent the injurious pathomechanics associated with injury to other body regions such as the shoulder and low back. Additionally, greater use of educational and behavioral modification strategies may further improve client outcomes after having participated in these programs (see Chapter 11).

Summary

Rehabilitation clinicians are basing more of their therapeutic exercise program design decisions on scientific evidence. Rehabilitation clinicians are gaining appreciation of the importance of proprioception, kinesthesia and motor control during resistance training in addition to the basics of muscular strength, hypertrophy, endurance and power. Regardless of whether the program is designed to improve client strength, power, endurance, balance, or kinesthesia, or some combination of these components, the rehabilitation clinician ultimately must be concerned about the functional relevance of their selections and the extent to which their choices will actually help minimize the client's disability level. Greater appreciation for how motor control and motor learning concepts and behavioral change strategies can be used to better facilitate therapeutic exercise program goals is needed and rehabilitation clinicians are advised to pay particular attention to advances in these areas. (see Chapter 8 and 11).[154]

Therapeutic exercise program benefits may only be optimally realized when clients build their confidence level by successfully completing new, unfamiliar tasks that they perceive as being important to them in addition to previously difficult to perform ADLs or IADLs. Concentrated focus on isolated muscle or muscle group activities (for example, core stabilization programs, isolated rotator cuff exercises) is often the emphasis of traditional therapeutic exercise programs. However, activities that integrate appendicular and core function during the performance of functionally relevant movement patterns may ultimately need to be mastered for the client to minimize their disability level. While allowing the client to consciously plan their movements is appropriate during the early stages of therapeutic exercise program participation, it is equally as important for the client eventually to perform spontaneous activities with minimal time for pre-planning in preparation for the challenges of their daily life. The rehabilitation clinician has an ideal opportunity to educate the client as to the rationale behind each component of their therapeutic exercise program, increase their appreciation for lifelong fitness and joint preservation, and foster the enthusiasm necessary to enhance program compliance. With proper education the client is better prepared to make appropriate decisions in selecting home exercise equipment.

References

1. American College of Sports Medicine. Position Stand: The recommended quantity and quality of exercise for developing and maintaining cardiorespiratory and muscular fitness, and flexibility in healthy adults. *Med Sci Sports Exerc.*1998;30:975–991.

2. American College of Sports Medicine. Position Stand: Progression models in resistance training for healthy adults. *Med Sci Sports Exerc.* 2002;34(2): 364–380.

3. Stone MH, Fleck SJ, Triplett NT, Kraemer WJ. Health- and performance-related potential of resistance training. *Sports Med.* 1991;11(4):210–231.

4. Bryant CX, Peterson JA, Graves JE. Muscular strength and endurance. *In ACSM's Resource Manual for Guidelines for Exercise Testing and Prescription*, 3rd ed. Baltimore: Williams & Wilkins, 1998.

5. Evans WJ, Patton JF, Fisher EC, Knuttgen HG. Muscle metabolism during high intensity eccentric exercise. *In Biochemistry of Exercise, Symposium, 1982.* Champaign, IL: Human Kinetics, 1983, pp. 225–228.

6. Byrnes WC, Clarkson PM. Delayed onset muscle soreness and training. *Clin Sports Med. 1986; 5(3): 605–614.*

7. Baker D, Wilson G, Carlyon R. Generality versus specificity: A comparison of dynamic and isometric measures of strength and speed-strength. *Eur J Appl Physiol.* 1994;68:350–355.

8. Heyward VH. *Advanced Fitness Assessment and Exercise Prescription*, 3rd ed. Champaign, IL:Human Kinetics; 1991, p. 122.

9. Davies G. Assessment of strength (ch. 10). In T Malone, T McPoil, AJ Nitz (eds): *Orthopaedic and Sports Physical Therapy*, 3rd edition. St. Louis: Mosby Year Book, Inc., 1997.

10. Voloshin I, DiGiovanni BF, Baumhauer JF. Plantar heel pain: making a difficult diagnosis: The variety of possible causes and treatments poses a challenge. *J Musculoskel Med.* 2002;19(9):373-376, 378–380.

11. Kraemer WJ, Ratamess NA. Fundamentals of resistance training: Progression and exercise prescription. *Med Sci Sports Exerc.* 2004;36(4):674–688.

12. Kraemer WJ, Hakkinen K, Newton RU. Effects of heavy-resistance training on hormonal response in younger vs. older men. *J Appl Physiol.* 1999;87(3): 982–992.

13. Sale DG. Neural adaptation to strength training. *In Strength and Power in Sports*, PV Komi (ed.), 2nd ed. Malden, MA: Blackwell Science, 2003, pp. 281-314.

14. Kraemer WJ, Patton J, Gordon SE, et al. Compatibility of high intensity strength and endurance training on hormonal and skeletal muscle adaptations. *J Appl Physiol.* 1995;78(3):976–989.

15. Campos GER, Leucke TJ, Wendeln HK, et al. Muscular adaptations in response to three different resistance-training regimens: Specificity of repetition maximum zones. *Eur J Appl Physiol.* 2002;88: 50–60.

16. Fleck S, Kraemer WJ, *Designing Resistance Training Programs*, 2nd ed. Champaign, IL:Human Kinetics, 1997, p. 98.

17. Fleck SJ. Periodized strength training: A critical review. *J Strength Cond Res.* 1999;13:82–89.

18. Marx JO, Ratamess NA, Nindl BC, et al. Low-volume circuit versus high-volume periodized resistance training in women. *Med Sci Sports Exerc.* 2001; 33(4):635–643.

19. Hakkinen K, Kallinen M, Komi PV, Kauhanen H. Neuromuscular adaptations during short-term "normal" and reduced training periods in strength athletes. *Electromyogr Clin Neurophysiol.* 1991;31:35–42.

20. Bosco C, Colli R, Bonomi R, et al. Monitoring strength training: neuromuscular and hormonal profile. *Med Sci Sports Exerc.* 2000;32(1):202–208.

21. Newton RU, Hakkinen K, Hakkinen A, et al. Mixed-methods resistance training increases power and strength of young and older men. *Med Sci Sports Exerc.* 2002;34:1367–1375.

22. Bobbert MA, Van Soest AJ. Effects of muscle strengthening on vertical jump height: A simulation study. *Med Sci Sports Exerc.* 1994;26:1012–1020.

23. Gambetta V. Rebuilding the athlete completely . . . Building the complete athlete. Course Notes. Chicago, IL: Optimum Sports Training, Inc., 1992.

24. Semmler JG, Enoka RM. Neural contributions to changes in muscle strength. *In* VM Zatsiorsky (ed.), *Biomechanics in Sport: The Scientific Basis of Performance.* Oxford, UK: Blackwell Science, *Exerc Sport Sci Rev.* 2000, pp. 3–20.

25. Zhou S. Chronic neural adaptations to unilateral exercise: Mechanisms of cross education. *Exerc Sport Sci Rev.* 2000;28:177–184.

26. Housh DJ, Housh TJ. The effects of unilateral velocity-specific concentric strength training. *J Orthop Sports Phys Ther.* 1993;17(5):252–256.

27. Vuori I, Heinonen A, Sievanen H, et al. Effects of unilateral strength training and detraining on bone mineral density and content in young women: A study of mechanical loading and deloading on human bones. *Calcif Tissue Int.* 1994;55:59–67.

28. Hortobagyi T, Scott K, Lambert J, et al.. Cross-education of muscle strength is greater with stimulated than voluntary contractions. *Motor Control.* 1999;3:205–219.

29. Yue G, Cole KJ. Strength increases from the motor program: A comparison of training with maximal

voluntary and imagined muscle contractions. *J Neurophysiol.* 1992;67:1114–1123.

30. Siff MC. *Supertraining*, 5th ed. Denver, CO: Supertraining Institute, 2000, p. 298.

31. Morgan RE, Adamson GT. *Circuit Training.* London: G. Bell and Sons Ltd., 1957.

32. Fyfe I, Stanish WD. The use of eccentric training and stretching in the treatment and prevention of tendon injuries. *Clin Sports Med.* 1992;11:601–624.

33. Guide to Physical Therapist Practice. *Phys Ther.* 2001; 81(1):S1–S738.

34. U.S. Department of Health and Human Services. *Healthy People 2010: Understanding and Improving Health*, 2nd ed. Washington, DC: U.S. Government Printing Office, November 2000.

35. *Taber's Cyclopedic Medical Dictionary*, 19th ed. Philadelphia: F.A. Davis Company, 2001.

36. Fernel JF. *De naturali parte medicinae* (On the natural parts of medicine), Paris, 1542.

37. Lieber RL. *Skeletal Muscle Structure and Function: Implications for Rehabilitation and Sports Medicine.* Baltimore: Williams & Wilkins, 1992.

38. Gray G. Chain reaction: Successful strategies for closed chain and open chain testing and rehabilitation. Course notes. Adrian, MI: Wynn Marketing, 1993.

39. Salter RB. General principles and specific methods of musculoskeletal treatment, Chap.3. *In Textbook of Disorders and Injuries of the Musculoskeletal System*, 3rd ed. Baltimore, MD: Williams & Wilkins, 1999, pp. 91–116.

40. Beevor CE. *The Croonian Lectures, on Muscular Movements and Their Representation in the Central Nervous System.* London: Adlard and Son, 1904.

41. Wallis EL, Logan GA. *Figure Improvement and Body Conditioning Through Exercise.* Englewood Cliffs: Prentice Hall, 1964.

42. Gray GW. Team reaction: Lower extremity functional profile. Adrian, MI: Wynn Marketing, 1995.

43. Logan GA, McKinney WC. *Anatomic Kinesiology*, 3rd ed. Dubuque, IA: Wm. C. Brown Company, 1982.

44. Sahrman SA. *Diagnosis and Treatment of Movement Impairment Syndromes.* St. Louis, MO: Mosby, 2002.

45. Kendall FP, McCreary EK, Provance PG. *Muscles Testing and Function, with Posture and Pain*, 4th edition. Baltimore, MD: Williams & Wilkins, 1993.

46. Saliba VL, Johnson GS. Vertical compression test. In *Therapeutic Exercise: Techniques for Intervention*, WD Bandy, B Sanders (eds.), Baltimore, MD: Lippincott Williams & Wilkins, 2001.

47. Kaplan FS, Hayes WC, Keaveny TM, et al. Form and function of bone. *In* SR Simon (ed.), *Orthopaedic Basic Science.* Rosemont, IL: AAOS, 1994, pp. 127–184.

48. Snyder-Mackler L. Scientific rationale and physiological basis for the use of closed kinetic chain exercise in the lower extremity. *J Sport Rehabil.* 1996;5:2–12.

49. Mueller MJ, Maluf KS. Tissue adaptation to physical stress: A proposed "physical stress theory" to guide physical therapist practice, education, and research. *Phys Ther.* 2002;82:383–403.

50. Dye SF. The knee as a biologic transmission with an envelope of function: A theory. *Clin Orthop.* 1996; 325(1):10–18.

51. Borg GAV. Psychophysical bases of physical exertion. *Med Sci Sports Exerc.* 1982;14:377–87.

52. Sale DG. Neural adaptation to resistance training. *Med Sci Sports Exerc.* 1988;20:S135–S145.

53. Chu DA: *Jumping into Plyometrics.* Champaign, IL: Human Kinetics, 1992.

54. Fry AC, Kraemer WJ. Resistance exercise overtraining and overreaching. *Sports Med.* 1997;23 (2):106–129.

55. Kraemer WJ, Nindl BC. Factors involved with overtraining for strength and power. *In* Krieder RB, Fry AC, O'Toole ML (eds.), *Overtraining in Sport.* Champaign, IL: Human Kinetics, 1998, pp. 69–86.

56. Aristotle. *Progression of Animals.* (Peck AL, Forster ES, trans.) Cambridge: Harvard University Press, 1968.

57. Higgins S. Movement as an emergent form: Its structural limits. *Hum Mov Sci.* 1985; 4:119–148.

58. Palmitier RA, An KN, Scott SG, Chao EYS. Kinetic chain exercises in knee rehabilitation. *Sports Med.* 1991;11:402–413.

59. Grood ES, Suntay WT, Noyes FR, et al. Biomechanics of the knee-extension exercise. Effect of cutting the anterior cruciate ligament. *J Bone Joint Surg.* 1984;66A:725–734.

60. Henning CE, Lynch MA, Glick KR. An in vivo strain gauge study of elongation of the anterior cruciate ligament. *Am J Sports Med.* 1985;13:22–26.

61. Shelbourne KD, Nitz P. Accelerated rehabilitation after anterior cruciate ligament reconstruction. *J Orthop Sports Phys Ther.* 1992;15(6):256–264.

62. Steindler A. *Kinesiology of the Human Body Under Normal and Pathological Conditions.* Springfield, IL: Charles C Thomas, 1955.

63. Wilk KE., Reinold M. Closed-kinetic-chain exercise and plyometric activities, pp. 179–211. *In* WD Bandy, B Sanders (eds), *Therapeutic Exercise: Techniques for Intervention.* Baltimore, MD: Lippincott Williams & Wilkins, 2001.

64. Lefever-Button, S. Closed kinetic chain training (Chapter 15, pp. 252–273). *In* CM Hall, L Thein-Brody (eds.), *Therapeutic Exercise: Moving Toward Function.* Philadelphia: Lippincott Williams & Wilkins, 1999.

65. Dillman CJ, Murray TA, Hintermeister RA. Biomechanical differences of open and closed chain exer-

cises with respect to the shoulder. *J Sport Rehabil.* 1994;3:228–238.

66. Wilk KE, Naiquan Z, Glenn SF, et al. Kinetic chain exercise: Implications for the anterior cruciate ligament patient. *J Sport Rehabil.* 1997;6:125–140.

67. Panariello RA, Backus SI, Parker JW. The effect of squat exercise on anterior-posterior knee translation in professional football players. *Am J Sports Med.* 1994; 22:768–773.

68. Graham VL, Gehlsen GM, Edwards JA. Electromyographic evaluation of closed and open kinetic chain rehabilitation exercises. *J Athl Train.* 1993;28(1):23–30.

69. Snyder-Mackler L, Ladin Z, Schepsis AA, Young JC. Electrical stimulation of the thigh muscles after reconstruction of the anterior cruciate ligament. *J Bone Joint Surg.* 1991;73-A(7):1025–1036.

70. Snyder-Mackler L, Delitto A, Bailey SL, Stralka SW. Strength of the quadriceps femoris muscle and functional recovery after reconstruction of the anterior cruciate ligament. *J Bone Joint Surg.* 1995;77-A(8):1166–1173.

71. DiFabio RP. Making jargon from kinetic and kinematic chains. Editorial. *J Orthop Sports Phys Ther.* 1999;29(3):142–143.

72. Levangie PK, Norkin CC. *Joint Structure and Function: A Comprehensive Analysis*, 3rd ed. Philadelphia: F.A. Davis, 2001.

73. English AW, Wolf SL, Segal RL. Compartmentalization of muscles and their motor nuclei: The partitioning hypothesis. *Phys Ther.* 1993;73:857–867.

74. Klein KK. The deep squat exercise as utilized in weight training for athletes and its effect on the ligaments of the knee. *J Assoc Phys Ment Rehabil.* 1961;15(1):6–11.

75. Chandler TJ, Stone MH. The squat exercise in athletic conditioning: A review of the literature. *National Strength Conditioning Assoc J.* 1991;13(5):52–58.

76. Powers CM, Ward SR, Fredericson M, et al. Patellofemoral kinematics during weight-bearing and non-weight-bearing knee extension in persons with lateral subluxation of the patella: a preliminary study. *J Orthop Sports Phys Ther.* 2003;33(11):677–685.

77. Powers C. Rehabilitation of patellofemoral joint disorders: A critical review. *Phys Ther.* 1998;28(5):345–354.

78. Steinkamp LA, Dillingham MF, Markel MD, et al. Biomechanical considerations in patellofemoral joint rehabilitation. *Am J Sports Med.* 1993;21:438–444.

79. Hungerford DS, Barry M. Biomechanics of the patellofemoral joint. *Clin Orthop.* 1979;144:9–15.

80. Fitzgerald GK. Open versus closed kinetic chain exercise: Issues in rehabilitation after anterior cruciate ligament reconstructive surgery. *Phys Ther.* 1997;77(12):1747–1754.

81. Beynnon BD, Fleming BC, Johnson RJ, et al. Anterior cruciate ligament strain behavior during rehabilitation exercises in vivo. *Am J Sports Med.* 1995;23(1):24–34.

82. Escamilla RF, Fleisig GS, Naiquan Z, et al. Effects of technique variations on knee biomechanics during the squat and leg press. *Med Sci Sports Exerc.* 2001;33(9):1552–1566.

83. Gracovetsky S. *The Spinal Engine.* New York: Springer-Verlag, 1988.

84. Farfan HF. Muscular mechanisms of the lumbar spine and the position of power and efficiency. *Orthop Clin North Am.* 1975;6:135–144.

85. Bergmark A. Stability of the lumbar spine: A study in mechanical engineering. *Acta Orthop Scand.* 1989;230:1–54.

86. Kavic N, Grenier S, McGill SM. Determining the stabilizing role of individual torso muscles during rehabilitation exercises. *Spine.* 2004;29(11):1254–1263.

87. Cholewicki J, McGill S. Mechanical stability of the in vivo spine: Implications for injury and chronic low back pain. *Clin Biomech.* 1996;11:1–15.

88. Axler CT, McGill SM. Low back loads over a variety of abdominal exercises: Searching for the safest abdominal challenge. *Med Sci Sports Exerc.* 1997;29:804–811.

89. McGill SM. Low back exercises: Evidence for improving exercise regimens. *Phys Ther.* 1998;78:754–765.

90. McGill SM, Grenier S, Kavcic N, Cholewicki J. Coordination of muscle activity to assure stability of the lumbar spine. *J Electromyogr Kinesiol.* 2003;13:353–359.

91. Myers TW. *Anatomy Trains: Myofascial Meridians for Manual and Movement Therapists.* Edinburgh: Churchill Livingstone, 2001.

92. Nitz AJ, Nyland J, Brosky T, Caborn D. Neurosciences. *In* B Brownstein, S Bronner, (eds.), *Evaluation, Treatment, and Outcomes: Functional Movement in Orthopaedic and Sports Physical Therapy.* New York: Churchill Livingstone, 1997.

93. Peck D, Buxton DF, Nitz AJ. A comparison of spindle concentrations in large and small muscles acting in parallel combinations. *J Morphol.* 1984;180:243–252.

94. Bastide G, Zadeh J, Lefebvre D. Are the little muscles what we think they are? *Surg Radiol Anat.* 1989;11:255–256.

95. Nitz AJ, Peck D. Comparison of muscle spindle concentrations in large and small human epaxial muscles acting in parallel combinations. *Am Surg.* 1986;52:273–277.

96. Saunders HD. *Assessing Flexibility and Strength in Industrial Workers.* Chaska, MN: The Saunders Group, 1995, pp. 12–16.

97. Soncrant J. Core stability training: The core six-pack. Course notes. Orthopaedic Section, American

Physical Therapy Association, Combined Sections Meeting, Boston, MA, 2002.

98. Gambetta V, Odgers S. *The Complete Guide to Medicine Ball Training.* Sarasota, FL: Optimum Sports Training, 1991.

99. Gambetta V, Soncrant J. *Building and Rebuilding the Athlete Seminar.* Sarasota, FL: Gambetta Sports Training Systems, 2002.

100. Timm KE. A new model for functional outcomes measurement in sports physical therapy: Determination on return to competition. *J Rehabil Outcomes Meas.* 1997;1(1):35–44.

101. Radcliffe JC, Farentinos RC. *Plyometrics: Explosive power training, 2nd ed.,* Champaign, IL: Human Kinetics, 1985.

102. Hewett TE, Lindenfeld TN, Riccobene JV, Noyes FR. The effect of neuromuscular training on the incidence of knee injury in female athletes: A prospective study. *Am J Sports Med.* 1999;27(6):699–706.

103. Hewett TE. Neuromuscular and hormonal factors associated with knee injuries in female athletes: Strategies for intervention. *Sports Med.* 2000;29 (5):313–327.

104. Elftman H. Biomechanics of muscle. *J Bone Joint Surg.* 1966;48:363.

105. Albert M. *Eccentric Muscle Training in Sports and Orthopaedics.* New York: Churchill Livingstone, 1991.

106. Gambetta V. Plyometric training explained. *Sports Coach.* 2003;26(3):15–17.

107. Gray GW. Dumbbells are Smart. Course notes. Adrian, MI: Wynn Marketing, 1991.

108. Foran B. *High-Performance Sports Conditioning.* Champaign, IL: Human Kinetics, 2001.

109. Barrow HM, McGee R, Tritschler KA. *Practical Measurement in Physical Education and Sport,* 4th ed. Philadelphia: Lea and Febiger, 1989.

110. Brosky JA, Nitz AJ, Malone TR, et al. Intrarater reliability of selected clinical outcome measures following anterior cruciate ligament reconstruction. *J Orthop Sports Phys Ther.* 1999;29(1):39–48.

111. Bandy WD, Rusche KR, Tekulve FY. Reliability and limb symmetry for five unilateral functional tests of the lower extremities. *Isokinet Exerc Sci.* 1994;4:108–111.

112. Greenberger HB, Paterno MV. The test-retest reliability of a one-legged hop for distance in healthy adults. *J Orthop Sports Phys Ther.* 1994;19: 61 [Abstract].

113. Booher LD, Hench KM, Worrell TW, Stikeleather J. Reliability of three single-leg hop tests. *J Sport Rehabil.* 1993;2:165–170.

114. Mangine RE, Noyes FR, Mullen MP, Barber SD. A physiological profile of the elite soccer athlete. *J Orthop Sports Phys Ther.* 1990;12:147–152.

115. Noyes FR, Barber SD, Mangine RE. Abnormal lower limb symmetry determined by functional hop test after anterior cruciate ligament rupture. *Am J Sports Med.* 1991;19:512–518.

116. Hu HS, Whitney SL, Irrgang JJ, Janosky J. Test-retest reliability of the one-legged vertical jump test and the one-legged standing hop test. *J Orthop Sports Phys Ther.* 1992;15:51 [Abstract].

117. Lephart SM, Perrin DH, Fu FH, et al. Relationship between selected physical characteristics and functional capacity in the anterior cruciate ligament insufficient athlete. *J Orthop Sports Phys Ther.* 1992; 16:174–181.

118. Lephart SM, Perrin DH, Fu FH, Minger K. Functional performance tests for the anterior cruciate ligament insufficient athlete. *J Athl Train.* 1991; 26:44–50.

119. Risberg MA, Ekeland A. Assessment of functional tests after anterior cruciate ligament surgery. *J Orthop Sports Phys Ther.* 1994;19:202–217.

120. Barber SD, Noyes FR, Mangine RE, et al. Quantitative assessment of functional limitations in normal and anterior cruciate ligament deficient knees. *Clin Orthop.* 1990;255:204–214.

121. Hubley CL, Wells RP. A work-energy approach to determine individual contributions to vertical jump performance. *Eur J Appl Physiol.* 1983;50: 247–254.

122. Luhtanen P, Komi PV. Segmental contribution to forces in vertical jump. *Eur J Appl Physiol.* 1978; 38:181–188.

123. Robertson DGE, Fleming D. Kinetics of standing broad jump and vertical jumping. *Can J Sport Sci.* 1987;12:19–23.

124. Gray G. *Lower Extremity Functional Profile.* Adrian, MI: Wynn Marketing, 1995.

125. Harman E, Garhammer J, Pandorf C. Administration, Scoring, and Interpretation of Selected Tests. *In* TR Baechle, R Earle (eds.), *Essentials of Strength Training and Conditioning,* 2nd ed. Champaign, IL: Human Kinetics, 2000.

126. Williams D. Sport specific functional testing. Lecture notes. Carroll College, Waukesha, WI, August 12, 1998.

127. Hortobagyi T, Katch FI. Role of concentric force in limiting improvement in muscular strength. *J Appl Physiol.* 1990:68:650–658.

128. *Strength Training and Aging.* Fresno, CA: Keiser Corporation, 1998.

129. Faigenbaum AD, Kraemer WJ, Cahill B, et al. Youth resistance training: Position statement paper and literature review. *J Strength Cond.* 1996;18(6): 62–75.

130. Nachemson A. The load on lumbar disks in different positions of the body. *Clin Orthop.* 1966;45:107–122.

131. Nachemson AL. Disc pressure measurements. *Spine.* 1981;6:93–97.

132. Nachemson A, Morris JM. In vivo measurements of intradiscal pressure. *J Bone Joint Surg Am.* 1964; 46:1077–1092.

133. Chaffin D, Anderson G, Martin BJ (eds). *Occupational Biomechanics.* Hoboken, NJ: John Wiley and Sons, 1984.

134. DiVeta J, Walker M, Skibinski B. Relationship between performance of selected scapular muscles and scapular abduction in standing subjects. *Phys Ther.* 1990;70(8):470–476.

135. Blackburn TA, McLeod WD, White B, Wofford L. EMG analysis of posterior rotator cuff exercises. *J Athl Train.* 1990;25(1):41–45.

136. Townsend H, Jobe FW, Pink M, Perry J. Electromyographic analysis of the glenohumeral muscles during a baseball rehabilitation program. *Am J Sports Med.* 1991;19(3):264–272.

137. Moseley JB, Jobe FW, Pink M, et al. EMG analysis of the scapular muscles during a shoulder rehabilitation program. *Am J Sports Med.* 1992;20(2): 128–134.

138. Chu DA. *Plyometric Exercises with the Medicine Ball.* Livermore, CA: Bittersweet Publishing Company, 1989.

139. Patterson RM, Stegink Jansen CW, Hogan HA, Nassif MD. Material properties of Thera-band™ tubing. *Phys Ther.* 2001;81(8):1437–1445.

140. Simoneau GG, Bereda SM, Sobush DC, Starky AJ. Biomechanics of elastic resistance in therapeutic exercise programs. *J Orthop Sports Phys Ther.* 2001; 31:16–24.

141. Hislop HJ, Perrine JJ. The isokinetic concept of exercise. *Phys Ther.* 1967;47:114.

142. Wilk KE. Dynamic muscle strength testing. *In* LR Amundsen (ed.), *Muscle Strength Testing: Instrumented and Non-Instrumented Systems.* New York: Churchill Livingstone, 1990.

143. Davies GJ. *A Compendium of Isokinetics in Clinical Usage,* 3rd ed. Onalaska, WI: S & S Publishers, 1987.

144. Kanehisa H, Miyashita M. Specificity of velocity in strength training. *Eur J Appl Physiol.* 1983;52(1): 104–106.

145. Irion JM. Aquatic therapy. *In* WD Bandy, B Sanders (eds.), *Therapuetic Exercise: Techniques for Intervention.* Baltimore, MD: Lippincott Williams & Wilkins, 2001.

146. Thein-Brody L. Aquatic physical therapy. *In* CM Hall, L Thein-Brody (eds.), *Therapeutic Exercise: Moving Toward Function.* Baltimore, MD: Lippincott Williams & Wilkins, 1999.

147. Harrison RA, Hillman M, Bulstrode S. Loading the lower limb when walking partially immersed: Implications for clinical practice. *Physiother.* 1992;78: 164–166.

148. Harrison R, Bulstrode S. Percentage weight bearing during partial immersion in the hydrotherapy pool. *Physiother Practice:* 1987;3:60–63.

149. Carrière B. *The Swiss Ball: Theory, Basic Exercises, and Clinical Applications.* New York: Springer-Verlag, 1998.

150. Klein-Vogelbach S. *Functional Kinetics.* New York: Springer-Verlag, 1990.

151. Caraffa A, Cerulli G, Projetti M, et al. Prevention of anterior cruciate ligament injuries in soccer. A prospective controlled study of proprioceptive training. *Knee Surg Sports Traumatol Arthrosc.* 1996;4(1): 19–21.

152. Silvers HJ, Mandelbaum BR. Preseason conditioning to prevent soccer injuries in young women. *Clin J Sport Med.* 2001:11(3):206.

153. Keshner, E. Controlling stability of a complex movement system. *Phys Ther.* 1990;70(12):844–854.

6

Training for Joint Stability

TIMOTHY F. TYLER

MICHAEL MULLANEY

Objectives

The reader will be able to:

- Describe the important influence of joint structures on maintaining joint stability.

- Explain the contributions of both contractile and non-contractile structures to joint stability.

- Describe the influence of age and gender on joint stability.

- Identify contemporary therapeutic exercise interventions to enhance dynamic joint stability.

- Describe the utility of bracing and taping techniques to enhance joint stability.

Outline

INTRODUCTION

Joint stability is an essential component of human movement. The purpose of joint stability is to maintain weight bearing and non–weight bearing posture so that purposeful movement can occur. Proximal joint stability is essential to achieve distal joint mobility. This concept is evident in the client with Duchenne's muscular dystrophy who is unable to feed himself. Such a client lacks scapular stability, which is necessary to enable the more distal muscles of the arm to move. So this client, because of scapular instability, is unable to move the hand to the mouth and so cannot feed himself. Similarly, the absence of an anterior cruciate ligament (ACL) contributes to knee joint instability. In this case, however, function may or may not be affected depending on factors related to dynamic contractile tissue and the joint stability provided by other non-contractile (capsuloligamentous) restraints. The local components of joint stability include the topography, or architecture, of the joint, non-contractile soft tissues (joint capsules and ligaments) and contractile tissues (musculotendinous structures). However, postural influences occurring some distance away from a specific joint may also influence joint stability. For example, the chain reaction associated with sitting with the trunk in a slumped posture can position the scapula in a protracted and downward alignment, thereby increasing laxity at the glenohumeral joint.

Rehabilitation clinicians are often called upon to restore dynamic joint stability following injury. Contributing to task difficulty are the inherent stability differences between differing joints, and between individuals, in addition to the influence of gender on capsuloligamentous tissues. Therefore, the rehabilitation clinician must draw from a myriad of treatment techniques to achieve dynamic or contractile joint stability in the presence of disease or injury.

THE ORGANIZATION OF JOINT STABILITY

Joint Structure and Design

The foundation of all joint stability lies in the structural design of the particular joint. The structural design of a joint will in turn, determine its functional nature. If a joint is designed primarily for mobility, it will differ in structure from a joint designed for stability. To discuss joint stability, we must first investigate the structural foundation for each type of joint. Joints are categorized according to their structural design and fit into one of the following groups: synarthroses, amphiarthroses, or diarthroses.

The *synarthrodial joints* are traditionally known for their articulating joint stability and lack of mobility. Synarthrodial joints utilize fibrous tissue as the connective material between the bony components. A synarthrodial joint that is

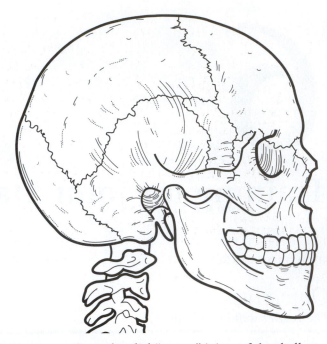

Figure 6.1   Synarthrodial "suture" joints of the skull.

designed as interlocking edges connected by fibrous tissue is called a suture joint. Located in the skull (**Figure 6.1**), this joint design allows for minimal movement during early childhood, but fusion of the two bony edges occurs during maturation. This design enables early mobility for cranial passage during the birthing process, but is truly designed to provide protection to the central nervous system (CNS).

Amphiarthrodial joints are known for their articulating cartilaginous surfaces. These joints will connect two bony surfaces together by either fibrocartilage or hyaline cartilage. The symphysis pubis joint utilizes fibrocartilage to join the two pubic bones together. This joint is designed for extreme weight bearing stability; however, during pregnancy this fibrocartilage softens in response to fluctuating hormone levels to allow joint mobility for cranial passage. An amphiarthrodial joint, which utilizes hyaline cartilage between two bony components, is termed a synchondrosis. These joints, such as the first sternocostal joint, connect two ossifying centers of bone. Once again, designed for early mobility, these joints ossify with maturation and develop into a stable bony union.

The final joint design categorization is the *diarthodial joints*. Until now, our description of primary joint function has centered on stability of simplistically designed human articulations. Our discussion will now introduce a more complexly designed joint categorization that considers mobility a primary component of function. As with synarthrodial and amphiarthrodial joints, diarthrodial joints vary in size and function according to location along the kinetic chain.

The structure of diarthrodial joints differs from that of previously discussed joint articulations in that their bony components move freely in relation to one another (**Figure 6.2**). In contrast to the stable cartilaginous syarthrodial and amphiarthrodial joints, diarthrodial joints articulate indirectly within a joint capsule. The articular capsule consists of an outer fibrous capsule and an inner synovial membrane that is responsible for the production of synovial fluid. The articular hyaline cartilage lining of the bony ends of the two bones that contribute to a diarthrodial joint and the synovial fluid that reduces joint friction and provides joint nutrition are found within the joint capsule (**Figure 6.3**). Diarthodial joints present an environment that sacrifices primary anatomical stability for active mobility.[1]

Key Point:

The basis of joint stability lies in its structural design. Three primary joint structure categories include synarthrodial, amphiarthrodial and diarthrodial. Diarthrodial joints often sacrifice stability for active mobility.

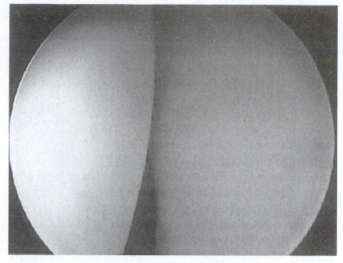

Figure 6.3   Arthroscopic view of articular hyaline cartilage.

Diarthrodial Joint Designs

There are six major diarthrodial joint designs throughout the human body. The anatomical architecture of each joint is considered its primary stabilizing characteristic, corresponding directly with its function. For example, a large weight bearing joint like the hip (**Figure 6.4**) possesses considerable bony congruency and structural stability. In contrast, smaller non–weight bearing joints, such as the acromioclavicular and glenohumeral joints of the shoulder (**Figure 6.5**), rely more on secondary stabilization from adjacent capsuloligamentous structures due to their inherent lack of bony stability. In learning about joint movements, the concept of *mechanical degrees of freedom* should be appreciated. For example, a joint that rotates primarily around one axis is said to have one degree of freedom (uniaxial). From an osteokinematic standpoint, anatomical joints have between one degree (uniaxial) and

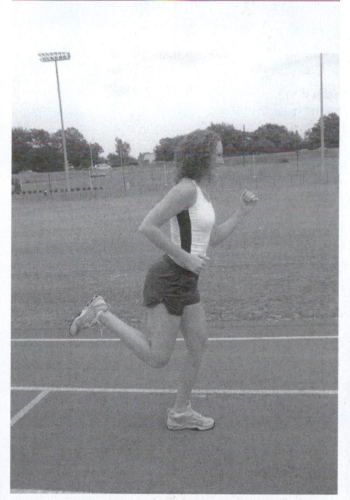

Figure 6.2   Upper and lower extremity diarthrodial joint movements when running.

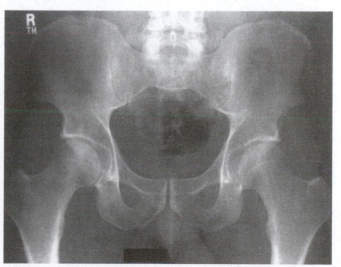

Figure 6.4   Radiograph of the pelvis and hip joints.

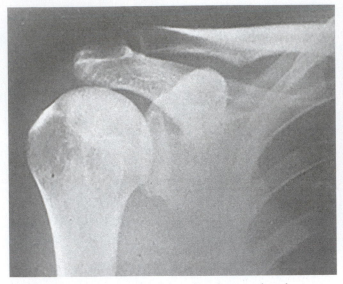

Figure 6.5   Radiograph of the glenohumeral and acromioclavicular joints.

three degrees (triaxial) of freedom. However, joint motion descriptions that combine osteokinematic (rotational) and arthrokinematic (translatory) joint movements enable certain joints (such as the hip and glenohumeral joints) to be described as having up to six degrees of joint freedom. Understanding the arthrokinematic contributions to joint function becomes increasingly important when the rehabilitation clinician intervenes with manual therapy techniques.

Plane Joints.   Plane joints are considered to have three degrees of rotational freedom (triaxial), are numerous throughout the body, have smooth articular surfaces, and possess poor primary structural stability from bone architecture. The carpal joints of the hand **(Figure 6.6a)** and the tarsal joints of the foot are examples of plane joints. Plane joints place a high demand on secondary stabilization from capsuloligamentous structures and tertiary stabilization from musculotendinous structures.

Condyloid Joints.   Condyloid joints are considered to have two degrees of freedom (biaxial), allowing flexion–extension in the sagittal plane, *abduction–adduction* (movement away from and toward the midline, respectively) in the frontal plane, and *circumduction* (arc-like combination of frontal and sagittal plane motion). These joints are seen in the metocarpophalangeal joints of the hand **(Figure 6.6b)**. This structural design sacrifices stability from bony architecture in favor of increased joint mobility, placing greater importance on the secondary (capsuloligamentous) and tertiary (musculotendinous) stabilizers.

Saddle Joints.   Saddle joint surfaces are anatomically designed with both a convex and a concave bony architecture at each joint end. Most noted of these joints is the

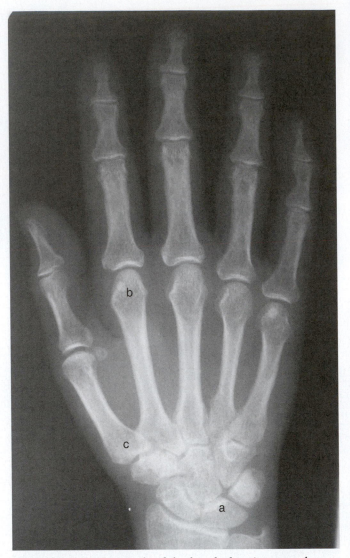

Figure 6.6   Radiograph of the hand, showing carpal (a), metacarpophalangeal (b), and carpophalangeal (c) joints.

carpometacarpal joint of the thumb **(Figure 6.6c)**. These joints have two degrees of rotational freedom (biaxial). The joint is highly mobile by design, allowing for flexion–extension, abduction–adduction, and *opposition* (ability to bring the thumb tip in contact with the palmar surface of the other digits). The highly mobile function available at these joints dictates that the surrounding secondary capsuloligamentous stabilizers enhance stability.

Hinge Joints.   Hinge joints are considered to have primarily one degree of freedom (uniaxial) and allow for *flexion* (joint angle becomes smaller with movement) and *extension* (joint angle becomes larger) movements. Most noted of these joints is the elbow **(Figure 6.7)**. The primary structural stability of the elbow joint is provided by the bony architecture between the concave olecranon and coronoid processes of the ulna and the convex trochlea of the distal humerus.

articulates within the shallow glenoid fossa. The gleno-humeral head is considerably larger than its articulating glenoid surface and is designed with a loose, mobile joint capsule to further enhance its functional mobility. Due to the poor bony architectural design, secondary (capsuloligamentous) and tertiary (musculotendinous) stabilizers are essential to maintain glenohumeral joint stability.

Pivot Joints.   Pivot joints have one degree of rotational freedom (uniaxial). Most noted of these joints is the atlantoaxial joint of the cervical spine. This articulation between the odontoid process of the second cervical vertebra (axis) and the first cervical vertebra (atlas) possesses minimal inherent bony stability, being strictly dependent on secondary ligamentous stabilization. This lack of structural stability in such a vulnerable region should be noted when evaluating injuries to the cervical region.

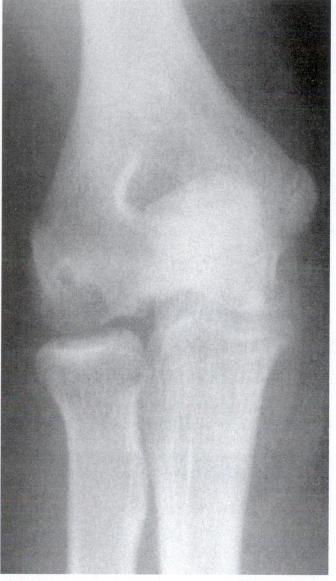

Figure 6.7   Radiograph of the elbow (ulnohumeral "hinge" and radiohumeral joints).

Ball and Socket Joints.   Ball and socket joints have three degrees of rotational freedom (triaxial) and are highly mobile. The overall structural design of these joints includes a spheroidal surface moving within the socket of the adjoining articular surface. Most noted of these joints are the hip and the glenohumeral joint of the shoulder; however, the stability of the bony architecture of these two joints varies greatly. As mentioned earlier, the weight bearing hip joint possesses an inherently stable structural design. The spherical head of the femur articulates deeply within the acetabulum. In contrast, the glenohumeral joint also possesses a high degree of mobility, but sacrifices its structural stability. The articular glenoid surface is typically oriented in a superior, anterior direction during overhead functional activities. The hemispherically shaped humeral head

> ## Key Point:
> The anatomical architecture of each joint corresponds with its function. The stability of many diarthrodial joints depends on secondary stabilization from capsuloligamentous (non-contractile) and tertiary stabilization from musculotendinous (contractile) tissues.

Non-Contractile Stability

Restraints involved in providing joint stability are categorized as being either non-contractile or contractile. Non-contractile restraints include the capsule, ligaments, fascia, skin, meniscus, and the design of the joint surfaces. Non-contractile structures are interdependent, beginning with the design of the joint surfaces. In contrast, contractile stabilizers (musculotendinous tissues) provide dynamic joint stability. (**Figure 6.8**)

Joint Capsule.   The joint capsule is composed of two layers, an outer layer called the stratum fibrosum and an inner layer called the stratum synovium. The stratum fibrosum is a dense fibrous capsular tissue which completely surrounds the ends of the bony components of the joint. The stratum synovium is attached to the periosteum of the component bones by *Sharpey's fibers*, (organized collagen bundle attachments) receiving further reinforcement from ligamentous and musculotendinous structures that cross the joint. Together these layers combine to provide the joint with its first soft tissue component of joint stability.[2] Encapsulated within the joint capsule are a variety of mechanoreceptors which transmit information about the status of the joint to the CNS (see Chapters 7 and 8).[3,4] These mechanoreceptors are sensitive to different stimuli such as compression, tension, vibration, and rate and

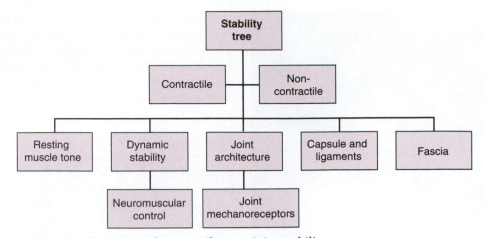

Figure 6.8   Structures that contribute to joint stability.

direction of motion. Probably the most functionally important mechanoreceptors for joint stability are the Golgi ligament organs and the Golgi-Mazzoni corpuscles. The Golgi ligament organs are sensitive to ligament stretching, providing CNS feedback to help facilitate immediate dynamic joint stability when a joint is being forced into an unstable position. The Golgi-Mazzoni corpuscles are located within the inner joint capsule layer, providing feedback during joint capsule compression. These mechanoreceptors communicate with the surrounding muscles to provide joint protection via enhanced dynamic joint stability.[3,4] If injured, the joint capsule has an adequate blood supply and the potential to heal.

Ligament.   A ligament is connective tissue that connects a bone to a bone. The ultrastructure of ligaments depends on where the ligament is located in the body. In general, a ligament is composed of extracellular matrix, fibroblasts, collagen, and elastin.[5] The arrangement of the collagen fibers and the collagen to elastin fiber ratio determines the relative ability of the ligament to provide stability to a particular joint.[6] The collagen fiber orientation in ligaments is varied in relationship to the topographic bony architecture, providing differing levels of joint stability depending upon the direction of the applied joint forces.[7] In the spine, the ligamentum flavum has more elastin fiber content than collagen fiber content. Therefore, it is much more elastic, contributing to the mobility needed to reach down and touch one's toes, for example. In contrast, the ACL has a considerably higher collagen content and is more likely to rupture before its stretches. Research using animal models have revealed that mechanoreceptors found in the ACL are linked to dynamic knee joint stability.[8,9] Gardner[9] demonstrated a direct reflex connection between the ACL and muscle reflex initiation at the knee joint. It is essential to remember that no single ligament functions independently in providing non-contractile joint stability when muscles are not activated around a joint. Rather, each of the ligaments of any joint (in addi-

tion to the other non-contractile stabilizers previously mentioned) provide at least minimal stability contributions when confronted with applied joint forces.

Joints that provide a variety of functional motions such as the glenohumeral joint at the shoulder require a complex arrangement of ligaments for stability. For example, the vertebral column not only has movement at individual segments but also has large amounts of combinational mobility. Combinational mobility warrants a spinal ligamentous system consisting of two parts: the *intrasegmental system* and the *intersegmental system*. Although the ligaments alone cannot independently support a joint, both of these systems directly contribute to overall joint stability during functional movements.[10]

The intrasegmental system connects individual or adjacent vertebrae to each other. The ligamentum flavum, the interspinous and the intertransverse ligaments are the foundation of the intrasegmental system. The ligamentum flavum is located within the vertebral canal from the second cervical vertebra to the sacrum, connecting the spinal lamina of each adjoining vertebra. This ligament adds to total joint stability by providing a compressive tension on the intravertebral disks in the neutral position.[1] The interspinous ligament of the intrasegmental system runs from the spinous processes of the adjacent vertebra. This ligament maintains stability primarily in the lumbar spine by preventing excessive separation of spinous processes during flexion. Like the interspinous ligaments, the intertransverse ligaments are well developed in the lumbar spine. These paired ligaments run from each pair of transverse processes and resist side-bending movements. These ligaments work like collateral ligaments, where the left intertransverse ligament will be stressed during right side bending and the right intertransverse ligament will be slacked.

The primary components of the intersegmental system include the anterior longitudinal ligament (ALL), the posterior longitudinal ligament (PLL), and the supraspinous ligament (**Figure 6.9**). The ALL, located on the anterior

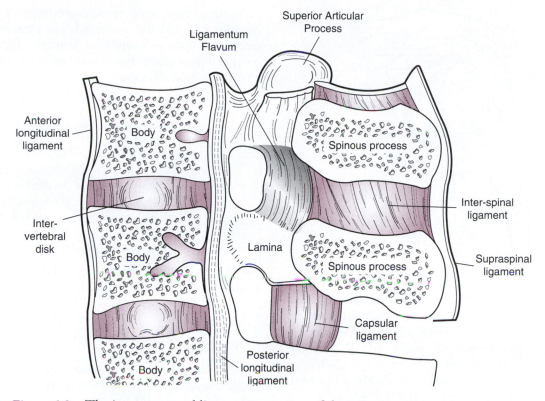

Figure 6.9   The intersegmental ligamentous system of the spine.

surfaces of the vertebral bodies, possesses superficial fibers that bridge multiple vertebral segments and deep fibers that attach individual vertebrae and disks. This anterior support not only provides static vertebral stability but also offers dynamic stability during back extension. This stability may be compromised following a decrease in disk height or vertebral bone mineral density.

The PLL is located along the posterior surfaces of the vertebral bodies, within the vertebral canal. As with the ALL, the superficial fibers bridge multiple vertebrae together and the deeper fibers attach to the intervertebral disks. The PLL provides tension and stability during spinal flexion and the ligament becomes slack with spinal extension. The PLL is an essential support for preventing posterior disk prolapse; however, its resistance to axial tension, especially in the lumbar region, is notably weaker compared to the ALL.

The final triad of the intersegmental ligaments is the supraspinous ligaments. These ligaments are attached to the tip of each spinous process. Originating in the cervical region as the ligamentum nuchae, these ligaments run down each spinous process and blend into the lumbar musculature. The supraspinatus ligaments provide stability during flexion by preventing separation between each spinous process. These ligaments are often the first ligaments to fail during an extreme hyperflexion injury episode.

Spinal stability requires a complex mixture of both uniplanar and multiplanar combinational movements. This complexity is addressed through the important combinations of intrasegmental and intersegmental ligamentous systems. However, these elaborate ligamentous systems are designed to assist the other non-contractile and contractile joint stabilization contributors with spinal stability, not to serve as the sole or primary spinal stability source. All complex ligamentous systems depend on a combination of stabilizing factors, including joint design (as mentioned earlier) in addition to the trainable dynamic joint stability provided by musculotendinous contributions.

While the spinal ligamentous system is a complex matrix of strong stabilizing forces, the glenohumeral ligamentous system is considerably different. The glenohumeral ligaments are considered thickenings of an already slack glenohumeral capsule. The fibrous capsule has a volume that is twice that of the humeral head.[11] This laxity allows for a highly mobile joint with a lack of intrinsic non-contractile stability. The angular alignment of the glenoid fossa is often associated with shoulder instability. Saha et al.[12] reported that 80 percent of unstable shoulders displayed an anteriorly tilted glenoid fossa. The glenohumeral ligaments are designed to add stability to the highly mobile joint capsule. Each of the three glenohumeral ligaments is designed to check or become taut at specific glenohumeral joint range of motion locations.

The idea of a *circle stability concept*, introduced by Bowen and Warren,[13] proposed that humeral head translation is resisted by capsular restraints on all sides of the

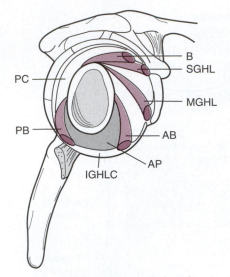

Figure 6.10   The circle concept of glenohumeral joint stability (PC = posterior capsule, AB = anterior band of the inferior glenohumeral ligament, PB = posterior band of the inferior glenohumeral ligament, MGHL = middle glenohumeral ligament, B = biceps tendon, SGHL = superior glenohumeral ligament, AP = aponeurosis, IGHLC = inferior glenohumeral ligament complex). (From MK Bowen, RF Warren. Ligamentous control of shoulder stability based on selective cutting and static translation experiments. *Clin Sports Med.* 1991;10:757-782.)

joint (**Figure 6.10**). While the coracohumeral ligament and the superior glenohumeral ligament provide non-contractile support against inferior motion, the inferior glenohumeral ligament is the primary restraint for anterior humeral head migration. This restraint is strongly evident as the glenohumeral joint is abducted and externally rotated.[14] The inferior glenohumeral ligament possesses a sling effect as the glenohumeral joint is externally and internally rotated during abduction. With this motion the anterior band and axillary pouch of the inferior ligament are pulled taut to protect from anterior humeral head migration. In contrast, as the glenohumeral joint is internally rotated from this position, the posterior band and the axillary pouch of the inferior ligament are pulled taut to prevent posterior humeral head migration.[14]

These designs of a circle concept or a sling effect to provide glenohumeral joint stability are relatively primitive. The glenohumeral joint provides considerable functional mobility. To enable this mobility, the capsuloligamentous stabilizing component of the glenohumeral joint requires a simplistic design. This need for mobility and lack of inherent structural non-contractile stability leaves this joint highly vulnerable to subluxation, dislocation or structural disruption. Once again, the need for the

supporting contractile musculotendinous stabilizers to enhance joint stability is stressed. The glenohumeral ligamentous complex depends on joint design, joint alignment and musculotendinous contractile structures to offer a functionally stable joint.

> ## Key Point:
> Non-contractile and contractile tissues in addition to joint architecture contribute to joint stability. The stratum fibrosum and stratum synovium of the joint capsule provide non-contractile tissue stability. Many joints, like the vertebral column joint system, have a complex arrangement of ligaments to provide non-contractile joint stability.

Contractile Stability

Muscle Tone. Before we can have dynamic joint stability produced by muscular activation we must have muscle tone. *Muscle tone* is the firmness to palpation that a healthy muscle exhibits at rest, which provides joint stability. This firmness is present even in the most relaxed subjects but is lost once the motor nerve supplying the muscle is cut. The muscle tone of normally innervated, relaxed muscles appears to be a function of the non-contractile components of the muscles (epimysium, perimysium, endomysium) in combination with muscular sensory receptors called muscle spindles that are responsible for conveying resting muscle length and stretch-state feedback to the CNS. Muscle tone sets the stage for muscle activation (see Chapter 2).

Muscle Activation. The most important characteristic of a muscle is its ability to develop tension and exert a force to produce dynamic joint stability and purposeful movement. Muscle activity begins in the motor cortex of the CNS with impulses traveling down the corticospinal tract until they reach the anterior horn cells of the gray matter in the spinal cord segment correlating to the muscles, which are being activated. The anterior horn cell bodies, together with their axon and all the muscle fibers they innervate, form a *motor unit*. To a certain extent, an individual can control the degree of dynamic joint stability by regulating muscle activation gradation. When activated, a motor unit stimulates all of the muscle fibers it innervates. However, by stimulating variable numbers of motor units one can control the muscle activation force. Smaller motor units are generally activated first, followed by the activation of progressively larger motor units. By increasing the frequency of stimulation of individual motor units, the percentage of time that each activated muscle fiber develops maximum tension is increased. Not only can muscle force gradation be controlled to provide varying amounts of dynamic joint stability, but the activation of entire muscle group synergies can be modulated to enhance dynamic joint stability (see Chapter 2).

> ## *Key Point:*
>
> Force gradation of an individual muscle or of synergistic muscles can be modulated to enhance contractile or dynamic joint stability.

Dynamic Joint Stability

Stability is defined as the state of being unchanged, even in the presence of forces that would normally change that condition. Riemann and Lephart[15] define joint stability as the state of a joint remaining or promptly returning to proper alignment through an equalization of forces.[15–17] Dynamic or contractile joint stability is the ability to gradate muscle forces and activation modes to prevent joint injury.[18,19] The basic types of muscle activation are isometric (constant length), concentric (shortening), and eccentric (lengthening). Concentric activations display decreased force production with increasing activation velocity. Conversely, eccentric activations display increased force production with increasing activation velocity (see Chapter 5). Isometric muscle activations occur when there is no observable joint movement, thereby providing the joint with maximum stability. Dynamic joint stability requires a well blended combination of muscle activations both proximal and distal to the joint. The client must be able to display dynamic joint stability against multiplanar joint stresses. Functional exercise programs generally increase in difficulty by progressing from more isolated, uniplanar, single segment function to more integrated, multiplanar, multiple segment function (see Chapter 5). The memory of the muscular activation pattern sequence used to enhance dynamic joint stability is a form of neuromuscular control (see Chapter 8).[20]

Neuromuscular Control

Specific neuromuscular activation patterns are essential to dynamic joint stability during function.[21] Riemann and Lephart[15] defined *neuromuscular control* as the unconscious activation of dynamic restraints occurring in preparation for and in response to joint motion and functional joint stability. By stimulating both afferent receptors and CNS control centers, unconscious motor responses can be trained to improve dynamic joint stability.[20,22] The continual processing of afferent information and activity pattern re-adjustments during movement is known as *feedback control*. Proprioceptive information from both non-contractile (capsuloligamentous) and contractile (musculotendinous) tissues is vital to this feedback control mechanism (see Chapters 7 and 8). *Proprioception* refers to the use of sensory input from receptors in muscle spindles, tendons, meniscus, skin, and capsuloligamentous structures to discriminate joint position and movement, including direction, amplitude and velocity, as well as relative tendon tension. Of equal importance to neuromuscular control is the feed-forward mechanism of human movement. *Feed-forward control* has been described as anticipatory actions occurring before the sensory detection of joint stability disruption. Increased muscle tone prior to athletic competition maybe the result of a feed-forward mechanism. Increasing neuromuscular control is an important component of practice for the rehabilitation clinician who treats clients who desire increased dynamic joint stability.[23–25] Motor control concepts are discussed in greater detail in Chapter 8.

> ## *Key Point:*
>
> Muscle tone is the foundation for contractile tissue contributions to dynamic joint stability. Neuromuscular control proficiency directly influences dynamic joint stability. Dynamic joint stability requires neuromuscular contributions both proximal and distal to the joint. Proprioceptive input contributes to neuromuscular control via both feedback and feed-forward systems.

Generalized Joint Hypomobility vs. Hypermobility

Vast differences in soft tissue composition enable some clients to display hypermobile joints while others are hypomobile. Joint hypermobility is also a well recognized characteristic of collagen tissue disorders such as Marfan syndrome and Ehlers-Danlos syndrome. The literature documenting the relationship between generalized joint mobility and injury is divided.[26–29] In a study of 58 boys and 80 girls (age range 10.3–13.3 years), Kujala et al.[26] reported that joint hypermobility was not associated with a higher incidence of low back pain. In a study of 377 male and female ballet dancers, Klemp et al.[27] reported that dancers who were characterized as having hypermobile joints using Beighton's mobility score (see Chapter 3, and discussed later in this chapter) displayed a direct relationship between the dancer's age and the duration of dance training. Nicholas,[28] who examined the association between the knee injury incidence of "tight" and "loose-jointed" professional football players, reported that hypermobile players were significantly more likely to damage their knee ligaments, while hypomobile players were more likely to sustain muscle strains. In a prospective study of 147 male and 163 female college lacrosse players, Decoster et al.[29] reported an increased rate of ankle injuries among hypermobile subjects and an increased rate of strains among hypomobile subjects, however significant differences were not evident for overall injury rates. What is lacking in each of these studies is knowledge of the capacity for the study subjects to display dynamic joint stability. None of the previous referenced studies examined the relationship between capsuloligamentous joint laxity, dynamic joint stability and joint injuries. Since literature on this subject is lacking, we can only hypothesize that the hypermobile individual would attempt to enhance their poor non-contractile joint stability with increased dynamic joint stability. To decrease injury likelihood the client with joint hypermobility would be better served being "hypermobile with neuromuscular activation efficiency" than "hypermobile with inefficient neuromuscular activation" for dynamic joint control. However, this does not guarantee that acquired joint laxity will not occur.

Key Point:

Literature on the relationship between injury rates and joint hypermobility is divided; however, it can be hypothesized that the client with poor joint stability from non-contractile tissue would benefit from enhanced contractile tissue neuromuscular activation efficiency to improve dynamic joint stability.

Intrinsic vs. Acquired Joint Laxity

Intrinsic joint laxity refers to the amount of laxity or hypermobility an individual is born with.[30] An individual can evaluate his or her relative hypermobility by performing a series of five screening tests described by Beighton et al.[31] This method, later validated by Bird et al.,[32] uses a zero to nine point system to score hypermobility by evaluating the client's ability to hyperextend the knees and elbows past 10°, to passively extend the fingers so they are parallel to the forearm, to passively abduct the thumb so it touches the forearm, and to forward bend down with the knees locked in extension and touch the palms to the floor (**Figure 6.11**) (see Chapter 3). This hypermobility assessment can be used in both non-impaired clients and those who have congenital collagen tissue disorders.

Intrinsic joint laxity is most often observed in people with disorders like Marfan's syndrome. Marfan's syndrome is a congenital disorder often associated with musculoskeletal, cardiovascular and vision impairments. Clients with Marfan's sydrome often appear taller and thinner than other members of the same family and possess marked inherent joint laxity. These clients are most affected by the cardiovascular abnormalities associated with this syndrome. Mitral valve prolapse develops early in life and progresses with age. The vision changes take many forms in these clients; most characteristic is the subluxation or dislocation of the lens. All of these defects are associated with connective tissue deficiencies and must be considered during therapeutic exercise program planning. Intrinsic joint laxity adds to client care complexity and needs to be addressed, regardless if it is the primary or a secondary, underlying condition.[33,34]

Acquired joint laxity occurs from the plastic deformation associated with injury pathomechanics. In the shoulder the glenohumeral capsuloligamentous structures provide a static check against excessive humeral translation at extreme positions.[14,35–40] The glenohumeral joint ligaments are distinct capsular thickenings (as shown in **Figure 6.10**). However, considerable anatomical variation exists between clients. Non-impaired elasticity of the superior, middle and inferior glenohumeral ligaments is essential to non-contractile glenohumeral joint stability.[40,41] Bigliani et al.[36] reported that the inferior glenohumeral ligament was prone to plastic deformation before disruption, concluding that deformation occurred during injuri-

9-Point Beighton Scoring System for Joint Hypermobility
1 point on each side for......
• Passive dorsiflexion of the fifth metacarpophalangeal joint to 90°
• Opposition of the thumb to the flexor aspect of the forearm
• Hyperextension of the elbow > 10°
• Hyperextension of the knee > 10°
1 point for......
• Forward trunk flexion placing hands flat on floor with knees extended.
Maximum score = 9

Figure 6.11   Beighton scoring system.

ous loading without actual ligamentous detachment.[36] The result of acquired glenohumeral joint laxity may be an increased likelihood of humeral head subluxation or dislocation.

Acquired joint laxity also commonly occurs in the knee joint. Capsuloligamentous knee joint stability can be evaluated with clinical ligament stress testing.[42] Anterior cruciate ligament laxity (ACL deficiency) can be evaluated with an anterior drawer test, the Lachman test, an instrumented Lachman test using an arthrometer (**Figure 6.12**), or radiographic measurements with a weight providing anterior tibial translation. Posterior knee joint laxity (posterior cruciate ligament deficiency) can be tested with the posterior drawer test or posterior sag sign. The varus stress test (tibiofemoral joint adduction) is used to evaluate lateral knee joint stability. The valgus stress test (tibiofemoral joint abduction) is used to evaluate medial knee joint stability. Knee joint laxity is graded for each of these tests using a one to four scale. In this scale one represents approximately five mm of joint space opening. Two represents between five and ten mm of joint space opening, while a grade of three or four represents approximately 10–15 mm and 15–20 mm of joint space opening, respectively.[42]

Key Point:

A clinical hypermobility screening exam can aide in detecting a client with joint hypermobility. Intrinsic joint hyperlaxity is often associated with congenital disorders like Marfan's syndrome. Acquired joint laxity from plastic deformation of the non-contractile tissues is usually associated with a violent force at the joint or with repetitive submaximal joint loading forces.

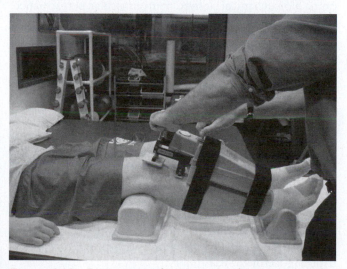

Figure 6.12 Instrumented anterior Lachman's test with an arthrometer.

Spinal Stability

According to Panjabi,[43] spinal stability is the combination and relationship between three subsystems of the body: the spinal column, the spinal musculature, and the neural network. Together these subsystems work in coordination to promote non-impaired, pain free function. The spinal column makes up a non-contractile stabilization subsystem incorporating the osseous and articular vertebral structures in addition to their capsuloligamentous stabilizers. The spinal muscles make up an active subsystem that relies on the force generating capacity of muscles to stabilize the spinal column, not only in neutral or resting positions, but also during dynamic activities. The neural component of this system is termed the control subsystem, which must recognize and respond to sensory (afferent) feedback from the previous two subsystems by enabling a motor (efferent) muscular response to any situation. To a certain extent, each one of these subsystems is considered an interdependent spinal stabilization component, capable of compensating for the other. However, these compensations, if prolonged, may lead to further dysfunction within the spinal stabilization system.

The structure and articular arrangement of the spinal column is designed as a first line of stability. If this subsystem is compromised, stabilization may be compromised if the other subsystems cannot fully compensate. The most common structural instabilities are spondylolysis and spondylolisthesis. Spondylolysis is considered a stress or fatigue fracture of the pars interarticularis, often caused by repetitive trauma associated with trunk flexion and hyperextension. This condition is often seen and can be exacerbated by gymnastics, football, weightlifting, and diving. If this condition is exacerbated, or if further separation occurs at the defect, slippage of the vertebral segment may occur. In this case, the defect is referred to as spondylolisthesis.

Definitive diagnosis can be achieved through an oblique radiograph showing what is referred to as "a Scottie dog with a collar" pattern (spondylolysis) (**Figure 6.13**) or "a Scottie dog decapitated" pattern (spondylolisthesis). There defects are most commonly observed in young, active clients and athletes. These clients will present with back pain, muscle spasm, loss of lordotic curve and limited straight leg raise ability. These clinical signs are all associated with the compensatory mechanisms of the other subsystems. Fractures such as these may take up to 16 months to heal with conservative treatment, including rest, intermittent traction, possible spinal orthosis, and dynamic stability training of the lumbo-pelvic region musculature. If conservative treatment fails, spinal stabilization surgery may be needed.[43–45]

The structural stability of the spine may also be affected by high velocity facet joint injuries. These "whiplash" injuries often involve articular locking or ligamentous disruption of the facet joint. Spinal fractures

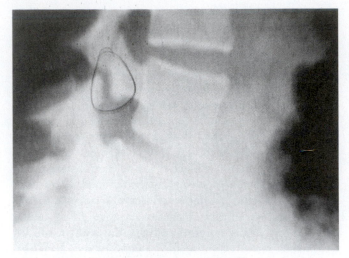

Figure 6.13   Radiographic view of the "Scotty dog" lesion at the pars region of the lumbar spine.

such as burst fractures or an unstable vertebral fracture may also create spinal instabilities that often require surgical fusion for spinal stabilization.

In the active or contractile subsystem, the spinal musculature is responsible for maintaining spinal stability both during resting posture and during dynamic movements. Bergmark[46] categorized the trunk muscles into local and global muscle systems, according to their particular stabilization role. The *local muscle system* is located deep, attaching distally or proximally to the lumbar vertebrae. The local muscle system is responsible for controlling the stiffness and intervertebral relationship of the spinal segments, as well as for maintaining lumbar spine posture. The *global muscle system*, as described by Bergmark,[46] encompasses the larger, more superficial trunk muscles. These muscles are responsible for spinal movement and transferring loads directly between the thoracic cage and the pelvis. The local and global muscle systems work together as external loads are accepted by the global muscles, enabling the local muscle system sufficient time to respond to functional loads and maintain spinal stability.

This muscular subsystem is essential for spinal stability, but it can be compromised with overuse, fatigue or by an inhibitory neural feedback response from muscular spasm or pain. Type II (fast twitch) muscle fiber atrophy[47–49] and pathologic inner structural changes[49] have been reported among clients who experience low back pain. These muscular changes may explain why clients who experience low back pain may have similar strength as non-impaired clients, but the endurance of their low back musculature is compromised.[50,51] Suboptimal muscular subsystem function may be the weak link that creates a primary spinal stabilization system deficiency, or it may result as a secondary factor following compromised non-contractile stabilization system function.

The neural subsystem for spinal stabilization requires coordinated trunk muscle co-contractions or co-activations. Co-contraction is an essential component to stabilization at all joints; however, it is of no greater necessity than at the spine. Co-contraction relies on neural programming to decrease reciprocal inhibition (see Chapter 2) and direct antagonistic muscles to increase their activity in unison.[52] The neural control subsystem must continually monitor and re-evaluate spinal position, external loading, neuromuscular activity, and spinal mobility. The neural component acts as the "glue" for the spinal stabilization system. The neural control subsystem links together the non-contractile subsystem (spinal column) and the active contractile subsystem to effectively maintain spinal stability.

> ## *Key Point:*
> The spinal column, musculature, and neural network are subsystems that work together to maintain spinal stability. Poor low back muscular endurance, not poor strength, is more often associated with clients who experience low back pain. Although the co-contraction of muscular agonists and antagonists enhance stability at all joints, it is of potentially its greatest value in maintaining dynamic spinal stability.

Increased Joint Laxity in Females: Fact or Fiction?

Recent interest in joint laxity has focused on the knee joint of athletic female subjects. Studies have shown that women are two to eight times more likely to sustain an ACL tear than their male counterparts.[53,54] This influx of injuries has been attributed to four major areas: anatomical or biomechanical design, neuromuscular performance, joint laxity, and hormonal influences. Reflecting on these four contributing factors and considering gender differences, few if any of these can be altered. It has been established that women have greater anterior-posterior knee joint displacement than men during arthrometric measurements.[55–57] Although it has been established that females have a greater degree of ACL laxity, it is still uncertain how much of a role laxity plays in the increased rate of female ACL lesions. Many have investigated the relationship between knee joint laxity and ligamentous injury among athletes, only to find contrasting information.[28–30,58–60] In a study that compared characteristics of 31 clients who had sustained bilateral ACL ruptures with 23 non-impaired control subjects, Harner et al.[59] concluded that increased ligamentous laxity was not a contributing factor to ACL injury.

The hormonal differences between genders are often scrutinized when discussing female joint laxity. The identification of estrogen and progesterone receptors in the fibroblasts of the human ACL suggests that these hormones play a role in ligamentous consistency.[61] Unlike their male counterpart, the menstruating female undergoes a cyclical hormone level change throughout her reproductive years. Heitz et al.[62] reported that ACL laxity increased with peak estrogen and progesterone levels.[62] These alterations in ACL cellular metabolism may change the ACL composition, rendering it more susceptible to injury. In a recent study by Wojtys et al.,[63] it was concluded that women had a higher percentage of ACL injuries during the midcycle ovulatory phase and a reduced injury percentage during the luteal phase. Interestingly, this study also found that subjects who took oral contraceptives had a decreased rate of ACL injury during the ovulatory phase.

As mentioned earlier, many potential factors may influence the predisposition of ACL injuries among females. However, the influence of hormonal changes on the collagen metabolism of connective tissues among females should not be overlooked. While testosterone levels in males tends to increase collagen metabolism, female sexual hormones tend to decrease both the collagen content and the fibril diameter of connective tissues.[64] Although the female hip and knee joints may be most susceptible to injuries associated with connective tissue degradation, sudden fluctuations in the levels of these sexual hormones may affect the dynamic stability of all joints.

The glenohumeral joint is also commonly affected by gender-related joint laxity. However, in a generalized laxity study of 124 preadolescent and adolescent males and females (6–18 years of age), Marshall et al.[65] concluded that females had significant looseness in some joints but not the shoulder. Additionally, they reported that overall joint laxity or "total looseness" was not related to gender, but more of a characteristic of the individual. Other studies have suggested that, contrary to expectations, generalized joint laxity does not correlate with shoulder laxity in females.[66] Contrarily, Beighton et al.[31] described females as possessing more glenohumeral joint range of motion than males at any age, although range of motion for both males and females decreases with age. Glenohumeral joint laxity studies of both high school and college athletes concluded that females had greater laxity than their male counterparts.[67,68] Conflicting reports of the influence of gender on glenohumeral joint laxity underscores the need for continued research in this area, with particular interest focusing on the joint laxity changes that occur during and after puberty.

Gender-related laxity should be considered during the evaluative process and when designing a therapeutic exercise program, particularly among athletically active female clients. Regardless of the contradicting gender-related joint laxity studies, it is well known that females have a proportionally greater incidence of ACL lesions than males. By considering the demographics of our client populations, we can design the most efficacious therapeutic exercise program for each individual client.

> ## Key Point:
> Factors that contribute to an increased ACL injury incidence among females may include differences in anatomical design, neuromuscular performance, joint laxity, and hormonal effects. The influence of gender on the laxity of specific joints should be considered during therapeutic exercise program planning.

Joint Stability Changes Across the Lifespan

Over the lifespan, from fetal development through adulthood, soft tissue consistency and composition changes. These changes related to aging represent a complex situation involving not only physiological considerations, but also activity-induced "wear and tear."[69] The soft tissue aging process may also be influenced by occupation, habitual activities of daily living and behavioral patterns.

Elastin fibers are present in many compliant connective tissues (including hyaline cartilage)[70] serving a joint protection function. Elastin fibers first appear as microfibril scaffolds in the developing fetus, maturing as the fetus develops and continuing to proliferate during childhood. Mature elastin fibers have a long half-life in connective tissues and are replaced largely in response to local injury.[70] High elastin fiber content contributes to the pliability and flexibility of the joints of children.

Joint capsules are predominantly composed of Type I collagen. Collagen is the most abundant protein in the human body, comprising 90 percent of ligament and joint capsule composition.[71] The ultrastructure of collagen consists of molecules arranged in a highly ordered extended triple helix with a specific composition and molecule orientation in differing ligaments based on their unique functional characteristics. The remaining portion of capsuloligamentous structures consists of water, proteoglycans, fibronectin, elastin, and glycoproteins. During the aging process there may be a selective increase of type II collagen fibers, particularly at capsular attachments.[72] Histological degenerative changes often appear as early as the third decade.[73,74] The anterior glenohumeral joint capsular structures are reportedly stiffer in later decades.[41] These aging effects have been noted in the overall flexibility of soccer players in their thirties, when compared with younger players.[75] Although age-related flexibility decreases are clinically obvious, such changes have not been studied extensively.

Age-induced soft tissues changes that directly affect joint stability are difficult to categorize. As rehabilitation clinicians, we must consider the vocational, athletic, and psychobehavioral characteristics of our aging clients. As seniors and "*baby boomers*" (clients born between 1946 and 1964) become increasingly active, rehabilitation clinicians must realize that individuals place different demands on their joints, largely dictated by their lifestyle. During the aging process, muscular strength, size, and type II (fast twitch) muscle fiber content tend to be reduced.[76] Each of these age-related degenerative changes, combined with knowledge of a client's physical demands, must be considered when developing a therapeutic exercise program.

> ### *Key Point:*
> Although joints are primarily composed of collagen fibers, elastin fibers give connective tissue its pliability. As we age, collagen composition and elastin content begin to change, contributing to increased joint stiffness.

TREATMENT TECHNIQUES

Neuromuscular Training

Neuromuscular training may include any therapeutic exercise activity that attempts to facilitate a coordinated neuromuscular response. Conceptually, neuromuscular training provides dynamic stability through muscle coordination and *kinesthetic sense* (the musculotendinous tissue contribution to proprioception) during movement.[16,25,26,77,78] Neuromuscular training can be used to increase dynamic or contractile stability at many joints. Neuromuscular training to increase lumbo-pelvic stabilization is similar in philosophy to that used when treating the client who has ACL deficiency at a knee or who has glenohumeral joint instability. Following capsuloligamentous joint injury or surgical intervention, healed non-contractile joint restraints are insufficient to adequately restore functional joint stability because the coordinated neuromuscular control mechanisms required during activities of daily living and sports are still lacking. A joint with poor dynamic stability also generally has delayed neuromuscular reactivity to sudden loads, leading to episodes of recurrent joint instability. Several methods of neuromuscular training have been described in the literature, including wobble board training, perturbation training, agility training, stabilometry, multiplanar functional training (jumping and landing), and neuromuscular reactive training. The basic concepts behind these training methods is that by repetitively challenging an individual's ability to maintain dynamic joint control in specific positions or during specific tasks, neuromuscular reactivity and, subsequently, dynamic joint stability are improved.[78–80]

Wobble board or balance board training emphasizes the ability to maintain a balanced three-dimensional posture to enhance dynamic joint stability. Rehabilitation clinicians should design therapeutic exercises that challenge the client to focus on three-dimensional dynamic postural awareness and the position of the body in space, with the aim of maintaining balance without changing the base of support. Balance exercises are generally initiated from a stable surface using double limb support before progressing to single limb support on progressively more unstable surfaces (**Figure 6.14, Table 6.1.**) (see Chapter 9). Dynamic three dimensional postural awareness training using wobble boards and a Bosu ball can increase dynamic ankle joint stability (**Figure 6.15a–b**).[80,81] Tropp et al.[81] evaluated the effect of a 10-week dynamic ankle joint stability program using an "ankle disk" on 65 male soccer players with a history of ankle instability compared to a non-impaired control group (with no previous ankle injury) over the course of a soccer season. Following participation, the training group displayed an ankle joint re-injury risk that was equivalent to the primary ankle injury risk of the non-impaired control group.[82] Caraffa et al.[83] performed a similar study in an attempt to prevent ACL injury among soccer players. The researchers instructed one group of 300 soccer players to perform traditional training, while an experimental group of 300 players added dynamic three dimensional postural awareness training using a wobble

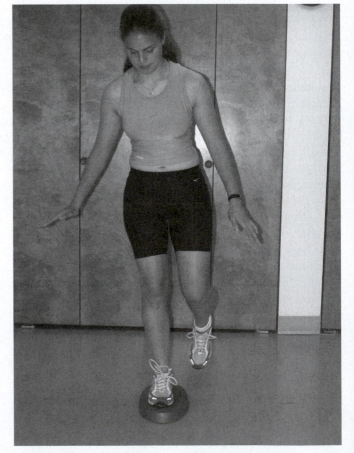

Figure 6.14   Single lower extremity support on an unstable surface.

TABLE 6.1   Neuro-reactive stability training progression

I. Double-limb balance
   a. Eyes opened
   b. Eyes closed
   c. External challenges

II. Single-limb balance
   a. Eyes opened
   b. Eyes closed
   c. External challenges

III. Soft foam stability trainer
   a. Double-limb
   b. Single-limb
   c. Eyes opened
   d. Eyes closed
   e. External challenges

IV. Wobble board
   a. Double-limb
   b. Single-limb
   c. Eyes opened
   d. Eyes closed
   e. External challenges

board to their program. Over a period of three consecutive soccer seasons, the athletes in the experimental group displayed an incidence of ACL injury that was one-seventh that observed in the traditional training group. Dynamic postural awareness training using a wobble board can be a useful method of enhancing three dimensional dynamic joint stability to both prevent joint injury and rehabilitate joints following injury.

Another type of neuromuscular training combines three dimensional dynamic postural awareness training on a roller board, progressing to maintaining posture during the application of sudden perturbations. The intent behind adding perturbations is to improve the acuity of the neuromuscular responses by exposing the client to unexpected dynamic three-dimensional joint control and balance challenges. Conceptually, perturbation training enables clients to develop the protective neuromuscular reactions needed to avoid moving into unstable joint positions, thereby protecting the joints from injury (see Chapter 7). In a randomized trial, Fitzgerald et al.[84] studied perturbation training among 26 subjects with knee joint instability associated with ACL deficiency. They treated one group with traditional rehabilitation and the experimental group received additional perturbation training. The group that received additional perturbation

training had significantly greater success in returning to high level sporting activities without experiencing symptoms of knee instability. Fitzgerald et al.[85] also examined the effect of perturbation training on a physically active 73-year-old woman with knee osteoarthritis. After 12 treatment sessions and a home therapeutic exercise program utilizing perturbation training, the client was able to walk on level surfaces and stairs and return to golf and tennis without episodes of knee instability and with reduced pain. Pintsaar et al.[86] evaluated the benefits of perturbation training to increase postural control during single limb stance among female soccer athletes. Subjects with dynamic ankle joint instability displayed greater use of a *hip postural control strategy* (**Figure 6.16**) when medially directed perturbations of the support surface were administered during single limb stance. Following an eight-week duration perturbation training program, subjects displayed greater use of a more appropriate *ankle postural control strategy* (**Figure 6.17**) in response to the same perturbation.

Recently, the use of lower extremity plyometrics and jump training has received attention as a possible aid in the prevention of non-contact ACL injuries.[87] While it is still early in terms of research that has focused on postural control during athletic movements, appropriately administered plyometric training may turn out to be a crucial ACL injury reduction factor, especially among females (see Chapters 5 and 11). A growing body of evidence is linking ACL injuries to poor neuromuscular control and faulty technique during jumping, landing, stopping, and running directional changes. Neuromuscular control must be developed in three dimensional (frontal, sagittal and transverse motion planes), functionally relevant patterns, to reduce ACL stresses by transferring the local loading forces to proximal and distal synergistic musculotendinous stabilizers. Proper plyometric training can decrease knee joint reaction forces.[87] The movement patterns, muscle stretch-shortening cycles, and proprioception associated with plyometric activities can be easily and effectively integrated into therapeutic exercise programs designed to prevent knee injuries. These same exercises can be applied to a functionally unstable upper extremity with diminished proprioception.

Hewett et al.[87] examined the effects of a six-week duration plyometric training program on landing mechanics and lower extremity strength among 11 adolescent female athletes involved in jumping sports. The plyometric training program was designed to decrease landing forces via improved lower extremity neuromuscular control during jump landing. Peak landing forces during a volleyball block jump decreased by 22 percent. Horizontal forces acting upon the knee during landing were reduced approximately fifty percent. Hamstring: quadriceps femoris peak torque ratios increased 26 percent on the non-dominant lower extremity and 13 percent on the dominant lower extremity. Hamstring power increased 44 percent

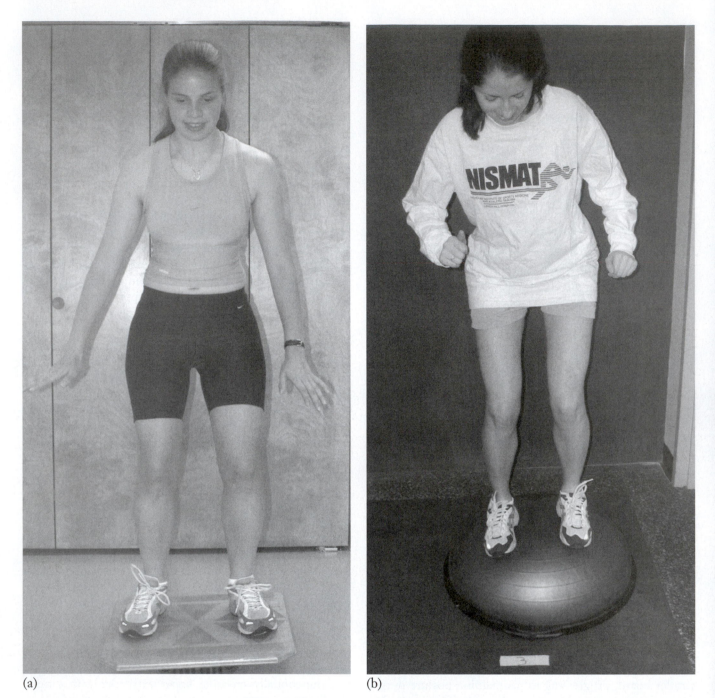

(a)   (b)

Figure 6.15   Dynamic three dimensional postural awareness training. (a) wobble board training; (b) Bosu ball training.

on the dominant lower extremity and 21 percent on the non-dominant lower extremity. Mean vertical jump height increased by 10 percent overall. These results suggest that a properly performed plyometric training regimen may help prevent knee injury among female athletes involved in jumping sports such as volleyball by increasing dynamic knee joint stability during landing and by improving neuromuscular control. Appropriately administered, plyometric jump training may also help correct torque imbalances between the hamstring and quadriceps femoris muscle groups.

While the improved vertical jumping aspect of plyometric training is important for athletic conditioning, it is the method of jump landing that is most important in the prevention of knee injuries. Landing technique is crucial in order to avoid placing the knee into combined hyperextension, valgus, and external rotation, "the point of no return" (see Chapter 11). Essentially, the athlete needs to jump land softly and quietly while using the knees and hips as shock absorbers with the shoulders positioned over the knees during landing. Equally important to prevent ACL injury is the avoidance of an upright posture and

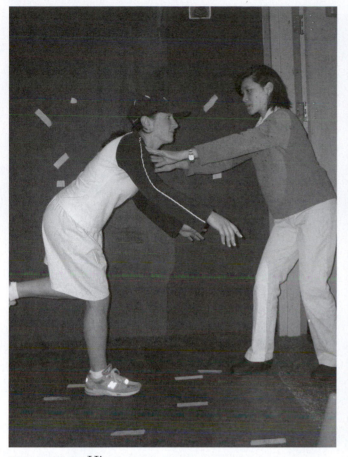

Figure 6.16   Hip strategy.

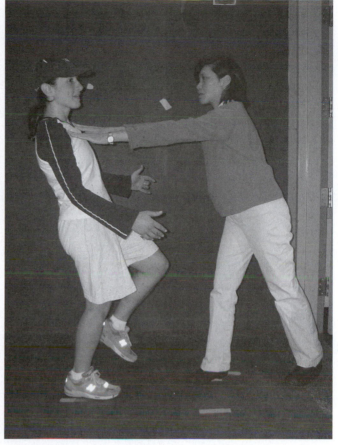

Figure 6.17   Ankle strategy.

knee joint hyperextension during activities that involve sudden directional changes such as cutting, jump landings, and running accelerations-decelerations (see Chapters 9 and 11). When performing plyometric activities the subject should be able to "stick and hold" the landing for five to six seconds without having to take additional steps (**Figure 6.18**). More recently, this type of neuromuscular training was used to prospectively evaluate its effect on the incidence of knee injury among female athletes. Hewett et al.[88] compared two groups of female athletes with one group of male athletes throughout their high school soccer, volleyball, and basketball seasons. One group of female athletes received structured six week duration plyometric training prior to sports participation, while the other female group and the male group did not receive training. Weekly reports included the number of practice and competition exposures and injury mechanisms. There were 14 serious knee injuries among the 1,263 athletes tracked throughout the study. Ten of 463 untrained female athletes sustained serious knee injuries (eight non-contact), two of 366 trained female athletes sustained serious knee injuries (zero were non-contact), and two of 434 male athletes sustained serious knee injuries (one was non-contact). Untrained female athletes had a 3.6 times higher knee injury incidence than trained female athletes and 4.8 times higher

knee injury incidence than male athletes. The knee injury incidence of trained female athletes was not significantly different from that of untrained male athletes. There was a significant difference in the incidence of non-contact knee injuries between the female groups. This prospective study reported a decreased knee injury incidence among female athletes who participated in a structured plyometric training program. Activities used during the technique, fundamentals, and performance phases of this program are listed in **Table 6.2**.

Reactive neuromuscular training (RNT) is a therapeutic exercise regimen that emphasizes kinesthetic or proprioception input and places less emphasis on verbal and visual input from the rehabilitation clinician.[89] This type of training asks only that the client respond to a stimulus created by an external force (e.g., being pulled by elastic tubing). The initial emphasis is not on improving strength, but rather on developing dynamic joint stability, proprioception, and postural awareness when confronted with changes in equilibrium. Foundational to RNT is the use of neuromuscular activation to maintain postural alignment during functional activities. Through the activation of muscular synergists, abnormal joint translations are controlled. These activities are designed to emphasize movement quality over quantity (repetitions/sets, etc).[90]

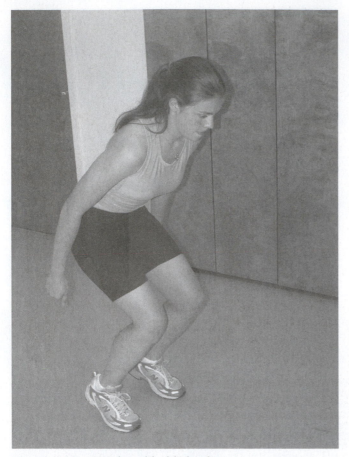

Figure 6.18   "Stick and hold" landing.

Currently, there are no studies that have tested the validity or reliability of this treatment method.

Stabilometry is commonly used to measure an individual's ability to balance on a single lower extremity (**Figure 6.19**). Stabilometry or balance training has been shown to improve dynamic ankle joint stability.[21] Using an electronic stabilometer, Rozzi et al.[91] reported that single leg balance training is an effective method of improving joint proprioception among subjects with unstable and with non-impaired ankle joints. Zatterstrom et al.[92] reported that clients with chronic knee instability who performed one year of stabilometry training during single limb stance in addition to standard rehabilitation displayed significantly better postural stability during single leg stance than a group that received standard rehabilitation alone. The ability to maintain balance during single leg stance tends to decrease with age. Therefore, rehabilitation clinicians should consider the ability of an older client to maintain single leg stance prior to therapeutic exercise program planning, and when necessary, incorporate stabiliometry or balance training early into the program (see Chapters 9 and 10).[93]

Supplementing standard therapeutic exercise programs with any of the neuromuscular treatment interventions described previously may improve the dynamic joint sta-

bility of clients with joint instability, thereby decreasing their disability level and improving their function. Obtaining sufficient dynamic joint stability to overcome capsuloligamentous insufficiency is an inherently complex and complicated physiologic process. In the absence of capsuloligamentous joint stability, the fact that many individuals return to pre-injury levels of function without surgical intervention suggests that compensatory mechanisms can be developed within the neuromuscular system structures of the involved joint in addition to motor adaptations at proximal and distal segments to provide varying levels of supplemental dynamic joint stability.[94] This suggests the importance of both higher and lower level CNS organization to optimize dynamic joint stability.

> ## *Key Point:*
> Neuromuscular training provides dynamic joint stability by improving proprioception and coordination. Using sudden perturbations with a neuromuscular training program helps the client develop protective reactions. A properly designed plyometric training program may help prevent knee injuries by improving dynamic joint stability.

Proprioceptive Neuromuscular Facilitation

Dynamic joint stability can also be enhanced using *proprioceptive neuromuscular facilitation (PNF)* patterns and techniques designed to place specific demands on the client to achieve specific desired neuromuscular responses.[95] By stimulating or hastening the response of the neuromuscular system through proprioceptor stimulation the ultimate purpose of PNF is to improve proximal and peripheral dynamic joint stability.[96–99] Shimura and Kasai[100] reported increased motor evoked potentials in upper extremity muscles following PNF intervention. Joint approximation is a commonly used PNF technique. By applying joint compression or approximation, isometric neuromuscular activity around a joint is enhanced, thereby improving dynamic joint stability. A clinical application of joint approximation occurs when the rehabilitation clinician has a client who is status-post knee surgery and who would benefit from lateral weight shifting activities to increase dynamic knee joint stability prior to ambulation[4,32,96] (**Figure 6.20**).

Rhythmic stabilization uses an isometric activation of a *muscular agonist* (the prime mover or muscle(s) most influential in bringing about a movement) immediately followed by an isometric activation of the *muscular antagonist* (muscle(s) that slow down or stop a movement) to facilitate dynamic joint stability (**Figure 6.21**). *Rhythmic initiation* is a PNF technique that takes the client's upper or

TABLE 6.2 Jump training program.

Descriptions		Repetitions or Time	
Phase I: Technique		**Week 1**	**Week 2**
Wall jumps	Hop up and down on toes next to wall with knees slightly flexed and arms raised overhead	20 seconds	25 seconds
Tuck jumps*	From a standing position, jump, and bring both knees up to chest as high as possible, repeat quickly.	20 seconds	25 seconds
Broad jumps ("stick the landing")	Two-footed jump as far as possible. Hold landing for five seconds.	5 reps	10 reps
Squat jumps*	Standing jump raising both arms overhead, land in squatting position touching both hands to the floor.	10 seconds	15 seconds
Double leg cone jumps*	Double leg jump over cones with feet together.	30 seconds (side-to-side) 30 seconds (back-to-front)	30 seconds (side-to-side) 30 seconds (back-to-front)
180° jumps	Two footed jump. Rotate 180° in midair. Hold landing for two seconds, then repeat in the opposite direction.	20 seconds	25 seconds
Bounding in place	Jump from one leg to the other straight up and down, progressively increasing rhythm and height.	20 seconds	25 seconds
Phase II: Fundamentals		**Week 3**	**Week 4**
Wall jumps		30 seconds	30 seconds
Tuck jumps*		30 seconds	30 seconds
Jump, jump, jump, vertical jump	Three broad jumps with a vertical jump immediately after the final broad jump.	5 reps	8 reps
Squat jumps*		20 seconds	20 seconds
Bounding for distance	Start bounding in place and slowly increase distance with each step, keeping knees high.	1 run	2 runs
Double leg cone jumps*	Begin in stride position with one foot well in front of the other. Jump up, alternating foot positions in midair.	30 seconds (side-to-side) 30 seconds (back-to-front)	30 seconds (side-to-side) 30 seconds (back-to-front)
Scissor jump		30 seconds	30 seconds
Hop, hop, stick the landing	Single leg hop. Stick the second landing for five seconds. Increase hop distance as technique improves.	5 reps/side	5 reps/side

(continued)

TABLE 6.2 Jump training program. (Continued)

Phase III: Performance	Descriptions	Repetitions or Time	
		Week 5	Week 6
Wall jumps		30 seconds	30 seconds
Step, jump up, down, vertical	Two-footed jump onto a 6–8 inch step. Jump down from step with two feet, then perform a vertical jump.	5 reps	10 reps
Mattress jumps	Two-footed jump on a mattress, trampoline, or other padded surface.	30 seconds (side-to-side) 30 seconds (back-to-front)	30 seconds (side-to-side) 30 seconds (back-to-front)
Single-legged jumps for distance	One-legged hop for distance. Hold landing with knees flexed for five seconds.	5 reps/side	5 reps/side
Jump into bounding	Two-footed broad jump. Land on single leg, then progress into bounding for distance.	3 runs	4 runs
Hop, hop, stick the landing		5 reps/side	5 reps/side

(Fifteen to twenty minutes of stretching, two laps of skipping, and two laps of side shuffles preceded jumping exercises. * = Performed on an exercise mat).

(Reprinted with permission from Hewett TE, Stroupe AL, Nance TA, et al. Plyometric training in female athletes. Decreased impact forces and increased ham-string torques. *Am J Sports Med.* 1996;24(6):765-773.)

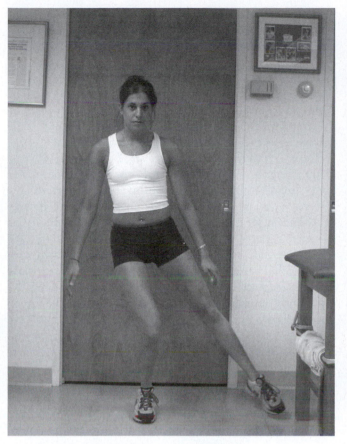

Figure 6.19   Single lower extremity balance.

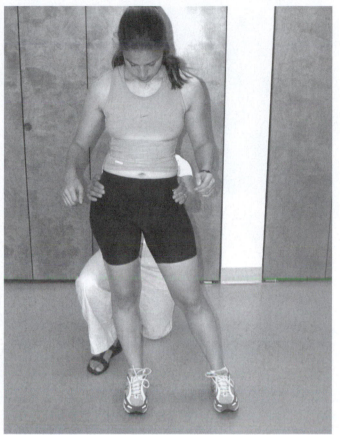

Figure 6.20   Joint approximation in standing.

lower extremity initially through a progression of passive joint range of motion, progressing towards active-assistive range of motion, and finally active movement through the agonist pattern ultimately achieving joint stability. Rhythmic initiation can be used for a wide variety of clients with musculoskeletal or neurological impairments, including those who have sustained a cerebrovascular accident (CVA) and display a functional limitation with their inability to initiate a hand-to-mouth movement. One of the best applications of this PNF technique is at the shoulder, where dynamic stability is at a premium secondary to the humeral head being much larger than the glenoid fossa. During rhythmic initiation with a client who has sustained a CVA, the rehabilitation clinician may first use manual contact to passively move the client's hand toward their mouth while simultaneously providing joint approximation at the scapulothoracic articulation, glenohumeral joint and elbow joint to help facilitate dynamic joint stability prior to progressing to active-assistive shoulder range of motion. For the client who has glenohumeral joint instability due to capsuloligamentous injury, the rehabilitation clinician may want to begin strengthening the shoulder musculature in unstable positions using rhythmic stabilization techniques to regain dynamic glenohumeral joint stability at or near the position of instability or ap-

prehension. Rhythmic stabilization techniques can also be used on a more global scale with clients who present with poor postural control ranging from mild muscle tone reductions that tend to resolve spontaneously to incapacitating sitting and standing balance deficiencies secondary to various neurological impairments. A PNF program that uses rhythmic stabilization may begin with having the client attempt to maintain a sitting position on the edge of a bed. Following this, rhythmic stabilization can be applied in anterior/posterior, medial/lateral or diagonal directions to challenge the client's ability to maintain dynamic postural stability of the trunk while in a sitting position. The same progression can be used while the client is standing to improve his or her standing balance prior to gait instruction.[101]

Repeated contractions is a PNF technique that uses a series of isometric activations performed during a concentric activation of a muscular agonist throughout a specific range of motion to increase dynamic joint stability. This technique may help increase dynamic joint stability during the performance of purposeful movements. The rehabilitation clinician uses this technique when they facilitate isometric muscle activation at different elbow joint flexion angles during concentric muscle activation to improve dynamic joint stability. The rehabilitation clinician

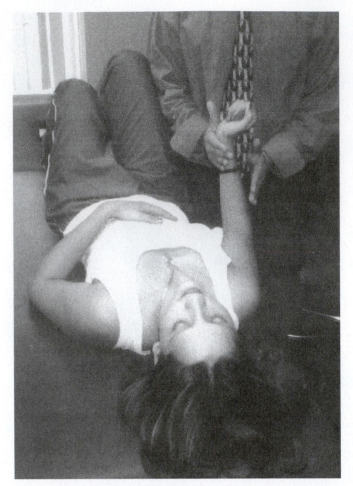

Figure 6.21   Rhythmic stabilization of the upper extremity.

begins this PNF technique by placing the clients elbow in extension. The client is then asked to flex the elbow. During elbow flexion, the rehabilitation clinician provides enough resistance to stop the motion at various points within the range of motion eliciting a series of isometric muscle activations.

Slow reversal and *slow reversal hold* are two PNF techniques that involve activation of a muscular agonist followed immediately by muscular antagonist activation. These PNF techniques are often used when rehabilitation clinicians treat clients who have impaired balance. Treatment using this PNF technique may begin with having the client attempt to maintain a sitting posture on the edge of a bed as the rehabilitation clinician applies either slow reversal or slow reversal hold techniques. The application of these techniques may continue as the client attempts to maintain correct sitting posture with reaching, and finally during standing and walking. Use of PNF treatment methods to improve gait following a CVA has been shown to be beneficial.[102] There are also *mass movement* PNF techniques that combine rotational (spiral) and

diagonal upper or lower extremity movements that closely resemble functional movement patterns to facilitate dynamic joint stability. These spiral and diagonal movements are intended to simulate the natural spiral and rotatory characteristics of the musculoskeletal system (see Chapter 5). These movements are intended to be performed in harmony with the longitudinal alignment and structure of the muscles from origin to insertion. Each diagonal PNF pattern has a flexion and an extension component.

Upper extremity flexion diagonal 1 is initiated with scapular elevation, abduction and upward rotation, combining relative glenohumeral joint flexion, adduction and external rotation, while the elbow may move into flexion or extension, or may remain in extension throughout the movement pattern. The wrist and fingers flex and deviate toward the radial side and the thumb adducts. When performing this pattern, the client moves the upper extremity away from their side as if about to "bring food toward the mouth" (**Figure 6.22a**) to a position where the upper arm is aligned across the chin (**Figure 6.22b**). *Upper extremity extension diagonal 1* is exactly the opposite movement, beginning with the upper extremity positioned across the chin and moving it back down toward the client's side. Upper extremity extension diagonal 1 is initiated with scapula depression, adduction, and downward rotation, combining relative glenohumeral joint extension, abduction, and internal rotation, while the elbow may move into flexion or extension, or may remain extended throughout the movement pattern. The wrist and fingers extend and deviate toward the ulnar side and the thumb abducts. *Upper extremity flexion diagonal 2* is the other rotatory and diagonal PNF movement pattern. Upper extremity flexion diagonal 2 begins with scapular elevation, adduction, and upward rotation, combining relative glenohumeral joint flexion, abduction and external rotation. The elbow may move into flexion or extension, or may remain extended throughout the movement pattern while the wrist and fingers extend and deviate toward the radial side and the thumb extends. Clients are instructed to "pull the sword from the scabbard" near their opposite side front pants pocket (**Figure 6.23a**) and finish in a position "like they are carrying a pizza" (**Figure 6.23b**). *Upper extremity extension diagonal 2* is the opposite movement, beginning with scapular depression, abduction, and downward rotation, combining glenohumeral joint extension, adduction and internal rotation. The elbow may move in flexion or extension, or may remain extended throughout the movement pattern. The wrist and fingers flex and deviate toward the ulnar side and the thumb opposes the fingers. The use of PNF treatment techniques have been shown to improve the upper extremity function of clients with long term hemiplegia.[103] Comprehensive information regarding these upper extremity diagonal patterns is presented in **Table 6.3.** There are also lower extremity PNF movement pat-

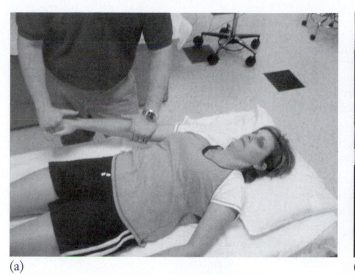 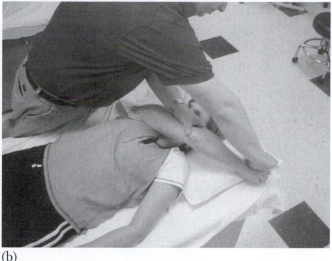

(a) (b)

Figure 6.22 Upper extremity flexion diagonal 1 pattern (D1). (a) initiation; (b) completion.

terns that facilitate dynamic joint stability. *Lower extremity flexion diagonal 1* begins with pelvic protraction while combining hip flexion, adduction, and external rotation (**Figure 6.24a–b**). During this pattern, the knee may move into flexion or extension, or may remain extended, while the ankle dorsiflexes and inverts and the toes extend. The opposite movement pattern occurs for *lower extremity extension diagonal 1*, where the pelvis begins with pelvic retraction while combining hip extension, abduction, and internal rotation. The knee may move into flexion or extension, or may remain extended, while the ankle plantar flexes and inverts and the toes flex. *Lower*

extremity flexion diagonal 2 begins with pelvic elevation while combining hip flexion, abduction, and internal rotation (**Figure 6.25a–b**). The knee may move into flexion or extension, or may remain extended, while the ankle dorsiflexes and everts and the toes extend. *Lower extremity extension diagonal 2* is the opposite pattern, with pelvic depression in combination with hip extension, adduction, and external rotation. The knee may move into flexion or extension, or may remain extended, while the ankle plantar flexes and inverts and the toes flex. Comprehensive information regarding these lower extremity diagonal patterns is presented in **Table 6.4.**

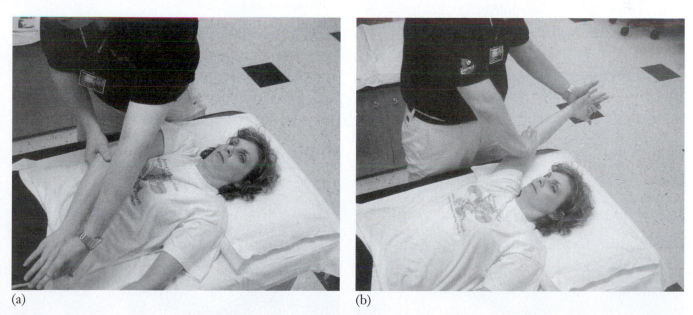

(a) (b)

Figure 6.23 Upper extremity flexion diagonal 2 pattern (D2). (a) initiation; (b) completion.

TABLE 6.3   Upper extremity PNF joint motions

	Scapula	**Glenohumeral**	**Elbow**	**Wrist/fingers**
D1 flexion	Elevation Abduction Upward rotation	Flexion Adduction External rotation	Flexion or extension	Flexion Radial deviation
D1 extension	Depression Adduction Downward rotation	Extension Abduction Internal rotation	Flexion or extension	Extension Ulnar deviation
D2 flexion	Elevation Adduction Upward rotation	Flexion Abduction External rotation	Flexion or extension	Extension Radial deviation
D2 extension	Depression Abduction Downward rotation	Extension Adduction Internal rotation	Flexion or extension	Flexion Ulnar deviation

D1 = diagonal 1; D2 = diagonal 2.

These diagonal and rotational upper and lower extremity PNF patterns can be advanced to a higher level by incorporating the diagonal 1 (D1) and diagonal 2 (D2) patterns with the other PNF techniques introduced earlier, or by performing the activities on an unstable surface such as that provided by a Swiss ball. These advancements may also be seen by re-introducing rhythmic stabilization into a D1 or D2 pattern. For example, while resisting a client during an upper extremity flexion D1 movement, the rehabilitation clinician may stop the movement at various locations in the glenohumeral joint range of motion to incorporate rhythmic stabilization. This technique will challenge dynamic joint stability throughout the range of motion. Diagonal and rotational PNF patterns are designed for functional strengthening, so rehabilitation clinicians are encouraged to integrate these techniques creatively into the therapeutic exercise programs they design.

Key Point:

PNF was created to improve both proximal and distal dynamic joint stability. Rhythmic stabilization, compression, slow reversal, and slow reversal hold are examples of PNF techniques designed to stimulate co-activation of muscular agonists and antagonists. Diagonal and rotatory PNF techniques promote the development of functionally relevant dynamic joint stability.

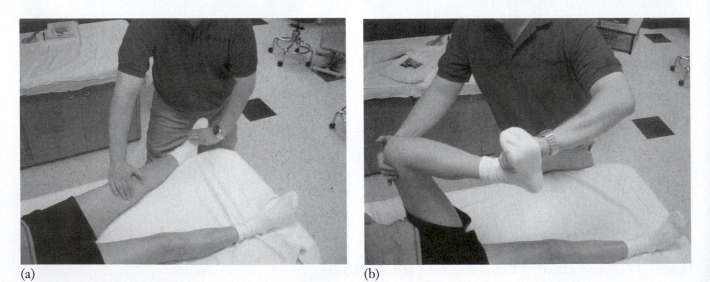

(a)   (b)

Figure 6.24   Lower extremity flexion diagonal 1 (D1). (a) initiation; (b) completion.

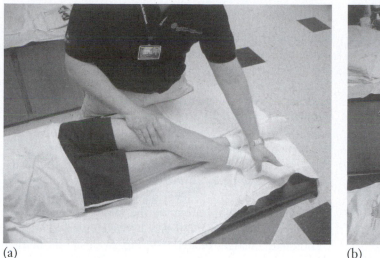
(a)

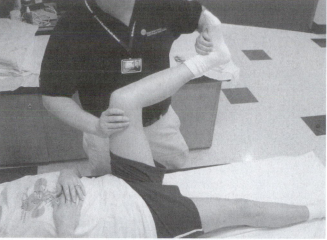
(b)

Figure 6.25   Lower extremity flexion diagonal 2 (D2) (client with limited knee flexion). (a) initiation; (b) completion.

Biofeedback

Biofeedback is a motor learning tool that can be used to measure and train dynamic joint stability. Clients can be taught the tactile appreciation of an activated vastus medialis muscle or biofeedback can be attained via electromyographic (EMG) instrumentation. Specifically, EMG sensors record the level of bioelectrical activity produced by an activated muscle. Biofeedback is commonly used to facilitate vastus medialis muscle activation to increase dynamic knee joint stability in standing or to improve patellar alignment (**Figure 6.26**). Biofeedback has also been used to improve dynamic glenohumeral joint stability during postural adjustments among clients who have experienced a stroke and who have sustained capsuloligamentous glenohumeral joint injury. Even when a client has sensory impairments and cannot voluntarily move an

extremity, appropriately adjusted biofeedback can often detect some level of bioelectrical muscle activity, thereby providing a benchmark for additional volitional muscle activations. The EMG biofeedback device amplifies the bioelectrical activity emitted from the paralyzed extremity, and as the client becomes aware of the activity via an audio or visual cue, he or she is encouraged to achieve even greater muscle activation levels to improve dynamic joint stability.

Biofeedback has been studied and used clinically for a number of years to enhance client recovery following a CVA and to improve both volitional muscle activation and relaxation levels among clients who have sustained a spinal cord injury. Petrofsky[104] used EMG biofeedback to correct Trendelenburg gait patterns among 10 subjects after spinal cord injury. Subjects who received conventional therapy alone had a 50 percent reduction in "hip drop" during gait

TABLE 6.4   Lower extremity PNF joint motions

	Pelvis	Hip	Ankle	Toes
D1 flexion	Protraction	Flexion Adduction External rotation	Dorsiflexion Inversion	Extension
D1 extension	Retraction	Extension Abduction Internal rotation	Plantar flexion Eversion	Flexion
D2 flexion	Elevation	Flexion Abduction Internal rotation	Dorsiflexion Eversion	Extension
D2 extension	Depression	Extension Adduction External rotation	Plantar flexion Inversion	Flexion

D1 = diagonal 1; D2 = diagonal 2.

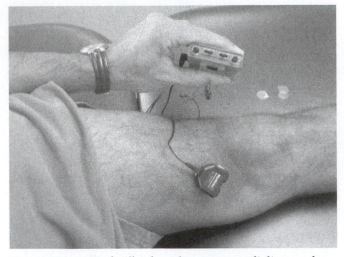

Figure 6.26   Biofeedback at the vastus medialis muscle.

while the group that used biofeedback was able to eliminate the Trendelenburg gait completely over the same treatment duration. While appealing conceptually, the actual efficacy of biofeedback in other areas of the body remains in dispute. Existing research has provided conflicting results, and there is no consensus at present as to whether this technique should be used routinely, selectively, or not at all.

Key Point:

Biofeedback is a useful motor learning tool to both measure and train dynamic joint stability. The cues received by the client during biofeedback use encourages them either to activate or relax the target muscles. However, research that strongly supports the use of biofeedback as a therapeutic exercise modality is sorely lacking.

Lumbar Stabilization Training

The underlying basis for lumbar stabilization training is to minimize the spinal degeneration that occurs from the repetitive loading forces associated with activities of daily living across the lifetime, particularly when the client's body fat percentage has also increased. This degeneration is usually not a painful process. Sometimes it will result in temporary, relatively minor pain that usually resolves in a day or two. Sometimes the consequences are more significant, but usually, in several weeks the pain is gone. Eventually this essentially pain-free cumulative microtrauma may progress to such a level of degeneration that spinal segments are unable to tolerate the forces associated with activities of daily living and may become unstable in association with changes related to aging. At this point neither therapeutic exercise positioning routines, like Williams flexion exercises (**Figure 6.27a–b**) or McKenzie extension exercises (**Figure 6.28a–b**), nor modalities like heat, massage, or joint mobilization may have any lasting effect on improving the client's function.

To improve dynamic lumbar spinal stability and avoid this progression of disability, clients must learn to locate their neutral spine position and develop the ability to maintain this position during activities of daily living. The neutral spine position is the spinal alignment in which maximal bony congruence occurs, allowing for maximal mechanical force tolerance and relatively equal distribution of vertical forces across the weight bearing spinal surfaces. This exact location of neutral spinal alignment can be different for different clients and it may be influenced by the sacral angle or by sacroiliac joint function. To offset the pain associated with the bony lesion, a client with spondylitis or spondylolisthesis may display a slightly more flexed neutral spine position, while a client with a severe lumbar disc herniation may display a more extended neutral spine position to prevent the disc from compressing a nerve root. The most common neutral spine position is

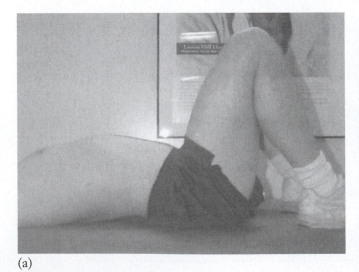

(a)   (b)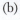

Figure 6.27   Posterior pelvic tilt. (a) start; (b) completion.

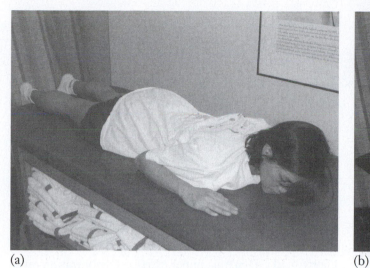

(a)

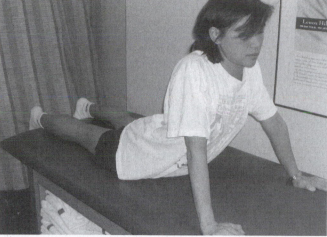

(b)

Figure 6.28   Prone trunk extension. (a) start; (b) completion.

midway between their flexion and extension range of motion. This is the position that the client should maintain to achieve spinal stability when significant forces act on the spine. Significant forces on the lumbar spine occur during sitting, standing for long periods of time, getting in and out of a car, moving around in bed, pushing, pulling, and reaching. Lumbar stabilization training attempts to place the lumbar spine in its most anatomic, pain-free, and balanced alignment and facilitates maintaining that position by using dynamic trunk muscle activation during the performance of functional tasks (see Chapter 5).

The amount of muscular effort needed to maintain neutral spinal alignment depends upon the magnitude of the external forces that are acting upon the spine. Maintaining neutral spinal alignment while standing, walking at an easy pace, or while sitting in proper alignment may take very little effort. However, heavy manual work, weightlifting, and contact sports may, at times, require considerable trunk muscle activation and neuromuscular control to effectively brace the spine to prevent injury. For neutral spinal positioning to be practical and efficient, the client must learn to use only the minimal amount of neuromuscular effort needed in a given situation. Poor hip flexor, paraspinal, hamstring and hip extensor muscle flexibility and/or obesity may make maintenance of neutral spinal alignment difficult or impossible.

Probably the most important component of a spinal stabilization program is incorporating the neutral spine position into functional movement training. Efficient functional movements require power and the body's most effective power source is the lower extremities. Traditional instruction in body mechanics emphasizes maintaining the spine in a vertical position and keeping the feet under the trunk during lifting tasks. If this were the most powerful method of moving, we would throw a ball with the feet planted directly under us and use only the arm. To generate lower extremity power and transfer that power to the upper

extremities, as we must do for many activities of daily living, we must transfer our body weight from one lower extremity to the other, and transmit the force generated from the lower extremities through the trunk to the upper extremities. Unless the lumbar spine is in its optimum stable position to transmit these forces and the trunk musculature (particularly the abdominals) are sufficiently braced to dynamically stabilize the spine, the spine will not tolerate this kind of action well and may be injured. By using the abdominals to stabilize the lumbar spine dynamically, a wide variety of powerful functional movements are possible. With lumbar stabilization training, it is not difficult to achieve short term success for most clients; however, maintaining long term success requires the client to implement the lessons taught by the rehabilitation clinician. The creation of long term positive behavioral changes in the client is needed for positive outcomes to be attained (see Chapter 11). Ideally, lumbar stabilization training should be initiated long before the development of a chronic spine condition where the ultimate goal is avoiding surgery. Ideally, lumbar stabilization training is incorporated into games and functional movement challenges during childhood to prevent spinal injury during adulthood.

> ## *Key Point:*
> The client needs to understand and recognize their neutral spinal alignment at rest and during lifting task performance. The magnitude of the muscle recruitment needed to maintain neutral spine alignment is dependent on the external forces that are applied. The ultimate goal of lumbar stabilization training is to decrease the risk of degenerative spinal changes by instilling in the client positive behavioral changes or healthy back behaviors.

Swiss Ball Therapy for Lumbar Stabilization

The unstable surface provided by a Swiss ball provides a useful multi-purpose therapeutic exercise tool. The enhanced muscular endurance obtained by training on an unstable surface is believed to strengthen the core trunk stabilizing muscles and reduce the likelihood of injury due to repetitive stresses (see Chapters 5, 8, 9, 11). The shape of the ball also facilitates multi-angle training with the client overcoming resistance in various movement plane combinations to enhance dynamic trunk stability. The Swiss ball can also be used as a multi-purpose platform when performing therapeutic exercises designed for upper and lower extremity function in conjunction with lumbar stabilization exercises. For example, alternate upper extremity and lower extremity raises can be performed while lying on the ball to enhance lumbar stabilization during functionally relevant movements (**Figure 6.29**). By having to continually weight shift to maintain dynamic trunk stabilization on the ball, the client has to recruit postural trunk muscles that are not normally used during traditional weight training exercises, (**Figure 6.30**). Ultimately, these core trunk stabilizers become stronger and more endurant, enhancing dynamic trunk stabilization in the process.

Conventional strength training using resistance machines and to a certain extent training with free weights like dumbbells or barbells on stable platforms predominantly train dynamic joint stability in only one primary movement plane. During the performance of three dimensional functional movement patterns the unstable surface provided by a Swiss ball might more effectively facilitate trunk muscle recruitment for dynamic stabilization in a functionally relevant manner. Examples of the benefits of dynamic trunk stability occur when a football lineman or a ballet dancer powerfully uses both lower and upper extremities through the core to move an opponent or to lift a dance partner, respectively.

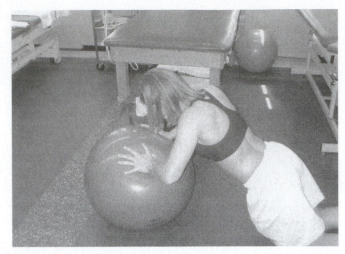

Figure 6.30   Dynamic upper extremity stabilization on a Swiss ball.

The spherical shape of the Swiss ball enables clients to train muscles through a greater range of motion than provided by flat surfaces. For example, while lying with the lower back on the center of a Swiss ball, clients can perform abdominal crunches beginning with the abdominal muscles in the stretched position (**Figure 6.31**). This stretched position cannot be achieved while lying on a horizontal surface as is commonly used when performing traditional bent knee sit-ups. The muscular pre-stretch that is mediated by the rounded surface may create an environment that optimally increased dynamic proximal and core stability, thereby improving distally joint mobility.

Gantchev and Dimitrova[105] reported that muscle activation patterns change when arm elevations are performed while standing on an unstable surface. Compared to the same maneuver on a stable surface they observed increased co-activation between antagonistic postural muscles in addi-

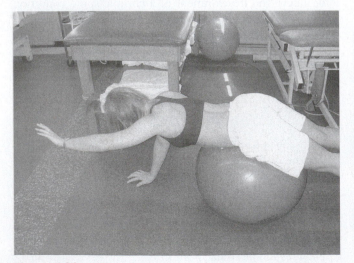

Figure 6.29   Alternate upper extremity raises on a Swiss ball.

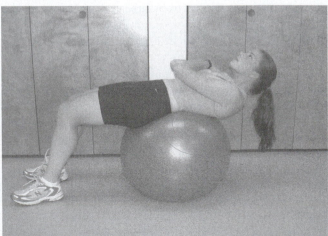

Figure 6.31   Abdominal crunches on a Swiss ball.

tion to changes in trunk muscle activation timing to enhance dynamic stability. They concluded that postural control when balancing on an unstable surface consists of adapting the neuromuscular program to maintain stability, while the overall postural strategy is maintained. Gantchev and Dimitrova's[105] findings supports the use of devices like the Swiss ball to increase dynamic joint stability through enhanced postural muscle activation levels. The dynamic joint stability gained from training on devices like the Swiss ball is most likely due to the improved neuromuscular coordination achieved by training in movement patterns that deviate from traditional therapeutic exercises. Additionally, the unstable surface provides a useful "pallet" from which the creative rehabilitation clinician can better integrate upper and lower extremity function through the trunk.

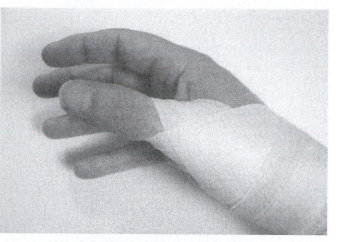

Figure 6.32   Spica athletic taping for gamekeeper's thumb.

> ## Key Point:
> Training on an unstable surface such as a Swiss ball is believed to increase dynamic stability of core trunk muscles with and without upper and lower extremity integration. Training on surfaces like that provided by a Swiss ball enables a greater therapeutic exercise range of motion enabling more effective three dimensional, functionally relevant movements.

Taping for Joint Stability

Taping can help prevent joint injury or facilitate an injured client's return to function by providing non-contractile joint stability and possibly by enhancing muscle activation to provide dynamic joint stabilization. Tape provides joint stability by limiting abnormal or excessive joint mobility of the sprained joint while also protecting the injured soft tissue structures. An added value of taping may be the enhanced proprioceptive feedback that is provided during activity.[106] An example of athletic tape application to enhance non-contractile joint stability is spica taping to protect an ulnar collateral ligament injury at the thumb (gamekeeper's thumb) (**Figure 6.32**). Taping provides stability around the injured joint and proprioceptive feedback as the tape becomes tighter on the skin when the joint approaches motion extremes at which capsuloligamentous injury most often occurs.

Tape can also be used in conjunction with a therapeutic exercise program to treat a client who has patellofemoral pain. The evaluation and treatment of patellofemoral alignment is important in order to enhance normal patellar tracking within the femoral trochlea, thereby increasing the likelihood of therapeutic exercise program effectiveness.[107–109] Four positional components have been described for examining patellar orientation in relation to the femur. These positions are described as: 1) medial-lateral

tilt, 2) medial-lateral glide, 3) internal-external rotation in the frontal plane, and 4) anterior-posterior tilt in the sagittal plane.[110–115] Once patellar malalignment has been identified, taping with an inflexible tape can be used to correct alignment or provide proprioceptive feedback to enable pain-free therapeutic exercise performance.

One of the most commonly observed patellar malalignments is a lateral tilt. The taping technique to correct this malalignment is a medially directed pull from lateral to medial (**Figure 6.33**). Kowall et al.[116] used a prospective randomized study that tested the efficacy of patellar taping in the management of patellofemoral joint pain versus a standard therapeutic exercise program. Results on a visual analog pain scale revealed that both groups reported similar decreases in patellofemoral pain. However, the authors of this study did not identify the true etiology of the patellofemoral pain, nor did they select the client population that received taping intervention based on patellofemoral

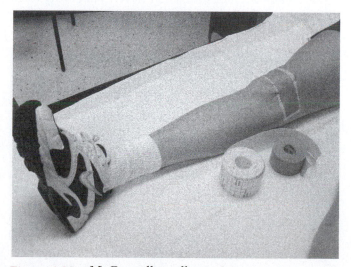

Figure 6.33   McConnell patellar taping.

alignment. The absence of patellofemoral pain reduction differences between groups could be attributed to the lack of proper patellofemoral malalignment identification prior to taping intervention.[113] Bockwrath et al.[117] examined the effect of patellar taping on anterior knee pain and used a Merchant radiographic view (**Figure 6.34**) to assess its affect on malalignment. Although clients who were taped reported decreased pain, patellar alignment changes were not evident during the performance of isometric quadriceps femoris muscle activation. Our experience suggests that patellar taping is an effective method of relieving patellofemoral pain when used in conjunction with an appropriate therapeutic exercise program. The exact mechanism by which patellar taping alleviates pain is unknown. Perhaps subtle changes to patellar alignment help to reduce contact pressures and synovial tissue compression, providing temporary pain relief. Conversely, the positive influence of patellar taping may be the result of enhanced proprioceptive feedback.[116,118,119]

Kinesio Taping® uses a stretchy tape to reduce muscle pain, decrease lymphadema, increase muscular performance, and enhance dynamic joint stability.[120] Although research evidence supporting the use of Kinesio Taping® is lacking, testimonials supporting its applications have been highly promoted. Conceptually, this treatment method applies stretchy tape in the pattern of muscle fiber orientation to support muscle function and joint stability, improve lymphatic drainage, increase joint range of motion and decrease muscle pain. This taping method may be a useful treatment option for a client who presents with glenohumeral joint instability secondary to neuromuscular dysfunction. The lack of neuromuscular control associated with a CVA often leads to a painful hemiplegic shoulder. When a client who has sustained a CVA reaches the flaccid stage, impaired proprioception, poor muscle tone and paralysis reduce the dynamic glenohumeral joint stability that is normally provided by the rotator cuff muscles. This paralysis now increases the glenohumeral joint stabilization demands of the non-contractile capsuloligamentous tissues. The continual distraction force from gravity often creates a painful shoulder condition. Conceptually, Kinesio Taping® may be used initially to substitute for rotator cuff muscle function, helping to prevent the development of a "painful shoulder syndrome" due to the effects of unconstrained gravitational glenohumeral joint distractive forces. Eventually, this taping method may also support and facilitate rotator cuff muscle activation during therapeutic exercise performance. To perform this technique, the elbow is flexed to 90° and the upper arm is raised to 90° abduction. Following this a Y shaped piece of stretchy tape is applied proximally from the middle aspect of the lateral upper arm with the proximal anterior and posterior tape segments secured in line with the anterior and posterior deltoid muscle fibers (**Figure 6.35**).

Kinesio Taping® may also enhance joint stability among clients with dyskinetic or unstable dynamic scapulothoracic movement patterns. Altered scapulo-thoracic movement patterns and related scapular muscle weakness are often associated with impaired shoulder function. Kinesio Taping® may be useful in combination with a neuromuscular re-education therapeutic exercise program designed to correct for scapulo-thoracic dyskinesia. Conceptually, by taping along the fiber lines of the rhomboid muscles, the tape will assist these muscles as well as the subscapularis in approximating the scapula to the thorax during exercise and functional activity performance. By improving proximal joint stability at the scapulo-thoracic articulation, distal upper extremity mobility may be improved. Controlled research using both electromyographic and kinematic techniques is needed to validate the use of Kinesio Taping®. Nonetheless, the novel use of tape for facilitation of dynamic muscle function warrants consideration.

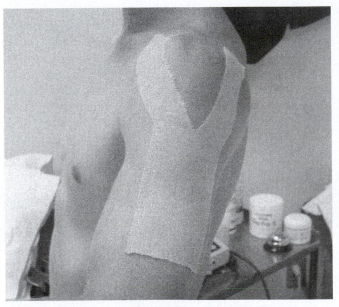

Figure 6.35   Kinesio Taping™ to assist deltoid and supraspinatus muscle function.

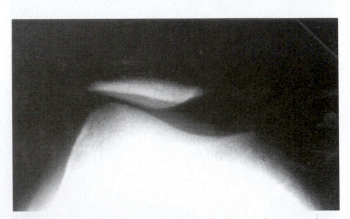

Figure 6.34   Merchant's view patellofemoral joint radiograph.

Although its use has been questioned, conventional athletic taping remains a commonly used method to enhance joint stability during athletic participation, particularly to prevent injury (prophylactic) or to protect existing injuries (functional) to the lateral capsuloligamentous structures of the ankle joint. The ankle joint is highly mobile, presenting an anatomical structure and arrangement of bones, muscles, and ligaments that predisposes it to instability during athletic endeavors.[121] With proper application, including heel locking, athletic taping can reduce the forces that act on the lateral capsuloligamentous ankle structures, while simultaneously enhancing ankle joint proprioception.

The use of athletic taping following an ankle injury is a common practice that is used to increase joint stability and improve proprioceptive feedback. The notion that athletic tape can improve joint proprioception has been debated and studied for years.[122–124] However, of greater concern are the potential ill effects of prolonged or extended use of athletic tape at a particular joint. Lohrer et al.[124] reported decreased electromyographic latencies immediately following athletic tape application, followed by increased latencies 20 minutes later. Rehabilitation clinicians must consider the adaptive changes that may occur with prolonged or extended reliance on athletic taping to provide joint stabilization. As with long term orthosis (brace) use, prolonged reliance on athletic taping for joint stabilization may decrease dynamic joint stability from muscle activation. The importance of performing therapeutic exercises as indicated without concurrent athletic tape use cannot be over emphasized.

Athletic taping can be instrumental in preventing ankle joint re-injury.[125] Conflicting studies suggest that ankle taping may or may not have an effect on functional performance.[126–131] There is equivocal evidence of the effect of athletic taping on ground reaction forces, balance and ankle muscle strength. One concern with athletic ankle taping is that after only 30 minutes of athletic activities, the majority of the benefits of restriction of inversion and eversion ranges of motion that are observed immediately post-taping are lost. Although range of motion restrictions are lost and functional performance study results are conflicting, taping may give a strong psychological reminder, so the athlete is consciously moderating lower limb–loading behavior.[121]

Mulligan[132] has described a novel series of taping interventions using inflexible tape to correct for dysfunction associated with ankle, knee, and spinal joint impairments. Following injury to the lateral capsuloligamentous structures of the ankle, Mulligan described a method of using tape to re-position the distal fibula after application of a dorso-cranially directed mobilization force (**Figure 6.36**). For clients with knee joint osteoarthritis patello-femoral pain, and restricted flexion range of motion, Mulligan combines knee flexion and internal rotation mobilization or automobilization of the tibia with knee taping to maintain tibial internal rotation during function. For clients

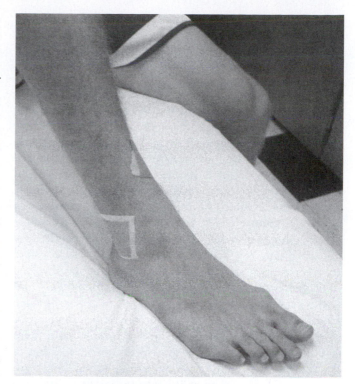

Figure 6.36   Mulligan taping for distal tibiofibular joint instability.

with cervical joint dysfunction secondary to postural malalignment, Mulligan uses tape to stabilize the shoulder girdle in a retracted position to enable relatively pain-free active cervical spine mobility.

Further evidence is needed to substantiate the claims made by proponents of different joint taping regimens. To effectively implement any of these taping intervention strategies in conjunction with an appropriate therapeutic exercise regimen, the reader is advised to further study the evaluative and diagnostic criteria used by the proponents of each method. From this information, clinical evidence can be gathered to provide further support for combined therapeutic exercise-taping interventions.

Key Point:

Taping can facilitate function by supplementing non-contractile joint stability. Patellar taping using inflexible tape, Kinesio Taping®, and Mulligan Taping may be useful adjuncts to a well designed therapeutic exercise program. Prolonged reliance on conventional athletic taping may promote decreased dynamic joint stability; therefore, supplemental therapeutic exercises are recommended without tape support to facilitate neuromuscular responses for dynamic joint stability.

Post-Operative Joint Stabilization Training

When conservative methods of retraining joint stability fail, surgical stabilization is the last option. A well designed post-operative joint stabilization therapeutic exercise program is essential to complement the surgical intervention. Careful consideration of many factors is indicated when designing such a program. Some of these factors include the biomechanical and biological sequelae associated with the surgical procedure, the involved anatomical region, and the client's inherent capsuloligamentous laxity, functional goals and aspirations. Consideration of the architectural topography of the primary and secondary joints affected by the surgical stabilization procedures should also be considered in the therapeutic exercise program. The rehabilitation clinician must consider the congruency and functional mobility of the involved joint. For example, the glenohumeral joint is a highly mobile component that is often subjected to primarily open kinetic chain activities. A post-operative therapeutic exercise program should include both relatively static joint stability training in neutral joint positions in addition to dynamic joint stability training with external forces applied at multiple functionally relevant points within the total range of joint motion. Utilizing PNF techniques such as rhythmic stabilization early, and plyometric-type activities during the later stages of a therapeutic exercise program may be effective strategies (see Chapter 7).

Rehabilitation clinicians often overlook the inherent capsuloligamentous joint laxity a client displays. In extreme cases like Marfan's syndrome or Ehlers Danlos syndrome, joint laxity is obvious during the clinical examination. However, the general capsuloligamentous joint laxity of each client should be evaluated using the five screening tests highlighted by Beighton et al.[31] (see **Figure 6.11**). By evaluating the client's joint laxity and evaluating the contralateral joint involved, the rehabilitation clinician will obtain needed insight regarding both the emphasis and the timing of joint range of motion progressions. A client who displays excessive generalized joint laxity warrants a "red flag," suggesting the need to progress slowly through the range of motion restoration phase of the therapeutic exercise program.

Finally, the rehabilitation clinician must be aware of the individual client's functional goals and aspirations. This is an essential component to achieving a successful outcome following therapeutic exercise program intervention. For example, a post-operative therapeutic exercise program that focuses on the restoration of dynamic glenohumeral joint stabilization may differ between the client who is an overhead-throwing athlete, and the client who has experienced a traumatic glenohumeral joint dislocation following a recreational motorcycle accident. A client whose livelihood is dependent on the mobility of the shoulder should have a therapeutic exercise program designed to help them reach their functional goals. Each client will present with different goals and aspirations, and the rehabilitation clinician must design each therapeutic exercise program on an individual basis with these considerations in mind.

Key Point:

The restoration of dynamic joint stability is vital to the long term health of a surgically repaired or reconstructed joint. The generalized joint laxity of each client should be considered when designing a therapeutic exercise program, particularly for the client who has undergone surgery. The goals and aspirations of each individual client should be considered and when indicated should be incorporated into the therapeutic exercise program.

Functional, Prophylactic, and Post-Operative Orthoses

Orthosis (brace) use has been considered an integral part of joint stabilization not only following surgical intervention, but also prophylactically for injury prevention, neuromuscular re-education, and to reduce the pain associated with joint instability.[133,134] As part of a therapeutic exercise program, braces may be prescribed to supplement weak or healing musculotendinous or capsuloligamentous tissues. The most common lower leg brace employed following ankle neuromuscular dysfunction is an AFO (ankle foot orthosis) (**Figure 6.37**), which

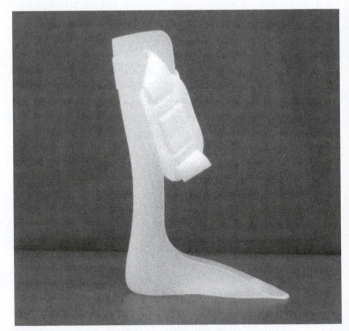

Figure 6.37   Ankle-foot orthosis (AFO).

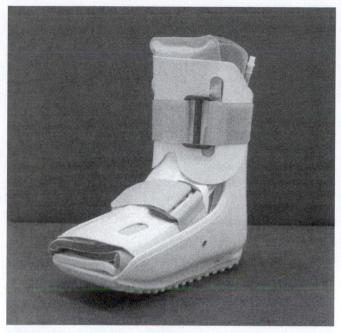

Figure 6.38   Short walking boot.

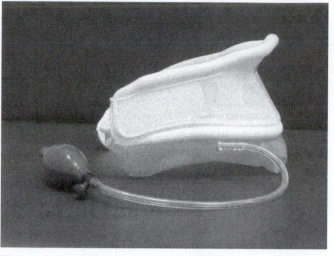

Figure 6.40   Inflatable cervical orthosis.

is a plastic or metal brace extending from below the knee to the foot. Following acute ankle injury a more rigid walking boot is often prescribed (**Figure 6.38**). Other commonly seen orthoses include a hand-wrist splint with additional thumb control to alleviate symptoms related to tenosynovitis conditions (**Figure 6.39**) and an inflatable

neck orthosis to protect the cervical region following acute injury (**Figure 6.40**). Following lumbar region injury or surgery, a neoprene orthosis is often prescribed to prevent aggravating the condition (**Figure 6.41**). There are many different types of braces to choose from when attempting to improve patellofemoral joint stability. Palumbo[135] examined the use of a dynamic patellar brace on 58 clients (62 knees) with patellofemoral pain and subluxation, reporting that 93 percent of the clients reported that the brace alleviated or reduced symptoms associated with patellar subluxation or patellofemoral arthritis. Levine and Splain[136] reported that 77 percent (54 of 70) of clients with anterior knee pain reported decreased pain

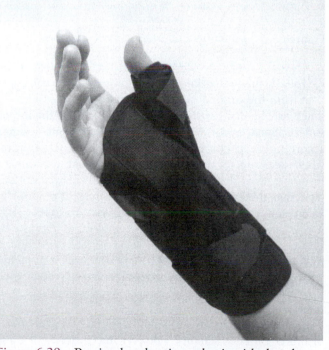

Figure 6.39   Resting hand-wrist orthosis with thumb support.

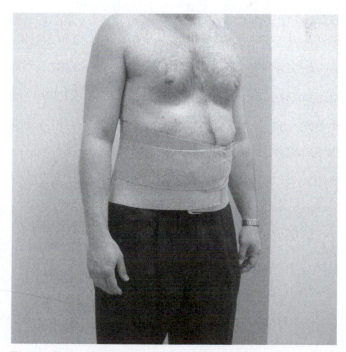

Figure 6.41   Neoprene lumbar orthosis.

with the use of an infrapatellar strap (**Figure 6.42**). Using magnetic resonance kinematic imaging to confirm patellar position, Shellock et al.[137] evaluated the effectiveness of a new patellar realignment brace. Improved patellar alignment was observed among 76 percent (16 of 21 knees) of the knees studied during brace use. Using magnetic resonance imaging to verify patellar alignment, Worrell et al.[138] reported that patellar taping and bracing were both able to influence the patella congruence angle and lateral displacement angle at 10° of knee flexion. Based on the findings of these studies it is evident that bracing can influence patellofemoral alignment and reduce symptoms. The OnTrack™ brace (DJ-Orthopaedics Inc., Vista, CA) was originally designed to mimic patella taping in a brace form. It is described as a patellofemoral pain brace. There are no peer review publications examining the effectiveness of the OnTrack™ brace for its ability to change patellofemoral alignment. The developer of the brace has reported on a series of clients with lateral tracking and found the brace to effectively reduce lateral tilt on Merchant views. In addition, clients reported significantly less pain during the performance of 10 functional activities during brace use compared to clients with a standard brace or no brace.[139]

Functional and prophylactic knee bracing was introduced into the spotlight when Dr. James A. Nicholas introduced the Lenox Hill brace to address Joe Namath's knee instability.[140] The purpose of these braces is both to add stability to an inherently unstable joint and to prevent excessive loading to knee structures (**Figure 6.43**). In theory, these braces help control range of motion during high impact sports. However, research has shown that these braces contribute little to injury prevention and may change the kinematics of the joint that is wearing the orthosis as well joints immediately proximal and distal to that joint.

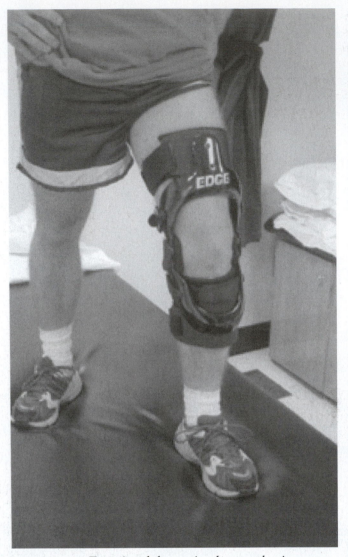

Figure 6.43   Functional derotation knee orthosis.

Today's functional knee braces have evolved considerably from the original derotation brace of Lenox Hill.[141] They can be custom fit or off the shelf, hard shelled or soft strapped, and they come in many different designs, according to client needs. An important consideration when deciding to recommend that a client use one of these braces is that more then 90 percent of wearers believe that the braces are beneficial, helping to reduce the frequency and severity of giving way episodes.[142,143] These studies suggest improved subjective ratings by clients. The perceived sense of security that these braces provide may lead to a possible increase in the risk-taking behavior of the client. This aggressiveness may be of concern when we investigate biomechanical, proprioceptive, metabolic, and epidemiological studies.

Several studies have evaluated the biomechanical effects of braces on knee stability; however, the majority of these studies were performed on cadaveric models.[144–146] Additionally, studies supporting the effectiveness of these

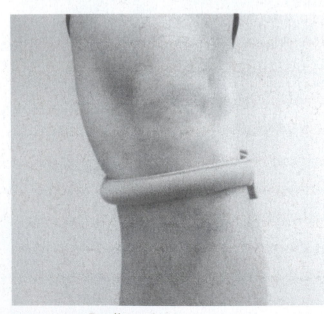

Figure 6.42   Patella tendon strap.

braces in controlling anterior tibial translation or valgus loading have been performed under loading conditions that are considerably lower and at velocities that are slower than those commonly encountered during normal activities. Although subjective scores have been shown to be increased among brace wearers, Risberg et al.[147] revealed that functional knee bracing had no effect on proprioception among clients who had undergone ACL reconstruction, or among non-impaired clients. In a later study, Risberg et al.[148] reported no significant differences between braced and unbraced clients following ACL reconstruction for knee joint laxity, range of motion, muscle strength, functional knee tests, or pain.

The metabolic costs of brace wearing should be considered when deciding on bracing. Houston and Goemans[149] reported a significant increase in oxygen consumption and heart rate and a 40 percent increase in blood lactate concentration during a bicycle ergometer endurance test. These blood lactate level increases also suggest increased muscle effort secondary to bracing. Prolonged knee brace use may also promote altered neuromuscular recruitment patterns that promote quadriceps femoris muscle group atrophy. Isokinetic testing evaluations have revealed a 15 percent decrease of knee flexion–extension velocity when clients are tested while wearing a functional knee brace.[149] There has been little evidence to support the idea that functional brace use increases athletic performance. While investigating the speed of running and turning, running and jumping and accuracy of landing, Wu et al.[150] revealed decreased speeds during both functional knee brace use and during the use of a mechanical placebo brace when compared to control subjects.

When considering the use of a functional or prophylactic knee brace, the rehabilitation clinician should consider the findings of well designed epidemiology studies. Taft et al.[151] suggested that a reduction in medial collateral ligament knee injury frequency was associated with football players wearing lateral hinge knee braces. Hewson et al.,[152] however, reported no difference between functional knee brace users and non-users over four college seasons. The number of season ending injuries was similar between groups. A study by Rovere et al.[153] suggested that the use of such braces may actually increase the knee injury rate of an athlete. A prospective randomized study of intramural football players using prophylactic bracing revealed a similar severity of ligament injury between groups. However, non-braced players had a greater number of medial collateral ligament and anterior cruciate ligament injuries then those who wore a brace.[154] The role of functional and prophylactic knee bracing remains controversial. As rehabilitation clinicians we must understand the tradeoffs associated with recommending brace use for dynamic joint stability.

Although similar tradeoffs may be present with the use of functional ankle braces, research more abundantly suggests that ankle brace use reduces the risk of inversion ankle

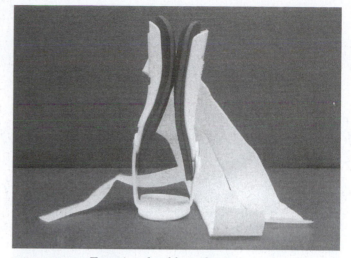

Figure 6.44 Functional ankle orthosis.

sprains (**Figure 6.44**).[127–132,155] Functional ankle braces primarily reduce the risk of inversion ankle injury by decreasing the available range of motion. If functional ankle braces are to be used, they should be used during practices and during competitions, and they should be supplemented with out of brace dynamic joint stability exercises.

The use of foot orthoses (orthotics) is also considered a means of prophylactic bracing (**Figure 6.45**). The basis of the kinetic chain begins at the highly complicated foot. The foot possesses many joints that are designed for stability with a mild degree of mobility; however, hypermobility due to an over mobile (pronated foot) or hypomobility due to a more rigid (supinated foot) may lead to problems more proximally up the kinetic chain. An appropriately designed orthotic applied to a neutrally aligned

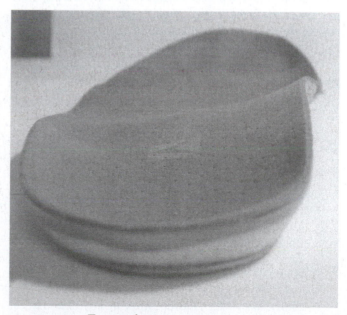

Figure 6.45 Foot orthotic.

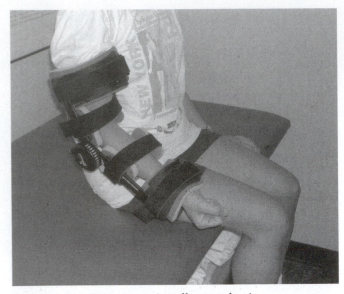

Figure 6.46   Post-operative elbow orthosis.

foot attempts to "build the ground up to the foot" with materials of differing rigidity to either increase the stability (pronated foot) or increase the cushioning (supinated foot) to prevent injury either at the foot or more proximally up the kinetic chain. Improved lower extremity alignment attained from orthotic use may help the client better withstand the loads commonly associated with a progressively more intense closed kinetic chain therapeutic exercise regimen.

Post-operative bracing is imperative following a surgical stabilization procedure. During the immediate post-operative period, the brace provides the stability that the healing muscles and capsuloligamentous structures are unable to provide. Depending upon the extent and timing of the surgery, the procedure that was performed, the method of surgical fixation, the client's general health, and the tissue(s) used for reconstructive procedures, different levels of joint protection are indicated. Post-operative bracing is commonly used following spinal stabilization, knee reconstruction, glenohumeral joint stabilization, and ulnar collateral ligament reconstruction procedures (**Figure 6.46**).

Key Point:

Bracing for patellofemoral pain syndrome can decrease symptoms and improve patellar alignment. Functional knee braces have little or no effect on proprioception and have been shown to increase metabolic rates, decrease agility, and decrease knee flexion–extension speed. Functional braces designed to enable early return to athletics may give the client a false sense of security. Functional ankle braces are a good option to protect against inversion ankle sprains.

Summary

There are many components to achieving and maintaining joint stability. We are constantly challenged by pathology and dysfunction to provide therapeutic exercise interventions that either maintain or improve joint stability. Over the course of this chapter, we touched on a few of the therapeutic exercise interventions such as PNF, dynamic lumbar stabilization, and neuromuscular training.

We also explored ways to provide static joint stability restraints in the form of bracing and taping. New therapeutic exercise strategies are constantly evolving and rehabilitation clinicians must continue to critique the level of evidence that supports the particular interventions that they select.

References

1. Norkin C, Levange P. *Joint Structure and Function: A Comprehensive Analysis.* Philadelphia: FA Davis Company, 1992.
2. Kaltsas DS. Comparative study of the properties of the shoulder joint capsule with those of other joint capsules. *Clin Orthop.* 1983;173:187–197.
3. Wyke B. The neurology of joints. *Ann R Coll. Surg Engl.* 1967;41:25–50.
4. Zinny ML. Mechanoreceptors in articular tissues. *Am J Anat.* 1988;182:16–32.
5. Frank C, Woo SL-Y, Amiel D, et al. Medial collateral ligament healing: A multidisciplinary assessment in rabbits. *Am J Sports Med.* 1983;11:379–389.
6. Parry DA, Barnes GR, Craig AS. A comparison of the size distribution of collagen fibrils in connective tissues as a function of age and a possible relation between fibril size distribution and mechanical properties. *Proc Roy Soc Lond.* 1978;B203:305–321.

7. Frank C, Schachar N, Dittrich D. Natural history of healing of the repaired medial collateral ligament. *J Orthop Res*. 1983;1:179–188.

8. Schultz RA, Miller DC, Kerr CS, Micheli L. Mechanoreceptors in human cruciate ligaments: A histological study. *J Bone Joint Surg*. 1984;66A: 1072–1076.

9. Gardner E. Reflex muscular responses to stimulation of articular nerves in the cat. *Am J Physiol*. 1950;161:133–141.

10. Peacock EE. *Wound Repair*, 3rd ed. Philadelphia: W.B. Saunders, 1984.

11. Rothman RH, Marvel JP Jr., Heppenstall RB. Anatomic considerations in the glenohumeral joint. *Orthop Clin North Am*. 1975;6(2):341–352.

12. Saha AK. Dynamic stability of the glenohumeral joint. *Acta Orthop Scand*. 1971;42:491–505.

13. Bowen MK, Warren RF. Ligamentous control of shoulder stability based on selective cutting and static translation experiments. *Clin Sports Med*. 1991;10:757–782.

14. Turkel SJ, Panio MW, Marshall JL, Girgis FG. Stabilizing mechanisms preventing anterior dislocation of the glenohumeral joint. *J Bone Joint Surg*. 1981; 63A:1208–1217.

15. Riemann BL, Lephart SM. The sensorimotor system, part I: The physiologic basis of functional joint stability. *J Athl Train*. 2002;37(1):71–79.

16. Riemann BL, Myers JB, Lephart SM. Sensorimotor system measurement techniques. *J Athl Train*. 2002; 37(1):85–98.

17. Riemann BL, Lephart SM. The sensorimotor system, part II: The role of proprioception in motor control and functional joint stability. *J Athl Train*. 2002;37(1):80–84.

18. Lear LJ, Gross MT. An electromyographical analysis of the scapular stabilizing synergists during a push-up progression. *J Orthop Sports Phys Ther*. 1998;28(3):146–157.

19. Lentell GL, Katzman LL, Walters MR. The relationship between muscle function and ankle stability. *J Orthop Sports Phys Ther*. 1990;11:605–611.

20. Williams GN, Chmielewski T, Rudolph KS, et al. Dynamic knee stability: Current theory and implications for clinicians and scientists. *J Orthop Sports Phys Ther*. 2001;31(10):546–566.

21. Richie DH Jr. Functional instability of the ankle and the role of neuromuscular control: A comprehensive review. *J Foot Ankle Surg*. 2001;40(4): 240–251.

22. Hakkinen A, Hakkinen K, Hannonen P, Alen M. Strength training induced adaptations in neuromuscular function of premenopausal women with fibromyalgia: Comparison with healthy women. *Ann Rheum Dis*. 2001;60(1):21–26.

23. Forwell LA, Carnahan H. Proprioception during manual aiming in individuals with shoulder instability and controls. *J Orthop Sports Phys Ther*. 1996; 23(2):111–119.

24. Lloyd DG. Rationale for training programs to reduce anterior cruciate ligament injuries in Australian football. *J Orthop Sports Phys Ther*. 2001;31 (11):645–654.

25. Risberg MA, Mork M, Jenssen HK, Holm I. Design and implementation of a neuromuscular training program following anterior cruciate ligament reconstruction. *J Orthop Sports Phys Ther*. 2001;31: 620–631.

26. Kujala UM, Salminen JJ, Taimela S, et al. Subject characteristics and low back pain in young athletes and nonathletes. *Med Sci Sports Exerc*. 1992; 24: 627–632.

27. Klemp P, Stevens JE, Isaacs S. A hypermobility study in ballet dancers. *J Rheumatol*. 1984;11:692–696.

28. Nicholas JA. Injuries to knee ligaments: Relationship to looseness and tightness in football players. *JAMA*. 1970;212:2236–2238.

29. Decoster LC, Bernier JN, Lindsay RH, et al. Generalized joint hypermobility and its relationship to injury patterns among NCAA lacrosse players. *J Athl Train*. 1999;34:99–105.

30. Acasuso Diaz M, Collantes Estevez E, Sanchez-Guijo P. Joint hyperlaxity and musculoligamentous lesions: Study of a population of homogeneous age, sex, and physical exertion. *Br J Rheumatol*. 1993;32:120–122.

31. Beighton P, Solomon L, Soskolne C. Articular mobility in an African population. *Ann Rheum Dis*. 1973;32:413–418.

32. Bird HA, Brodie D, Wright V. Quantification of joint laxity. *Rheumatol Rehabil*. 1979;18:161–166.

33. Cotran RS, Kumar V, Robbins SL. *Robbins Pathologic Basis of Disease*, 4th ed. Philadelphia: WB Saunders, 1989.

34. Isselbacher KJ, Braunwald E, Wilson JD, et al. *Harrison's Principles of Internal Medicine*, 13th ed. New York: McGraw-Hill, 1994.

35. Bigliani LU, Kelkar R, Flatow EL, et al. Glenohumeral stability: Biomechanical properties of passive and active stabilizer. *Clin Orthop*. 1996; 330:13–30.

36. Bigliani LU, Pollock RG, Soslowsky LJ, et al. Tensile properties of the inferior glenohumeral ligament. *J Orthop Res*. 1992;10(2):187–197.

37. O'Brien SJ, Arnoczky SP, Warren RF, et al. Developmental anatomy of the shoulder and anatomy of the glenohumeral joint. *In* CA Rockwood, Jr., FA Matsen III (eds). *The Shoulder*. Philadelphia: WB Saunders, 1990, chap. 1, vol. 1, pp. 1–33.

38. O'Brien SJ, Neves MC, Arnoczky SP, et al. The anatomy and histology of the inferior glenohumeral ligament complex of the shoulder. *Am J Sports Med*. 1990;18(5):449–456.

39. Schwartz R, O' Brien SJ, Warren RF. Capsular restraints to the anterior-posterior translation of the

shoulder. A biomechanical study. *Orthop Trans.* 1987;18:409–417.

40. Warner JP, Deng XH, Warren RF, et al. Static capsuloligamentous restraints to superior-inferior translation of the glenohumeral joint. *Am J Sports Med.* 1992;20:675–685.

41. Reeves B. Experiments on tensile strength of the anterior capsular structures of the shoulder in man. *J Bone Joint Surg.* 1968;50B:858–865.

42. Zachazewski J, Magee DJ, Quillen W. *Athletic Injuries and Rehabilitation.* Philadelphia: WB Saunders, 1996.

43. Panjabi MM. The stabilising system of the spine: Part I. Function, dysfunction, adaptation and enhancement. *J Spinal Disorders.* 1992;5:390–397.

44. Pizzutillo PD, Hummer CD. Nonoperative treatment for painful adolescent spondylolysis or spondylolisthesis. *J Pediatr Orthop.* 1989;9:538–540.

45. Micheli LJ, Hall JE, Miller ME. Use of modified Boston brace for back injuries in athletics. *Am J Sports Med.* 1980;8:351–356.

46. Bergmark A. Stability of the lumbar spine. A study in mechanical engineering. *Acta Orthop Scand Suppl.* 1989;230:1–54.

47. Fidler MW, Jowett RL, Troup JDG. Myosin ATPase activity in multifidus muscle from cases of lumbar spinal derangement. *J Bone Joint Surg.* 1975;57B:220–227.

48. Ford D, Bagnall KM, McFadden KD, et al. Analysis of vertebral muscle obtained during surgery for correction of a lumbar disc disorder. *Acta Anat.* 1983;116:152–157.

49. Rantanen J, Hurme M, Falck B, et al. The lumbar multifidus muscle five years after surgery for a lumbar intervertebral disc herniation. *Spine.* 1993;18:568–574.

50. Jorgensen K, Nicolaisen T. Trunk extensor endurance. Determination and relation to low back trouble. *Ergonomics.* 1987;30:259–267.

51. Nicolaisen T, Jorgensen K. Trunk strength, back muscle endurance and low back trouble. *Scand J Rehab Med.* 1985;17:121–127.

52. Nielson J, Kagamihara Y. The regulation of disynaptic reciprocal Ia inhibition during co-contraction of antagonistic muscles in man. *J Physiol.* 1992;456:373–393.

53. Arendt EA, Agel J, Dick R. Anterior cruciate ligament injury patterns among collegiate men and women. *J Athl Train.* 1999;34:86–92.

54. Arendt EA, Dick R. Knee injury patterns among men and women in collegiate basketball and soccer: NCAA data and review of literature. *Am J Sports Med.* 1995;23:694–701.

55. Rozzi SL, Lephart SM, Gear WS, Fu FH. Knee joint laxity and neuromuscular characteristics of male and female soccer and basketball players. *Am J Sports Med.* 1999;27:312–319.

56. Huston LJ, Wojtys EM. Neuromuscular performance characteristics in elite female athletes. *Am J Sports Med.* 1996;24:427–436.

57. Anderson AF, Snyder RB, Federspiel CF, Lipscomb AB. Instrumented evaluation of knee laxity: A comparison of five arthrometers. *Am J Sports Med.* 1992; 20:135–140.

58. Lysens RJ, Ostyn MS, Vanden Auweeley Y, et al. The accident-prone and overuse prone profiles of the young athlete. *Am J Sports Med.* 1989; 17:612–619.

59. Harner CD, Paulos LE, Greenwald AE, et al. Detailed analysis of patients with bilateral anterior cruciate ligament injuries. *Am J Sports Med.* 1994; 22:37–43.

60. Godshall RW. The predictability of athletic injuries: An eight-year study. *J Sports Med.* 1975;3:50–54.

61. Liu SH, Al-Shaikh RA, Panossian V, et al. Estrogen affects the cellular metabolism of the anterior cruciate ligament: A potential explanation for female athletic injury. *Am J Sports Med.* 1997;25(5): 704–709.

62. Heitz NA, Eisenman PA, Beck CL, Walker JA. Hormonal changes throughout the menstrual cycle and increased anterior cruciate ligament laxity in females. *J Athl Train.* 1999;34(2):144–149.

63. Wojtys E, Huston L, Boynton MD, et al. The effect of the menstrual cycle on anterior cruciate ligament injuries in women as determined by hormone levels. *Am J Sports Med.* 2002;30(2):182–188.

64. Hama H, Yamamuro T, Takeda T. Experimental studies on connective tissue of the capsular ligament. *Acta Orthop Scand.* 1976;47:473–479.

65. Marshall JL, Johanson N, Wickiewicz TL, et al. Joint looseness: A function of the person and the joint. *Med Sci Sports Exerc.* 1980;12:189–194.

66. Emery RJH, Mullaji AB. Glenohumeral joint instability in normal adolescents: Incidence and significance. *J Bone Joint Surg.* 1991;73B:406–408.

67. McFarland E, Campbell G, McDowell J. Posterior shoulder laxity in asymptomatic athletes. *Am J Sports Med.* 1996;24:468–471.

68. Grana WA, Moretz JA. Ligamentous laxity in secondary school athletes. *JAMA.* 1978;240:1975–1976.

69. Brewer BJ. Aging of the rotator cuff. *Am J Sports Med.* 1979;7:102–110.

70. Byers P. The biology of normal connective tissue. *In* V McKusick, *Heritable Disorders of the Connective Tissue.* St. Louis: CV Mosby, 1972.

71. Kaltsas DS. Comparative study of the properties of the shoulder joint capsule with those of other joint capsules. *Clin Orthop.* 1983;173:20–26.

72. Ralphs JR, Benjamin M. The joint capsule: Structure, composition, ageing and disease. *J. Anat.* 1994 June;184 (Pt3):503–509.

73. DePalma AF. *Surgery of the Shoulder.* Philadelphia: JB Lippincott, 1950.

74. Olsson O. Degenerative changes of the shoulder joint and their connection with shoulder pain: A morphological and clinical investigation with special attention to the cuff and biceps tendon. *Acta Chirurg Scand Suppl.* 1953;181:1–130.

75. McHugh MP, Magnusson SP, Gleim GW, et al. A cross-sectional study of age-related musculoskeletal and physiological changes in soccer players. *Med Exerc Nutr Health.* 1993;2:261–268.

76. Wilmore JH. The aging of bone and muscle. *Clin Sports Med.* 1991;10(2):231–244.

77. Strojnik V, Vengust R, Pavlovcic V. The effect of proprioceptive training on neuromuscular function in patients with patellar pain. *Cell Mol Biol Lett.* 2002;7(1):170–171.

78. Gentile AM. Skill acquisition: Action, movement, and neuromotor processes. *In* JH Carr, RB Shepherd (eds.). *Movement Science: Foundations for Physical Therapy in Rehabilitation.* Rockville, MD: Aspen Publishers, 1987, pp. 93–154.

79. Ihara H, Nakayama A. Dynamic joint control training for knee ligament injuries. *Am J Sports Med.* 1986;14(4):309–315.

80. Hoffman M, Payne VG. The effects of proprioceptive ankle disk training on healthy subjects. *J Orthop Sports Phys Ther.* 1995;21:90–93.

81. Tropp H, Askling C, Gillquist J. Prevention of ankle sprains. *Am J Sports Med.* 1985;13:259–262.

82. Tropp H, Ekstrand J, Gillquist J. Stability in functional instability of the ankle and its value in predicting injury. *Med Sci Sports Exerc.* 1984;16:64–66.

83. Caraffa A, Cerulli G, Projetti M, et al. Prevention of anterior cruciate ligament injuries in soccer. A prospective controlled study of proprioceptive training. *Knee Surg Sports Traumatol Arthrosc.* 1996;4:19–21.

84. Fitzgerald GK, Axe MJ, Snyder-Mackler L. The efficacy of perturbation training in nonoperative anterior cruciate ligament rehabilitation programs for physically active individuals. *Phys Ther.* 2000; 80(2):128–140.

85. Fitzgerald GK, Childs JD, Ridge TM, Irrgang J. Agility and perturbation training for a physically active individual with knee osteoarthritis. *Phys Ther.* 2002;82 (4):372–382.

86. Pintsaar A, Brynhildsen J, Tropp H. Postural corrections after standardized perturbations of single limb stance: Effect of training and orthotic devices in patients with ankle instability. *Brit J Sports Med.* 1996;30(2):151–155.

87. Hewett TE, Stroupe AL, Nance TA, Noyes FR. Plyometric training in female athletes. Decreased impact forces and increased hamstring torques. *Am J Sports Med.* 1996;24(6):765–773.

88. Hewett TE, Lindenfeld TN, Riccobene JV, Noyes FR. The effect of neuromuscular training on the in-cidence of knee injury in female athletes: A prospective study. *Am J Sports Med.* 1999;27:699–706.

89. Voight ML, Cook G. Clinical application of closed kinetic chain exercise. *J Sport Rehabil.* 1996;5:25–44.

90. Cook G, Burton L, Fields K. Reactive neuromuscular training for the anterior cruciate ligament-deficient knee: A case report. *J Athl Train.* 1999;34 (2):194–201.

91. Rozzi SL, Lephart SM, Sterner R, Kuligowski L. Balance training for persons with functionally unstable ankles. *J Orthop Sports Phys Ther.* 1999;29(8):478–486.

92. Zatterstrom R, Friden T, Lindstrand A, Moritz U. The effect of physiotherapy on standing balance in chronic anterior cruciate ligament insufficiency. *Am J Sports Med.* 1994; 22:531–536.

93. Lin SI, Woollacott MH. Postural muscle responses following changing balance threats in young, stable older, and unstable older adults. *J Mot Behav.* 2002; 34(1):37–44.

94. Kamm K, Thelen E, Jensen JL. A dynamical systems approach to motor development. *Phys Ther.* 1990;70:763–775.

95. Johnson GS. PNF and knee rehabilitation. *J Orthop Sports Phys Ther.* 2002;30(7):430–431 [comment].

96. Voss DE. Proprioceptive neuromuscular facilitation. *Am J Phys Med.* 1967; 46:838–899.

97. Stockmeyer SA. An interpretation of the approach of Rood to the treatment of neuromuscular dysfunction. *Am J Phys Med.* 1967; 46:900–961.

98. Semans S. The Bobath concept in treatment of neurological disorders; neurodevelopmental treatment. *Am J Phys Med.* 1967;46: 732–788.

99. Knott M, Voss DE. *Proprioceptive Neuromuscular Facilitation*, 2nd ed. New York: Harper & Row, 1968.

100. Shimura K, Kasai T. Effects of proprioceptive neuromuscular facilitation on the initiation of voluntary movement and motor evoked potentials in upper limb muscles. *Hum Mov Sci.* 2002;21(1):101–113.

101. Wilson E. Central facilitation and remote effects: Treating both ends of the system. *Manual Therapy.* 1997;2(2):165–168.

102. Wang RY. Effect of proprioceptive neuromuscular facilitation on the gait of patients with hemiplegia of long and short duration. *Phys Ther.* 1994;74 (12):1108–1115.

103. Kraft GH, Fitts SS, Hammond MC. Techniques to improve function of the arm and hand in chronic hemiplegia. *Arch Phys Med Rehabil.* 1992; 73(3): 220–227.

104. Petrofsky JS. The use of electromyogram biofeedback to reduce Trendelenburg gait. *Eur J Appl Physiol.* 2001;85(5):491–495.

105. Gantchev GN, Dimitrova DM. Anticipatory postural adjustments associated with arm movements during balancing on unstable support surface. *Int J Psychophysiol.* 1996;22:117–122.

106. Perlau R, Frank C, Fick G. The effect of elastic bandages on human knee proprioception in the uninjured population. *Am J Sports Med.* 1995;23: 251–255.

107. Cutbill JW, Ladly KO, Bray RC, et al. Anterior Knee Pain: A Review. *Clin J Sports Med* 1997;7:40–45.

108. Ficat RP, Hungerford DS. *Disorders of the Patello-Femoral Joint*, 2nd ed. Baltimore: Williams & Wilkins, 1990.

109. Doucette SA, Goble EM. The effect of exercise on patellar tracking in lateral patellar compression syndrome. *Am J Sports Med.* 1992;20(2):434–440.

110. Fulkerson JP. *Disorders of the Patellofemoral Joint*, 3rd ed. Baltimore: Williams & Wilkins, 1997.

111. Fulkerson JP. Evaluation of the peripatellar soft tissues and retinaculum in patients with patellofemoral pain. *Clin Sports Med.* 1989;8:197–202.

112. Fulkerson JP. Office evaluation of patients with anterior knee pain. *Am J Knee Surg.* 1997;10: 181–183.

113. Fitzgerald GK, McClure PW. Reliability of measurements obtained with four tests for patellofemoral alignment. *Phys Ther.* 1995;75(2):84–92.

114. McConnell J. *Patellofemoral treatment plan: Course notes.* McConnell Institute, Marina del Rey, CA, 1989.

115. McConnell J. The management of chondromalacia patellae: A long term solution. *Aust J Physiother.* 1986;32(4):215–225.

116. Kowall MG, Kolk G, Nuber GW, et al. Patellar taping in the treatment of patellofemoral pain: a prospective randomized study. *Am J Sports Med.* 1996;24(1):61–66.

117. Bockrath K, Wooden C, Worrell T, et al. Effects of patella taping on patella position and perceived pain. *Med Sci Sports Exerc.* 1993;25:989–992.

118. Gilleard W, McConnell J, Parsons D. The effect of patellar taping on the onset of vastus medialis oblique and vastus lateralis muscle activity in persons with patellofemoral pain. *Phys Ther.* 1998; 78:25–32.

119. Callaghan MJ, Selfe J, Bagley P, Oldham JA. The effects of patellar taping on knee proprioception. *J Athl Train.* 2002;37(1):19–24.

120. Hecimovich J. *Introduction to Kinesio Taping.* New York: Keep Pace Seminars, 2002.

121. Hume PA, Gerrard DF. Effectiveness of external ankle support: Bracing and taping in rugby union. *Sports Med.* 1998;25(5):285–312.

122. Refshauge KM, Kilbreath SL, Raymond J. The effect of recurrent ankle inversion sprain and taping on proprioception at the ankle. *Med Sci Sports Exerc.* 2000;32(1):10–15.

123. Jerosch J, Bischof M. The effect of proprioception on functional stability of the upper ankle joint with special reference to stabilizing aids. *Sportverletz Sportschaden.* 1994;8(3):111–121.

124. Lohrer H, Alt W, Gollhofer A. Neuromuscular properties and functional aspects of taped ankles. *Am J Sports Med.* 1999;27(1): 69–75.

125. Garrick JG, Requa RQ. Role of external support in the prevention of ankle sprains. *Med Sci Sports.* 1973;5(3):200–203.

126. Bocchinfuso C, Sitler MR, Kimura IF. Effects of two semi-rigid prophylactic ankle stabilizers on speed, agility, and vertical jump. *J Sport Rehabil.* 1994;3(2):125–134.

127. Gross MT, Everts JR, Roberson SE, et al. Effect of Donjoy Ankle Ligament Protector and Aircast Sport-Stirrup orthoses on functional performance. *J Orthop Sports Phys Ther.* 1994;19(3):150–156.

128. Macpherson K. Effects of a semi-rigid and a soft-shell prophylactic ankle stabilizer on performance (microfiche). Eugene, OR: University of Oregon Microform Publications, 1995.

129. Coffman JL, Mitze NL. A comparison of ankle taping and the Aircast Sport Stirrup on athletic performance. *J Athl Train.* 1989;24(2):123.

130. Greene TA, Wight CR. A comparative support evaluation of three ankle orthoses before, during, and after exercise. *J Orthop Sport Phys Ther.* 1990; 11(1):453–466.

131. Burks RT, Bean BG Marcus R, Barker HB. Analysis of athletic performance with prophylactic ankle devices. *Am J Sports Med.* 1991;19(2):104–106.

132. Mulligan BR. *Manual Therapy* ("NAGS," "SNAGS," "MWMS," etc.), 4th ed. Hutcheson Bowman & Stewart Ltd: Wellington, New Zealand, 1999.

133. BenGal S, Lowe J, Mann G, et al. The role of the knee brace in the prevention of anterior knee pain syndrome. *Am J Sports Med.* 1997;25:118–122.

134. Beynnon BD, Good L, Risberg MA. The effect of bracing on proprioception of knees with anterior cruciate ligament injury. *J Orthop Sports Phys Ther.* 2002;32:11–15.

135. Palumbo PM. Dynamic patellar brace: a new orthosis in the management of patellofemoral disorders: A preliminary report. *Am J Sports Med.* 1981;9:45–49.

136. Levine J, Splain S. Use of the infrapatellar strap in the treatment of patellofemoral pain. *Clin Orthop.* 1979;139:179–181.

137. Shellock FG, Mink JH, Deutsch AL, et al. Effect of a patella realignment brace on patellofemoral relationships: Evaluation with kinematic MR imaging. *J MRI.* 1994;4:590–594.

138. Worrell T, Ingersoll CD, Bockrath-Pugliese K, Minis P. Effect of taping and bracing on patella position as determined by MRI in patients with patellofemoral pain. *J Athl Train.* 1998;33:16–20.

139. Grace K. New method for patellofemoral pain and clinical implications. *J Orthop Sports Phys Ther.* 1991;25:86 [abstract].

140. Branch T, Hunter R. Functional analysis of anterior cruciate ligament braces. *Clin Sports Med.* 1990;9:771–797.
141. Nicholas JA. Bracing the anterior cruciate ligament deficient knee using the Lenox Hill derotation brace. *Clin Orthop.* 1983;172:137–142.
142. Colville MR, Lee CL, Ciullo JV. The Lenox Hill brace: An evaluation of effectiveness in treating knee instability. *Am J Sports Med.* 1986;14:257–261.
143. Mishra DK, Daniel DM, Stone ML. The use of functional knee braces in the control of pathologic anterior knee laxity. *Clin Orthop.* 1989;241:213–220.
144. Anderson K, Wojtys EM, Loubert RV, Miller RE. A biomechanical evaluation of taping and bracing in reducing knee joint translation and rotation. *Am J Sports Med.* 1992;20:416–421.
145. Branch T, Hunter R, Reynolds P. Controlling anterior tibial displacement under static load: A comparison of two braces. *Orthopedics.* 1988;11:1249–1252.
146. Cawley PW, France EP, Paulos LE. Comparison of rehabilitative knee braces. A biomechanical investigation. *Am J Sports Med.* 1989;17:141–146.
147. Risberg MA, Beynnon BD, Peura GD, Uh BS. Proprioception after anterior cruciate ligament reconstruction with and without bracing. *Knee Surg Sports Traumatol Arthrosc.* 1999;7(5):303–309.
148. Risberg MA, Holm I, Steen H, et al. The effect of knee bracing after anterior cruciate ligament reconstruction: a prospective, randomized study with two years follow up. *Am J Sports Med.* 1999;27(1):76–83.
149. Houston ME, Goemans PH. Leg muscle performance of athletes with and without knee support braces. *Arch Phys Med Rehabil.* 1982;63:431–432.
150. Wu GK, Ng GY, Mak AF. Effects of knee bracing on the functional performance of patients with anterior cruciate ligament reconstruction. *Arch Phys Med Rehabil.* 2001;82(2):282–285.
151. Taft TN, Almenkinders LC. The dislocated knee. *In* F Fu (ed.), *Knee Surgery.* Baltimore: Williams & Wilkins, 1994.
152. Hewson GF Jr, Mendini RA, Wang JB. Prophylactic knee bracing in college football. *Am J Sports Med.* 1986;14(4):262–266.
153. Rovere GD, Haupt HA, Yates CS. Prophylactic knee bracing in college football. *Am J Sports Med.* 1987;15:111–116.
154. Sitler M, Ryan J, Hopkinson W, et al. The efficiency of a prophylactic knee brace to reduce knee injuries in football. A prospective, randomized study at West Point. *Am J Sports Med.* 1990;18(3):310–315.
155. Rovere GD, Clarke TJ, Yates CS, Burley K. Retrospective comparison of taping and ankle stabilizers in preventing ankle injuries. *Am J Sports Med.* 1988;16(3):228–233.

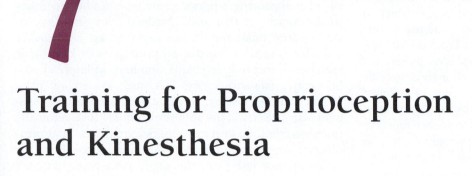

7

Training for Proprioception and Kinesthesia

WILLIAM K. OGARD

Objectives

The reader will be able to:

- Define proprioception and discuss variations of the definition.
- Describe the methods and procedures used to measure proprioception.
- Critically review the literature related to measurement of and interventions for proprioception of the trunk, neck, and limbs as applied to individuals with and without musculoskeletal injuries and dysfunction.

- Discuss the efficacy of proprioceptive exercise and training.
- Describe the proprioceptive aspects of therapeutic exercises commonly used to treat for various injuries and movement dysfunctions of the musculoskeletal system.

Outline

INTRODUCTION

As movement specialists, the challenge for physical therapists and other rehabilitation clinicians involved in examination and evaluation of, and intervention in, movement dysfunction, is the restoration and/or maintenance of functional movement and quality of life. The use of various therapeutic exercise approaches is advocated for complete restoration of function, from low level passive and active single joint exercises to high level, activity specific, multi-joint exercises with significant "limits of stability" challenges. Musculotendinous and capsuloligamentous structures provide mechanical and neurosensory functions at joints during movement, including proprioceptive information that contributes to movement control by providing information about the status of the moving limbs.[1]

It has been speculated that capsular or ligamentous injuries result in loss of proprioception that may lead to further compromise of joint neuromuscular function, injury, and reinjury.[2–8] However, the varied results of proprioceptive studies have resulted in equivocal conclusions regarding the effect of injury on proprioceptive function and functional outcomes after rehabilitation. Also, the role of ligamentous and capsular mechanoreceptors in proprioception may, in fact, be limited from a neurophysiologic standpoint. The muscle spindle, providing sensory feedback from the muscles to all levels of the central nervous system (CNS), is now considered to be the primary source of position and motion information[1,9–15] (see Chapters 2 and 8).

The use of specific proprioceptive or kinesthetic exercises as a component of therapeutic exercise for rehabilitation has been advocated for many musculoskeletal dysfunctions, especially in the lower extremity, as an important means of addressing proprioceptive deficits and restoring normal function after injury and surgery.[3,4,8,16,17] With regard to anterior cruciate ligament (ACL) injuries, Hardin[18] has stated, "It is universally accepted" that proprioceptive deficits exist, and that it is an "accepted practice" to incorporate activities that enhance proprioceptive ability following ACL injury and/or reconstruction. Irrgang[2] states that therapeutic exercise interventions for clients with ACL deficiency or who are status–post ACL reconstruction should be based on sound scientific principles, and this would be true for therapeutic exercise programs designed for clients who display other types of musculoskeletal dysfunctions.

While many therapeutic exercise programs emphasize proprioceptive or kinesthetic training as a necessary component for restoration of normal function,[19,20] the evidence is unclear as to whether reported proprioceptive deficits actually result in clinically or functionally significant movement deficits.[14,21–23] Also, there is no unequivocal scientific evidence that demonstrates that joint proprioception, as currently assessed in the literature, actually improves as a direct result of specific proprioceptive or kinesthetic exercise.[14,21] Ashton-Miller et al.,[14] in a comprehensive review and discussion of the issues regarding the efficacy of proprioceptive exercise, concluded that "despite their widespread acceptance, current exercises aimed at improving proprioception have not been demonstrated to achieve that goal." Nashner[21] suggests that somatosensory input for various motor tasks, like balance activities, commonly cited as proprioceptive or kinesthetic exercises, is lost only in clients who have widespread proprioceptive (somatosensory) loss, such as cerebral palsy and Parkinson's disease, or other neuropathic or neuromuscular diseases. This author also notes that automatic reactions from the lower extremities are driven by proprioceptive inputs received from locations throughout the extremity, not just from the single joint being tested.[21] Nashner concludes that there is no evidence supporting (or refuting) proprioceptive losses at the ankle or knee that disrupt motor responses or result in injury.[21] Further, given the equivocal nature of the evidence on proprioception, Ashton-Miller et al.[14] suggested that the relevant studies determining whether proprioception, as currently assessed, can be improved by exercise have yet to be conducted.

> # Key Point:
> Proprioception is not clearly defined in the literature.

Proprioceptive testing methods generally evaluate this sensory modality at a single joint, disregarding the fact that joints seldom function in isolation during functional activity and receive sensory information from muscles acting at all joints to provide appropriate limb position and motion information. The question then becomes, does a loss of sensory input from a single structure at a single extremity joint (e.g., ACL rupture or reconstruction), or in the spine, result in a functionally significant movement dysfunction? Or can the neuromuscular system adequately compensate for this change with no apparent loss of overall sensory input, resulting in maintenance of function?

Addressing the issues and controversy surrounding deficits of proprioception and proprioceptive therapeutic exercise or training is essential for validation of current rehabilitation methods and intervention. The purpose of this chapter is to describe and delineate the nature and appropriateness of current proprioceptive assessment and intervention, to assist rehabilitation clinicians in determining the actual efficacy and effectiveness of therapeutic proprioceptive or kinesthetic exercise, and to describe therapeutic exercises that may be used to accomplish the goals of optimum functional outcome and improved quality of life.

WHAT IS PROPRIOCEPTION?

Proprioception (*proprio:* one's own; *ception:* to receive), as a component of the sense of touch, has been generally defined as the ability of the CNS to sense the position and movement of body segments in space.[24–27] Sherrington[24] used this term to describe sensory input from vestibular, joint, and muscular receptors to the CNS. *Kinesthesia* (*kinesis:* movement; *aisthesis:* sensation), or movement sense, is a component of proprioception. Boscoe and Poppele define kinesthesia as the conscious sense of position and motion,[28] synonymous with the general definition of proprioception noted above. In an 1888 publication entitled *The "Muscular Sense," Its Nature And Cortical Localization*, Bastian[29] used kinesthesia to describe both position and motion sensations of the limb. Gandevia et al.[11] define kinesthesia (synonymous with proprioception) as encompassing three main sensations: movement and position of joints, force, and sense of effort or heaviness associated with muscular contractions. This definition includes a kinetic component attributed to the forces generated by active movements. Weiler and Awiszus[30] state that position sense, sense of movement detection, sense of force, and sense of effort are the four parameters of proprioception and are essential for goal-directed movements and locomotion. Finally, Beard et al.[31] state that "There is no accepted definition of proprioception . . ." and considers proprioception to consist of the following three components: 1) static awareness of joint position, 2) kinesthetic awareness (detection of movement and acceleration), and 3) closed-loop efferent activity that is required for the reflex response and the regulation of muscle stiffness.

Given these varied definitions, proprioception would seem to be a complex sensory function for processing kinetic and kinematic information from the trunk, head, and limbs, conveyed to, and processed at, all levels of the CNS, resulting in accurate placement and movement of body segments in space. As a sensory system, proprioception appears to provide an important mechanism that contributes to motor control[1] (see Chapter 8).

> ## Key Point:
> Proprioceptive sensation includes position, displacement, velocity, acceleration, muscular effort (force) and/or sense of heaviness.

NEUROANATOMIC AND NEUROPHYSIOLOGIC BASIS FOR PROPRIOCEPTION

Control of human movement, including volitional actions and responses to perturbations, is mediated at all levels of the CNS, utilizing peripheral sensory information to monitor movement tasks in an efficient and effective manner. Feed-forward and feedback control is utilized to initiate, monitor, and alter movement patterns for a given task within a specific environment[15] (**Figure 7.1**). While purposeful volitional movement per se is not dependent on peripheral sensory information, the loss or alteration of visual, vestibular, and proprioceptive input[12] can affect the accuracy and precision of movement. These sensory inputs provide information to effect limb positioning, balance, and posture during normal human movement.[3,6,21,32] It has been speculated that disruption or loss of sensory input from any one component, including proprioceptive (somatosensory) input, as a result of injury, surgery, or disease of the musculoskeletal system may result in a change in the sense of position and movement, possibly affecting function and resulting in disability or re-injury.[3] However, as noted previously, the relationship between proprioception and movement dysfunction after musculoskeletal injury is unclear at this time.

Sensory organs in cutaneous, articular, and musculotendinous tissues provide peripheral sensory information about the relative motion and position of body segments during static and dynamic activity. Muscle spindles, Golgi tendon organs (GTO), and various articular (capsuloligamentous) and skin mechanoreceptors are the specific sensory organs within the body tissues that subserve proprioceptive function[12] (**Table 7.1**) (see Chapters 2, 6, and 8). These mechanoreceptors transduce mechanical energy into electrical signals that are processed at several levels of the CNS, including the spinal cord, brainstem, midbrain, cerebellum, and cerebral cortex (see Chapter 8).

> ## Key Point:
> Proprioception subserves the accurate placement and movement of the limbs, trunk, and head in space.

Conscious proprioceptive information is carried to appropriate CNS levels via the dorsal columns of the spinal cord (**Figure 7.2**). The spinal lemniscal system, including the *fasciculus gracilis* (lower extremities) and *fasciculus cuneatus* (upper extremities), projects through the midbrain via the medial lemniscus to the somatosensory cortex. Unconscious proprioception is mediated in the

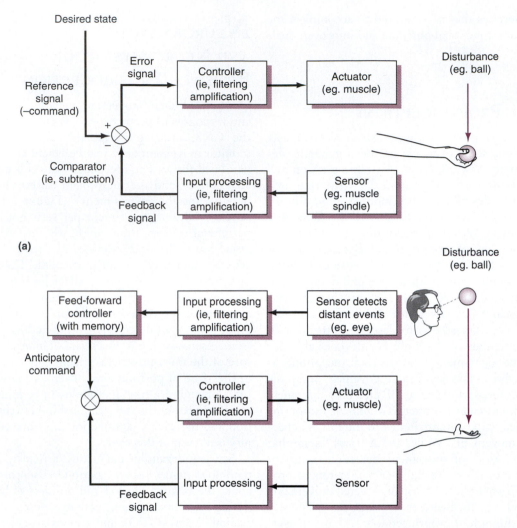

Figure 7.1   (a) Feedback control: Command specifies desired state; (b) feed-forward control: Command specifies response. (Redrawn from ER Kandel, JH Schwartz, TM Jessell. (eds.), *Principles of Neural Science*, 4th ed. New York: McGraw-Hill, 2000.)

TABLE 7.1   Classification and description of proprioceptive mechanoreceptors

Class	Description	Fiber type(s)	Fiber groups	Function
Cutaneous	Ruffini	II (SA)	Aα β	Skin stretch (e.g., distal interphalangeal joint)
Joint	Ruffini	I	A β	Joint angle, excessive force or stress, deep pressure
	Pacinian	II		
	GTO-like	III		
	Free nerve endings	IV	Aδ	Stretch-sensitive free endings
Muscle	Spindle	Ia, II	Aα, Aβ	Muscle length and rate of length change
	GTO	Ib	Aα	Muscle contractile force

From: Rothwell[132], Kandel et al[15], Newton[44], Hogervorst & Brand.[45]

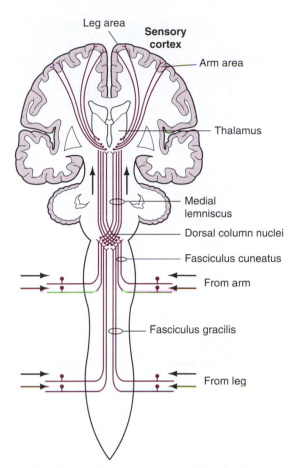

Figure 7.2   Central nervous system dorsal column-medial lemniscus pathways for proprioception. (Redrawn from SG Waxman. *Clinical Neuroanatomy*, 24th ed. New York: McGraw-Hill, 2000.)

cerebellum via afferent signals from the ventral and dorsal spinocerebellar tracts (lower extremities) and the cuneocerebellar and rostral spinocerebellar tracts (upper extremities). Finally, reflexes are mediated at the level of the spinal cord via large afferents in the muscle. As a result of afferent input to the CNS, particularly from muscle spindles, efferent signals are generated to direct and/or modify muscular responses that result in appropriate body segment motions for the accomplishment and control of a given movement task within a specific environment.[14,15]

MUSCLE RECEPTORS: MUSCLE SPINDLE AND GOLGI TENDON ORGAN (GTO)

The *muscle spindle* is most likely the primary source of proprioceptive information. These fusiform-shaped intrafusal muscle fibers lie in parallel with extrafusal (skeletal) mus-

cle fibers and contain a number of specialized structures (**Figure 7.3**) (see Chapters 2 and 8). There are two types of intrafusal muscle fibers: nuclear bag (subtypes dynamic and static) and nuclear chain (static only). The central regions are non-contractile, while the polar ends are contractile. Type Ia afferent (primary) endings innervate the central portions of nuclear bag and chain spindle fibers. Type Ia endings monitor absolute muscle length and rate of muscle length change. Type II afferents, or secondary endings, supply the polar regions of the nuclear chain and static nuclear bag fibers and monitor only absolute muscle length. Motor supply to the polar ends of intrafusal fibers is supplied by dynamic and static gamma efferent fibers. The gamma efferents adjust intrafusal fiber length as a result of shortening of extrafusal fibers in order to maintain spindle sensitivity. A second type of efferent ending, a beta efferent, innervates both intrafusal and extrafusal fibers. In general, the muscle spindle is a very sensitive muscle length detector capable of providing critical information for determining position and motion of body segments.

Golgi tendon organs (GTOs) are sensory receptors located at the junction between muscle fibers and tendon. They are connected in series to a group of skeletal muscle fibers. Stretching of the GTO straightens the collagen fibers, thus compressing the nerve endings and causing them to be activated. Whereas muscle spindles are most sensitive to changes in muscle length, GTOs are most sensitive to changes in muscle tension. The average level of activity in a population of GTOs in a given muscle–tendon unit is a fairly good measure of the total force produced by the contracting muscle (**Figure 7.4**) (see Chapters 2 and 8). This mechanoreceptor is innervated by type Ib afferent fibers and responds to changes in muscle contractile force (tension) and, to a lesser extent, changes in muscle length.[15] Rymer and D'Almeida[33] suggest that afferent discharges from the GTO as a result of muscle force contribute to proprioception. Dietz and Duysens[34] also suggest that the GTO significantly contributes sensory information to the regulation of stance and gait. Several investigators have found differences in weight bearing vs. non–weight bearing knee joint position sense, at varied joint angles, and during active vs. passive knee joint position sense as determined by reproduction of position.[35–38] However, the extent and exact nature of the GTO contribution to current proprioception measures, as well as the possible combined influence of the muscle spindle, is not clearly established at this time and warrants more extensive study in the future.

Key Point:

The primary receptor for proprioception is the muscle spindle.

A Muscle spindle

Intrafusal
muscle
fibers

Capsule

Sensory
endings

Afferent
axons

Efferent
axons

Gamma
motor
endings

B Intrafusal fibers of the muscle spindle

Dynamic nuclear
bag fiber

Static nuclear
bag fiber

Nuclear
chain fiber

II

Ia

Static

Dynamic

C Response of Ia sensory fiber to selective
activation of motor neurons

200

Imp/s

0   Stretch alone

Dynamic response

Steady-state response

200

Imp/s

0

Stimulate static gamma fiber

200

Imp/s

0

Stimulate dynamic gamma fiber

Stretch   6

0

0.2 s

Figure 7.3   (a) Muscle spindle; (b) intrafusal fibers of the muscle spindle; (c) response of Ia sensory fiber to selective activation of motor neurons. (Reprinted with permission from ER Kandel, JH Schwartz, TM Jessell. (eds.), *Principles of Neural Science*, 4th ed. New York: McGraw-Hill, 2000.)

ARTICULAR RECEPTORS: CAPSULAR AND LIGAMENTOUS MECHANORECEPTORS

A number of investigators have identified several types of mechanoreceptors within human joint articular structures, including joint capsules and ligaments.[39–42] In the knee joint, *Ruffini receptors* are slowly adapting (SA) low threshold type I receptors that are believed to act as stretch receptors and are located in the superficial fibrous layer of the joint capsule (see Chapters 6 and 8).[9,41,43–45] *Pacini receptors* are rapidly adapting (RA) type II receptors that respond to compression (pressure) within the joint, although Zimny notes that they also are active at onset and cessation of movement and thus can detect acceleration and deceleration.[41] GTO-like type III receptors have been identified in ligaments as well as the joint capsule.[15,46] Type III free nerve endings act as high threshold mechanoreceptors, and actually become more sensitive (decreased threshold) in the presence of inflammation, and as local effectors by releasing neuropeptides.[43–45,47] In the human ACL, the preponderance of evidence points to the presence of Ruffini (two types) and Pacini endings, and free-nerve endings (see Chapters 6 and 8).[40,41,45]

Given the known mechanical sensitivity of these joint mechanoreceptors, the question then arises as to the their specific role in proprioception. Grigg[9,10,47] states that joint and ligament receptors act primarily as motion limit detectors since they are activated primarily at the limits of joint rotation. Thus they are unlikely to serve as primary position and motion detectors during normal locomotion when joint displacement occurs within normal physiologic limits. However, other investigators have found limited evidence for mid-range mechanoreceptor activity, at least in animal studies.[48,49]

Microneurographic studies of the afferent nerves of the human hand seem to provide evidence that, at least for the distal interphalangeal joint, adequate position sense can occur in the absence of agonist-antagonist muscle length (spindle) input during very slow, small, passive angular displacements.[1,11,13,50] However, with more rapid movements (within the range of active physiologic movement) of the finger joints, the loss of muscle spindle input results in impairment of position sense. For joints of the lower extremity, however, detection of slow, small displacements seems to be dependent on muscle spindle input.[11,15,51] It is likely that capsular and ligamentous receptors can and do provide important position and motion sensations in the joints of the lower extremity,[11,40] although it is likely secondary to the input of the muscle spindle, especially

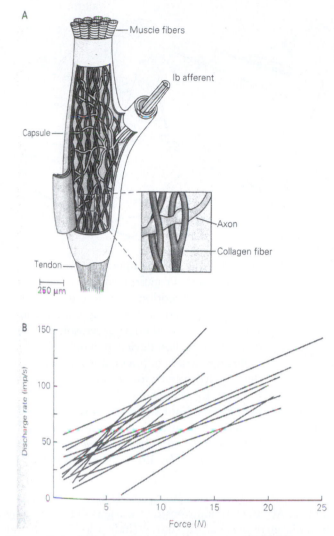

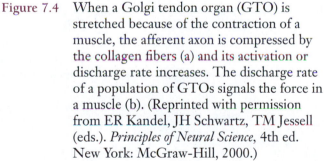

Figure 7.4 When a Golgi tendon organ (GTO) is stretched because of the contraction of a muscle, the afferent axon is compressed by the collagen fibers (a) and its activation or discharge rate increases. The discharge rate of a population of GTOs signals the force in a muscle (b). (Reprinted with permission from ER Kandel, JH Schwartz, TM Jessell (eds.). *Principles of Neural Science*, 4th ed. New York: McGraw-Hill, 2000.)

EVIDENCE FOR A PRIMARY SOURCE OF AFFERENT INFORMATION FOR PROPRIOCEPTION

The argument regarding the primary source of proprioceptive information has continued over many years. During the 1950s and 1960s, the predominant view based on experimental evidence was that articular receptors were the primary source of proprioceptive information.[52] During the 1960s, evidence began to point to the muscle spindle as an important and primary source of sensory information regarding movement. From the 1970s to present, the primary importance of the muscle spindle contribution to proprioception has been more firmly established.

Several lines of evidence point to muscle spindles as the primary source of proprioceptive information.[11,15] First, muscle vibration studies demonstrate perceptual errors of position and motion in the opposite direction of the action of the vibrated muscle.[53] These perceptual errors have been demonstrated in the trunk and limbs during functional and experimental activities, and, in clients with sensory deficits from peripheral neuropathy (e.g., diabetes), the effects of vibration are diminished during joint angle reproduction testing.[54] Second, proprioception is not altered in clients who have undergone total joint replacement with resulting capsulectomy or elimination of intraarticular ligaments.[55–57] Third, articular anesthesia fails to diminish or eliminate, to any significant level, accurate active movement patterns. Barrack et al.[58] demonstrated that intraarticular anesthesia of the knee joint did not alter gait parameters or proprioception in normal subjects, suggesting that proprioception is mediated by the muscle rather than joint or ligamentous receptors. Fourth, muscle fatigue appears to result in deficits of proprioception, as measured by both reproduction of position and threshold to detection of passive motion methods.[59–62] Finally, movement enhances kinesthetic acuity, indicating a primary role of muscle spindles.[11] However, it again must be noted that there are varying types and amounts of proprioceptive information available to the CNS and this sensory information may be dealt with in a manner that will provide the relevant information for determination of segment position and motion for a particular task.

during active physiologic motion. Gandevia et al.[11] conclude that "coherent" discharges from muscle, articular, and cutaneous mechanoreceptors will be used by the CNS in some capacity to encode limb movement and position. The manner in which the CNS encodes and processes this ensemble information to produce precise position and motion information is not clearly understood.

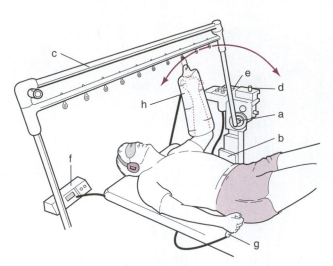

TESTING PROPRIOCEPTION

In the literature, proprioception is primarily determined by the ability to detect a change in limb position, and/or accurately position a limb at a specified joint angle. *Threshold to detection of passive motion* determines the smallest angular displacement that is necessary for the detection of a change in limb position, measured in degrees. In a normal population, this movement is often in the range of one to two degrees, or less.[14,52] The limb is moved passively at very slow angular velocities (range 0.1° to 2.0°/second). Subjects are tested in a seated (**Figure 7.5**) or supine (**Figure 7.6**) position and there is no visual or auditory input to augment somatosensory information. *Reproduction of position* determines the accuracy of positioning the limb with respect to an index or initial joint angle that is then matched by repositioning the same or opposite limb. Reproduction of position may be per-

Figure 7.6   Testing device for the upper extremity internal and external rotation (threshold to detection of passive motion). a. rotational transducer, b. motor, c. moving arm, d. control panel, e. digital microprocessor, f. pneumatic compression device, g. hand-held disengage switch, h. pneumatic compression sleeve. (Reprinted with permission from SL Lephart. Reestablishing Proprioception, Kinesthesia, Joint Position Sense, and Neuromuscular Control in Rehabilitation. In WE Prentice (ed.). *Rehabilitaion Techniques in Sports Medicine.* St. Louis: Mosby, 1994.)

formed passively and/or actively in both components of the test. Accuracy of joint position sense is determined by the difference between the initial (index) joint angle and the reproduced joint angle. Absolute angular error (magnitude only), real or constant error (magnitude and direction), and variable error (standard deviation or error variability) are the variables determined for reproduction of position. Absolute angular error is the most consis-

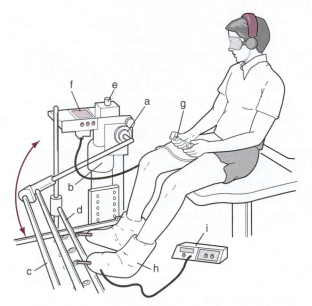

Figure 7.5   Testing device for lower extremity proprioception (threshold to detection of passive motion). a. rotational transducer, b. motor, c. moving arm, d. stationary arm, e. control panel, f. digital microprocessor, g. hand-held disengage switch, h. pneumatic compression sleeve, i. pneumatic compression device. (Reprinted with permission from SL Lephart. Reestablishing Proprioception, Kinesthesia, Joint Position Sense, and Neuromuscular Control in Rehabilitation. In WE Prentice (ed.). *Rehabilitaion Techniques in Sports Medicine.* St. Louis: Mosby, 1994.)

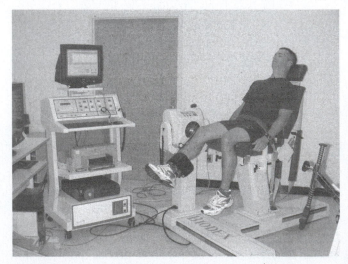

Figure 7.7   Proprioceptive testing on an isokinetic device.

tently recorded measure. Subjects may be seated, recumbent, or standing during testing depending on methods, with visual cues eliminated (**Figure 7.7**). Normal reproduction of position error is generally in the range of 1° to 5°. Reproduction of position also can be tested by perceived knee position using a goniometric visual analog knee model. The client replicates a knee joint flexion angle on a goniometer after the test knee has been placed at an index angle. The difference between the replicated goniometric angle and actual knee angle is the absolute angular error as perceived by the client.[63,64]

Authors often describe threshold to detection of passive motion as a measure of motion sense or kinesthesia and reproduction of position as a measure of joint position sense.[3] These two measures may be subserved by different neural mechanisms, but the neurophysiologic mechanism for, and relationship between, these two methods of determining proprioception have not been clearly determined. Skinner et al.[65] reported a significant but weak correlation between threshold to detection of passive motion and reproduction of position (r = 0.29, r^2 = 0.084), indicating that very little of the variance in reproduction of position error can be attributed to threshold measures.

Muscle reflex latency has been used to test unconscious proprioception in the lower extremity. Beard et al.[31,66,67] have tested reflex hamstring contraction latency as a measure of knee joint proprioception. During their testing, an anterior translation force was imposed on the tibia and electromyographic recordings of the latency of the reflex firing of the hamstrings was noted. Increased latency was interpreted as a deficit of proprioception at the spinal level. Beard et al. has noted increased latencies in subjects with ACL deficiency as well as improved (decreased) reflex hamstring contraction latency after proprioceptive training.[31,66,67] However, in similar experiments, Jennings and Seedholm,[68] and Klein et al.,[69] were unable to replicate these findings. Reflex latencies of leg muscles in response to sudden inversion perturbations also have been measured in order to determine proprioceptive deficits at the ankle.[70]

While the validity of threshold to detection of passive motion and reproduction of position has not been discussed in the literature, these methods are generally the accepted "gold standard" for testing proprioception. While most studies do not report test-retest reliability for threshold to detection of passive motion, at least one study has reported an intraclass correlation coefficient (ICC) value of r = 0.92.[71] Test-retest reliability for reproduction of position also is not often reported. The reliability of reproduction of position has been questioned because of moderate to poor ICC values in those studies that have determined test-retest reliability for reproduction of position,[35,36,72-75] suggesting that reproduction of position may not be a very precise test of proprioception. Marks[75] suggested that use of the ICC may be inappropriate for reproduction of position reliability and advocates the use of standard error of measurement (SEM) as a

more appropriate measure. He found the SEM of repeated reproduction of position error measures to be within the 95 percent confidence interval of initial error scores (or within expected variability). Ogard[36] determined test-retest reliability of weight bearing reproduction of position to be poor (ICC 2,1, r = 0.36) but also noted that SEM values were within the expected variability of the error scores, in agreement with Marks' findings. In view of these findings, conclusions concerning proprioceptive deficits from reproduction of position studies must be interpreted carefully and with caution.

Key Point:

Common proprioception tests include threshold to detection of passive motion performed at slow angular velocities in non-weightbearing, and reproduction of position performed passively and/or actively in non-weight bearing and weight bearing positions.

KNEE JOINT PROPRIOCEPTION

Proprioception studies are commonly reported for the knee, ankle, and shoulder, and less commonly for other extremity joints and the spine. Reproduction of position procedures used to measure knee joint proprioception, particularly with active reproduction of position, with few exceptions generally demonstrate no significant change in proprioception in clients who are ACL deficient, those with patellofemoral pain, or those who have undergone ACL reconstruction. In contrast, studies utilizing threshold to detection of passive motion as a method of measuring proprioception have demonstrated mixed findings. These differing findings may be the result of methodological differences and thus cast some doubt on the clinical or functional significance of changes in proprioception. Furthermore, the results of these studies are difficult to compare given differences in methodology.

Barrack et al.[76] published one of the earliest studies on the effects of ACL deficiency on knee joint proprioception. Threshold to detection of passive motion (a measure of "joint position sense" in their paper) was diminished in the injured knee of subjects when compared to the uninjured knee and to a control group. The between-knee difference was approximately one degree (2.57° ± 0.59° vs. 3.56° ± 1.22°).[76] Testing was initiated at a knee flexion angle of 30°–40°. More recently, Borsa et al.[71] tested subjects with ACL deficiency using threshold to detection of passive motion and found diminished thresholds only when starting at 15° of knee flexion and moving toward full extension. Threshold to detection of passive motion at 45° moving toward either flexion or extension, and from 15° extension moving into flexion, was not affected in these subjects. The magnitude of threshold measures was lower in their study (approximately 0.8 to 1.1°), compared to those of Barrack et al.[76] Borsa et al.[71] noted that threshold to detection of passive motion was significantly more sensitive at 15° flexion moving to extension than into flexion (difference approximately 0.2°). Borsa et al.[71] did not test a control group, while Barrack et al.[76] did. The method of determining angular displacement was different in each study as well; however, test angular velocity was the same in both studies (0.5°/sec).

Key Point:
Results of proprioceptive tests of the knee following injury or surgery demonstrate varied results.

These results point to other possible variables involved in testing proprioception. In the above studies, it appears that joint angle may affect threshold acuity. Lephart et al.[77] noted similar findings to those of Borsa et al.[71] in a study of subjects who had undergone ACL reconstruction. The results seem to suggest the importance of the ACL in sensing end-range motion or as limit detectors, as described by Grigg.[9] Borsa et al.[71] also found a significant but modest negative correlation between single-leg hop distance and threshold to detection of passive motion, suggesting a functional relationship between the two measures. This finding is interesting in that threshold to detection of passive motion is assessed passively at limb velocities well below those of functional movements, in non–weight bearing, and at a single joint. This particular relationship has not been investigated in other knee proprioception studies. However, Gauffin and Tropp[78] have noted altered knee biomechanics and muscle activation patterns during single-leg hop for distance in subjects with ACL deficiency who were more than 10 years post-injury, suggesting altered or compensatory movement patterns to decrease capsuloligamentous loads after ACL injury. Whether this is a result of adaptations in motor function or the result of sensory deficits is not known and requires further study. Other authors have noted adaptive functional changes in lower limb biomechanics after injury and have speculated that these changes might be related to proprioceptive deficits or neuromuscular adaptations.[79–82]

Corrigan et al.[83] found differences in threshold to detection of passive motion between subjects with ACL deficiency and non-impaired control subjects, although no statistical analysis was performed comparing group means. Start position for testing was 35° of knee flexion, similar to that of Barrack et al.[76] Threshold measures of the injured knee were smaller than those noted by Barrack et al.[76] and similar to those noted by Borsa et al.[71] Friden et al.[84,85] also found significant threshold to detection of passive motion increases in subjects with acute ACL deficiency, but these changes were not significant by one month post-injury or when compared to a non-impaired control group. In addition, subjects with ACL deficiency had no differences in active or visual analog reproduction of position tests. Wright et al.[86] were unable to find any significant difference in threshold to detection of passive motion in subjects with ACL deficiency utilizing methods similar to those of Corrigan et al.[83] MacDonald et al.,[87] while finding differences in threshold to detection of passive motion when comparing the injured and uninjured knees of subjects with unilateral ACL deficiency, were unable to identify differences compared to a control group. Beynnon et al.[88] determined that subjects with ACL deficiency had significant deficits in threshold to detection of passive motion averaging 0.28°, but questioned the clinical significance of such small deficits. They did not test a control group. Pap et al.,[89] while finding no difference in the magnitude of threshold to detection of passive motion between non-impaired control group subjects and subjects with ACL deficiency, found that the ACL deficient group was less capable of recognizing the onset or end of motion than control group subjects. Failure rates declined (i.e., proprioception improved) with increasing velocity of test movements (0.1° to 0.85°/sec), demonstrating the influence of velocity on threshold to detection of passive motion. The authors concluded that threshold to detection of passive motion tests alone are inadequate for proprioceptive testing, while determining the failure rate for detecting movement onset is essential to test proprioception. These conflicting results with threshold to detection of passive motion reveal that conclusions as to proprioceptive deficits in clients with ACL deficiency are inconclusive at best.

Threshold to detection of passive motion testing also has been performed on subjects with ACL reconstructed knees. Lephart et al.[77] found deficits only at a start position of 15° knee flexion when subjects moved into either flexion or extension, with no changes at 45°, similar to the findings in the ACL deficient subjects reported by Borsa et al.[71] The deficits reported by Lephart et al.[77] were small, approximately 1° or less between knees, and a control group was not tested. MacDonald et al.[87] also found no significant deficit in threshold to detection of passive motion in subjects who had undergone ACL reconstruction when compared to a non-impaired control group, with small between-knee differences averaging less than 0.2°.[87] Co et al.[90] reported a significant difference in threshold to detection of passive motion in subjects following unilateral ACL reconstruction when comparing the injured and uninjured knees. However, compared to a control group, the ACL reconstruction group demonstrated no significant difference in threshold to detection of passive motion. Pooled data were then analyzed and results indicated that threshold to detection of passive motion measures were actually significantly smaller (increased acuity) in the ACL reconstruction group. The magnitude of between knee differences was no larger than 0.75°. These studies indicate that proprioceptive deficits clearly are not universal after ACL reconstruction or ACL deficiency, and the clinical or functional significance of these small differences, although statistically significant, are not known. Establishing the point at which single-joint deficits result in significant loss of function is critical to the efficacy of proprioceptive testing.

> ## Key Point:
> For proprioceptive deficits measured via single-joint testing to be meaningful, the point at which they result in a significant loss of function must be determined.

Passive and active reproduction of position tests for knee joint proprioception generally demonstrate no significant change after injury to, or reconstruction of, the ACL. Co et al.[90] found no differences in either passive or relative (opposite limb) reproduction of position in subjects who had undergone ACL reconstruction. Harter et al.[91] and Dvir et al.[92] similarly found no errors for varied conditions of reproduction of position in subjects who had undergone ACL reconstruction. Ogard[36] demonstrated no loss of proprioception for standing weight bearing or non–weight bearing reproduction of position in subjects who had undergone ACL reconstruction.

Conflicting results have been noted with visual analog reproduction of position measures of proprioception for subjects with ACL deficiency or following ACL reconstruction. Barrett[63] reported significant differences in perception of actual knee joint position in subjects with ACL deficiency or following ACL reconstruction. Measurement reliability was reported to be good (r = 0.81).[63,64] Barrett[63] also noted a strong correlation between visual analog reproduction of position errors, client satisfaction and a subjective measure of knee joint function (r = 0.90 and 0.84 respectively). In contrast, Friden et al.[84] failed to find visual analog reproduction of position error differences in subjects who had acute ACL deficient knees.

> ## Key Point:
> Varied methodology limits the interpretation and comparison of results between studies.

Proprioceptive tests of subjects with other knee pathologies have yielded more consistent results. In a study of clients with total knee arthroplasty (TKA), Barrett et al.[64] again used visual analog reproduction of position and found smaller errors after TKA compared to aged-matched subjects with osteoarthritis, but higher errors compared to subjects without osteoarthritis and younger subjects. The passive reproduction of position test results reported by Skinner et al.[56] for clients having undergone TKA for osteoarthritis were very similar to those of Barrett et al.[64] These results suggest that the visual analog method may in fact be a valid method for testing proprioception (position sense). Pai et al.[93] also noted proprioceptive (threshold to detection of passive motion) deficits in subjects with osteoarthritis compared to age-matched control subjects and younger subjects, also noting a correlation with proprioception and disease-specific functional status, although functional status score only accounted for approximately 16 percent of the variability in threshold to detection of passive motion (r = 0.397, r^2 = 0.158). Age was positively correlated with proprioception deficits in these studies. Apparently age and osteoarthritis are two factors that consistently reflect at least some change in joint function related to changes in proprioception. However, the functional significance of these deficits has not been determined.

In contrast to these findings, Pap et al.[94] reported poorer threshold to detection of passive motion measures, as well as failure to detect onset or end of motion, in subjects with TKA compared to subjects with arthrosis and non-impaired control subjects. Also, there was no correlation between clinical outcome measures and threshold to detection of passive motion measures, noting that subjects who had undergone TKA significantly improved function scores compared to subjects with arthrosis.[94] The authors concluded that removal of diseased joint receptors as a result of TKA diminished proprioception, but improved function. Interestingly, total hip arthroplasty in which capsulectomy has been performed has not been shown to result in proprioceptive deficits.[55,57]

Jerosch and Prymka[95] noted proprioceptive deficits (visual analog reproduction of position) in subjects who had sustained a patellar dislocation when compared to a non-impaired control group. Smaller errors were noted at the extremes of knee motion (10° and 80° knee flexion) than at mid-range (60° flexion). These results confirm the findings of Borsa et al.[71] and Lephart et al.[77] regarding the joint angle specificity of proprioception related to acuity. Surprisingly, no studies have been performed that compare pre- and post-proprioceptive therapeutic exercise regimens in subjects who demonstrate deficits in threshold to detection of passive motion. Two studies comparing weight bearing (standing) and non–weight bearing (sitting) reproduction of position in subjects with patellofemoral pain syndrome demonstrate conflicting findings. Kramer et al.[74] reported no significant differences in reproduction of position for clients with patellofemoral pain syndrome, while Baker et al.[96] determined that subjects with patellofemoral pain syndrome did have significant reproduction of position errors under both test conditions. These conflicting results might be explained by differing methods of measuring knee joint angle. Baker et al.[96] concluded that based on their findings, proprioceptive re-education should be included when managing clients with patellofemoral pain syndrome. However, the authors provided no evidence that proprioception could actually be improved through the use of proprioceptive exercise with these clients.

Summarizing the findings regarding proprioceptive deficits at the knee, these statements seem appropriate: 1) Proprioception, as assessed by reproduction of position and threshold to detection of passive motion, seems to be affected by age and fatigue; 2) proprioception may be affected in subjects with osteoarthritis, and TKA appears to attenuate the proprioceptive deficit; 3) evidence for statistically, functionally, and clinically relevant proprioceptive deficits following ACL injury, ACL deficiency, ACL reconstruction, and patellofemoral pain syndrome is equivocal at best; and 4) while several authors recommend that therapeutic exercise programs include specific proprioceptive exercises in addition to traditional strengthening exercises, there is no direct scientific evidence provided that demonstrates improved proprioception as a result of proprioceptive exercise when treating clients with knee joint problems.

Key Point:

Evidence of functional limitations at the knee based on proprioceptive deficits is equivocal at best and warrants further study.

SHOULDER JOINT PROPRIOCEPTION

Proprioceptive deficits also have been described at the shoulder.[97–102] Warner et al.[97] noted significant changes in threshold to detection of passive motion in subjects with glenohumeral instability. Threshold to detection of passive motion methods were similar to those utilized for testing the knee. As in the knee joint, deficits were more notable at the extremes of joint motion (toward external rotation) rather than at middle ranges. Between-limb differences were in the range of 0.6° to 1.3°, depending on condition, when compared to a non-impaired control group or the uninjured limb. Reproduction of position was noted to be less accurate in subjects with shoulder instability. Error averaged approximately one degree.[97] When subjects were tested after shoulder stabilization surgery, threshold to detection of passive motion and reproduction of position measures returned to normal values; however, there was no indication as to whether these deficits related to any functional changes at the shoulder. Lephart et al.[102] had nearly identical findings in their study of clients with shoulder instability and subsequent surgical stabilization. Smith and Brunolli[100] also found proprioceptive differences for active reproduction of position and threshold to detection of passive motion after shoulder dislocation. Between-limb differences were slightly higher (mean difference 1.57°) for threshold to detection of passive motion

than those reported by Lephart et al.[102] and Warner et al.[97] Generally these studies only examined internal and external rotation, excluding motion in the sagittal and frontal plane.

More recently, Lephart et al.[99] were only able to find a significant difference in one variable of active joint repositioning (humeral displacement) in subjects who had undergone thermal capsulorraphy for capsuloligamentous shoulder instability. The authors had hypothesized that thermal energy would result in damage to capsular mechanoreceptors resulting in proprioceptive deficits, but their results did not support this hypothesis. Active humeral rotation, passive reproduction of position, threshold to detection of passive motion, and motion path reproduction all were normal.[99] These subjects were not tested to determine whether deficits existed prior to thermal capsulorraphy. No data were reported regarding clinical stability, although all subjects had high scores (> 90/100) on a questionnaire rating shoulder function.[99] Histological findings were not provided, so it is unclear whether capsuloligamentous mechanoreceptors were affected by the thermal procedures.

Brindle et al.[103] studied latent muscle reaction times as a component of proprioception in throwing athletes. Results determined that throwing athletes had significantly different patterns of latent muscle timing compared to non-throwing control subjects, specifically in the infraspinatus and teres minor muscles, in response to sudden perturbation. The authors concluded that this change represented an acquired neuromuscular imbalance, but that the data could not be generalized to actual throwing activities since testing was performed at speeds that were unrelated to throwing.[103] These results would appear to be related to reflex activity rather than higher level CNS proprioceptive activity (unconscious or conscious). The authors suggested further studies were necessary to interpret the findings.

Dover et al.[101] examined the effect of overhead throwing on reproduction of position in asymptomatic female softball athletes compared to non-throwing athletes. Reproduction of position was measured at four different positions of the shoulder: internal rotation, external rotation, flexion and extension. A significant difference in reproduction of position was only found at the externally rotated position with an error difference of approximately 1.5°. The softball athletes had no known shoulder pathology or clinical findings that might explain the difference. Since there was no functional change in the softball players, it is unlikely that this deficit had any effect on performance. The authors speculated about a possible relationship between proprioception and injury, as well as the use of proprioceptive exercises, either closed or open kinetic chain, to prevent injury. However, there is no definitive research to support that speculation.

Finally, Voight et al.[61] tested reproduction of position at the shoulder before and after a fatiguing protocol. The results demonstrated significant errors in active and passive repositioning after the fatiguing protocol. Passive repositioning errors were very large compared to active error (30.4° vs. 3.3°, respectively) for the dominant extremity, and there was no difference between the dominant and non-dominant extremity. The authors concluded that fatigue is a factor affecting glenohumeral proprioception. However, no definitive conclusions about the functional significance of these findings were noted. Since most upper extremity activities are performed actively, it is difficult to interpret how a difference of 3.3° in shoulder rotation positioning might affect hand or elbow position during reaching activities, or even accuracy of throwing. Pederson et al.[104] also demonstrated changes in detecting varying movement velocity of the shoulder after fatiguing exercise in non-impaired subjects. No other proprioceptive variables were measured. In contrast, Sterner et al.[105] were unable to demonstrate any proprioceptive deficits for varied reproduction of position and threshold to detection of passive motion tests of the shoulder after a fatiguing protocol in non-impaired subjects. Overall, as with proprioception studies of the knee, these studies of shoulder proprioception are inconclusive with regard to functionally significant changes after fatigue, injury, surgery, and rehabilitation. Further, there are no studies that demonstrate direct changes in proprioception as a result of specific proprioceptive therapeutic exercise intervention.

> ## Key Point:
> There is some evidence that proprioceptive differences exist at the glenohumeral joint of the shoulder under varied conditions including injury; however, the clinical and functional significance of these differences is unclear.

Ankle Joint Proprioception

A number of ankle proprioception studies have been performed on subjects demonstrating chronic ankle instability or functional instability. Freeman et al.[106] suggested that changes in afferent information from ankle joint mechanoreceptors after injury resulted in decreased single leg stance stability in subjects with functional instability of the ankle joint. Given the fact that joint receptors are not the primary source of proprioceptive input, it is questionable whether changes in proprioception at the ankle after injury are actually attributable to damage to these receptors. Garn and Newton[107] and Glenncross and Thornton[108] demonstrated decreased threshold to detection of passive motion and reproduction of position function, respectively, in subjects after unilateral ankle sprains. However, Gross[109] and Refshauge et al.[110] reported no changes

in ankle joint proprioception in subjects with recurrent ankle sprains. Konradsen and Ravn[111] detected changes in reflex latencies of the peroneal muscles in subjects with chronic ankle instability. However, Osborne et al.[70] were not able to detect any changes in peroneus longus muscle reflex contraction latencies in subjects with a history of ankle sprains either before or after ankle disc training. Methodological differences may explain the differences in results in these studies, but any conclusions as to the extent and nature of proprioceptive deficits resulting from ankle sprains and functional instability must be interpreted with caution and skepticism.

Other investigators have noted increased postural sway in subjects with functional ankle instability.[112] Friden et al.[113] noted differences in frontal plane sway characteristics in subjects with functional ankle instability, but not sagittal plane differences. However, Tropp and Odenrick[114] were unable to demonstrate differences in postural sway in a comparison of soccer players with and without previous ankle sprains. Other factors such as fatigue and specific athletic activities have been shown to have an effect on proprioceptive acuity and accuracy of ankle joint proprioception.[115,116] Aydin et al.[116] noted that young gymnasts had better passive and active reproduction of position measures than non-gymnasts. Their conclusion was that gymnastics training might have had a positive effect on position sense. However, given that the study was retrospective in nature, the only conclusion that can be made is that gymnasts appear to have more accurate position sense than non-gymnasts, but not necessarily as a result of their specific training.

As noted in studies of the knee and shoulder, results of proprioceptive studies of the ankle have resulted in somewhat conflicting findings, possibly as a result of methodological differences. Based on the evidence, it is difficult to determine the effect of ankle ligamentous injuries on proprioception, and whether these reported changes have any effect or causal relationship to injury or recovery from ligamentous injury to the ankle or functional instability.

> ## Key Point:
> From existing evidence it is difficult to determine the effect of ankle ligamentous injuries on proprioception, and whether the changes that have been reported have any effect or casual relationship to injury, recovery from the injury, or functional instability.

The Spine and Proprioception

In comparison to the upper and lower extremities, fewer proprioceptive studies have been performed on the spine, with most focusing on the lumbar spine. Lam et al.[117]

were unable to detect any kinesthetic deficits in subjects with low back pain using active reproduction of position in a sitting position; however, subjects with low back pain tended to overshoot the target position more often than asymptomatic subjects. Koumantakis et al.[73] tested reproduction of position in a group of subjects with low back pain and a control group and were unable to detect any differences in multi-plane position testing. They concluded that poor reliability of the testing methods did not allow for identification of subjects with low back pain on the basis of proprioceptive deficits.

It has been speculated that proprioceptive deficits may lead to joint injury or re-injury and should be a significant focus of therapeutic exercise programs. Parkhurst and Burnett[118] examined relationships between proprioception and factors related to low back injury in a large group of firefighters (n = 88). Age and years of experience displayed a weak relationship with proprioception measures (r < 0.36). Injuries also correlated with proprioceptive changes for movements in single and multiple planes, but these factors were poorly correlated, with injury accounting for no more than 0.05 percent (r ≤ 0.22) of the variability in proprioception as determined by threshold to detection of passive motion, reproduction of position, and direction of motion perception. The authors concluded that impaired proprioception "may degrade lumbar motor function," leading to an increased risk of injury.[118] However, there is no direct evidence that proprioceptive deficits result in injury or re-injury to the lumbar spine. They recommended that a therapeutic exercise program goal should be the restoration of proprioception, but their results provide little evidence that proprioception had a significant role in low back injuries among the subjects they studied. Overall, evidence remains unclear with regard to changes in proprioception after injury to the spine or the relationship between proprioception and low back pain.

Key Point:
The relationship between changes in proprioception after injury to the lumbar spine region and the relationship between proprioception and low back pain remains unclear.

EFFECTS OF TRAINING/EXERCISE ON PROPRIOCEPTION

Proprioceptive or kinesthetic exercises are commonly recommended as an indispensable component of therapeutic exercise programs for improving proprioception after injury and/or preventing re-injury.[2,4,6,8] However, there is little evidence to suggest that proprioception, as determined by reproduction of position or threshold to detec-

tion of passive motion, can be improved by specific proprioceptive exercises. Ashton-Miller et al.,[14] in a comprehensive literature review on proprioception and proprioceptive therapeutic exercise, concluded that, "despite their widespread acceptance, current exercises aimed at 'improving proprioception' have not been demonstrated to achieve that goal." However, it is clear that sensory information from the muscle spindles of muscles involved in movement do contribute to movement control at all CNS levels.[1] Based on current neurophysiologic findings, active and passive motions throughout a joint's range motion should elicit appropriate levels of sensory input from cutaneous, capsuloligamentous, and musculotendinous mechanoreceptors.[11,12] The exact mechanisms of how proprioceptive input from these receptors influences motor output are complex, and various models exist that might explain the processes involved[1,12,14] (see Chapter 8). In general, motor commands are noted to be modifiable via muscle spindle input throughout the CNS, while signals from joint and cutaneous receptors provide sensory information at subcortical levels (**Figure 7.8**). Combined information from these receptors about position and motion, both during and after motion, provides a basis for efficiency and plasticity of the motor control system in regulating goal-oriented movement for a given task within a specific environment.[1,12] Whether therapeutic exercises modify these mechanoreceptors either morphologically or neurophysiologically, is a question that still needs to be answered.

No studies have directly measured the effects of specific proprioceptive training protocols on measures such as reproduction of position and threshold to detection of passive motion at the knee joint. Lephart et al.[77] determined that subjects with ACL reconstructions had statistically significant end range extension threshold deficits and recommended that these subjects engage in functional, weight bearing therapeutic exercise activities to improve proprioception. However, threshold to detection of passive motion testing is performed in a non–weight bearing position at a very slow velocity without muscle activation, thereby displaying little similarity to functional activities, especially in a highly athletic population. Borsa et al.[71] were able to identify a relationship between single leg hop for distance, a commonly used knee function test, and threshold to detection of passive motion (r = 0.54), which was highest at a mid-range test position (45° flexion) where subjects with ACL deficiency had no proprioceptive deficit. Proprioception was less correlated to single leg hop at near-full knee extension (r = 0.45) where subjects demonstrated a significant deficit in threshold to detection of passive motion measurements.

Bernier and Perrin[119] tested both active and passive reproduction of position in subjects with ankle instability before and after commonly used balance and coordination therapeutic exercise protocols to improve proprioception and postural sway. There was no significant change in any

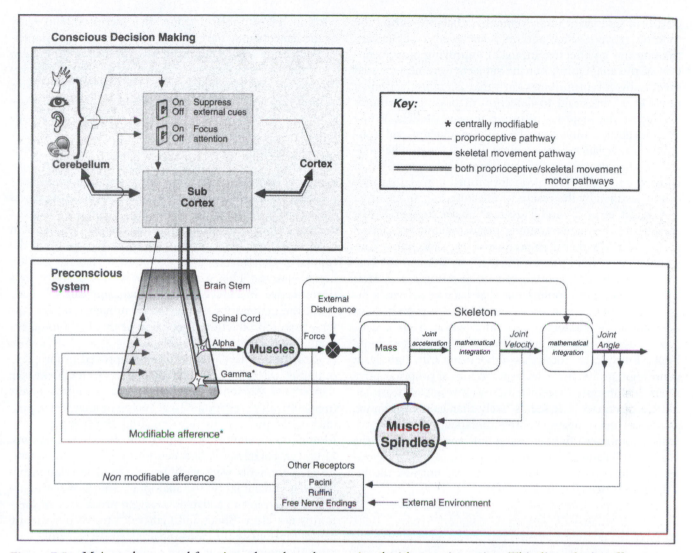

Figure 7.8   Main pathways and functions thought to be associated with proprioception. Thin lines depict afferent pathways that subserve proprioception, and thick lines depict efferent pathways subserving motor actions and skeletal movement. To optimize proprioception, the higher central nervous system structures (Conscious Decision Making box) that control attention and motivation may have to suppress tactile, visual, auditory and vestibular cues and up-regulate the cerebellar and reticular system structures that control arousal. These structures then modulate the rubrospinal and rubro-bulbospinal pathways that help modulate muscle spindle output via gamma system recruitment. The system that directly subserves proprioception (Preconscious System box) includes motor pathways (bold lines) that generate skeletal movements and sensory feedback on those forces emanating from the Golgi tendon organs and position feedback provided primarily by the muscle spindles whose output is centrally modifiable via the gamma motor neurons. (Reprinted with permission from JA Ashton-Miller et al. Can proprioception be improved by exercise? *Knee Surg Sports Traumatol Arthrosc.* 2001;9(3):128–136.)

measure of reproduction of position after the training regimen; however, subjects did demonstrate improvement in postural sway control.[119] The mechanisms underlying the improvement in sway control are not identifiable based on the methods and results of this study. Rozzi et al.[120] were able to demonstrate a similar effect for balance training in both non-impaired subjects and subjects with functional ankle instability. Presumably, the control group subjects had normal proprioception at the ankle joint, demonstrating that balance can be improved even in subjects without sensory impairments. All subjects trained with a balance device that provided visual feedback for maintaining position during single limb stance and vestibular cues were not blocked. However, both groups displayed significant improvements in balance during the training period. The authors concluded that balance training was an effective means of improving proprioception of the ankle joint, but the subjects were never tested specifically for proprioception—that is, reproduction of position or threshold to detection of passive motion, as utilized in the majority of proprioceptive studies. While proprioceptive input may be utilized during, and contribute to, balance training activities, it cannot be concluded that proprioception was improved as a result of balance training. Only a conclusion of improved balance can be justified by the results of the study.

Gauffin et al.[121] and Nashner[21] have suggested that these types of balance training protocols improve central motor control rather than peripheral proprioception. This would seem to hold true for the study by Bernier and Perrin,[119] since there was improvement in postural sway after training. Nashner[21] points out that balance activities involve more than single joint control, including multi-joint neuromuscular strategies and information from a wide distribution of proprioceptive inputs to maintain stability limits. Further, he notes that only clients with significant neurologic problems or widespread loss of proprioceptive input demonstrate destabilization as a result of disrupted muscle responses.[21] It seems likely that balance training, as used in many proprioceptive therapeutic exercise programs, combines multiple sources of input to improve the control of balance, including sensory input from proprioceptors throughout the lower extremity, not just the involved joint (see Chapters 9 and 10).

Key Point:

Proprioceptive or kinesthetic exercises are commonly included in therapeutic exercise programs for treating upper and lower extremity injuries.

Several studies have shown more accurate proprioceptive function in trained athletes than in non-impaired control subjects without the same sports training, including gymnasts[116,122,123] and ballet dancers.[124] The subjects in these studies had years of training in specific sports that included motor skills related to balance and precise movement control. The results of these studies seem to suggest that proprioceptive acuity can be affected by long term specific training activities. However, the specificity principle might be evident with regard to the test procedures, i.e., accuracy of position and sensing of proper position. Further, the dancers in the study by Barrack et al.[124] were better in only one parameter of proprioceptive measures—threshold to detection of passive motion—compared to non-dancers, who were more accurate in reproduction of

position. The authors presumed that increased joint laxity of the dancers may have played a role in the proprioceptive differences, but joint laxity was not measured. Finally, all studies were retrospective in nature, so pre-training reproduction of position or threshold to detection of passive motion measurements were not made. Consequently, no effect can be claimed for the training, only that the groups were different in the measures.

Lephart et al.[122] found that gymnasts had a more sensitive threshold to detection of passive motion than non-gymnasts, but also noted that their response times (i.e., stopping the passive motion when change of position was sensed) were significantly better, by 74 percent, than the control group. The authors did not discuss this factor in relation to their findings, and it was not factored into the results of the threshold to detection of passive motion measurements. This study, like those noted above, was retrospective in nature, so no conclusion can be made about the gymnastics training as an influence on the difference in reproduction of position or threshold to detection of passive motion.

Two studies have demonstrated improved proprioception after warm-up activities for muscles (see Chapter 3). Bartlett and Warren[125] reported significant improvements ($p = 0.005$) in perception (visual analog of knee) for reproduction of position in non-impaired subjects after performing four minutes of jogging and stretching exercises. However, correlations between the pre- and post-warm-up measurements were weak ($r = 0.58$). The relationship between perceptual (visual analog) measures of reproduction of position and active or passive reproduction of position is not clear. Bouet and Gahery[126] tested passive and active kinesthesia in non-impaired subjects before and after 10 minutes of stationary cycling on the test leg only. Warm-up resulted in improved active knee reproduction of position measurements, but no improvement in passive reproduction of position or visual analog reproduction of position measurements. While not speculating on the mechanism of improvement, the authors concluded that enhanced motor performance might be due to improved muscle mechanical properties and kinesthetic sensibility.

Beard et al.[31,67] demonstrated that reflex hamstring contraction latency as a measure of unconscious proprioception in a group of subjects with ACL deficiency could be improved by proprioceptive therapeutic exercise to a greater extent than by traditional therapeutic exercises (muscle strengthening). While both exercise groups improved their reflex hamstring contraction latency, the improvement was significantly greater in the proprioceptive exercise group. The question remains however, as to whether reflex hamstring contraction latency actually is a true measure of proprioception or reflects only changes in reflex activation sensitivity. Jennings and Seedhom,[68] and Klein et al.,[69] found no changes in reflex hamstring contraction latency among subjects with ACL deficiency, casting some doubt on the results of Beard et al.[31,67] Osborne et al.[70] demonstrated a significant decrease in anterior tibialis muscle activation latency with ankle disk training in both experimental and control (contralateral) ankles. There was no change in peroneus longus, posterior tibialis, or flexor digitorum longus muscle activation latency. The reason for a change in only one muscle is unclear, but results may have been affected by a small sample size and methodology.[70] Subjects in the study were asymptomatic and had no evidence of instability, so the benefit of the effect is unclear. Further, it is not clear whether the training effects are strictly sensory in nature or include motor control and motor learning aspects, as noted by Nashner[21] (see Chapter 8). These limited and equivocal findings suggest the need for future investigations to determine the specific effects of therapeutic exercise program intervention on proprioceptors and proprioceptive function, and better methods of testing proprioception.

> ## *Key Point:*
> A direct relationship between improved proprioceptive measurements and participation in a proprioceptive or kinesthetic sense based therapeutic exercise program has not be conclusively demonstrated.

Fitzgerald et al.[127] implemented a neuromuscular training program in a select number of subjects with ACL deficient knees, enabling them to return to high level activity without ACL reconstruction. Athletes with ACL deficiency were divided into training groups that included standard ACL rehabilitation methods, including therapeutic exercise activities that are typically termed proprioceptive, and a group that additionally utilized various perturbation therapeutic exercise activities.[127] Subjects who had the additional perturbation training were able to return to their previous high level of activity to a more significant extent, were able to postpone ACL reconstruction, and had fewer episodes of the knee joint giving way than subjects who had not undergone perturbation training. The authors could not explain the mechanism of the perturbation effects based on the study design, so the question remains as to the exact neurophysiologic, neuromuscular, and sensorimotor nature and effect of the perturbation component of the therapeutic exercise protocol.

Proprioceptive exercises have been recommended as a means of preventing ACL injuries.[128,129] Cerulli et al.[128] suggested that implementation of therapeutic exercises such as proprioceptive neuromuscular facilitation (PNF) (see Chapter 6) and activities utilizing various balance (wobble) boards resulted in a decreased incidence of ACL injuries. Caraffa et al.[129] prospectively studied the effect of proprioceptive training on the incidence of ACL injuries in Italian soccer players. Soccer players who underwent proprioceptive training, as described by Cerulli et al.,[128] had significantly fewer ACL injuries than players who underwent only traditional training. However, they noted that proprioception (awareness of limb position) was not tested before or after the training protocol, so no statement as to the effect of the training on proprioception could be made. While exercises or activities such as these almost certainly elicit proprioceptive responses, there is no evidence that proprioception actually improves as result of the exercises. The neurophysiologic and neuromuscular mechanisms that result in fewer injuries to the ACL are not clear and are only speculative at this time.

Hamstring muscle group training after ACL injury and deficiency has been noted to improve symptoms of knee instability.[130,131] Giove et al.[131] were able to improve function in subjects with ACL deficiency after participation in a therapeutic exercise program that emphasized hamstring strengthening through isometric, isotonic and isokinetic exercises. All subjects returned to some level of sports activity, with 59 percent able to return to pre-injury participation levels.[131] Ihara and Nakayama[130] were able to effect changes in dynamic hamstring function as measured by isokinetic variables in subjects with varying levels of ACL deficiency. None of the subjects exhibited a positive Lachman test for anterior instability. Hamstring training was accomplished by imposing rapid resistance to knee flexion while subjects positioned themselves on various unstable surfaces. Subjects with ACL deficiency (n = 4) demonstrated improved dynamic hamstring function on isokinetic testing compared to five non-injured control group subjects. Subjects did not undergo any other testing procedures, although all four noted decreased episodes of giving way and were able to return to some level of sports activity.[130] The small sample size and lack of a control group of subjects with ACL deficiency limits the generalizability of these results with regard to the training effect. Certainly a casual comparison can be made to the results of Fitzgerald et al.[127] The studies by Giove et al.[131] and Ihara and Nakayama[130] suggest that neuromuscular control can be changed through specific training and that stability can be improved during the performance of motor skills at a high level. However, a relationship to proprioceptive function cannot be ascertained from these results.

> ## *Key Point:*
> Although neuromuscular control can be enhanced with a properly designed therapeutic exercise program, improved proprioception has not been clearly demonstrated.

One of the limitations with studies that advocate the benefits of proprioceptive therapeutic exercises or training is that there are relatively few outcome measures that directly measure proprioceptive changes. Studies have not consistently measured reproduction of position or threshold to detection of passive movement both pre- and post-treatment to demonstrate significant changes in these measures. Further, correlations with improvement in these measures and functional outcome measures have not been clearly demonstrated, or show only limited relationships.[71] Examples of functional outcome measures include various single leg hop tests, agility tests, or single leg vertical jump tests (see Chapters 5, 9, and 11). Other sports specific functional tests (timed) that include dynamic stability also have been developed.[132] Again, the relationship of these tests to traditional proprioceptive measurement methods is unclear.

Client self-report outcome measurements also might be used to determine relationships between proprioceptive measures. Region specific tools (e.g., the Cincinnati Knee Rating Scale) and general health outcome tools (e.g., SF-36) can serve as appropriate measures of functional outcome or general health (see Chapter 11). A significant relationship has been demonstrated between Cincinnati Knee Rating Scale scores and weight bearing reproduction of position ($r = -0.40$, $p = 0.03$), although the correlation is weak, this suggests that clients with less perceived symptoms displayed smaller position reproduction errors.[36] Other authors have demonstrated a relationship between proprioceptive measures (visual analog reproduction of position), client satisfaction (visual analog measure) and functional outcome (activity level).[63]

> ## Key Point:
> The proprioceptive system has a direct influence on motor skills through influences at all CNS levels.

ASPECTS OF THERAPEUTIC EXERCISE AND TRAINING WITH UTILIZATION OF PROPRIOCEPTIVE INPUT

Based on current evidence, there is little scientific basis for specific proprioceptive or kinesthetic training or therapeutic exercises that directly improve proprioception.[14] The theoretical and practical basis for therapeutic exercises must then be based on the assumption that their performance will result in appropriate proprioceptive input for posture, balance and stability, whether static or dynamic, and guiding or controlling movement, resulting in successful completion of a specific motor task in a given environment. Philosophically, it is imperative to note that, while we may not be directly training and/or improving proprioception through exercise, the exercises performed are eliciting proprioceptive information that influence, control, and/or enhance motor output.[14] Therefore, motor learning and improved motor control occurs as a result of practicing motor skills or activities, hopefully resulting in improved performance and decreased risk of injury or re-injury. The number and variety of therapeutic exercises and activities that can be used is considerable. Therapeutic exercises should be selected according to the nature and extent of the specific injury and impairment, and the effects on the client's function or disability, with appropriate goals for returning the client to optimum function and quality of life in a reasonable time frame.

Therapeutic exercise prescription and progression should attempt to match activities with the specific needs and goals of the client. This progression involves, but is not exclusive to, addressing pathology (e.g., muscle strain), impairments (e.g., loss of strength or range of motion), loss of function (e.g., inability to ascend or descend stairs), and disability (e.g., inability to perform job). The therapeutic exercise program is aimed at re-establishing motor control through motor learning and skill acquisition (see Chapter 8). With these assumptions and aims in mind, various examples of exercises and activities can be described to successfully achieve program goals from initial examination and evaluation, to discharge and return to activity.

Several authors have outlined therapeutic exercise programs specific to enhancing or re-establishing proprioception.[6,17,19,20,128,129] The majority of these programs focus on lower extremity injuries, specifically ACL deficiency or reconstruction. Lephart[6] describes four phases for proprioceptive (kinesthetic) training and neuromuscular control as applied to the lower extremity. Phase I aims are to re-establish balance, dynamic joint stability, and a "kinesthetic" running gait. Phase II activities emphasize change of direction, i.e., cutting and turning movements (see Chapters 5 and 9). Phase III activities emphasize activities to promote return to activity, or sports specific activity (see Chapter 11). Phase IV emphasizes integration of proprioceptive elements refined in the first three phases into functional activities (e.g., sport specific activities, work activities). Several activities specific to each of these phases are listed in **Table 7.2**.

Voight and Cook[17] advocate the use of what is termed *reactive neuromuscular training* for the restoration of neuromuscular control and proprioception, subserved by proprioceptive, visual, and vestibular input. Reactive neuromuscular training is designed to facilitate return to activity by complementing traditional strength and endurance activities, and with balance and proprioceptive training.[17] Three phases of the reactive neuromuscular activities emphasize minimal joint motion and isometric muscle activity, primarily in weight bearing (e.g., single limb stance), with weight shifting and varying resistance

TABLE 7.2   Typical activities for lower extremity proprioceptive training

Phase I	Phase III
• Walk/run on stable, flat surface	• Running
• Balance activities	• Shuttle run
• Two feet, unstable surface	• Kinesthetic/agility training
• Eyes open	• Shuttle run
• Multi-directional	• Carioca
• Eyes closed	• Cutting drills
• Multi-directional	• Eccentric loading
• One foot, unstable surface	• Plyometric activities
• Eyes open	**Phase IV**
• Unidirectional	• Sport specific activities
• Multidirectional	• Four-corner running while dribbling basketball
• Eyes closed	• Carioca while defending
• Unidirectional	• Sport specific drills isolated from team setting
• Multidirectional	• Basketball layups
• Passive and active joint repositioning	• Fielding ground balls—baseball
• Eccentric loading	• Pass patterns for football
• Stairs: up, down, forward backward	• Defensive maneuvers for specific sports
Phase II	
• Running	
• Decreasing circle diameter, varied speeds	
• Kinesthetic training	
• Co-contraction lateral slides	
• Mini-trampoline: hopping, jogging	
• Lateral slide board activities	
• Active joint repositioning	
• Eccentric loading	
• Stair climbing	
• Plyometric activities	

(adapted from Lephart S.[6])

applied through elastic bands or cords, and varied surface stability to modify proprioceptive input (**Figure 7.9**). Activities can be performed with eyes closed to eliminate visual references for balance and increase dependence on somatosensory and vestibular inputs. Phase II (*transitional stability*) exercises emphasize movement through full range of motion, including resisted concentric and eccentric contractions, during various weight bearing activities such as walking and running, lunges, and lateral movements (**Figure 7.10**). Phase III activities increase the demands on the neuromotor system, increasing joint loads and velocity of motion through impact and ballistic exercise. Resisted running (**Figure 7.11**) or bounding (plyometric) (**Figure 7.12a–c**) exercises would be an example of Phase III activities.

Hewett et al.[20] describes a similar series and progression of exercises, and activities aimed at re-establishing proprioception and neuromuscular control after ACL deficiency or reconstruction. Included are six phases and a return to sports component, each relating to the post-operative course of treatment, with emphasis on restoring or enhancing proprioception and/or neuromuscular function. The exercises range from weight shifting during the early post-operative days to high level motor activities, including plyometrics and balance challenges during activity and sport specific exercises.[20]

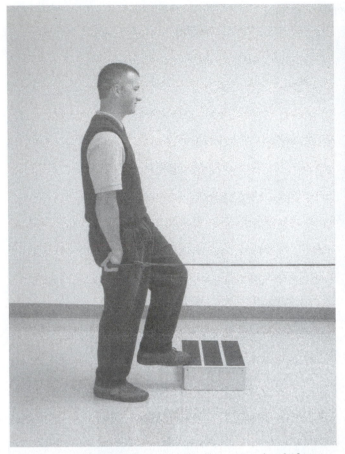

Figure 7.9   Phase I, static stabilization: weight shifting with resistance.

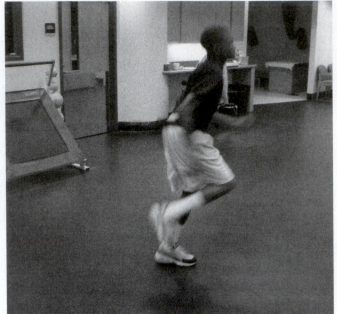

Figure 7.11   Phase III, dynamic stabilization: resisted running.

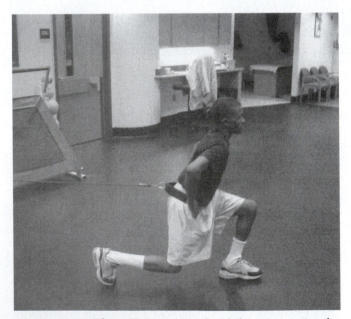

Figure 7.10   Phase II, transitional stabilization: resisted lunge technique.

Finally, Wilk et al.[19] describes two therapeutic exercise programs for clients following ACL reconstruction, one for young athletic clients and a second, slower program for older clients who participate in recreational activities. The authors state that the primary difference between the two programs is the rate of progression.[19] Emphasis is placed on restoring proprioception, dynamic stability, and neuromuscular control.[19] Many of the activities and therapeutic exercises described are similar, if not the same, as those described by other authors. Again, the distinctions between proprioceptive, neuromuscular control and dynamic stability exercise are not clear. The authors list proprioceptive training and proprioceptive drills as therapeutic exercises included during various phases of the programs, but do not describe the specific aspects/nature of these exercises.[19] However, any of the active exercises listed will elicit proprioceptive input to the CNS, and the neurophysiologic basis for a training effect has not been definitively established.

Although not as extensively or specifically addressed in the literature, therapeutic exercise for training the upper extremity would include the principles noted previously for the lower extremity, excluding activities or movements specific to the lower extremity. Early phase activities for the shoulder might include proprioceptive neuromuscular facilitation (PNF) techniques (e.g., rhythmic stabilization) for stability, range-specific strengthening and motor activities, and weight bearing (closed kinetic chain) bilateral and single upper extremity activities (**Figure 7.13** and **Figure 7.14**) to promote joint stability. Later phases may include activities through specified ranges using weights, elastic tubing (**Figure 7.15**), or manual resistance, including PNF diagonals, plyometrics (**Figure 7.16a–f**), and ac-

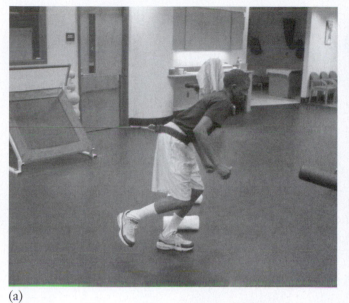

(a)

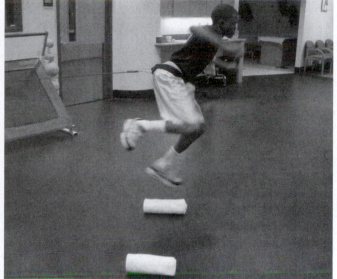

(b)

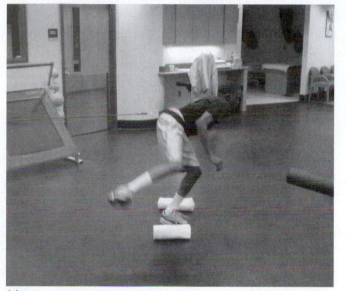

(c)

Figure 7.12   Phase III, dynamic stabilization: lateral bounding with resistance. (a), start; (b), mid-jump; (c), finish.

tivity/sport specific exercises (**Figure 7.17a–b**). Final phases of therapeutic exercise activity would increase the level of intensity of previous phases, again including exercises specific to work, recreation, or sports, and finally return to those activities.

The previously mentioned therapeutic exercise programs emphasizing proprioception or kinesthesia demonstrate a wide range of activities that can be used for intervention in musculoskeletal dysfunction. Many of the above strategies can be modified in numerous ways to provide the desired effect based on therapeutic exercise training principles. In addition, numerous types of equipment can be used to promote or enhance desired exercise effects. It is important to realize that these therapeutic exercises are not proprioceptive or kinesthetic per se, but are

exercises that require proprioceptive input during their execution. Proprioceptive input from the muscles to the CNS has significant influences on motor output,[1] but the extent to which prorioception is improved or that sensory receptors are altered through the performance of these exercises has not been established.[14]

> ## Key Point:
> Active exercise at all levels of intensity will elicit appropriate sensory input from proprioceptors in the muscle, providing information for motor skill performance.

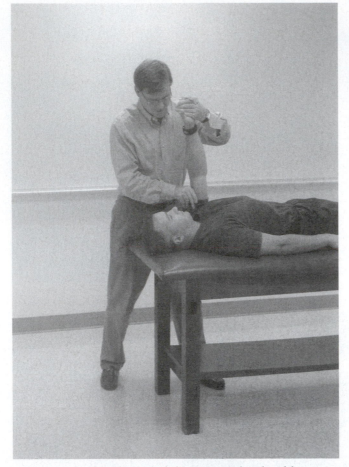

Figure 7.13   Rhythmic stabilization at the shoulder to enhance proximal stability.

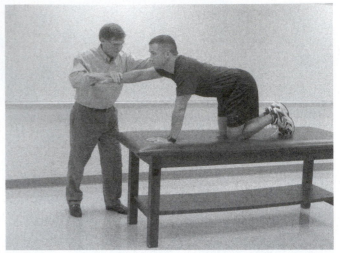

Figure 7.14   Upper extremity stabilization and weight shift in quadruped posture.

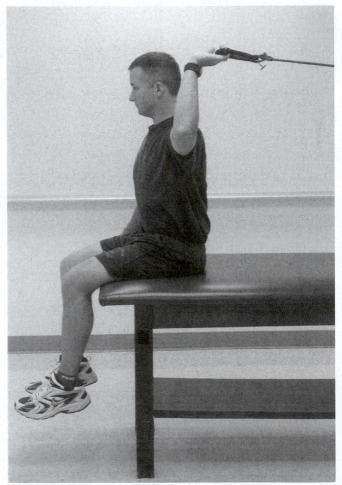

Figure 7.15   Use of surgical tubing for concentric-eccentric loading of the shoulder during internal rotation.

The initial stages of the rehabilitation process may involve management of acute or sub-acute symptoms and re-establishment of volitional muscle contraction within available range of motion, as may be evidenced, for example, by poor quadriceps recruitment after TKA or following ACL reconstruction. Quadriceps setting may be an appropriate therapeutic exercise at this early stage of rehabilitation.[19] The sensation of the contraction may be subserved by proprioceptors in the muscle. Mini-squats can be performed in weight bearing through a specific range in bilateral or single limb stance (e.g., 5°–20° knee flexion), requiring sensory information about ankle, knee, and hip motion and position during execution of the activity.[19] Alternatively, clients can perform seated, non–weight bearing knee flexion and extension in a prescribed range of motion and at a prescribed velocity. An example at the shoulder would be performing abduction in the scapular plane in a specified range of motion. In general, active range of motion exercises will elicit position and motion sensation from the muscle spindle primarily, as well as other proprioceptors. Increasing resistance by adding weight would require increased recruitment of motor units, resulting in increased sense of effort.

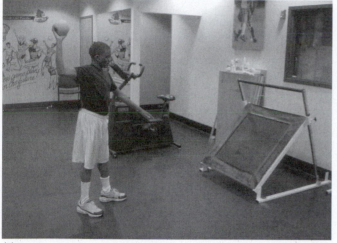

(a)

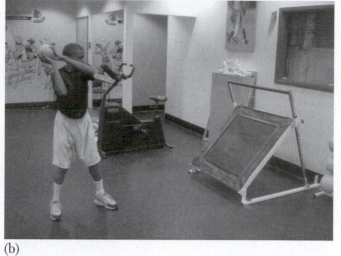

(b)

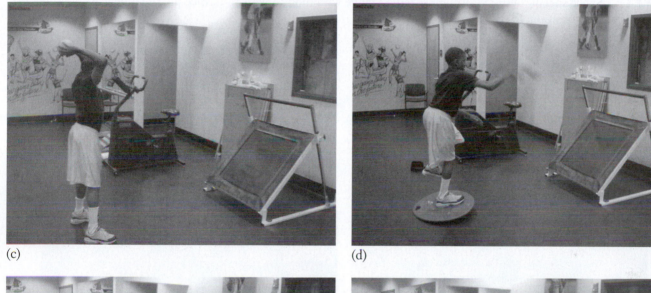

(c)

(d)

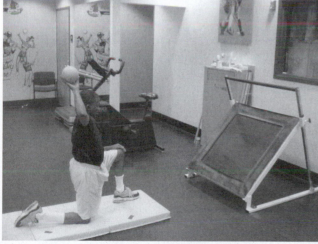

(e)

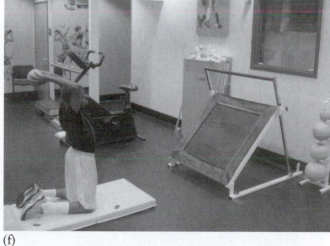

(f)

Figure 7.16   Plyometric activities for the upper extremity with varied postures, static and dynamic, using plyoball and rebounder. (a) single arm toss; (b) two-arm toss, trunk rotation; (c) two-arm overhead toss; (d) single-arm toss, unstable surface; (e) kneeling single-arm toss; (f) kneeling two-arm overhead toss.

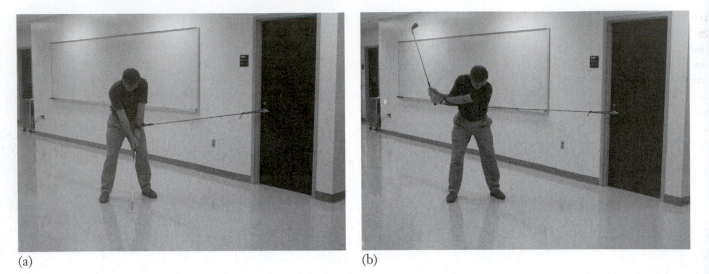

(a)   (b)

Figure 7.17   Sport-specific activity through specified range with motion with resistance provided by elastic tubing. (a) start position; (b) finish position.

As the therapeutic exercise program continues, higher level, activity or sports specific exercises can be included, requiring higher level motor skills and continued integration of sensory information at multiple CNS levels. These exercises may include multi-joint movement at varied ve- locities and ranges of motion. Upper extremity activities may involve moving objects of varied mass to different heights in a given time period, or with a specified degree of accuracy. Lower extremity exercises may utilize changes of direction, acceleration and deceleration during walking,

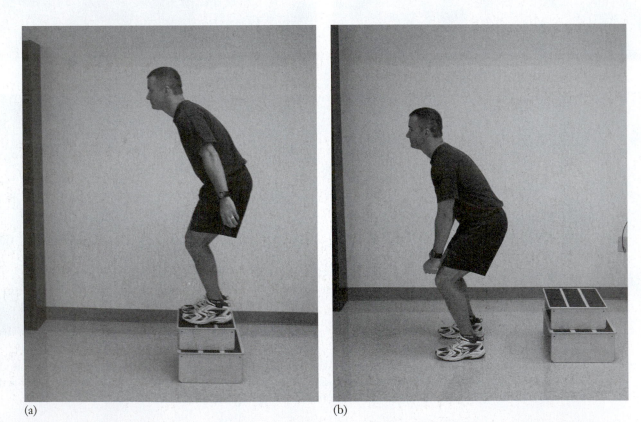

(a)   (b)

Figure 7.18   Plyometric drop jumps from elevated surface. (a) take-off; (b) landing. Landing phase (b) is followed by vertical jump and landing.

fast walking and running. Varied loading responses can be elicited by plyometrics (stretch-shortening activities) (**Figure 7.18a–b**) (see Chapters 5 and 8). Single limb stance activities on varied surfaces with or without perturbations (**Figure 7.19**), can be used for balance, dynamic stability, or recovery from perturbed stance. Foam pads and various types of balance boards (e.g., BAPS™ board) (**Figure 7.20a–b**), rocker boards (**Figure 7.21a–b**) or roller boards (**Figure 7.22**) are commonly used for this purpose[19,127] (see Chapter 6). Perturbations such as multidirectional resistance to the board or unexpected body or limb perturbations can add to sensory inputs utilized by the neuromuscular system, ultimately contributing to limb and joint stability.[127] Integration of other activities along with the exercise, such as dribbling or catching a basketball while performing agility drills or maneuvering through an agility course, will integrate skills that are performed during sports specific activities. This integrated activity can provide changes in attention levels from cognitive to automatic during the execution of multiple motor tasks.[14]

Balance activities are commonly used or recommended as proprioceptive exercises.[6,17,19,20,129] However, it must be remembered that balance, i.e., maintenance of the center of mass within one's base of support, is subserved by the somatosensory, vestibular, and visual systems, with the primary system in adults being the sensorimotor system.[15,32] If the client's balance has been diminished as a result of injury and/or surgery, varied levels of balance activities and challenges can be included in the therapeutic exercise program, including strengthening of the leg muscles. Single leg stance activities with eyes open and closed, (**Figure 7.23a–b**) with or with added resistance (**Figure 7.24a–b**) and with a soft or unstable support surface can significantly add to balance challenges (see Chapter 9).

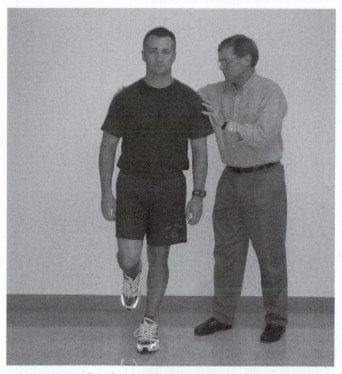

Figure 7.19   Single leg stance with perturbations.

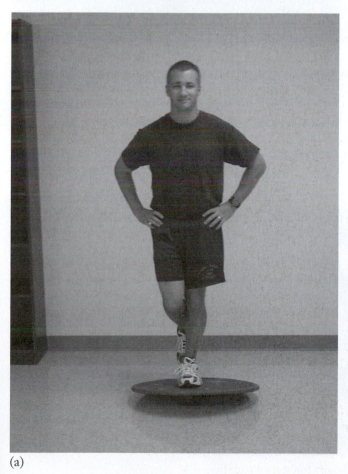

(a)

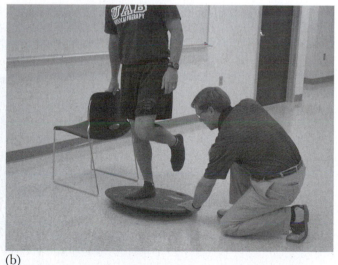

(b)

Figure 7.20   (a) single leg balance activities on BAPS™ board; (b) resistance or perturbations applied to BAPS™ board during single leg balance activities.

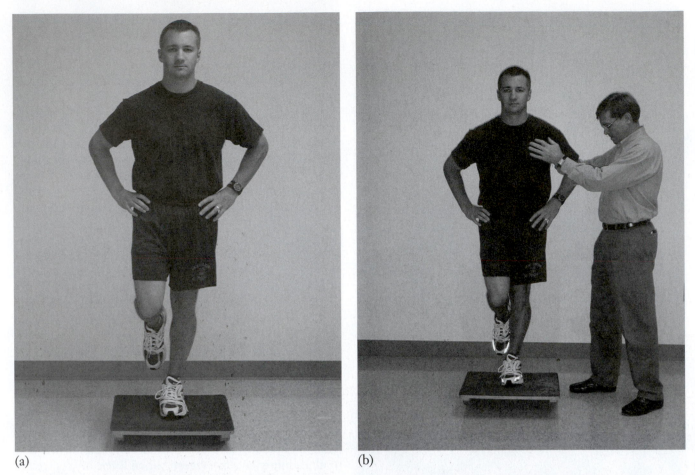

(a)   (b)

Figure 7.21   Single leg stance on rocker board, sagittal plane, (a) without perturbation; (b) with perturbation.

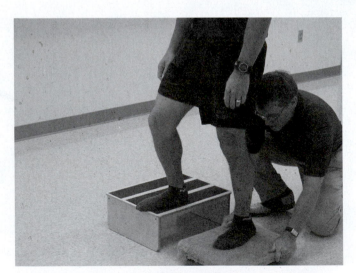

Figure 7.22   Use of a roller board for stance stability.
Resistance or perturbations can be applied
from multiple directions.

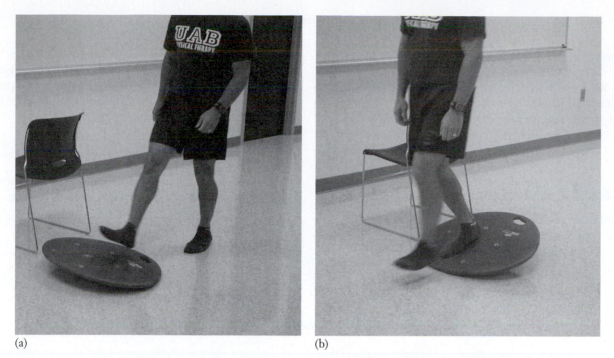

(a)　　　　　　　　　　　　　　　　　　(b)

Figure 7.23　Dynamic balance activity: stepping across unstable surface using BAPS™ board. (a) stance initiation; (b) terminal stance.

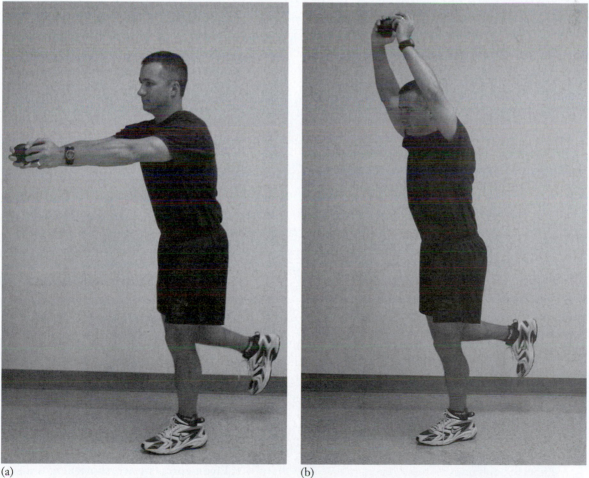

(a)　　　　　　　　　　　　　　　　　　(b)

Figure 7.24　Single leg stance with weighted upper extremity movements to impose perturbations. Dumbbell held in forward position (a), and moved overhead (b), while maintaining balance. Velocity of movement and weight of dumbbell can be varied to change challenge of task.

Commercially available dynamic balance systems also can be used to develop improved balance, providing feedback to clients, as well as varied levels of challenge to both single and double limb stance. However, these systems do not provide a measure of proprioception, but a measure of maintaining the center of mass within the base of support.

Exercise and Training Guidelines

A number of therapeutic exercise programs that are commonly used for proprioceptive or kinesthetic training and the basic principles of the varied phases are the basis for the guidelines for a progressive range of exercises presented in **Table 7.3** and **Table 7.4**. These paradigms are meant to be a principled guide to designing a comprehensive therapeutic exercise program and not an all inclusive or exhaustive list of exercises.

> ## *Key Point:*
> Activities must be selected on the basis of accepted therapeutic exercise principles with consideration for the client's physical condition, needs, and goals related to the desired functional outcome.

TABLE 7.3   Guidelines for exercise and training in the lower extremity to re-establish neuromotor control

- Non–weight bearing (open chain) exercises
  - Traditional range of motion and strengthening exercises (e.g., quad sets, TKEs, SLRs; isokinetics)
    - Varied loads, velocities, types of contraction, and ranges of motion (reproduction of position)
- Weight bearing (closed chain) exercises
  - Bilateral stance activites: eyes open or eyes closed, varied foot positions
    - Weight shifting
      - Side-to-side, forward and back
    - Mini-squats
      - Varied loads, velocities, types of contraction, and ranges of motion (reproduction of position)
  - Perturbations
    - Expected, unexpected
    - Isometric resistance to trunk, pelvis in all planes
  - Single limb stance activities: eyes open or eyes closed
    - Stable surface
      - Movement of the non-stance limb to various targets
        - Varied loads, velocities
      - Movement of the upper limbs
        - Varied loads, velocities
      - Perturbations
        - Expected and unexpected
        - Isometric resistance to trunk, pelvis in all planes
    - Unstable surfaces (altered somatosensory inputs): foam pads (varied densities), balance boards, roller boards
      - Perturbations to body or surface
      - Manual, tubing, changes in free limb positions (includes upper extremity)
      - Resistance applied to body or surface
- Functional activities (work, recreational, or sports activities)
  - Specific tasks performed in the appropriate environment
  - Performance of the specific task in the appropriate environment
    - Utilize performance measures
      - Time constraints
      - Load constaints
      - Spatial constraints
      - Velocity constraints
      - Appropriate frequency, intensity and duration
    - Walking, jogging, running; forward and backward
    - Stairs and ramps; ascending, descending
    - Hopping, jumping, cutting
    - Agility; side-to-side, carioca, figure-of-eight
      - Changes of body position, direction, velocity
      - Imposed upper extremity skills during activity (e.g., catching a ball)
  - Plyometrics (stretch-shortening drills)
  - Return to activity

TABLE 7.4   Guidelines for exercise and training in the upper extremity to re-establish neuromotor control

- Non–weight bearing (open chain) exercises
  - Traditional range of motion and strengthening exercises (e.g., thrower's ten, PREs in planes of motion; dumbbells, tubing; isokinetics)
    - Varied loads, velocities, types of contraction, and ranges of motion (reproduction of position)
- Weight bearing (closed chain) exercises
  - Bilateral activities: varied hand positions
    - Weight shifting
      - Side-to-side, walk hands forward or back
    - Push-up, push-up plus
      - Varied loads, velocities, types of contraction, and ranges of motion (reproduction of position)
    - Perturbations
      - Expected, unexpected
      - Isometric resistance to trunk, pelvis in all planes
  - Single limb activities
    - Stable surface
      - Movement of the non-support limb to various targets
        - Varied loads, velocities
    - Perturbations
      - Expected and unexpected
      - Isometric resistance to trunk, pelvis in all planes
  - Unstable surfaces (altered somatosensory inputs): foam pads (varied densities), balance boards, roller boards
    - Perturbations to body or board
      - Manual
- Functional activities (work, recreational, sports)
  - Performance of the specific task in the appropriate environment
    - Utilize performance measures
      - Time constraints
      - Load constraints
      - Spatial constraints
      - Velocity constraints
      - Appropriate frequency, intensity and duration
  - Object manipulation
    - Lifting, pushing, throwing
    - Plyometrics (stretch-shortening activities with a weighted object or other form of resistance)
  - Return to activity

Summary

The use of exercise to improve proprioception assumes that clients with musculoskeletal dysfunction actually have a significant and functionally limiting proprioceptive deficit as a result of injury, surgery or disease. This assumption is not supported by the literature. Further, there is no credible evidence that exercise in any form can change the histologic or neurophysiologic nature of the muscle spindle, the primary source of proprioceptive input, or secondary sources of input such as joint and cutaneous mechanoreceptors, for determination of motion and position of the body in space. The terminology proprioceptive or kinesthetic exercise or training should not be utilized until definitive and unequivocal information is found to substantiate these assumptions. Exercise utilized for the treatment of musculoskeletal pathology, impairment, and functional loss will elicit varied responses from proprioceptors that then transmit sensory information to all three levels of the CNS to control and enhance motor responses for the completion of a specific task by an individual within a specific environment. Exercises and training methods should be chosen based on accepted standards and principles, and information gathered from the examination of the client, evaluation of signs and symptoms, determination of a diagnosis and prognosis, and implementation of an appropriate intervention.

References

1. Park S, Toole T, Lee S. Functional roles of the proprioceptive system in the control of goal-directed movement. *Percept Mot Skills.* 1999; 88(2): 631–647.

2. Irrgang JJ. Modern trends in anterior cruciate ligament rehabilitation: Nonoperative and postoperative management. *Clin Sports Med.* 1993; 12(4): 797–813.

3. Lephart SM, Pincivero DM, Giraldo JL, Fu FH. The role of proprioception in the management of athletic injuries. *Am J Sports Med*. 1997; 25(1): 130–137.

4. Voight ML. The balance component of orthopedic rehabilitation. *Orthop Phys Ther Clin N Am*. 2002; 11(1):17–29.

5. Wallman HW. Balance and the functionally unstable ankle. *Orthop Phys Ther Clin N Am*. 2002; 11(1): 33–48.

6. Lephart S. *Reestablishing Proprioception, Kinesthesia, Joint Position Sense, and Neuromuscular Control in Rehabilitation. In* WE Prentice (ed.), *Rehabilitation Techniques in Sports Medicine*. St. Louis: Mosby, 1994, pp. 118–137.

7. Lephart SM, Pincivero DM, Rozzi SL. Proprioception of the ankle and knee. *Sports Med*. 1998; 25(3):149–155.

8. Cavanaugh JT, Mox RJ. Balance and postoperative lower extremity joint reconstruction. *Orthop Phys Ther Clin N Am*. 2002; 11(1):75–97.

9. Grigg P. Articular neurophysiology. *In* JE Zachazewski, DJ Magee, WS Quillen (eds.), *Athletic Injuries and Rehabilitation*. Philadelphia: W.B. Saunders Company, 1996; pp. 152–169.

10. Grigg P. Peripheral neural mechanisms in proprioception. *J Sport Rehabil*. 1994; 3:2–17.

11. Gandevia SC, McCloskey DI, Burke D. Kinaesthetic signals and muscle contraction. *Trends Neurosci*. 1992; 15(2):62–65.

12. Gandevia SC, Burke D. Does the nervous system depend on kinesthetic information to control natural limb movements? *Behav Brain Sci*. 1992; 15: 614–632.

13. McCloskey DI, Prochazka A. The role of sensory information in the guidance of voluntary movement: Reflections on a symposium held at the 22nd Annual Meeting of the Society for Neuroscience. *Somatosensory Motor Res*. 1994; 11(1):69–75.

14. Ashton-Miller JA, Wojtys EM, Huston LJ, Welch-Fry D. Can proprioception really be improved by exercise? *Knee Surg Sports Traumatol Arthrosc*. 2001; 9(3):128–136.

15. Kandel ER, Schwartz JH, Jessell TM. *The Organization of Movement. Principles of Neuroscience*. New York: McGraw-Hill, 2000: 653–673.

16. Safran MR, Caldwell GL, Fu FH. Proprioception considerations in surgery. *J Sports Rehabil*. 1994; 3:105–115.

17. Voight ML, Cook G. Impaired neuromuscular control: Reactive neuromuscular training. *In* WE Prentice, ML Voight (eds), *Techniques in Musculoskeletal Rehabilitation*. New York: McGraw-Hill, 2001, pp. 93–124.

18. Hardin JA., Predisposing factors to non-contact anterior cruciate ligament injury. *Sports Physical Therapy Section Newsletter*, (Summer Issue) 2000;9–11.

19. Wilk KE, Reinhold MM, Hooks TR. Recent advances in the rehabilitation of isolated and combined anterior cruciate ligament injuries. *Orthop Clin N Am*. 2003; 34:107–137.

20. Hewett TE, Paterno MV, Meyer D. Strategies for enhancing proprioception and neuromuscular control of the knee. *Clin Orthop*. 2002; 402:76–94.

21. Nashner LM. The anatomic basis of balance in orthopedics. *Orthop Phys Ther Clin N Am*. 2002; 11(1): 1–15.

22. Good L, Beynnon BD, Gottlieb DJ. Joint position is not changed after ACL disruption. *Trans Orthop Res Soc*. 1995; 20:95.

23. Good L, Roos H, Gottlieb DJ, et al. Joint position sense is not changed after acute disruption of the anterior cruciate ligament. *Acta Orthop Scand*. 1999; 70(2):194–198.

24. Sherrington CS. *The Integrative Action of the Nervous System*. New Haven: Yale University Press, 1906.

25. Madey SM, Cole KJ, Brand RA. The sensory role of the anterior ligament. *In* DW Jackson (ed.), *The Anterior Cruciate Ligament: Current and Future Concepts*. New York: Raven Press, Ltd., 1993, pp. 23–33.

26. Fredericks CM. Basic sensory mechanisms and the somatosensory system: Touch and proprioception. *In* CM Fredericks, LK Saladin (ed.), *Pathophysiology of the Motor Systems*. Philadelphia: FA Davis, 1996, pp. 96–101.

27. Gillquist J. Knee ligaments and proprioception. *Acta Orthop Scand*. 1996; 67(6):533–535.

28. Bosco G, Poppele RE. Proprioception from a spinocerebellar perspective. *Physiolog Rev*. 2001; 81(2): 539–568.

29. Bastian H. The "muscular sense," its nature and cortical localisation. *Brain*. 1888; 10(1):5–137.

30. Wieler H, Awiszus F. Influence of hysteresis on joint position sense in the human knee joint. *Exp Brain Res*. 2000; 135:215–221.

31. Beard DJ, Kyberd PJ, Fergusson CM, Dodd CAF. Proprioception after rupture of the anterior cruciate ligament. *J Bone Joint Surg*. 1993; 75-B: 311–315.

32. Shumway-Cook A, Woollacott M. Postural control. *In Motor Control: Theory and Practical Applications*. Philadelphia: Lippincott, Williams & Wilkins, 2001, pp. 163–191.

33. Rymer WZ, D'Almeida A. Joint position sense: The effects of muscle contraction. *Brain*. 1980; 103:1–22.

34. Dietz V, Duysens J. Significance of load receptor input during locomotion: A review. *Gait Posture* 2000; 11(2):102–110.

35. Bullock-Saxton J, Wong W, Hogan N. The influence of age on weight-bearing reposition sense of the knee. *Exp Brain Res*. 2001; 136:400–406.

36. Ogard WK. The effect of weight bearing and joint position on knee joint position sense after anterior

cruciate ligament reconstruction. Doctoral dissertation. University of Iowa, 2000.

37. Birmingham TB, Kramer JF, Inglis TJ, et al. Effect of a neoprene sleeve on knee joint position sense during sitting open kinetic chain and supine closed kinetic chain tests. *Am J Sports Med.* 1998; 26(4): 562–566.

38. Anderson AF, Snyder RB, Federspiel CF, Lipscomb AB. Instrumented evaluation of knee laxity: A comparison of five arthrometers. *Am J Sports Med.* 1992; 20(2):135–140.

39. Schutte MJ, Dabezies EJ, Zimny ML, Happel LT. Neural anatomy of the human anterior cruciate ligament. *J Bone Joint Surg.* 1987; 69-A(2):243–247.

40. Zimny ML, Schutte M, Dabezies E. Mechanoreceptors in the human anterior cruciate ligament. *Anat Rec.* 1986; 214:204–209.

41. Zimny ML. Mechanoreceptors in articular tissues. *Am J Anat.* 1988; 182:16–32.

42. Halata Z, Haus J. The ultrastructure of sensory nerve endings in human anterior cruciate ligament. *Anat Embryol.* 1989; 179:415–421.

43. Grigg P, Hoffman AH. Properties of ruffini afferents revealed by stress analysis of isolated sections of cat knee capsule. *J Neurophysiol.* 1982; 47(1): 41–54.

44. Newton RA. Joint receptor contributions to reflexive and kinesthetic responses. *Phys Ther.* 1982; 62(1):22–29.

45. Hogervorst T, Brand RA. Current concept review: Mechanoreceptors in joint function. *J Bone Joint Surg.* 1998; 80-A(9):1365–1378.

46. Schultz RA, Miller DC, Kerr CS, Micheli L. Mechanoreceptors in human cruciate ligaments. *J Bone Joint Surg.* 1984; 66-A(7):1072–1076.

47. Grigg P. Mechanical factors influencing response of joint afferent neurons from cat knee. *J Neurophysiol.* 1975; 38:1473–1484.

48. Ferrell WR. The adequacy of stretch receptors in the cat knee joint for signaling joint angle throughout a full range of movement. *J Physiol.* 1980; 299:85–99.

49. Ferrell WR, Gandevia SC, McCloskey DI. The role of joint receptors in human kinaesthesia when intramuscular receptors cannot contribute. *J Physiol.* 1987; 386:63–71.

50. Burke D, Gandevia SC, Macefield G. Responses to passive movement of receptors in joint, skin and muscle of the human hand. *J Physiol.* 1988; 402: 347–361.

51. Clark RJ, Horch KW, Bach SM, Larson GF. Contributions of cutaneous and joint receptors to static knee-position sense in man. *J Neurophysiol.* 1979; 42(3):877–888.

52. Williams WJ. A systems-oriented evaluation of the role of joint receptors and other afferents in position and motion sense. *CRC Crit Review Biomed Eng.* 1981;(December):23–77.

53. Brumagne S, Lysens R, Swinnen L, Verschueren S. Effect of paraspinal muscle vibration on position sense of the lumbosacral spine. *Spine* 1999; 24(13):1328–1331.

54. van Duersen WM, Sanchez MM, Ulbrecht JS, Cavanaugh PR. The role of muscle spindles in ankle movement perception in human subjects with diabetic neuropathy. *Exp Brain Res.* 1998; 120:1–8.

55. Grigg P, Finerman GA, Riley LH. Joint-position sense after total hip replacement. *J Bone Joint Surg.* 1973; 55-A(5):1016–1025.

56. Skinner HB, Barrack RL, Cook SD, Haddad RJ. Joint position sense in total knee arthroplasty. *J Orthop Res.* 1984; 1(3):276–283.

57. Ishii Y, Tojo T, Terajima K. Intracapsular components do not change hip proprioception. *J Bone Joint Surg.* 1999; 81-B:345–348.

58. Barrack RL, Skinner HB, Brunet ME, Haddad RJ. Functional performance of the knee after intraarticular anesthesia. *Am J Sports Med.* 1983; 11(4): 258–261.

59. Marks R, Quinney HA. Effect of fatiguing maximal isokinetic quadriceps contractions on ability to estimate knee-position. *Percept Mot Skills.* 1993; 77: 1195–1202.

60. Skinner HB, Wyatt MP, Hodgdon JA, et al. Effect of fatigue on joint position sense of the knee. *J Orthop Res.* 1986; 4(1):112–118.

61. Voight ML, Hardin JA, Blackburn TA, et al. The effects of muscle fatigue on and the relationship of arm dominance to shoulder proprioception. *J Orthop Sports Phys Ther.* 1996; 23(6):348–352.

62. Carpenter JE, Blazier RB, Pellizon GG. The effects of muscle fatigue on shoulder joint position sense. *Am J Sports Med.* 1998; 26(2):262–265.

63. Barrett DS. Proprioception and function after anterior cruciate reconstruction. *J Bone Joint Surg.* 1991; 73-B:833–837.

64. Barrett DS, Cobb AG, Bentley G. Joint proprioception in normal, osteoarthritic, and replaced knees. *J Bone Joint Surg.* 1991; 73-B:53–56.

65. Skinner HB, Barrack RL, Cook SD. Age-related decline in proprioception. *Clin Orthop.* 1984; 184: 208–211.

66. Beard DJ, Kyberd PJ, O'Conner JJ, et al. Reflex hamstring contraction latency in anterior cruciate ligament deficiency. *J Orthop Res.* 1994; 12(2): 219–228.

67. Beard DJ, Dodd CAF, Trundle HR, Simpson AH. Proprioception enhancement for anterior cruciate ligament deficiency. *J Bone Joint Surg.* 1994; 76-B:654–659.

68. Jennings AG, Seedhom BB. Proprioception in the knee and reflex hamstring contraction latency. *J Bone Joint Surg.* 1994; 76-B:491–494.

69. Klein B, Blaha JD, Simons W. Anterior cruciate ligament deficient knees do not have altered proprioception. *Orthop Trans.* 1992; 15:539.

70. Osborne MD, Chou LS, Laskowski ER, et al. The effect of ankle disc training on muscle reaction time in subjects with a history of ankle sprain. *Am J Sports Med.* 2001; 29(5):627–632.

71. Borsa PA, Lephart SM, Irrgang JJ, et al. The effects of joint position and direction of joint motion on proprioceptive sensibility in anterior cruciate ligament-deficient athletes. *Am J Sports Med.* 1997; 25(3):336–340.

72. Brumagne S, Lysens R, Spaepen A. Lumbosacral position sense during pelvic tilting in men and women without low back pain: Test development and reliability assessment. *J Orthop Sports Phys Ther.* 1999; 29(6):345–351.

73. Koumantakis GA, Winstanley J, Oldham JA. Thoracolumbar proprioception in individuals with and without low back pain: Intratester reliability, clinical applicability, and validity. *J Orthop Sports Phys Ther.* 2002; 32:327–335.

74. Kramer J, Handfield T, Kiefer G, et al. Comparisons of weight-bearing and non-weight-bearing tests of knee proprioception performed by patients with patello-femoral pain syndrome and asymptomatic individuals. *Clin J Sports Med.* 1997; 7(2): 113–118.

75. Marks R. The reliability of knee position sense measurements in healthy women. *Physiother Can.* 1994; 46(1):37–41.

76. Barrack RL, Skinner HB, Buckley SL. Proprioception in the anterior cruciate deficient knee. *Am J Sports Med.* 1989; 17(1):1–6.

77. Lephart SM, Kocher MS, Fu FH, et al. Proprioception following anterior cruciate ligament reconstruction. *J Sport Rehabil.* 1992; 1:188–196.

78. Gauffin H, Tropp H. Altered movement and muscular-activation patterns during the one-legged jump in patients with an old anterior cruciate ligament rupture. *Am J Sports Med.* 1992; 20(2): 182–192.

79. Berchuck M, Andriacchi TP, Bach BR, Reider B. Gait adaptations by patients who have a deficient anterior cruciate ligament. *J Bone Joint Surg.* 1990; 72-A(6):871–877.

80. Wojtys EM, Huston LJ. Neuromuscular performance in normal and anterior cruciate ligament-deficient lower extremities. *Am J Sports Med.* 1994; 22(1):89–104.

81. Ciccotti MG, Kerlan RK, Perry J, Pink M. An electromyographic analysis of the knee during functional activities: The normal profile. *Am J Sports Med.* 1994; 22(5):645–650.

82. Ciccotti MG, Kerlan RK, Perry J, Pink M. An electromyographic analysis of the knee during functional activities: The anterior cruciate ligament-deficient and -reconstructed profiles. *Am J Sports Med.* 1994; 22(5):651–658.

83. Corrigan JP, Cashman WF, Brady MP. Proprioception in the cruciate deficient knee. *J Bone Joint Surg.* 1992; 74-B:247–250.

84. Friden T, Zatterstrom R, Lindstrand A, Moritz U. Proprioception after an acute knee ligament injury: A longitudinal study on 16 patients. *J Orthop Res.* 1997; 15(5):637–644.

85. Friden T, Roberts D, Zatterstrom R, Moritz U. Proprioceptive defects after an anterior cruciate ligament rupture-the relation to associated anatomical lesions and subjective knee function. *Knee Surg Sports Traumatol Arthrosc.* 1999; 7:226–231.

86. Wright SA, Tearse DS, Brand RA, Gabel RH. Proprioception in the anteriorly unstable knee. *Iowa Orthop.* 1995; 15:156–161.

87. MacDonald PB, Hedden D, Pacin O, Sutherland K. Proprioception in anterior cruciate ligament-deficient and reconstructed knees. *Am J Sports Med.* 1996; 24(6):774–778.

88. Beynnon BD, Ryder SH, Konradsen L, et al. The effect of anterior cruciate ligament trauma and bracing on knee proprioception. *Am J Sports Med.* 1999; 27(2):150–155.

89. Pap G, Machner A, Nebelung W, Awiszus F. Detailed analysis of proprioception in normal and ACL-deficient knees. *J Bone Joint Surg.* 1999; 81-B(5):764–768.

90. Co FH, Skinner HB, Cannon WD. Effect of reconstruction of the anterior cruciate ligament on proprioception of the knee and the heel strike transient. *J Orthop Res.* 1993; 11(5):696–704.

91. Harter RA, Osternig LR, Singer KM, et al. Long-term evaluation of knee stability and function following surgical reconstruction for anterior cruciate ligament insufficiency. *Am J Sports Med.* 1988; 16(5):434–442.

92. Dvir Z, Koren E, Halperin N. Knee joint position sense following reconstruction of the anterior cruciate ligament. *J Orthop Sports Phys Ther.* 1988; 10(4):117–120.

93. Pai Y, Rymer WZ, Chang RW, Sharma L. Effect of age and osteoarthritis on knee proprioception. *Arthritis Rheum.* 1997; 40(12):2260–2265.

94. Pap G, Meyer M, Weiler H, et al. Proprioception after total knee arthroplasty: A comparison with clinical outcome. *Acta Orthop Scand.* 2000; 71(2): 153–159.

95. Jerosch J, Prymka M. Knee joint proprioception in patients with posttraumatic recurrent patella dislocation. *Am J Knee Surg.* 1996; 4(1):3–8.

96. Baker V, Bennell K, Stillman B, et al. Abnormal knee joint position sense in individuals with patellofemoral pain syndrome. *J Orthop Res.* 2002; 20:208–214.

97. Warner JJP, Lephart S, Fu FH. Role of proprioception in pathoetiology of shoulder instability. *Clin Orthop.* 1996; 330:33–39.

98. Blasier RB, Carpenter JE, Huston LF. Shoulder proprioception effect of joint laxity, joint position, and direction of motion. *Orthop Rev.* 1994;45–50.

99. Lephart SM, Myers JB, Bradley JP, Fu FH. Shoulder proprioception and function following thermal capsulorrhaphy. *Arthroscopy.* 2002; 18(7):770–778.

100. Smith RL, Brunolli J. Shoulder kinesthesia after anterior glenohumeral joint dislocation. *Phys Ther.* 1989; 69(2):106–112.

101. Dover GC, Kaminski TW, Meister K, et al. Assessment of shoulder proprioception in the female softball athlete. *Am J Sports Med.* 2003; 31(3):431–437.

102. Lephart SM, Warner JP, Fu FH. Proprioception of the shoulder joint in normal, unstable, and surgically repaired individuals. *J Shoulder Elbow Surg.* 1994; 3:371–379.

103. Brindle TJ, Nyland J, Shapiro R, et al. Shoulder proprioception: Latent reaction times. *Med Sci Sports Exer.* 1999; 31(10):1394–1398.

104. Pedersen J, Ljubisavljevic M, Bergenheim M, Johansson H. Alterations in information transmission in ensembles of primary muscle spindle afferents after muscle fatigue in heteronymous muscle. *Neurosci.* 1998; 84(3):953–959.

105. Sterner RL, Pincivero DM, Lephart SM. The effects of muscular fatigue on shoulder proprioception. *Clin J Sports Med.* 1998; 8(2):96–101.

106. Freeman MAR, Dean MRE, Hanham IWF. The etiology and prevention of functional instability of the foot. *J Bone Joint Surg.* 1965; 47B:678–685.

107. Garn GN, Newton RA. Kinesthetic awareness in subjects with multiple ankle sprains. *Phys Ther.* 1988; 68(11):1667–1671.

108. Glencross K, Thornton E. Position sense following joint injury. *J Sports Med Phys Fitness.* 1981; 21: 23–27.

109. Gross MT. Effects of recurrent lateral ankle sprains on active and passive judgments of joint position. *Phys Ther.* 1987; 67(10):1505–1509.

110. Refshauge KM, Kilbreath SL, Raymond J. The effect of recurrent ankle inversion sprain and taping on proprioception at the ankle. *Med Sci Sports Exer.* 2000; 32(1):10–15.

111. Konradson L, Ravn JB. Ankle instability caused by prolonged peroneal reaction time. *Acta Orthop Scand.* 1990; 61:388–390.

112. Cornwall AW, Murrell P. Postural sway following inversion sprain of the ankle. *J Am Podiatr Med Assoc.* 1991; 81:243–247.

113. Friden T, Zatterstrom R, Lindstrom A, Moritz U. A stabilometric technique for evaluation of lower limb instabilities. *Am J Sports Med.* 1989; 17(1):118–122.

114. Tropp H, Odenrick P. Postural control in single-limb stance. *J Orthop Res.* 1988; 6:83–89.

115. Forestier N, Teasdale N, Nougier V. Alteration of the position sense at the ankle induced by muscular fatigue in humans. *Med Sci Sports Exer.* 2002; 34(1): 117–122.

116. Aydin T, Yildiz Y, Yildiz A, Kaylon TA. Proprioception of the ankle: A comparison of female teenaged gymnasts and controls. *Foot Ankle Int.* 2002; 23(2): 123–129.

117. Lam S, Jull G, Treleaven J. Lumbar spine kinesthesia in patients with low back pain. *J Orthop Sports Phys Ther.* 1999; 29(5):294–299.

118. Parkhurst T.M. Burnett CN. Injury and proprioception in the lower back. *J Orthop Sports Phys Ther.* 1994; 19(5):282–295.

119. Bernier JN, Perrin DH. Effect of coordination training on proprioception of the functionally unstable ankle. *J Orthop Sports Phys Ther.* 1998; 27(4): 264–275.

120. Rozzi SL, Lephart LM, Sterner R, Kuligowski L. Balance training for persons with functionally unstable ankles. *J Orthop Sports Phys Ther.* 1999; 29(8): 478–486.

121. Gauffin H, Tropp H, Odenrick P. Effect of ankle disc training on postural control in patients with functional instability of the ankle joint. *Int J Sports Med.* 1988; 9:141–144.

122. Lephart SM, Giraldo JL, Borsa PA, Fu FH. Knee joint proprioception: A comparison between female intercollegiate gymnasts and controls. *Knee Surg Sport Traumatol Arthrosc.* 1996; 4(2):121–124.

123. Vuillerme N, Teasdale N, Nougier V. The effect of expertise in gymnastics on proprioceptive sensory integration in human subjects. *Neurosci Lett.* 2001; 311(2):73–76.

124. Barrack RL, Skinner HB, Cook SD. Proprioception of the knee joint: Paradoxical effect of training. *Am J Sports Med.* 1984; 63(4):175–181.

125. Bartlett MJ, Warren PJ. Effect of warming up on knee proprioception before sporting activity. *Br J Sports Med.* 2002; 36:132–134.

126. Bouet V, Gahery Y. Muscular exercise improves knee position sense in humans. *Neurosci Lett.* 2000; 289(2):143–146.

127. Fitzgerald GK, Axe MJ, Snyder-Mackler L. The efficacy of perturbation training in nonoperative anterior cruciate ligament rehabilitation programs for physically active individuals. *Phys Ther.* 2000; 80(2): 128–140.

128. Cerulli G, Benoit DL, Caraffa A, Ponteggia F. Proprioceptive training and prevention of anterior cruciate ligament injuries in soccer. *J Orthop Sports Phys Ther.* 2001; 31(11):655–660.

129. Caraffa ACG, Projetti M, Aisa G, Rizzo A. Prevention of anterior cruciate ligament injuries in soccer: A prospective controlled study of proprioceptive training. *Knee Surg Sports Traumatol Arthrosc.* 1996; 4:19–21.

130. Ihara H, Nakayama A. Dynamic joint control training for knee ligament injuries. *Am J Sports Med.* 1986; 14(4):309–315.

131. Giove TP, Miller SJ, Kent BE, et al. Nonoperative treatment of the torn anterior cruciate ligament. *J Bone Joint Surg.* 1983; 65-A(2):184–192.

132. Rothwell J. Proprioceptors in muscles, joints and skin. In: *Control of Human Voluntary Movement*, 2nd Ed., pp 86–126, 1994, London: Chapman and Hall Publishers.

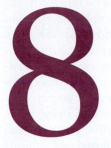

Training for Neuromuscular Coordination and Re-Education

TIMOTHY J. BRINDLE

Objectives
The reader will be able to:

- Explain basic central nervous system function for motor control.
- Describe the various methods used for evaluating human movement.
- Identify the components that contribute to motor program development.
- Compare and contrast different theories of motor control and motor learning.

- Describe the influence of therapeutic exercise intervention on motor control as we age.
- Select population specific neuromuscular function evaluation and training techniques.

Outline

INTRODUCTION

Terminology such as neuromuscular coordination is vague because the term neuromuscular could imply any adaptations in either the nervous or muscular system. Operative definitions of the exact nature and location of these adaptations within the nervous or muscular systems are needed. For example, increases in strength are initially brought about by adaptations of the central nervous system (CNS) but with persistent training morphological changes in the muscle account for increased strength. Both of these adaptations are within the neuromuscular system; however, the mechanism behind each of these changes is drastically different. Similarly, movement is typically created via muscle activation either shortening (concentric) or elongating (eccentric) its length (see Chapters 2 and 5). Muscle can also activate isometrically with no appreciable change in length, which adds dynamic stability to joints associated with certain segmental movements (see Chapters 5, 6, 7). Ultimately it is the CNS that coordinates all of this muscle activity in order to generate movements. The emphasis of this chapter is exploring CNS adaptations to motor coordination because without proper planning for even simple movements we would not be able to function optimally. Thus motor coordination is dependent upon a plan generated from higher CNS levels. Complex movements that require greater coordination are primarily the product of CNS motor programs. These programs generate movement patterns that can vary from relatively simple, isolated, single joint movements to the complex, integrated, multiple joint limb movements associated with many functional tasks.

Neuromuscular coordination is dependent on the ability of the CNS to generate the correct motor program in order to accomplish the appropriate task. The motor program is the generation of neural impulses sent to muscles (neuromuscular) to execute purposeful movements. Movement characteristics, such as speed, variability and repeatability, will vary as movement complexity increases. Neuromuscular control, or more appropriately the ability of the CNS to generate the appropriate motor program, becomes more important as task complexity increases. A more complex motor program is needed for skilled movements. However, even simple, single joint movements such as elbow flexion can be quite complicated because of the numerous parameters that the CNS needs to control. *Control parameters* include which muscle(s) to activate (synergist or antagonist), for how long (duration) and with how much intensity (amplitude). Other information due consideration when evaluating purposeful movements includes the mechanical properties of muscle, the starting position of the limb, and the desired terminal position. The CNS monitors the mechanical properties of limbs continuously during movement. External environment input regarding the movement target or goal and per-ceived ways to avoid obstacles must also be relayed to the motor program. This is generally accomplished by input from *exteroreceptors* such as that provided by vision to make target position identification easier. Peripheral musculotendinous (see Chapters 2 and 7) or capsuloligamentous joint (see Chapters 6 and 7) mechanoreceptors provide information regarding initial muscle length, contraction velocity, joint angle, and overall limb orientation. Vestibular input signals maintain stable postures and whole body orientations. All of this external and internal information is needed for optimal motor program generation to occur. The overlapping peripheral afferent information can increase the complexity of even simple movement tasks. Bernstein termed all of these internal movement control parameters as *degrees of freedom.*[1] This use of the term degrees of freedom, which differs from the previously discussed mechanical perspective, will be discussed later in this chapter. *Coordination* is achieved by reducing the number of these control parameter degrees of freedom and integrating it with peripheral feedback, thereby making movement control as simple and efficient as possible for the CNS. This is one of the concepts we will explore as a means of movement control.

Movements can range from single joint, fast reflexive movements to slower, complex, multi-joint skills that require higher levels of CNS involvement (**Table 8.1**). This chapter will discuss the purposeful movements that require motor program development to coordinate individual joint contributions to movement. To optimize their efficiency and to avoid wasted energy, purposeful movements are generally performed with a specific goal. The context of a movement helps to identify its relative success or failure for attaining the goal. For example, walking is a common lower extremity movement task. This lower extremity movement would be considered successful if one can get to the desired location in an efficient time frame with minimal energy cost, and without any major incident such as tripping. Lower extremity movements are usually rhythmical and do not require much conscious effort in order to complete the task; however, ambulating on an icy surface may require a greater conscious effort. The CNS control of coordination for upper extremity movements requires accurate, discrete movement patterns in order to manipulate objects in our environment, which generally necessitate a greater conscious effort. Appropriate CNS motor program execution or coordination is relative to the required function.

Key Point:

To manipulate objects in the environment, upper extremity tasks are generally more discrete, requiring more conscious effort than lower extremity tasks.

TABLE 8.1 Example of different movements and characteristics associated with these types of movements

Simple ←——————————————————————————————→ Complex

	Reflexive		Voluntary			
	Single-joint	Multi-joint / single limb	Single-joint	Multi-joint / single limb	Multi-limb / inter-limb coordination	Highly practiced / skilled movement
Characteristics	Predictable, repeatable and stereotypic		Predictable, stereotypic / task dependent, adaptable			Task dependent, adaptable, highly specialized with training
Tasks	Response to stimuli, discrete		Discrete, simultaneous		Rhythmic or simultaneous, repetitive, and sequential	A combination of rhythmic/ simultaneous, repetitive/sequential
Speed of movement	Fast		Task dependent			
Level of control	Spinal cord		Upper levels of CNS control of speed, force and limb trajectory			
Accuracy	Not important		Level of accuracy dependent on task and movement speed			
Examples	Deep tendon reflex	Flexor withdrawal reflex	Research paradigm	Reaching for object	Ambulation	Athletic or performing artist
Contribution to functional tasks	Physiologic	Safety / protection	Minimal	Minimal–Moderate	High	Extremely high

External stimuli like verbal or visual commands and cues or written instructions can prompt movements. Purposeful movements can also be driven by environmental factors such as attempting to locate an object in a poorly illuminated external environment. Unprompted, internally motivated movements involve tasks such as reaching for an object like a glass of water. Both prompted and unprompted movements are goal directed, requiring CNS motor planning. As stated previously, the CNS takes into account present body position in relation to the spatial orientation of an object in order to create a motor program to manipulate an object or to move toward an object. The CNS relies on previous movement experiences as the foundation for creating the desired motor program.

This chapter will also discuss the neuromuscular system contributions that provide for coordinated, controlled movements. The mechanisms that control motor coordination include input from peripheral receptors, the CNS motor planning centers, and the implementation and output of these plans through neuromuscular activity which, when properly activated, should enable smooth and efficient, purposeful movements. Thus, "*neuromuscular coordination*" is the ability of the CNS to generate the appropriate motor programs or plans in a manner that produces appropriate movement sequences in a timely, efficient manner.

> ### Key Point:
> Neuromuscular coordination is the ability of the CNS to generate the appropriate motor programs or plans in a manner that produces appropriate movement sequences in a timely, efficient manner.

To fully comprehend coordination and motor performance, an understanding of neuroanatomy, neurophysiology, motor learning, motor control and biomechanics is necessary. We will look at this process from an input-to-output perspective, where afferent information (input) is analyzed by the CNS, and assimilated to form a motor program that will be executed in the form of an actual movement output. Movements can be described through kinematic, kinetic, and neuromuscular activation characteristics. This input-to-output perspective will be used to examine the process of motor coordination. Input to the CNS includes visual and other peripheral feedback (i.e., auditory, joint, muscle, and/or vestibular) to locate an object in space and determine the initial state or body position prior to purposeful movement initiation. The CNS devises a coordinated motor program based on this peripheral information, the effectiveness of similar or previous movement experiences and the overall movement goal. Previous movement history and overall success of

those movements serve as the template on which help to organize new or modified motor programs is based. Ongoing modulation from visual, tactile, and proprioceptive receptors can help influence the motor program outcome. The processing portion of the motor program requires assimilation of the peripheral feedback in context with higher CNS levels. The output of the model is the execution of the motor program from the CNS and the actual movement performance. Proprioceptive feedback can affect a motor program via changes in muscle length and from activated mechanoreceptors within a joint capsule or ligament when stresses or strains are applied. Changes in movement speed, the presence of an object that may obstruct the movement, and unexpected positional or postural changes can all affect coordination, requiring motor program modifications.[2] *Motor control* refers to the CNS commands of the motor program or plan to execute a movement. *Motor learning* refers to the adaptations of these programs over time and practice to develop new or novel movements. Conceptually, motor control theory describes how the CNS controls movements, *motor programs or plans* are the instructions regarding specific movements, and motor learning involves motor program adaptations to produce new movement patterns. In order to develop optimal movement strategies, it is important for the rehabilitation clinician to understand how movement control is related to the learning of movements.

This chapter will review the relevant anatomy of the neuromuscular system and it's contribution to coordinated movements, via the implementation of the motor program. Upon completion of this chapter the reader should have an improved understanding of the motor control theories that provide a construct for how movements take place. Additional objectives of this chapter are to enhance the readers understanding of foundational neuroanatomy, and movement control information in order to implement motor control training strategies in therapeutic exercise programs. Both traditional and non-traditional (see Chapter 10) approaches to the restoration of movement coordination will also be reviewed.

MOVEMENT

The characteristics of simple movements will be discussed prior to examining more complex movements. As mentioned previously, movement is generally goal directed and can range from simple single plane, one joint movements to complex, multi-planar movements encompassing contributions from multiple joints. An initial challenge is how movement characteristics or motor program changes can be measured or quantified. With increasing movement complexity there is an almost exponential increase in the number of variables that need to be controlled. Even seemingly simple, primarily uniplanar, single joint movements can be complex because of all the degrees of freedom[1] or movement variables that need to be considered.

Movement measurements can vary from relatively simple, stationary goniometric measurements of single joint range of motion to the high speed, three dimensional whole body movement measurement and analysis commonly used with motor control research, especially during the study of motor coordination. Movements are routinely evaluated using kinematic, kinetic, and neuromuscular activation analysis. *Kinematic analysis* describes position, displacement, velocity, and acceleration (**Figure 8.1**). *Kinetic analysis* describes the contribution of forces to a movement, and *neuromuscular activation analysis* using electromyography (EMG) provides a description of muscle activation patterns including onsets and sequencing during movement execution. During unfatigued conditions, the EMG signal from a muscle is also considered to be representative of the level of CNS drive to the muscle. Analysis and processing EMG signals is more tedious; however, knowledge of muscle activity in relation to kinematic and kinetic measurements is crucial to understanding motor control. Kinematics, kinetics, and EMG are considered movement outputs and are relatively easy to measure. Exactly how the CNS controls these outputs to coordinate movement is more complicated, and is not fully understood. The goal of *motor control analysis* is to understand the controls that enable coordinated movements. First we will examine the neuroanatomical basis of motor control and then progress to some contemporary theories of how the CNS controls movement.

> ## Key Point:
> Kinematics, kinetics, and EMG are considered outputs of movement patterns and are easily measured. How the CNS controls these variables is not completely understood and is of particular interest when exploring the concepts of the ability of the CNS to control the creation and execution of a motor program.

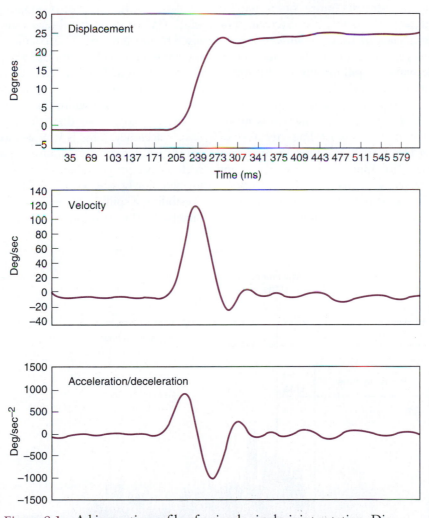

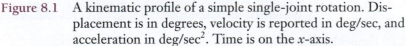

Figure 8.1   A kinematic profile of a simple single-joint rotation. Displacement is in degrees, velocity is reported in deg/sec, and acceleration in deg/sec^2. Time is on the *x*-axis.

The most commonly studied movements during motor control studies are *prompted or goal directed movements* that occur in response to an external signal or cue. To help identify different areas of CNS processing relative to the movement, prompted or goal directed movements can be broken down into discrete phases (**Figure 8.2**). *Pre-motor time* is the time between the initial motor command to the onset of EMG activity in a muscle. *Motor time* is the time between the initiation of EMG activity and actual movement. *Reaction time* is the combination of pre-motor time and motor time. Reaction time is thought to represent CNS processing for a given movement. *Movement time* is the duration between the initiation and cessation of a total movement. *Response time* is reaction time and movement time combined.

MOVEMENT ACCURACY

Successful motor program completion is relative to the *context* or goal of the particular movement. Upper extremity movements are generally discrete, requiring accuracy, while lower extremity movements more often require rhythmical movement patterns to traverse a terrain. For example, reaching for a glass of water in order to get a drink would be considered successful if the glass gets to the mouth accurately without spilling any of the water, while achieving the task in a reasonable amount of time. In contrast, runners rely on repetitious movement cycles of hundreds or thousands of strides, where success is measured in the time needed to cross a finish line. Accuracy of foot placement during lower extremity movements is not considered as important as upper extremity placement during upper extremity movements like reaching for a glass of water. Generally, these faster, more powerful lower extremity movements do not require as much accuracy as

fine upper extremity movements that tend to be performed at slower velocities. From observations made while subjects moved a stylus between two targets over a given time, Fitts et al.[3] demonstrated an inverse linear relationship between speed and accuracy where movement accuracy decreased as movement speed increased. From these data they developed a formula for *index of difficulty (ID)*, which is calculated from movement amplitude or distance between the two targets (A) and target width (W):

$$ID = Log_2\left(\frac{2A}{W}\right)$$

Movement time (MT) is equal to the index of difficulty (where *a* and *b* are empirical constants) as follows:

$$MT = a + b(ID)$$

Plotting movement time versus target width results in a linear logarithmic relationship between target distance and target width (**Figure 8.3**). Conceptually, it is more important to appreciate that movement time (MT) is dependent on the distance or amplitude (A) and the target width (W) or in practical terms the "margin of error" for discrete movements. The coefficients *a* and *b* represent the *y* intercept and slope from a regression analysis of the above equation. *Fitts' law* states that movement time increases as a result of either increasing movement distance or decreasing target width. As the complexity of the motor program increases so does the CNS processing time to ensure accuracy. This is why we do not move at very fast speeds when activities require great accuracy. An activity such as bringing a glass of water to the mouth is performed slowly with considerable control to decrease the possibility of spilling the water or missing the mouth completely. In this example, velocity and accuracy represent

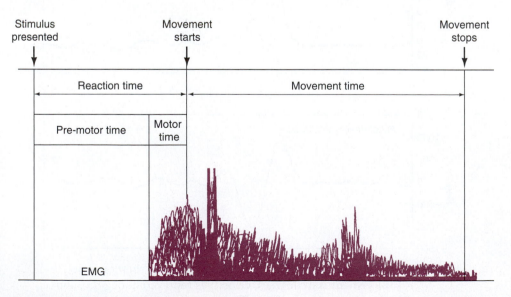

Figure 8.2   Events leading to movement.

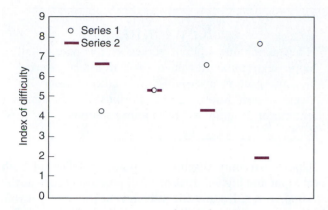

Figure 8.3   Demonstration of Fitts law. Movement time is estimated by the relationship between the amplitude of movement and the target width. As amplitude of movement is increased (constant target width), estimated movement time increases (Series 1). As target width is increased (constant movement amplitude), estimated movement time is decreased (Series 2).

two of many other degrees of freedom that need to be controlled during this movement. Movement time alone, however, is not a complete performance indicator. Other methods of measuring the relative success or failure of movements will be discussed later in this chapter.

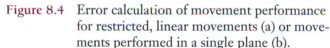

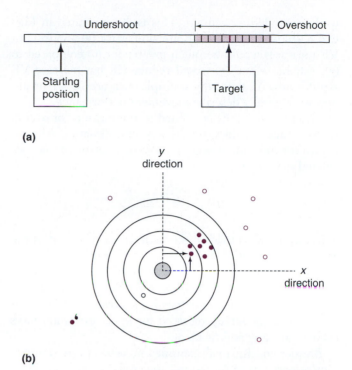

Figure 8.4   Error calculation of movement performance for restricted, linear movements (a) or movements performed in a single plane (b).

> ## Key Point:
> Fitts' law states that movement time increases as a result of either increasing movement distance or decreasing target width.

Movement Errors

To make adjustments to existing motor programs, feedback variables that identify the relative success or failure of discrete goal directed movements are needed. Motor learning is the process of incorporating these adjustments and it will be discussed later; however, errors must be measured so that success or failure can be quantified for various types of movements. Constricted, single-joint movements are measured relative to under (−) or over (+) shooting a target with error measures in only one dimension (**Figure 8.4a**). Single plane or two dimensional movements require measures in two dimensions, typically an x and a y direction (**Figure 8.4b**). Measures of error can include constant error, variable error, and absolute error. Each of these error measurements is believed to identify different aspects of motor performance, so it is

important to understand how these measurements complement each other, and to consider them in combination. *Constant error (CE)* is calculated as follows:

$$CE = \frac{\sum (x_i - T)}{n}$$

where x_i is the final position of a single trial, T is the actual target position and n is the number of trials. Constant error is the average mean difference error relative to the target position or bias of the score relative to the target position. This value can be misleading because movement scores with large variability can still display relatively low constant error scores (see below). To combat this, the measure of score inconsistency or *variable error (VE)* for a given individual over multiple trials can be calculated as follows:

$$VE = \sqrt{\frac{\sum (x_i - \overline{X})^2}{n}}$$

where x_i is the final position of a trial, n is the total number of trials and $\overline{X}$ is the average accuracy of all the trials ($\overline{X} = (x_1 + x_{i+1} + \cdots + x_n)/n$). With VE, subjects may miss the target consistently but with low variability (refer to **Figure 8.4b**). Variable error is most affected by learning, whereas bias or constant error will remain relatively unchanged after the first few trials.[4] Ideally, reporting both of these error measurements will provide a better description of the success or failure of the motor program relative to the intended movement. This is demonstrated in **Figure 8.4b**, where scores CE are similar for (•) and (o), but VE measures would be much greater for (o) compared to (•). Adding (•') to (•) would reduce CE but increase VE significantly. This is why multiple measures of error are necessary to fully describe movement performance.

Absolute error (AE) is defined as the measure of overall performance accuracy or the absolute deviation without regard for movement accuracy. Absolute error can be calculated as follows:

$$AE = \frac{\sum |x_i - T|}{n}$$

where x_i is the individual scores from each trial, T is the actual target position and n is the number of repetitions.

Absolute and constant error measurements are believed to evaluate similar aspects of performance.[5] These are just some of the measures to determine success of a movement plan and are generally reserved for upper extremity tasks such as pointing and reaching.

Messier and Kalaska[6] identified movement errors in two dimensions: extent (over- and under-shooting), and direction (movement error that occurs perpendicular to the intended movement path). However, measurements for complex three dimensional movements do not presently exist. Having a better understanding of standard three dimensional error among non-impaired subjects could help provide greater insight into the motor control of complex movement patterns and the true deficits that exist when motor control processes are impaired. More importantly, rehabilitation clinicians need to incorporate measures of accuracy as indicators of movement pattern success or failure.

POINTING OR REACHING WITH THE UPPER EXTREMITY

Reaching is a task usually performed by the upper extremity as mentioned during our previous example of reaching for a glass of water when one is thirsty. Studies of upper extremity movement characteristics have been examined for reaching or pointing both with and without the use of visual feedback. Pointing at an object in space is similar to reaching because both movements require similar precision for successful completion. Even though there is increased complexity in three dimensional reaching versus single plane reaching similar strategies are used to perform these common tasks. Kinematically these movements demonstrate similar hand movement velocities. The velocity curve of the hand segment displays a typical bell shaped curve, with maximum velocity achieved approximately halfway through the movement and maximum acceleration and deceleration at equal sides of the maximum velocity point (**Figure 8.1**). Let's first examine pointing or reaching movements and see how we would go about analyzing the coordination of this type of movement.

> ## Key Point:
>
> The glenohumeral joint serves as the base of all upper extremity movement and transfers external (linear) space to internal (joint rotations) space. All linear afferent information is transposed to the efferent motor program to create joint rotations.

Upper extremity reaching or pointing relies on both local input and higher areas of CNS processing such as the cerebral cortex. Locally the stretch reflex may play a role during relatively simple movements because it is influenced by higher CNS centers and also subject to a certain amount of pre-planning. Movement modifications are usually achieved via the cerebellum through peripheral feedback from local mechanoreceptors and exteroreceptors such as the eyes. Changes imposed on an upper extremity movement can provide insight as to how the movement is controlled during single plane movements. Initial hand position even with single plane movements plays an important role in controlling upper extremity reaching.[7] Koshland and Hasan.[8] and Hocherman et al.[9] suggested that the initial motor program is encoded in terms of external target position or an external reference, not on internally derived joint position or displacement information. One method of determining the success of an initial movement is to study how it changes from its original state over repeated trials. The center of both simple and integrated upper extremity function is believed to be at the glenohumeral joint during reaching. Using the glenohumeral joint as an internal reference, there is an intrinsic association between visual space and kinesthetic space during three dimensional movements. In other words a linear world as observed visually is transferred into joint rotations beginning at the shoulder during upper extremity movements regardless of the number of planes in which a movement occurs.[10–12] After the internal characteristics of the body with respect to the environment have been determined, the CNS initiates movement. Flanders et al.[13] reported that an initial burst of EMG activity specified both movement magnitude and direction during vertical reaching. Others, however, contend that movement time is more important to the local influence of movement control than the intensity of the observed EMG activity.[14]

Upper extremity movements may be planned in reference to an external or linear coordinate system, producing straight hand paths, or an internal joint reference system producing curved hand paths. Gielen et al.[11] and others[15,16] reported that curvilinear movement paths are the result of a transformation between the visual or external reference system to coordinated joint rotations during upper extremity movements. During voluntary movements there appears to be a link between visual feedback, an internal reference frame, and limb dynamics. *Perturbations*, or temporary alterations of a limb's trajectory during reaching movements, have been used to test the *equilibrium trajectory hypothesis*.[17] This hypothesis, discussed in detail later, essentially states that internal muscle forces and the mode of getting to a position or movement trajectory is consistent among trials. Soechting[17] has stated it is not just the ability of muscles to generate force during movements but it is also length information provided by all of the muscles acting at the moving joint that enhances feedback about limb position. Typically EMG activity is greater during the earlier phases of movement, suggesting that most of the efferent information (motor command) is contained in the initial muscle activation sequence. After movement initiation, EMG activity and afferent feedback become more of a factor. When muscle belly vibration was introduced, Forwell and Carnahan[18] reported diminished movement accuracy among subjects with shoulder instability who had visual feedback denied via a blindfold. They suggested that decreased movement accuracy demonstrated the importance of the muscle spindles to kinesthetic feedback during reaching movements.[18]

> ## Key Point:
> Successful reaching can be measured in terms of accuracy and smoothness of the trajectory. Effective task performance is directly related to appropriate muscle activation onset timing, sequencing, and magnitude of force production.

LOCOMOTION

We have shown that spatial accuracy or precision is an important measure of upper extremity movement. Lower extremity movements generally only have to be accurate enough to transport oneself as efficiently as possible without stumbling or falling. In contrast to discrete upper extremity reaching and pointing movements, gait is a rhythmic, repetitive movement pattern. Motor control from the CNS during rhythmic locomotion is believed to occur from lower CNS levels such as central pattern generators (discussed later). A review of walking and running gaits are reviewed in Chapter 9.

Measurement of neuromuscular coordination should consider both the movement pattern or task and whether the upper or lower extremity is the segment of interest. Whether these measurements take place in a research laboratory or in a clinic, upper extremity movement studies should include measures of accuracy because this aspect is of particular importance to upper extremity function. Quantification of movement errors can also help detect control parameters following reaching and pointing tasks. Movement precision measurements alone do not address the efficiency in which one would accomplish the discrete task. Therefore, CNS control of motor programs (neuro-

muscular coordination) requires the processing of many parcels of information or what Bernstein[1] refers to as degrees of freedom, in order to develop the most efficient way to accomplish a desired task.[1] Although accuracy measurements can help identify the success of a movement, they tend to neglect the "online" modifications associated with making a movement smooth, coordinated, and thereby efficient. Assessing proper foot placement may be a useful indicator of the smoothness or efficiency of locomotion. Optimization is another way to describe smoothness and typically relates to a kinematic measure such as velocity or acceleration. Other important gait characteristics will be discussed in detail in Chapter 9.

> ## Key Point:
> The parameters for measuring successful locomotion are somewhat different than those used to define the success or failure of upper extremity movements.

INPUT TO THE CENTRAL NERVOUS SYSTEM

Peripheral feedback from afferent fibers comes from a number of receptors providing a vast array of input to the CNS. Input that often influence movements include haptic (tactile), vision, vestibular or balance sense (see Chapter 9), proprioception and kinesthesia (see Chapter 7). These senses can all contribute position sense information from a limb segment. Although at first it seems inefficient to dedicate all input sources to this responsibility, it is useful to have this overlap. The term redundancy, with reference to Bernstein, will be used frequently in this chapter because of system overlap.[1] The influence of *peripheral receptor redundancy* on movement is important because the elimination of any single sensory modality, through injury or disease, can often be compensated for by some of the other feedback senses. The CNS in essence learns to adapt if one of the feedback mechanisms are disrupted. This learning can also be called "*neural plasticity*" because further biological changes can lead to additional adaptations, particularly if the therapeutic exercise environment provides ample opportunity.

> ## Key Point:
> The CNS "learns" to adapt if one of its feedback mechanisms is disrupted. This learning can also be called "neural plasticity" because further changes can lead to additional adaptations, particularly if the therapeutic exercise environment provides ample opportunity.

Visual Feedback

The CNS has the ability to independently detect object form from object motion, if the object is indeed moving.[19–23] Undoubtedly it would take both form and motion information, processed in parallel, to create precise estimates of motion. This would be particularly important for catching a ball in flight or hitting a baseball. To transform this visual information to spatial representation for motor program creation, CNS processing must occur. The connection between eye-hand coordination is unclear, but it is necessary to complete saccadic eye movements prior to initiation of future movement tasks, suggesting discrete motor program formulations.[19] *Saccadic eye movements* are abrupt, high speed, lateral eye movements that link visual feedback information, motor program generation, and eye-hand coordination. The completion of saccadic eye movements appears to be necessary prior to the initiation of a new motor program. Upper extremity movement accuracy decreases with delayed visual feedback; however, this delay does not prevent the ability to learn new tasks.[20] Although movement accuracy can be diminished with delayed visual feedback, blind subjects have demonstrated straighter hand paths during reaching movements than blindfolded, non-impaired subjects.[21] This suggests that although vision is necessary for movement precision, it is not essential for the learning and completion of highly consistent movements.

As stated earlier, the overlap of afferent information that must be processed by the CNS creates an interaction between object form and object motion information that makes it difficult to parcel out subtle movement control responsibilities. Goodbody and Wolpert[22] determined that motor programs are partially derived from an internal estimate of intrinsic coordinates and visual information. Kinesthetic information from movements influences the processing of visual information during upper extremity movement tasks.[24] Once deficiencies from any of these feedback systems are identified they can be corrected rather quickly. Prolonged exposure to visual disturbances such as wearing prism glasses that distort visual information creates plastic changes in the CNS. These changes can occur within a few repetitions (depending upon the disturbance) and will last until the distortion is removed. For example, if prism glasses tended to shift visual feedback laterally, the CNS can adapt to enable movement patterns that display similar accuracy to when normal feedback was received. Prolonged exposure to visual disturbances creates plastic corrections within the CNS, meaning that these adaptations are not permanent, eventually returning to their original state. Pick et al.[25] reported that visual distortion of the movement of one limb can affect the trajectories of the contralateral limb, referring to this process as transfer. *Transfer* and *plasticity* are examples of how afferent information and the processing of this information by the CNS can influence motor programs and, ultimately, movements. Unfortunately, the precise mechanisms by which these CNS adaptations occur are not clearly understood.

> ## *Key Point:*
> Visual feedback plays an important, maybe even a dominant, role in determining movement success. However, connections with the CNS can help maintain movement accuracy when vision is poor or absent.

Mechanoreceptors

Mechanoreceptors include both capsuloligamentous joint (see Chapters 6 and 7) and musculotendinous receptors (see Chapters 2 and 7). Haptic or tactile skin mechanoreceptors are not generally believed to have much influence on movement planning. Capsuloligamentous joint mechanoreceptors influence movement by providing proprioceptive feedback to the CNS.[26–29] Feedback from peripheral skin, muscle, and joint receptors contribute to provide overlapping or redundant proprioceptive information to the CNS. Attempts at isolating the function of any one of these individual proprioception information sources, whether in the laboratory or in the clinic, have proven to be difficult, if not impossible. Sherrington[30] first identified the role of mechanoreceptors in proprioception, but it wasn't until 1967 that Freeman and Wyke[31] used a cat knee model to classify four basic joint mechanoreceptor types based on size, location and functional characteristics.

Joint Receptors. Type I joint receptors (Ruffini endings, Golgi-Mazzoni endings, Meisner corpuscles or spray endings) are generally small (100 × 40 μm) and slowly adapting with a low threshold to stimulus. These receptors are generally located in the fibrous joint capsule. Type II joint receptors (Pacinian corpuscles, Paciniform corpuscles, Golgi-Mazzoni bodies, or club-like endings) are slightly larger (280 − 120 μm), more rapidly adapt to stimulus and have a low activation threshold. These receptors are also located predominantly in the fibrous joint capsule, but in a deeper layer, closer to blood vessels. Type III joint receptors (Golgi endings, Golgi-Mazzoni corpuscles) are much larger (600 × 100 μm), are slow adapting to stimuli, and have a high activation threshold. These receptors are located in ligaments and tendons.[31,32] Type IV joint receptors are nociceptive receptors (respond to pain stimulus), are very small (1–5 μm) because they are unmyelenated and are located throughout most joint capsules, tendons, muscles and ligaments. Collectively, these receptors are believed to contribute to joint position sense, especially at end range of motion.

Muscle Receptors.

A muscle will usually have two types of kinesthetic receptors, *muscle spindles* (see Chapter 2) and *Golgi tendon organs (GTO)* (see Chapter 7). Both of these receptors provide feedback to the CNS, but the morphological differences between them and their location within the musculotendinous unit determines their exact contribution to kinesthesia. Muscle spindles are located within the muscle belly itself and provide feedback on muscle length and the change in muscle length. GTO are located at the musculotendinous junction and provide feedback on muscle and tendon tension.

Muscle Spindles.

Intrafusal muscle fibers or muscle spindles do not generate tension like extrafusal muscle fibers, but regulate muscle spindle excitability via the *gamma motor neuron system*. There are two types of muscle spindle receptors, *nuclear bag fibers* (primary, larger Ia fibers) and *nuclear chain fibers* (secondary, possessing both larger Ia fibers and smaller type II fibers). Both of these afferents are arranged in parallel with the extrafusal muscle fibers. The nuclear bag fibers are wider, are innervated with primary or dynamic gamma motor neurons, and respond to dynamic changes in muscle length or velocity of movement. Nuclear chain, or secondary fibers, however, are innervated by static gamma motor neurons, responding primarily to muscle length changes.[33] Because of their parallel orientation to extrafusal muscle fibers, intrafusal fibers can be temporarily put on slack as muscle length shortens. The gamma motor system helps take up the slack within the muscle spindle receptors as the extrafusal muscle fibers shorten. Concurrently, the GTO that are arranged in series with the extrafusal muscle fibers respond to the tension generated by a stretch by either stretching or by facilitating active muscle shortening. This makes the spindles more sensitive to position and velocity information than the GTO. Although greater proprioceptive acuity has been reported near end range joint motion because of greater capsuloligamentous deformation,[34,35] Rossetti et al.[36] reported reduced proprioceptive acuity near the end of joint range of motion during reaching due to subject discomfort. Their results suggest that input from pain receptors could be interfering with proprioceptive feedback near the end ranges of joint motion.[36]

Houck et al.[37] suggested that nuclear bag fibers are better suited for motion detection than for signaling the velocity of a muscle stretch. Higher muscle spindle discharge rates are observed at shorter muscle lengths and diminish with longer lengths. Vallbo and al-Falahe[38] demonstrated significantly greater muscle spindle activity during active compared to passive finger movements, suggesting greater feedback contributions during active movements. Kinesthetic information from muscle spindles appears to be the dominant feedback source at mid-range joint movements while capsuloligamentous joint mechanoreceptors provide more substantial contributions at the end ranges.

The gamma motor neuron is the effector side of the muscle spindle stimulating the intrafusal muscle fibers to take up muscle spindle slack, especially at shorter muscle lengths. Likewise, these motor neurons enhance the sensitivity and dynamic responsiveness of nuclear bag and nuclear chain fibers. As recently as 30 years ago, muscle spindles were thought by some to initiate movement; however, Vallbo[39] reported 10–50 ms delays in muscle spindle activation onset timing relative to the onset of EMG activity. This was roughly identical to the nerve conduction latency traveling from the spinal cord to a muscle.[39] Due to this delay, Vallbo[39] concluded that muscle spindle activation did not contribute directly to movement initiation, but rather played a more significant role during later movement phases. This information effectively negated the servomotor theory of motor control (discussed later).[40] Kakuda et al.[41] demonstrated a coupling between muscle spindle activation (fusimotor drive) and actual EMG activity during functional upper extremity movements. This coupling was considered to be representative of peripheral kinesthetic feedback to the CNS. Rymer[42] observed that fusimotor system activation occurred simultaneously with alpha motor neuron activation, suggesting a greater role in motor control.

Computer simulations of muscle spindle function have demonstrated the enhanced position sense capabilities of muscles that cross two or more joints when its spindles are more concentrated in the proximal aspect of the muscle.[43,44] Scott and Loeb[43] suggested that this arrangement helped to minimize background noise during movement, with errors tending to occur during movements away from the body where muscle spindle receptors were the least sensitive. This has not yet been investigated in human or animal studies.

> ## Key Point:
>
> Nuclear chain fibers are more sensitive to muscle length changes, whereas primary endings or nuclear bag fibers are more sensitive to the rate of change in muscle fiber length or movement velocity.

Golgi Tendon Organs (GTO).

GTO are located in series with the extrafusal muscle fibers, primarily at the musculotendinous junction. This afferent fiber is entwined within the collagen of the muscle tendon. During shortening muscle activation (concentric) an increased load on the collagen will deform this receptor, thereby signaling tension within the muscle–tendon unit. Crago et al.[45] and Houck et al.[46] observed that individual GTO responded to specific stretch activation thresholds and were generally more sensitive to active muscle shortening than to the lengthening created by passive muscle stretching. Afferent information from the GTO is related to external stimuli, or musculotendinous tension with the activation threshold sensitivity set by the CNS. Averaged signals from the activation of several GTO help the CNS eliminate extraneous information or noise from this feedback mechanism. This does not make the afferent information from the GTO any less important than other afferent feedback. The GTO alone do not provide enough information for kinesthetic awareness, but the CNS clearly uses this information in concert with other peripheral feedback in order to assist with movement control.

It is the morphology, orientation, and neurophysiology of each of the contributing afferent receptors that dictate their roles as movement control feedback mechanisms. During passive muscle stretching GTO and muscle spindles increase their activation frequency. During shortening muscle activations the activation frequency of GTO will increase, while muscle spindle activation frequency will decrease. This is due to the parallel arrangement of the muscle spindles. Shortening muscle activation will stimulate the GTO to unload the muscle spindle by inhibiting feedback from this receptor. Muscle spindle and GTO feedback also overlap with the proprioceptive output from capsuloligamentous joint receptors that signal changes in joint position or movement velocity. In the case of simple reflexes, this afferent information is relayed monosynaptically directly back to the muscle of origin, or polysynaptically to alpha motor neurons that innervate other muscles. This enables afferent information from one motor unit to be transferred to other local muscles, which could affect movement patterns. All proprioceptive and kinesthetic information is transferred up the spinal cord and processed within the higher CNS centers. The redundancy of the information from various receptors requires the CNS to process all of this information to increase movement accuracy.

Key Point:

Mechanoreceptors provide local information such as tensions within a joint or muscle-tendon structure, or movement onset, contributing considerably to overall proprioceptive information.

CENTRAL NERVOUS SYSTEM: MOTOR PROCESSING

The motor system allows us to move and manipulate our environment. In the late 1800s, Hughling-Jackson[47] originally described a *three tier level of control for coordinated*

movements. The first level is from the pons, medulla and the spinal cord to control the simple mechanics of relatively automatic movements such as ambulation. The second level of CNS control, the primary motor area of the motor cortex, is able to provide basic commands to limbs for movement. The third level of control, the supplementary motor cortex, commands the least automatic movements or movements that require the greatest skill. Spatiotemporal information is supplied by the parietal lobe to ensure proper displacements and orientations of the specific motor programs. Although intimate connections between these brain regions are present, their specific interactions are not well understood. These higher order executive centers provide guidance to the subcortical and spinal regions via facilitation and inhibition of each of their specific capabilities. Ghez[48] described a four level control system for movement coordination. The first level is the spinal cord that controls reflex mechanisms, followed by the brain stem that coordinates both ascending sensory information and descending motor commands. The motor cortex is the third hierarchical level where motor commands originate. The highest level of motor control is the premotor cortex, which is responsible for identifying objects in space and choosing a course of action. Two other structures are important for controlling motor function: the cerebellum and the basal ganglia. The cerebellum adjusts the intended motor output to the sensory feedback that occurs as a result of a movement, while the basal ganglia scales movement and is associated with motor learning.

Spinal Cord

The first level of movement control is at the local segment level of the spinal cord (**Figure 8.5**). This control encompasses the monosynaptic reflex such as the stretch reflex from muscle spindles. Sensory afferents carry proprioceptive and kinesthetic information into the spinal cord through the dorsal horn, and can connect directly onto an alpha motor neuron in the ventral horn to make up the monosynaptic reflex (see Chapter 2). Indirect connections to second order nerve fibers are completed via interneurons. The incoming afferent fibers can also send branches to other areas of the motor neuron pool in the *ventral horns*. These branches, called *columns*, usually extend over two to four spinal segments. Therefore, afferent information can have an effect on spinal segments at many levels. These columns are generally arranged to serve a functional role where the medial side of the column controls axial muscle function and the lateral column controls limb muscle function. The ventral aspect of the column controls muscles that extend joints and the dorsal aspect of the column controls muscles that flex joints. The spinal cord region between the dorsal and ventral horns, known as the *intermediate region*, is where most interneurons are located. The lateral portion of the interneurons project ipsilaterally

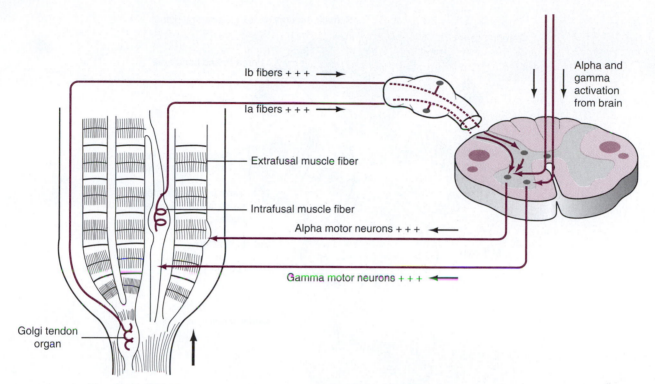

Ib fibers + + + →
Ia fibers + + + →
Extrafusal muscle fiber
Intrafusal muscle fiber
Alpha motor neurons + + + ←
Gamma motor neurons + + + ←
Golgi tendon organ
Alpha and gamma activation from brain

Figure 8.5   Local control of movement through simple reflexes that is influenced by higher CNS centers. Reflexive action is created by stimulation of afferent nerves (Ia, II) into the dorsal horn and synapse on to local alpha motorneurons that stimulate the extrafusal fibers. The Golgi tendon organ (Ib afferent) also influences local excitability. Descending control from higher CNS centers can influence the excitability of both the alpha and gamma motor neurons and the influence of this reflex activity. (Reprinted with permission from KE Wilk, et al. Stretch-shortening drills for the upper extremities: Theory and clinical application. *J Orthop Sports Phys Ther*. 1993;17:225–239.)

to the dorsolateral motor neurons and control the limb muscles. The medial portion projects contralaterally to control muscles on the opposite side. Interneurons will also travel in the white matter of the spinal cord a couple of segments distally or proximally. These inter-connecting interneurons make up part of the propriospinal tract and can influence motor program execution.

Descending commands from higher CNS levels transmitted to the spinal level of motor control usually control complex actions. This higher order of influence on local spinal circuitry is achieved through spinal interneurons. Direct connections between local afferent and efferent neurons are utilized for reflexive movements such as the withdrawal reflex. These interneurons located in the spinal cord have also demonstrated the ability to generate simple flexion and extension movements that are seen in tasks such as locomotion.[48] Rhythmical movements generated in the spinal cord from *central pattern generators (CPG)* are associated with automatic movements that do not require conscious effort such as gait.

Peripheral afferent information enters the *dorsal horns* of the spinal cord. *Pain and general touch information* typically synapse at the local spinal cord segment before crossing to the contralateral side and ascending up toward the

brain (**Figure 8.6**). The anterolateral pathway transmits general sensory information such as pain and sharp/dull sensation. Fine touch and proprioceptive information synapse at the local spinal cord segment before ascending ipsilaterally up toward the brain (**Figure 8.7**). The *dorsal columns* consist of the *gracile fascicle* and the *cuneate fascicle* that transmit proprioceptive information to the brain stem and cerebral cortex. The cuneate fascicle contains neurons predominantly from the upper extremities and upper thoracic regions, while the gracile fascicle contains neurons predominantly from the ipsilateral lower extremity, sacral, lumbar and lower thoracic regions. Martin[49] reported that proprioceptive information from the upper extremities traveled to the cuneate fascicle. Afferent fibers from mechanoreceptors located in the skin, capsuloligamentous and musculotendinous tissues will initially synapse in the dorsal root ganglion. Neurons from the upper extremity continue traveling ipsilaterally within the dorsal column until they synapse in the cuneate nucleus, located in the medulla. Neurons now cross or decussate in the medulla at the sensory decussation and travel within the medial leminiscus until they reach the *ventral portion of the lateral nucleus* of the thalamus or the posterior nucleus of the thalamus. The thalamus relays this proprioceptive

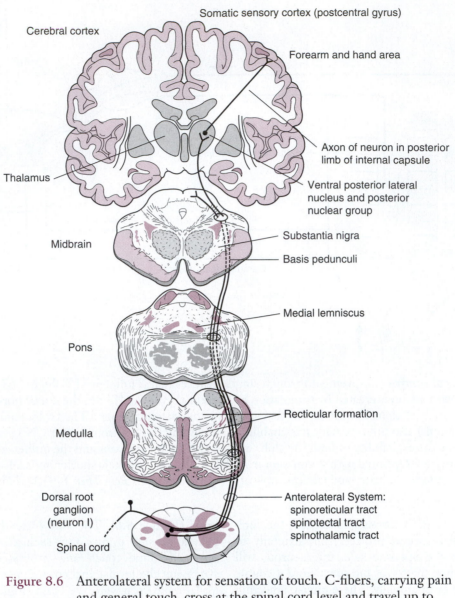

Somatic sensory cortex (postcentral gyrus)

Cerebral cortex

Forearm and hand area

Axon of neuron in posterior limb of internal capsule

Thalamus

Ventral posterior lateral nucleus and posterior nuclear group

Midbrain

Substantia nigra

Basis pedunculi

Medial lemniscus

Pons

Medulla

Recticular formation

Dorsal root ganglion (neuron I)

Anterolateral System: spinoreticular tract spinotectal tract spinothalamic tract

Spinal cord

Figure 8.6 Anterolateral system for sensation of touch. C-fibers, carrying pain and general touch, cross at the spinal cord level and travel up to the brain through the anterolateral tract. Conscious awareness of pain occurs in the sensory part of the cerebral cortex. (Redrawn with permission from ER Kandel and JH Schwartz (eds.). *Principles of Neuroscience*, 2nd ed. New York:Elsevier, 1985, Figure 24-10, p. 311.)

information to the somatic sensory cortex via the posterior limb of the internal capsule.

Brain Stem

The next level of control in the hierarchical system is located in the brain stem—specifically it is the *basal ganglia* and the *cerebellum*, both of which can provide direct and indirect connections to higher cortical structures. Unfor-

tunately, the definitive way each of these structures contributes to movement control is not totally understood.

Basal Ganglia. The major components of the basal ganglia are the *caudate nucleus*, *putamen* and *globus palladus*, with the caudate nucleus and putamen making up the *striatum*. The basal ganglia does not have direct (afferent or efferent) connections with the spinal cord, it connects

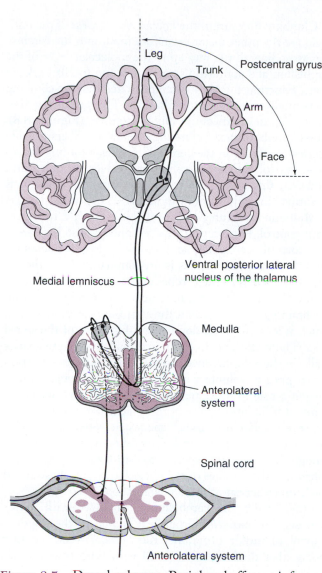

Figure 8.7   Dorsal columns. Peripheral afferent information such as that from proprioceptors or fine touch immediately ascend in the spinal cord in the dorsal columns and finally cross at the midbrain. The medial lemniscus transfers this information to the cortex, where it can influence movement. (Reprinted with permission from ER Kandel and JH Schwartz, (eds.). *Principles of Neuroscience*, 2nd ed. New York:Elsevier, 1985, Figure 25-1A, p. 317.)

mainly with the cerebral cortex via the thalamus. Therefore, influence on movement control rests with higher motor programming levels. A series of complex loops connect the cerebral cortex with the basal ganglia and the thalamus when regulating movement and motor learning. The striatum receives afferent information from most areas of the cerebral cortex, including the sensory and limbic centers. The striatum then sends connections to the globus palladus, which in turn relays information to the thalamus via the substantia nigra and the ansa lenticu-

laris. Limb movement information is sent to the *ventral anterior nucleus* of the thalamus and is relayed back to the pre-motor cortex via the ansa lenticularis.

The basal ganglia and cerebellum are both intimately involved with motor programs, but delineation of their exact roles is difficult. Contreras-Vidal[50] suggested dis-inhibition of thalamocortical pathways as a way to control movement. Turner and Delong[51] believed that the basal ganglia was primarily involved in specification, responding to a small range of stimuli when communicating with the primary motor cortex. Hayes et al.[52] suggested that the basal ganglia is involved in filtering relevant instructions in order to perform a specific task. This set switching is part of the executive function of movement control and is usually performed in concert with the cerebral cortex. We presently do not know whether or not the primary function of the basal ganglia is movement specification, selection, preparation, or retention. Suri et al.[53] reported that musculoskeletal system information involved with movement parameter computation is stored in the "motor" basal ganglia-thalamocortical circuit. Using magnetic resonance imaging to study brain function, Jueptner et al.[54] and Jueptner and Weiller[55] reported that the basal ganglion was more active during motor learning than it was during motor performance. The identification of greater areas of frontal cortex activation during complex movements that required greater central processing reinforced the connections between the cerebral cortex, basal ganglia and thalamus during movement tasks.[55] These studies also reported minimal basal ganglia activation during movements that required sensory feedback.

Cerebellum.   The cerebellum has by far the greatest influence on the motor control of movement from a proprioceptive feedback standpoint; therefore, this is where we will spend most of our discussion. Cerebellar lesions will generally not produce deficits of neuromuscular strength or sensation. The *cerebellum* however plays a crucial role in adjusting the output of the major descending motor systems from the brain. The cerebellum has three major functional components; the *vermis*, the *intermediate hemisphere*, and the *lateral hemisphere*. The vermis and intermediate hemisphere make up the spinocerebellum, while the lateral hemisphere is also called the cerebrocerebellum.

The vermis of the spinocerebellum receives afferent information from axial or proximal upper extremity muscles, the face, and visual and auditory receptors. These ipsilateral afferents enter the cerebellum through the spinocerebellar tract from the spinal cord and synapse in the vermis of the cerebellum before exiting the cerebellum from the superior peduncle and crossing over at the decussation eventually terminating at the motor cortex representing axial or proximal upper extremity muscles. This region of the cerebellum (vermis with spinocerebellum) has the greatest impact on upper extremity movement execution.

Key Point:

The spinocerebellum region of the cerebellum which is primarily responsible for monitoring motor programs sends output to the red nucleus of the midbrain and the motor cortex.

The intermediate hemisphere of the spinocerebellum receives input from the spinocerebellar tract and also from pontine nuclei in the midbrain area. This information is relayed to the *globose and emboliform nuclei*, which together are referred to as the interposed nucleus. The output from these nuclei travels either to the red nucleus in the brain stem or directly to the cerebral cortex. The functional significance of this pathway is believed to be for distal motor control and on-going or instantaneous motor program execution.[57] The lateral hemisphere of the cerebrocerebellum receives cortical afferents from the pontine nuclei and relays information to the dentate nucleus. These fibers cross immediately and are either relayed directly to the red nucleus or continue up to the cerebral cortex synapsing at the thalamus. This pathway is involved in the initiation, planning and timing of a motor program.[56]

Key Point:

The cerebrocerebellum region of the cerebellum is involved in motor program planning, timing, and initiation, also sending output to the red nucleus and cerebral cortex.

Afferent neurons to the cerebellum include *mossy fibers* and *climbing fibers*. Mossy fibers are more numerous arising mainly from the cerebral cortex and the spinal cord. Mossy fibers excite deep cerebellar nuclei and parallel fibers via granule cells. The parallel fibers also stimulate inhibitory neurons such as the stellate, basket, and Golgi cells which then synapse directly on to the Purkinje fibers. Parallel fibers also course perpendicularly at the molecular level of the cerebellum and connect with numerous (approximately 200,000) Purkinje fibers, providing convergent information. Stellate and basket cells, located in the molecular layer of the cerebellum receive excitatory connections from the parallel fibers and inhibit surrounding Purkinje fibers. Parallel fibers stimulate a continuous row of Purkinje fibers along the surface of the cerebellum; however, the inhibitory cells provide "surround inhibition" of Purkinje fibers on either side of the excited parallel fibers helping to concentrate areas of axon activation and improve motor control localization.[56] Mossy fibers provide direct stimulation to deep nuclei in addition to inhibition of deep nuclei supplied by the Purkinje fibers. These loops of information are believed to provide enhanced methods of movement control.

Climbing fibers from the *inferior olive nucleus* of the midbrain are the other major excitatory input into the cerebellum ascending all the way up to the molecular layer of the cerebellum and stimulating only a few (up to 10) Purkinje fibers. Functionally, Marr[57] demonstrated that the climbing fibers modify the response of Purkinje fibers to mossy fiber input, therefore affecting motor control (**Figure 8.8**). Mossy (inhibitory) and climbing (excitatory) fibers provide a series of affects on the cerebellum, thus affording movement control through a scaling or modulation of actions. However, this motor control is not complete unless it is performed in conjunction with higher CNS levels.

Midbrain structures also contribute directly to movement control. For example, the red nucleus also has extensive cortical, cerebellar, and inferior olive connections. Input from the red nucleus is predominantly from the interposed nucleus of the cerebellum and the somatosensory cortex. Efferents from the red nucleus cross midline within the brain stem and descend through the rubrospinal tract, which is located in the dorsolateral funiculus of the spinal cord. These efferents from the red nucleus synapse ipsilaterally in the inferior olive nucleus. Red nucleus activation occurs prior to voluntary upper extremity movements, suggesting a role in movement planning. The red nucleus is believed to be involved with movement pattern dynamics. However, Keifer and Houk[58] suggested evidence of its role in movement velocity and force direction control. Although the results are expected to transfer to human motor control, to date studies of red nucleus functions have relied solely on either cat or primate animal models.

Functionally, the cerebellum is involved with motor learning, but more importantly it is vital to the ongoing control of motor programs. Kan et al.[59] reported that mossy fiber discharge correlated with limb position and

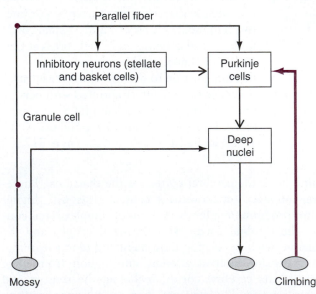

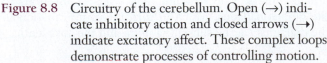

Figure 8.8   Circuitry of the cerebellum. Open (→) indicate inhibitory action and closed arrows (→) indicate excitatory affect. These complex loops demonstrate processes of controlling motion.

movement velocity. The cerebellum is capable of providing feedback for relatively slow movements, but as limb movement speed increases, direct feedback is impossible due to limitations in peripheral nerve conduction velocities and in CNS processing.[60] The CNS utilizes a feedback mechanism to control slower movements while a feed-forward mechanism is used to control fast movements. Knowledge of results after a movement is performed will enable adjustments to be implemented the next time a similar movement strategy is needed. This is a feed-forward paradigm that will be discussed later in the chapter. Schweighofer et al.[61] demonstrated through model simulations that the cerebellum learns through inverse dynamics, providing a template for future movements to compensate for inadequate feedback. Contreras-Vidal et al.[62] suggested that the cerebellum modifies movement velocity through antagonist muscle activation. Sensory feedback to the cerebellum in the form of ongoing modulation via peripheral feedback or the feed-forward paradigm influences future movement patterns.[55,63]

Thalamus.

The *thalamus* is considered the "gatekeeper" in serving as the the final relay of sensory information before the cerebral cortex. Different nuclei within the thalamus receive information from specific tracts and then relay this information to different parts of the cerebral cortex. The *ventral posterior nuclei* receive input from the medial and spinal lemniscus and relay that information to the somatic sensory area of the cerebral cortex (**Figure 8.9**). There are inhibitor neurons within these nuclei that can regulate the flow of sensory input and motor feedback to the cerebral cortex. The *ventral lateral nuclei* of the thalamus receives input from the dentate nucleus of the cerebellum via the cerebello-thalamic pathway and sends it to the primary motor cortex. The ventral lateral nuclei also decode sensory information for targeted limb movements. The ventral anterior nucleus receives input from the globus palladus of the basal ganglion and relays this information to the premotor cortex in the frontal lobe. It is important to distinguish that the ventral posterior nuclei are involved with somatic sensation that can influence movement and the ventral lateral and ventral anterior nuclei of the thalamus are involved with motor function. The *lateral geniculate nucleus* receives visual information form the optic nerve and is therefore involved with the processing of visual information that can influence movements. Ilinsky and Kultas-Ilinsky[64] described these afferent projections as inhibitory, with the exception of excitatory connections from the ventral anterior nuclei of the corticothalamic fibers.

Cerebral Cortex

The primary motor area of the *cerebral cortex* is the next level of motor control. The motor portion of the cortex is believed to be associated more with voluntary, skilled movements and less with automatic or reflexive movements. Organizational patterns of the motor and sensory portions of the cerebral cortex are described as a homunculus where the feet are represented superiorly and the upper extremities are located more laterally. The upper extremity is generally located more laterally, but Lotze et al.[65] reported that during complex, or multi-joint upper extremity movements a broader activation area can be observed. Cortical loops to the cerebellum, basal ganglia and thalamus provide multiple movement control layers, with the cortex responsible for the highest level of control.

The highest CNS motor control levels include the *premotor* and *supplementary* cerebral cortex regions in association with adjacent areas that assist with motor program creation. The frontal cortex contains both the pre-motor and supplementary motor regions. Scott[66] recorded impulses in the primary cortex of monkeys prior to shoulder and elbow movements indicating its function as a control area for upper extremity movements. Rather than controlling specific muscle activations, this region appeared to be broadly activated during upper extremity movements. Armstrong and Drew[67] demonstrated in cats that shoulder movements were associated with coronal gyrus activation in the cerebral cortex. Using a monkey model, Schieber[68] reported that the premotor cortex is crucial in determining how an object will be grasped. The supplementary motor area is believed to be involved with the preparatory phase of self-paced, complex movements.[69,70] Jenkins et al.[71] further subdivided the supplementary motor area into the *rostral* (toward the front of the brain) section, involved more with movement preparation and the *caudal* (toward the back of the brain) section, which is more involved with motor execution. Ball et al.[72] reported that decreased posterior supplementary motor cortex activation triggers the primary motor area to send a motor command. Ball et al.[72] also reported activation of the anterior cingulate motor area, intermediate supplementary motor area, and the inferior parietal lobe prior to changes in posterior supplementary motor area activation.

Another cortical area that assists with motor program planning is the parietal lobe. The parietal lobe and supplementary cerebral cortex areas are the locations for the critical step of information processing and spatial representation for movement initiation. Feedback information from the periphery appears to be processed earlier through the cerebellum.

> ## *Key Point:*
> Motor commands originate from the motor region of the cerebral cortex; however intimate connections exist with the parietal lobe, cerebellum and basal ganglia.

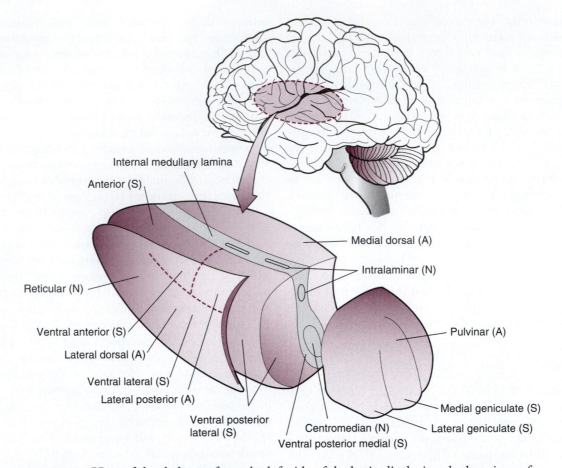

Internal medullary lamina

Anterior (S)

Medial dorsal (A)

Intralaminar (N)

Reticular (N)

Pulvinar (A)

Ventral anterior (S)

Lateral dorsal (A)

Ventral lateral (S)

Lateral posterior (A)

Ventral posterior lateral (S)

Centromedian (N)

Medial geniculate (S)

Lateral geniculate (S)

Ventral posterior medial (S)

Figure 8.9   View of the thalamus from the left side of the brain displaying the locations of the major thalamic nuclei. The internal medullary lamina divides the thalamus into the anterior, lateral, and medial groups of nuclei. The lateral group is divided into a dorsal and ventral tier. The ventral tier is composed of the ventral anterior, ventral lateral, and ventral posterior nuclei. The lateral geniculate nucleus, which is concerned with vision, and the medial geniculate nucleus, which is concerned with hearing, are often classified as components of the ventral tier. The nuclei of the dorsal tier are the lateral dorsal, lateral posterior, and the pulvinar. The medial dorsal nucleus is the largest of the medial group. The ventral tier nuclei are specific nuclei, while the dorsal tier and the medial group project to the association cortex. The intralaminar nuclei lie within the internal medullary lamina, while the reticular nucleus caps the lateral aspect of the thalamus. The functional class of each nucleus is indicated parenthetically: Specific relay (S), association (A), and nonspecific (N). (Redrawn with permission from ER Kandel and JH Schwartz (eds.). *Principles of Neuroscience,* 2nd ed. New York: Elsevier, 1985, Figure 20-10, p 233.)

CENTRAL NERVOUS SYSTEM OUTPUT

The *corticospinal tract* is considered the final direct output from the primary motor cortex. However, divergent motor neuron pools and the presence of interneurons can complicate specific motor control output patterns from the cerebral cortex. Pearce et al.[73] described motor cortex excitability and re-organization changes supporting the plasticity of its influence on motor control. It is not presently understood if these excitability changes are located solely within the cortex or in adjacent areas that interact with the cortex, such as the cerebellum or basal ganglia. MacKay[74] suggested that initial activity in both the frontal cortex and parietal cortex associated with limb movement reflects the cerebellum's influence on the cortex via the thalamocortical circuitry. This limb movement activity subsides with movement onset, supporting the importance of peripheral feedback during movement.

Regardless of the exact cerebral cortex area or other structures involved in motor control, it is uncertain what the precise functional relationship is between brain activity and motor outputs. Fuchs et al.[75,76] reported a strong correlation between movement velocity and cerebral cortex activation amplitude, thus providing a link between the equilibrium point hypothesis (discussed later) and cerebral cortex activity. This suggests that a motor program to control movement amplitude located in the cerebral cortex could be selectively activated depending on the speed of the movement task. Marsden et al.[77] demonstrated coherence of both spatial and frequency output during similar movements, suggesting the presence of only one mechanism for motor control within the cerebral cortex.

By processing the spatial information of targets in space, *Brodmann's area number 7*, located in the posterior parietal cortex, is considered to be crucial for movement task performance. Lesions to Brodmann's area number 7 causes *apraxias*, or the inability to execute learned movement sequences.[48] Preliminary information to specify target location whether provided visually or proprioceptively is usually processed in this brain region and then communicated with the motor cortex. This information may be all that is needed for motor plan initiation to occur. Visual and proprioceptive feedback are then used to make movement adjustments in order to successfully reach the desired target. The *pre-frontal cortex* is active during periods of learning a new motor command, while the cerebellum is more involved with on-line or on-going corrections of movement, or feedback.[77–79]

> ## *Key Point:*
> The pre-frontal cortex is active during learning, while the cerebellum is more involved with on-line or on-going movement corrections, or feedback.

The major descending pathway that ultimately carries the CNS commands to the muscles is the corticospinal tract. This tract is the continuation of the pyramids at the midbrain traveling within the anterior portion of the spinal cord to synapse with alpha motor neurons.[48] Alpha motor neurons activate the muscles they innervate, thereby allowing the movement sequence to be performed. During ipsilateral hand muscle activation, Kosarov and Christova[80] observed similar activation patterns in contralateral hand muscles, suggesting the existence of supraspinal control of similar contralateral muscles.

BACKGROUND OF MOVEMENT CONTROL AND MOTOR LEARNING

To better understand current opinions of how movements are controlled, a basic understanding of common motor control theories is necessary. The CNS controls our ability to create movements, maintain appropriate postures, and manipulate objects in our environment. Many daily tasks are performed without much conscious awareness and with reasonable accuracy. The CNS assimilates information from multiple peripheral receptors such as the visual, haptic (skin), proprioceptive and vestibular systems and combines it with the past motor history to create the desired movement. It is difficult to determine how the CNS combines past information about posture and movement control with current on-line peripheral afferent information in order to maintain a given posture or movement pattern.

Successful upper extremity movements are particularly interesting because these discrete, goal-directed movements typically require locating an object, reaching for the object, and manipulating objects in space. Successful coordination of these upper extremity movements would be relative to both spatial and temporal accuracy in addition to proper muscle force timing at different segments in order to generate the correct movement pattern efficiently. The lower extremities function to provide both stability and mobility. Lower extremity movements are typically rhythmical and involve walking or traversing changing terrains where the need to generate force is greater than generally observed during upper extremity functions. Precise movement accuracy is generally less of a concern for lower extremity movements; however, force modulation is still critical. Precise lower extremity placement in space may not be critical, but proper force modulation and avoidance of obstacles is necessary to avoid tripping and falling. Coordinated lower extremity movement patterns should be measured both for efficiency and proper obstacle avoidance.

Upper extremity movements can be performed under an almost infinite combination of muscle contributions to joint movements (degrees of freedom), which lead to significant challenges in studying movement control.[1] Controversies exist regarding the contributions of numerous motor control factors. As mentioned earlier, the study of motor control generally describes kinematic, kinetic and/or EMG changes during movements relative to different tasks and environmental conditions. Stein[81] suggested separate control for individual factors such as muscle force, muscle length, and velocity of contraction, joint stiffness, joint viscosity or any combination of these factors.

> ## Key Point:
> Stein[81] suggested that effective movement control depended on appropriate muscle force, appropriate control of muscle contraction velocity, control of muscle length, and joint viscosity.

Appreciating these factors and their interactions helps to understand the available degrees of freedom in the study of movement control and the great amount of information that must be controlled during motor programming.[81] Constraining one of these factors during specific movements and observing outcomes (kinematic, kinetic and EMG) enables the development of a theory on how the CNS organizes neural signals and controls movement. However, it remains difficult to study motor control because of the many variables that can confound movements in addition to the factors that Stein has suggested.[81] As movement control is becoming better understood for constrained conditions, we may develop a better understanding of the coordination of appropriate motor commands under any condition.

This section is dedicated to the review of some contemporary motor control theories and how they relate to motor coordination. There exists no single unifying motor control theory, which makes it difficult to understand specific CNS control of muscle coordination. Moreover, these theories tend to deal with the highest level of CNS control, neglecting the specifics of how the motor program itself is carried out.

EQUILIBRIUM POINT HYPOTHESIS

Two versions of the equilibrium point hypothesis (the original alpha version and an expanded lambda version) describe different controls of limb position and trajectory. Equilibrium in this context refers to movement trajectories and forces involved with the control of limb position and movement. This section will discuss some of the basic tenets of these two movement theories (alpha and lambda) to better understand how they contribute to the control of coordination. Original equilibrium hypothesis control

theories stipulate final position control, whereby the CNS specifies a terminal position and relegates details of the movement to local controllers.[82–84] Viscoelastic properties of muscle and inertial limb characteristics are taken into consideration by the CNS as muscle stiffness is modulated in the absence of peripheral feedback. Sugarman and Tiran[85] suggested that it is the final position, and not movement amplitude, that the motor program controls, even for finger movements. This positional control dictates appropriate force/length interactions between agonist and antagonist muscles with the final muscle force/length interaction generating the motor program.

The idea of higher CNS levels only having to specify final position, allowing lower control centers (such as the spinal cord) to regulate muscle stiffness in order to generate movement, is attractive because this allows higher CNS centers to attend to other cognitive functions. In reality, multiple CNS levels are involved in movement control as will be discussed later. Sanes and Evarts[86] demonstrated that the equilibrium point hypothesis works well for large movements, but this hypothesis is not appropriate for fine motor tasks in which a premium is placed on accuracy. Final position control for movements that function under an open loop feedback paradigm is a reasonable theory, yet Sanes and Evarts[86] claim that there is no peripheral feedback mechanism to make adjustments during movement.

Limb control trajectory is another theory of characterizing limb movement.[87–89] Trajectory is the orientation of the limb in space (like the arm during a reaching task) and the speed of movement from initial to final position. Upper extremity movements demonstrate some invariant kinematic characteristics in which hand paths are generally straight and the tangential velocity profile of the segment resembles a bell curve (refer to **Figure 8.1**). The CNS devises a movement strategy in which it determines limb trajectories from a visual coordinate system and transforms this information to a motor coordinate system. Characterization of hand path velocities is a useful method to limit the degrees of freedom in order to control movement and yield optimal performance.[90] Optimal performance for this model is determined by minimizing the mathematical derivative of acceleration, or jerk, creating smooth movement. This model describes movements, but neglects the effect of changes in load or the role of peripheral feedback in altering movements. Consistent with the equilibrium point hypothesis, Uno et al.[91] stated that joint torques are optimized to control upper extremity movements, where efficient movements are identified as those that require the least amount of integrated torques over the movement time. Regardless of whether motor control focuses on joint torques or limb trajectory, once the motor program is initiated, local control of muscle force and joint torque is regulated at the spinal cord level, thereby sparing the CNS from having to compute individual joint parameters.

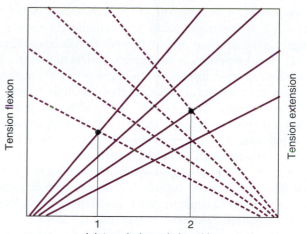

Figure 8.10   Equilibrium point hypothesis. Bizzi's model demonstrates the relationship between muscle length and force and how this can help guide movements. Solid lines represent flexors and broken lines represent extensors. Extensor muscles are longer at joint angle 1 and force of extensors must be increased to move limb to joint angle 2, in order to shorten the extensor's length. (Reprinted with permission from Bizzi et al. Arm trajectory formation in monkeys. *Exp Brain Res.* 1982;46:139–143.)

The Alpha Model

Bizzi's[82] *alpha model* of the equilibrium point hypothesis suggests that the CNS generates signals to specify a new position that is ultimately achieved through changes between agonist and antagonist muscle forces. This is similar to the classical equilibrium point hypothesis except that it also incorporates force and positional control, and local movement control based on the spring-like properties of muscles. The CNS determines joint position by the ratio between agonist and antagonist muscle tension surrounding the joint. This feed-forward mechanism allows the higher CNS levels to relegate lower orders of processing to the spinal cord so it can command the new positions. The alpha model suffers from the same criticism as other equilibrium point hypotheses in that it does not consider the contributions of feedback to the CNS during movement.

Bizzi et al.[92] studied monkey movements and determined that movement is accomplished through the interaction of muscle activity and inertial and viscoelastic muscle properties. Simple movements are controlled by changes in the equilibrium point position. The length-tension properties of both agonist and antagonist muscles are represented for a fixed range of motion (**Figure 8.10**). As a joint is extended from 30° flexion to 0° flexion increased tension is produced in the flexors because they are lengthened or stretched. The equilibrium point is where the slopes of extensor and flexor muscle stiffness meet. Changes in agonist or antagonist muscle torques will lead to changes in position. Thus if an external force induces a position change to another joint angle, the increased force from the viscoelastic stiffness of one of the muscles will cause the joint to regain the original position after a brief movement away from the original equilibrium point.

Human upper extremity movements demonstrate segmented curved paths in three-dimensional space, where mean movement duration is longer than the mean for straight paths.[93] This appears to be related to the limb control trajectory theory already discussed; however it is the length-tension ratio of involved muscles rather than the path of trajectory of the limb that acts as the primary control mechanism. Abend et al.[93] and Bizzi et al.[94] concluded that muscle length and internal force information were the only inputs needed to achieve target position in the absence of peripheral feedback during movement. This model stipulates that joint position is the main parameter controlled by higher CNS levels, and the length-tension properties of muscles are modulated at lower CNS levels.

In summary, the alpha model also neglects feedback information during movement and is concerned with regulation of muscle stiffness to generate movements. In reality, pre-existing motor programs are seldom used for instantaneous movement execution, but are used more for motor learning, where they are adjusted based on feedback from previous movements.

The Lambda Model

The *lambda model* is an expanded version of the equilibrium point hypothesis where Feldman[83] also stated that limb position or posture was the result of equilibrium between length dependent agonist and antagonist muscle forces. One difference between the lambda and alpha models is that only the lambda model considers the mechanical forces exerted by agonist and antagonist muscles about a joint via gamma motor neuron modulation at the spinal cord level. Feldman[83] measured length-tension curves for antagonist muscles and proposed that the position of a joint is controlled by the CNS through manipulation of the length-tension curves, referred to as *invariant characteristics*. The invariant characteristic modulated by the CNS is the relationship between muscle force and length in descending output control or lambda (**Figure 8.11**). The framework of the lambda model of motor control resulted from the observation that while maintaining posture the antagonistic muscles about a single joint produce a restoring force toward an equilibrium position when a perturbation is applied. Feldman[83] suggested that manipulation of the length-tension curves of muscles occur through changes in the motor neuron activation thresholds. Motor neuron activation thresholds are modified directly by neural signals descending from the brain and indirectly through negative position feedback from muscle spindles. Feldman[83] formulated the lambda model to explain the observed characteristics and relate them to known neural pathways. The lambda model was later extended to include velocity sensitive muscle spindle feedback as a modulating factor for motor neuron activation threshold levels.

The lambda model incorporates both spring-like and viscoelastic muscle properties (see Chapter 3) and motor control where the CNS regulates agonist and antagonist activation in order to create movement. The CNS controls local reflexes, internal muscle stiffness and external loads in order to generate movements via the output that is referred to as lambda (**Figure 8.12a–c**). The lambda is generated by the CNS by comparing muscle spindle output to alpha motor neuron activity. The lambda model is part of the equilibrium point hypothesis where the CNS is seeking equilibrium between the afferent and efferent information. Shifting lambda along the *x*-axis, which ultimately changes the invariant or force-length characteristics of local muscle, generates voluntary movements. The internal drive to change position is the result of changes in the gamma motor neuron activation of a muscle. The gamma motor neuron drive adjusts internal muscle tension, creating enough force to generate movement until it reaches the equilibrium point position between the agonist and antagonist muscles.

The major difference between the alpha and lambda models of motor control is that peripheral feedback is only incorporated into the lambda model. In the lambda model, central commands influence alpha motor neurons and modulate stretch reflex activation thresholds.[95] The

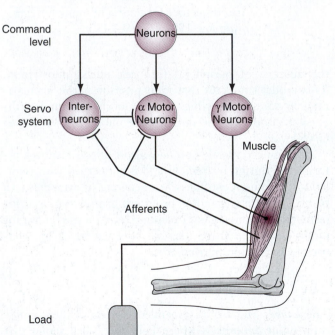

Figure 8.11   Equilibrium hypothesis λ model: Anatomical model. Descending control (command level neurons) can influence muscle afferents, which indirectly can affect the alpha motor neuron via the interneurons. (Redrawn with permission from AG Feldman. Once more on the equilibrium point hypothesis (lambda model) for motor control. *J Mot Behav*. 1986;18:17–54.)

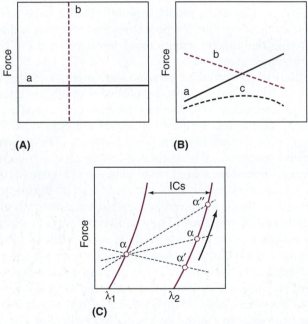

Figure 8.12   Equilibrium point hypothesis (λ) model. A. Isotonic load (a) and isometric load (b) B. Loads can have different gradients; positive (a), negative (b), or variable (c). C. Invariant characteristics (IC) are shifted according to length (λ) and EMG (α) is scaled with load movement. (Reprinted with permission from AG Feldman. Once more on the equilibrium point hypothesis (lambda model) for motor control. *J Mot Behav* 1986;18:17–54.)

equilibrium or set point is regulated relative to muscle length, and muscle force is calculated from

$$F = f(x - \lambda)$$

where F is the desired muscle force, f is the muscle force at the current equilibrium point, x is muscle length, and λ is new muscle length. The lambda (λ) model requires direct feedback to modulate movements; therefore any discrepancies between extrafusal muscle fiber function and the intrafusal fiber function of the gamma motor system (γ) are used to correct position. In the lambda model the CNS seeks equilibrium between the current joint angle and the desired joint angle. Feed-forward signals from the CNS control changes in the equilibrium of a resting muscle's length, and movement occurs through local gamma motor system control, based on the newly set equilibrium point. This is accomplished by the difference between the gamma motor neurons and alpha motor neurons.[83,96] This method of control is less specific regarding direct muscle control because it does not suggest control parameters such as muscle activation onset timing, duration or amplitude.

> ## Key Point:
> The major difference between the alpha and lambda motor control models is that peripheral feedback is only considered in the lambda model.

The lambda model was derived from the *servo-reflex model* postulated by Merton in 1953.[40] The servo-reflex model defined a length-error signal that the CNS identifies via the gamma motor system. However, in the lambda model, movement is initiated by a central command.[40] Vallbo et al.[97] found an EMG burst to precede muscle spindle activity by at least 10 ms for voluntary movements, thus disproving the servo-reflex model and possibly indicating a greater role for the central command of movement, further supporting the lambda model. The lambda model does not suggest that any feedback information is transferred to higher CNS processing centers, but rather its influence remains local at the spinal cord level, sparing any higher order CNS processing.

Gottlieb[98] challenged the physiologic assumptions of the equilibrium point hypothesis, such as the damping of muscle reflexes, and the addition of reciprocal and co-activation commands to muscles. Other microneurographic studies by Burke et al.[99] have demonstrated that fusimotor or intrafusal muscle fiber drive could not be maintained with the stretch reflex during slower movements. More recently, however, Adamovich et al.[100] demonstrated an increased stretch reflex mechanism gain during fast elbow movements. This change in the gain of the stretch reflex supports the lambda model for fast movements, because of the influence of the descending control on the fusimotor drive. The discrepancy noted between the studies of Burke et al.[99] and Adamovich et al.[100] could rest in the movement speed. The stretch reflex is not activated at slower speeds but could influence movements at faster speeds. As we have already discussed, as movement speed increases it can get to the point where even the stretch reflex is also rendered unusable for providing movement feedback because it can not respond adequately.

The essence of these three motor control theories (trajectory, alpha, or lambda) based on the equilibrium point hypothesis is that central commands are transmitted as virtual trajectories and joint positions are represented by a combination of muscle lengths and joint angles. The CNS must remember these positions in order to generate the command to change position, because peripheral feedback is believed to be too slow to account for the changes that occur with fast movements. Questions remain about how the CNS assesses joint stiffness under various movement conditions and the specific role of both central and peripheral processes.

> ## Key Point:
> Motor control theories (trajectory, alpha and lambda) based on the equilibrium hypothesis consider the reflexive properties of muscle as a major factor in the control of voluntary movements.

AMPLITUDE AND DURATION CONTROL

The speed of movement is one of the major decisions that the CNS must employ when creating a motor program. Various investigators[101–105] have used differing terminology to describe the relationship between movement speed and how movement speed is controlled. Lestienne[101] originally used the term *pulse control* to describe characteristics of simple single joint movements that change as movement speed is increased. Corcos et al.[102] and Gottlieb et al.[103,104] have further developed this concept and defined a *dual strategy hypothesis*: a *speed sensitive strategy* used for fast movements and a *speed insensitive strategy* used for slower movements.[102–104] In their *pulse-height model* of movement control, Gordon and Ghez[105] reported that the rise time of force generation is modulated for fast movements. Subtle differences between these theories will be presented here; however, in aggregate, velocity control of a predetermined motor program is a critical aspect of movement control.

Corcos et al.[102,106] and Gottlieb et al.[103,104,107] evaluated active elbow flexion movements toward targets under various conditions that included changes in load, distance and speed. They developed a dual hypothesis of motor control where slower movements are controlled by duration of pulse activity and the initial activity is held constant. Pulses represent CNS activation of the alpha motor neuron and, ultimately, muscle activity patterns. Pulses of activity are initially selected with consideration of the entire task, but initial alpha motor neuron activity is independent of changes that occur later in a movement or task. Once amplitude is selected it remains invariant over changes in task variables such as distance and inertial load. In the speed insensitive strategy, although speed is affected by the task, the initiation of the movement is not.[103,104] Keeping task duration constant, modulation of motor neuron excitation amplitude, and ultimately kinematic characteristics creates a speed sensitive strategy. The initial rate of motor neuron recruitment is adjusted to adapt to changes in specific tasks. Kinematic movement characteristics are scaled with additional loads. Specifically, measures like burst of muscle activity, torque rise time and acceleration are used to separate movements performed under the speed insensitive strategy.[102] The speed insensitive strategy, or pulse duration modulation, is described as the default strategy, only utilizing the speed sensitive strategy at faster movement speeds.[104] Corcos et al.[102] and Gottlieb et al.[104] discussed the influence of load and distance on antagonist muscle activity whereby the addition of a load to a movement provided earlier antagonist activation while movement distance did not affect antagonist muscle activity. Agonist activity was increased as movement velocity increased, unless a load was added to the limb, which tended to slow a movement and create a movement modulated by pulse duration, not amplitude.

used for the generation of lesser forces. Muscles antagonistic to the primary mover are also controlled by this dual hypothesis incorporating a combination of both a speed sensitive and a speed insensitive strategy. Gottlieb et al.[107] reported increased antagonistic muscle activation latency delays with greater agonist activation during slower movements than usually occurs during faster movements. The antagonist muscle is also sensitive to increased load during slower movements as these loads further slow the movements and increase the duration of (or delay) antagonist muscle activation latencies. As mentioned earlier, the dual control theory suggests that the overall amount of agonist muscular activation may increase over the task duration, but the initial burst of EMG activity is attenuated. An interesting relationship exists between movement speed, the addition of loads to movements and muscle activity, where the addition of a load will cause movement speed to decrease, overall muscle activity will be greater, but initial burst activity will remain unchanged.[107] This is contrary to changes in speed where an initial burst of activity will result in changes in movement speed for both agonist and antagonist muscles.

Key Point:
The addition of a load will cause movement speed to decrease and overall muscle activity will be greater, but initial burst activity will remain unchanged. This is contrary to changes in movement speed when an initial burst of activity will result in changes in movement speed for both agonist and antagonist muscles.

Key Point:
The CNS modulates muscle activity duration during self-paced movements, but modulates amplitude of muscle activity for fast movements, while duration remains relatively constant.

Corcos et al.[106] evaluated this control strategy for isometric elbow muscle activations, whereby faster maximal agonist muscle activations resulted from a speed sensitive control strategy, while slower sub-maximal muscle activations used a pulse duration control strategy. They concluded that isometric torque pulses are similar to forces that are needed during isotonic movements; this means that the speed sensitive strategy is also used for the generation of larger forces while the speed insensitive strategy is

In evaluating their pulse-height control model, Gordon and Ghez[105] required subjects to develop a pre-determined force as accurately or as quickly as possible at the elbow joint. They measured rate of rise of the force produced at the elbow and described similar modulation of EMG and joint torque outputs as those reported by Corcos et al.[106] and Gottlieb et al.[107] during simple elbow movements. Since force rise time was more closely associated with reduced variability during this elbow task they concluded that pulse amplitude control was preferred when fast, accurate movements are generated.[105] From these findings they suggested that this is one way the CNS simplifies movement control, thereby decreasing the degrees of freedom associated with movements or tasks.[105] Both agonist and antagonist muscle activation patterns display pulse amplitude and/or duration control, suggesting that a coupling of these mechanisms may help to further decrease available degrees of freedom. Allum[108] suggested a pulse-like proprioceptive feedback control, particularly in antagonist muscles to oppose upper extremity perturbations. Allum's hypothesis[108] suggested that responses to perturbations also appear to be under the same organization as motor programs.

Most studies cited here use movements that are restricted to a single plane. Almedia et al.[109] challenged the notion that unconstrained movements behave differently than constrained (single joint or single plane) movements. Specifically, they identified both speed sensitive and speed insensitive strategies during both constrained and unconstrained upper extremity movements. Almedia et al.[109] further identified scaling differences between movements opposed to gravity compared to movements where gravity was eliminated. Nonetheless, the overall pattern of control remained consistent. This further suggests a central control of similar movements regardless if the movement is constrained or unconstrained.

Khan et al.[110] also described a similar modulation of EMG amplitude and duration and movement kinematics as velocity increased when movement was a function of target size. Larger targets allowed faster movements, while smaller targets had less tolerance for error and dictated slower movements. The addition of a load during movement, especially when small targets were used created slower movements but had little effect on the muscle burst activity. This suggested that while there was a change in movement speed there was no change in muscle burst activity, thus the findings of Khan et al.[110] are consistent with the speed insensitive strategy reported by Gottlieb et al.[104] Lestienne[101] demonstrated that the principle of a pulse control also applied to antagonist muscles that terminate elbow movement. The speed selected by the subject before starting the movement was critical in pre-determining the timing of agonist and antagonist muscle activations. However, these pre-determined commands such as the stretch reflex could be modified locally.[101] Lestienne[101] reported that overall muscle activation amplitude was related to movement velocity with activation timing remaining constant. This relationship was maintained when a load was added, with muscle activation amplitude displaying a scaled increase.

Motor program segmentation based on the control of movement speed is especially desirable because of the relationship between the reduced amounts of peripheral feedback that can be utilized during fast versus slow movements. Incorporation of fast movements with the pulse control or a speed sensitive theory represents a *feedforward strategy*. After the initial part of the motor program is completed, slower movements can incorporate information from peripheral feedback, or the *closed feedback loop*. Motor control theories discussed in this section incorporate peripheral feedback at the end of a movement, with regards to movement error, in order to determine how the CNS organizes an appropriate movement pattern. Peripheral feedback includes mechanical factors such as position, load, movement speed, and all of the internal dynamics previously discussed. Peripheral feedback of mechanical factors such as position, load, and speed of movement as well as internal muscle dynamics affect the motor program output.

Key Point:

Pulse duration and muscle activation amplitude identify different movement strategies based on the CNS control of muscle activity.

CENTRAL NERVOUS SYSTEM CONTROL OF MOVEMENT

To understand the actual coordination of movement it is necessary to be familiar with CNS mechanisms responsible for movement control. Although knowledge of neuroanatomy helps us understand the location of information processing, it does not tell us how movements are controlled. For example, we know the cerebellum is important for helping control movement but we have not described precisely how it monitors and controls motion in non-impaired subjects. Parameters controlled by the cerebellum may include position, trajectory, energy, velocity or any number or combinations of these movement variables. However, there is probably some optimum use of neural control signals by the cerebellum, with excess information being too demanding to be of any use to the CNS. To simplify the complex nature of how the CNS controls movement we look at the process from an input-output model; where peripheral information is sent into the CNS, the information is processed, and movement characteristics are the output. This permits us to evaluate the complex nature of motor coordination and motor programs.

MOTOR PLANNING: INPUT

Identifying the anatomical location of motor programs and the physiology of the CNS in relation to movement control regulation is important. Conceptually, however, it is difficult to identify how interacting variables such as movement velocity, coordination, and accuracy interact as sub-components within the overall motor program. Longer duration movements use peripheral feedback to influence movement accuracy and efficiency. Shorter duration movements do not have the time to use peripheral feedback. There simply isn't enough time for the information to travel along the nervous system to provide any assistance. Peripheral input plays a role in motor program execution when there is sufficient time for the information to be incorporated into the movement. There are also other open loop feedback mechanisms to assist with movement control, especially during fast movements.

Closed Loop Control

Closed loop movements rely on peripheral feedback to ensure accuracy (**Figure 8.13**). Peripheral input from visual, auditory, and vestibular systems, and from capsuloligamentous and musculotendinous mechanoreceptors and haptic (tactile sense, skin) receptors provide specific information to the CNS. Information from all of these receptors is assimilated by the CNS and used to adjust movement programs. This on-line comparison provides constant movement modulation relative to the goal of the motor program. In addition, closed loop feedback can occur after higher CNS levels have compared the actual movement outcome to the expected movement goal. Information regarding the error between the actual and the expected movement is input to the CNS so that motor program corrections can be implemented for future use. The goal of the closed loop system is to minimize the error or the difference between the reference movement pattern and the actual movement.

Regulation of closed loop movements requires a significant amount of CNS processing to appropriately use all of the external information provided by the peripheral receptors. As movement time increases, more time is available for the CNS to process peripheral feedback creating more coordinated and accurate movements. Woodworth[111] originally addressed the relationship between movement time and accuracy over 100 years ago when he defined two phases of movement, the initial impulse phase and the current control phase. The *initial impulse phase* represented the original motor program, devoid of peripheral feedback. The second movement phase, the *current control phase*, used peripheral feedback to adjust the initial motor program provided there was sufficient time. Woodworth[111] examined the movement time and error of subjects as they moved a pencil between targets on paper at slow and fast movement speeds. At the fast movement speeds there was no difference in movement error whether or not subjects used visual feedback. When vision was used for feedback, movements were much more accurate when movement time durations were greater than 215–250 ms.[111] More recently, in a similar study Keele and Posner[112] randomly denied visual feedback as subjects moved a stylus toward a target at pre-determined veloci-

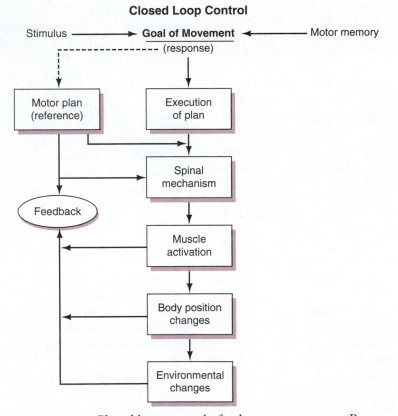

Figure 8.13   Closed loop control of voluntary movement. Peripheral feedback has direct consequences on the ongoing motor program that can affect movement outcome.

ties. The probability of hitting the target was unchanged, unless movement time durations were greater than 190–260 ms, at which point visual feedback was believed to be utilized to enhance movement accuracy.[112] There is not sufficient time for peripheral information to be used in movements that are less than approximately 200 ms in duration. Therefore closed loop feedback does not influence movements that are completed in less than 200 ms.

> ## *Key Point:*
> Peripheral feedback that is not conscious plays an important role in movement control, but the precise physiological significance of its signals are hard to determine.

> ## *Key Point:*
> While closed loop feedback needs movements to last at least 200 ms, visual information can be processed in as little as 135 ms.

Others have reported that less time is needed to use visual feedback for continuous movement. Carlton[113] blocked visual feedback during the initial 75 percent of movement toward a target and reported that the CNS could process visual information during movements as small as 135 ms in duration. Carlton's[113] study precluded the use of visual feedback during the initial impulse phase of a movement, but visual feedback was used during the current control phase. Sudden changes in target position during movement execution can create corrections for movement durations as small as 100 ms. Changes in target size also necessitate the need for longer processing times, due to Fitts' law.[114,115] Fitts' law is intimately related to target width; narrowing the target will prolong movement time duration. Peripheral feedback such as that provided by vision is believed to be the primary source of information for movement corrections. Movements shorter than 150–200 ms in duration are thought to make greater use of the error between the desired and actual final positions, visual feedback or not, to correct the motor program prior to the next time it is used.

In a study by Dewhurst,[116] subjects were required to hold their elbow in a fixed position while an unexpected resistance was added to the forearm. The added weight temporarily changed (perturbed) the elbow position but subjects were able to return to the original position in about 250 ms. Using EMG latency measurements subjects used two distinct muscle activation patterns to change arm positions. A monosynaptic-like initial burst of EMG activity occurred 30 ms after perturbation (*short reflex loop*), and a second, larger burst occurred 50 ms after perturbation (*long reflex loop*). The long reflex loop was believed to be modulated by higher CNS control. The authors believed that descending control signals from the long reflex loops helped to modulate motor output.[116] Because the longer reflex loop appeared to be under some level of supraspinal control it was believed to be more plastic or flexible, playing a greater role in movement adjustments.

All of the studies presented to this point have relied on relatively simple movement models, requiring minimal CNS processing. The greater CNS processing associated with more complex tasks can alter or prolong the long reflex loop latency. Using a spring-loaded apparatus, Henry[117] studied force modulation, or the ability to adjust upper extremity force output. Subjects were able to respond to subtle tension changes when given the instructions to maintain pressure, but when they had to identify changes in tension and then respond to the apparatus, sensitivity decreased.[117] Higher order CNS processing, in this case the ability to identify muscle tension changes, appears to decrease the overall acuity of locally processed information. This suggests that conscious awareness of certain stimuli could actually decrease motor performance. Long duration movements can utilize peripheral feedback to enhance movement accuracy and efficiency. During short duration, high velocity movements, there is not enough time to make adjustments unless they are pre-programmed.

High velocity movements can be influenced by local, intermediate feedback. The Ia afferent activity is influenced by muscle fiber length, rate of length change, and the amount of tension within the intrafusal muscle fibers. This information is relayed back to the spinal cord, thereby influencing the alpha motor neuron output to the muscle. Alpha motor neuron output may be modulated by both descending control from higher CNS control center systems and feedback from gamma motor neurons. Using signals from supraspinal centers and Ia afferents, alpha and gamma motor neurons are co-activated to improve motor coordination strategies.[118,119]

Stiffness, or the amount of tension required to increase muscle length, is strongly influenced by the muscle spindle (see Chapters 2 and 7). Nichols and Houck[120] demonstrated the importance of muscle spindles for providing postural control via increased muscle stiffness when a muscle is stretched. The viscoelastic mechanical properties of muscle, in conjunction with the muscle spindle firing patterns, enable almost immediate responses to postural or position changes. This strategy appears to be less important during voluntary, unprompted movements. Researchers have shown that movements in excess of 200 ms duration require peripheral feedback to be executed accurately. Other muscle properties can also contribute to movement coordination.

The Stretch Reflex and Its Contribution to Motor Control

Since the myotatic stretch reflex is modulated locally at the spinal cord level, it has been widely studied as a motor control component (see Chapter 2). Soechting et al.[88] demonstrated that this reflex is related more to the physical properties of the limb and less on muscle activity during movements. Since inertial properties do not change quickly, over a short period of time, the stretch reflex of a particular limb should remain very stable. The presence of a late stretch response does not contribute to the control of fast movements because these movements occur too quickly. Lacquaniti and Soechting[121] postulated that it is torque from a perturbation that initiates the stretch reflex. Regardless of the external force that caused a perturbation, reactions from peripheral mechanoreceptors would take too long to reach the spinal cord before the efferent portion of the stretch reflex influenced movement. Only with sufficiently slow movements can the effects of a stretch reflex influence ongoing motor program execution. Faster movements occur too rapidly to be affected by the stretch reflex.

Stretch reflex modulation has also been shown to occur locally and from higher CNS control centers. Capaday[122] reported decreased local stretch reflexes and muscle stiffness in cats following baclofen injection into the alpha motorneuron, as a mechanism of local inhibition. Baclofen is a neurotransmitter-blocking agent that impairs muscle output following injection. It is possible that spinal interneurons, such as *Renshaw cells*, provide some type of local stretch reflex inhibition (see Chapter 2). Using cat models, other investigations have demonstrated the ability to diminish stretch reflex responsiveness by stimulating the red nucleus region of the CNS.[123,124] Allum[108] suggested that slow speed shoulder movements are regulated predominantly by muscle viscoelastic properties, while fast movements use a combination of muscle viscoelastic properties and short and long loop antagonist muscle activation latencies. Long EMG activation latencies (60–120 ms) following perturbation appear to be influenced by movement direction.[125] This suggests some type of higher CNS influence on later muscle activation following perturbation.

Many motor control factors may affect the stretch reflex. The stretch reflex might appear to be a crucial component in arresting movement, but Brooke et al.[126] reported *H-reflex* attenuation during both passive and active upper extremity movements. The H-reflex was pro-duced by electrically stimulating gamma motor neurons with an electrical impulse to monosynaptically activate alpha motor neurons in a manner similar to the stretch reflex. Although the stretch reflex may be under some form of higher level CNS modulation when the terminal position is known, it is not clear how this modulation can affect movement control. Simple monosynaptic reflexes do not appear to play a major role in the coordination of movement but they do help maintain muscle function during these movements.

MOTOR PLANNING: CENTRAL PROCESSING

Open Loop Control

Open loop control of movement occurs when a command is given to execute a movement and no feedback is provided to make motor program adjustments (**Figure 8.14**). Woodworth[111] previously described this as the *initial impulse control strategy* of movement. As stated previously, shorter duration movements do not have sufficient time to

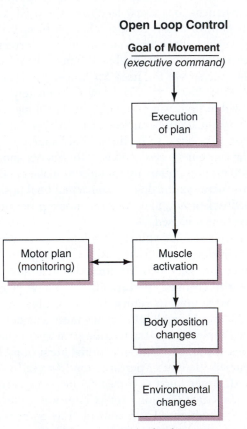

Figure 8.14   Open loop control of voluntary movement. Peripheral feedback does not immediately impact the ongoing motor program. Knowledge of the results, or motor learning can change the motor program.

receive and respond to peripheral feedback. A feed-for-ward, open loop strategy is used for movements that are completed in less than 200 ms. This strategy is achieved by more than the original motor program that was sent to the CNS portion to execute the motor program. An efferent copy of this program is also sent to the same brain region so that the actual movement outcome can be compared to the original motor program. Peripheral feedback does not have to be individually processed. Only the results of the movement can be compared to the original efferent copy of the motor program, thus sparing extensive CNS processing.

The relationship between motor programs and peripheral feedback has been demonstrated in previous upper extremity studies.[127–129] Perception of roughness is diminished when the fingers are passively moved over sandpaper but not when subjects actively rub sandpaper.[127] Enhanced kinesthetic information during active movements supports the intimate relationship between afferent and efferent information in the CNS. Preparatory postural responses to sudden upper extremity movements also occur 60 ms prior to limb movement, meaning that the open loop command must consider postural changes to center of gravity location and make adaptations prior to movement execution.[128] Following movement initiation, ongoing motor program adjustments take about 90 ms, clearly faster than any peripheral feedback mechanism.[129] Changes in the motor program could be the result of relationships between central feedback loops and the efferent copy of the motor program in the sensory portion of the CNS. Certain peripheral feedback variables can trigger motor program adjustments. These triggers can be from anticipated changes in the environment, and can be "pre-wired," substantially shortening the motor program adaptation time.

Key Point:

Adaptations based on previous movement outcomes are incorporated into the open loop motor program to enable adjustments for subtle environmental changes. These adaptations can be accomplished by proprioceptive feedback, visual feedback, or knowledge of the results of the movement.

In contrast to the closed loop control system, the open loop system of motor control is executed without any feedback or information about the consequences of the movement. Support of this control method comes from de-afferentation studies, where peripheral feedback is eliminated. Using a primate model, Taub[130] and Taub and Berman[131] observed near normal gross upper extremity movements following de-afferentation; however, fine ma-

nipulation deficiencies were evident. Based on these findings, peripheral feedback appears to be more involved with fine motor control, which according to Fitts' law would require slower movement velocities, while gross movements are under more open loop control influence from the CNS.

The gamma loop may play a role in the fine motor control of upper extremity movement. When joint mechanoreceptors are destroyed during finger arthroplasty procedures, clients have minimal or no loss of finger movement accuracy.[84] Anesthetic block of the upper extremity gamma afferents reportedly has little affect on dart throwing accuracy and grip strength tasks in humans when vision is not obscured.[132] Unobscured vision was powerful enough to overcome gamma motor neuron feedback deficits. Peripheral feedback mechanism redundancies are robust enough to overcome impairment of the gamma afferents, especially when vision is present.

If an open loop system is used to control movements, from where do these commands come? The CNS has many control mechanisms that can greatly influence movements. These range from local viscoelastic (see Chapter 3) and reflexive (see Chapter 2) muscle properties to very complex motor programs that are generated in the higher orders of the CNS to create complex movement patterns. *Central pattern generators* (CPG) located in the spinal cord represent an intermediate level of movement control during gross rhythmical movements. Cats have been shown to maintain locomotion despite receiving surgically induced brain lesions or spinal cord de-afferentation.[133–135] At least in cat models, CPGs located in the spinal cord have been shown to produce pre-wired, unconscious control of rhythmical or oscillatory movement patterns. Of course these reports are from studies using quadruped animal models; these findings have not yet been directly related to the control of bipedal human locomotion. The presence of spinal cord based CPGs have not been proven in primates or humans. Other investigations postulate that bipedal primates or humans have lost the ability to generate autonomous, unconscious movements and must rely on higher CNS centers to provide control over movement pattern generation, maintenance, and termination.[136–140]

Key Point:

Open loop feedback typically comes after the movement has ended, but motor program adjustments can still be made based on the knowledge of results.

Motor Programs.   It would require considerable CNS processing to control efficiently all motor program parameters such as the information provided by individual joints and muscles. Motor programs are thought to control or inventory the organization of the intricacies of the parameters as they influence movement patterns. There is nearly an infinite amount of information to control what Bernstein referred to as *degrees of freedom*.[1] Motor programs are the highest level of movement planning, usually involving the development of movement strategies and control of all the variables (degrees of freedom) that may influence a particular movement. Bernstein further described redundancy of all the degrees of freedom, where there are many more options to movement control than are actually needed to perform the movement itself.[141] Degrees of freedom such as joint angle information supplied by joint mechanoreceptors and muscle length information provided by muscle spindles provide similar limb position information, creating redundant afferent input to the CNS. Decreasing this redundancy to make movements more efficient is believed to be one of the major tasks of motor programs.

Bernstein's[1] use of the term degrees of freedom is different than mechanical degrees of freedom, which typically describe joint movement complexity. Simple, single joint, uniplanar movements only have two mechanical degrees of freedom (flexion-extension, anterior-posterior translation, for example). Ball and socket joints such as the glenohumerol joint possess six degrees of mechanical freedom when both rotational and translational movements in all three cardinal motion planes are considered (see Chapter 6). The actual mobility of a segment is then related to the joint surface architecture, capsuloligamentous restraints, and musculotendinous attachments. In addition to the mechanical degrees of freedom of a body segment there are other factors the CNS must control, including the activation of specific muscles with varying length tension properties and their insertion angles which change with movement, internal forces created by capsuloligamentous and tendinous attachments, and external forces acting on each body segment. A motor program controls individual degrees of freedom and is influenced by the environment in which a given task is performed.

> ## Key Point:
> Once initiated, the motor program itself monitors the individual degrees of freedom of specific movements.

Specifically, the motor program is initiated by higher level CNS centers based on the previous movement outcome. This frees the higher order CNS centers for extensive processing allowing greater attention to be placed on the ensuing tasks and on additional incoming environmental information. It is presently not clear how the CNS globally controls motor program variables in relation to the specific degrees of freedom that a given movement requires when performed in a specific environment. Minimizing degrees of freedom would entail restricting motion (limiting planes of motion) and/or limiting muscles involved with a motor program and/or changing the neurological drive toward the muscle involved with the motor program. With motor programs it is believed that there are certain characteristics that remain constant or invariant and other variant parameters that change depending on the task.

Hierarchy of Motor Programs.   Due to the complex nature of controlling movements a combination of open and closed loop motor control mechanisms work together. It is conceivable that closed loop control is embedded in the open loop control structure, or visa versa. In such a case, peripheral information could terminate in an open loop command and initiate a closed loop motor program. Essentially a motor program is a string or repertoire of motor commands that are only influenced by the peripheral environmental or peripheral feedback when the program includes a closed loop process. The open loop programs are independent of peripheral feedback. Sensory information can alter certain movements, if errors are detected with respect to the motor program. Green[87] suggested that the command to shoot a basketball is a general, centralized motor command that has little to do with actual muscle activation. The higher order CNS levels of movement control pass along the individual processes to lower control levels to generate specific, coordinated muscle activation patterns. Initially the motor program is not specific, but becomes more specific at the local level. This explains how alterations in existing motor programs does not require much processing time. Switching motor programs completely is more computationally difficult and requires considerably more processing time.

Sensory Input to Motor Programs.   Evidence for closed loop control of movements of sufficient duration suggests that motor programs are not as rigid as previously believed, but are robust enough to be modified as situations change. There is always the possibility for overlap between both open and closed loop motor control systems. The motor program has a higher order CNS level that formulates the plan, and local muscular and spinal reflex activity that modifies the plan, whether it is an open or closed loop system. Afferent information from peripheral receptors is less capable of influencing motor programs that are performed at faster velocities and shorter durations. While slower, more accurate movements require feedback to ensure a successful outcome, faster velocity movements cannot be corrected on-line as in the case of a baseball pitcher, where he cannot make performance adjustments until he knows the task outcome. This occurs after the event has been completed. Afferent information can influence movements both prior to and after a particular movement. Position awareness is vital to movement initiation. Using a monkey model, Polit and Bizzi[142] reported that simple movements such as flexing the elbow joint 45° from a fully extended position creates changes in peripheral information such as muscle length, joint position, and the number of joints and muscles involved. All of this peripheral information influenced the initial movement parameters of the motor program. Typically, single joint movements affect adjacent limb segments, causing compensatory changes either distally or proximally to the single joint movement described. There are two major factors that contribute to these compensations: the action of two joint muscles on surrounding joints and changes in the limb's moment of inertia. The biceps brachii moves the elbow to the 45° flexed position, which also affects the shoulder more proximally. This influence on the shoulder can be offset by activation of the triceps brachii to stabilize the shoulder dynamically during elbow flexion. In addition, by flexing the elbow, the moment of inertia from the upper extremity segment changes, thereby changing the upper extremity dynamic stabilization demands.[142] On a more practical level, in order to initiate proper weight shifting to start walking, the motor control system must comprehend which foot has most of the weight during stance in order to either shift weight to the opposite foot, or to begin walking with the contralateral extremity. Afferent information provided from even simple movements can influence motor programming. For example, extending an elbow joint 45° produces information on muscle length, joint position, how many joints are involved, how many muscles are involved with the movement, and any other compensatory actions that can influence initial movement parameters of a motor program. The relationships between all of these parameters for even simple movements are not necessarily linear, which make it difficult to predict movement control. The CNS, however, appears to be efficient at minimizing the conscious effort needed to control most movements.[143,144] Error information at the end of a movement or the knowledge of the success of the results is sent back to the CNS and could be utilized to improve the efficiency of future movements.

Summary of Motor Programs. Motor programs are complex by nature because of all the movement variables that need to be controlled either individually or collectively. Part of the goal of this chapter has been to organize some of these motor program concepts so the rehabilitation clinician can better understand how the CNS controls non-impaired motion. The concept of a motor program, as a single algorithm, which contains in memory all the information necessary to create movements is believed to be too restrictive. As demonstrated by the ability of the CNS to use peripheral feedback to modify existing programs, it is possible that some motor programs are amenable to on-line changes during task execution.[145]

This is especially true during longer duration, more complex movements where the use of peripheral feedback is essential and especially when instructed movements are beyond the short term memory capabilities of the CNS.

Henry and Harrison[146] claimed that motor programs are pre-programmed for relatively simple, short duration, high velocity movements. Others have demonstrated that reaction times increase as task complexity increases.[147] Motor program execution during sufficiently complex movements may utilize planning after the movement starts. This planning may arise from continuous feedback on the executive command from either previous motor programs or peripheral feedback. This type of strategy has been demonstrated when motor programs exceed CNS motor memory capabilities or when one element of a movement is complex enough to necessitate adjustment of the existing motor program.[148–150] While motor program characteristics have been described in previous sections, motor programs themselves adapt based on imposed movement constraints, and may demonstrate different characteristics depending on the constraints presented.

MOTOR PROGRAM: OUTPUT

Motor program outputs are the measurable variables, which allow theories to be developed on how movement control is organized by the CNS. The rehabilitation clinician should be aware of these motor program output variables, as they can be indicators of improved motor coordination following injury and therapeutic exercise program intervention. In this section the measurable outcomes from motor programs are presented so that rehabilitation clinicians can better understand their usefulness as evaluation tools during therapeutic exercise program intervention. Some motor program characteristics appear to be adaptable, while others remain fixed. The two components of programs include invariant features that are relatively stable, and variant parameters that tend to be more modifiable. Invariant motor program features remain relatively consistent between repeated trials. Variant movement parameters are adaptable and change during repeated trials even with subtle motor program changes. Motor program coordination in healthy, non-impaired adults is the result of proper CNS organization, adaptability and execution during activities of importance to the client (activities of daily living, grooming, recreational activities, etc.).

Invariant Movement Parameters

Invariant parameters are generally more global with respect to the movement and are fundamentally linked with the overall motor program. These invariant parameters may be linked to a higher order of movement control, remaining stable or relatively unchanged regardless of the movement.

Burst Activity or the Initial Impulse.

Burst or initial impulse activity represents the initial burst of muscle activity that occurs near a muscle's activation onset (typically in an agonist) and the beginning of observable segment movement. The burst activity pattern tends to be a stable and consistent measure of muscle activity across nearly identical tasks. The initial burst of antagonistic muscles during similar tasks has also been found to behave in a consistent manner where the onset of the antagonist muscle burst is usually delayed until after movement initiation.[111] Although the CNS probably does not control specific agonist and antagonist activity, initial burst or initiation of activity might be important enough to be under direct CNS control via a set motor program. Initial burst or impulse of muscular activity is the first invariant characteristic of motor programs. It is not clear if this level of processing is initiated at a lower reflexive level, or at some higher CNS level. For short duration, high velocity movements there is not enough time for higher CNS centers to execute antagonist muscle activity in response to agonist activation. Therefore, antagonist activity is either preplanned or under some local control. Henry and Harrison[146] suggested that the entire motor program was pre-programmed because subjects were only able to alter a planned movement sequence 110 ms into the reaction time phase of a task when they were asked to stop during various parts of the movement. Interestingly, the stop command presented at 190 ms after the cue to initiate movement had no affect on the original motor program command. The stop command typically occurred just 24 ms prior to the onset of movement. This suggests complete motor control pre-programming.[118]

This *initial impulse-timing theory* for motor programs proposes that the CNS provides pulses of activity to create movements. This activity, measured as EMG signal amplitude, increases and translates into muscle action. The impulse-timing theory proposes that these pulses influence initial muscle activation duration, timing, and amplitude, which can all affect motor programs. Unfortunately it is difficult to comprehend how these pulses can consider all of the peripheral information, such as muscle lengths, number of muscles involved with the task and other neurologic factors that can influence muscle dynamics. As movements become more complex, relevant peripheral information increases exponentially, and it becomes increasingly difficult to explain how something as simple as an initial pulse or EMG burst can account for the entire motor program. The order of events within a movement task appears to be a major influence on motor program execution. The impulse-timing hypothesis assumes the correct sequencing of events in order to achieve the appropriate movement. In studying handwriting, Lashley[151] demonstrated that, while some aspects of movement such as amplitude and frequency varied, the order of the letters remained constant, suggesting that once task order is controlled, other motor control parameters must be included for effective movement coordination.

Phasing of muscle activity.

Phasing of muscle activity is the temporal sequencing of muscle activation patterns relative to the total movement time or a percentage of its contribution to movement execution. Phasing remains invariant with the duration of muscle activity accounting for movement changes. The correct muscle activation sequence is also needed to maintain the proper order of movement events. A specific task can be accomplished by a variety of muscle activation patterns. A motor program for a task can be expanded in time; however, the relative phasing of the muscle contributions to the motor program will remain constant, provided the movements remain similar. Muscle activity phasing may vary with changes in movements. Simple, single plane movements demonstrate a triphasic burst of agonist and antagonist muscle activity. The agonist muscle is activated first, followed by an antagonist muscle burst, and then a second agonist burst is observed near the end of the movement. In 1923, Wacholder[152] originally demonstrated that agonist muscle activity is present at the initial movement onset and near movement termination. Synergists display similar activation patterns as the primary agonist and are not dependent on spinal reflexive mechanisms for movement initiation.[153] The influence of CNS control is therefore evident for all muscles, the primary agonist, synergists and antagonists involved in motor program execution.

Evaluation of EMG activity during movements can demonstrate temporal muscle activity patterns. Normalizing phases of individual muscle activity to total movement time provides an index of the relative muscular contributions. This is similar to gait studies where a client's gait characteristics such as stance or swing phase are normalized to the percentage of the gait cycle (see Chapter 9). The magnitude of muscle activity may change relative to the movement time, but the portion of relative muscle activity tends to remain invariant or fixed.

Relative Force of Muscle.

The force a specific muscle contributes to the overall forces generated at a specific joint is referred to as its *relative force*. Relative force involves the magnitude of the force produced, not the duration of muscle activity during a movement, as demonstrated by the previous invariant characteristic, relative phasing duration. Overall relative muscle force contributions remain fixed as force demands increase or decrease for a specific task. For example, the biceps brachii and brachialis both flex the elbow and if they each contribute 50 percent of the overall force during a specific task, this ratio tends to remain fixed regardless of the load required for that specific motor program to flex the elbow. This part of the motor program assumes relatively fixed initial muscle impulses and phasing. In other words the initial muscle burst activity and phasing for each of the contributing muscles would have to remain constant for the relative force at each muscle to remain at the 50 percent level.

These three invariant characteristics (burst activity, phasing, and relative muscle force) assume stability of each of the other characteristics. The generation of initial muscle impulses occurs under the assumption of invariant muscle temporal phasing and invariant relative force contributions to the motor program. Changes in relative muscle force in order to modify a motor program assume there is a fixed or consistent initial burst and phasing (duration and sequence) of muscle activity where increased effort will be accomplished by changes in the relative force. The invariant nature of the initial burst of EMG activity and temporal contribution to increased elbow flexion force would be due to the increased effort. This increased effort would be provided by all of the muscles that contribute to the overall force with the relative contribution of each component remaining fixed or invariant. The same relationship exists for relative force production with regard to the motor program. These relationships typically remain unchanged, regardless of movement or instructions, and are thus invariant.

Key Point:

Muscle burst, muscle phasing, and relative force are motor program characteristics that remain fairly constant for a specific movement. Alterations in the external environment, such as the addition of a weight, will change variable movement parameters, while the invariant characteristics will remain unchanged.

Variable Movement Parameters

While the invariant movement parameters are generally more stable relative to the motor program, *variable movement parameters* change depending on the specific motor program used, overall movement task duration, the overall muscle force needed to accomplish the task, and the interaction between muscle force and movement task duration. Variable movement parameters tend to change according to the specific movement task goals. These parameters include: overall movement duration, overall force needed to accomplish the task, specific muscle activations and related inhibition of particular muscles. Overall duration of movement directly affects movement velocity and displacement, while relative force can account for increased effort with similar movement characteristics. Specific muscle activation or inhibition is difficult to separate com-

pletely from muscle sequencing or phasing as an invariant feature. All of these parameters occur under the assumption that the invariant features of a motor program remain relatively fixed. Significant alterations or variations from a set movement suggest that a different motor program was implemented or that the existing motor program was modified via motor learning.

Duration of Movement.   Duration is the overall time from the beginning to the end of the performance of a specific movement task or skill. The motor program contains information in terms of muscle activation duration that is relative to the task duration. If two movements are from the same motor program, except that one is of longer duration, phasing of muscle activity will remain fixed or invariant. The motor program duration can be relatively short or long, whereby muscle activation phasing is condensed or extended to meet the duration of the movement. Using a series of elbow pronation and supination movements at fast and slow velocities in which the proportion of time between pronation and supination remained relatively constant to the total movement time, Shapiro[154] reported that subjects displayed compressed muscle activation phasing at intentionally faster speeds with decreased overall movement durations. The temporal muscle activation characteristics of a movement were compressed as the overall movement duration decreased. Learning variables such as knowledge of results can affect relative movement task timing or overall movement duration. Wulf et al.[155–157] demonstrated that although increased task variability led to improved relative timing, the dissociation it produced between motor program scaling and timing actually degraded the ability to replicate the task. This suggests that training which focuses solely on either temporal parameters (duration) or invariant characteristics (relative muscle force) can disassociate the overall motor program.

Overall Force.   Overall force refers to the sum of all muscle forces generated by individual muscles to create movement at a specific joint. Overall force modification is a vital component of motor programming due to the wide variety of movement tasks. Humans typically perform tasks that require subtle force changes such as holding a glass of water and tasks that require comparatively higher forces, such as going up or down stairs. Using handwriting studies in which word size was increased, Hollerbach[158] reported that temporal patterns remained similar but overall force was increased to create the bigger letters. Others have demonstrated increased friction between the pen and paper when writing size was increased.[159] These studies suggest similar force control patterns for this motor program.

Schmidt et al.[160] suggested that in order to determine the correct movement duration, one initially determines the movement time and then modulates the force necessary to complete the task. It presently remains unclear how the orders in which variable and invariant movement parameters are modulated to formulate a motor program.

Muscle Selection.

Muscle selection is the activation of specific muscles in the sequence needed to generate a co-ordinated motor program. An example of this phenomenon is the proximal to distal activation of muscles during common tasks such as reaching. However, this parameter can be more complex than simple proximal to distal activations because many muscles have overlapping functions, creating many different ways that a given movement task can be accomplished. Shapiro[154] reported that subjects who trained one extremity in an elbow supination and pronation task displayed similar movement characteristics when the contralateral extremity was tested. This suggests that a motor program originally designed for one extremity may be easily replicated at the contralateral extremity. The motor program is therefore "abstract" in nature, and the final parameters for movement specifics have to be implemented later, regardless of which extremity is used.

Inhibition.

Inhibition is the ability of the CNS to terminate muscle activity. Inhibition plays an important motor control role because it assists with the timing of agonist and antagonist muscle activation and contributes to the precision of finely graded movements. While initial impulse and muscle phasing are invariant characteristics that deal with motor program initiation, inhibition is a mechanism that terminates muscle activity to modulate joint forces. Inhibition assists with the temporal characteristics of muscle activity, basically limiting muscle activation duration. Although inhibition can be controlled centrally as part of the motor program, it is also influenced by peripheral monosynaptic or polysynaptic reflex pathways. Furthermore, descending CNS control can modulate reflexes and control the excitation threshold of alpha motor neurons.[122] Inhibition is therefore affected by local reflexive activity, but is ultimately under the guidance of descending influence by the CNS. In extreme cases such as CNS injury, lack of inhibition can lead to spasticity due to intermittent prolonged agonist and antagonist muscle co-activation.

In his 1932 Nobel Lecture entitled "Inhibition as a Co-ordinative Factor," Sherrington[161] appreciated that it was equally important that muscle activity be initiated and inhibited. In statements that were revolutionary for their time, Sherrington[161] described how the CNS actually uses inhibition as a means of organizing movement. He stated that CNS inhibition of muscle action is as important as muscle excitation for movement initiation, and inhibition is continually modulated with muscle activation to create smooth movements. In simple movements cyclical excitation of an agonist muscle is followed by activation of the antagonist, where the agonist muscle is briefly inhibited.

When movements are sufficiently slow, the inhibition of antagonist muscles may be complete.

While all of these features are under CNS control, the invariant characteristics typically are more difficult to modify in the short term, while variable movement parameters are very adaptable. The change in invariant characteristics over time essentially represents the development of a new motor program. Once invariant characteristics have been defined, they remain as permanent motor program characteristics. To adapt the motor program to specific movement, invariant parameter scaling is required by the CNS. Additionally, task dependence has been demonstrated on peripheral inhibition, which could result in changes in the quality of movement.[162] Proper movement coordination may be achieved through the balanced relationship between force modulation and movement duration. Therapeutic exercise may influence this relationship by changing the motor program's parameters, but it has little effect on the invariant characteristics. In order to change a movement strategy, a new motor program must be created and this would involve a new set of invariant characteristics.

> ### Key Point:
> Variable parameters such as duration of activity, overall force, and muscle selection-inhibition provide mechanisms for adjustments in motor program presentation and a vehicle of change for the creation of new motor programs.

Muscle Output

Synchronization.

Synchronization is the close activation relationship within or between muscles that contribute to a specific task. Synchronization may indicate a common CNS drive to the muscles involved with a movement and could represent a single motor program created at higher decision making centers of the CNS. This section deals with motor program outcomes that are typically measured by EMG signal characteristics and kinematic analysis of joint movement patterns.

The distribution of motor units throughout a muscle is a complicating factor to movement control that is not well understood. Fortunately, there are some techniques that help explore the relationship between motor unit function and movement control. Higher CNS control areas stimulate targeted alpha motor neurons in the spinal cord. This common CNS drive should produce consistency of the EMG output or synchrony. Synchronization of motor unit activity within a muscle may represent intra-muscle coordination in addition to the inter-muscle coordination described previously such as the relationship between agonists and antagonists. Bremner et al.[163] reasoned that total synaptic drive from common neurologic input may influence muscle activity. Synchronization was measured via the cross correlation of discharge times between two active motor units as determined with fine wire EMG electrodes within a muscle (**Figure 8.15a–d**). Therefore, synchronization of motor unit activity between muscles could be due to the common drive from a motor program. Inter- and intra-muscle motor unit synchronization has been demonstrated in multiple lower extremity muscles during ambulation representing common synaptic drive for short duration activities.[164] This suggests that there is common CNS drive, possibly via the pyramidal tracts, that contribute to the brief motor activity seen during non-impaired ambulation. Semmler and Nordstrom[165] examined the effect of habitual activity on motor unit synchronization in the first dorsal interosseous muscles of five musicians, five weight lifters and six untrained age-matched control subjects.[165] Synchronization was greatest in the hands of the weight lifters and least in the hands of the musicians on the side that was highly trained. The authors suggest less dependence on higher CNS centers after extensive training for relatively simple tasks such as index finger movements. This control strategy, convergence of motor commands via synchronization tends to free up the higher CNS centers for more complex tasks should the need arise.

> ## Key Point:
> Electromyography provides a method of measuring common CNS drive during movements by the level of muscle synchronization that occurs.

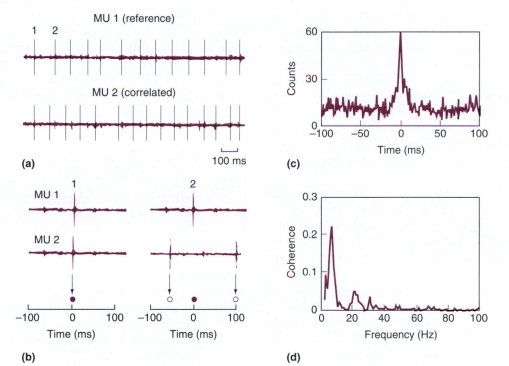

Figure 8.15   Quantification of motor unit (MU) synchronization. (a) train of single MU action potentials from two motor units. (b) construction of cross-correlation histogram for the first two discharges from the reference MU1 in panel A. The discharge times from the reference MU1 are placed at time 0 in the histogram and relative discharges of MU2 are plotted at the appropriate time with respect to MU1. Closed circles represent MU2 with respect to MU1. Open circles represent the time of MU with respect to the second discharge of MU1. This continues for each discharge of MU1. (c) an example of this histogram from a 2-min recording. (d) an example of a common coherence pattern, generally between 1 and 12 Hz and 16 and 32 Hz, for isometric finger abduction. (From JG Semmler. Motor unit synchronization and neuromuscular performance. *Exerc Sport Sci Rev.* 2002;30(1):8–14.)

Muscle Macro- and Microscopic Architecture. Muscle architecture is defined as the arrangement of muscle fibers within a muscle relative to the axis of force generation.[166] Macroscopic evaluation of muscle architecture has included the influence of muscle length and muscle fiber orientation on the ability to generate force. Muscles that act together and create similar movement patterns are called *synergists*. Functionally grouping muscles, based on a specific task, is one method of reducing the complexity of movement control. For example, synergistic biceps brachii, brachialis, and brachioradialis muscle activation flexes the elbow. The biceps brachii also crosses the shoulder joint, influencing motion at both the elbow and shoulder. The brachioradialis, similar to the brachialis, only crosses the elbow joint but has a much different angle of pull on the radius because of its orientation to the elbow joint. The brachialis is ideally suited to providing a rotatory force component at the elbow to create movement while the brachioradialis provides more joint compression, thereby contributing more to joint stability. Therefore, although both the brachialis and brachioradialis cross the elbow joint the influence of each at the joint is markedly different based on the sites of their origins and insertions. This kinesiological classification has been described as either a *spurt* or *shunt* muscle type.[167–169] Muscles that have similar actions across a joint are called synergists because of similarities in only one area of function, but the true contribution of each muscle to joint movement is much more complex than any simple classification system.

The similar functional outcomes displayed by synergistic muscle activation make it difficult to determine how an individual muscle contributes to a specific task. This is true for both *agonists* that initiate a specific motion or *antagonists* that attempt to arrest or stop the motion. *Co-activation* or activity of both agonist and antagonist muscles across a joint has been demonstrated for bi-articular muscles during tasks that required high degrees of stability or accuracy.[170–173] Muscle synergies and co-activation helps to create well executed motor programs. Identifying the relationship between these control schemes can help us form a better understanding of coordinated movements.

Based on cat studies, mono-articular muscles appear to be designed to provide postural stability, while multi-articular muscles produce forces that appear to be better suited for propulsion and medio-lateral joint stability.[174,175] Descriptions of muscle function should include even minor force contributions during specific tasks such as multi-planar dynamic joint stabilization contributions. Describing muscles as the major providers of propulsion in addition to assisting with medio-lateral joint stability provides more detail regarding the specific contribution of a muscle to a specific task.

Muscle architecture deals with muscle fiber distribution and orientation and CNS recruitment of these fibers in order to create movement. *Motor units* are the collection of muscle fibers that are innervated by the same nerve. A single motor neuron can innervate as few as three to six muscle fibers in the hand for fine motor control. In larger muscles, such as the gastrocnemius, a single motor neuron may innervate up to 2,000 muscle fibers.[176] Large muscles may contain up to 300 motor units, while smaller muscles may contain as few as 50 motor units, thereby providing enhanced fine control.[177] Small muscle fibers are generally slow twitch or fatigue resistant fibers (type I) and the larger muscle fibers are more fast twitch or fatigable (type II). Motor units or the number of muscle fibers innervated by a single nerve also present with different physiological properties (see Chapter 2). Motor units that can be activated at higher frequencies and have fast conduction velocities usually innervate fast twitch muscle fibers. Henneman and Mendell[178] described the size principle of motor unit recruitment, whereby smaller, slower conducting slow twitch motor units are activated first, followed by the larger, faster conducting fast twitch motor units.[178] Muscle fibers from a given motor unit may be localized within a muscle, or may be widely distributed, inter-mingling with muscle fibers from other motor units.[178–180] When motor units are activated, a mosaic of active regions within a given muscle help to distribute force across the entire muscle, enabling smooth, controlled muscular force generation.

> # *Key Point:*
> The location and type of a motor unit within a muscle can influence motor program output.

Compartmentalization of motor units within a muscle contributes to the overall function of that muscle (see Chapter 2). In smaller mammals slow twitch fibers tend to predominate in deep layers of muscle and fast twitch fibers tend to predominate in more superficial layers, but this is not as apparent in humans.[181–183] With compartmentalization, particular muscle regions can be used to provide specific functions. For example, two branches of the innervating nerve to the flexor carpi ulnaris, four branches to the extensor carpi ulnaris, and eight branches to the flexor digitorum profundus have been identified, suggesting compartmentalized function.[184] The biceps brachii muscle also provides an example of compartmentalized function, as medially orientated motor units within the muscle can influence supination as well as elbow flexion, while the pure elbow flexors are located more laterally.[185,186] Synergies between individual muscles are relatively easy to appreciate; however, synergy between motor units within a muscle adds multiple layers of complexity to the ability to control movements. For example, Herrmann and Flanders[187] suggested directional spatial tuning of single motor units based on the preferred direction of upper extremity force generation. This suggests that motor units demonstrate a preference toward activation when movement is intended in a specific direction. They surmised that these synergistic motor units were broadly distributed across a muscle contrary to the compartmentalization concept. Whereas compartmentalization indicates that areas within a muscle provide subtle muscle action direction or force differences, the existence of spatially tuned motor units dispersed throughout a muscle makes functional compartmentalization less likely. Spatial activation of motor units does not necessarily violate the temporal activation pattern proposed by Henneman and Mendell.[178] The spatial distribution of these motor units would help minimize fatigue by reducing the workload within specific muscle regions, in addition to ensuring consistency of force vectors from the whole muscle. While this debate is beyond the scope of this chapter, Fuglevand and Segal[188] modeled blood perfusion to motor units within muscle and determined a broad distribution of apparently synergistic motor unit activity in a muscle. Physiologic, not necessarily neural, control benefits of this arrangement include perfusion of the whole muscle even at low levels of activation, thus avoiding oxygen debt as workload increases.

Complex analysis of muscle recruitment patterns during tasks is believed to provide information regarding the CNS organization of motor programs. It is necessary for rehabilitation clinicians to understand these principles when evaluating movements. Temporal organization within a muscle or between muscles suggests common CNS temporal motor drive. Spatial distribution of motor units within a muscle, or compartmentalization, also adds to the complexity of controlling motion. The CNS must take all of these factors into consideration when implementing a motor program to optimize the movement. Errors in motor programs must be identified so that movements can be performed optimally the next time a specific motor program is implemented.

MOTOR LEARNING

Up to this point we have focused on the neuroanatomy and motor control theory behind enhancing movement patterns. *Motor learning* is the process of acquiring the capability for executing skilled movements. The motor learning process cannot be directly observed. Rather, behavioral changes reflecting the effects of motor learning are observed. These changes are considered to be plastic, meaning that they are constantly being modified, getting worse with inactivity and improving with appropriate, movement repetitions. Traditionally, once adequate joint range of motion and muscle strength have been achieved, therapeutic exercise programs begin to focus more on the development of new and more efficient movement patterns. However, motor learning considerations should be foundational to early therapeutic exercise program design and be embedded in early, simple activities and tasks. Ultimately, the goal of the rehabilitation clinician is to ensure proper movement dynamics, which means proper neuromuscular coordination. This is accomplished by providing a therapeutic exercise environment that is ideally suited to facilitate motor learning (see Chapter 5). This may include the use of modalities such as biofeedback (see Chapter 6) to assist movement and motor learning. Biofeedback devices amplify the EMG signal providing an audio or visual cue to the client as to their physiological muscle activation characteristics during movements.

There are entire disciplines dedicated to application of motor learning principles. One theory in particular is based on the motor programs that have been already discussed in this chapter. Schmidt[189] formulated a theory based on the abstract memory representation or schema as described by Bartlett[190] and Head.[191] Schmidt adapted these schema principles to motor learning.[189] Schema describes two types of memory, *recall* and *recognition*. Recall memory is responsible for accessing the correct motor program and all necessary peripheral information in order to generate the correct *schema*. This peripheral information includes internal feedback mechanisms such as proprioceptive information and exteroreceptive information such as visually locating an external object. Recognition memory would be the evaluation of success or failure of the specific motor program relative to the goal of the intended movement and any adaptations that might need to be made to ensure better accuracy or quality for the next time this motor program is needed. Recognition memory is responsible for the motor learning aspect of this theory, while the motor program and its feedback are dependent on recall memory.

> ## Key Point:
> According to motor learning theory schema, recall memory is responsible for accessing the motor program, and recognition memory is responsible for learning based on the outcome of previously recalled motor programs.

Developing a skill involves learning how and when to implement numerous movement control factors related to muscle activation (when, how long, how strong, etc.). Motor program adjustments require knowledge of the schema information: initial state, movement parameters, movement outcomes and accessory feedback. Adaptations to the original motor program are driven by feedback from the eventual movement outcome. The schema theory applies to movements performed under closed loop or open loop feedback. Missing information such as knowledge of results may delay motor learning. Incorporating all of the needed information that influences movement into motor learning strategies allows for optimal motor program development. *Practice* (the use of many repetitions of a specific movement pattern) is also necessary to fine tune the movement or decrease variability. In that way errors can be minimized during motor program execution.[192]

Training helps make movements more automatic, thereby decreasing CNS executive control. In this hierarchical system lower CNS levels control more automatic movements and higher CNS centers control movements that require more cognitive information processing. This model frees higher levels of conscious activity during more automatic movements for other associated tasks. After many practice trials, the motor program is initiated and cognitive interference on the motor program is minimized. Driving a motor vehicle is an example of automatic movements, where simple movements such as moving the foot from the accelerator pedal to the brake pedal are generally automatic. This frees higher cognitive centers for other information processing like avoiding other vehicles. This makes the simpler movements more automatic and decreases movement times. Compare the simple movement just mentioned (moving foot from accelerator to brake) to shooting basketball free throws. Some of the best basketball players spend hours practicing this skill and still only achieve an 80–90 percent success rate. Success rates are usually never perfect because of errors within the system (selection and execution) or external environmental factors. For the basketball players, external environmental factors may include subtle changes in gymnasium lighting, dimensions of the interior building (background), or fans waving and cheering from the stands. Success rates may drop precipitously without continued practice.

Fitts et al.[3] demonstrated this hierarchical adaptation system during their object tracking studies. Subjects initially responded to object position, but with training, they became more adept at adjusting to the velocity and/or acceleration information of the object being tracked. However, under duress, subjects relapsed and ignored the more complex information (velocity/acceleration) resorting to a reliance on simpler position information. Exactly where these hierarchical adaptations occur in the CNS remains unknown.

We have not yet discussed how new motor programs are actually created. Most likely it is a constant evolution of motor programs that are modified into new programs. Considerable ambiguity exists between existing motor programs and the creation of new motor programs. Put another way, CNS plasticity allows for an existing motor program to be continuously updated, until it is changed sufficiently enough to be considered a separate or new motor program. Newer motor programs initially demonstrate greater movement pattern (kinematic, EMG) variability. Linking together individual motor programs or *convergence* is also a method of creating larger motor programs. Individual sub-programs that previously existed for simpler movements may converge during more complicated movement tasks. These simple motor programs are then sequenced together to form the larger or giant motor programs that are needed for more intricate, complex tasks. For example, complex tasks like throwing a ball can be composed of sub-routines that link the movements of the lower extremities through the trunk to the upper extremity.

These routines can be interchanged based on the conditions in which the throw is occurring. A baseball pitcher will have a set program for pitching because the starting position remains constant. However, an infielder must either adapt his throwing strategy based on how he fields the ball (an interchangeable lower extremity and trunk strategy coupled with a consistent upper extremity strategy) or create an almost infinite number of throwing programs. Practice is considered valuable when linking or interchanging these sub-programs in order to create larger motor programs. In essence, it could be argued that the evolution of all movements that occur later in life stem from gross movements that occur as an infant. These programs are continually developed and changed as differing and more complex task demands are encountered over a lifetime.

Key Point:

Convergence occurs when a series of sub-programs are connected to create a larger or giant motor program for accomplishing more complex movement tasks.

Motor learning occurs from many practice repetitions and feedback from movement outcomes. While motor learning is a complex process, some basic principles are necessary for proper movement coordination. The ability to refine or generate a new or modified motor program through repetitious practice and feedback is dependent on the status of an existing motor program. The two major feedback sources regarding the outcome of a motor program include *knowledge of results* and *knowledge of performance*. Knowledge of performance can be feedback ranging from simple comments from a coach or rehabilitation clinician to complex computer generated reports of kinematic, EMG, kinetic energy expenditure, and functional activity measures.[193] As a method of improving performance, knowledge of performance is not as powerful as knowledge of results.[193–195] Knowledge of results is more likely to improve human performance.[196–199] Knowledge of results is also referred to as positive reinforcement between a motor program and a successful outcome.[200] Most important is the continued presentation of knowledge of results so that the appropriate learned movement pattern is reinforced (see Chapter 11). Appropriate reinforcement increases the likelihood that the improved movement pattern will be maintained. In the absence of reinforcement (knowledge of results), there is the chance that performance will degrade. This suggests that knowledge of the results of performance such as an understanding of hand placement accuracy are more important to motor learning than the feedback provided by knowledge of performance such as an understanding of proper hand velocity.

Key Points:

Knowledge of results refers to the use of feedback regarding the success of a performance to adapt the existing motor program. Knowledge of performance refers to the use of feedback during the actual performance (i.e., biofeedback) to adapt an existing motor program.

When teaching new motor skills, it is common to break down complex movements and create a series of simple movement tasks requiring mini–motor programs (see Chapters 5 and 6). Once all of the pieces, or mini-programs, are learned, they can be linked to create the desired overall movement outcome. These mini-programs should be taught with adequate feedback (visual, proprioceptive and knowledge of results) to ensure that the correct motor sequence is being performed.

To enhance learning, the movement task should be performed initially at slower than normal speeds or over longer durations. Once this has been completed successfully, the task can be normalized to its natural characteristics. Special equipment may be needed to address the parameters that were discussed in the motor program section. For example, EMG biofeedback, kinematic and/or kinetic data might be used to determine if movement, force and phasic muscle activations are performed appropriately during a movement task (see Chapter 9). Ultimately, high repetition training progressions using slow to fast speeds and using less isolated or component movements and more composite or integrated movements are considered to be the most important aspects of improving or updating motor programs.

Basic motor learning paradigms usually start out with slow, controlled or simple movements and progress to faster, more complex movement patterns when sufficient coordination is present. Based on present knowledge, many techniques can be used for this type of training such as verbal instructions with positive feedback, visual feedback with a mirror, and video analysis with or without biofeedback using EMG signals to indicate successful movement pattern performance.

Motor Program Errors

Errors from motor program are difficult to assess, but this feedback is necessary in order to make corrections. Successful movements might be evaluated as either the ability to complete the task (for example, reaching for an object) or how efficiently one can accomplish a task. Movement errors can be classified either as an error in *selection* or an error in *execution*. An error in selection occurs when either a wrong movement pattern is selected for a specific situation, or the right movement pattern is selected with the wrong spatial-temporal characteristics. An error in execution occurs when the correct movement pattern is selected, but an external event renders the movement unsuccessful. A baseball batter who incorrectly guesses the pitch, swings and misses the pitch is an example of a selection error. When the same batter correctly guesses the pitch but misses anyway, this is an example of an execution error. In the selection error the batter used the wrong spatial-temporal patterns necessary to hit the ball, while with the execution example the motor program was not initiated correctly to hit the ball. This feedback information is necessary so that the batter can make the appropriate motor program corrections the next time they come up to hit. Intent of the action in conjunction with error measurements, as discussed earlier, will determine the degree of inaccuracy and whether the error was of selection or execution. This information will help identify solutions to any faulty motor program outcomes.

Key Point:

Selection errors occur when the wrong motor program is executed. Execution error uses the correct motor program, but a mistake was made due to human error. Practice can help minimize both of these errors.

AGE AND TRAINING

As one ages there are measurable decreases in motor performance such as overall strength, nerve conduction velocity, metabolic rate, perceptual skills and proprioception, memory and attention as they relate to motor performance.[190,201–207] Muscle atrophy affects mainly fast twitch fibers (type II), where the loss of motor units can lead to decreased muscle mass, functional strength, and the ability to perform functional tasks.[202]

The contributions of the CNS to strength and coordination are necessary to maintain function through the aging process, but changes in motor unit recruitment can affect both strength and coordination.[207] The relationship between strength and proper motor program execution is not clearly defined; if strength impairments are sufficient they may interfere with the ability to generate forces in a coordinated activity pattern.[204] Effective therapeutic exercise programs can reverse much of the strength losses and "dis-coordination" that have been associated with aging. However, these gains do not persist if training is halted. Neural factors are key during the initial period of therapeutic exercise program intervention, and it is reasonable to assume that these neural processes, still present in the elderly, can provide gains in both strength and coordination.[201] The ability to generate greater muscle activation and joint torques occurs primarily from improved neuromuscular firing rates, more synchronized neural drive, and improved coordination of the CNS signal.[206] Therapeutic exercise programs which focus on foundational strength training are often the best first step to improve function among the elderly, particularly with functionally relevant movement patterns that require appropriate force modulation via an effectively executed motor program. However, principles of motor control and/or motor learning should be embedded in these programs even at early levels.

Key Point:

Neural factors are key during the initial period of therapeutic exercise program intervention, as increased muscle strength occurs primarily from improved neuromuscular firing rates, more synchronized neural drive, and improved coordination of the CNS signal.

For effective motor program implementation, the elderly client must not only be able to generate maximal strength, but must also be able to efficiently modulate or scale muscle forces. Therapeutic exercise movements must be scaled to specific functional tasks or goals in conjunction with the environment in which the movement must occur. An example of this is the amount of force required to hold and stabilize a grasped object. An object with a rough surface has a high coefficient of friction, while a smooth surface object has a low coefficient of friction. When the weight of two objects is equivalent, more force is needed to hold the smooth object as compared to the object with the rough surface. Cole[208] studied pinch force variability for both smooth and rough surfaces and found that elderly subjects demonstrated greater pinch force regardless of the surface. Younger subjects were able

to adjust pinch force regardless of the order of presentation of the surfaces, while older subjects tended to maintain greater force levels even with rougher surfaces. Elderly subjects used greater pinch forces to accommodate sensory system impairments, even when they switched from a smooth to a rough surface. Younger subjects tuned their pinch forces to the appropriate surface, thereby optimizing the forces generated; this is a form of energy conservation. Cole[208] and Johannson and Cole[209] concluded that age tends to negatively influence the feedforward mechanisms, which are used to integrate peripheral feedback and movement memory, which in turn creates motor programs.

Increased force fluctuations produced at the distal end of an extremity among the elderly could result from the loss of low threshold motor units, an increase in the innervation ratio of some motor units, or an increase in motor unit synchronization. Keen et al.[210] suggested that fluctuations in the activation of individual motor units did not relate to variations in the ability to generate force. Individual motor units are activated or deactivated during sustained activity.[201] There remains uncertainty regarding changes in the innervation ratio of some motor units and the synchronization of these units. *Synchronization* is indicative of common motor drive of intra-muscular or inter-muscular motor units for both agonist and antagonist muscles. During aging, there is a reduction of motor neurons within the CNS with increased collateral sprouting, which increases the number of muscle fibers that are controlled by a single alpha motor neuron. This creates a loss of fine motor control with these larger motor units, but this concept and the possible positive influence of therapeutic exercise intervention remains to be fully explored. Motor unit synchronization has been studied and described earlier in this chapter, but it has not been examined as a factor affecting motor programs among elderly subjects.

Key Point:

To improve function, therapeutic exercise programs designed for elderly clients should incorporate basic motor learning principles. Due to their greater likelihood of having perception deficits, performance feedback may be especially important among the elderly to reinforce positive behavioral changes.

Falls among the elderly are a major concern, due to the high morbidity associated with both the primary injury and the prolonged bed rest commonly associated with them (see Chapter 1).[211] Decreased strength can contribute to falls; however, impaired vestibular system function may contribute more significantly to the incidence of falls among this population (see Chapter 9). Neuromuscular coordination training to prevent falls focuses on the ability to react to the sudden external forces or perturbations that can disrupt balance. Elderly clients may display impaired reaction times, or more specifically delayed muscle activation times that contribute to a decreased capacity for responding to sudden external forces.[203] If CNS processing deficits are contributing to falls among elderly clients, muscular strength gains alone would be of limited benefit in decreasing their incidence of falls. Lassau-Wray and Parker[205] identified delayed muscle activation latencies among 10 elderly women compared to 10 younger women when they attempted to combine walking with another task, suggesting a CNS processing problem when confronted with dual tasks.

Therapeutic exercise programs that focus on improving neuromuscular control in addition to strength may be particularly beneficial among elderly clients who are at increased risk of falling.[212] Appropriately designed therapeutic exercise programs rarely isolate one aspect of performance. Rather, these interventions are usually multifactorial, addressing balance, strength, endurance and cognitive processing, making it difficult to evaluate only neuromuscular contributions to function. Because they stress both the vestibular and proprioceptive systems, balance and postural control training would be especially beneficial among the elderly.[203] (See Chapters 6, 7, and 9) Alternative therapeutic exercise interventions such as Tai Chi Chuan (see Chapter 10) have strong appeal because these techniques emphasize neuromuscular control principles with inter-system training (musculoskeletal, vestibular and proprioceptive). Controlled movements, with emphasis on quality rather than on overall volume (sets-repetitions), should be emphasized during all types of exercises in an effort to establish effective motor learning. For example, a simple therapeutic exercise such as a straight leg raise should be instructed with specific verbal instructions and specific performance criterion. Prior to lifting their lower extremity, clients should be instructed first to maximally activate their quadriceps femoris muscle. After lifting their leg, clients should be instructed to maintain this muscle group activation while returning their lower extremity to the treatment table in order to ensure maximal stability across the knee and maximize muscle activation. Effective instructions and cues are vital to ensuring appropriate therapeutic exercise movements and motor program creation or modification (see Chapter 11).

> ## *Key Point:*
> Physical impairments among the elderly may be attributed to a more sedentary lifestyle. Therapeutic exercise programs that emphasize motor learning and awareness in addition to strength and balance can be particularly effective among this group.

NEUROMUSCULAR TRAINING/ EVALUATION AND TECHNIQUES

Rehabilitation clinicians commonly observe impaired movement patterns or impaired coordination among clients either as a result of primary injury or from associated compensatory maladaptations that occur following injury onset. In most cases, these compensations contribute further to the injury sequelae and functional limitations, and need to be corrected. The CNS may make short term adaptations to restore early function at the expense of long term recovery. For example, altered gait following acute knee injury may place increased valgus forces on the knee leading to pathological osseous adaptations at the tibial surface and patellofemoral joint mal-tracking. These secondary changes, if left uncorrected, could prove to be as or more debilitating than the original knee injury. Managing these secondary changes following injuries is of critical importance to rehabilitation clinicians, who must determine which movement adaptations need to be corrected.

Once adequate joint range of motion and muscle strength have been sufficiently restored, the creation of appropriate functional movement patterns becomes a greater focus of therapeutic exercise programs. Traditional clinical measurements typically evaluate strength and/or range of motion across one joint, but functional movement patterns are much more complex (see Chapter 5). Factors such as balance and neuromuscular coordination can also affect function. Traditional clinical measurements of impairment are of limited value in predicting functional capability. Functional capability measurements assess gross movements as diverse as walking speed, the amount of time to get out of a chair, and crossover hopping speed. These measurements are typically selected based on the needs and ultimate functional expectations of the client. Functional measurements for elderly clients may include the time it takes to get up from a chair, while young, athletically active clients might be evaluated for a *single leg standing broad jump* or a *6 meter timed hop* (see Chapter 5). Client goals also play an important part in what functional measurements should be used. An elderly client may have a realistic goal of walking without assistance. A performance measurement may include the *timed get up and go test* (see Chapter 9) where clients are timed from the point of arising from a chair, walking 10 m, turning, walking back, and sitting back down in the chair (see Chapter 9). This would be a combined measure of the client's ability to perform a sit to stand transfer and to ambulate a standardized distance. Athletic injuries require evaluation of complex movement patterns that are similar to what the client would encounter during competition. In this case, an obstacle course that requires a run and cut would be specific for sports that require sudden running directional changes such as basketball, soccer, and football. Tests such as the single leg hop and the 6 meter timed hop have been developed to simulate the demands placed on lower extremity function during some sporting activities. These types of tests are usually implemented after appropriate joint range of motion has been restored and isolated muscle or muscle group strength has been adequately re-established.[213–215] Once clients are able to perform tests such as these to establish a functional baseline, repeated tests can be used to chart progress until they are ready to return to athletic competition (see Chapter 11). To develop the skills necessary for specific work or sporting activities, more frequent practice sessions are often needed; therefore, the terminal stages of a therapeutic exercise program often focuses primarily on facilitating the motor learning process during vocation or sport specific skill performance.

CRITICAL TRACKING TASKS

New microelectronic devices and software that can measure and analyze body motion, physical activity, client behavior patterns, and estimate energy expenditure in a free-living situation on 24-hr basis display tremendous potential for evaluating the efficacy of therapeutic exercise program intervention (**Figure 8.16**). The ultimate neuromuscular coordination goal is to produce efficient functional movements during tasks ranging from routine activities of daily living to sport specific movements.

Computer based training systems to teach control of joint force or position are also a relatively new addition to therapeutic exercise programs following injury. Some of this technology is based on critical tracking tasks that were

developed in the 1950s by the U.S. Air Force to investigate the ability of pilots to control steering devices.[216] This technology has also been used by the transportation industry as a reliable method of determining the effect of fatigue on motor performance.[217] The idea behind this type of intervention is to start implementing motor control strategies early in the therapeutic exercise program. A critical tracking system incorporates the use of a mechanical control element that interfaces with a computer (such as a joystick) as the client attempts to control the position of an object on a video screen. The object on the screen undergoes a series of oscillations at greater speeds until the client can no longer control the position of the object.

A critical tracking device has recently been developed to assess specific joint function through task performance as a way of measuring motor control. A mechanical interface to a computer was developed to assess shoulder internal-external rotation (**Figure 8.17a**) or knee flexion and extension as the client attempts to correct for the unpredictable oscillations of a cursor on the video screen. The client must actively stabilize a progressively unstable element (faster movements) until they lose control of the device. This task is analogous to balancing a broomstick in the palm of an open hand with the broomstick becoming progressively shorter until control is no longer possible. Dynamic stability is increased via visual feedback as acceleration is gradually increased until the user is no longer able to keep the on-screen cursor within the prescribed field. The *critical level* (that instant where the client loses control) is proportional to the client's time delay and is used for future comparisons.[216] The critical level is also defined as the point at which the movement is sufficiently fast that the user can no longer control the cursor.

Critical tracking tasks can be started as early as the initial post-operative day, with very little movement or force, as the client uses fine motor control to maintain the cursor position on a video screen. As the therapeutic exercise program progresses, this fine motor coordination can be made progressively more challenging by performing the activity within different ranges of motion, and with different isolated and integrated joint positions, with greater movement amplitude or with the addition of external weights to the extremity to provide greater resistance. These devices may help facilitate the return of muscle memory for sport specific tasks. Measures of coordination appear to be similar for high performance athletes and recreational athletes suggesting that this device could be used with a variety of client populations.[218] Outcomes from this type of task are typically related to movement velocities and neglect joint or muscle contributions to a specific task. While these devices claim to enhance the coordination of muscle activity, they provide no direct measurement of muscle activity. In addition, some critical tracking task devices only measure performance of one isolated joint, neglecting muscle contributions from other parts of the kinematic chain. While joint isolation is ideal early in the therapeutic exercise pro-

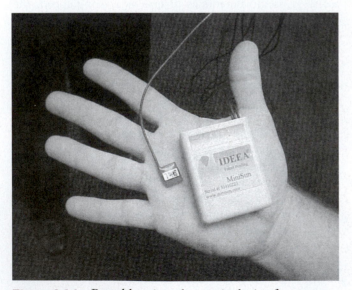

Figure 8.16   Portable microelectronic device for measuring daily physical activity, gait analysis, energy expenditure, and functional capacity during "free living." (IDEEA® Intelligent Device for Energy Expenditure and Activity, MiniSun, LLC).

gression, eventually the incorporation of multi-joint complex movements is necessary. The CNS control behind this task is complex, but as the client learns to control simple linear displacements, their performance adjustments should become automatic. Functionally, critical tracking is based on a closed loop feedback system where adjustments to movement changes are limited by the inherent delays in conduction velocities and central processing that was discussed previously (in the closed loop section). When cursor movement becomes sufficiently fast, the point at which motor responses cannot keep up with the movement changes provides a measure of coordination. The ultimate limitation to the responses is the actual transmission time of the neural impulses and activation of the muscles to react to the movements. Once clients are sufficiently trained with this device, the actual motor program is presented and a reduced cognitive response from higher CNS control centers is needed for cursor control.

Critical tracking tasks require responses to linear displacements on a video screen (in two dimensions) and one would have to question how responses to a two dimensional system would transfer to a visual system that usually functions in three dimensions. While a loaded device during movements would provide increased overload, thus strengthening the muscles, it would be interesting to measure the client's neuromuscular responses to changes in these forces during the performance of a functionally relevant tracking task. Force modulation is essential for re-establishing normal muscle coordination (as part of invariant characteristic of a motor program); therefore, force tracking tasks may provide greater insight into the modulation of motor programs. Simple movements arise from the slow cursor displacements and as the client can handle increased movement speeds with similar accuracy, their progress becomes self-evident. The upper extremity critical tracking device we discuss only calculates movement duration. Overall movement force and muscle activation

selection or inhibition cannot presently be determined with this device, suggesting that claims of improved motor coordination may be exaggerated, especially since only single joints are evaluated in a non-functional movement pattern context. The Functional Squat System provides composite lower extremity force, work and speed of movement information during a series of computerized movement challenges.(**Figure 8.17b**).

Medicine Ball and Plyometric Exercises from a Motor Control Perspective

Plyometric exercises make use of the stretch shortening cycle or the elastic properties of the musculotendinous unit. The stretch shortening cycle occurs when concentric (shortening) muscle activation follows eccentric (lengthening) muscle action. Lower extremity plyometric exercises include activities such as jumping (see Chapter 5 and 7) and upper extremity plyometric activities include activities such as medicine ball tossing and catching (see Chapter 7). Examples of upper extremity plyometric exercises include the use of a medicine ball or a plyo-ball where clients catch the ball using eccentric (lengthening) muscle control to decelerate the ball, followed by immediate concentric (shortening) activation to throw the ball. Between the eccentric and concentric phases there is a transient amortization phase where electromechanical delay is responsible for the shifting muscle activity.[219] Cordasco et al.[220] described three upper extremity medicine ball plyometric exercise phases including the cocking phase, followed by the acceleration phase and lastly the deceleration phase. The cocking phase involved catching the ball and taking the arms and ball back as far as possible. The acceleration phase began as the ball accelerates

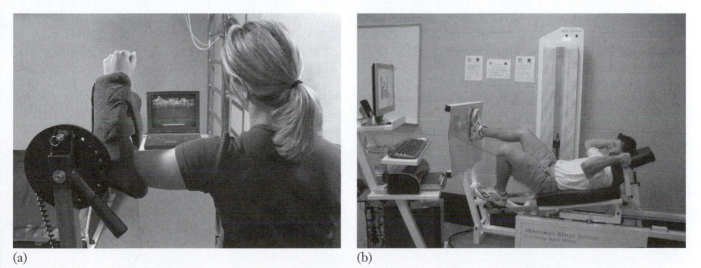

(a)   (b)

Figure 8.17   Critical tracking tasks. (a) shoulder internal-external rotation motor control (Performance Health Technologies, Boulder, CO). (b) lower extremity motor control (CDM Sport, Fort Worth, TX).

forward, and the deceleration phase occurs from the point of release until the arms slow down.[220] Cordasco et al.[220] demonstrated increased muscle activation patterns during the acceleration phase of overhead throwing with a medicine ball. Plyometric exercises are heavily dependent on increasing the stretch rate so that elastic energy is used during the concentric portion or acceleration phase of the movement rather than being dissipated as heat. Incorporating these variables into a motor program and modulating these factors are necessary for movement control.

Plyometric exercises are used to acclimate clients to the greater forces that commonly occur during athletic activities. Plyometric exercises are also thought to facilitate a more efficient use of the stretch reflex in order to enhance muscle stiffness. Plyometric exercises make use of the elastic properties of muscle and desensitization of the Golgi tendon organs, which inhibit muscle activity to enhance neuromuscular coordination.[219,221] While there are temporal limits to the stretch reflex, gamma motor neuron activation can increase muscle stiffness during extremely fast movements.[222] It remains unclear, however, if plyometric training improves the viscoelastic properties of the musculotendinous unit or even enhances muscle contractile properties.[223–225] The factor most likely influenced by plyometric training is optimized muscle activation timing or phasing of muscle activity between the cocking, acceleration and deceleration phases.

When used with properly performed functional movement patterns, plyometric exercises provide motor control characteristics that should enhance neuromuscular control or coordination. Plyometric exercises can be similar to exercises performed during the advanced stages of Pilates or Tai Chi exercise programs (see Chapter 10). It is the explosive, power dependent nature of these plyometric exercises that makes motor control difficult, necessitating the need for preliminary training prior to starting a plyometric exercise regimen. There is a limit, however, to how slow plyometric exercises using a medicine ball can be performed while still employing the stretch-shortening cycle, and the strong eccentric component involved in their appropriate performance mandates appropriate technique, adequate recovery time, and careful manipulation of resistance training variables (see Chapter 5). Since athletically active clients routinely have to employ integrated function at high intensities, therapeutic exercises that make use of plyometric training principles may have numerous applications.

Plyometric training is usually initiated during the terminal part of a therapeutic exercise program to ensure that adequate tissue healing, joint range of motion, and foundational strength has been restored so the client can adequately withstand the high forces associated with this method of training. Initial therapeutic exercises using plyometric principles should be performed slowly with limited resistance, making sure that form or technique is optimal. The specific movement can even be broken into sub-routines similar to the sub-motor programs discussed earlier and then can be put back together into larger, more complex motor programs. For example, overhead plyometric medicine ball exercises can be broken into three sub-routines representing each of the phases and then the phases can be combined to create the whole movement pattern. Once the entire motor program has been re-assembled, the rehabilitation clinician is still able to control some exercise program parameters, such as task position or posture (seated, standing, etc.), medicine ball velocity, and resistance in addition to therapeutic exercise volume components (sets, reps, rest intervals, frequency, etc.). Specific motor program parameters such as activity duration are linked to the mechanical constraints of the task, meaning that increasing the medicine ball resistance will slow down the movement, thus increasing the task duration. In addition to increased power, enhanced neuromuscular coordination would be a likely adaptation to plyometric training with a medicine ball, but this has not been reported. As with strength training, neuromuscular adaptations occur within the first few weeks of plyometric training program initiation, while morphological changes in the musculotendinous and bone structures take much longer.

Even commonly performed tasks can display considerable performance variability both within and between clients, making it difficult to establish the optimal performance method. For example, there are many different baseball pitching techniques; what could be an optimal motor program for one pitcher might not be optimal for another. It is crucial to re-establish the movement pattern that a client performed with high efficiency prior to their pain or injury (see Chapter 11). An excellent method of doing this would be to have a video record of their performance technique prior to injury. This knowledge of performance could also serve as a teaching tool for enhancing neuromuscular control during therapeutic exercise program intervention and in designing component therapeutic exercise program tasks. It is particularly important that clients not develop maladaptive coping strategies following injury. Plyometric exercises may enhance the stress accommodation and force and power generation capabilities for specific movement patterns. However, proper technique and postural control are essential or neuromuscular coordination will not improve.

Summary

The re-establishment of neuromuscular control is an essential part of function, however one chooses to define neuromuscular control. Ultimately the knowledge of motor learning strategies and motor control theories, in conjunction with the presented techniques, should help the rehabilitation clinician to better understand neuromuscular control during therapeutic exercise performance.

During the early stages of post-injury therapeutic exercise program participation, clients should perform slow, controlled movements, where knowledge of results and performance are essential to correcting the motor program. These movements should be simple and have easily attainable goals. Once the client can master slow, simple movements that do not require great coordination, strength, or power demands they can progress to tasks that make use of greater movement velocities and imposed forces. Knowledge of results and performance and other peripheral feedback is needed to facilitate the progression from slow, simple movements to faster, more complex tasks. Tools such as EMG, kinetic and kinematic analysis can help identify the re-establishment of normal movement parameters.

Non-traditional therapeutic exercise approaches using Pilates and Tai Chi (see Chapter 10) incorporate movement pattern progressions that begin with slow movements and move to fast movements, and also use techniques such as meditation and breathing to facilitate motor learning. Specialized training is needed for both of these therapeutic exercise modes in order to become competent as a provider. Critical tracking requires special equipment and exercises that incorporate plyometric training principles should only be used near the final stages of the therapeutic exercise progression once non-impaired joint range of motion and foundational muscle strength have been re-established. The breakdown of complex movements into multiple smaller motor programs early during therapeutic exercise program participation is essential so that clients can focus more on isolated joint movement and muscle group strength deficiencies. Optimal neuromuscular training can be achieved with appropriate movement progressions, using feedback to enhance performance and many repetitions to fully install an effective motor program in the CNS.

References

1. Bernstein N. *The Coordination and Regulation of Movements*. Oxford, U.K.: Pergamon Press; 1967.
2. Reimann BL, Lephart SM. The sensorimotor system, Part II: The role of proprioception in motor control and functional joint stability. *J Athl Train*. 2002;37:80–84.
3. Fitts PM, Bahrick HP, Noble ME, Briggs GE (1959). Skilled performance (Ohio State University Final Report for Contract AF 41[657]-70). Dayton, OH: Wright Air Development Center, Wright-Pattern Air Force Base.
4. Schmidt RA, McGown C. Terminal accuracy of unexpectedly rapid aiming movements: Evidence for a mass spring mechanism in programming. *J Mot Behav*. 1980;12:149–161.
5. Smoll FL, Schutz RW. Relationships among measures of preferred tempo and motor rhythm. *Percept Mot Skills*. 1978;46:883–894.
6. Messier J, Kalaska JF. Differential effect of task conditions on errors of direction and extent of reaching movements. *Exp Brain Res*. 1997;115:469–478.
7. Vindras P, Desmurget M, Prablanc C, Viviani P. Pointing errors reflect biases in the perception of the initial hand position. *J Neurophysiol*. 1998;79:3290–3294.
8. Koshland GF, Hasan Z. Selection of muscles for initiation of planar, three-joint arm movements with different final orientations. *Exp Brain Res*. 1994;98: 157–162.
9. Hocherman S, Aharonson D, Medalion B, Hocherman I. Perception of the immediate extrapersonal space through proprioceptive inputs. *Exp Brain Res*. 1988;73:256–262.
10. Baud-Bovy G, Viviani P. Pointing to kinesthetic targets in space. *J Neurosci*. 1998;18:1528–1548.
11. Gielen CC, Vrijenhoek EJ, Flash T, Neggers SF. Arm position constraints during pointing and reaching in 3-D space. *J Neurophysiol*. 1997;78: 660–673.
12. Sullivan MP, Christina RW. Target location and visual feedback as variables determining accuracy of aiming movements. *Percept Mot Skills*. 1983;56: 355–358.
13. Flanders M, Pellegrini J, Geisler S. Basic features of phasic activation for reaching in vertical planes. *Exp Brain Res*. 1996;110:67–79.
14. Buneo C, Soechting J, Flanders M. Muscle activation patterns for reaching: The representation of distance and time. *J Neurophysiol*. 1994;71: 1546–1558.
15. Morasso P. Spatial control of arm movements. *Exp Brain Res*. 1981;42:223–227.
16. Atkeson C, Hollerbach J. Kinematic features of unrestrained vertical arm movements. *J Neurosci*. 1985;5:2318–2330.

17. Soechting JF. Effect of load perturbations on EMG activity and trajectories of pointing movements. *Brain Res.* 1988;451:390–396.

18. Forwell LA, Carnahan H. Proprioception during manual aiming in individuals with shoulder instability and controls. *J Orthop Sports Phys Ther.* 1996; 23:111–119.

19. Carey DP. Eye-hand coordination: Eye to hand or hand to eye? *Curr Biol.* 2000;10:416–419.

20. Carnahan H, Hall C, Lee T. Delayed visual feedback while learning to track a moving target. *Res Q Exerc Sport.* 1996;67:416–423.

21. Sergio LE, Scott SH. Hand and joint paths during reaching movements with and without vision. *Exp Brain Res.* 1998;122:157–164.

22. Goodbody SJ, Wolpert DM. The effect of visuomotor displacements on arm movement paths. *Exp Brain Res.* 1999;127:213–223.

23. Ross J, Badcock DR, Hayes A. Coherent global motion in the absence of coherent velocity signals. *Curr Biol.* 2000;10:679–682.

24. Tillery SIH, Flanders M, Soechting JF. A coordinate system of the synthesis of visual and kinesthetic information. *J Neurosci.* 1991;11:770–778.

25. Pick HL, Warren DH, McIntyre C, Appel L. Transfer and the organization of perceptual-motor space. *Psych Forchburg.* 1972;35:163–177.

26. Millar J. Joint afferent fibers responding to muscle stretch, vibration and contraction. *Brain Res.* 1973; 63:380–383.

27. Newton RA. Joint receptor contributions to reflexive and kinesthetic responses. *Phys Ther.* 1982;62: 22–29.

28. Chambers M, Andres KH, Duering MV, Iggo A. The structure and function of the slowly adapting type II mechanoreceptors in hairy skin. *Q J Exp Physiol.* 1972;57:417–445.

29. Jones LA. Peripheral mechanisms of touch and proprioception. *Can J Physiol Pharmacol.* 1994;72: 484–487.

30. Sherrington CS. *The Integrative Action of the Nervous System.* Cambridge: Cambridge Press, 1948.

31. Freeman MAR, Wyke B. The innervation of the knee joint: An anatomical and histological study in the cat. *J Anat.* 1967;101:505–532.

32. Skoglund S. Anatomical and physiological studies of knee joint innervation in the cat. *Acta Physiol Scand.* 1956;36:7–101.

33. Carew TJ, Ghez C. Muscles and muscle receptors. *In* ER Kandel, JH Schwartz (eds.), *Principles of Neural Science.* New York: Elsevier, 1985; pp. 443–456.

34. Clark FJ, Burgess RC, Chapin JW, Lipscomb WT. Role of intramuscular receptors in the awareness of limb position. *J Neurophysiol.* 1985;54:1529–1440.

35. Gandevia S, McCloskey D. Joint sense, muscle sense, and their combination as position sense, measured at the distal interphalangeal joint of the middle finger. *J Physiol.* 1976;260:387–407.

36. Rossetti Y, Meckler C, Prablanc C. Is there an optimal arm posture? Deterioration of finger localization precision and comfort sensation in extreme arm-joint postures. *Exp Brain Res.* 1994;99: 131–136.

37. Houck JC, Rymer WZ, Crago PE. Dependence of dynamic response of spindle receptors on muscle length and velocity. *J Neurophysiol.* 1981;46: 143–166.

38. Vallbo A, al-Falahe N. Human muscle spindle response in a motor learning task. *J Physiol (Lond).* 1990;421:553–568.

39. Vallbo A. Muscle spindle response at the onset of isometric voluntary contractions in man. Time difference between fusimotor and skeletomotor effects. *J Physiol (Lond).* 1971;318:405–431.

40. Merton PA. Speculations on the servo-control of movement. In GEW Wolstenholme (ed.), *CIBA Foundation Symposium, The Spinal Cord.* London: Churchill, 1953; pp. 247–255.

41. Kakuda N, Miwa T, Nagaoka M. Coupling between single muscle spindle afferent and EMG in human wrist extensor muscles: Physiological evidence of skeletofusimotor (beta) innervation. *Electroencephalogr Clin Neurophysiol.* 1998;109:360–363.

42. Rymer WZ. Spinal mechanisms for control of muscle length and force. In PM Conn (ed.), *Neuroscience in Medicine.* Philadelphia: J.B. Lippincott Co., 1995; pp. 369–400.

43. Scott SH, Loeb GE. The computation of position sense from spindles in mono- and multiarticular muscles. *J Neurosci.* 1994;14:7529–7540.

44. Wallace KR, Kerr GK. A numerical simulation of muscle spindle ensemble encoding during planar movement of the human arm. *Biol Cybern.* 1996; 75:339–350.

45. Crago PE, Houck JC, Rymer WZ. Sampling of total muscle force by tendon organs. *J Neurophysiol.* 1982;47:1069–1083.

46. Houck JC, Singer JJ, Henneman E. Adequate stimulus for tendon organs with observations on mechanics of the ankle joint. *J Neurophysiol.* 1971;34: 1051–1065.

47. Jackson JH. A study of convulsions. *Transactions St. Andrews Medical Graduates Association.* 1870;iii:162.

48. Ghez C. Introduction to motor systems. In ER Kandel, JH Schwartz (eds.), *Principles of Neural Science.* New York: Elsevier, 1985; pp. 428–442.

49. Martin JH. Anatomical substrates for somatic sensation. In ER Kandel, JH Schwartz (eds.), *Principles of Neural Science.* New York: Elsevier, 1985; pp. 301–315.

50. Contreras-Vidal JL. The gating functions of the basal ganglia in movement control. *Prog Brain Res.* 1999;121:261–276.

51. Turner RS, DeLong MR. Corticostriatal activity in primary motor cortex of the macaque. *J Neurosci.* 2000;20:7096–7108.

52. Hayes AE, Davidson MC, Keele SW, Rafal RD. Toward a functional analysis of the basal ganglia. *J Cogn Neurosci.* 1998;10:178–198.

53. Suri RE, Albani C, Glattfelder AH. A dynamic model of motor basal ganglia functions. *Biol Cybern.* 1997;76:451–458.

54. Jueptner M, Frith CD, Brooks DJ, et al. Anatomy of motor learning: II. Subcortical structures and learning by trial and error. *J Neurophysiol.* 1997;77:1325–1337.

55. Jueptner M, Weiller C. A review of differences between basal ganglia and cerebellar control of movements as revealed by functional imaging studies. *Brain.* 1998;121:1437–1449.

56. Ghez C, Fahn S. The cerebellum. In ER Kandel, JH Schwartz (eds.), *Principles of Neural Science.* New York: Elsevier, 1985; pp. 502–521.

57. Marr D. A theory of cerebellar cortex. *J Physiol.* 1969;202:437–470.

58. Keifer J, Houk J. Motor function of the cerebellorubrospinal system. *Physiolog Rev.* 1994;74: 509–542.

59. Kan PLE, Gibson AR, Houk JC. Movement related inputs to intermediate cerebellum of the monkey. *J Neurophysiol.* 1993;69:74–94.

60. Grill SE, Hallett M, McShane LM. Timing of onset of afferent responses and of use of kinesthetic information for control of movement in normal and cerebellar-impaired subjects. *Exp Brain Res.* 1997; 113:33–47.

61. Schweighofer N, Spoelstra J, Arbib MA, Kawato M. Roles of the cerebellum in reaching movements in humans. II. A neural model of the intermediate cerebellum. *Eur J Neurosci.* 1998;10:95–105.

62. Contreras-Vidal JL, Grossberg S, Bullock D. A neural model of cerebellar learning for arm movement control: Cortico-spino-cerebellar dynamics. *Learn Memory.* 1997;3:475–502.

63. Grill SE, Hallett M, Marcus C, McShane L. Disturbances of kinaesthesia in patients with cerebellar disorders. *Brain.* 1994;117:1433–1447.

64. Ilinsky IA, Kultas-Ilinsky K. The basal ganglia and the thalamus. In PM Conn (ed.), *Neuroscience in Medicine.* Philadelphia: J.B. Lippincott, 1995; pp. 343–367.

65. Lotze M, Erb M, Flor H, et al. MRI evaluation of somatotopic representation in human primary motor cortex. *Neuroimage.* 2000;11:473–481.

66. Scott SH. Comparison of onset time and magnitude of activity for proximal arm muscles and motor cortical cells before reaching movements. *J Neurophysiol.* 1997;77:1016–1022.

67. Armstrong DM, Drew T. Topographical localization in the motor cortex of the cat for somatic afferent responses and evoked movements. *J Physiol (Lond).* 1984;350:33–54.

68. Schieber MH. Inactivation of the ventral premotor cortex biases the laterality of motoric choices. *Exp Brain Res.* 2000;130:497–507.

69. Erdler M, Beisteiner R, Mayer D, et al. Supplementary motor area activation preceding voluntary movement is detectable with a whole-scalp magnetoencepalography system. *Neuroimage.* 2000; 11:697–707.

70. Ohara S, Ikeda A, Kunieda T, et al. Movement-related change of electrocorticographic activity in human supplementary motor area proper. *Brain.* 2000;123:1203–1215.

71. Jenkins IH, Jahanshahi M, Jueptner M, et al. Self-initiated versus externally triggered movements. II. The effect of movement predictability on regional cerebral blood flow. *Brain.* 2000;123: 1216–1228.

72. Ball T, Schreiber A, Feige B, et al. The role of higher-order motor areas in voluntary movement as revealed by high resolution EEG and fMRI. *Neuroimage.* 1999;10:682–694.

73. Pearce AJ, Thickbroom GW, Byrnes ML, Mastaglia FL. Functional reorganization of the corticomotor projection to the hand in skilled racquet players. *Exp Brain Res.* 2000;130:238–243.

74. MacKay WA. Cooperative structures for visually guided reach. *Can J Physiol Pharmacol.* 1996;74: 463–468.

75. Fuchs A, Jirsa VK, Kelso JAS. Theory of the relation between human brain activity (MEG) and hand movements. *Neuroimage.* 1999;11:359–369.

76. Fuchs A, Jirsa VK, Kelso JAS. Issues in the coordination of human brain activity and motor behavior. *Neuroimage.* 2000;11:375–377.

77. Marsden JF, Werhahn KJ, Ashby P, et al. Organization of cortical activities related to movement in humans. *J Neurosci.* 2000;20:2307–2314.

78. Beppu H, Nagaoka M, Tanaka R. Analysis of cerebellar motor disorders by visually-guided elbow tracking movement. *Brain.* 1987;110:1–18.

79. Day BL, Thompson PD, Harding AE, Marsden CD. Influence of vision on upper limb reaching movements with cerebellar ataxia. *Brain.* 1998; 121:357–372.

80. Kosarov D, Christova L. Time relations between the impulses of two motor units from symmetrical muscles upon voluntary control. *Acta Physiol Pharmacol Bulg.* 1991;17:59–66.

81. Stein R. What muscle variable(s) does the nervous system control in limb movements. *Behav Brain Sci.* 1982;5:535–577.

82. Bizzi E. Central and peripheral mechanisms in motor control. In GE Stelmach, J Requin (eds.),

Tutorials in Motor Behavior. Amsterdam, Holland, 1980; pp. 131–144.

83. Feldman AG. Functional tuning of the nervous system with control of movement or maintenance of a steady posture: II. Controllable parameters of the muscles. *Biophysics.* 1966;11:565–578.

84. Kelso JAS, Holt KG, Flatt AE. The role of proprioception in the perception and control of human movement: Toward a theoretical reassessment. *Percept Psychophys.* 1980;28:45–52.

85. Sugarman H, Tiran J. A novel approach to the amplitude vs. position control controversy. *Brain Cogn.* 2000;43:407–412.

86. Sanes JN, Evarts EV. Effects of perturbations on accuracy of arm movements. *J Neurosci.* 1983;3: 977–986.

87. Green PH. Problems of organization of motor systems. In R Rosen, FM Snell (eds.), *Progress in Theoretical Biology.* New York: Academic Press, 1972.

88. Soechting JF, Durfesne JR, Laquaniti F. Time-varying properties of myotatic response in man during some simple motor tasks. *J Neurophysiol.* 1981;46: 1226–1243.

89. Saltzman E. Levels of sensorimotor perception. *J Math Psychol.* 1979;90:91–163.

90. Flash T. The control of hand equilibrium trajectories in multi-joint arm movements. *Biol Cybern.* 1987;57:257–274.

91. Uno Y, Kawato M, Suzuki R. Formation and control of optimal trajectory in human multijoint arm movement. Minimum torque-change model. *Biol Cybern.* 1989;61:89–101.

92. Bizzi E, Accornero N, Chapple W, Hogan N. Arm trajectory formation in monkeys. *Exp Brain Res.* 1982;46:139–143.

93. Abend W, Bizzi E, Morasso P. Human arm trajectory formation. *Brain.* 1982;105:331–348.

94. Bizzi E, Accornero N, Chapple W, Hogan N. Posture control and trajectory formation during arm movement. *J Neurosci.* 1984;4:2738–2744.

95. Feldman AG. Once more on the equilibrium-point hypothesis (lambda model) for motor control. *J Mot Behav.* 1986;18:17–54.

96. St-Onge N, Adamovich S, Feldman A. Control processes underlying elbow flexion movements may be independent of kinematic and electromyographic patterns: Experimental study and modeling. *Neuroscience.* 1997;79:295–316.

97. Vallbo A, Hagbarth K, Torebjork H, Wallin B. Somatosensory, proprioceptive, and sympathetic activity in human peripheral nerves. *Physiolog Rev.* 1979; 59:919–957.

98. Gottlieb GL. Rejecting the equilibrium point hypothesis. *Motor Control.* 1998;2:10–12.

99. Burke D, Gandevia S, Macefield G. Responses to passive movement of receptors in joint, skin and muscle of the human hand. *J Physiol.* 1988;402: 347–361.

100. Adamovich S, Levin M, Feldman A. Central modifications of reflex parameters may underlie the fastest arm movements. *J Neurophysiol.* 1997;77: 1460–1469.

101. Lestienne F. Effects of inertial load and velocity on the braking process of voluntary limb movements. *Exp Brain Res.* 1979;35:407–418.

102. Corcos D, Gottlieb G, Agarwal G. Organizing principles for single-joint movements: II. A speed-sensitive strategy. *J Neurophysiol.* 1989;62:358–368.

103. Gottlieb G, Corcos D, Agarwal G. Organizing principles for single-joint movements: I. A speed-insensitive strategy. *J Neurophysiol.* 1989;62:342–357.

104. Gottlieb G, Corcos D, Agarwal G, Latash M. Organizing principles for single joint movements: III. Speed-insensitivity strategy as a default. *J Neurophysiol.* 1990;63:625–636.

105. Gordon J, Ghez C. Trajectory control in targeted force impulses. *Exp Brain Res.* 1987;67:241–252.

106. Corcos D, Agarwal G, Flaherty B, Gottlieb G. Organizing priciples for single-joint movements: IV. Implications for isometric contraction. *J Neurophysiol.* 1990;64:1033–1041.

107. Gottlieb G, Latash M, Corcos D, et al. Organizing principles for single joint movements: V. Agonist-antagonist interactions. *J Neurophysiol.* 1992; 67:1417–1427.

108. Allum JH. Responses to load disturbances in human shoulder muscles: The hypothesis that one component is a pulse test information signal. *Exp Brain Res.* 1975;22:307–326.

109. Almedia G, Hong D, Corcos D, Gottlieb G. Organizing principles for voluntary movement: Extending single-joint rules. *J Neurophysiol.* 1995;74: 1374–1381.

110. Khan M, Garry M, Franks I. The effect of target size and inertial load on the control of rapid aiming movements. *Exp Brain Res.* 1999;124:151–158.

111. Woodworth RS. The accuracy of voluntary movement. *In Psychological Review Monographs,* vol. 13, 1899.

112. Keele SW, Posner MI. Processing of visual feedback in rapid movements. *J Exp Psychol.* 1968;77: 155–158.

113. Carlton LG. Processing visual feedback information for movement control. *J Exp Psychol Hum Percept Perform.* 1981;7:1019–1030.

114. Pelisson D, Prablanc C, Goodale MA, Jeannerod M. Visual control of reaching movements without vision of the limb. II. Evidence of fast unconscious processes correcting the trajectory of the hand to the final position of double-step stimulus. *Exp Brain Res.* 1986;62:303–311.

115. Paulignan Y, Jeannerod M, MacKenzie C, Marteniuk R. Selective perturbations of visual input during prehension movements: 2. The effects of changing object size. *Exp Brain Res.* 1991;87: 407–420.

116. Dewhurst DJ. Neuromuscular control system. *IEEE Trans Biomed Eng.* 1967;14:167–171.

117. Henry FM. Dynamic kinesthetic preception and adjustment. *Res Q Exerc Sport.* 1953;30:176–187.

118. Granit R. *The Basis of Motor Control.* New York: Academic Press, 1970.

119. Rothwell J. *Control of Human Voluntary Movement.* London: Chapman and Hall, 1994.

120. Nichols TR, Houck JC. Improvement of linearity and regulation of stiffness that results from actions of stretch reflex. *J Neurophysiol.* 1976;39:119–142.

121. Lacquaniti F, Soechting JF. Behavior of the stretch reflex in a multi-jointed limb. *Brain Res.* 1984; 311: 161–166.

122. Capaday C. The effects of baclofen on the stretch reflex parameters of the cat. *Exp Brain Res.* 1995; 104:287–296.

123. Feldman AG, Orlovsky GN. The influence of different descending systems on the tonic stretch reflex in the cat. *Exp Neurol.* 1972;37:481–494.

124. Nichols TR, Steeves JD. Resetting of resultant stiffness in ankle flexor and extensor muscles in the decerebrate cat. *Exp Brain Res.* 1986;62:401–410.

125. Koshland GF, Hasan Z. Electromyographic responses to a mechanical perturbation applied during impending arm movements in different directions: One-joint and two-joint conditions. *Exp Brain Res.* 2000;132:485–499.

126. Brooke JD, Peritore G, Staines WR, et al. Upper limb H-reflexes and somatosensory evoked potentials modulated by movement. *J Electromyogr Kinesiol.* 2000;10:211–215.

127. Brodie EE, Ross HE. Jiggling a lifted weight does aid discrimination. *Am J Psych.* 1985;98:469–471.

128. Cordo PJ, Nashner LM. Properties of postural adjustments associated with rapid arm movements. *J Neurophysiol.* 1982;47:287–302.

129. Angel RW, Higgins JR. Correction of false moves in pursuit tracking. *J Exp Psychol.* 1969;82:185–187.

130. Taub E. Movement in nonhuman primates deprived of somatosensory feedback. *Exerc Sports Sci Rev.* 1976;4:335–374.

131. Taub E, Berman AJ. Movement and learning in the absence of sensory feedback. In SJ Freedman (ed.), *The Neuropsychology of Spatially Oriented Behavior.* Homewood, IL: Dorsey Press, 1968.

132. Smith JL, Roberts EM, Atkins E. Fusimotor neuron block and voluntary arm movements in man. *Am J Phys Med.* 1972;5:225–239.

133. Marder E, Calabrese RL. Servo-action in human vountary movement. *Nature.* 1996;238:140–143.

134. Grillner S. Locomotion in vertebrates: Central mechanisms and reflex interaction. *Physiolog Rev.* 1975;55:247–304.

135. Grillner S, Wallen P, Brodin L, Lansner A. Neuronal network generating locomotion behavior in lamprey: Circuitry, transmitters, membrane properties and stimulation. *Annu Rev Neurosci.* 1991;14:169–248.

136. Bussel B, Roby-Brami A, Azouvi P, et al. Myoclonus in a patient with spinal cord transection. Possible involvement of the spinal stepping generator. *Brain.* 1988;111:1235–1245.

137. Denny-Brown D, Yanagisawa N, Kirk EJ. The localization of hemispheric mechanisms of visually directed reaching and grasping. In KJ Zulch, O Creutzfledt, EC Galbraith (eds.), *Cerebral Localization.* New York: Springer-Verlag, 1975, pp. 63–75.

138. Forssberg H. Ontogeny of human locomotor control: I. Infant stepping, supported locomotion and transition to independent locomotion. *Exp Brain Res.* 1985;57:480–493.

139. Lawrence DG, Kuypers HGJM. The functional organization of the motor system in the monkey: I. The effects of bilateral pyramidal lesions. *Brain.* 1968;91:1–14.

140. Lawrence DG, Kuypers HGJM. The functional organization of the motor system in the monkey: II. The effects of lesions of the descending brain-stem pathways. *Brain.* 1968;91:15–36.

141. Bernstein N. Biodynamics of locomotion. *In* HTA Whiting (ed.), *Human Motor Actions: Bernstein Reassessed.* New York: Elsevier, 1984, pp. 171–222.

142. Polit A, Bizzi E. Characteristics of motor programs underlying arm movements in monkeys. *J Neurophysiol.* 1979;42:183–194.

143. Partridge LD. Muscle properties: A problem for the motor physiologist. In RE Talbott, DR Humphrey (eds.), *Posture and Movement.* New York, Raven, 1979.

144. Partridge LD. Neural control drives a muscle spring: A persisting yet limited motor theory. *Exp Brain Res Suppl.* 1983;7:280–290.

145. Massaro DW, Cowan N. Information processing models: Microscopes of the mind. *Annu Rev Psychol.* 1993;44:383–425.

146. Henry FM, Harrison JS. Refractoriness of a fast movement. *Percept Mot Skills.* 1961;13:351–354.

147. Christina RW, Fischman MG, Vercruyssen MJP, Anson G. Simple reaction time as a function of response complexity: Memory drum theory revisited. *J Mot Behav.* 1982;14:301–321.

148. Garcia-Colera A, Semjen A. Distributed planning of movement sequences. *J Mot Behav.* 1988.

149. van Mier H, Hulstijn W, Petersen SE. Changes in motor planning during the acquisition of movement patterns in a continuous task. *Acta Psychol.* 1993;82:291–312.

150. Smiley-Oyen AL, Worringham CJ. Distribution of programming in a rapid aimed sequential movement. *Q J Exp Psychol A.* 1996;49A:379–397.

151. Lashley KS. The problem of serial order in behavior. In LA Jeffress (ed.), *Cerebral Mechanisms in Behavior: The Hixon Symposium.* New York: Wiley, 1951, pp. 112–136.

152. Wacholder K. Beitrage zur physiologie der Willkurlichen Bewegungen: III. Uber die Form der Muskeltatigkeiten bei der Ausfuhrung einfacher

willkurlicher, 2. Die Antagonisten. *Pflugers Arch.* 1923;200:266–285.

153. Wacholder K, Altenburger H. Beitrage zur physiologie der Willkurlichen Bewegungen: IV. Uber die Form der Muskeltatigkeiten bie der Ausfuhrung einfacher willkurlicher Einzelbewegungen, 3. Die Synergisten. *Pflugers Arch.* 1926;209: 286–300.

154. Shapiro DC. A preliminary attempt to determine the duration of a motor program. In DM Landers, RW Christina (eds.), *Psychology of Motor Behavior and Sport.* Champaign, IL: Human Kinetics, 1977.

155. Wulf G, Lee T. Contextual interference in movements of the same class: Differential effects on program and parameter learning. *J Mot Behav.* 1993; 25:254–263.

156. Wulf G, Lee T, Schmidt RA. Reducing knowledge of results about relative versus absolute timing: Differential effects on motor learning. *J Mot Behav.* 1994;26:362–369.

157. Wulf G, Weigelt C. Instructions about physical principles in learning a complex motor skill: To tell or not to tell. *Res Q Exerc Sport.* 1997;68:362–367.

158. Hollerbach JM. A study of human motor control analysis and synthesis of handwriting. In *AI Technical Report 534.* Cambridge, MA: MIT Artificial Intelligence Laboratory, 1980.

159. Denier van der Gon JJ, Thuring JP. The guiding of human writing movements. *Kybernetik.* 1965;2: 145–148.

160. Schmidt RA, Zelaznik HN, Hawkins B, et al. Motor-output variability: A theory for the accuracy of rapid motor acts. *Psycholog Rev.* 1979;86:415–451.

161. Sherrington CS Inhibition as a coordinative factor. Nobel Lecture. In *Nobel Foundation,* Stockholm: 1932, pp. 278–289.

162. Lavoie BA, Devanne H, Capaday C. Differential control of reciprocal inhibition during walking versus postural and voluntary motor tasks in humans. *J Neurophysiol.* 1997;78:429–438.

163. Bremner FD, Baker JR, Harrison LM, et al. Activity in branches of last order common stem presynaptic input fibers to motorneurone pools: A mechanism for muscle synergy? In A Taylor, MH Gladden, R Durbaba (eds.), *Alpha and Gamma Motor Systems.* New York: Plenum Press, 1994, pp. 187–194.

164. Hansen NL, Hansen S, Christensen LO, et al. Synchronization of lower limb motor unit activity during walking in human subjects. *J Neurophysiol.* 2001;86:1266–1276.

165. Semmler JG, Nordstrom MA. Motor unit discharge and force tremor in skill and strength-trained individuals. *Exp Brain Res.* 1998;119:27–38.

166. Lieber RL. *Skeletal Muscle Structure and Function: Implications for Physical Therapy and Sports Medicine.* Baltimore, MD: Williams and Wilkins, 1992.

167. MacConaill MA. Anatomical note: Spurt and shunt muscles. *J Anat.* 1978;126:619–621.

168. Drukker J, Van Mameren H. Spurt muscles and shunt muscles: A critical evaluation and an extension of the concept. *Acta Morphol Neurol Scand.* 1976;14:255–256.

169. Stern JT Jr. Investigations concerning the theory of "spurt" and "shunt" muscles. *J Biomech.* 1971; 4: 437–453.

170. van Ingen Schenau GJ, Boots PJM, de Groot G, et al. The constrained control of force and position in multijoint movements. *Neuroscience.* 1992;46: 197–207.

171. Bobbert MF, van Ingen Schenau GJ. Coordination in vertical jumping. *J Biomech.* 1988;21:249–262.

172. Buchanan TS, Roval GP, Rymer WZ. Strategies for muscle activation during isometric torque generation at the human elbow. *J Neurophysiol.* 1989; 62:1201–1212.

173. Flanders M, Soechting JF. Arm muscle activation for static forces in three dimensional space. *J Neurophysiol.* 1990;64:1818–1837.

174. Lawrence JH. The 3-dimensional mechanics of the cat ankle joint. Doctoral Dissertation: Emory University 1994 [publication number AAT 942485].

175. Lawrence III JJ, Nichols TR, English AW. Cat hindlimb muscles exert substantial torques outside the sagittal plane. *J Neurophysiol.* 1993;69:282–285.

176. Rowland LP. Disease of the motor unit: The motor neuron, peripheral nerve, and muscle. In ER Kandel, JH Schwartz (eds.), *Principles of Neural Science.* New York: Elsevier Science, 1985.

177. Burke D. Motor units: Anatomy, physiology and functional organization. In *The Handbook of Physiology: The Nervous System, Motor Control.* Bethesda, MD: American Physiological Society, 1981, pp. 345–422.

178. Henneman E, Mendell LM. Functional organization of motor neuron pool and its inputs. In *Handbook of Physiology: The Nervous System, Motor Control.* Bethesda, MD: American Physiological Society, 1981, pp. 423–507.

179. Bodine SC, Roy RR, Eldred E, Edgerton VR. Maximal force as a function of anatomical features of motor units in the cat tibialis anterior. *J Neurophysiol.* 1987;57:1730–1745.

180. Totosy de Zepetnek JE, Zung HV, Erdebil S, Gordon T. Innervation ratio is an important determinant of force in normal and reinnervated rat tibialis anterior muscles. *J Neurophysiol.* 1992;67:1385–1403.

181. Armstrong RB, Laughlin MH. Metabolic indicators of fiber recruitment in mammalian muscles during locomotion. *J Exp Biol.* 1988;115:201–213.

182. Johnson MA, Polgar D, Weightman D, Appleton D. Data on the distribution of fiber types in thirty-six human muscles: An autopsy study. *J Neurol Sci.* 1973;18:111–129.

183. Lexell JD, Downham D, Sjostrom M. Distribution of different fibre types in human skeletal muscles: Fibre type arrangement in m.vastus lateralis from three groups of healthy men between 15 and 83 years. *J Neurol Sci.* 1986;72:211–222.

184. Segal RL, Catlin PA, Krauss EW, et al. Anatomical partitioning of three human forearm muscles. *Cell Tissues Organs.* 2002;170:183–197.

185. Ter Haar Romeny BM, Denier van der Gon JJ, Gielen CC. Relation between location of a motor unit in the human biceps brachii and it critical firing levels for different tasks. *Exp Neurol.* 1984;85:631–650.

186. Ter Haar Romeny BM, Denier van der Gon JJ, Gielen CC. Changes in recruitment order of motor units in the human biceps muscle. *Exp Neurol.* 1982;78:360–368.

187. Herrmann U, Flanders M. Directional tuning of single motor units. *J Neurosci.* 1998;18: 8402–8416.

188. Fuglevand AJ, Segal SS. Simulation of motor unit recruitment and microvascular unit perfusion: Spatial considerations. *J Appl Physiol.* 1997;83:1223–1234.

189. Schmidt RA. A schema theory of discrete motor skill learning. *Psychol Rev.* 1975;82:229–261.

190. Bartlett FC. *Remembering: A Study in Experimental and Social Psychology.* Cambridge, Eng.: The University Press, 1932.

191. Head H. *Aphasia and Kindred Disorders of Speech.* New York: Hafner, 1963.

192. Shapiro DC, Schmidt RA. The schema theory: Recent evidence and developmental implications. In JAS Kelso, FJ Clark (eds.), *The Development of Movement Control and Co-ordination.* New York: Wiley, 1982, pp. 113–150.

193. Gentile AM. A working model of skill acquisition with application to teaching. *Quest.* 1972;17:3–23.

194. Holding DH, Newell A. Skill learning. *Human Skills.* New York: Wiley, 1981.

195. Ross D, Bird AM, Doody SG, Zoeller M. Effects of modeling and videotape feedback with knowledge of results on motor performance. *Human Mov Sci.* 1985;4:149–157.

196. Reeve TG, Dornier LA, Weeks DJ. Precision of knowledge of results: Consideration of the accuracy requirements imposed by the task. *Res Q Exerc Sport.* 1990; 61:284–290.

197. Magill RA, Wood CA. Knowledge of results precision as a learning variable in motor skill acquisition. *Res Q Exerc Sport.* 1986;57:170–173.

198. Bennett DM, Simmons RW. Effects of precision of knowledge of results on acquisition and retention of a simple motor skill. *Percept Mot Skills.* 1984;58: 785–786.

199. Towbridge MH, Cason H. An experimental study of Thorndike's theory of learning. *J Gen Psych.* 1932;7: 245–260.

200. Thorndike EL. The law of effect. *Am J Psych.* 1927; 39:212–222.

201. Enoka RM. Neural strategies in the control of muscle force. *Muscle Nerve.* 1997;5 (Suppl):s66–s69.

202. Williams HG. Aging and eye-hand coordination. In C Bard, M Fleury, L Hay (eds.), *Development of Eye-Hand Coordination across the Life Span.* Columbia, SC: University of South Carolina Press, 1989, pp. 327–357.

203. Manchester D, Woollacott M, Zederbauer-Hylton N, Marin O. Visual, vestibular and somatosensory contributions to balance control in the older adult. *J Gerontol.* 1989;24:169–178.

204. Kelso JAS. Concepts and issues in human motor behavior: Coming to grips with the jargon. In JAS Kelso (ed.), *Human Motor Behavior: An Introduction.* Hillsdale NJ: Lawrence Erlbaum Associates, 1982, pp. 21–58.

205. Lassau-Wray ER, Parker AW. Neuromuscular responses of elderly women to tasks of increasing complexity imposed during walking. *Eur J Appl Physiol Occup Physiol.* 1993;67:476–480.

206. Connelly DM, Carnahan H, Vandervoort AA. Motor skill learning of concentric and eccentric isokinetic movements in older adults. *Exp Aging Res.* 2000;26:209–228.

207. Erim Z, Beg MF, Burke D, DeLuca CJ. Effects of aging on motor-unit properties. *J Neurophysiol.* 1999;82:2081–2091.

208. Cole KJ. Grasp force control in older adults. *J Mot Behav.* 1991;23:251–258.

209. Johannson RS, Cole KJ. Sensory-motor coordination during grasping and manipulative actions. *Curr Opin Neurobiol.* 1992;2:815–823.

210. Keen DA, Yue GH, Enoka RM. Training-related enhancement in the control of motor output in elderly humans. *J Appl Physiol.* 1994;77:2648–2658.

211. Kochera A. Falls among older persons and the role of the home: An analysis of cost, incidence, and potential savings from home modification. *Issue Brief (Public Policy Inst (Am Assoc Retired Pers)).* 2002: 1–14.

212. Sinaki M, Lynn SG. Reducing the risk of falls through proprioceptive dynamic posture training in osteoporotic women with kyphotic posturing: A randomized pilot study. *Am J Phys Med Rehabil.* 2002;81:241–246.

213. Bolgla LA, Keskula DR. Reliability of lower extremity functional performance tests. *J Orthop Sports Phys Ther.* 1997;26:138–142.

214. Novak PJ, Bach BR Jr., Hager CA. Clinical and functional outcome of anterior cruciate ligament reconstruction in the recreational athlete over the age of 35. *Am J Knee Surg.* 1996;9:111–116.

215. Wilk KE, Romaniello WT, Soscia SM, et al. The relationship between subjective knee scores, isoki-

netic testing, and functional testing in the ACL-reconstructed knee. *J Orthop Sports Phys Ther.* 1994;20:60–73.

216. Jex HR, McDonnell JD, Phatak AV. A "critical" tracking task for man-machine research related to the operator's effective delay time: I. Theory and experiments with a first-order divergent controlled element. NASA CR-616. *NASA Contract Rep NASA CR.* 1966:1–105.

217. O'Hanlon JF. Critical tracking task (CTT) sensitivity to fatigue in truck drivers. In BJ Osborne, JA Levis (eds.), *Human Factors in Transportation Research.* London: Academic Press Inc., 1981.

218. Syms J, Paden J, Moeckel K, et al. Shoulder coordination as measured by the SportsRac apparatus: A comparison between professional baseball players and recreational athletes. http://www/ptjournal.org/abstracts/pt2002/abstractspt2002.cfm?pubno=po-rr-110-f.

219. Wilk KE, Voight ML, Keirns MA, et al. Stretch-shortening drills for the upper extremities: Theory and clinical application. *J Orthop Sports Phys Ther.* 1993;17:225–239.

220. Cordasco FA, Wolfe IN, Wooten ME, Bigliani LU. An electromyographic analysis of the shoulder during a medicine ball rehabilitation program. *Am J Sports Med.* 1996;24:386–392.

221. Voight ML, Draovitch P. Plyometrics. In M Albert (ed.), *Eccentric Muscle Training in Sports and Orthopaedics.* New York: Churchill Livingstone, 1991, pp. 45–73.

222. Trimble MH, Kukulka CG, Thomas RS. Reflex facilitation during the stretch-shortening cycle. *J Electromyogr Kinesiol.* 2000;10:179–187.

223. Aura O, Komi PV. Effects of prestretch intensity on mechanical efficiency of positive work and on elastic behavior of skeletal muscle in stretch-shortening cycle exercise. *Int J Sports Med.* 1986;7:137–143.

224. Bosco C, Tarkka I, Komi PV. Effect of elastic energy and myoelectrical potentiation of triceps surae during stretch-shortening cycle exercise. *Int J Sports Med.* 1982;3:137–140.

225. Strojnik V, Komi PV. Fatigue after submaximal intensive stretch-shortening cycle exercise. *Med Sci Sports Exerc.* 2000;32:1314–1319.

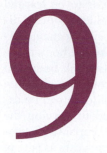

9

Training for Agility and Balance

CLAUDIA ANGELI

Objectives

The reader will be able to:

- Identify the components of agility and balance.
- Describe the mechanical factors that influence agility and balance.
- Explain the mechanical differences between walking, running, and directional change movements.
- Explain the concepts of agility, speed and balance from a biomechanical perspective.

- Describe commonly used agility screening methods.
- Discuss similarities and differences between commonly used clinic and laboratory based methods of balance testing.

Outline

INTRODUCTION

Among the ultimate characteristics of the perfect athlete, undoubtedly we include *agility*, the ability to rapidly and accurately change the position of the body in space. The football player who is running around the defense to make the spectacular catch that wins the game has to demonstrate agility. The basketball player who fakes out an opponent to drive by her and dunk the basketball has to demonstrate agility.

Key Point:

Agility is defined as the ability to rapidly and accurately change the position of the body in space.

Agility falls within the *Sports Related Fitness Domain of Physical Fitness*. Other components of this domain are balance, coordination, power, reaction time, and speed. These components are acknowledged to be important requirements to successful competitive and recreational sports performance; however, their contributions to routine activities of daily living may be underappreciated.

COMPONENTS OF AGILITY

Agility cannot be achieved in isolation. Many of the components of sports-related fitness are linked, and training for one component can enhance the execution of the other components. Many of the drills developed to measure agility are based on time. The fastest time and the larger number of movements within a given period are both valid measures of agility. Agility requires a combination of *body awareness* (the ability to perceive body position and orientation in space), *spatial awareness* (the ability to perceive where objects are in relation to one another, or to one's self), neuromuscular coordination (see Chapter 8), *reaction time* (time between stimulus onset and movement initiation), and *power* (strength/time) in addition to speed (see Chapter 5).

Key Point:

Agility requires a combination of body and spatial awareness, neuromuscular coordination, reaction time, speed, and power (strength/time).

Space is a concept that we have trouble understanding as young children. The idea of moving the body in a rapid and accurate way is something that needs to be learned. Young children have trouble making sudden stops or direction changes. Why is this? In part, they lack the necessary neuromuscular coordination to make the body move in such a complex pattern. Children also lack body and spatial awareness, which makes the concept of agility much more difficult for them. Before children can be expected to demonstrate agility they need to develop the concepts of spatial and body awareness. Emphasis on spatial awareness is usually taught in the early years as part of physical education. However, most children will learn *body awareness* without formal teaching of these concepts. The other important aspect associated with the lack of agility at an early age is the link with neuromuscular control (see Chapter 8). Once awareness and a high level of neuromuscular control is acquired, moving the body rapidly and accurately is simplified. But as with any other characteristics that define elite athletes, only a selected few have the perfect combination of neuromuscular control and body awareness.

A further analysis of the definition of agility leads us into the concept of speed, which is the ability to perform an action in a very small amount of time. Speed is usually classified as another component of sports related physical fitness. You can be fast without being agile, but the opposite is not as typical. The next question that comes to mind: "Is reaction time a requirement for agility?" First we need to differentiate between speed and reaction time.

Key Point:

Speed is the ability to perform an action in a very short amount of time. Reaction time is the duration between a stimulus and the response to the stimulus.

As was previously mentioned, agility is measured by time. If a client's reaction time is slow, then it will take them longer to perform the task, therefore being classified as less agile than the client whose reaction time is quicker and who performed the task given the same speed and body awareness. Reaction time is the duration between a stimulus and the response to the stimulus. The influence of reaction time during an agility drill often has to do with the millisecond difference between being very good and being excellent. Young et al.[1] investigated the relationship between concentric muscle power (isokinetic squat), *reactive strength* (the ability to change quickly from an eccentric to a concentric muscle activation) using drop jumps, and speed (eight meter straight sprint) to agility (eight meter sprint with various directional changes) among 15 non-impaired men. Their results showed a low correlation between concentric muscle power and straight line running speed. A moderate correlation however was found between reactive strength and speed while changing direction.

Key Point:

Both speed and reaction time will have a significant influence on agility drill performance.

Conflicting results can be obtained when examining the importance of each component of agility to the overall result of the task. Strength and speed have been examined in some detail. Hilsendager et al.[2] examined the influence of training for speed and strength on the development of agility using the Illinois Agility Test. Investigators developed a six-week training program administered to four groups, plus a control group not involved in any physical training. Three groups trained to improve agility, speed, or strength, in isolation. The fourth group combined speed and strength training. The results indicated that the Illinois Agility Test was most effective in discriminating differences between groups. The speed group scored higher than the agility group in the 10-second squat thrust (described later). The strength and speed, and strength groups combined did not surpass the scores of the agility group in any of the seven agility test components of the Illinois Agility Test. The results of this study show the need for sport/skill specific training, which will be discussed in more detail in the training section of this chapter. Training for the components of agility independently will not assure a complete transfer to the complex tasks evaluated in agility tests. Equally, running numerous agility tests will not assure the transfer of this skill to the playing field.

CHANGES ACROSS THE LIFESPAN

Agility changes across the life span. Previously, we discussed the developmental changes associated with body awareness. Further analysis of the overall changes in agility will be presented in this section. From the time we begin to walk to the early elementary school years, agility is dependent on body awareness and neuromuscular coordination. During this development period the agility components of speed and reaction time are hampered by the overall lack of body awareness and neuromuscular coordination. Once sufficient body awareness and neuromuscular coordination have been achieved, speed and reaction time begin to become the primary factors that influence agility. Most notable agility increases usually occur between middle childhood (7–12 years of age) and early adulthood (18–38 years of age). The activities and sports we become involved in are often related to our agility

level. Here we can briefly consider the concept of self-selection in sports. In football, why does the linebacker become a linebacker and not a wide receiver? Maybe there is a family tradition of linebackers, but most likely not. First there was the decision to play football. Once the child has selected a sport, a number of factors contribute to the position and particular role the child will play on the team. Additionally, but no less important, are personal experience and sports psychological factors that are beyond the scope of this book. Leaving the influence of parents and coaches aside, there is a large component of *self-selection*. During practice and camps the child realizes that he has more difficulty than others on some of the drills that require agility. Even though he can train and practice this component, he will never be able to achieve the same agility level as other players. Is this an indication that he will never be a good athlete? Of course not; he may excel at other components and became an integral part of the team. He may be better suited for a position that does not require agility, but rather muscular power to be successful. One can train to improve agility, however, just like any sport-related component how good one becomes is in part determined by genetics.

The selection and classification of athletes has become popular in both high school and college sports. Thissen-Milder and Mayhew[3] evaluated the use of a battery of six general characteristics and tests (height, weight, percent body fat, agility run, vertical jump, and two flexibility maneuvers) and four specific tests (overhead volley, forearm pass, wall spike, and self bump/set) with 50 high school volleyball players to differentiate their ability levels. They reported that the combination of scores on performance tests for the forearm pass, overhead volley, vertical jump and weight correctly classified 68 percent of the players to their team level. The combination of bump-set, height, weight, and shoulder flexibility allowed correct classification of 78 percent of the starters and nonstarters.[3] A skill-specific volleyball agility test was designed by Schall,[3] which evaluated changes in direction, and rapid, anterior-posterior and lateral movements. Other measures included: height, weight, body composition, vertical jump, sit and reach and shoulder flexibility. They reported that varsity players performed better in the vertical jump and agility tests, than the junior varsity and freshman players. Specific skill tests were also included in the evaluation, with starters displaying both greater agility and better ball-handling skills than non-starters.

Aging seems to have a detrimental affect on agility. We can continue training for agility but we will ultimately observe a slower performance time with increasing age. Are we losing speed or are we losing body awareness? Our decrease in agility is usually more strongly influenced by a decrease in speed. However, a decrease in body awareness is not completely out of the question, especially during the senior years. Consider how postural body control and balance are affected by age. Even though we have not yet discussed balance and its influence on agility, it is a critical component of body awareness and postural control. Judge et al.[4] reported on the sensory function changes that are likely to influence gait. *Visual acuity* (the ability to visually distinguish details and shapes), *contrast sensitivity* (the ability to differentiate between an object and its background), and *edge detection* (the ability to distinguish where one object ends and another object starts) decrease with age and have been found to be risk factors for falls and fractures. It has been shown that physical and functional fitness deteriorates with age. When assessing the fitness of individuals 60 years of age and older, the evaluative focus should change from physical fitness as a separate entity to physical fitness that directly relates to function. The primary goal of a therapeutic exercise program among this population should be to maintain independence in the performance of everyday tasks. Functional fitness, however, can be measured by the same components as physical fitness, but with several adaptations in the focus of the tests. Netz and Argov[5] evaluated the functional fitness of older adults using a battery of tasks that focused on coordination, balance, arm strength, upper extremity flexibility, lower extremity flexibility, agility, lower extremity strength, and walking. As expected, the results of all tests showed a decline with age. A slalom-walking task, performed around eight cones placed one meter apart, was used to measure agility in this particular study. A factor analysis showed that agility is highly influenced by neuromuscular performance and strength. Flexibility did not have as much influence on agility. Balance was a task represented in the neuromuscular performance category which was shown to influence agility.

Key Point:

As individuals age, balance becomes the component that most dramatically influences the ability to maintain a functional level of agility.

Without static and dynamic balance, all other components of agility become trivial. Changes associated with age have also been found in tasks as simple as walking.[6] Step length and time spent in single leg support (defined later) also tend to decrease as age increases. A decrease in range of motion at the hip and ankle were also found to be characteristic of older individuals. The effects of therapeutic exercise and physical fitness have been studied in the aging population as a method to prevent or slow down disease.[7,8] Bravo et al.[7] reported the benefits of physical activity among 124 women between 50 and 70 years of age who were diagnosed with osteopenia. The therapeutic exercise program included a 25-minute walk, step climbing, localized muscle strengthening, stretching, and neuromuscular coordination exercises. Functional fitness was assessed through a battery of tests that measured flexibility, coordination, agility, strength/endurance and cardiorespiratory endurance. All tests were modified to accommodate the older adult's functional abilities. The modified agility test was a walking time trial around a set of cones. The test started from a seated position; the client was asked to rise from a chair and walk around a cone placed to the right of the chair and return back to a full-seated position. Once in a full-seated position, the client was instructed to rise from the chair and walk around the cone placed to the left of the chair. The time needed for a subject to complete the course served as their agility measurement. Agility improved at 6 and 12 months for the physically active group. This study demonstrated the use of functionally relevant tests to measure the influence of physical fitness training. For the older adult a sit to stand task and gait initiation are important functional components and valid agility measurements. Bravo et al.[8] used the same modified agility test to assess the effects of a water based therapeutic exercise program on the same population. They observed improvements in flexibility, agility, strength/endurance, and cardiorespiratory endurance for the group after they had participated in the program for three days/week over a 12-month period.[8]

Injury mechanisms often differ between the older adult population and the more physically active younger population. Among older individuals, injuries from falls increase dramatically. Environmental factors contribute to approximately 44 percent of the falls experienced by individuals of 75 years of age or older.[9] Understanding the environmental factors that lead to falls might be useful to help develop functionally relevant agility training tasks among this population to reduce their fall risk.

BIOMECHANICS OF AGILITY

Ultimately the successful performance of an agility drill is dependent on a combination of postural control and body awareness. The body under certain inertial characteristics will have to respond to an external stimulus as quickly as possible. Let's examine the mechanics of balance and equilibrium. *Balance* is a state of equilibrium. Mechanically, we can be under equilibrium in both static and dynamic situations. *Static equilibrium* is defined as the resistance to linear and angular motion. For this condition to occur, the sum of all the forces must be equal to zero, and the sum of all of the moments also must equal zero. During static equilibrium, the system is balanced with no net forces or moments.

Dynamic equilibrium, which relates more strongly to agility, refers to a system in motion under a constant velocity and direction. The equations used to describe dynamic equilibrium are similar to those used for static equilibrium, with the added component of an *inertia vector* (the mechanical state of the body as it resists any forces that try to move

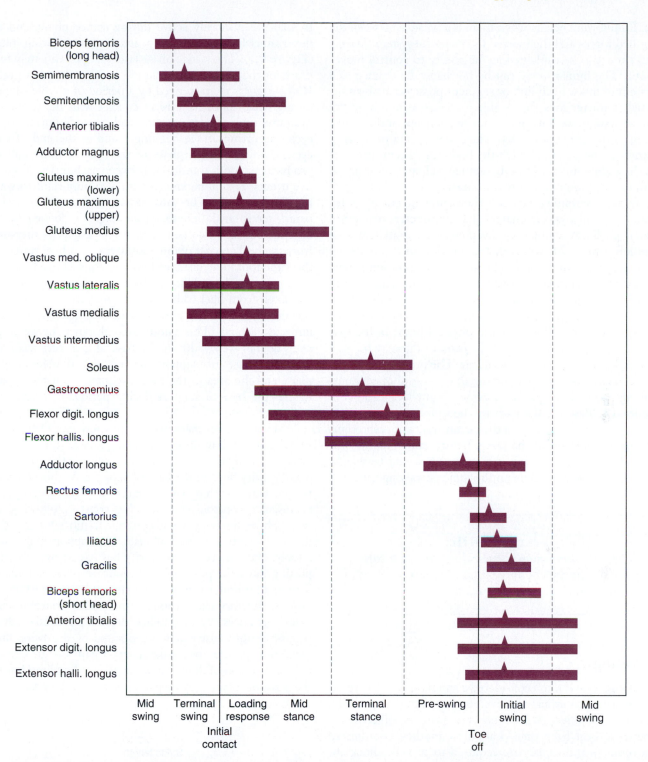

Figure 9.1   Lower extremity muscle activation sequence during walking gait. (Used with permission from J. Perry *Gait Analysis: Normal and Pathological Function.* Thoroughfare, NJ: Slack, Inc, 1992, Figure 9.9, p. 159.)

it). Equilibrium occurs when there is a balance between the applied forces and the inertial forces of the system. *Balance* can then also be explained as the ability to control movement. The human body can be mechanically defined as a system of links. Each link or segment possesses its own inertial characteristics. To be able to describe motion of the entire system, we must introduce the concept of the center of mass or center of gravity. The *center of mass* or *center of gravity* is the point at which the body (or system) balances in three dimensions. As body segments change position, so will the location of the center of mass.

In the anatomical position the center of gravity is located centrally, approximately five centimeters above the pelvic girdle. A segmental movement such as abduction of the left arm to 90° will shift the location of the center of gravity up and to the left. The arm in this position generates a larger moment relative to the other segments; therefore, it has a greater influence on the location of the center of gravity. Body position can cause the position of the center of gravity to fall outside the physical body. In the case of a "flop-style" high jumper, the center of gravity passes a few millimeters underneath the bar. The jumper arches the back to clear the bar, positioning the center of gravity outside the body. Changes in the center of gravity location can be used to describe the path the body follows as it moves through space. The path of the center of gravity represents the overall motion of the body. Before examining a complex skill such as running and cutting it would be worthwhile to spend some time on the topic of walking gait.

> ## Key Point:
> Dynamic equilibrium occurs when there is a balance between the applied forces and the inertial forces of the system.

Walking

Walking, even though considered a simple task, is the result of a series of coordinated movements of both the upper and lower extremities. Aside from the primary objective of transportation from one location to another, coordinated movements and signals are required to provide shock absorption, maintain an erect posture, and maintain balance. Propulsive gait, which is the most efficient gait pattern, is usually not achieved until a child reaches four years of age. Walking is usually studied with reference to a particular series of repetitive events commonly referred to as a gait cycle. The *gait cycle* is divided into two phases: a *stance phase* and a *swing phase*. The stance phase is initiated when a foot makes contact with the ground and ends at toe-off. The swing phase is the period in time when the limb swings freely through space. The extensor muscles of the lower ex-

tremity are primarily active during stance phase, and the flexor muscles are primarily active during swing phase (**Figure 9.1**). The stance phase lasts for approximately two-thirds of the entire gait cycle (58 to 62 percent of cycle). *Walking gait* is characterized by a period of double support during which both feet are in contact with the ground at the same time. There are two such periods during a gait cycle, occurring at the beginning and at the end of each cycle. Timing of each phase of the cycle is important for producing smooth transitions between each series of repetitive events. Spatial parameters are also important to walking (**Figure 9.2**). The most commonly measured spatial parameter is stride length. *Stride length* is defined by the distance between two consecutive foot contacts, measured from the heel contact of one foot to the next heel contact of the same foot. The distance between consecutive foot contacts of contralateral limbs defines a step. *Step length* is measured from heel contact of one foot to heel contact of the opposite foot. In normal gait, step lengths between limbs are equal. The side-to-side distance between the heels defines step width or the base of gait. *Step width* defines the base of support during the double support phase and the area of the foot in contact with the ground defines the base of support during periods of single limb stance.

Walking can be characterized as a series of "falling forward" phases followed by a "catching phase." During swing phase, the body is propelled forward, shifting the body's center of gravity beyond the base of support. At this point, the body is falling with dynamic equilibrium facilitated by neuromuscular control. Without this control following the swing phase, the body would continue to move forward over the stance limb and eventually fall. The support limb acts as a lever; once the center of gravity has passed over the supporting limb, the push-off, or propulsive phase is initiated. The support limb has been shown to act as a passive contributor to the forward motion of the body. Neuromuscular control is necessary to stabilize the limb and take advantage of the propulsive action generated by the swing limb. Once the opposite foot makes contact with the ground and there is a period of double support, the trailing limb finishes the push-off phase and prepares for swing. The *path of the*

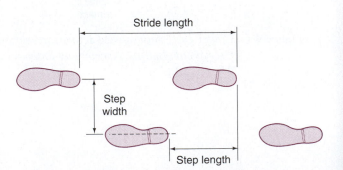

Figure 9.2   Spatial characteristics of the gait cycle.

center of gravity (**Figure 9.3**) illustrates this perpetual falling and catching series as the rising and falling characteristics indicate. Mathematically, the rising and falling of the center of gravity can be written using equation [1]. This equation represents a sinusoidal curve. The variable y_o is the height of the center of gravity of the body and C is the amplitude of the displacement of the center of mass.[10]

$$y(t) = C \cos(2\pi t - \pi) + y_o \qquad [1]$$

Key Point:

The path of the center of gravity illustrates the perpetual falling and catching series that occurs during the gait cycle as shown by the sinusoidal pattern of the curve.

A double differentiation of equation [1] will determine the acceleration of the center of mass during walking. Equation [2] is the result of the double differentiation of equation [1].

$$a(t) = -4\pi^2 C \cos(2\pi t - \pi) \qquad [2]$$

The displacement (**Figure 9.4a**) and acceleration (**Figure 9.4b**) patterns are opposite to each other. At the point of *double support* during walking gait, the center of gravity of the body is at its lowest point, while it is at its highest point during single limb stance.

Ground Reaction Forces

Ground reaction forces provide a very detailed description of the mechanical characteristics of the stance phase of the gait cycle. Ground reaction forces measured via a force platform are the result of *Newton's third law of motion*. In simple terms, this law states that "for every action there is an equal and opposite reaction." During walking the action is generated by the combination of body mass and gravity (weight) exerting a force on the ground as contact is made at heel strike. The ground therefore has to exert an equal and opposite force on the body to maintain equilibrium. Since the ground reaction forces are a reaction to the motion of the center of mass and bodyweight, they are very useful in the description of body mechanics. There are three components of the ground reaction force that can be measured: vertical, anterior-posterior and medial-lateral. Each component possesses its own characteristics, but, they are somewhat dependent on each other.

The *vertical ground reaction force* follows the vertical displacement of the center of gravity of the body (**Figure 9.5**). As the foot makes contact with the ground the loading response is initiated. The body weight is transferred to the limb, as the body is decelerated from the falling period. This maximum deceleration can reach magnitudes of 100 to 150 percent body weight. Peak deceleration coincides with toe-off of the opposite foot. At this point the limb is the single support of the body, the absorption period has ended and the center of gravity rises as the opposite leg is propelled forward during swing. The rising of the center of gravity causes movements of the bodyweight in the opposite direction than gravity; therefore, during midstance the vertical ground reaction force magnitude falls below bodyweight. As the opposite leg passes the support leg the falling period is initiated again. The center of gravity accelerates downward, reaching maximum velocity at the time of contralateral foot contact. The pattern of the vertical ground reaction force is governed by *Newton's second law of acceleration*, which states that "the acceleration of an object as produced by a net force is directly proportional to the magnitude of the net force, in the same direction as the net force, and inversely proportional to the mass of the object." During double support, the ground reaction force is greater than body weight, while during single support the ground reaction force is less than bodyweight.

The *anterior-posterior ground reaction force* component represents the *braking* and *propulsive* forces generated during walking (**Figure 9.6**). The objective of ambulation is to progress forward; therefore, force generation in the direction of motion is critical. The braking force is a component of the "catching" of the body. The body is decelerated in the vertical as well as the anterior directions. Foot placement has an influence on the magnitude of vertical or anterior deceleration that occurs. A foot that is placed at a large angle with the ground, is usually associated with longer stride lengths, and will generate larger braking force magnitudes than a shorter stride length where the foot movement has a larger vertical braking force magnitude component. Adaptations seen in the vertical ground reaction force are usually compensated for by adaptations in the anterior-posterior force pattern. For typical walking, the initial 50 percent of the stance phase is spent braking, followed by a propulsive force of the same magnitude and duration. Slower loading rates for

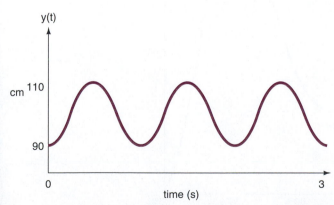

Figure 9.3   Vertical displacement characteristics of the center of gravity during walking gait.

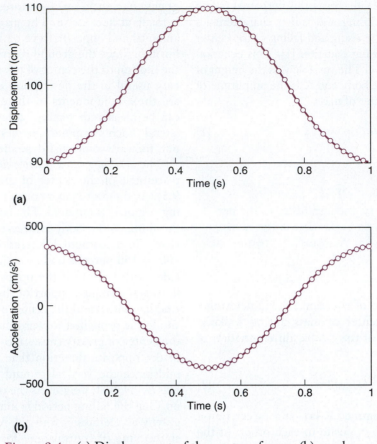

Figure 9.4   (a) Displacement of the center of mass; (b) acceleration of the center of mass.

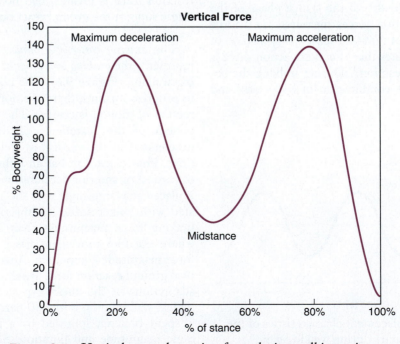

Figure 9.5   Vertical ground reaction force during walking gait.

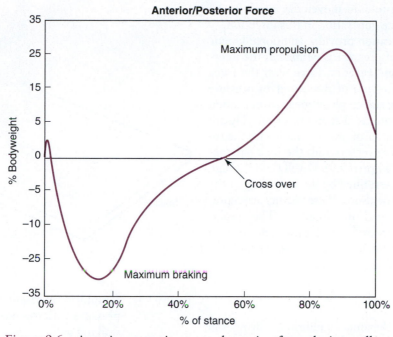

Figure 9.6   Anterior-posterior ground reaction force during walking gait.

the vertical force are compensated by higher anterior-posterior forces generated over shorter time periods. Asymmetries found in the vertical ground reaction force curve are usually mirrored by asymmetries in the anterior-posterior force curve.

The *medial-lateral ground reaction force* is related to balance during walking (**Figure 9.7**). This component is gen- erally the one with the lowest force magnitude. In cases in which balance during walking is compromised, the medial-lateral force increases. Occasionally this compromise is accompanied by an increase in step width. As the center of gravity of the body moves in the line of progression, there is some medial-lateral oscillation associated with pelvic rotation and foot placement. To optimize energy efficiency

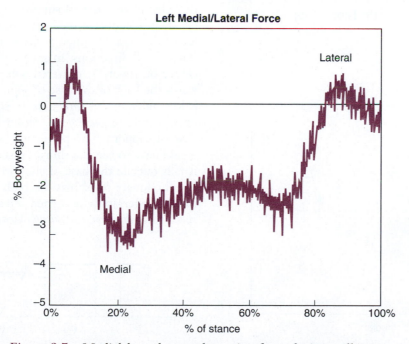

Figure 9.7   Medial-lateral ground reaction force during walking gait.

during walking, this side-to-side movement needs to be reduced, reducing the force generation in this direction.

The *center of pressure* location provides additional kinetic information. The center of pressure is defined as the intercept of the resolved ground reaction force with the force plate surface.[11] The progression of the center of pressure path along the foot during stance phase gives an indication of any medial-lateral deviations that might occur (**Figure 9.8**). The overlay of the center of pressure path with the resolved ground reaction force vectors adds the time parameter to the analytical tools (**Figure 9.9**). Dwell time through the stance phase can be determined by the frequency of the ground reaction force vectors, since these vectors are represented at predetermined equal time intervals. The combination of high loads, increased dwell time, and sudden directional changes over a small foot area suggests high demands in that area, increasing injury risk.

Base of Support

During walking we are in dynamic equilibrium. Changes in the base of support during walking will have an influence on the mechanical pattern of the task. The characteristics of the base of support will determine our ability to maintain equilibrium during static and dynamic situations. The base of support is formed by the perimeter around the parts of the body that are in contact with the supporting surface(s). Stability can be increased by increasing the area of the base of support, or by placing the location of the center of gravity closer to the base of support (**Figure 9.10**). In this graphical representation, shape (b) is more stable than shape (a) because it has a wider (larger) base of support. Shape (c) is the least stable of the group because it has the smallest base of support and shape (d) is more stable than shape (a) because its center of gravity is close to the base of support.

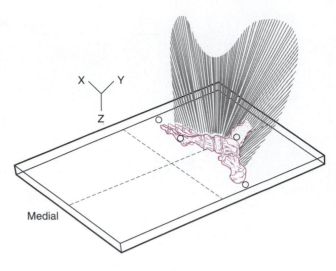

Figure 9.9   Graphical representation of the center of pressure with force vector overlay during walking gait.

> # *Key Point:*
> The characteristics of the base of support will determine a client's ability to maintain equilibrium during static and dynamic situations.

The body is most stable in the direction in which the projection of the center of gravity is furthest away from the edge of the base of support (**Figure 9.11**). In square (a), the projection of the center of gravity falls in the center of the base of support; therefore, the body is equally stable in all directions. In square (b) the projection of the center of gravity is centered side-to-side, but it falls towards the back of the base of support; therefore, the body is less stable in this direction. In square (c) the projection of the center of gravity falls closer to the right edge of the base of support. The projection of the center of gravity would have to travel a shorter distance to the right before it falls outside the base of support and loses equilibrium. Finally, square (d) shows the body to be equally unstable in the posterior-right corner. This concept is sometimes referred as *directional stability*. Most agility drills require a

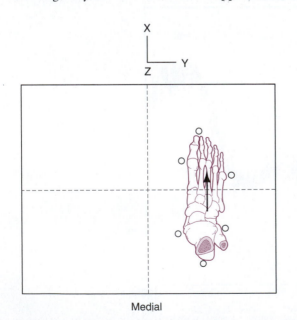

Figure 9.8   Graphical representation of the center of pressure path during walking gait.

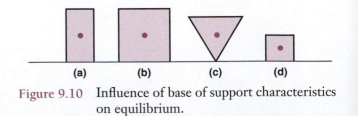

Figure 9.10   Influence of base of support characteristics on equilibrium.

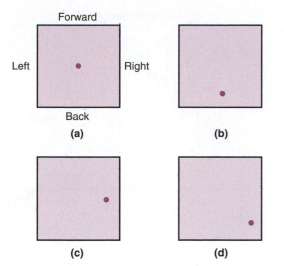

Figure 9.11   Graphical representation of directional stability.

constant changing of direction. During these direction changes, the projection of the body's center of gravity will move around the base of support and in many cases will fall outside the boundaries of the base. If the projection of the center of gravity falls outside the base of support the body will start into free fall. Neuromuscular activation will correct this free fall condition and return the body to a state of dynamic equilibrium. The time between when the body starts falling and the neuromuscular activation that counteracts the fall is only a few milliseconds in non-impaired clients. This demonstrates body awareness and neuromuscular coordination working in combination to provide postural control. The difference between the falling action that occurs during walking and the falling action that occurs during an agility drill is primarily the speed of motion. The faster the movement, the greater the inertia that needs to be overcome to maintain the body in a state of dynamic equilibrium.

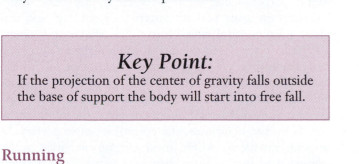

Key Point:

If the projection of the center of gravity falls outside the base of support the body will start into free fall.

Running

One of the most obvious differences between walking and *running gait* is speed. An increase in speed increases the inertia the body carries in the direction of movement. As was shown with walking, running can be characterized by a series of falls. At each step the lower extremity has to slow down the momentum of the body, absorb the shock of the step, and then convert it into positive energy to continue propelling the body forward. The vertical component of

the ground reaction forces changes significantly (**Figure 9.12**), both as it relates to the pattern as well as the magnitude of force, when compared to walking. Running is characterized by a flight period, when neither foot is in contact with the ground. This free fall allows the force of gravity to accelerate the body toward the ground. Due to the greater inertia the body carries, the magnitude of the vertical ground reaction force increases by a factor of two or three times body weight. The absence of a double support phase turns the typical M ground reaction force curve pattern observed during walking into a one-peak curve. The significant increase in force during running occurs in approximately one-third the time of walking.[12]

The anterior/posterior force pattern of running maintains the symmetrical attributes of a walking gait (**Figure 9.13**). During the contact phase of each foot the objective remains the same: Stop the falling action of the body and propel the body forward. The impulse of each of the two phases (braking and propulsion) should be equal, assuming a constant movement velocity (**Figure 9.14**). The concept of equal braking and propulsive impulses is simple to understand. As the body enters the flight phase, it carries the impulse generated by the stance limit during propulsion. During the flight phase, the body is unable to change this impulse value, due to the lack of contact with the ground. During landing, the opposite limb has to brake the impulse, which should be equal to the impulse generated by the "initial" propulsion.

A similar increase in medial-lateral ground reaction forces is apparent during running (**Figure 9.15**). The shear forces generated during running increase due to the more demanding balance requirements associated with a smaller base of support. Out of plane motion occurring at the hip joint can also affect the medial-lateral force magnitude. *Circumduction* (extremity movement where the proximal end be-

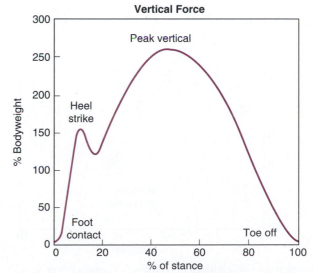

Figure 9.12   Vertical ground reaction force during running gait.

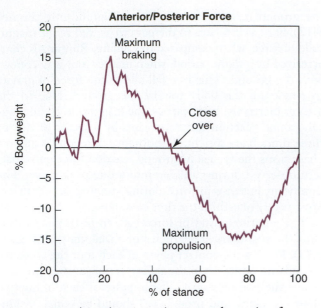

Figure 9.13   Anterior-posterior ground reaction force during running gait.

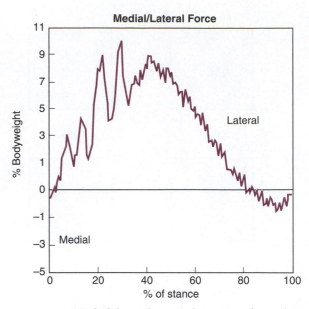

Figure 9.15   Medial-lateral ground reaction force during running gait.

comes relatively fixed and the distal end moves in a circular pattern) at the hip during the swing phase will change the initial contact pattern of the foot, creating a more lateral to medial approach. This change in hip biomechanics will increase the initial medial ground reaction force.

Cutting

The biomechanical demands of cutting activities are very similar to running. The primary difference between running and cutting is the added component of an abrupt change in

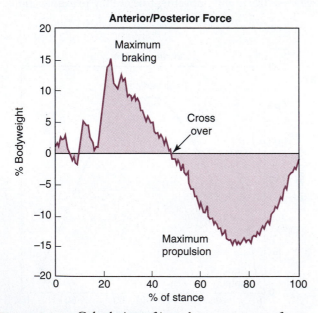

Figure 9.14   Calculation of impulse-momentum from shear force during running.

direction (**Figure 9.16a–c**). The laws of physics prevent us from changing direction in mid-air. Therefore, the cutting action has to occur when the foot is in contact with the ground. At this time Newton's third law of motion, "the generation of an action will cause an equal and opposite reaction," can be appreciated. If the objective is to cut to the left, we push to the right. Up to the point of contact with the ground the body displays the same mechanics of running, free fall. The deceleration of the body in the vertical direction does not change; therefore, the vertical ground reaction force curve remains the same (**Figure 9.17**).

Cutting displays different anterior-posterior (**Figure 9.18**) and medial-lateral ground reaction forces than running (**Figure 9.19**). The degree of the cut will determine the distribution of forces between the direction of motion and its perpendicular angle. A 90° cut should theoretically maintain the same braking pattern as a running task, and show a symmetrical lateral force. The symmetry between the braking force and the lateral force is the result of the propulsion phase being performed at an angle 90° to the initial direction of motion. Similarly, one could calculate the exact distribution of forces between the anterior-posterior and medial-lateral directions given the angle of the cut. However, neuromuscular control is not so perfect. In athletic situations, where most cutting activities occur, players tend to anticipate their next move. Foot position will usually determine the degree or angle of the cut. The foot is positioned at an angle away from the initial direction of motion to facilitate the cut. This change in foot position will generate a different distribution of medial-lateral forces and reduce the braking forces observed during early stance phase. The graphic example (**Figure 9.19**) shows a significant increase in the lateral ground reaction

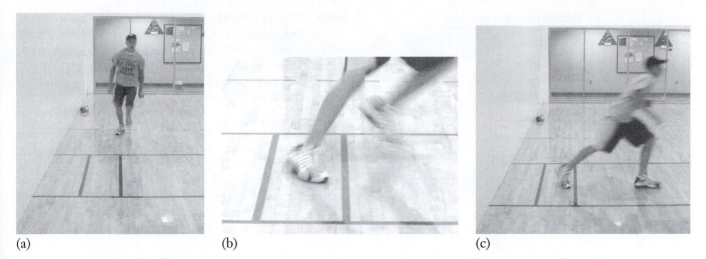

(a)   (b)   (c)

Figure 9.16   Side-step cutting maneuver. (a) approach; (b) plant-pivot; (c) cut.

forces, when compared to the running example. The increase in lateral ground reaction forces are accompanied by a reduction and loss of symmetry in the propulsive force. The braking component of the cutting maneuver is prolonged, suggesting a greater need for body control associated with the drastic change in direction.

During most agility drills, the client will be required to change direction, sometimes abruptly, without losing speed. This statement is a biomechanical paradox, since every change in direction requires a period of zero velocity. If we constrain the task to one dimension, the problem becomes easier to understand. Assume that during a shuttle run, a female athlete's horizontal velocity is five m/s when she is two meters away from the touchline. In order for her to change directions, her body has to undergo a deceleration period until the horizontal velocity reaches 0 m/s. One instant of time after the linear velocity is zero the body can change directions and start accelerating again. When we compare this situation with a bouncing ball, the concept is exactly the same. The ball decelerates on the way up, as a result of the force of gravity, reaches a velocity of zero at peak height, changes direction and accelerates, again as a result of the force of gravity, on the way down (**Figure 9.20**). So as we discuss the mechanisms that are required for agility, we have to understand the mechanical implications associated with speed and changes in direction to determine which components become most critical during training.

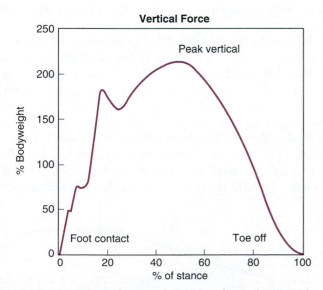

Figure 9.17   Vertical ground reaction force during side step cutting.

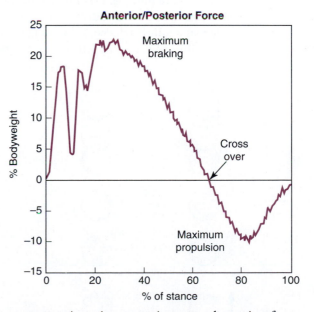

Figure 9.18   Anterior-posterior ground reaction force during side step cutting.

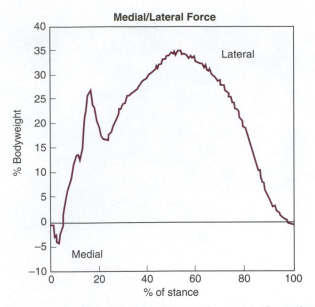

Figure 9.19   Medial-lateral ground reaction force during side step cutting.

Key Point:

Abrupt directional changes without losing speed are mechanical paradoxes, since every change in direction requires a period of reduced velocity.

A mechanical factor that will influence the performance of all agility tasks is inertia. Agility drills are designed to test the ability of the body to change directions. These changes in direction may require, as explained above, the body to reach zero absolute velocity during some portion of the drill, or they may require a deceleration of the body along a curvilinear path. As the body turns, the compo-

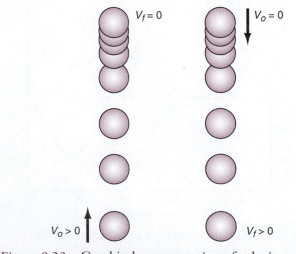

Figure 9.20   Graphical representation of velocity values during directional changes.

nents of linear velocity serve different purposes. Curvilinear motion possesses a tangential and a normal component, e_t and e_n respectively (**Figure 9.21**). Two force components can also be defined for all motions along a curve. Equations [3] and [4] (below) are the tangential (F_t) and normal force (F_n) equations respectively (m = mass, s = displacement, t = time, $\frac{ds}{dt}$ = first derivative, $\frac{d^2s}{dt}$ = second derivative, ρ = radius). The tangential component is influenced by velocity, which is defined by the distance along the curve. The normal force is dependent on velocity as well as the radius of curvature.[10]

$$F_t = m\frac{d^2s}{dt^2} \qquad [3]$$

$$F_n = \frac{m}{\rho}\left(\frac{ds}{dt}\right)^2 \qquad [4]$$

Key Point:

When making a cut around a cone there are two basic components that will determine the success of the task: (1) the velocity upon initiating the cut and (2) the angle of approach or attack.

If a runner carries too much velocity into a turn and attempts a sharp turn, lack of friction between the footwear and the running surface may cause them to fall. The friction force has to be greater than the centrifugal force generated during the turn. The optimal angle of lean during the cut is directly proportional to the ratio between the linear velocity squared and the radius of the turn times gravity.

Walker[13] examined the ability of the spotted boxfish to maneuver in the water. The results showed the rigid-bodied fish could perform 180° turns with a minimum turning radius (high maneuverability or agility); however, defining maneuverability as the area required to turn, the more rigid boxfish was considered to be less agile than more flexible fish. The flexible fish is able to overcome inertia and other external forces more efficiently. The spotted boxfish, although able to perform the 180° turns with a minimum turning radius (change in body position/body

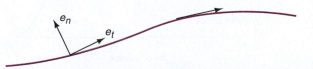

Figure 9.21   Vector representation in a curvilinear path. (e_n = normal component vector, e_t = tangential component vector)

control) is not able to maintain the speed component (rapid change in position) that is characteristic of agility. The limited agility of the boxfish was related to the inability of the body to overcome the external mechanical impositions applied to the body.[13] Even though human movement or locomotion is significantly different from that of fish, the mechanical factors that need to be overcome during quick maneuvers are the same. In the same manner, certain body characteristics in humans lead to some clients being more agile than others.

The last mechanical concept that one must understand when addressing the demands of an agility task is moments. Previously in the chapter, we examined ground reaction forces in some detail. Those ground reaction forces generate moments about joint centers. *Moments* or *torques* are turning forces. Within the definition of equilibrium, (the resistance to linear or angular motion) we see the importance of moments in the generation of motion. A force that is applied out of line with the center of rotation of an object will generate a moment. This moment will generate angular motion. The simplest example is to look at a box, when a force is applied in line with the center of the box, the box will slide (**Figure 9.22a**). However, when a force is applied off line from the center of the box, the box will rotate (**Figure 9.22b**). In the first example, the box moved in a linear pattern, as it translated along the plane. In the second example, the box moved in an angular pattern.

Joint Moments

Moments about joints are produced throughout the different phases of a movement. Very seldom will we encounter the situation, during motion, when all forces are applied in line with all joint centers. The importance in understanding joint moments comes from the need to understand neuromuscular control during activities that place high demands on the body, such as agility drills. There are two types of moments that will act simultaneously at each joint. External moments are those produced by the ground reaction forces or external forces, and internal moments are those produced by the body, primarily

caused by muscle forces. A muscle can be activated to counteract the external moment, generating the opposite action (concentric), or the muscle can act to slow down (eccentric) the action generated as a result of the external moment. **Figure 9.23a–c** represents a simple example to help you understand the difference: The elbow joint is the center of rotation, the 20 lb dumbbell is the external force generating an external extension moment about the elbow, the elbow flexors are the muscle group of interest. If the elbow flexors act to counteract the external moment with sufficient force, the elbow will flex against the resistance (concentric action). If the muscle group acts to slow down, but not stop, the action, visually we see extension of the elbow; however, the elbow flexors are contracting to control the movement (eccentric action). If no elbow flexor muscle action occurs, the elbow will extend rapidly, potentially creating a severe injury. The elbow will extend as a result of the external moment created by the weight of the dumbbell, placed away from the center of rotation. The greater the force, in this case the weight of the dumbbell, and the greater the distance away from the center of rotation, in this case the longer the forearm, the larger the external moment that is generated.

During walking, external moments are generated by the ground reaction forces about the joints of the lower extremities (**Figure 9.24a–b**). Muscle activations, both concentric and eccentric, will be generated to produce the desired motion. As speed increases, forces increase; therefore, external moments increase in magnitude. Movements that occur in the same plane in which these moments function generally do not produce an increased lower extremity injury risk. However, "multi-planar" tasks (function outside of the cardinal movement planes) (see Chapter 5) and unexpected conditions require higher levels of neuromuscular coordination and postural control.

Take the situation of someone who is jogging at night in a poorly lit area and almost misses the curb with his stride leg after he crosses the street. At the instant his foot hits the curb less than one-third of his foot is on the curb and the rest of his foot is without a base of support. Since his center of mass is not over the curb, his weight is placed posterior to his base of support. The external force of gravity acts on his bodyweight, generating an external dorsiflexion moment about the ankle. If the jogger succumbs to gravity without appropriate muscle activations, the ankle will dorsiflex maximally over the curb and he will eventually fall backwards. However, as soon as the jogger feels the external moment attempting to take over, he sends a signal to the brain to activate his ankle plantar flexors. Only a maximum contraction of the ankle plantar flexors will be able to overcome the external moment that is driven by the inertia of the body. Depending on how fast the ankle plantar flexors can be activated is how much ankle dorsiflexion can be counteracted, placing his foot back in a biomechanically advantageous position. For many recreational joggers, this situation will result in an Achilles tendon rupture. Maximal activation of the ankle

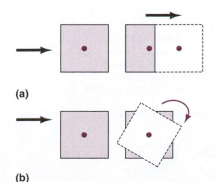

(a)

(b)

Figure 9.22   Graphical representation of linear (a) and angular (b) motions.

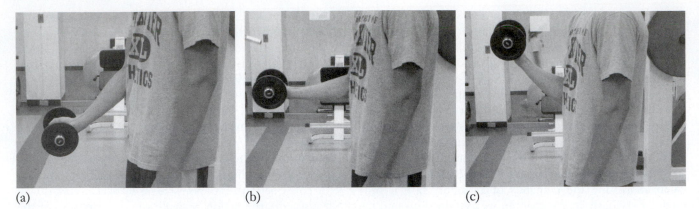

(a)   (b)   (c)

Figure 9.23   Biceps curl. (a) start; (b) mid-way; (c) completion.

plantar flexors at a very fast rate creates an extremely high internal joint moment to overcome the high magnitude external joint moment. Controlled applications of negative or eccentric ankle plantar flexor loads have been used successfully as a form of therapeutic exercise to treat Achilles tendinosis.[14,15]

Reaching and Grasping

Agility is not limited to running or cutting tasks. The same biomechanical concepts described in previous sections can be applied to upper extremity motion. A fast and accurate change in position of the arms and trunk should also be considered under the definition of agility. Reaching and grasping tasks may mechanically isolate the upper extremity and trunk (**Figure 9.25**). Upper extremity joint trajectories have been studied in relation to trunk movements during reaching and grasping tasks.[16,17] Upper extremity joint trajectories during fast movements tend to be more curved when compared to slower movements; however, higher movement speeds do not seem to affect upper extremity joint rotations.[16] The pattern of upper extremity inter-joint coordination changes when trunk motion is restricted.[18] Changes in coordination and trajectories are a result of the different interactions of internal joint moments that are generated as a result of imposing constraints to the system. Reach and grasp tasks

are highly dependent on the neuromuscular coordination of joint movements (see Chapter 8).[19] Increased internal joint moments are produced at the proximal upper extremity joints as the arm moves through space when reaching. The moments and inertial parameters have to be counteracted by appropriate neuromuscular activations to produce a controlled and accurate result. Neuromuscular activations have to follow a particular sequence to create a smooth trajectory toward the objective.

Movement coordination during the performance of a reach and grasp task is similar to throwing. Throwing is a higher velocity movement than a reaching task, but it requires a similar level of neuromuscular coordination. The correct sequencing of each kinetic chain component from the foot-ground interface, through the instant of ball release is critical to a successful throw (**Figure 9.26a–d**). The kinetic chain provides a sequence of movements from the proximal to the distal segments. Maximal angular and linear velocities need to be reached by the proximal segment prior to the distal segment reaching maximal resultant velocity. A high level of neuromuscular control and coordination is needed during throwing to generate the correct timing of neuromuscular activations and joint rotations.

The kinetic chain provides a system for momentum transfer from the lower extremity to the throwing arm. The larger segments, the lower extremities and trunk, will initiate the rotational motion and force generation prior

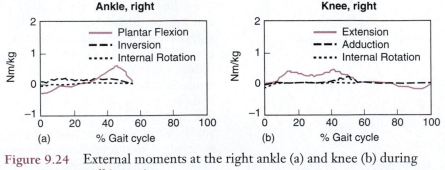

Figure 9.24   External moments at the right ankle (a) and knee (b) during walking gait.

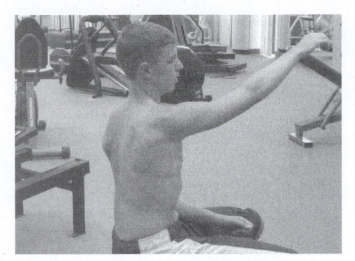

Figure 9.25   Upper extremity reaching task.

to the upper extremity. A summation of forces occurs from the larger segments to the more distal segments. This sequencing of rotations allows for the most efficient transfer of momentum from the larger to the smaller segments. In an overhead throw, the kinetic chain is initiated by the forward step toward the target. This step generates the movement of the lower extremities, followed by trunk rotation, shoulder rotation, elbow rotation, and finally wrist rotation. The most forceful and efficient overhead throw is one in which a step toward the target is taken, and both feet remain on the ground during the force production phase. A child learning to throw a ball tends to not take advantage of this kinetic chain force generation, limiting all rotations to the upper extremity.

AGILITY TRAINING PROGRESSIONS

Training for agility should follow the classic simple to complex pattern (see Chapter 5 and 8). During the early stages of an agility training program, tasks should be re-stricted to a single plane beginning with smaller movements, with a limited number of position changes. The tasks can become progressively more difficult until efficient performance of larger movement sequences are achieved. As explained earlier, agility cannot be achieved in isolation.

While training for agility the therapeutic exercise program should focus on subcomponents including balance, proprioception-kinesthesia (see Chapter 7), postural control, and speed. Consideration for each of these subcomponents during therapeutic exercise program planning will build a stronger foundation for the performance of more complex tasks. Joint proprioception-kinesthesia is directly linked with body control. Understanding joint position and sensing movement will enable a faster reaction time to the external stimulus. Good proprioception/kinesthesia in the lower extremity joints might prevent injury in cases in which the client has misjudged the maximum velocity or the angle of attack during a turn. If either of these two factors is too high and combined with a low friction coefficient between the shoe and the playing surface, neuromuscular control will be required to prevent the foot from slipping under the runner. Having an accurate sense of foot position and the initial movement generated by the external force better facilitates a signal to the brain for lower extremity position corrections in non-impaired clients. This reaction time is critical to the client's ability to overcome the inertia of the body and prevent injury.

With slight modifications, the same basic agility task can be used for different purposes. Each drill can be adapted to focus on a different component (**Figure 9.27a–c**). In (a), the cones are spaced out and placed in a straight line; this drill can be classified as an agility drill focused on speed. The placement of the cones allows the runner to gain linear velocity and requires minimum changes in direction. When the cones are placed closer together (b), there is a greater focus on postural control; now the runner is required to make sharper turns to clear

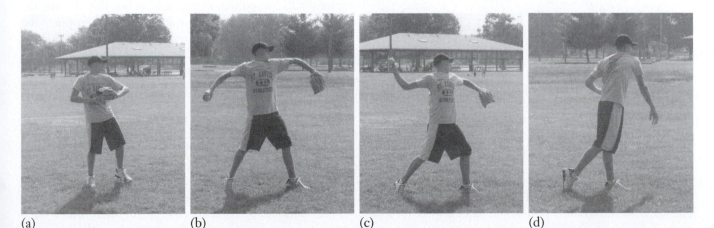

(a)   (b)   (c)   (d)

Figure 9.26   Throwing a baseball. (a) wind-up; (b) cocking; (c) acceleration; (d) follow through.

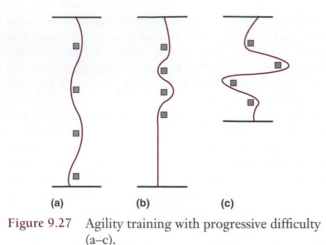

Figure 9.27 Agility training with progressive difficulty (a–c).

the cones, which will cause a reduction in the linear velocity that can be achieved. The spacing of the cones laterally (c) has a further effect on the postural control component. The cones are spaced out laterally but maintained in a short linear displacement; therefore, sharper turns are required and greater control of velocity changes is critical to the successful performance of the task. Speed of movement can also be adjusted in the drill. In the initial stages of the agility phase of therapeutic exercise program intervention, the activities should be performed at approximately one-half full speed. The reduction in speed will allow the neuromuscular system more time to control the movement generated by the inertia of the body. As the client becomes more comfortable with the tasks, they can be performed at faster speeds. Manipulating the number of directional changes and the speed of the test can also be combined with changing the objective for each run: 1) run as fast as you can, 2) run through the circuit without touching any of the cones, 3) run as close to the cones as possible (see **Figure 9.27**).

Key Point:

Understanding joint position and sensing joint movement will allow for a faster reaction time to an external stimulus.

Young et al.[20] studied the relationship between straight sprint speed (30 m) training to six agility tests with various directional change angles among 36 college age men after sprint and agility training. Following the initial test, the subjects were divided in three groups: One group trained for speed, a second group trained for agility, and the third group served as the control. The training consisted of specific exercise movements performed twice a week for a period of six weeks. Subjects repeated the same agility tests following the training period. As might be expected, there were no significant improvements in any of the tasks for the control group. The speed training group showed improvements in two tasks, while the agility training group improved in all tasks except one. The researchers pointed out that increased agility task difficulty correlated with an increase in the performance time. They reported that the more complex the agility task, the less transfer was observed from the speed training to the agility task. Conversely, the agility training resulted in significant improvements in the change of direction tests, while significant performance improvements were not observed in straight sprint performance. They concluded that speed and agility training methods were specific and produced limited transfer between each other.[20]

As agility task complexity increases, either due to the number of directional changes or changes in the approach angle, neuromuscular control and task biomechanics also change. The direction of the primary ground reaction forces change from anterior-posterior during a full sprint to medial-lateral during a side-step cut. Greater deceleration and acceleration periods are required to perform the required changes in direction, which in turn result in an increase in the overall time for task performance.

AGILITY DRILL EXAMPLES

The *shuttle run* was developed by the American Alliance of Health, Physical Education and Recreation (AAHPER) in 1976 as part of a battery of tests given to school-aged children to test their speed and agility (**Figure 9.28a–c**). The goal of the test is to retrieve two blocks, placing then behind the starting line, in the least amount of time. The test requires three changes in direction, and full speed running between the two lines placed 30 feet apart. This test emphasizes the speed component of agility, usually the fastest runners will have greatest success. Directional changes of 180° occur at the end of the 30-foot sprints. By drawing a couple of rectangular boxes with chalk behind the starting line, the drill can be easily modified to integrate a skill component to the task. When this is done, the client has the added requirement of having to place the block within its appropriate rectangle. This adaptation requires vision, as well as motor control of the upper extremity as critical components during the test. With this adaptation coordination between the upper and lower extremities through the trunk or core become critical components of successful task performance.

Another common test used to measure agility that was developed in 1951 is the Illinois Agility Run Test. This test includes the same components as the shuttle test, speed and uni-dimensional directional changes, with the addition of a more complex zig-zag component. Four cones positioned 10 feet away from each other in a straight line create the zig-zag pattern. As with the shuttle run, the Illinois Agility Run Test can be modified to in-

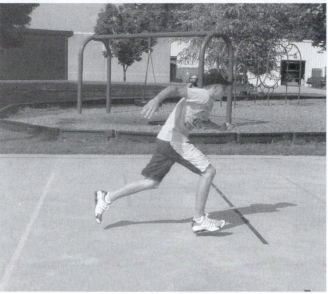

(a)

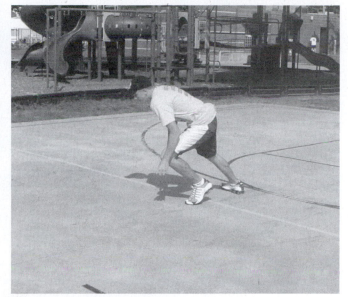

(b)

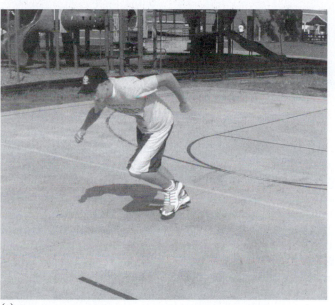

(c)

Figure 9.28   Shuttle run. (a) running approach; (b) directional change; (c) return.

crease the level of complexity. More cones can be added, larger cones or other impediments can be used, or a different cone configuration can be used to increase the difficulty associated with the directional changes.

The two previous tests were designed with a running emphasis; however, agility testing does not have to rely on running speed. The *side stepping test* was developed by the State of North Carolina in 1977. During the performance of this test the client moves laterally between two lines positioned 12 feet apart. As the client side steps laterally between the lines, the feet are not allowed to cross each other. Over a 30 second interval the client is scored for their ability to move laterally as quickly as possible. A touch is counted every time the lead foot touches or

crosses the line. The number of touches completed by the client during the 30 second interval determines the score. This is another drill that focuses on uni-dimensional changes in direction. All movements occur in one primary motion plane (frontal or coronal).

Another popular agility test is the *squat thrust* or *Burpee maneuver* (**Figure 9.29a–c**). This test measures the ability of the client to quickly change body positions. This test does not rely on running speed, as some of the other drills do, but is based on strength, postural control, neuromuscular coordination, and body awareness. Modifying the characteristics of the surface on which these movements are performed can add to the joint proprioception/ kinesthesia component.

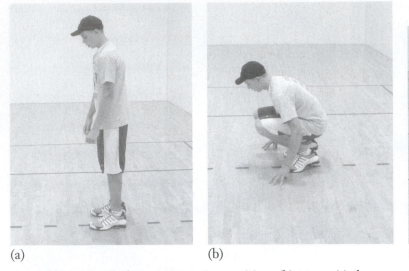
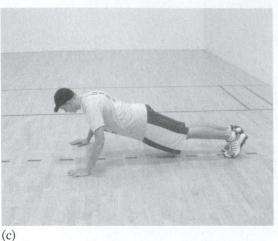

(a)   (b)   (c)

Figure 9.29   Squat thrust. (a) starting position; (b) squat; (c) thrust.

AGILITY AS A THERAPEUTIC EXERCISE

Agility is often the last thing the rehabilitation clinician thinks about during therapeutic exercise program planning. We all too often do not think about agility at all unless we are attempting to return a client back to sports that require this component of physical fitness. However, the improved neuromuscular control and reaction time that can be gained from agility training makes it a potentially critical component of injury prevention for a wide variety of clients of all ages.

Traditionally, strength training has been emphasized as the most critical component of therapeutic exercises designed to protect the knee joint from injury. It has been shown that in anterior cruciate ligament (ACL) deficient knees, instability can be controlled when clients have quicker dynamic neuromuscular reaction times.[21] Wojtys et al.[22] investigated the effects of three different training programs on the neuromuscular activation reaction time and time to peak torque of the muscles that cross the knee joint of 32 non-impaired adults (16 men, 16 women). Healthy subjects trained 30 minutes, three times a week for six weeks in one of the following programs: isokinetic, isotonic, agility, or control. The agility training group performed five exercises as part of the program: 1) slide-boarding, 2) unilateral bouncing "box hop" jumps, 3) *carioca, or grapevine* stepping, which involves sideways jogging while alternating a cross over and a cross under step, 4) figure 8 runs, and 5) backward runs. The results revealed that in the agility trained group a spinal level reflex in response to anterior translation of the tibia was generated 13.8 to 15.4 milliseconds earlier than that displayed by the other groups. The agility trained group also showed the largest improvement in time to peak knee extensor and flexor torque during isokinetic testing.

The United States Military Academy has a therapeutic exercise program that emphasizes strength, agility and aerobic fitness.[23] This program includes six phases: pre-surgery, postoperative, early healing, late healing (water training), healing (land training) and competition. Agility training is initiated during the land training stage and continues through the competition phase. Sample drills of the healing (land training) phase include: toe-rises, upside-down bicycling, hopping on one foot, rope skipping, backward running, stair climbing and vertical jumping. When the drills of each of these phases are mastered, the program continues with simple games played in a controlled environment. Timed events are the last component of the healing (land training) phase. Examples of these drills are: shuttle running, circle running, figure 8 running, straight ahead running and timed vertical jumping.

Functional therapeutic exercise programs have become increasingly popular over the past 10 years, especially for the rehabilitation of ACL injuries. These programs have been compared with traditional (non–weight bearing, open kinetic chain, slow progression) and accelerated (early weight bearing, closed kinetic chain, fast progression) programs and have shown some benefits. Shelbourne et al.[24] studied the changes in ACL graft laxity following reconstruction and the initiation of a functional sports agility program at four weeks post-surgery. Subjects were tested for knee laxity prior to the start of the program. Each client had a functional agility program designed according to their sporting goals. The results revealed no graft elongation as a result of the early return to physical activity. One of the goals of the functional agility programs designed in the study by Shelbourne et al.[24] was to promote the return of knee joint proprioception (see Chapter 7). The link between agility and proprioception and kinesthesia was mentioned earlier in this chapter. Sensory information about knee joint position and movement velocity are critical components for the successful execution of an agility related task.

Sailors et al.[25] evaluated the effects of agility tests on the anterior laxity of the knee joint following ACL reconstruction. For this purpose, they designed an agility course that combined sprinting, jogging, and zig-zag running. Subjects were asked to run the course for 30 minutes at 70 to 85 percent of their maximum heart rate (see Chapter 4). A knee arthrometer was used to measure anterior tibial translation pre- and post-run (see Chapter 6). The results of the study showed no significant differences between the laxity values for the ACL reconstructed knee and the non-impaired knee (control). The forces generated during running were expected to stress the ACL graft beyond the normal ranges and therefore induce a change in laxity; however, differences were not observed.

Even in cases in which an ACL injury is not treated surgically, therapeutic exercise program interventions include lower extremity muscular strength and endurance activities, knee joint mobility, agility, and sports specific training. Fitzgerald et al.[26] compared a standard therapeutic exercise program for clients who had unilateral ACL deficiency with one that also included perturbation training. Agility training was initiated at slow speeds and progressed to full speed activities by the end of the program. Once clients reached full speed agility training without pain, swelling or hesitation, sport specific skills were added. The sport specific skill progressions began without opposition, progressing to one-on-one play, and ended with unrestricted play with the entire team.

Risberg et al.[27] described a neuromuscular training program for clients who were status-post ACL reconstruction. Their program was divided into six phases, which include balance exercises, dynamic joint stability activities (see Chapters 5, 6 and 7), plyometric (see Chapters 5 and 8) and agility drills and sport specific exercises. Each phase lasted between three and five weeks. Once the client mastered balance, coordination, and dynamic joint stability, the focus shifted to increased overall agility of movement during the last two phases. Henriksson et al.[28] studied the effect of a functional therapeutic exercise program that included a component of proprioception and agility on postural control. Subject groups consisted of clients who were status post–unilateral ACL reconstruction and a non-impaired control group. Even though anterior knee joint laxity was greater in the ACL reconstructed group, postural control was within normal ranges. These results suggest that a functional therapeutic exercise program has a positive influence on the restoration of dynamic knee joint stability. In a study that evaluated the knee joint function of clients who underwent unilateral ACL reconstruction using an augmented double-looped hamstring graft, Nakayama et al.[29] reported that agility and sports specific training enabled return to full sports competition at an average of 8.1 months after surgery.

BALANCE

Balance and body control were identified as components of agility and discussed earlier in this chapter. When discussing changes in agility across the lifespan, balance was mentioned as a key component affecting the functional level of agility at both ends of the spectrum. In this section, we will discuss the mechanisms affecting balance in more detail and the quantification of balance deficiencies in the clinic.

First we will revisit the states of equilibrium (static, dynamic). *Static balance* is defined as resistance to linear and angular motion. All tests evaluating static balance will consist of maintaining a predetermined posture for a length of time. Quantification of static balance is based on how well the client is able to resist motion. Maintaining the center of gravity over the base of support is the first requirement in sustaining balance.

> ## Key Point:
> Maintenance of the center of gravity over the base of support is the first requirement in sustaining balance.

The easiest situation to illustrate balance would be quiet standing with the feet shoulder width apart and the eyes open. Young healthy adults can maintain this posture for long periods of time without losing postural control. However, closer observation of the control mechanisms provides us with clues that posture is maintained through controlled sway of the body during the task. Body sway during quiet standing is generated by neuromuscular control mechanisms necessary to maintain the center of gravity in line with the center of pressure. Movement of the center of gravity results in a movement of the center of pressure. Perfect alignment is not achieved during quiet standing; instead, the center of gravity and center of pressure chase one another, resulting in body sway. The closer the chase, the lesser the amount of body sway and the better the balance. In young healthy adults the body responds by moving the center of gravity toward the center of the base of support and away from the limits of stability.[30]

The vestibular, somatosensory, and visual systems each contribute to balance. To display balance, the client must have at least two out of the following three systems providing accurate information to the cerebral cortex: 1) visual confirmation of their position, 2) non-visual confirmation of their position from proprioceptive and vestibular input and 3) a normally functioning cerebellum. If the client loses his or her balance during the *Romberg Test* (standing with feet together and arms at sides) while standing still with the eyes closed, but is able to maintain balance with eyes open, then there may be a lesion in the cerebellum (see Chapter 8). This would be a positive Romberg Test. The traditional Romberg Test has been modified to include differing foot positions: feet at shoulder width apart, semi-tandem stance (heel to instep) and tandem stance (heel to toe) (**Figure 9.30**) and single leg stance (**Figure 9.31**). It is essential that the rehabilitation clinician discern the specific Romberg test style employed when reviewing and comparing the results of research reports.

A comprehensive balance assessment will systematically evaluate each contributing system to identify the source(s) of the deficits. Several tools exist for the assessment of balance deficits with their selection being dependent on setting, equipment options, and the magnitude of the deficit. Force platforms are typically used to calculate the center of pressure during standing. The movement path of the center of pressure and the velocity at which it moves are the parameters of interest in the assessment of balance. The tighter the oscillation of the center of pressure location, the better the balance; the larger the radius of center of pressure displacement, the worse the balance (**Figure**

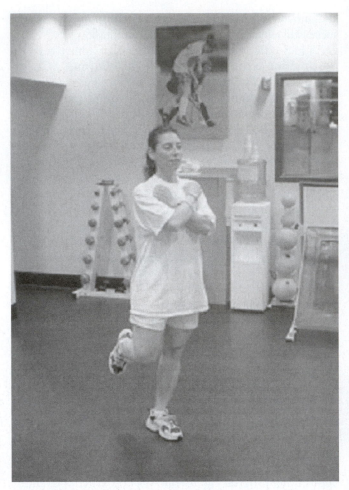

Figure 9.31   Single Leg Stance Test.

9.32a–b). However, a complete assessment of balance needs to also include the velocity component.

Neuromuscular control during quiet standing requires very fast, precise correction of the relative difference between the center of gravity and the center of pressure locations. Changes in relative center of gravity and center of pressure locations have to be identified through the vestibular and somatosensory systems. The neuromuscular system must respond to these changes. The inability to detect a shift in the center of pressure as it moves toward the boundaries of the base of support may cause the center of gravity to move outside of the base of support, resulting in a fall. When a center of pressure location shift is detected, motor control mechanisms provide a high velocity adjustment to maintain equilibrium (see Chapter 8). As a client stands with the feet positioned at shoulder width apart and moves the body slowly through a large circle, the center of pressure representation would show a large radius of displacement, but the slow velocity and well controlled center of pressure location change would allow for the maintenance of good balance. Effective balance evaluations should include measurement of both center of pressure locations and the velocities at which they change. Abrupt center of pressure location and velocity changes

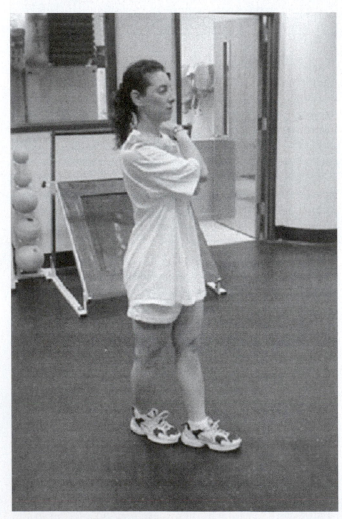

Figure 9.30   Romberg Test in tandem stance.

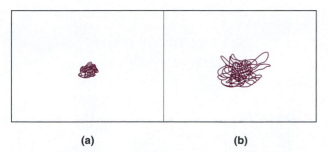
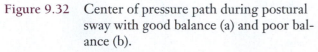

Figure 9.32 Center of pressure path during postural sway with good balance (a) and poor balance (b).

may be the most indicative components of a balance deficit. Neuromuscular responses and sudden center of pressure location changes should be evident when the client is confronted with a balance loss even when the neuromuscular system cannot successfully correct the deficit. *Induced sway* through applied perturbations results in larger sway amplitudes than spontaneous sway.[31–33] However, measurements of induced sway under an eyes open condition have not been shown to produce better prediction of clients who are at risk for sustaining a fall than spontaneous sway measurements.[31]

> ### Key Point:
> Changes in the location of relative center of gravity and center of pressure have to be perceived by the vestibular, somatosensory, or visual system before the neuromuscular system can respond.

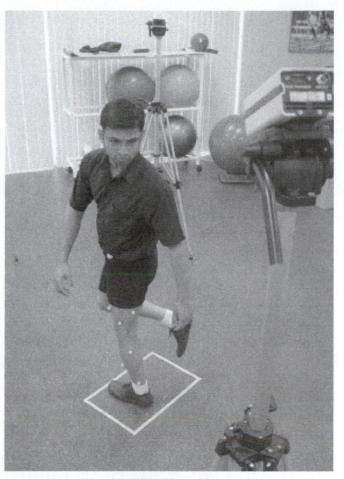

Figure 9.33 Combined kinetic and kinematic data collection during a crossover pivot maneuver.

Balance assessment through the use of a force platform can be enhanced with synchronized motion capture of kinematic data. The addition of kinematic analysis to balance evaluations enables investigators to have a better understanding of how compensatory body movements occur in an attempt to maintain balance (**Figure 9.33**).[34,35] In a comparison of static postural control between young adults (20.1 ± 2.4 years of age) and older adults (70.1 ± 4.3 years of age), Amiridis et al.[34] reported a significant difference in the maximum range of ankle, knee, and hip motion during quiet standing, with older adults displaying larger angular displacements at each joint. Similar results were observed during Romberg test performance and during one-leg stance. The hip joint displayed the greatest angular displacement difference between groups and electromyographic data at the hip displayed greater activity for the older population, suggesting greater reliance on the hip region for postural control.[34]

Other technology is available to quantify balance deficits. The EquiTest® system (NeuroCom International, Clackamas, OR) has the ability to evaluate postural stability under changing environmental conditions. The system is able to alter surface angles as well as the vertical surroundings (**Figure 9.34**). The Balance Master® (NeuroCom International, Clackamas, OR) allows for the assessment of center of pressure symmetry during quiet standing as well as during dynamic tasks such as walking, sit to stand, step over, and other tasks (**Figure 9.35**). A similar device is the Chattecx Balance System, which allows multi-planar perturbation during balance assessments.[36] Most laboratory based devices are designed to assess the influence of each of the contributing physiological systems that might create a balance deficit. A characteristic of the Balance Master® is the integration of visual biofeedback technology to enhance the training component of balance during functionally relevant activities (**Figure 9.36**).

The high cost of equipment and specialized laboratory settings may limit the use of high-technology equipment in the clinical setting. Development of clinical tests should focus on simple, low cost evaluations that can be performed in a variety of settings with considerations for the

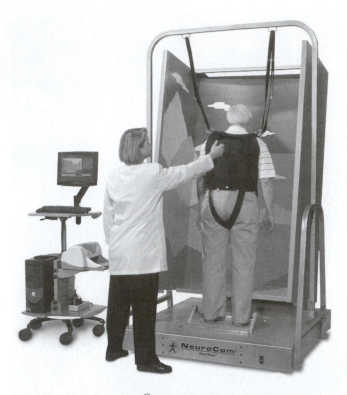

Figure 9.34   EquiTest® Computerized Dynamic Posturography. Courtesy of Neurocom International. Clackamas, Oregon, 97015.

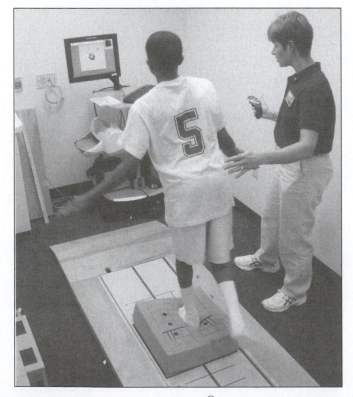

Figure 9.35   The Balance Master® system being used to train postural control during unilateral stance on a foam block.

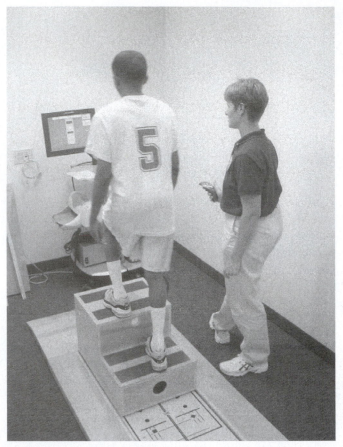

Figure 9.36   Balance Master® being used to train reciprocal stairclimbing.

clientele of primary interest. Tests and scales that have been developed for clinical use are mostly used with the purpose of initially identifying a balance deficit or assessing improvements in balance during or following therapeutic exercise program intervention. Clinical tests have limited ability to identify the systematic components that contribute to a balance disorder. A referral for a laboratory based assessment of balance complements the initial assessment and provides the rehabilitation clinician with comprehensive results identifying the cause of the balance deficiency. Examples of commonly used clinical tests often include the single leg stance test, Romberg and modified Romberg tests, the functional reach test, the Berg scale, and the Activity Specific Balance Confidence scale.

The *Single Leg Stance Test* measures static balance. Clients are timed while maintaining a predetermined posture. Modifications to this test can include changes in surface, changing head positions, changing arm positions (standard to have arms crossed in front) and including conditions with eyes open and eyes closed. This test can also be used for balance training in the clinic. Unexpected perturbations can be added to the training to challenge the individual to correct for increased displacement of the center of gravity (**Figure 9.37**).

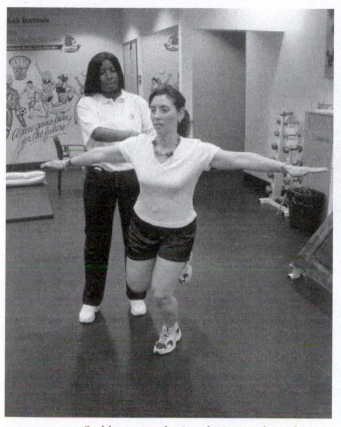

Figure 9.37   Sudden perturbation during unilateral stance.

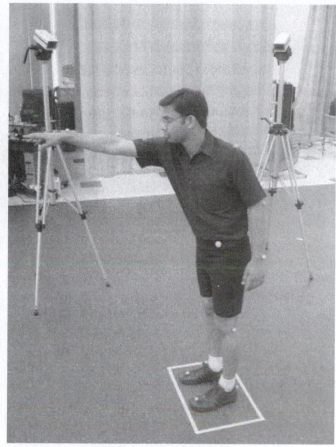

Figure 9.38   Instrumented Functional Reach Test.

The Romberg Test also measures static balance and can use modified foot placement to change the base of support, thereby increasing the difficulty of the test. All foot positions can be performed with eyes opened and eyes closed to assess the influence of the visual system during the balance task.

The *Functional Reach Test* measures balance by challenging the client to shift their center of gravity forward as they reach without losing their balance (**Figure 9.38**). The functional reach test was developed as a clinical tool to evaluate dynamic postural stability.[37] To perform this test, a yardstick or tape measure is placed parallel to the floor on a wall at the height of the client's dominant acromion process. With the client standing with the feet positioned at a comfortable distance apart, they are asked to make a fist and flex the dominant shoulder to approximately 90°. While in this position, the client is instructed to reach forward as far as possible without taking a step or touching the wall. The distance between the start and end points is measured using the head of the third metacarpal as the reference point.[37] Normative values for males and females have been reported (20–40 yrs of age: males = 16.73 in., females = 14.64 in.; 41–49 yrs of age: males = 14.98 in., females = 13.81 in.; 70–87 years of age: males = 13.16 in., females = 10.47 in.).[37] This test has been shown to be sensitive to improvements in balance following reha-

bilitation.[38] Duncan et al.[39] reported that the functional reach test displayed predictive validity for identifying recurrent fallers among elderly males; however, other studies have suggested that the functional reach test is not effective for clinically differentiating clients who are at risk for falling versus those who are not.[40–42] Wallmann[40] suggested that a decreased ability to lean forward correlated better with decreased balance than a decreased ability to reach forward.

The *Berg Functional Balance Scale* is based on 14 tasks that require different levels of dynamic balance as well as strength and flexibility. Scores for each task can range from 0 to 4 (**Table 9.1**).[43]

The *Activity Specific Balance Confidence Scale (ABC)* is a 16 item questionnaire that examines perceived confidence in mobility for some common household and community functional tasks. Subjects rate mobility confidence by circling a percentage between 0 and 100 for each of the functional activities, with higher scores indicating greater confidence in performing tasks of daily living.[44] In a study that evaluated the difference in reaction time with the Berg Functional Balance Scale scores and ABC scores of clients with and without a history of falling, Lajoie et al.[45] reported that clients with a history of falling had significantly lower scores in all three measures when compared to clients who did not have a history of falling.

TABLE 9.1   Components of the Berg Functional Balance Scale (highest possible score = 56/56)

1. _____Sit unsupported	4 = able to sit safely and securely for 2 minutes
	3 = able to sit 2 minutes with supervision
	2 = able to sit for 30 seconds
	1 = able to sit for 10 seconds
	0 = unable to sit unsupported
2. _____Sit to stand	4 = able to stand, no hands, stabilize independently
	3 = able to stand independently using hands
	2 = able to stand using hands more than one try
	1 = minimal assist to stand or stabilize
	0 = moderate to maximum assist
3. _____Stand unsupported	4 = able to stand safely for 2 minutes
	3 = able to stand 2 minutes with supervision
	2 = able to stand 30 seconds unsupported
	1 = able to stand 30 seconds after several tries
	0 = unable to stand 30 seconds unassisted
4. _____Stand eyes closed	4 = able to stand safely for 10 seconds
	3 = able to stand 10 seconds with supervision
	2 = able to stand for 3 seconds
	1 = able to stand for less than 3 seconds
	0 = needs help to keep from falling
5. _____Stand with feet together	4 = able to place feet together and stand for 1 minute
	3 = able to place feet together and stand 1 minute with supervision
	2 = able to place feet together and stand for 30 seconds
	1 = needs help to attain position but can hold for seconds
	0 = can't perform
6. _____Forward reach (arm at 90°) (_____number of inches)	4 = can reach forward confidently > 10 inches
	3 = can reach forward safely > 5 inches
	2 = can reach forward safely > 2 inches
	1 = can reach forward but needs supervision
	0 = needs help to keep from falling
7. _____Retrieve object from floor	4 = able to pick up object and stand safely and easily
	3 = picks up object but needs supervision
	2 = unable to retrieve, but within 1–2″ and maintains balance
	1 = unable to retrieve, needs supervision while trying
	0 = can't perform
8. _____Turn to look behind left and right shoulders	4 = looks behind both sides, good weight shift
	3 = looks behind one side only
	2 = turns sideways only, but maintains balance
	1 = needs supervision when turning
	0 = needs assistance to keep from falling
9. _____Turn 360°	4 = able to turn 360° safely in < 4 seconds, either direction
	3 = able to turn 360° safely in < 4 seconds, one direction only
	2 = able to turn 360° safely but > 4 seconds

TABLE 9.1   (Continued)

		1 = needs close supervision or verbal cueing
		0 = can't perform
10. _____	Alternating stool touch	4 = safely completes 8 steps in < 20 seconds
		3 = safely completes 8 steps in > 20 seconds
		2 = safely completes 4 steps
		1 = completes 2 steps, needs supervision or minimal assist
		0 = can't perform
11. _____	Heel/toe stance	4 = able to independently place feet in tandem, hold 30 seconds
		3 = able to get one foot in front of the other, hold 30 seconds
		2 = able to take small step independently, hold 30 seconds
		1 = needs help to place feet, holds for 15 seconds
		0 = can't perform
12. _____	Stand on one foot	4 = able to lift one leg and hold > 10 seconds
		3 = able to lift one leg and hold 5–10 seconds
		2 = able to lift one leg and hold for 3–5 seconds
		1 = able to lift leg but can't hold for 3 seconds
		0 = can't perform
13. _____	Stand to sit	4 = sits safely with minimal or no use of hands
		3 = controls descent with use of hands
		2 = uses back of legs against chair to control descent
		1 = sits independently but has uncontrolled descent
		0 = needs assistance to sit
14. _____	Transfers	4 = able to transfer safely with minor use of hands
		3 = able to transfer safely, must use hands
		2 = able to transfer with verbal cues or supervision
		1 = one person to assist
		0 = two person assist

From KO Berg, SL Wood-Dauphinee, JI Williams, Maki B. Measuring balance in the elderly: validation of an instrument. *Can J Public Health.* 1992,83:S7–S11.

Client balance tests can be modified by changing the surface material the client stands on. Variable density foam blocks or incline/decline slant boards can be used effectively to modify the testing environment. Slight modification of the environment is a common tactic used clinically when training and evaluating a client's balance. Since the visual and auditory systems are involved in postural control, the influence of sensory integration in the assessment of balance has received greater attention in recent years.

Sensory systems are affected with age, leading to a decrease in postural control and an increase risk of falls. As a result of a 30 percent incidence of community-dwelling older subjects over 65 years of age falling at least one time per year, research has focused on identifying the mechanisms that contribute to the high risk of fall among this group and the development of prediction models that will help identify clients who are specifically at risk. Some of the previously mentioned technologies have been used to study postural control in the older population; however, dynamic postural control can also play a substantial role in understanding the decline in balance with age. Several studies have evaluated the relationship between static measurements of balance with gait related measures.[46,47] Older clients often refer to the reduction of dynamic balance as unsteadiness. By revisiting the requirements of normal gait, one can understand the complexity of the neuromuscular coordination required to maintain a steady gait pattern.

As an individual gets older there tends to be a reduction in the range of motion at all joints; there is also a reduction in the ground reaction force generation and a slower response to postural changes. Mechanical adaptations result from the combination of all of these factors, leading to slower gait, shorter stride length, and wider step width. Research has shown a high correlation between clinical measures of balance and active and passive ankle range of motions.[48] A reduction in ankle range of motion might lead to use of other joints as primary controllers of postural sway (see Chapter 6). An M-shaped vertical ground reaction force in elderly females with knee joint osteoarthritis was shown to correlate with superior functional reach test scores and timed up and go test scores.[49] The mechanical adaptations that lead to a less dynamic gait pattern may also lead to a decrease in overall function, including a decrease in balance performance.

Key Point:

The mechanical adaptations that lead to a less dynamic walking gait pattern may also suggest decreased overall function, including impaired balance, particularly among older individuals.

Abnormal posture in gait has also been shown to correlate with poor functional reach scores and timed up and go test scores in the elderly.[50] The *Get Up and Go test* was developed by Mathias and Nayak[51] as a quick tool to detect balance problems among elderly clients. The test involves rising from a chair, walking 3 m (118.11 inches), turning, and returning to the chair. The client is scored on a scale of one to five, with one being normal and five being severely abnormal. A score of three or higher suggests an increased fall risk. The *Timed Up and Go test* is essentially the same test, but with proficiency based on the time required to complete the circuit.[52] Neurologically non-impaired adults who are independent in balance and mobility skills are able to complete the course in less than

10 seconds.[53] Adults who take longer than 30 seconds to complete the test tend to be dependent in most activities of daily living and mobility skills. Placing the individual in challenging environments allows the rehabilitation clinician to gain a better understanding of how dynamic balance might be affected.

Some research has focused on obstacles or changes in surfaces, requiring the client to change motion patterns to adjust to the environment.[54,55] The *Emory Functional Ambulation Profile* (E-FAP) measures time to walk over an array of different surfaces and obstacles. In a study to evaluate the reliability and validity of this test among clients who had experienced a stroke, the results showed a strong negative correlation between the E-FAP and timed 10-meter walk test scores and Berg Functional Balance Scale scores.[55]

The impact of the visual system on balance has been shown through movement adaptations during single leg stance test performance. Auditory stimuli have also been shown to affect balance in the elderly population with a laterally moving auditory signal producing an increase in lateral sway.[56]

Balance and strength training and exercise can improve balance among the elderly population. However, it is a good idea to perform a *Mini-Mental State Examination* (MMSE) among clients over 65 years of age to evaluate their level of cognition prior to designing a specific therapeutic exercise intervention to improve balance.[57]

Balance training has been shown to improve static balance function, while gait training has been shown to improve dynamic balance.[58] Among clients with osteoarthritis, decreased lower extremity strength and decreased proprioception-kinesthesia lead to decreased static and dynamic balance. Strength training (Chapter 5) and aerobic walking (Chapter 4) have been shown to decrease body sway in clients who have lower extremity osteoarthritis.[59] Tai Chi training has also been found to improve balance control and functional mobility among older adults (see Chapter 10).[60,61]

Summary

Agility requires a combination of body and spatial awareness, neuromuscular coordination, reaction time, speed, and power (strength/time). These components have different influences in overall agility throughout the life span. Static balance is the ability to resist linear and angular motion. A high level of neuromuscular coordination and balance are necessary to maintain a smooth pattern of movement during the performance of activities that require agility.

Biomechanical demands on the lower extremities increase as a result of speed and more acute directional changes. Agility tasks that combine sprinting and sharp di-

rectional changes greatly increase the biomechanical demands placed throughout the lower extremities. Agility and balance training programs should include exercises that improve proprioception-kinesthesia (see Chapter 7), postural control (see Chapters 5, 6, and 7), speed control, and acceleration-deceleration control. During the early stages of a therapeutic exercise program, agility activities should be performed slowly and initiated only after the client has demonstrated that they are capable of passing static balance tests. With the appropriate progression, the client can advance to activity specific agility tasks at full speed.

References

1. Young WB, James R, Montgomery I. Is muscle power related to running speed with changes of direction?. *J Sports Med Phys Fitness.* 2002;42:282–288.

2. Hilsendager DR, Strow MH, Ackerman KJ. Comparison of speed, strength and agility exercises in the development of agility. *Res Q.* 1969;40:71–75.

3. Thissen-Milder M, Mayhew JL. Selection and classification of high school volleyball players from performance tests. *J Sports Med Phys Fitness.* 1991; 31:380–384.

4. Judge JO, Ounpuu S, Davis III RB. Effects of age on the biomechanics and physiology of gait. *Clin Geriatr Med.* 1996;12:659–679.

5. Netz Y, Argov E. Assessment of functional fitness among independent older adults: A preliminary report. *Percept Mot Skills.* 1997;84:1059–1074.

6. Turner CH. Toward a cure for osteoporosis: Reversal of excessive bone fragility. *Osteoporo Int.* 1991;2:12–19.

7. Bravo G, Gauthier P, Roy P, et al. Impact of a 12-month exercise program on the physical and psychological health of osteopenic women. *J Am Geriatr Soc.* 1996;44:756–762.

8. Bravo G, Gauthier P, Roy P, et al. A weight-bearing, water based exercise program for osteopenic women: Its impact on bone, functional fitness, and well-being. *Arch Phys Med Rehabil.* 1997;78:1375–1380.

9. Kerschan-Schindl K, Uher E, Grampp S, et al. A neuromuscular test battery for osteoporotic women. *Am J Phys Med Rehabil.* 2001;80:351–357.

10. Soutas-Little RW, Inman DJ. *Engineering Mechanics: Dynamics.* Upper Saddle River, NJ: Prentice Hall, 1998.

11. Soutas-Little RW. Center of pressure plots for clinical use. *The Winter Annual Meeting of the American Society of Mechanical Engineers Proceedings,* 1987.

12. Mann RA. *Biomechanics of Running:* In Nicholas JA Hershman EB (ed.). *The Lower Extremity and Spine in Sports Medicine* (2nd ed.), vol. 1. St. Louis: Mosby, 1995.

13. Walker JA. Does rigid body limit maneuverability? *J Exp Biol.* 2000;203:3391–3396.

14. Alfredson H, Pietla T, Jonsson P, Lorentzon R. Heavy-load eccentric calf muscle training for the treatment of chronic Achilles tendinosis. *Am J Sports Med.* 1998;26(3):360–366.

15. Ohberg L, Lorentzon R, Alfredson H. Eccentric training in patients with chronic Achilles tendinosis: Normalized tendon structure and decreased thickness at follow-up. *Br J Sports Med.* 2004;38(1):8–11.

16. Pigeon P, Bortolami SB, DiZio P, Lackner JR. Coordinated turn-and-reach movements: II. Planning in an external frame of reference. *J Neurophysiol.* 2003; 89:290–303.

17. Adamovich SV, Archambault PS, Ghafouri M, et al. Hand trajectory invariance in reaching movements involving the trunk. *Exp Brain Res.* 2001; 138:288–303.

18. Ghafouri M, Archambault PS, Adamovich SV, Feldman AG. Pointing movements may be produced in different frames of reference depending on the task demand. *Brain Res.* 2002;929:117–128.

19. Alberts JL, Saling M, Stelmach GE. Alterations in transport path differentially affect temporal and spatial movement parameters. *Exp Brain Res.* 2002; 143:417–425.

20. Young WB, McDowell MH, Scarlett BJ. Specificity of sprint and agility training methods. *J Strength Cond Res.* 2001;15:315–319.

21. Wojtys EM, Huston LJ. Neuromuscular performance in normal and anterior cruciate ligament deficient lower extremities. *Am J Sports Med.* 1994; 22:89–104.

22. Wojtys EM, Huston LJ, Taylor PD, Bastian SD. Neuromuscular adaptations in isokinetic, isotonic and agility training programs. *Am J Sports Med.* 1996;24:187–192.

23. Curl WW, Markey KL, Mitchell WA. Agility training following anterior cruciate ligament reconstruction. *Clin Orthop.* 1983;172:133–136.

24. Shelbourne KD, Davis TJ. Evaluation of knee stability before and after participation in a functional sports agility program during rehabilitation after anterior cruciate ligament reconstruction. *Am J Sports Med.* 1999;27:156–161.

25. Sailors ME, Keskula DR, Perrin DH. Effect of running on anterior knee laxity in collegiate-level female athletes after anterior cruciate ligament reconstruction. *J Orthop Sports Phys Ther.* 1995;21: 233–239.

26. Fitzgerald GK, Axe MJ, Snyder-Mackler L. The efficacy of perturbation training in nonoperative anterior cruciate ligament rehabilitation programs for physically active individuals. *Phys Ther.* 2000;80:128–140.

27. Risberg MA, Mork M, Jenssen HK, Holm I. Design and implementation of a neuromuscular training program following anterior cruciate ligament reconstruction. *J Orthop Sports Phys Ther.* 2001;31:620–631.

28. Henriksson M, Ledin T, Good L. Postural control after anterior cruciate ligament reconstruction and functional rehabilitation. *Am J Sports Med.* 2001;29 (3):359–366.

29. Nakayama Y, Shirai Y, Narita T, et al. Knee functions and a return to sports activity in competitive athletes following anterior cruciate ligament reconstruction. *J Nippon Med Sch.* 2000;67:172–176.

30. Nichols DS, Glenn TM, Hutchinson KJ. Changes in the mean center of balance during balance testing in young adults. *Phys Ther*. 1995;75:699–706.

31. Maki BE, Holliday PJ, Fernie GR. Aging and postural control. A comparison of spontaneous and induced-sway balance tests. *J Am Geriatr Soc*. 1990;58:1–9.

32. Wollacott MP, Shumway-Cook AT, Nasher LM. Changes in the postural response system with aging. *Soc Neurosci Abstr*. 1982;8:838.

33. Wolfson LI, Whipple R, Amerman P, Kleinberg A. Stressing the postural response a quantitative method for testing balance. *J Am Geriatr Soc*. 1986; 34:845–850.

34. Amiridis IG, Halzitaki V, Arabatzi F. Age-induced modifications of static postural control in humans. *Neurosci Let*. 2003;350:137–140.

35. Hahn ME, Chou L. Can motion of individual body segments identify dynamic instability in the elderly? *Clin Biomech*. 2003;18:737–744.

36. Rogind H, Simonsen H, Era P, Bliddal H. Comparison of Kistler 9861A, force platform and Chattecx Balance System for measurement of postural sway: Correlation and test-retest reliability. *Scan J Med Sci Sports* . 2003;13:106–114.

37. Duncan PW, Weiner DK, Chandler J, Studenski S. Functional reach: A new clinical measure of balance. *J Gerontol*. 1990;45:M192–197.

38. Weiner DK, Bongiorni DR, Studenski SA, et al. Does functional reach improve with rehabilitation? *Arch Phys Med Rehabil*. 1993;74:796–800.

39. Duncan PW, Studenski S, Chandler J, Prescott B. Functional reach: Predictive validity in a sample of elderly male veterans. *J Gerontol*. 1992;47:M93–98.

40. Wallman HW. Comparison of elderly nonfallers and fallers on performance measures of functional reach, sensory organization and limits of stability. *J Gerontol*. 2001;56A:M580–M583.

41. Wernick-Robinson M, Krebs DE, Giorgetti MM. Functional reach: Does it really measure dynamic balance? *Arch Phys Med Rehabil*. 1999;80:262–269.

42. Cho CY, Kamen G. Detecting balance deficits in frequent fallers using clinical and quantitative evaluation tools. *J Am Geriatr Soc*. 1998; 46:426–430.

43. Berg KO, Wood-Dauphinee SL, Williams JI, Maki B. Measuring balance in the elderly: Validation of an instrument. *Can J Public Health*. 1992;83:S7–S11.

44. Powell LE, Myers AM. The Activities-specific Balance Confidence (ABC) Scale. *J Gerontol A Biol Sci Med Sci*. 1995;50A(1): M28–34.

45. Lajoie Y, Girard A, Guay M. Comparison of the reaction time, the Berg Scale and the ABC in non-fallers and fallers. *Arch Gerontol Geriatr*. 2002;35:215–225.

46. Cho CY, Kamen G. Detecting balance deficits in frequent fallers using clinical and quantitative evaluation tools. *J Am Geriatr Soc*. 1998;46:426–430.

47. Whitney S, Wrisley D, Furman J. Concurrent validity of the Berg Balance Scale and the Dynamic Gait Index in people with vestibular dysfunction. *Physiother Res Int*. 2003;8:178–186.

48. Mecagni C, Smith JP, Roberts KE, O'Sullivan SB. Balance and ankle range of motion in community-dwelling women aged 64 to 87: A correlational study. *Phys Ther*. 2000;80:1004–1011.

49. Takahashi T, Ishida K, Hirose D, et al. Vertical ground reaction force shape is associated with gait parameters, timed up and go, and functional reach in elderly females. *J Rehabil Med*. 2004;36:42–45.

50. Hirose D, Ishida K, Nagano Y, et al. Posture of the trunk in the sagittal plane is associated with gait in community-dwelling elderly population. *Clin Biomech*. 2004;19:57–63.

51. Mathias S, Nayak U, Issacs B. Balance in elderly patients: The "Get-up and Go" Test. *Arch Phys Med Rehabil*. 1986;67:387–389.

52. Podsiadlo D, Richardson S. The timed "Up & Go": A test of basic functional mobility for frail elderly persons. *J Am Geriatr Soc*. 1991;39:142–148.

53. Mahoney RI, Barthel DW. Functional evaluation: The Barthel Index. *MD State Med J*. 1965;14:61–65.

54. Means KM. The obstacle course: a tool for the assessment of functional balance and mobility in the elderly. *J Rehabil Res Dev*. 1996;33:413–429.

55. Wolf SL, Catlin PA, Gage K, et al. Establishing the reliability and validity of measurement of walking time using the Emory Functional Ambulation Profile. *Phys Ther*. 1999;79:1122–1133.

56. Tanaka T, Kojima S, Tadeka H, et al. The influence of moving auditory stimuli on standing balance in healthy young adults and the elderly. *Ergonomics*. 2001;44:1403–1412.

57. Bravo G, Hebert R. Age- and education-specific reference values for the Mini-Mental and modified Mini-Mental State Examinations derived from a non-demented elderly populations. *Int J Geriatr Psych*. 1997;12(10):1008–1018.

58. Hiroyuki S, Uchiyama Y, Kakurai S. Specific effects of balance and gait exercises on physical function among the frail elderly. *Clin Rehabil*. 2003;17: 472–479.

59. Messier SP, Royer TD, Craven TE, et al. Long-term exercise and its effect on balance in older, osteoarthritic adults: Results from the fitness, arthritis and seniors trial (FAST). *J Am Geriatr Soc*. 2000; 48:131–138.

60. Tsang WN, Hui-Chan C. Effect of 4- and 8-wk intensive Tai Chi training on balance control in the elderly. *Med Sci Sports Exerc*. 2004;36:648–657.

61. Hartman CA, Manos TM, Winter C, et al. Effects of Tai Chi training on function and quality of life indicators in older adults with osteoarthritis. *J Am Geriatr Soc*. 2000;48:1553–1559.

10

Complementary and Alternative Approaches to Movement and Exercise

THERESA J. KRAEMER

Objectives

The reader will be able to:

- Define the terms complementary and alternative therapeutic exercise approaches.
- Explain the similarities and differences between traditional exercises and complementary and alternative therapeutic exercise approaches.
- Summarize the Structural Functional Integrative Movement approach to therapeutic exercise.
- Compare and contrast the various complementary and alternative therapeutic exercise approaches.

- Discuss indications, contraindications, and safety factors related to each of the complementary and alternative therapeutic exercise approaches.
- Describe the basic techniques associated with each complementary and alternative therapeutic exercise approach.
- List factors that can be varied in a progression of each complementary and alternative therapeutic exercise approach.
- Outline a sample complementary and alternative therapeutic exercise program for a given specific diagnosis.

Outline

(continued)

INTRODUCTION

After World War II, the field of physical medicine and rehabilitation evolved in response to the fact that mainstream medicine was not providing adequate care and treatment for clients who had sustained musculoskeletal and central nervous system injuries. Henry H. Kessler, a pioneering physician in physical medicine and rehabilitation, advocated the need for supplemental therapies, many of which today would be referred to as alternative or complementary.[1] Kessler not only included physical and dietary interventions in his multi-disciplinary approach, he also recognized the importance that spirituality played in the healing process. Unfortunately, the lack of scientific evidence for these non-conventional or unorthodox therapies tended to brand their usage as a form of less rigorous medical practice.[2]

Despite the conservative nature of mainstream, or so-called Western medicine, the role of complementary and alternative therapeutic exercise approaches in the practice of medicine and in the realm of health, wellness, prevention, and rehabilitation has gone from an almost non-existent presence just a decade or two ago to a rapidly increasing and sometimes controversial component of today's health care options and practices.[2] This change is, in part, a response to several recent trends in health care, including a heightened interest in, and intense scrutiny of, individualized client care plans, the need to address and incorporate client issues arising from cultural diversity,

the call for improved pain management, and the demand for control of spiraling health care costs.[1] Much of this change has occurred since 1991, when a national cross-sectional survey of United States residents was published. The survey reported that more than one-third of respondents were using non-conventional therapies, that they were paying more money out of pocket for alternative therapies than for traditional medical therapies, and that they made more visits to providers of non-conventional therapy than to all primary care physicians (family practitioners, pediatricians, and internists) combined.[3] Furthermore, the survey found that nearly 90 percent of people who sought alternative therapy did so without permission of their primary care physician and more than 60 percent of respondents did not tell their primary health care provider that they were using complementary, alternative, or nontraditional therapies. Seven years later, a follow-up survey discovered that these patterns persisted, but that the percentage of people using alternative therapies had increased, while the lack of disclosure to the primary physician remained about the same.[4]

The same trend can be seen in rehabilitation care, due in large part to the chronicity of the various conditions treated with physical and rehabilitative medicine. A survey in 1995 found that of 401 individuals who had recently used outpatient rehabilitation services in New York, 57 percent had used a complementary or alternative therapy, and their patterns of usage and non-disclosure to a primary care physician were similar to those reported in the other studies.[3,4] More recent studies have shown that two-thirds of people in the United States and Canada utilize some form of complementary and alternative therapy to prevent and treat disease.[5]

Shiflett et al[6] reported that clients who participated in long term rehabilitation consider trying complementary and alternative therapies for several reasons, including: 1) having experienced an adverse reaction with traditional Western medicine and its treatment approaches and interventions; 2) the extent of these symptoms and their disabling effects; and 3) a value system that involves participation in their own health care. Interestingly enough, dissatisfaction with conventional medical care was not a factor in the decision to seek out alternative interventions. Additional reasons for why clients seek out and use complementary and alternative therapies include 1) the fact that most are non-invasive; 2) the growing body of evidence supporting their utilization; 3) their use of a holistic approach, focusing on the whole person (not solely the signs and symptoms); 4) the fact that most practitioners create and tailor an individual client treatment plan; 5) the fact that most alternative treatments have few or no side effects; and 6) the feeling of many clients with chronic complaints, for whom traditional interventions have been ineffective, that they have nothing to lose.[5,7] Another reason for the surge in the utilization of complementary and alternative therapies stems from the shift in the health care system towards managed care and health maintenance organizations (HMOs). This shift has placed greater emphasis on the prevention of disease and on health maintenance.

Recent Events

In 1991, Congress mandated the establishment of the first government office, the Office of Alternative Medicine, to focus on alternative health care practices within the National Institutes of Health (NIH).[2,8] The original charge of the Office of Alternative Medicine was to: 1) encourage the study of the wide variety of complementary and alternative therapies; 2) begin separating fact from fallacy and evidence from chicanery; and 3) present this information to the public, policy makers, and professional communities. Since then, the office has established numerous research centers in academic and medical institutions in the

United States, to study and teach various complementary and alternative therapies. In 1998, the Office of Alternative Medicine, although still part of the NIH, was renamed the National Center for Complementary and Alternative Medicine (NCCAM).[8] The budget for NCCAM has steadily increased, and new research centers and projects continue to be established. **Table 10.1** provides examples of the research projects that have been funded, and **Table 10.2** lists some of the academic centers and their areas of research.

As part of its evolution from the Office of Alternative Medicine to the NCCAM, the NCCAM was given the authority to grant funding for projects within the NIH, which stimulated scholarly research and inquiry in a wide variety of areas. It also developed working relationships with a number of other NIH institutes, with focused interest on physical medicine and rehabilitation, including the National Institute of Neurological Disorders and Stroke (NINDS), the National Institute of Arthritis and Musculoskeletal and Skin Diseases (NIAMS), and the National Center of Medical Rehabilitation Research (NCMRR).[2]

In 2000, President Clinton created a White House Commission on Complementary and Alternative Modality Policy to consider complementary and alternative modality applications.[9] This policy included exploring the utilization, consistency, and quality of various complementary and alternative therapeutic interventions. One consequence of establishing this commission is that there now exists a need to develop clinically relevant policies, procedures, protocols, and tools as well as to locate appropriate funding resources. The operating budget for complementary and alternative medicine is expected to continue to grow with each fiscal year, but due to limited appropriations, the NCCAM prioritizes its research programs according to the relative use of a modality, the evidence supporting its value and safety, and the opportunities available to advance the relevant field of science. Current NCCAM projects are investigating Tai Chi exercise, biofeedback, Qigong, acupuncture, meditation, spirituality, various herbal remedies (i.e., ginkgo biloba), and Reiki (pronounced RAY-kee), just to name a few.

Over the past 20 years, complementary and alternative medicine has become big business, not just in terms of the government agencies that have been established, but also with respect to the preferences of the average American

TABLE 10.1   Between 1993 and 1997, the National Institutes of Health's Office of Alternative Medicine awarded grants for research on the following complementary and alternative movement therapies

Research	Condition
Dance and movement therapy	Cystic fibrosis
Qigong	Late stage complex regional pain syndrome
Tai Chi Chuan	Balance disorders
Yoga	Obsessive-compulsive disorder

TABLE 10.2   Research centers established by the NCCAM

Location of research center	Area of research
Harvard	General medicine
Columbia	Women's health
Stanford	Aging
University of Arizona	Pediatrics
University of Texas	Cancer
Bastyr University, Seattle, Washington	HIV/AIDS
Kessler Institute of Rehabilitation, West Orange, New Jersey	Neurological conditions/stroke
Hennepin County Hospital, Minneapolis, Minnesota	Addictions
University of Michigan	Cardiovascular conditions
University of Maryland and University of Virginia	Pain/back pain
University of California–Davis	Asthma/allergies/immunology

client and the ever-changing environment of health care. It is realistic to anticipate that the inclusion of complementary and alternative approaches will become more commonplace within the Western medical health care system. Therefore, the rehabilitation clinician must become familiar with some of the more common clinical complementary and alternative therapeutic movement approaches if he or she is to provide consistent care.

Terminology

Terms such as complementary, alternative, non-traditional and unconventional are often used interchangeably in the media and in medical literature to denote healing practices that have not typically been part of Western medical practice or taught in mainstream medical schools or allied health curriculums. Unfortunately, when pertaining to medical interventions, a number of different and often unintended meanings and connotations occur, leading to confusion and negative reactions. "Alternative" is an especially confusing term because it usually means "instead of," as in an intervention provided in place of traditional medical treatments[9] and has the connotation of being questionable, suspect, or bogus.[2] However, alternative medicine can also refer to a wide range of treatments and practices not traditionally used or recommended within the mainstream biomedical community. Criteria that define this status can include whether or not it is offered in medical settings, taught in medical schools, requires licensure to practice, and is reimbursed by third party payers.[2] While these standards worked well 10 years ago, they are quickly losing relevance as more and more health care professionals and medical settings are providing various complementary and alternative therapies to their clients. That is, more and more interventions formerly thought of as alternative have become accepted as "normal."[10] Some

examples of alternative interventions include dietary regimens (e.g., cancer treatment), the use of herbal supplements (e.g., to reduce arthritic pain or enhance memory), and massage therapy or chiropractic interventions (e.g., for vertebral disk problems).[9] The list of services that NCCAM considers complementary or alternative continues to expand as more interventions establish a track record of safe and effective use.

The term complementary has been recommended as a way to get around the unfortunate and often negative connotations associated with "alternative." However, historically, the term complementary was used to describe interventions that enhanced the effects of traditional medical modalities, interventions, and care by decreasing pain, easing discomfort, relieving anxiety, and reducing stress.[9] *Complementary medicine* therefore has been defined as the use of non-traditional modalities or interventions jointly with conventional medical approaches.

Other commonly used terms include unconventional and unorthodox. However, these terms have a critical and often derogatory connotation. In fact, there is no adjective that entirely or adequately describes "new" therapeutic approaches. Most practitioners of these therapies prefer the term complementary because they believe the other terms have negative connotations, implying the use of unproven practices. Some practitioners make the following distinction: They define *alternative therapies* as those that are used instead of conventional or mainstream therapy and *complementary therapies* as those used in conjunction with conventional therapy.

In today's medical environment, complementary and alternative therapeutic approaches utilized in conjunction with traditional medical interventions are preferably referred to as *integrative medicine* or *integrative approaches*[11,12] because these terms permit traditional health care professionals and complementary and alternative practitioners to recognize the value of one another's expertise; allow for collaboration in designing wide ranging, holistic, and comprehensive treatment plans; and not only realistically describe the integration of traditional and complementary approaches but also allow for scientific exploration and explanation of the physiological changes that occur as a result of participating in various complementary and alternative therapeutic interventions (**Table 10.3**).

CLASSIFICATION SYSTEM

Seven major categories or fields of practice for complementary and alternative therapeutic interventions have been identified by the NCCAM: 1) alternative medical systems; 2) mind-body interventions; 3) biologically based therapies; 4) manipulative, manual healing, and body-based methods; 5) bioelectromagnetic (energy-based) modalities; 6) herbal medicine; and 7) diet and nutrition therapies.[8,11] The first, *alternative medical systems*, include systems that, for the most part, existed before the development of the conventional Western approach to medical treatment. They include systems developed in the West (e.g., homeopathy), the Far East (e.g., Chinese medicine), and India (e.g., ayurveda) as well as naturopathy, homeopathy, osteopathy, and environmental medicine. The *mind-body domain* is based on the philosophical belief that there exists an overwhelming interconnectedness between the body and mind and that each can have an effect on the other. Examples of such therapies include biofeedback, meditation, hypnosis, Yoga, Tai Chi, Qigong, guided imagery, mental healing, prayer, psychotherapy, music therapy, dance therapy, and art therapy. *Biologically based therapies* encompass biological and pharmacological modalities through the invasive administration of active chemical or natural substances into the body. Examples include chelation therapy, shark cartilage and anti-neoplastons, and neural therapy. *Manipulative and body-based methods* are becoming more and more common and involve techniques in which the practitioner either touches or manipulates the body in some way to improve body structure and function. Examples include chiropractic manipulation, therapeutic massage, reflexology, therapeutic touch, Rolfing, Qigong, and the Alexander, Feldenkrais, and Trager techniques. *Bioelectromagnetic (energy) therapies* are based on the theory that changes in the body's electromagnetic field can produce specific changes in the body's tissues. Examples include bioelectromagnetic interventions, bio-field interventions, transcutaneous electrical nerve stimulation, transcranial electrostimulation, pulsed electromagnetic fields, Qigong, and Reiki.[9,11] *Herbal medicine* is one of the oldest methods of healing, involves natural remedies or products that stem from herbs and plants, and is still used by many cultures around the world. Examples include herbal medications, dietary supplements, special diets, and vitamin products. *Diet and nutrition therapy* involves diet changes from high fat, processed and refined foods to a diet centered on whole foods (foods that are not refined, extracted, processed or made with synthetic chemicals), fresh fruits, and vegetables. Examples include the various therapeutic diets aimed at treating or preventing cancer (i.e., Hoxsey, Gerson, Kelley, Livingston, macrobiotic), and heart disease (i.e., Pritikin, Ornish), fasting, juice therapy, and enzyme therapy.[11]

Several of the complementary and alternative therapeutic interventions cross domains, however. For example, Qigong falls into the categories of alternative medical systems, mind-body interventions, and energy-based modalities. Hence, a more accurate and current term to describe these cross-domain techniques is the *Structural Functional Integrative Movement* approach[8] that is referred to in the clinical environment as the complementary and alternative therapeutic movement approach.

The structural functional integrative movement approach gains its name from each of its individual components. It is very similar to applied kinesiology in that it sees a relationship between tissue reaction and disease in

TABLE 10.3   Complementary and alternative medical therapy approaches vs. conventional medicine

Complementary and alternative medical therapy approach	Conventional medical approach
Observational	Experimental (empirical)
Qualitative/quantitative	Quantitative
Vitalistic and naturalistic	Mechanical–technical
Holistic	Reductionist
Placebo effect is considered to be "evidence" of the mind's role in disease and healing	Placebo effect is considered to be "evidence" of the power of suggestion
Combined movements	Isolated movements
Functional patterns	Linear patterns

Information from *Nurse's Handbook of Alternative and Complementary Therapies*. Springhouse, PA: Springhouse Corp., 1998.

the body, believes in a triad of health (body structure, psychology, and nutrition), and meshes energy and meridian-based therapy (discussed later) into the treatment plan.[8] While applied kinesiology tests the balance between mechanically opposed muscles, structural functional integrative movement seeks to evaluate the body in functional postures, positions, actions, or motions. However, applied kinesiology and structural functional integrative movement approaches are similar in that they both seek to improve function of the entire body and are particularly useful in analyzing musculoskeletal problems.[8] "Structural" refers to the anatomical, biomechanical, physiological, and kinematic aspects of the movement. This component focuses on the anatomical and biomechanical interactions between the musculoskeletal and neuromuscular systems. It also calls for the rehabilitation clinician to consider the physiological implications of movement on various tissues, organs, and systems as well as the impact of fatigue, injury, and aging.

"Functional" refers to practical, efficient, purposeful, active, and organized ways of completing activities of daily living, including athletic events, via the utilization of one's own body weight. It also involves both the physiological systems and biomechanics, especially the kinetic chains (see Chapter 5).[13] It is the kinetic chains that play a major role in what is commonly referred to as function or skill.[13] The functional aspect of this approach deals with maintenance of both proximal and distal stability, mobility, and core stabilization with or without peripheral segment movement and the utilization of the kinetic chain (see Chapters 5 and 6). It also requires that multiple muscle groups and joint segments be used simultaneously. In addition, since every functional or athletic movement involves coordinated activity by various physiological and biomechanical systems, this component allows the rehabilitation clinician to observe the client as they complete particular movement patterns to identify any existing or residual biomechanical deficits, incomplete sequencing of specific motor control movement patterns (see Chapter 8), or insufficiencies and instabilities in the kinetic chain.

Alterations in the kinetic chain can result in changes in joint stability (see Chapter 6), alterations in the joint axis of rotation, changes in forces and application of forces across the joints, inefficient transfer of forces and energy, muscle adhesions, inadequate or poorly balanced muscle strength and force coupling across the joints, especially during functional activities. If the system is not adequately adjusted, anatomical and biomechanical deficits can result in injury, instability, maladaptive movement patterns, or impaired performance.[13] Once an injury, disease, or chronic dysfunction is evident, it is important to remember that the adaptations, which occur in the biomechanical system, take place not only locally, but distally. The identification of biomechanical or physiological deficits as well as normalization and functional restoration of movement are the key components of the structural functional

integrative movement approach to injury prevention and rehabilitation. Within this context, integrative refers to synergistic upper and lower body muscle activation through the core (see Chapter 5).

Integrative medicine was a term suggested by Dr. Andrew Weil to define a synergistic combination of complementary and conventional medical treatment approaches.[8] *Integrative* includes three factors. First, it involves synergistic activation of the entire body (as opposed to an isolated limb) and its effect on individual organs and systems during each therapeutic exercise movement. Second and central to the integrative concept is the mind-body-energy connection and the effect that movements have on it (discussed in greater detail later in this chapter). Third and perhaps most important, it refers to a process and method of care that uses both conventional diagnosis and treatment methods that are complementary and alternative. According to Sierpina,[12] the term *integrative* represents a paradigm shift from the traditional model of health care delivery. The concept of integrative health care includes: 1) patient- or client-centered care; 2) the joining of mind, body, and spirit, which are mutually essential to the healing of whole persons; 3) a goal of promoting vibrant health, wellness, and the highest potential for human beings, not just treating disease; 4) using natural, less invasive approaches whenever possible; 5) accepting that health and healing are individually determined and may be different for each person, and that a person may be healed without being cured; and 6) encouragement of self-care and personal responsibility for health. However, it also addresses the issues of openness to using complementary or alternative therapies that have a record of safety and efficacy but are outside of the conventional biomedical model and collaborative partnerships involving interdisciplinary teams of health-care providers and the client and the application of evidence-based, critical thinking skills when integrating alternative therapies with conventional therapies.

The structural functional integrative movement approach therefore not only includes a shift toward a more holistic therapeutic exercise philosophy by calling for the blending of traditional and complementary or alternative approaches, but it focuses on: 1) physical body structure (i.e., anthropometrics, posture, flexibility, functional strength, balance, coordination, control); 2) how the body moves as a whole; 3) the means by which the body and its subtle energy system integrates body awareness and body movement control in relation to gravity; and 4) the process by which the physical components of the body (i.e., muscles, joints), the neurological system, and the emotional framework balance as well as complement each other as the client completes both simple and complex functional movements.[8,12,13] Regardless of which structural functional integrative movement approach is used, all involve movement (mobility, stability, transitions), many entail enhancing the client's awareness of the physical body, several can be conducted in a group format using verbal instructions, and a few involve physical touch by a facilitator.

The benefits of using complementary and alternative movement therapies in the rehabilitation process is that they: 1) allow a comprehensive approach to rehabilitation; 2) encourage both local and distal segments in the kinetic chain to be restored; 3) promote the identification and resolution of biomechanical deficits; 4) support the normalization of inflexibility, muscle strength, and force coupling; and 5) reinforce the utilization of core stabilization throughout the entire process (see Chapters 5, 6, and 11). Functional activities also allow for the restoration of strength with balance and coordination during static positions and transitional movements, force generation and absorption, flexibility and proprioception, and retraining of the entire kinetic chain.

This chapter presents examples from some of today's more frequently utilized complementary and alternative therapeutic movement approaches, including dance therapy, Feldenkrais, Nickolaus, Pilates, Qigong, Tai Chi, and Yoga, all of which fall under the category of the Structural Functional Integrative Movement approach. All of the movement approaches discussed in this chapter are health based and focused on holistic, psychosomatic, and physical training techniques to promote good health, and restore physical strength, balance, coordination, prowess, and awareness levels for everyday life, prevention of injury, rehabilitation, and athletic performance. Each of these approaches calls for neuromuscular coordination, diaphragmatic breathing exercises, and mental concentration. All of the approaches discussed can be used in group and individual formats and are designed for completion on a non-clinical independent basis. The reader is forewarned, however, that most types of mind-body exercises such as these lack a strong research base. There are relatively few controlled studies and it is often difficult to draw strong conclusions regarding their clinical effectiveness because of conflicting data, poor study design quality, small sample sizes, lack of control or comparison groups, potential Hawthorne effects (behavior changes because the client knows they are being measured), or because some studies use multimodal interventions.[14]

Basic Concepts Behind Complementary and Alternative Movement Approaches

Mind-Body-Energy Connection

For thousands of years, the idea of addressing the body's subtle energy system, more commonly known now as electromagnetic energy, along with the need to enhance the client's level of consciousness has been an integral part of Eastern holistic healing (e.g., Tai Chi, Qigong, Yoga). More recently, complementary and alternative therapeutic movement approaches (e.g., Feldenkrais, Pilates) have begun to address this concept as well. Central to the concept of the body's subtle energy system is the idea of "invisible energy" located within and coursing through the body.[15,16] It is believed that this invisible energy can be enhanced, manipulated, redirected, or unblocked, a concept supported in Eastern medical systems by the idea that life energy flows throughout the body along channels.

Western health care has traditionally preferred to think of energy in terms of the electrochemical energy of the nerves and Western movement therapies have traditionally relegated energy to two groups: the application of energy to the body (i.e., transcutaneous electrical nerve stimulation) and the role of the electrochemical energy of nerves as related to a reprogramming of movement patterns. Research has scientifically verified that there are two primary electrical systems in the body.[15,16] The first is the alternating current of the nervous system and brain, which governs one's muscles, physical sensations, and hormones. The second is a continuous electromagnetic radiation, which allows for energy exchange between an individual and the environment. Many of the complementary and alternative therapeutic exercise movement approaches address both of the body's electrical systems in the rehabilitative process.

A rudimentary knowledge of energy pathways and centers is important for the rehabilitation clinician and client to harness the power of movement to unblock emotional energy and ease muscular tension, restore feeling, and heighten awareness. To understand the subtle energy forces involved in the complementary and alternative therapeutic movement approaches discussed in this chapter, it is necessary to look at several ancient concepts including the universal life force, chakras and chi points, channels and meridians, as well as the role they play in healing via movement.

Universal Life Force

Central to all of the ancient medical systems underpinnings regarding the body's subtle energy system is the concept of a universal life force.[15,16] Ancient Hindu texts referred to this universal life force as *prana*, whereas traditional Chinese medicine called it *qi (chi)*. This pool of energy, drawn from a series of points, flows into the various channels or meridians, and then is transformed into a particular movement pattern, postural or positional sense, level of consciousness, and emotional or psychological state.[15,16] This flow of energy can be thought of like a water faucet connected to a garden hose. Once the faucet is turned on, the water (energy) should flow smoothly throughout the hose (system). However, if there is a kink (movement dysfunction or energy blockage) or a bulge (excessive volume or overuse) in the hose, this impacts optimal functioning of the whole unit (the body). Unless the kink is fixed, disease and physical, glandular, or emotional dysfunctions will occur.

Chakras or Energy Centers

Both the ancient Hindu and Vedic healing systems and traditional Chinese medicine distinguish seven major energy centers located within the body, which are called chakras.[15,16] The word *chakra* comes from Sanskrit and means wheel or disk. In the clinical environment, chakras are more commonly described as vortices or spinning wheels of concentrated energy and are considered the focal points for the transmission and reception of energies.[15,16] In traditional Chinese medicine, they are thought of as points where the chi is more densely concentrated.

The Vedic equivalent to the vertebral column is the sushumna. The physiological function of the spinal cord is to relay impulses to and from the brain and other parts of the body; analogously, the purpose of the sushumna is to channel one's universal life force energy from the root (coccyx) to the crown (head) chakras and back again.[15,16] The seven chakras correspond to seven points along the spine; each encompasses or has dominion over a specific area of the body and controls a specific set of emotions and health conditions. Even though the existence of the chakras cannot be demonstrated scientifically, many of the effects of chakras have analogous explanations in mainstream medical physiology. **Table 10.4** summarizes the seven chakras. These primary energy centers link with the secondary centers, which are located in the center of the feet, knees, hips, shoulders, elbows, and palms and can be affected by movement.[15,16] Some complementary and alternative health care practitioners believe that there is an eighth chakra or energy center located approximately 18 inches above the top of the head. This chakra is often referred to as the aura, the luminous field that surrounds and interpenetrates the entire body. The aura is considered to be a protective shield that encloses the other chakras and protects an individual from incoming negativity and transmittable diseases. It is also believed to provide the client with the power to project their visions into reality.

Meridians or Channels

The philosophical belief of several Eastern medical systems is that every type of cell, tissue or organ, whether bone, muscle, cartilage, nerve, or heart, is saturated with the universal life force (prana or chi) carried along the channels called *meridians* or *nadis*.[15,16] It is this interconnectedness of the various chakras with the physical body that determines one's level of health or disease.[15,16] If there is too much or too little energy, imbalance will occur at all levels (e.g., cellular, tissue, organ). Imbalances in the body's subtle energy system may become evident in the form of disease, muscle tension, tissue or joint dysfunc-

tion, emotional distress, digestive problems, anxiety, skin lesions, or injury.

Energy Systems and Healing

When imbalances occur within the energy system or life force, deviations in normal movement and thought patterning, energy utilization, prior programming, and level of consciousness or awareness take place as well.[15,16] One way in which the body copes with injury is to adopt an alternate or compensatory movement pattern. Over time, the individual repeats the pattern, but on a more unconscious level, until it becomes the new normal movement pattern. Therefore, the objective of a therapeutic exercise program that uses techniques based on the idea of chakras is to have the client gain an internal sense of awareness through exploration, establish new neural pathways, and practice new movements that do not facilitate dysfunction with an enhanced sense of consciousness until the new patterns become comfortable and innate.[15,16] The intent is to change the inappropriate, old, dysfunctional patterns into highly efficient movements, thoughts, behaviors, and optimal levels of performance.

It is this combination of addressing the physical as well as metaphysical aspects of a client's rehabilitation that makes the complementary and alternative therapeutic movement approaches of interest to rehabilitation clinicians. Regardless of which complementary and alternative therapeutic movement approach is used, the goal is to identify the physical and metaphysical dysfunction and to restore equilibrium, thereby restoring optimal functioning and performance.

Mind-Body-Energy-Movement Relationship

The majority of the complementary and alternative therapeutic exercise movement approaches discussed in this chapter speak to the physical, mental, and energetic aspects of life as they relate to the role of breathing, the process of motor learning (See Chapter 8), and the completion of various movement exercises. Like a bridge between matter (the body and its internal systems) and consciousness (the mind), the process of breathing and the exercises themselves shape, adjust, and redistribute the body's energy field, keeping its channels clear and energizing them. In addition, each therapeutic exercise movement presents the opportunity and possibility for change to be brought about consciously by working with different aspects of the body as it pursues, maintains, and transitions from movement to movement. It is the combination of breathing and the therapeutic exercise movement that generates and gathers energy and encourages its circulation through the body, thereby enhancing both tissue and system functioning while simultaneously allowing the mind to focus or rest in tranquility.[15,16]

TABLE 10.4 Summary of the seven chakras

Chakra	Location	Description
Hui yin, base or root chakra	Sacrum, base of spine at coccygeal plexus	Associated with bones, teeth, nails, legs, feet, gonads, anus, rectum, colon, prostate gland, blood, and blood cells. Associated with vitality, the need to survive and reproduce, and material reality. A sample exercise to realign the chakra is a standard bridge movement. When the chakra is working well, the client feels confident, secure, and grounded.
Lower Tanien or sacral plexus	Lower back at sacral plexus (hara center), extending anteriorly to a point approximately two inches inferior to the navel	Associated with personal power, motion, flow, emotional balance, change and sexuality. Connected to relationships, violence, and addictions. Physically, it is associated with the first lumbar vertebrae, the adrenal glands pelvis, kidneys, bladder, and the reproductive organs as well as the sacred liquids (blood, lymph, gastric juices, sperm). Sample exercises to realign this chakra include a standing pelvic rock and supine double knee to chest movements. When this chakra is in balance the client is creative, imaginative, adaptable, and has a healthy sex life.
Chung Wan or solar plexus chakra	Just below the solar plexus at the sternum	Associated with the seventh and eighth thoracic vertebrae, pancreas and adrenal glands, liver, stomach, spleen, gall bladder, and lower back. This chakra is believed to allow "good energy" to move in and out, but prevents "bad energy" from entering the mind and body as well. Associated with power, fear, anxiety, personal empowerment, and introversion. Physical dysfunctions of the chakra include diabetes and stomach ulcers. An example of an exercise that realigns this chakra is a standing trunk rotation and sidestep movement with the arms abducted to 90°. When this chakra is in balance the client takes initiative, demonstrates courage, possesses perseverance, and can accomplish great deeds.
Middle Tantien or heart chakra	Pulmonary and cardiac plexi (between the shoulder blades and the center of the chest)	Associated with the fourth thoracic vertebrae, thymus gland, heart, lungs, breasts, upper back, arms, and hands. Often seen as a bridge between the physical and non-physical, playing a balancing role between our darker aspects (jealously, envy, hate) and our potential for love, compassion, honesty, truth, and healing. An example of an exercise for this chakra is a prone trunk extension movement (with or without use of the lower extremities). When this chakra is balanced, the client is able to experience "true love" as well as kindness, compassion, and selfless acts of giving.
Hsuan Chi or throat chakra	Pharyngeal plexus near the throat (between the larynx and the clavicle)	Associated with the third cervical vertebrae, the thyroid and parathyroid glands, throat, ears, nose, trachea, neck, shoulder and lungs. Believed to be the gateway between the inside and outside and therefore associated with communication, self-expression, will, and fluent thought. Acts as a bridge between the physical and spiritual energies and corresponds to the need for balance between the emotional expression of the heart and the rational, cerebral approach. An example of an exercise for this chakra is the yoga shoulder stand. When this chakra is in balance, the client is able to communicate with penetrating, true, and compassionate words as well as take responsibility for personal needs including creating what one needs and receiving what is given.
Upper Tantien or third eye	Carotid plexus	Associated with the first cervical vertebrae, the pituitary gland, the eyes and brain (cerebellum and central nervous system). Often linked to visualizing, imaging, dreaming, symbolism, insight, intuition, and understanding as well as sight. A common exercise to balance this chakra is visualization of colors one at a time until a complete rainbow or mandala is created. When this chakra is balanced, the client is able to visualize and understand mental concepts including how to see the world, how one should expect the world to respond to the client, and how to manifest visions that will benefit all.
Pai Hui or crown chakra	Top of the head in the cerebral cortex more commonly known in the Vedic system as the crown center	Associated with the pineal gland and the brain (cerebral cortex). Considered the center for effective functioning of emotional, mental, physical self and source for inspirational thoughts, wisdom, ideas, profound knowledge, and consciousness. An example of an exercise for this chakra is gentle thoracic region stretching and a headstand. When this chakra is balanced, the client is able to integrate their own personality with spirituality, develop their own unique type of spirituality, and understand what others are talking about when they speak of spiritual experiences.

Energy Balance and Movement

In the ancient Eastern complementary and alternative movement approaches, every posture or movement is a combination of seven basic qualities. Six of the qualities are polarities: *yin* and *yang* (the forces of change and harmony); open and closed; and full and empty. The seventh concept is central equilibrium.[15,16] Consciousness of these seven qualities pervades every aspect of a movement posture while it is being performed.

Movements are a sequence of postures in a state of perpetual transformation, a cycle of harmony and change, or yin and yang. For example, a movement posture begins, grows, reaches a fullness, and starts to empty. The emptying of one movement is the growth of the next movement posture. Each movement "ebbs and flows" from one posture to another, thereby creating a cyclical and functional process. It is equally important to remember that the postures move between the polarities of open and closed.[15,16] This concept can be illustrated in many aspects of the posture, for example in the shoulders and arms. Standing with the arms squeezed tightly against the ribs is an example of a *closed posture*. Lifting the arms and shoulders outward as if welcoming a friend is an example of an *open posture*. The polarities of full and empty, which give the body mobility, can be illustrated in the process of walking.[15,16] Most people tend to drop their weight onto the leg being moved. In the complementary and alternative therapeutic movement approaches, however, balance is held in one leg, leaving the other free to move. In other words, the weight empties from one leg and fills the other, thereby increasing mobility.

Central to all of the complementary and alternative therapeutic movement exercise approaches is the concept of equilibrium. When a movement posture is based on *central equilibrium*, the body is aligned and perfectly balanced. In addition, it will retain the qualities of alignment and central equilibrium regardless of how small or large a movement the body makes.[15,16] However, when an injury, impairment, disease, or dysfunction has occurred, the body's equilibrium is altered. In order to restore harmony (i.e., between yin and yang) and equilibrium, the movements of the form must be executed with the correct technique and *mindset* (mind intent or attitude).[15,16] For an inexperienced client or a novice to complementary and alternative therapeutic movement approaches, the body and mind may be too fully occupied with learning the sequence of movements and the technique to completely experience the qualities of each movement. For example, with respect to body position awareness, a beginner may not know exactly where to place a hand or foot or where their weight should be distributed at each moment in a posture. Paradoxically, clients who are highly trained may also encounter difficulty initially because they may try to dominate the movement instead of focusing their mind and becoming aware of new ways of moving in order to successfully complete complex movement postures and patterns in a flowing manner. Therefore, the rehabilitation clinician as well as the client should devote time to learning about various movements and the appropriate transitional considerations (i.e., shifting body weight from one foot to the other) as well as focus on moving in certain ways and experiencing the qualities in each movement.

TEN PRINCIPLES OF MOVEMENT QUALITY

Based on the aforementioned concepts, McPartlend and Miller[17] identified 10 principles of movement quality that can be applied in clinical therapeutic movement care.

1. The five Ss—slow, small, soft, smooth, and sensitive: *Slow* refers to the rate of movement that occurs when restrictions are encountered (e.g., range of motion, tissue, energy) and applies to both passive and active movement (i.e., kinesthetic awareness and motor control). When the speed of movement is decreased, proprioception, tactile sensitivity, and skill acquisition are enhanced while the use of momentum and ballistic-type movement is avoided. *Small* refers to decreasing the movement amplitude so that the client's proprioceptive detection of fine movements and ability to initiate and control fine movements, and progress from micro-movement to macro-movements are enhanced. *Soft* denotes the importance of decreasing the muscular effort in order to maximize sensitivity and movement efficiency to facilitate the use of deep postural muscles and to reduce the chance of tissue irritation or injury. *Smooth* pertains to avoiding jerkiness or uneven deceleration or acceleration of movement, thereby building motor control and preventing additional or unexpected injury. *Sensitive* relates to the client's ability to focus their attention on the feeling and quality of movement, rather than on the more quantitative mechanical aspects (range of motion, velocity, etc.).[17] This is particularly important for high performance athletics where it is equally as important to attend to the process as to the goal.

2. Initiation: This pertains to the starting position of any type of movement therapy. The starting position of any movement strongly influences how that movement will be executed. Hence, it is important that the client always begin in the best possible balanced posture or alignment, requiring the lowest level of muscle tone, and the greatest degree of relaxation.

3. Technique: Technique relates to using the best form possible at all times during movement execution.[17] In order for a client to perform any type of movement therapy with ease and maximum efficiency, it is beneficial that they attain a detached, non-emotional attitude. However, inherent to the successful and efficient execution of a motion or series of movements, it is important that the client use proper technique with a clear intention for movement direction (spatial intent), using the most efficient trajectory (movement pathway), and proper component sequencing, timing, and coordination.

4. Breathing: Breathing is both an unconscious and a conscious process that plays a vital role not only in completing specific movements, but in circulating the body's subtle energy (chi, qi, prana). In this principle, the client should be encouraged to breathe freely and easily using a normal, regular rhythm. Using a natural breathing pattern is important, as it lowers extraneous muscle tone, increases kinesthetic awareness, and enhances neuromuscular control. It may be helpful for the client to visualize breathing in terms of a three dimensional framework, specifically focusing on increasing one's internal volume, using diaphragmatic breathing, and incorporating the core muscles (i.e., lower abdominals, pelvic floor, lumbar spine region, posterior thoracic region) into the breathing process. The rehabilitation clinician should remind the client to synchronize the rhythm of their breathing with the specific body posture or the flow of the movements and to exhale during the exertion phase of the movement.

5. Head and neck control: This relates to allowing the head and neck to relax upward, avoiding any unnecessary tension or stiffening of the cervical musculature. Ideally, the cervical musculature should be dissociated from the rest of the body, allowing it to remain relaxed during physical activity.

6. Elongation: This pertains to allowing the body to lengthen at rest and with movement, which allows it to avoid any tendency toward unnecessary co-contraction or compression. Elongation can be achieved mentally by visualizing length, paying specific attention to alignment, direction, and relaxation. Physically, elongation can be achieved by reciprocal lengthening and shortening, which means relaxing the tissues on the away side and softening or folding the tissues on the side toward which one is bending.

7. Differentiation of movement: This principle pertains to a form of neuromuscular "re-programming," which is achieved through guided exploratory movement. The client is encouraged to accomplish this progression by exploring the non-habitual movement options of the desired movement(s).

8. Synkinetic phenomena: This principle involves using a naturally occurring physiological phenomenon to accomplish and enhance movement. Common examples are the association between head-neck and eye movements (cervico-ocular coupling), righting reflexes (the ability to assume optimal position when there has been a departure from it), and the rib and spinal movements that occur in rhythm with respiration.

9. Conceptual ideas for movement: The client is encouraged to conceptualize how the body (axial skeleton) or a specific segment (freely moving joint) could move if there were no soft tissue or articular restrictions. For example, the rib cage could be imagined as boneless, made of soft rubber or jelly, while the client completes a restricted movement.

10. Center or core awareness: This final principle refers to allowing one's awareness and "sense of being" to center into the very core of the body. In the movement therapies, the core is located at one's center of gravity, usually several inches below the navel. During the completion of a movement, it is important that the client fully relaxes into the lower abdomen, utilizes three-dimensional breathing, and makes all peripheral movements from the core (i.e., torso or trunk).

Each of the complementary and alternative therapeutic movement approaches discussed in this chapter focus on teaching the client to become aware of their existing dysfunctional motions, being sensitive to new movement patterns, and alert to existing imbalances within the mind-body-energy system.[15,16] The client is encouraged to become alert to the intelligence from within while learning and responding to what is happening to the body internally as well as externally.[15,16] In addition, each of the complementary and alternative therapeutic movement approaches is intended to teach the client to be patient, confident, alert but quiet, and to wait for the right moment to take action (i.e., purposeful motion) rather than react with impatience, force, irritation, impulsiveness, or non-action. When performed correctly, the exercises work to calm the psyche, focus the mind, and soothe the spirit, so that the mind-body-energy connection can work in harmony, thereby allowing optimal function and enhanced performance.

Healing Through Movement

Healing is a natural process that can be enhanced by a person's physically building and circulating life energy (chi, qi, or prana).[15,16] When practiced regularly, the combination of body positions or postures, mindset including visualization, and active movement create the proper conditions for streams of energy to flow through the energy centers (i.e., chakras or chi points), through the meridians or channels, and then vigorously throughout the entire body, thereby stimulating the internal organs and various systems necessary for healing to occur. The role of the client in the process is to try, through the various complementary and alternative therapeutic movement exercise approaches, to create the physical-mental-emotional-spiritual situation in which energy can flow and the body can heal itself.[15,16]

Many of the traditional Eastern complementary and alternative therapeutic exercise approaches discussed in this chapter are better known in the West as exercises that promote healing, maintain health, prevent degenerative illnesses, preserve or improve function, and encourage longevity.[15,16] In terms of specific physiological benefits, the exercises outlined in this chapter are intended to bolster the immune system, improve respiration, maintain and enhance circulation, nourish the neurological system, enrich the digestive system, stimulate the endocrine glands, maintain vital organs, fortify the skeletal system (dexterity, flexibility, integrity, articulation), and strengthen the muscular system (mobility, stability, control) by stimulating the subtle energy systems (chakras/chi energy centers, nadis/meridians) within the body.[15,16] In addition, the various complementary and alternative therapeutic movement approaches are believe to stimulate one's whole body energy (prana, chi, qi), which should improve one's overall health, coordination, control, function, awareness, balance, and performance. In terms of cognitive function, these approaches are reported to improve breathing, which revitalizes the body and stimulates the brain by training the mind to focus and concentrate.[15,16] Finally, with respect to emotional function, the therapeutic approaches are intended to broaden the client's awareness and enhance their sensitivity with respect to the body, mind, and spirit.

The list of mental (emotional) benefits for any given complementary and alternative therapeutic movement exercise approach can be extensive. Examples include improvements in attitude, more personalized feelings, enhancement of perspective, increased compliance with treatment, provision of companionship, freer expression of feelings, increased verbal communication, provision of a grieving outlet, release of emotions, increased mental focus, memory stimulation, increased mental imaging, reduced blood pressure, accelerated healing, improved pain management, decreased anxiety, relief of mental tension, relief of body tension, reduced stress, and provision of time for meditation.[12,14–15,17–20] This chapter will discuss dance therapy, the Feldenkrais Method, the Nickolaus technique, Pilates method, Qigong, Tai Chi, and Yoga as complementary and alternative approaches to movement and exercise.

DANCE THERAPY

Dance therapy is a major or large movement therapy that capitalizes on the direct relationship between body and mind. The music, rhythm, and synchronous movements associated with dance are believed to promote healing by improving mood, reducing social isolation, awakening old memories and feelings, and enhancing overall well being. The continuous interchange of non–weight bearing to weight bearing postures provided by dance enhances balance and integrates neuromuscular motor control and coordination.[8]

Background

Dance movement therapy is defined by the American Dance Therapy Association (www.adta.org) as "the psychotherapeutic use of movement as a process which furthers the emotional, cognitive and physical integration of the individual." Marian Chace, a dancer who worked with psychi-

atric clients during the 1940s, is credited with the foundation of dance as a medical therapy. The American Dance Therapy Association was founded in 1966. Although primarily thought of as a psychotherapeutic intervention, dance therapists and movement specialists also use dance or dance-like movements as the principal medium for facilitating therapeutic change in clients who have emotional, social, cognitive, or physical problems.[8,11]

Depending on the goal, dance therapy can be performed alone, with a partner, or in a group. For example, range of motion exercises can be set to music with elderly clients, or formal dance routines can be used in individual therapy, such as with an athlete. Within the rehabilitation setting, group dance movement sessions are the most common format utilized, as they allow people of different physical abilities to participate. Dance movement routines can range from simple clapping and swaying while the client is in a seated or supine position to intricate aerobic sessions performed in standing.[11]

Therapeutic Indications

The benefits of dance movement therapy include physical changes, promotion of socialization, increased sense of connectedness with one's body and with a group of similar or dissimilar clients, decreased shyness and improved self esteem as well as improvement in one's body image, movement control, and coordination.[8,11,18] Dance movement therapy is also indicated for a wide range of clients who would benefit from the improved flexibility, balance, agility, coordination, muscle strength, and cardiovascular and cardiopulmonary system function associated with therapeutic exercise program participation. However, dance therapy may also help clients with cancer express their loss; emotionally disturbed or learning disabled children to enhance communication, promote socialization and sense of self esteem; and enhance the communication abilities of clients with psychiatric disorders.[8,11,18]

Contraindications

Dance movement therapy is safe for most clients but there are some risk factors to consider, including poor cardiovascular status and a history of chronic obstructive pulmonary disease (COPD) or degenerative musculoskeletal conditions.[8,11] The client's level of obesity, muscular atrophy, substance abuse (alcohol, tobacco, drugs) and exercise history are also factors to consider prior to implementing a dance movement therapy program. Because dancing is an aerobic activity, clients may experience signs of cardiovascular compromise, such as dizziness, flushing, profuse sweating, and disorientation.[8] Dizziness may also be a result of rapid motion (i.e., when up and down movements are used).[8] Clients who exercise strenuously or vigorously during a session may experience muscle soreness or strain. At risk clients should be cleared by their physician prior to participation in a dance therapy program.

Evidence

Lewis and Scannel[19] studied 112 women between 18 and 69 years of age who actively participated in creative dance using the Multidimensional Body-self Relations Questionnaire. Subjects who were more experienced in creative dance movements were more satisfied with their appearance, fitness, and body parts than subjects with less than five years of experience. Heber[20] reported that dance therapy improved the emotional, psychological, and physical well being of psychiatric clients. Hanna[21] in a review paper, and Serlin et al.[22] in a study of women with breast cancer identified dance therapy as a useful treatment during the healing process that allowed clients to gain a sense of control over their lives. In a prospective study of 28 women with a mean age of 67 ± 2 years, Kudlacek et al.[23] reported that dancers who displayed signs of osteoporosis prior to study participation showed a significant increase in lumbar vertebral bone density over the 12-month dance program. Berrol[24] presented a case study describing dance movement therapy intervention for a client with severe brain injury. In a comparison between geriatric clients who participated in a movement therapy group with those who did not, Goldberg and Fitzpatrick[25] reported that the movement therapy group had greater improvement in total morale and attitude toward their own aging. Hamburg and Clair[26] studied the influence of a Laban based movement program on 36 non-impaired adults (10 men, 26 females) between 63 and 86 years of age. After five weeks, clients displayed statistically significant improvements in gait and balance characteristics. There was no evidence in the literature as to negative impact or outcomes to be found with respect to dance movement therapy.

Technique

Preparation.   During dance therapy, movements may be spontaneous or choreographed sequences.[8,11,18] As mentioned earlier, before starting a dance therapy program the client should be cleared by a physician, particularly if aerobic activity is included. The rehabilitation clinician should begin by assessing the client or group for the presence of risk factors.[11] The presence of one or more risk factors does not preclude the client from participating but may influence the rehabilitation clinician's decision making regarding the type of dance, dance movements, level of activity (low, moderate, or high/vigorous) and length of the session. The rehabilitation clinician should also assess the client's hearing, mobility, vision, and utilization of assistive devices as well as previous dance experience.[9]

Another consideration is the type of music. The rehabilitation clinician should select music and dance steps appropriate to the client(s) participating in the dance movement session. The music should be appropriate to the population both in pace and aesthetic appeal.[11] For example, a group of agile senior citizens may not enjoy fast moving rock and roll, rap, or hip hop, but prefer music from the big band era. Typically, faster music is used to stimulate the group while slower music is used to provide a calming effect and therefore requires more controlled, precise movement.[11] Examples of types of calming music include ballads, lullabies, symphonies, sonatas, opera, Native American flute pieces, meditation-type works, and some new age and classical compositions.

A third consideration is the selection of the dance style itself.[9] If the goal is to work on posture, balance, and gross motor control, the rehabilitation clinician may opt to have the individual client or group participate in ballet, ballroom dancing, waltz, or Viennese waltz. If the purpose of the session is to improve more isolated or fine motor control, balance, and lower extremity strength via slower and more flowing motions, the rehabilitation clinician may opt to have the client or group perform the tango, rumba, mamba, meringue, samba, or tap dance.[9] If the purpose is to attain lower extremity strength, improve posture, move with precision, accomplish faster reaction or quick response times, and work on the ability to complete diagonal pattern changes, the rehabilitation clinician may opt to have the client or group practice doing the fox trot, salsa, quick step, or a fast polka. If the intent is to have the client or group work individually on reciprocal motions, linear (forward-backward) steps, specific lower extremity lateral motions, as well as upper extremity movements, the rehabilitation clinician may decide to use line dancing, the hustle, conga, cha-cha, disco, swing, or country western dancing.[9]

Intervention.   Prior to beginning the session, the rehabilitation clinician should establish an environment conducive to both physical and emotional relaxation.[9] In conjunction with the client, decisions must be made regarding session duration and frequency, preferred music and dance styles. The client should be instructed to maintain focus and to take a relaxed approach to the dance therapy intervention. If the rehabilitation clinician is not familiar with the specific dance selected for use as the intervention, it may be necessary to arrange for an experienced dance instructor to be present during the session.[9] The environment should be arranged so clients can move freely without fear of inadvertently bumping into each other. Chairs may be arranged around the periphery of the dance floor area to better accommodate clients who cannot participate while standing, those who fatigue easily, or for those who demonstrate significant or unexpected changes in cardiovascular status. If a client experiences signs of cardiovascular compromise, the rehabilitation clinician should assist them to a seated position and obtain their vital signs.[8]

Finally, prior to the initiation of a dance therapy session the rehabilitation clinician should introduce all of the participants, explain the purpose of the session, and encourage each client to participate according to their ability level.[11] In addition, the rehabilitation clinician should have the client or group perform warm-up activities such as seated ankle circles, alternating elbow flexion-extension, alternating shoulder flexion to 90°, gentle active neck flexion-extension, and head circles.[9] It is important to remind the client at the initiation of the dance therapy session to perform all of the movements at their own comfortable pace, and to sit and rest when necessary.[9] The rehabilitation clinician should circulate through the area during the dance, providing encouragement, feedback, motivation and praise to the participants for their efforts.[11] This interaction may also allow the client to discuss the feelings they are experiencing with each movement.[8] After completion of the session, the rehabilitation clinician should document the type and duration of the activity that was performed and each client's response.[11] In addition, they should note the effects of the music and dancing on the client's ability to complete movements, emotional state, sense of being, focus, memory, and recall. It may be necessary to revise the dance therapy intervention plan to better match the needs of the group.[9]

Practitioner Training

Individuals who work in the field of dance therapy are expected to meet basic educational requirements, including a master's degree from an approved graduate program plus preparation in performance or liberal arts and have movement therapy experience qualifications. In order to teach and maintain a private practice, individuals must also meet advanced requirements and be a registered member of the Academy of Dance Therapists (ADTR). Information regarding specific training requirements can be obtained from the American Dance Therapy Association (www.adta.org).

Key Point:

Dance movement therapy. . . .
- Is one of the oldest forms used to heal the sick and injured.
- Can be used with a wide variety of clientele.
- Is a combination of movements and breathing that engages both mind and body.
- Results in a variety of physical and psychosocial benefits.

THE FELDENKRAIS METHOD

The Feldenkrais Method is a gentle method of bodywork, named after its inventor, Dr. Moshe Feldenkrais, that focuses on re-learning and re-programming basic neuromuscular movements.[8,11] The underlying concept of this approach is re-education of the body through movement and relief of structural and functional stress.[12] It uses self-exploration and self-awareness of movement and teaches proper body movement though gentle massage, stretches, and exercises.[27] Through systemic movement exploration, modifications and adaptations can be made in habitual movement strategies, and coordination, flexibility, range of motion, and function can be improved.[28]

The *Feldenkrais Method* consists of two main techniques: 1) *Functional Integration* (FI), which refers to the coherent organization of choices for functional movement patterns; and 2) *Awareness Through Movement* (ATM) in which the client, through the rehabilitation clinician's words and gentle touch, or through self-exploration, and self-discovery, becomes aware of existing maladaptive movement patterns and re-learns optimal ones. The hands-on aspect of the Feldenkrais Method is to communicate rather than directly control the client by having them explore each motion, enhance their awareness, alter movement forms, and modify postures, all in response to suggestions from the rehabilitation clinician.

The Feldenkrais Method is a behavioral-cognitive approach to learning.[15] In this technique, the philosophy is that, through self-discovery, the client will be able to learn or relearn new options and new patterns of movement, thereby improving self-image, reorganizing posture, increasing self-awareness, enhancing health, and developing a more direct relationship with the world. Feldenkrais' philosophy runs counter to the traditional neurophysiological paradigm. While traditional neurophysiology separates the sensory and motor systems, Feldenkrais believed that emotional and mental activity could strongly influence and disturb all aspects of movement and performance.

Background

Moshe Feldenkrais was born in Russia and lived, at various points in his life, in Israel, France, and England. While living in France, he became interested in judo and earned a black belt. While living in England during World War II, he sustained an athletic knee injury that left him severely impaired.[11,29] It was with the hope that he might be able to avoid surgery for this injury that Feldenkrais explored psychology, anatomy, neurophysiology, and psychoanalysis in search of a deeper understanding of the body and its functioning.[11,28,30] This self-imposed interest and exploration resulted in the development of an entire philosophy of life that today underlies the Feldenkrais Method.[11]

Judo is the foundation for Feldenkrais movement classes. Feldenkrais realized that judo was not just an activity or sport, but a principle of life that involved art, science, movement, and a means for both cultural and personal attainment.[28] This is evident in the use of the circle, a principle of judo, within the Feldenkrais Method.[15] Feldenkrais realized by observing his own adaptations and responses to his knee injury that clients have a choice about how they move.[29] For example, Feldenkrais noted that at the time of an acute injury, the limbic system is activated and creates muscular splinting and other secondary changes in the body (e.g., changes in breathing patterns, respiration rate). Feldenkrais also observed that the longer the pain remained, the more maladaptive changes and dysfunctional movement patterns occurred, resulting in inefficient and ineffective movements.[29] By applying his knowledge of physiology, anatomy, neurology, and psychology, along with his experience of martial arts, Feldenkrais successfully reversed his impairment and taught himself how to walk again without pain.[30]

Central to the theory and technique of the Feldenkrais Method is the notion of self image.[28,30] According to Feldenkrais, "Each one of us speaks, moves, thinks, and feels in a different way, each according to the image of himself that he has built up over the years. In order to change our mode of action, we must change the image of ourselves that we carry within us."[28] Habitual patterns of movement underlie both our self awareness and our emotional actions and reactions.[11] If the negative habitual patterns of movement are interrupted, the body can function with greater efficiency, ease, effectiveness, fluidity, and movement.[30] The end result is enhanced self image, increased awareness, and improved health.

Three observations made by Feldenkrais are important in his exercise method: 1) the regulation of breathing as an integral part of movement, because poor function and movement can impair breathing, and impaired breathing can in turn interfere with proper function of body systems, especially muscle; 2) the role of eye movement in movement and function, whereby uncoordinated eye movement can negatively affect movement; and 3) the belief that clients practice a skill only until they achieve a desired goal, thereby using only a small portion of their potential.[11,30] Feldenkrais eventually developed 600 different lessons. Since then, thousands of planned lessons have been devised, evolving as rehabilitation clinicians introduce applications with different client groups.

Therapeutic Indications

Feldenkrais saw his technique as a training method rather than a medical therapy,[11] but current practitioners believe that the method can benefit anyone, young or old, physically fit or physically challenged. The Feldenkrais Guild (http://www.feldenkraisguild.com) and the Feldenkrais Educational Foundation of North America (http://www.feldenkrais.com) suggest that the Feldenkrais Method is especially useful for clients who are experiencing acute or chronic pain (neck, shoulders, low back, hips, legs, knees); central nervous system disorders, including multiple sclerosis, cerebrovascular accident, cerebral palsy, Parkinson's disease; and post-traumatic stress disorders. It has also been shown to reduce perceived stress and lower anxiety levels.[8] According to the Feldenkrais Guild, the method is popular with professional athletes (e.g., Julius Erving) and musicians (e.g., Yehudi Menuhin and Yo-Yo Ma), who claim it improves their levels of performance.

Contraindications

The literature on this method does not mention any contraindications. However, there are a few precautions. Rehabilitation clinicians should avoid working near inflamed body regions, and pain should not be ignored. It is important to note that movements that are performed roughly can cause injury, and clients should be encouraged to work within their limits.

Techniques

Feldenkrais Method exercises are taught in either individual client (i.e., one on one) or group classes.[11] Typically FI sessions are private and individualized, whereas ATM sessions are conducted in a group format. The essence of the Feldenkrais method is to develop a personalized learning program for each client.[31] To do this, the rehabilitation clinician must establish a relationship of trust and set up learning experiments.[32] In other words, the rehabilitation clinician assists the client in discovering existing habitual patterns and responses. The entire interaction is used to discover optimal movements to enhance the client's posture, motion, and performance.

Functional Integration (FI).   The term functional integration (FI) refers to the coherent organization of choices for functional movement patterns.[12] FI is a one-to-one method that consists of gentle bodywork with learning occurring through guided touch and sometimes verbal feedback.[11,30] The rehabilitation clinician actively guides the client physically through patterns of movement that have been selected specifically to address their needs.[30] FI enables clients to develop their own internal awareness through sensing and feeling. It is very safe because the rehabilitation clinician moves with the client. The result ideally is more fluid movements and a reduction in restrictive patterns that create pain, tension, and stiffness.[11]

Because FI is designed to enable the client to learn, one of the first principles is comfort. A specially designed table is used because the weight of both the rehabilitation clinician and the client are transmitted though the clinician's skeletal frame. For example, the weight of the client's leg, trunk and head must be lifted with minimal strain, nominal energy expenditure, and maximum efficiency while pressures are applied. During the FI session, the client stays fully clothed and may lie on a table or be in a sitting or standing position.[11] Lessons may focus on a particular function, action, or client request. For example, an athletically active client may be interested in learning how to move with more power, enhance flexibility, or restore balance whereas a client with degenerative joint disease may be interested in learning how to move from a standing to a supine position without pain. A typical session lasts approximately 45–60 minutes.[11] The rehabilitation clinician should appreciate the influence of a client's self-image, self-education, self-direction and self-maintenance on their learned movement patterns over time. For example, a maladaptive pattern could be associated with protecting a previously injured area. This protective pattern eventually will become a way of being. Function and performance will be enhanced only through heightened awareness and movement re-education.

Awareness Through Movement (ATM). Awareness through movement (ATM) is usually taught in group classes. The rehabilitation clinician verbally leads the group through a series of therapeutic exercises in the form of directed movement sequences (rather than using a hands on approach). Feldenkrais believed that guiding movements via verbal instructions can also enable clients to progress and experience each step of a class without direct manual contact. The exercises are designed to help the clients become more aware of their bodies and to develop new patterns of movement. The exercises are performed in a slow, relaxed way, progressing from easy movements to movements of greater range and complexity.[11] The emphasis of this Feldenkrais Method is on enjoyment and the avoidance of pain. Clients are often placed in gravity alleviated positions such as lying on their side, supine or prone.[15] The classes are often well defined and structured, with the rehabilitation clinician attending to each client. During ATM lessons, constraints such as unusual skeletal formations, unusual movements goals, and proximity to the floor are introduced. Clients then begin to discover new ways to move trying to find acceptable neuromuscular solutions.

Unlike, for example, a step aerobics class, there is no teacher standing at the front demonstrating. Instead, each client is encouraged to find their own way. A typical ATM session lasts from 30 to 60 minutes[11] with several pauses or rest periods. The pause or rest time is given so that the client's kinesthetic system learns or imprints the new neuromuscular pathways and their recently gained awareness of body posture and new movement patterns.[11] Each ATM session follows a well defined structure and the rehabilitation clinician attends to each client throughout the entire session. Clients can then use an audio tape at home as a follow-up to attending a class. According to Ruth and Kegerreis,[32] these recorded instructions can enhance physical and perceptual changes but are most effective when the client already has some experience with the method and desired movements.

As stated previously, ATM lessons are highly structured, but emphasize the experience rather than the goal. Numerous lessons are available, each focusing on a different area of the body. The lesson selected is typically dependent upon the client's needs and can be based upon developmental movements, functional activities, or abstract explorations of joint, muscle, and postural relationships. As the client learns how to listen to the lesson, they develop an awareness of the subtle changes in habit and movement.[30]

Feldenkrais stated that ATM lessons are designed to improve mobility, "to turn the impossible into the possible, the possible into the easy, and the easy into the elegant."[28]

Evidence

Kerr et al.[33] in evaluating the ability of a 10 week duration ATM program to reduce anxiety of 13 new and 42 returning students, reported decreased State-Trait Anxiety Inventory scores after a single lesson for both groups and further reductions by the end of the program. New students also experienced significantly greater reductions. Malmgren-Olsson et al.[34] compared Feldenkrais, body awareness therapy, and conventional individual physiotherapy with respect to changes in psychological distress, pain and self-image in 78 clients (64 females, 14 males) with non-specific musculoskeletal disorders. Results showed significant positive changes over time in all three groups; however, effect size analysis suggested that body awareness therapy and Feldenkrais might be more effective than conventional treatment. In a pilot study, Smith et al.[35] evaluated the Feldenkrais Method's effect on pain and state anxiety in 26 subjects between 25 and 78 years of age who were experiencing low back pain. Subjects were divided into two groups, with one group of clients receiving a 30-minute ATM session, while the other listened to a narrative for the same duration. They found that the Feldenkrais intervention was effective for reducing the affective dimension of pain, but not the sensory or evaluative dimensions, nor state anxiety. Kolt and McConville,[36] in evaluating the effects of a Feldenkrais ATM program and relaxation procedures on a volunteer sample of 54 undergraduate physiotherapy students over a two week period who were randomly assigned to either a treatment or control group, reported that females in the Feldenkrais and relaxation group reported significantly lower anxiety scores on completion of the fourth treatment session. Lundblad et al.[37] investigated whether physiotherapy or Feldenkrais interventions resulted in a greater reduction of complaints from the neck and shoulder region of 97 female industrial workers. Subjects were randomized to one of three groups (standard physiotherapy, Feldenkrais group, or control group). The Feldenkrais group displayed significant decreases in complaints of pain intensity and prevalence from the neck and shoulders. They also reported less disability during leisure time. James et al.[38] studied the effects of the Feldenkrais Method on hamstring muscle length changes among 48 non-impaired students who were divided into either a Feldenkrais, relaxation or control group. After four treatment sessions, no significant differences were noted among groups. Johnson et al.[39] compared the effects of Feldenkrais bodywork to non-therapeutic bodywork over an eight week period among 20 subjects with multiple sclerosis who were randomly assigned to each group. Subjects in the Feldenkrais bodywork group displayed significantly reduced perceived stress and lower anxiety levels compared to the control group.

Equipment

Group classes require no special equipment. Private sessions require a table or chair on which the client can lie down or sit. Mats, pillows, blankets, and other props can be used to facilitate certain movements. Clients are encouraged to wear loose, comfortable clothing.

Example: A Spinal ATM Lesson

Figure 10.1a–d illustrates a client performing a movement described in a series of audiocassettes entitled *The Intelligent Body: Awareness Through Movement.*[40] This particular lesson is from "Tape #1: The Spine as a Chain Bridging." As with all ATM classes, the client should be dressed as comfortably as possible, lie in an area with ample cushion below the body, and have ample room to move the arms and legs. All lessons are approximately 45 minutes in length. If the lesson is too long, the client should stop halfway and continue on the next day.

Practitioner Training

Feldenkrais practitioners come from a variety of backgrounds. While it is possible for individuals to be self taught, it is recommended that they be trained by rehabilitation clinicians who have undergone formal Feldenkrais Method training and are accredited by the Feldenkrais Guild. Practitioners must complete 800 to 1,000 hours of education and training in the form of 200 hours per year over a four-year period.[11]

> ### *Key Point:*
> Feldenkrais is a complementary and alternative therapeutic exercise approach which. . . .
> - Utilizes two key components: Awareness through movement (ATM) and functional integration (FI).
> - Provides clients with the opportunity to explore and learn through self-directed movements. Involves slow, relaxed exercises and gentle body work—all of which are dependent on each client's needs.
> - Focuses on relearning and reprogramming basic motions into efficient and effective movements.
> - Requires clients to gain active awareness of the "forgotten" parts of the body.
> - Emphasizes neuromuscular organization, fluid functional movement, and reductions in restrictive patterns.
> - May help to improve range of motion, flexibility, coordination, body awareness, and self-image.

NICKOLAUS TECHNIQUE

The *Nickolaus technique* is a program of 30 sequenced exercises that incorporates the rhythm of breathing with stretching, strengthening, conditioning, co-contraction of specific muscle groups, and regaining balance and coordination.[41] Another vital component of this therapeutic exercise technique is its focus on the co-contraction of the lower abdominal muscles and the gluteal muscles. It improves body alignment by means of exercises performed almost entirely on the floor, using the client's own body weight as a resistance.[41]

Background

Richard Nickolaus and Bill Thompson developed the Nickolaus technique in the late 1960s, after Nickolaus had undergone rehabilitation for a fractured ankle. Nickolaus realized that he could utilize his experience as a dancer combined with his new knowledge and understanding of the body and its movements to create a system of exercises that would enhance dancers' training and performance.[41] Through a dance company formed by Nickolaus and Thompson, Nickolaus continued to experiment with the most effective way to train dancers by having them use springs and weights while exercising.[41] He eventually surmised that his technique could be effective as rehabilitation for the wide variety of orthopedic problems and injuries that dancers incur. In 1972 the first Nickolaus Exercise Center was opened in New York treating both dancers and non-dancers with predominately musculoskeletal impairments, and by 1978 there were more than 14 centers nationwide.[41]

Therapeutic Indications

The Nickolaus technique has been used as an alternative therapeutic exercise intervention following athletic injury, general orthopedic injuries, other musculoskeletal conditions, scoliosis, and multiple sclerosis.

Contraindications

No contraindications to this technique have been identified in the literature.

Equipment

The Nickolaus technique requires no specific equipment other than comfortable clothing and a room large enough to practice in. Clients often prefer to complete the exercises on a mat for comfort.[41]

Technique

Each Nickolaus technique movement is designed to exercise a specific part of the body, to tone and refine each

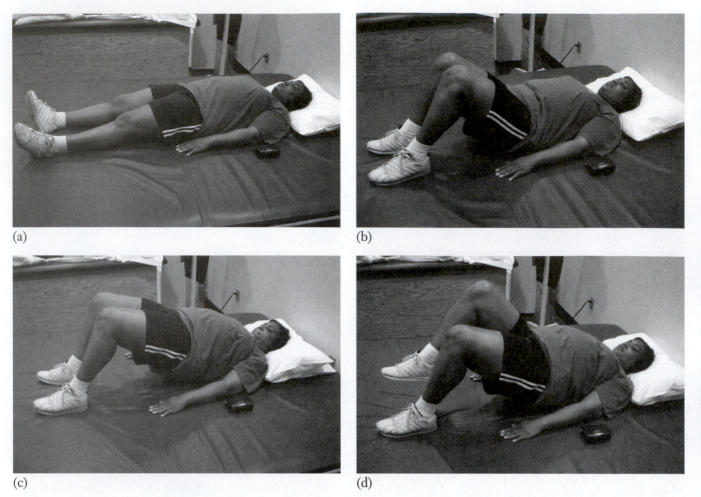

Figure 10.1   ATM using audiotape recording. (a) relax in supine position; (b) posterior pelvic tilt with knees flexed; (c) bridge; (d) single leg raise from bridge position.

muscle individually, and to enhance neuromuscular coordination between all muscles.[41] Performed properly and in the correct sequence and supported by deep breathing, the exercises can improve body alignment, tone muscles, and strengthen problem areas (e.g., lower back, knees), increase flexibility, and even reduce physical and mental tension.

Examples of Nickolaus Technique exercise movements include the single leg stretch (**Figure 10.2a–b**), the sitting arm and leg stretch (**Figure 10.3a–c**), the "V" (**Figure 10.4a–c**), the neck and upper back stretch (**Figure 10.5a–b**), the "bird" (**Figure 10.6**), the "bow" (**Figure 10.7**), the double thigh stretch (**Figure 10.8**) and the inner thigh stretch with spinal rotation (**Figure 10.9**).

Evidence and Practitioner Requirements

Published studies of this technique are lacking, as are published guidelines for practitioners. Anecdotally, however, the Nickolaus technique is a popular adjunct to other therapeutic exercise techniques and is used by many dancers as an exercise regimen to prevent injury and to enhance performance.

> ### *Key Point:*
> The Nickolaus technique. . . .
> ◆ Considers breathing its keystone.
> ◆ Involves a series of structured exercises.
> ◆ Focuses on stretching, strengthening, conditioning, co-contraction of specific muscle groups, and regaining balance and coordination.
> ◆ Encourages the enhancement of neuromuscular coordination.
> ◆ Has no published scientific evidence to support its efficacy.

PILATES

The Pilates Method of Movement was conceived approximately 90 years ago as a workout that could be performed by everyone, of any age and any level of ability, from basic to advanced, from the injured to the "super fit."[42] The

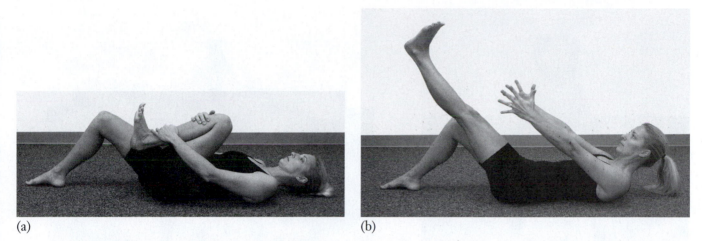

(a)   (b)

Figure 10.2   Single leg stretch. While in supine position (a) the knee is brought up to the chest, the back is kept flat on the floor, the hips as maintained as "square" as possible, the head is lifted up, the abdominal muscles are contracted, and the client exhales. As the client exhales, she extends the leg while simultaneously extending the arm (b). Following this, she inhales as she returns to the starting position. This exercise is designed to stretch the low back, neck, hips, shoulders, and knee regions and strengthen the abdominals and ankle dorsiflexors.

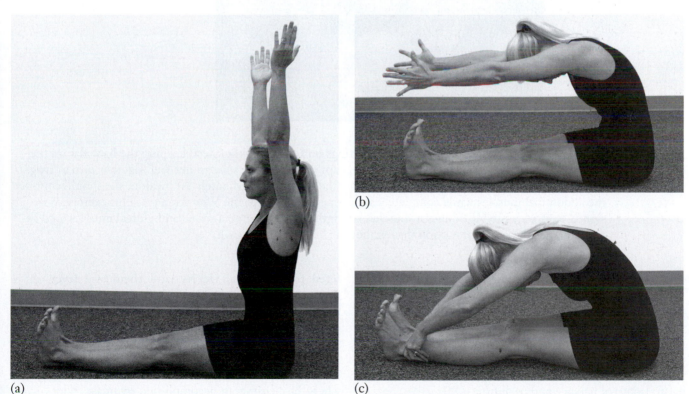

(b)

(a)   (c)

Figure 10.3   Sitting arm and leg stretch. While in long sitting the client inhales as she stretches her arms towards the ceiling (a). As she exhales, she contracts her lower abdominal muscles and reaches up even higher. In a controlled sweeping manner, she then brings her head down (chin to chest) and flexes her trunk, reaching with the fingers past the toes (b). To finish the movement, the client reaches with her hands and grasps her ankles to maintain the stretch position (c).

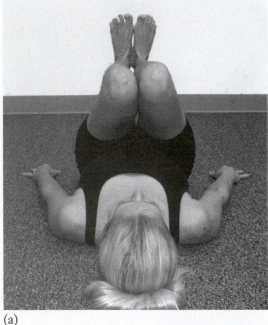

(a)

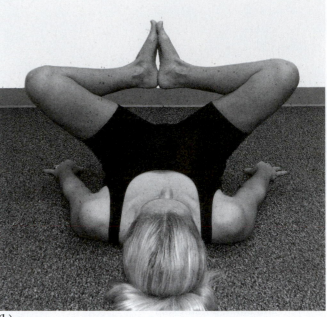

(b)

(c)

Figure 10.4   The V. While in supine position, the client brings both knees to the chest, keeping the back flat on the floor (a). As the client inhales, she abducts her hips and bring the soles of her feet together into a "frog-like" position (b). As she exhales, while keeping the hips at approximately 90° flexion, she should contract the abdominal muscles while completely abducting the hips into the V position (c). This exercise is designed to stretch the hip adductor muscles, strengthen the lower abdominal and gluteal muscles, and expand the natural range of motion throughout the lumbopelvic region.

Pilates Method combines Western and Eastern traditions, viewing the mind and body as working in complete harmony with one another. Pilates Method routines are considered to be biomechanically safe and non-impact in nature; the moves stretch and strengthen all of the major muscle groups without neglecting the smaller, weaker muscles—all with the focus on safely restoring the body's natural state of balance and total fitness.[42]

Background

Joseph H. Pilates (Pi-LAH-teez) was born near Dusseldorf Germany in 1880.[42] He was a sickly child who suf-

fered from asthma, rickets, and rheumatic fever. As a teenager, he began his lifelong quest to improve his health by studying ways to combat sickness through conditioning and strengthening the body. He actively participated in bodybuilding, diving, gymnastics, and skiing. The effect was so evident that by the age of 14, he began posing for anatomical charts. In 1912, Pilates moved to England, where he became an accomplished gymnast, skier, diver, boxer, and circus performer.[43] He initially earned a living as a circus performer and eventually as a self-defense trainer of English detectives. As World War I began, he was designated an "enemy alien" and interned with other Germans. During his imprisonment, Pilates became a

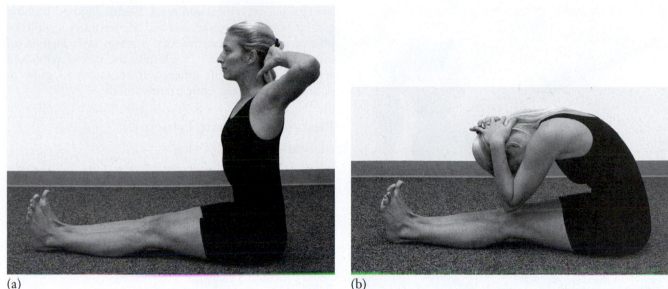

(a)   (b)

Figure 10.5   Neck and upper back stretch. While in an upright long sitting postion with the ankles dorsiflexed, the client clasps her hands behind the head, retracts the scapulae, and externally rotates and abducts the shoulders as she inhales (a). While exhaling, she should contract the abdominal muscles, flex the neck, bring the elbows closer together, bring the chin toward the chest, and flex the neck and trunk (b). This exercise is intended to decrease shoulder tension, increase cervicothoracic spine segmental motion, stretch the hamstrings and calf muscles, and strengthen both the ankle dorsiflexors and the abdominal muscles.

camp nurse working with bedridden and inactive clients, which gave him an opportunity to experiment with his exercise principles. He formulated a regimen that "develops the body uniformly, corrects faulty postures, restores physical vitality, invigorates the mind, and elevates the spirit." Pilates viewed fitness "holistically," taking into consideration the importance of the entire body working together as a healthy unit.[42–44] He recognized the need for a strong heart carrying oxygen-rich blood to the muscles and forcing accumulated waste out of the system. During this time, he invented exercise apparatuses and ways to exercise inmates' limbs, stretch their spines, and develop their core strength, for example, by attaching

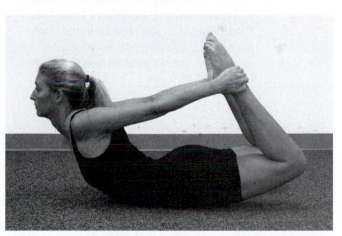

Figure 10.7   The Bow. While lying in prone with knees flexed, the client should grasp her ankles. While exhaling, she lifts the chest and knees off of the floor simultaneously. Once she has reached the top of the stretch, she should also extend her neck to stretch the anterior cervical and abdominal musculature. She should inhale as she returns to the starting position. This exercise helps to stretch the quadriceps muscles and facilitate lumbar spine flexibility.

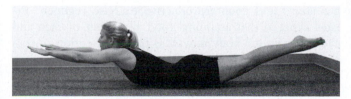

Figure 10.6   The Bird. While in a prone position with arms overhead, while exhaling, the client lifts her arms, head and legs slightly (2–4 in.) off the floor. As she inhales, she should slowly return to the start position. This exercise is intended to strengthen the lumbar paraspinal, gluteal, hamstring, scapular depressor, and cervical spine extensor muscles.

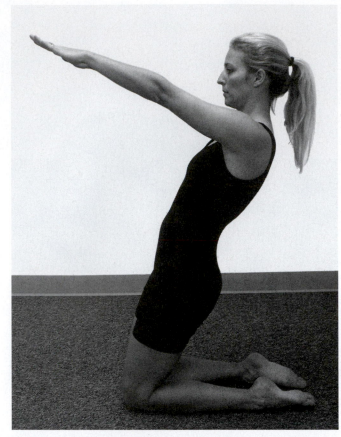

Figure 10.8   Double thigh stretch. While in a high kneeling position with the shoulders flexed 90°, the client exhales as she posteriorly tilts the pelvis, leaning back from the thighs while maintaining an upright trunk. She should inhale as she returns to the starting position. This exercise is intended to strengthen the lower abdominal muscles and the quadriceps.

springs to their hospital beds and bedside chairs. The equipment used during this time became the prototype of several pieces of equipment used today.

It was during the influenza epidemic of 1918 that his methods gained widespread recognition when none of the inmates under Pilates' care succumbed to influenza while thousands died throughout England.[42,43] Because of his success with the internees, Pilates was asked to train the most elite armed forces of the British military. After the war, Pilates continued his fitness training programs in Hamburg, Germany, where he honed his methods with the city's police force. In 1926, Pilates immigrated to the United States and established a fitness studio in New York City.[42,43] During the 1930s and 1940s, the Pilates Method was used by dancers, professional athletes, businessmen, and performing artists. Over time, Pilates went on to develop a series of exercise techniques and therapeutic exercise devices modified from gymnastics equipment such as

springs, pulleys, rings, and mats. Pilates Method training combines over 500 exercises and incorporates a philosophy of movement control that stresses coordination of mind, body and spirit.[42–44] Despite the lack of published evidence regarding its efficacy, it continues to grow in popularity as a therapeutic exercise method.

Pilates Eight Basic Principles of Body Conditioning

Contrology and the Basic Principles of Pilates Method. The *Pilates Method* involves a series of controlled movements that connect the mind and body (*contrology*) with the focus on body mechanics, posture and breathing patterns.[43,44] This method has eight basic principles: relaxation, concentration, control/alignment, centering, flowing movement, precision/coordination, breathing, and stamina.

Relaxation. The first goal of the Pilates Method is teaching the client to become aware of the presence and absence of tension throughout the entire body. Recognizing and releasing areas of unwanted tension is necessary before the client is to begin any type of workout. For example, if a client is not aware of muscles that are tense or holding tension, when the client begins to workout, the wrong muscles will be activated repeatedly, creating a cycle of poor posture, body mechanics, and movements which will result in pain, muscle imbalance, or dysfunction.

Concentration. The Pilates Method believes that the client must engage the mind with every movement. The client should be instructed to always think about each movement and notice how interrelated every motion is within the body. The client should visualize the next movement, as it will actually help his or her central nervous system choose the right combination of muscles to perform the exercise and its component movements.

Control / Alignment. Of fundamental importance to the Pilates Method is that all physical motion is controlled by the mind. Motion and activity without control leads to a haphazard and counterproductive exercise regimen. Pilates believed that attaining good alignment of each and every part of the body as well as paying attention to correct joint placement and proper muscle recruitment while completing any given exercise was essential to safety and to correcting muscle imbalances.

Centering. The human body has a physical center from which all motion proceeds. In Pilates, the single most important section of the body is the area between the bottom of the client's rib cage and the line across the hips. Pilates called this area the "*Powerhouse*" or the "*Girdle of Strength*". The center is located in the area of the abdomen, lower back, pelvic floor, and buttocks. Virtually all exercises in

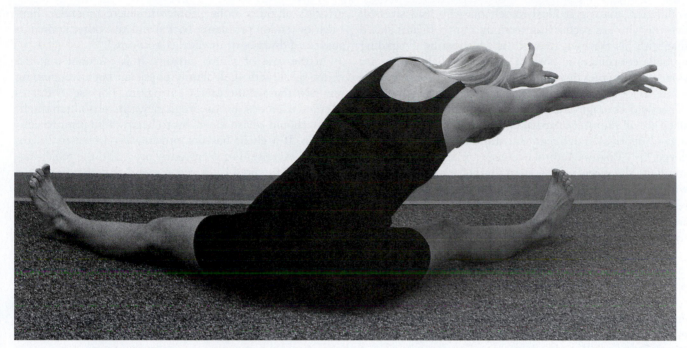

Figure 10.9   Inner thigh stretch with spinal rotation. While in a long sitting position with the hips abducted in as wide a V as comfortably possible, with the knees extended but not locked, the ankles dorsiflexed and the arms overhead, the client inhales and rotates the trunk until she faces her right or left leg. While exhaling, she brings the trunk toward the leg, reaching past the foot. This exercise is designed to stretch the hip adductors and the hamstrings. The spinal rotation component also facilitates segmental spinal mobility.

the Pilates Method work the Powerhouse. In order to create or work the Powerhouse, the client must "zip up" or lift the pelvic floor and hollow or take the navel to the spine. For example, as the client exhales he or she should draw up the muscles of the pelvic floor and tighten the abdominals.[42] Pilates believed one must create a strong center before doing any form of movement or exercise.

Flowing Movement.   Pilates believed in natural movements being performed correctly, gracefully, with control, and lengthening away from the strong core or center.[42] Clients should not rush through any step or movement, but rather move slowly, smoothly, and evenly, as damage and injury can occur by hurried movements. As soon as the client feels stress or strain they should stop the exercise and go on to the next exercise. Clients should also be instructed to avoid stiff or jerky movements.

Precision / Coordination.   Pilates said, ". . . concentrate on right movements each time you exercise or else you will do them improperly and lose their value." The intent with precision is to limit the client's movements while coordinating the specifics of each component for each movement. Once the client becomes familiar with the steps to each exercise, they should add the components together to create complex combinations (see Chapter 8), eventually seeking to replicate the precise sequence of

movements each time. When the movements become automatic and no longer feel awkward, then they have become a "muscle memory".

Breathing.   Pilates emphasized the importance of keeping the bloodstream pure. This purity comes as a result of proper breathing during the exercises, which oxygenates the blood and eliminates noxious gases. The client should be taught to coordinate breathing patterns with each movement of an exercise. As a general rule, the client should be instructed to inhale to prepare for a movement and exhale as the movement is being executed.

Stamina.   The final principle of the Pilates Method is to build endurance in key muscles and progressively challenge one's core stability. If the client has both stability and endurance, the end result will be efficient movement, enhanced performance, and improved energy conservation and utilization.

Therapeutic Indications

The Pilates Method claims that it can help the body becomes firmer and sleeker, with better shape, help a client to move more easily and quickly perform many tasks, acquire many desired physical skills, better prevent injury, and increase physical and mental strength as well as endurance, making it ideal for clients who lead stressful lives or who are recovering from an injury. Pilates stated that with his method, strength is added without building up bulk; coordination, posture, balance and alignment are corrected; fatigue, discomfort and pain are decreased; the mind becomes the body's master, increasing self-confidence and courage; muscle flexibility, joint mobility, and sleep are all improved; sexual enjoyment is increased; feelings of depression are reduced; and most back pain is relieved.[42–45] Pilates Method exercises are also purported to stimulate the circulatory system, oxygenate the blood, aid with lymphatic drainage, give the immune system a boost, release endorphins, and foster clearer thinking, faster reaction times, and enhanced memory by helping to speed transmission of nerve messages.[42–45]

Pilates Method exercises may benefit a host of non-impaired clients in addition to those who are experiencing or suffering from chronic pain, chronic joint stress/arthritis, pregnancy, both pre- and postnatal osteoporosis, and emotional stress.[42–45] Pilates also claimed that his exercise method is indicated for clients with 1) obesity, diabetes, heart disease and stroke, because it reduces the risk of these vascular diseases by lowering blood pressure, raising the level of protective, or "good" high-density lipoprotein cholesterol, reducing the risk of developing blood clots and diabetes and countering weight gain; 2) cancer, by reducing the risk of developing colon cancer, one of the leading causes of cancer deaths among men and women; and 3) osteoporosis, by increasing the client's bone density and reducing the risk of fractures.[42–45] This system is considered to be safe for most client groups, including senior citizens, and for pregnant and postpartum women, with some precautions.

Contraindications and Special Precautions

Common sense dictates that if a client has any physical disease or limitation, the rehabilitation clinician should consult with the client's physician before attempting any new exercise program. In addition, as a rehabilitation clinician who is new to the Pilates Method it is advisable to consult with a certified instructor to assess the client's problem areas and assist with creating a program that targets their specific needs. It is always advisable to instruct the client to discontinue any exercise that causes any discomfort or pain.

In general, clients younger than 35 years of age and in good health do not need a physical examination before beginning a Pilates Method exercise program. If the client is over 35 years of age and has been inactive for several years or has ever had any of the following medical conditions, both the client and the rehabilitation clinician should consult the client's physician prior to beginning any Pilates Method exercise program: high blood pressure, heart trouble, family history of stroke or heart attacks, frequent dizzy spells, extreme breathlessness after mild exertion, arthritis or other bone problems, severe muscular, ligament or tendon problems; back problems, other known or suspected diseases or medical conditions.[42–45]

In the case of senior citizens, it is essential that the client speak with their family physician before beginning any new therapeutic exercise program. For use of Pilates Method exercises during pregnancy, the rehabilitation clinician should advise the client to begin them prior to conception. If a client has not previously performed Pilates Method exercises but is currently pregnant, the rehabilitation clinician should not recommend that they initiate a Pilates Method exercise program. For clients who are versed in Pilates Method exercises prior to conception, Pilates offers nine recommended exercises specifically designed for the mom-to-be. Pilates Method exercises are believed to be excellent for post-partum recovery even if the client has not previously performed them.

Evidence

There is very little published scientific research available regarding the effectiveness of Pilates Method exercises. There is abundant research and theories regarding motor learning, biomechanics, and musculoskeletal physiology that can be applied to and help support the Pilates Method exercise approach, but this needs to be subjected to the rigors of research to better evaluate their efficacy for therapeutic exercise and wellness or injury prevention initiatives. A few published scientific studies do exist which explore the efficacy of Pilates Method exercise in the treatment of cardiovascular conditions,[46] general conditioning and fitness,[47–51] women's health,[52] and various orthopedic conditions and populations (i.e., patellofemoral joint dysfunction, anterior cruciate ligament injury, low back pain, frozen shoulder).[53–56] Hall[57] explored the effects of Pilates Method exercise on balance and gait in an elderly population. Thirty-one subjects ranging in age from 65 to 81 years of age completed a 10-week training program. Subjects were randomly assigned to one of three groups: a traditional strength plus flexibility group, a Pilates Method exercise group, and a control (no treatment) group. Pre- and post-treatment static and dynamic balance and Berg Balance Scale measurements were compared. The results revealed that Pilates Method exercises were effective for improving static postural balance. Hall[57] also indicated that Pilates Method exercise might improve dynamic balance in elderly adults.

Mallery et al.[58] examined the feasibility of performing resistance exercise with acutely ill hospitalized older adults. The participants were 39 acutely ill subjects over 70 years of age who were ambulatory prior to admission. In this study, subjects were randomized into one of two groups: a resistance training group ($n = 19$) or a passive range of motion group ($n = 20$). The resistance training group received a hospital-based resistance exercise program that incorporated both conventional exercises and

Pilates Method exercises that targeted the gluteals and lower extremities. In addition, principles of postural alignment, correct exercise technique, and proper breathing sequencing were emphasized. All therapeutic exercises were designed to be reproducible and easily performed in bed. The subjects completed each exercise for 3 sets of 10 repetitions for 3 times a week until hospital discharge or for a maximum of four weeks. The outcome measures were adherence and participation. The results found that participation was 71 percent among the resistance training group compared to 96 percent by the passive range of motion group. Adherence for the resistance training group was 63 percent compared to 95 percent for the passive range of motion group. Mallery et al.[58] concluded that acutely ill elderly subjects were generally able to comply with a simple and standardized resistance training program that included Pilates Method exercises.

Using a pre-test, post-test model, Kish[59] examined the effects of Pilates Method exercises upon pelvic alignment, stature, abdominal strength, and functional adductor and hip flexor flexibility among 17 college dancers of similar stature. Ten subjects completed a four-week Pilates Method exercise program, while seven served as control subjects. The results indicated that the Pilates group made significant improvements in abdominal strength, hip adductor, and flexor extensibility.

Using a randomized controlled study with a pre-test, post-test design and a 3, 6, and 12 month follow-up, Rydeard[60] investigated the efficacy of a specific therapeutic exercise program based on the Pilates Method among 39 physically active subjects with low back pain who were between 20 and 55 years of age. Subjects in the experimental group participated in a four week long Pilates program designed to train neuromuscular trunk stability while the control group received standard care and no specific treatment intervention. The experimental group displayed a significant reduction in average pain intensity compared to the control group. The experimental group also displayed decreased disability levels at 3 months post-treatment; however group differences were not evident at the 6 and 12 months follow-up.

Bryan and Hawson[61] used a case study format to explore the benefits of using Pilates Method exercises with a 48-year old subject who had been diagnosed with chronic low back pain. Pre- and post- intervention measurements included a Visual Analog Scale (VAS) for pain intensity and the Oswestry Scale for functional disability following six treatment sessions which incorporated Pilates Method exercise into standard treatment. At the end of the intervention they reported 81.5 percent, and 87.7 percent VAS score and Oswestry score improvements, respectively.

Hutchinson et al.[48] studied the efficacy of using Pilates Method exercises to improve the jumping ability of six elite rhythmic gymnasts who underwent an intense course of jump training. The experimental protocol included one month of aquatic training and Pilates method of body conditioning using spring controlled resistance followed by a nine-month duration maintenance program. Measurements of reaction time, jump height, and explosive leg power were obtained using a force plate on four occasions: pre-training, at the end of one month, at the end of four months, and at the end of one year. The results revealed that after one month of training, jump height improved 16.2 percent, ground reaction force timing improved 50 percent, and explosive power improved by 220 percent. They concluded that an intense course of jump training using aquatic training and Pilates Method exercises can safely and significantly improve leaping ability; however, no significant improvements occurred after the first month.[48] Subjects maintained their one-month gains at both the four-month and one-year post-tests, but they did not demonstrate any additional improvements despite continued jump training.

Equipment

Although many of the core exercises of the Pilates Method do not require special equipment, using instead available mats, boxes, springs, weights, ball, walls, barrels, and the "magic circle" (an exercise resistance ring made of soft rubber), it also makes use of spring resistance apparatus such as the Pilates Performer, Universal Reformer, Cadillac, Spine Corrector Barrel, Tower, Trapeze Table, and "the Chair."[42-45] Depending on the client's level and goals, the rehabilitation clinician can utilize various pieces of equipment to progress each client according to his or her ability and healing status and to achieve the desired functional or sport specific goals. Many clients prefer to complete their exercises on a mat, but a rug works fine. For some of the intermediate and advanced exercises, a 12–16 in. diameter ball is needed. Installing a set of springs or resistive tubing into any door frame can accommodate the need for wall springs. For exercises that require a Barrel, small and large pillows, or bolsters can be substituted. Pilates Method exercise apparatus and exercise videos are available from Pilates Studios and most can also be purchased online.

Technique

Nearly all of the approximately 500 exercises developed by Pilates involve a recumbent, or lying flat, position, which allows the client to exercise without strain to the heart, thereby taking advantage of a more natural, relaxed positioning of the internal organs.[42-44] However many Pilates exercises, especially those using the Reformer, can also be performed in sitting, supine, prone, or standing positions.

Pilates Method exercises concentrate on specific form and strengthening, beginning with little or no resistance and progressing to higher resistances as appropriate strength and awareness are developed. In the therapeutic exercise setting, most Pilates Method exercises are initially performed on a mat and progress to being performed on several types of apparatus.[62] Pilates Method exercise apparatus was developed to alter gravitational force alignment on the body with both springs and gravitational forces (i.e., position) being used to assist an injured client to be able to complete movements in a safe and successful manner. The end goal is to alter the spring tension and increase the effects of gravity by progressing the client into more functional positions (i.e., moving from supine to standing), that enable them to perform complete functional motions and activities of daily living in a non-impaired manner again (with the complete effects of gravity plus load).[62] Regardless of the exercise or position, Pilates Method exercises emphasize eccentric muscle activation as well as breathing that is coordinated with movement. Finally, depending on the client, the rehabilitation clinician can dictate the difficulty of the Pilates Method exercise program by selecting exercises and positions as well as progressing the client through three

phases: assisted movements, dynamic stabilization, and functional re-education.[62]

The initial Pilates Method exercise phase consists of assisted movements.[62] Exercises in this phase typically use a spring apparatus to avoid unwanted movements and muscle activity, which can be associated with pain, weakness, or muscular imbalances. Learning to isolate peripheral joint movements from trunk movements is also an essential part of the initial phase. This disassociation is necessary to focus concentration of movement control at specific joints and is accomplished by having movements occur on a relatively large base of support in order to minimize unwanted muscle guarding. Two commonly performed Pilates Method exercise progressions using specific apparatus are presented (**Figures. 10.10a–d and 10.11a–d**). The deep trunk and spinal muscles are thought to provide greater stabilization near the proximal upper or lower extremity segments, such as the hip and shoulder joints. This efficient use of the deep stabilizers and decreased guarding around the area of a lesion is consistent with Porterfield and DeRosa's[63] phase I of

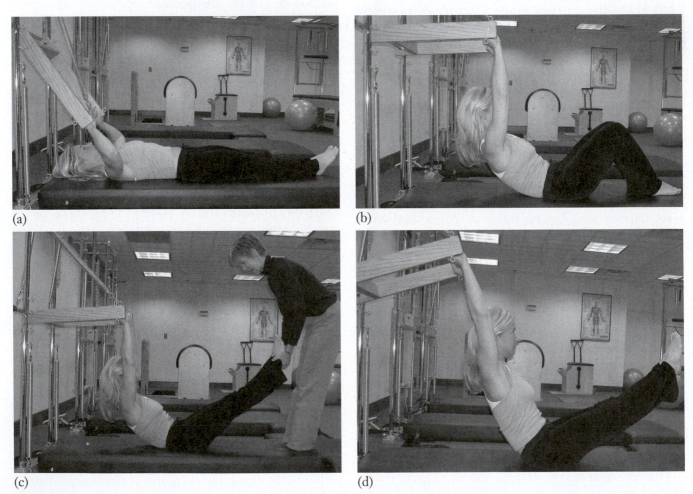

(a)   (b)   (c)   (d)

Figure 10.10 Pilates abdominal progression using the Wall System. Starting position with springs assisting abdominal curl-ups (a). Phase I has stable base of support with springs to assist movement (b). Instructor assists the progression to phase III (c). Phase III (d) performed with small base of support and decreased assistance provided by upper extremity apparatus.

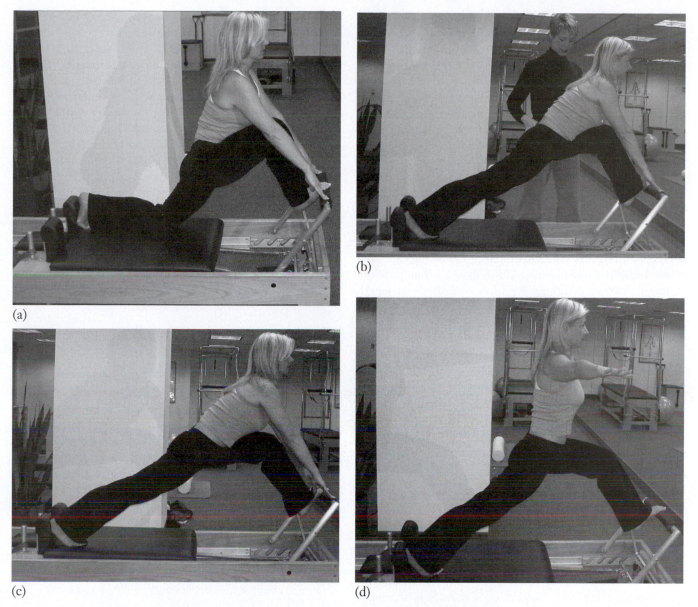

Figure 10.11   Progression of Pilates exercises using the Reformer. (a) Phase I starts with greater base of support and can be progressed by using springs to resist the movement. Progression to phase II (b) is performed with the assistance of instructor and use of springs to assist bed translation. Phase II (c) is performed with decreased base of support and upper extremity assistance. Phase III (d) relies heavily on balance and control of posture while the bed translates more easily, increasing the difficulty of the exercise due to greater demand of balance and stability while sliding the bed.

rehabilitation, the purpose of which is to control pain, encourage counseling on biomechanically correct technique, and provide assistance in the form of mobilization or restoring the desired movement properly without incurring additional injury. When using Pilates Method exercises, the rehabilitation clinician attempts to restore mobility by varying the effects of the gravitational forces that act on the client while using appropriate feedback and assistance to facilitate proper movements.[62]

During phase I (*assisted movements*), specific joint range of motion patterns are performed with spring-loaded assistance. By providing a 30 percent to 60 percent reduc-

tion in body weight, the spring-loaded apparatus is believed to provide movement feedback to the central nervous system (CNS) and assist in movement control. Even a minor reduction in body weight may be sufficient to alter force feedback and facilitate motor learning. A large base of support (see Chapter 9) and increased assistance from the springs makes phase I easier than the remaining exercises in the progression. Once appropriate movement is restored, it is believed that forces are then equally distributed to surrounding joints. Breathing is encouraged during this phase to facilitate the use of core dynamic trunk stabilizing musculature.

Phase II is called *dynamic stabilization*, and efficiency of movement is the goal.[62] This phase increases the challenges to stabilization and their associated movements. Once clients can adequately perform exercises during phase I, they are progressed to phase II. This can be as simple as maintaining a normal lordotic posture while both lower extremities remain flat on the ground. As exercises are advanced from phase I to phase II, assistance in the form of verbal or tactile cues from an instructor can provide guidance. Therapeutic exercise challenges increase with increases in the apparatus lever lengths, decreases in the base of support, or a decrease in the assistance provided by the spring apparatus.[62] These changes only occur when clients display non-impaired, efficient movement patterns. Decreasing the base of support provides challenges to stability. For example it is more difficult to perform exercises such as hip extension movements in a quadruped position than a prone position. Another example could involve increasing the lever length and progressing from an isolated movement across one joint (i.e., the shoulder) to more integrated joint movements across multiple body segments. Rhythmic breathing patterns change as the tempo of the movement changes, in an effort to maintain stability of the proximal segment. By incorporating the breathing and movement principles from phase I, the client is able to recruit secondary stabilizers (i.e., erector spinae, external and internal oblique abdominals, latissimus dorsi, deep pelvic musculature). In addition, this phase allows the rectus abdominus muscle to be trained for more ballistic functional movements.[62] Hence, the emphasis of the first two phases is movement control.

Phase III is called *functional re-education* and continues to emphasize balance and movement control as well as progressing from completing a specific task in a foreign environment to completing the same task in a familiar functional or recreational environment. The purpose of having the client initially complete a specific task in a "foreign environment" (i.e., supine vs. standing) is to ensure that the desired movement can be completed and repeatedly reproduced with less proprioceptive challenge, fewer destructive forces, the lack of desire to take the path of least resistance (i.e., the easy way), and the dissolution of old neuromotor patterns, poor training, or bad habits.[62] Once the client has successfully completed a specific task in a foreign environment, they are then challenged, encouraged, and provided both verbal and tactile cues to build adequate endurance and maintain efficiency of movement while completing the specific task in a familiar environment.[62] The most advanced phase of this exercise continuum occurs when the springs provide minimum assistance. Movements performed in this phase can also be performed in a foreign rather than a familiar environment. For example the client may not be ready to perform a one legged jump in their familiar standing environment, but may be ready to perform the jump in a foreign supine environment on a Pilates Method exercise apparatus with spring-loaded assistance. Exercise movements initially performed in a foreign envi-

ronment may not require the client to control for extraneous forces while executing the desired task.[62]

While the spring-loaded devices used in Pilates Method exercises provide unique environments, similar controls can possibly also be achieved without special equipment. Some examples of these movements are the open rocker (**Figure 10.12a–b**), the bridge with leg lift (**Figure 10.13a–b**), the reverse plank (**Figure 10.14**), the table top pose (**Figure 10.15**), and the forearm plank (**Figure 10.16**). Because of the wide range of movements that can be performed, clients can use Pilates Method exercise techniques with impairments ranging from low back pain to arthritis, or most movement disorders. Incorporation of Pilates Method exercises into conventional therapeutic exercise programs may be beneficial for many clients, although the rehabilitation clinician should attend a continuing education course to become more versed in specific techniques prior to adding them to the therapeutic exercise program that they design.

Practitioner Training

According to proponents of the Pilates Methods, the exercises are most effective when presented by a certified Pilates Instructor on specifically designed exercise equipment.[43,44] At this time there does not appear to be any clinical or scientific evidence that Pilates Methods are superior to or more harmful than other training methods, though there remains a great deal of enthusiasm surrounding this approach to conditioning, rehabilitation, and fitness. There are certified Pilates instructors located throughout the United States, Canada, and a growing number of countries around the world. Certification involves several hundred hours of theoretical and practical training. In addition, there are numerous books and training videos for beginners, intermediate and advanced students.

Key Point:

Pilates. . . .

- Is characterized by development of kinesthetic monitoring ability, especially in the trunk/pelvis and movement from a stable core.
- Is considered an awareness building technique, teaching the body to work as a whole.
- Contains eight principles of body conditioning.
- Has at its core the concept of contrology, the science and art of coordinated body-mind-spirit development through natural movements.
- Advocates conditioning of the entire musculoskeletal system.

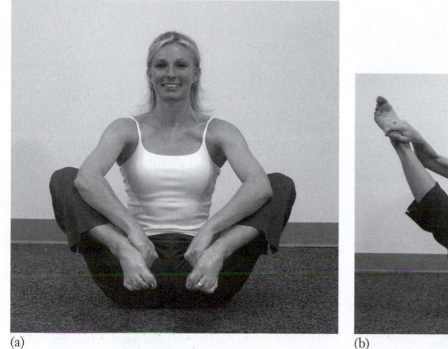
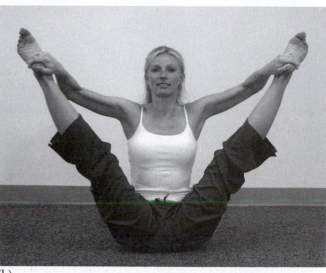

(a)   (b)

Figure 10.12   Open leg rocker. In sitting position, the client bends one knee at a time towards the chest, while inhaling, and grabs and holds onto the inside of the ankles (a). While exhaling, the client extends the legs, lifting them towards the ceiling to create a V, keeping the spine as straight as possible (b). The purpose of this exercise is to improve the client's coordination, strength, flexibility, sense of balance, and motion control.

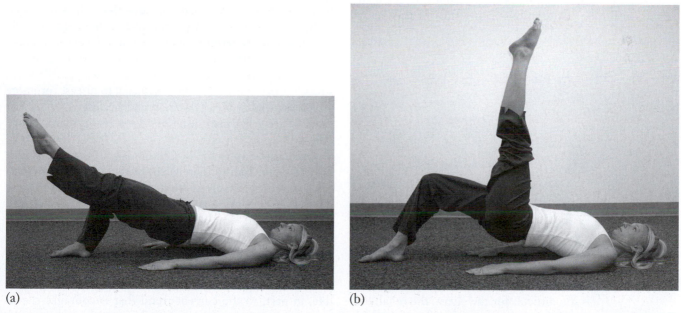

(a)   (b)

Figure 10.13   Bridge with leg lift. The client assumes a supine position with the knees flexed and the feet flat on the floor, approximately shoulder width apart. While exhaling, she initiates a posterior pelvic tilt and lifts the hips off the floor. The client then extends one knee, keeping the thighs parallel (a). Following this, she should inhale and extend the leg toward the ceiling (b). The client should exhale as she lower the leg back to the start position. This exercise strengthens the Powerhouse region.

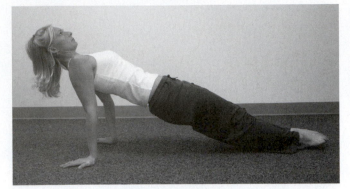

Figure 10.14   Reverse plank. From a long sitting position with the hands placed approximately 12 inches behind her, the client inhales as she lifts the pelvis toward the ceiling, pressing the chest up until the arms are straight. As she exhales, she should lift the pelvis up until the body forms a straight line. This exercise also trains the Powerhouse, the shoulders and the arms.

QIGONG

Qigong (pronounced "chee goong" and also known as Chikung or Chigong) is a branch of traditional Chinese medicine commonly described as the breathing exercise or energy work or exercise.[11] Qigong incorporates the concepts of *Qi*, the body's vital energy, and *Gong*, which indicates a level of prowess in some area of endeavor.[64–66] Practitioners believe that one's Qi is responsible for maintaining health.[11,65] Alterations in the flow of this energy

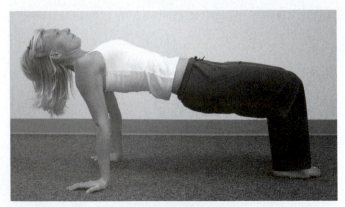

Figure 10.15   Table top pose. If pressing up to the reverse plank position with the legs straight is too difficult for the client, the rehabilitation clinician can have the client start with the knees bent and feet flat on the floor. As the client exhales she should press the hips and thighs up until they are in line with the shoulders, creating a table-like surface.

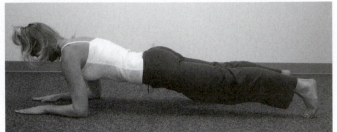

Figure 10.16   Forearm plank. Starting from a quadruped position, the client places her forearms parallel on the floor under the chest approximately shoulder width apart. Next, the client inhales, scooping the navel toward the spine and extending one leg back on the the ball of the foot, and then the other. As she exhales, she should lower the hips to shoulder height and hold the body in a straight line. Pressing firmly into the floor, the elbows should be under the chest, and the face should be over the hands. This exercise strengthens the chest, shoulders, upper core muscles, and improves pelvic and scapular stability.

results in states of excess or deficiency, which relates to subsequent disease or injury.[64,65] The practice of Qigong is believed to enhance the flow of Qi through breathing exercises, systematic movements, and intense concentration.[65] Qigong practitioners believe that when practiced daily, a series of actions or movements involving muscle coordination, breathing, and mental concentration can improve strength and flexibility, increase circulation, reverse damage due to injury or disease, relieve pain, reduce stress, restore energy, provide resistance to disease, promote awareness, and induce relaxation and healing.[15,27,30,65] For years Qigong has been used in China for its "anti-aging" effects.[67]

Qigong is similar to Tai Chi Chuan, in that it is physically less demanding than many of the exercise forms already discussed (such as Pilates or Nickolaus exercises). Therefore, it is more suitable for disabled clients, as well as clients of all ages and physical fitness levels.[11,30,65] It can be practiced while lying in bed, sitting, walking, or standing.[11,30,65] It can even be performed by clients who are confined to a wheelchair or bed.[30] The recent incorporation of Qigong into Western medical environments is due, in part, to the current trend that encourages clients to be independent consumers, active participants, and self-healers.[30] In addition, Qigong classes are gaining popularity in both public and private schools, corporate wellness programs, social agencies, and church and community recreation centers throughout the United States.[11,30,65]

Background

Qigong is one of the most ancient and traditional forms of Chinese therapies that have been passed down from generation to generation for over 3,000 years. Qigong's modern history began in the 1950s when research was established to investigate all forms of traditional Chinese medicine, which were being integrated into the health system in China after the establishment of the People's Republic of China in 1949.[68] Several Qigong centers were established throughout China in the 1950s[69]; however, during the Cultural Revolution (1966–1976), Qigong was officially prohibited and interest was strongly discouraged.[69] Only over the last 20 years has awareness regarding the medical benefits of Qigong become evident.[15] By 1996, more than 1,000 abstracts on the subject of Qigong had been published in English.[69] Over the past 20 years the numbers of people practicing Qigong has grown tremendously in all parts of the world.[8,69]

Principles

Historically, the goal of Qigong has been to gather Qi at the area of the body located below the navel known as the *Dantien*. Gathering energy in this area serves to protect the core of a client's strength. In medical and fitness environments, the goal is to promote tranquility enhanced by relaxation of the sympathetic nervous system and stimulation of the parasympathetic nervous system.[70]

Qigong is generally classified into five schools: Daoist, Buddhist, Confucian, martial art, and medical.[71] For many practitioners, the Daoist and Buddhist versions are the most common or "true" types. There are also two ways to practice the first four types of Qigong: actively and passively. Active Qigong, or Dong Gong, involves movements that are related to acupuncture points, meridians, and channels, and its purpose is to strengthen the internal organs.[8,71] Passive Qigong, or Jing Dong, consists primarily of meditation. It can be performed in sitting, lying, or standing and its purpose is to help cultivate and store Qi in the Dantien. Conceptually, this technique works on the internal body and in cleansing the mind.[8,71] The fifth type of Qigong, medical Qigong, usually involves the theoretical aspects but not the practical aspects associated with acupuncture points and channels.[71] Medical Qigong combines meditation, physical movements, and breathing exercises, similar to other Chinese therapies. The client who practices Qigong learns to identify stages of feeling related to awareness of Qi in the Dantien. The Qi has been described as a warm, tingling sensation, progressing to a liquid, pulsating feeling that passes through the body like blood.[71] Qigong masters achieve a state where their Qi becomes "crystal," and where they are said to be able to use their own Qi to help heal other people. At whatever stage a client is when practicing Qigong, controlling internal energy and learning to alter the flow of energy from areas of excess to areas of deficiency can enhance personal health and well being.[71]

Technique

There are three primary forms of Qigong: internal oriented, external oriented, and breathing exercise oriented.[27] Internal Qigong focuses on manipulating the Qi within one's own body to maintain health and self-healing and consists mainly of two forms: 1) quiescent or meditation oriented Qigong, which consists of meditation and breathing exercises; and 2) dynamic or movement oriented Qigong, which includes dance-like movements.[27,65]

Quiescent or meditation oriented Qigong focuses on inner serenity, control of one's own "micro-cosmic energy," and connection with the "macro-cosmic energy system."[27] This form can be practiced in standing, sitting, or lying down positions.[27] Body movements are kept to a minimum so that they do not interrupt the working of the mind. For example, the client might begin in sitting, focusing on inhaling while visualizing a concentration of Qi in the abdominal region. While exhaling they visualize the Qi leaving the abdomen and entering the abdominal organs, extremities, and various glands throughout the body.[11] It is with continual deep breathing, concentration, and relaxation that the Qi, as a healing energy, is believed to circulate through the body. In short, the client focuses on restoring homeostasis of the energy system, harmonizing the opposing Yin and Yang energies, removing any obstructions in the energy flow, and obtaining optimal energy functioning.[27]

In the external or movement oriented form of Qigong, the body is active while the mind is quiet and relaxed. This form originally involved simple body movements but has evolved into a series of slow, gentle, and supple dance-like movements. The purpose is to channel energy through blocked or stagnated areas, eliminate discomfort in affected parts or regions, and restore normal physiological function throughout the body.[27] This type of Qigong is also the province of Qigong masters, who have learned through years of practice to transmit the force of their Qi to others for healing purposes.[11]

The third form, breathing oriented exercises, were designed to increase energy levels, strengthen various organs, and expel the "unhealthy" or "ailing" Qi. For the practices of strengthening and invigorating Qi, one should practice daily breathing exercises, preferably in the morning, and for healing purposes; one should purposefully expel the ailing or unhealthy Qi and then enthusiastically inhale fresh, healthy air. The client should do this several times per day (particularly in the morning) for as long as it takes to restore sufficient energy to the body.[9] Then the client can use the restored energy to heal an injury or defeat illness.[27] There are several key concepts or components to Qigong, including mind training, breathing training, and body training.

Mind Training

The mind is an essential component to the practice of Qigong. During meditation, the client should be concentrating on the Dantien to ensure that the Qi will be stored there and should not be thinking of anything else. However, this can be difficult for the beginner. A beginning client should begin by just concentrating on relaxing and then slowly bring their mind to the Dantien.[71] The client should slowly work toward the goal of achieving "emptiness of mind." This state is described as being when "heaven and man become one."[71]

Some Qigong exercises require the client to concentrate on special areas of the body, for example on the *Yongquan point*, an acupuncture point on the sole of the foot. This point is connected to the kidneys and can benefit clients with hypertension or kidney disease.[71] Other Qigong exercises might concentrate on the *Laogong point*, the acupuncture point on the palm, which is related to the heart, circulation and to releasing negative Qi.[71] Some Qigong postures and movements might concentrate on the *Shangzhong point* for the heart and lungs.[71] It is important for the client to remember that any misdirection of Qi through the mind can easily cause a problem, resulting in improper movements, incorrect postures, and inadequate neurophysiological training, which may be difficult to correct.[71]

Breathing Training

Correct breathing in time with the movements is another important part of Qigong.[71] Inhaling brings the positive Qi into the body and is usually accompanied with an "opening" movement, while exhaling releases the negative Qi and accompanies a "closing" movement. This type of breathing is believed also to bring energy in through the skin, via the acupuncture points.[71] For many clients, breathing with the whole body may be a very new experience, requiring the rehabilitation clinician's assistance. Rising or elevating Qigong movements are linked with inhaling, while exhaling is linked with sinking or lowering movements. Movements to the left or right can be performed during either inhaling or exhaling breaths.[71]

There are also different ways to breathe during Qigong, including natural or normal breathing, and reverse breathing. Beginner Qigong practitioners should use natural or normal breathing which follow the body's movements or feelings without being aware of their breathing pattern.[71] During this type of breathing, the abdomen expands during inhalation and contracts during exhalation. This breathing method is connected with the Dantien, which, as mentioned before, is located in the area below the navel. Thus, the expanding and contracting of the abdomen in this manner stimulates the Dantien.[71]

Reverse breathing is the opposite of normal or natural breathing. When the client uses this breathing method, the abdomen contracts as they inhale and expands as they exhale. This method of breathing requires a slightly higher level of practice, because it makes the Dantien stronger and stimulates the *Ren* (front) and *Du* (back) channels.[71] Reverse breathing creates *fire* in the body and therefore the client should only use it at certain times and for a short while.[71] For example, a client may find it particularly effective during meditation. With practice, the client will forget the way that they breathe, and will unconsciously incorporate both normal and reverse breathing.

Body Training

In Qigong, the state of body postures and movements are just as important as the state of the mind. The standard posture for Qigong involves creating a straight line between the *Baihui point* or *Sky-door* (on the top of the head) and the *Huiyin point* (between the legs near the anus).[71] This posture allows the client to gather both the "heaven and earth" Qi and allow it to flow naturally. The advantage of this posture is that the client will not lose much energy or fatigue easily.[71] Keeping the mouth closed lets the Qi flow down to the Dantien, thereby allowing the negative Qi to sink down through the legs and release out to the earth. In turn, this lets the positive Qi rise up to the lungs, heart, forehead and Baihui point. Relaxing the joints helps the Qi pass through the entire body, allows more Qi to go to the organs, and allows negative Qi around a problem area to be released. This is believed to enhance blood circulation thereby helping to maintain normal blood pressure.[71] Use of faulty posture can have negative effects. For example, bending forward or backward suppresses the lungs, causes the breath to be short, and results in the individual losing Qi.[71] The body training aspect of Qigong incorporates many different movements, including closing the eyes, squeezing the toes, lifting up the anus, keeping the head upright, slightly bending forward, or keeping body weight shifted onto the left or the right foot.[71] Common to all of the movements is that the client must relax the mind and body, which will allow everything inside to work easily, efficiently, effectively, and naturally.

Direction and Time

One of the interesting features of Qigong is that practitioners believe the four points of the compass relate to different internal organs: east for liver, west for lungs, north for kidneys, south for the heart, and any direction for the stomach because it is the center. To address a health problem in any one of these areas, the client should face the appropriate direction.[8,71] It is also important to remember that according to Qigong, health problems are also connected to Yin and Yang. A low energy level reflects too much Yin, whereas excess energy reflects too much Yang.

Although Qigong can be performed at any time during the day, it is usually recommended that clients practice it during the *Zi* time (11 pm to 1 am) and the *Mao* time

(5 am to 7 am).[8,71] These times relate to the liver and the lungs. The liver is connected to the blood and circulation. The lungs are connected to breathing and Qi. No matter what time is chosen, it is important to remember that once the client has completed the active aspects of Qigong, they need to select a particular meditation to gather Qi.

Therapeutic Indications

Claims regarding the beneficial effects of Qigong include the following:

1. Initiating the "relaxation response," which is triggered by any form of mental concentration and "frees" the mind from distractions, thereby decreasing the sympathetic function of the autonomic nervous system. This, in turn, decreases heart rate and blood pressure, dilates the vascular capillaries, and optimizes the delivery of oxygen to tissues.

2. Altering the neurochemistry profile, moderating pain, depression, and addictive cravings, and optimizing immune system capability.

3. Enhancing the efficiency of the immune system through increased rate and flow of the lymphatic fluid and activation of immune cells.

4. Improving resistance to infection and disease by accelerating the elimination of toxic by-products from the interstitial spaces in the tissues, glands, and organs via the lymphatic system.

5. Enhancing cell metabolism efficiency and tissue regeneration through increased circulation of oxygen and nutrient-rich blood to the brain, and other tissues, and organs.

6. Coordinating right and left brain hemisphere dominance, promoting deeper sleep, reduced anxiety, and mental clarity.

7. Inducing alpha and, in some cases, theta brain waves, which reduces heart rate and blood pressure while facilitating relaxation, mental focus, and paranormal skills; this optimizes the body's self-regulative mechanisms by decreasing the activity of the sympathetic nervous system.

8. Moderating the function of the hypothalamus, pineal glands, and the cerebrospinal fluid system of the brain and spinal cord—all of which mediate pain, and mood, and accelerate immune function.[30]

Qigong has been used to treat such conditions as arthritis, asthma, constipation, depression, fatigue, headaches, digestive problems, and insomnia.[8,30] A number of studies have also reported its use in the treatment of hypertension, diabetes, coronary artery disease, kidney disorders, peripheral vascular disease, tuberculosis, neurasthenia, and a host of other chronic diseases.[15] It has been used to treat backaches, decrease neck problems, and enhance poor circulation.[8,30] Claims have also been made that Qigong can provide pain relief from the chronic pain associated with cancer and low back injury as well as prevent or cure cancer.[8] Other areas improved or influenced by Qigong exercises include general mobility, joint range of motion, reduced fall risk among the elderly, and reduction in mood disturbances (i.e., anger).[15]

Other claims regarding the practical benefits of practicing Qigong include enhanced youthfulness, weight loss and body toning, thereby allowing the client to return to a healthy size and shape; improved posture, attitude, improved coordination; maximized physical meditation performance; improved memory and attention to detail; increased problem solving ability and heightened awareness as well as receptivity via meditation; improved energy levels, strength, and health; enhanced self healing, stress reduction, and improved levels of calmness; improved sleep; and overall enhanced outlook on life.[8,71]

It is important to note that clients who practice Qigong can simultaneously participate in various athletic pursuits.[71] It is also important for the athlete and the rehabilitation clinician to realize that in contrast to Western based fitness training and traditional sports such as football or tennis, which involve external physical skills and performance, Qigong is focused on internal training connected with Qi, the blood, and internal organs.[71] Hence, clients practicing Qigong will not exhaust themselves as they would with recreational, collegiate, or professional sports. Instead the reverse will happen: The more the client practices Qigong, the more Qi they will have and the more energetic they will become.

Contraindications

When properly performed, Qigong is a gentle and invigorating exercise with no adverse effects.[11] There are no known physical health problem for which it is inadvisable to practice Qigong as long as the client relaxes while they practice, moving at their own self-selected pace, and within their tolerance levels. Clients should be aware that there is a so-called adjustment or adaptation period in which a number of unpleasant symptoms (i.e., muscle soreness, muscle aches, fatigue, pain) may occur from practicing Qigong.[27] These symptoms are usually temporary and minor, but do need to be managed properly. Likewise, Qigong exercises that are applied vigorously and consistently will need to be individualized and may need to be adapted to the client's needs, physical status, and current condition.[27]

During menstruation, Qigong can help circulation, ease headaches and cramps, and reduces emotional (mood) swings.[71] However, women experiencing a heavy menstrual cycle should change their meditation focus to the Shanzhong point. The Dantien, the usual focus point, is related to the womb area and focusing on it may overstimulate that area during a menstrual cycle.[71] By having the client concentrate on the Shanzhong point, which is related to the heart and lungs, the menstrual flow should not become heavier. During pregnancy, some of the movements and postures may need to be modified, eliminated, or practiced at the client's comfort level.[8] It is best not to practice Qigong on either an empty or a full stomach. As with other exercise approaches, the client should wait 30 minutes after eating before practicing Qigong.

Rehabilitation clinicians should be aware that clients with respiratory problems might not be able to perform the breathing exercises associated with Qigong.[11] In addition, some types of Qigong exercises (i.e., that focus on forehead concentration or that are similar to Tai Chi) may increase sympathetic tone and be may be contraindicated for clients with anxiety, angina, or hypertension.[27,30] Finally, clients with serious illnesses should be informed that Qigong may be a beneficial adjunct to conventional medicine, but should not be considered an acceptable substitute.[11]

Evidence

Over in the past 15 years, Chinese researchers have performed extensive research on the healing effects of Qigong and report success in treating asthma, insomnia, depression, anxiety, pain, diabetes, and hypertension in addition to aiding in cancer treatment.[11,66] Because the majority of the Chinese studies do not display the rigorous, controlled quantitative measurements that Western science demands, the current U.S. medical establishment generally does not accept many of the findings or claims of Qigong's effectiveness in treating specific diseases.[11] However, an increasing number of Western physicians believe that Qigong may be effective in reducing stress and anxiety, relieving pain from arthritis, improving sleep, and enhancing overall well being.[11] Only recently have the benefits of Qigong been recognized in Western cultures. Therefore, a lack of Western medical literature on this subject exists. What follows is a selective review of the available literature.

Cardiovascular System.   While there is a moderate body of research exploring the efficacy of Qigong and cardiovascular system function,[72–83] very few controlled studies exist. Several studies have indicated that practicing Qigong can have a positive effect on reducing hypertension.[72–75] Additional research has shown that clients who regularly practice Qigong display increased microcirculation,[76,77] reduced reactive catecholamine production and sensitivity,[78] increased cardiac output,[78] and reduced tissue ischemia,[76] enhanced lipolysis,[78,79] improved lipoprotein levels[80] and increased aerobic conditioning.[81] In comparing the effects of anti-hypertensive medications and Qigong, Wang et al.[82] reported that subjects who received medication and practiced Qigong techniques for 30 minutes twice a day displayed decreased blood pressure, a 20 percent reduction in stroke rates, and approximately a 16 percent reduction in mortality rates compared to a control group. Research from China involving several thousand hypertensive clients who had been instructed and participated in basic Qigong exercises showed that those who regularly complied with their training experienced dramatic improvements with respect to lowering their blood pressure, pulse rates, metabolic rates, and oxygen demand.[30] These studies indicated that Qigong triggers the body's relaxation response by reducing the level of dopamine, a neurotransmitter that controls neurological activity.[68] The longitudinal study of the positive effects of Qigong on lowering blood pressure performed by Wang et al.[73] among 242 clients concluded that Qigong plays a major role in improving self-regulation and alleviating multiple cerebrovascular and cardiovascular disease risk factors.

Pulmonary/Respiratory System.   Research exploring the effects of Qigong on the pulmonary system is minimal.[84–86] Qigong practice has been shown to increase respiratory volume and improve oxygen uptake and carbon dioxide exchange[84] and to be an effective treatment for asthma and emphysema.[85,86] Lim et al.[86] studied 10 nonimpaired volunteers who practiced Qigong in 20 minute group instructional sessions for 10 consecutive days. While the results of this study indicated no significant changes in heart rate or tidal volume, it did reveal a nearly 20 percent improvement in ventilatory efficiency. In a German study of Qigong used for treating asthma, Ruether and Aldridge[85] instructed 30 subjects with asthma in Qigong techniques and asked them to practice independently on a daily basis and to keep a diary of their symptoms. After one year, a significant number in the Qigong group, compared to the control group who did not practice Qigong, showed a decrease of at least 10 percent in peak flow variability (amount of air they could expire, an indication of airway obstruction). In addition, Qigong group participants displayed decreased hospitalization rates, used fewer sick days, had reduced antibiotic use, and fewer emergency consultations.

Nervous System.   The effect of Qigong on the nervous system has been reported in only a few clinical reports and studies.[87–89] Liu et al.[87] monitored the brainstem and cortical evoked responses in subjects before and after Qigong sessions and found an increase in brainstem auditory evoked responses and a decrease or depression of cortical responses from the baseline measurements. They surmised that Qigong might depress or lower the cortical control over brainstem responses, creating the potential for neural disinhibition.

Using electroencephalogram (EEG) recordings, Zhang et al.[88,89] studied the effects of Qigong on changes in brain electrical activity. A Qigong (experimental) group was divided by level of experience, creating a beginner level group and a masters level group. Statistically significant differences were observed in the EEG patterns of the masters level Qigong group. During the Qigong state, the alpha activity recorded among the masters level group predominantly occurred in the anterior half of the brain. These findings were not found in the beginner or control groups.[88] This study validated the effect of Qigong on brain activation patterns.

Endocrine System. Research exploring the effects of Qigong on the endocrine system is also limited.[90,91] Ryu et al.[90] examined stress hormone levels such as Beta-endorphin, adrenocorticotropic hormone (ACTH), cortisol, and dehydroepiandrosterone-sulfate (DHEA-S) among 20 healthy men and women Qigong trainees. In this study, blood samples were taken before, during, and after Qigong training periods to determine blood stress hormone levels. They reported no significant change in cortisol or DHEA-S levels. However, ACTH (adrenocorticotropic hormone) levels were found to decrease during Qigong training. In contrast, levels of Beta-endorphin, a hormone associated with pleasure, relaxation, and improved mental functioning, significantly increased during Qigong training. The authors inferred that Qigong exercises play a role in stress reduction, indicating a positive effect on the immune system, and suggesting an increase in pain relieving hormones levels.[90]

Skoglund[91] evaluated the effects of Qigong on reducing work-related stress. In this study, a comparison was made between a control group and an experimental (Qigong) group of adult computer operators. The purpose of this study was to measure some of the physiological changes that occur following a two-week period of Qigong training. Both the immediate responses and the long-term (five weeks) effects of practicing Qigong were measured. Qigong training reduced heart rate and noradrenaline excretion, thus indicating a reduced activity in the sympathetic nervous system.[91] This study also reported a reduction of spinal backache symptoms in the Qigong group. They concluded that Qigong exercises helped to reduce stress related to computerized work environments.[91]

Skeletal System. Kuang et al.[92] investigated bone density in men ranging in age from 50 to 60 years old. Between the two groups, those who practiced Qigong displayed an overall increase in bone density in comparison to their age-controlled counterparts who did not participate in Qigong. This study did not evaluate the effects of Qigong on bone density changes in women, which would have potentially carried more clinical significance.

Immune System. Research has also suggested that Qigong might be more effective than chemotherapy, acupuncture, and surgery for the prevention and treatment of disease by altering the client's Qi, thereby boosting their immune system.[93,94] Reduced side effects from chemotherapy and radiation during cancer treatment has

been claimed with Qigong use.[95] At the Kuangan Men's Hospital in Beijing, China, 93 subjects suffering with advanced malignant cancer were treated with a combination of drugs and Qigong exercises.[96] The control group, consisting of 30 subjects, who received only medication (drug) treatment. The results found that within the experimental Qigong group 81 percent gained strength, 63 percent had improved appetite, and 33 percent were free from diarrhea in comparison to improvements of only 10 percent, 10 percent, and 6 percent respectively by the control group.[96]

Pain Management. The efficacy of Qigong in the treatment of pain was studied by Wu et al.[97] at the Pain Management Center of Newark, NJ. Twenty-six subjects with complex regional pain syndrome, ranging in age from 18 to 65 years of age, were placed into two groups. The experimental group received Qi emission and Qigong instructions from a Qigong master, while the control group received a similar set of instructions from a "sham" master. Eighty-two percent of the Qigong (experimental) group reported less pain by the end of the first session, compared to only 45 percent of the control group.[97] At the end of the last training session, three weeks later, 91 percent of the Qigong (experimental) group reported pain relief, compared to only 36 percent of the control group. While anxiety decreased in both groups, its reduction was greater in the Qigong (experimental) group.[97]

Additional. Qigong may slow or reverse some of the effects of aging,[84,96,98–104] increase bone density,[101,102] increase estradiol levels in aging women,[102] reduce anxiety and fatigue,[103,104] improve cardiovascular function, and improve balance, and other age-related effects in normal elderly clients.[96] Zhou and Lian[105] examined the effects of Qigong therapy on 60 subjects with pregnancy-induced hypertension. In this study, the control group received the appropriate medications whereas the experimental group practiced Qigong exclusively. The results of this study revealed 90 percent improvement for the experimental Qigong group and only a 55 percent improvement for the control (medication only) group.[105] Jang and Lee[106] assessed the effects of Qigong therapy on premenstrual symptoms among 36 college age women with premenstrual syndrome (PMS) who were randomly assigned to either a Qigong therapy group or to a placebo control group. The Qigong therapy group displayed significant improvements in symptoms of negative feelings, pain, water retention, and total PMS symptoms compared to placebo.

Many other areas of Qigong effects have been presented in the literature. These reports however have lacked the controls of the previously mentioned studies. Eyesight,[11,30] sinus, allergies, hemorrhoids, and prostate problems,[11] and digestive problems, asthma, arthritis, insomnia, pain, anxiety, depression, cancer, heart disease, otitis media, neurosis, gastric ulcers, and HIV/AIDS[11,30,65] have all been reported to improve with Qigong therapy intervention.

Equipment

No special equipment is required. It is important to find a flat area in a quiet and peaceful environment either indoors or outdoors in which to practice. The client should make sure that they have plenty of fresh air and should wear comfortable clothing that is loose and allows for freedom of movement. During meditation, a light blanket can be used to prevent the client from getting cold.

Basic Techniques

To make the practice of Qigong more beneficial and accessible to the client who is just starting out, it is recommended that they: 1) Take it easy and do not rush. Excess effort and trying too hard go against the natural benefits of Qigong; 2) Always approach each practice with the intention to relax; direct the mind toward quiet indifference; and 3) Regulate breathing so that both the inhalation and exhalation are slow and deep, but not urgent or exaggerated.[30] It is important for the client to remember that results come over time, so they should not overdo it or expect too much too soon. Also, although Qigong may seem too easy to be beneficial, a dedication to these practices is believed to mobilize one's natural healing forces and if performed correctly, Qigong is safe to practice as often as desired. Finally, clients should feel free to create their own routine and to change the practices to suit their individual needs, likes, and limitations. For clients who are functionally limited, impaired, or disabled, the rehabilitation clinician should inform them that they might consider using postures other than standing (seated, supine, etc.).

Have the client prepare by rubbing their hands together to build up heat via friction. This is thought to increase the flow of Qi. Once the client's hands are warm they should stroke their palms across their face, eyes, and forehead in an upward motion towards the crown. The motion is similar to washing one's face except the client's hands only move in one direction. Continuing the movement, the client should slide their hands over the top and sides of the head, down the back of the neck, and forward along the shoulders (between the crease of the neck and the shoulder joint). Keeping the movement steady, the client should continue the motion by bringing the hands down over the anterolateral aspect of the rib cage, tracing around the waist to the back posterolateral to the spine (i.e., the hands should move over the kidneys), and down the back and sides of the legs (warming the gluteals, hamstrings, and gastrocnemius-soleus complex), continuing the motion on the lateral aspects of the feet. Using the same continuous motion, the client should continue tracing the meridian up the medial aspect of the feet, over the medial aspect of the arch, past the medial malleoli, continuing up the inner calf, past the medial knee, over the adductors, passing over the groin creases, and up the front of the torso, ending up back at the face.[11,30] After the preparation, the client begins exercises such as "Separating the Clouds" (**Figure 10.17a–c**), "Flying Wild Goose" (**Figure 10.18a–b**), and "Pushing the Wave" (**Figure 10.19a–c**).

Practitioner Requirements

There is no standard credentialing program for Qigong instructors.[9] Usually individuals who have practiced Qigong for a significant amount of time (i.e., years) choose to become instructors. Currently there are no state regulations for instructors. Qigong may be self-taught. There are also many classes for beginning, intermediate, and advanced clients. Though there are also many books and multi-media instructional materials on Qigong, classes should be taken with a qualified teacher. Teachers are often trained at centers that also teach Chinese philosophy. In the United States today, qualified instructors can be found in adult education centers, fitness centers, YMCAs, and even some hospitals teach Qigong.[11,15,30]

> ### *Key Point:*
>
> Qigong. . . .
> ◆ Represents a class of exercises that differ from the traditional routine of stretching and strengthening programs currently utilized in physical medicine and rehabilitation.
> ◆ Is a branch of Traditional Chinese Medicine of health practice that focuses on harnessing one's biological energy called *Qi*.
> ◆ Involves breathing exercises, slow, controlled movements, and mental concentration in the form of meditation.
> ◆ Ranges from simple callisthenic-type movements with breath coordination to more complex methods where brain-wave frequency, heart rate, and other organ functions can be intentionally altered.
> ◆ Can be performed by people of all ages, abilities, physical conditions, and levels of functional limitation, impairment, or disability.
> ◆ Should be practiced on a daily basis to achieve maximum benefits.
> ◆ Research appears promising although our understanding of the efficacy of this complementary and alternative therapeutic exercise approach and its techniques is clearly in the early stages.

Tai Chi

T'ai Chi Chuan (Tai Chi) is a martial arts form comprised almost entirely of movement control tasks. Tai chi literally means "supreme ultimate," the yin-yang symbol of har-

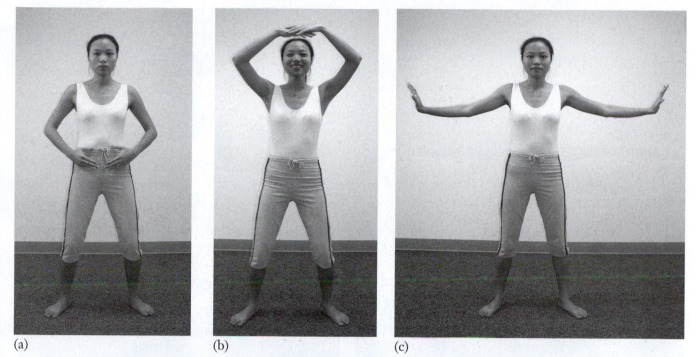

(a)   (b)   (c)

Figure 10.17   Separating the Clouds. With hips, knees, and ankles slightly flexed with hands in front of the Dantien (approximately 3 finger widths or 1.5 inches below the navel) (a), the client maintains a straight back and raises her arms overhead (b). As she inhales and extends ther hips and knees, the client turns her palms away (c), and circles her arms down and around back to the Dantien position as she flexes the hips, knees and ankles. This exercise trains both the upper extremities and lower extremities.

mony and balance, whereas chuan denotes "fist."[15] The practice of Tai Chi involves a sequence of movements, or forms, that require the whole body to move in a coordinated fashion, including the trunk, extremities, and breathing.[8,15] According to traditional Chinese beliefs, Tai Chi's unique combination of breathing, "intentional mind" or meditation, and slow, rhythmic exercise allows the body to take in essential elements, such as oxygen, iron, copper, zinc, and magnesium, and to rid itself of wastes and poisons. Tai Chi emphasizes self-awareness as well as circulating and balancing the body's internal energy or "Chi" or "Qi." Breathing assists the movement of chi around the body.

Although originally developed as a martial art, most people today practice Tai Chi for its reputed health benefits.[15] For centuries, Tai Chi has been practiced widely in China as a form of daily exercise, particularly among the elderly. Over the past several decades, Tai Chi has become best known in the West as a system of exercise to benefit health, prevent degenerative illness, promote longevity, enhance creativity and focus, and improve physical and mental vigor.

Background

The origins of Tai Chi are uncertain. It is thought to have originated in China thousands of years ago, around the 13th century A.D.[8] A popular legend is that Tai Chi was invented by a Taoist priest, Chang San Feng, after he witnessed a fight between a crane and a snake. It is based on Buddhism and the Taoist principle of yin and yang, which is the basis for the Chinese understanding of health and sickness. According to the Taoist views, a balance of opposing forces within the body is essential for good health.[8] If one or the other predominates, the result is sickness. It is this concept of opposites that is reflected in each Tai Chi movement.

Yang Ch'eng-fu is credited with establishing the *yang style* of Tai Chi as the dominant internal martial art system in China, having the greatest influence during the 1920s and 1930s. There are 108 forms in the traditional long form of yang style Tai Chi.[8] The yang style became the basis for the new "simplified" Tai Chi which was adopted in China in 1956. Perhaps Yang Ch'eng-fu's most famous student was Professor Cheng Man-ch'ing, who condensed the 128 postures in the long form into 37 postures, which are today known as the "yang style short form." In the 1940s Li T'ien-shih, at the request of the Wushu Council of China, devised the Beijing style, also referred to as the Peking style. The Beijing or Peking style consists of 24 steps from which the essential elements of the yang style are condensed. In addition, a 36-step form and an 88-step form exist, but are not as popular among the Chinese people. A 48-step style that combines the essential elements of Chen, Yang, Wu, and Hou styles, is a standard

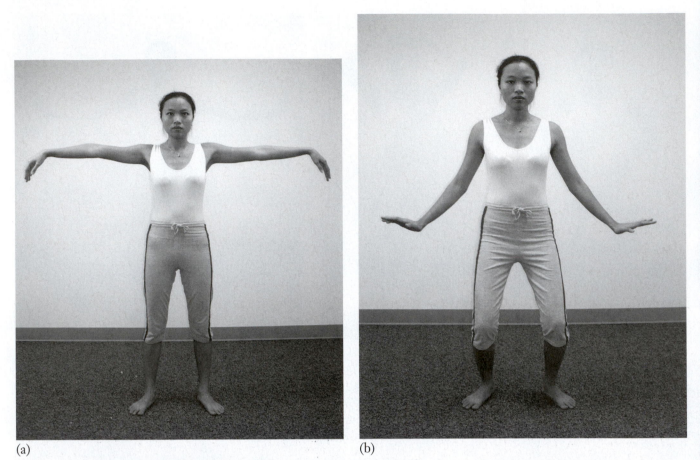

(a)   (b)

Figure 10.18   Flying Wild Goose. The client begins in a relaxed standing position. While inhaling, she abducts her shoulders to approximately 90° with her elbows extended, forearms pronated, wrists flexed, and fingers relaxed (a). While exhaling, the client should slowly flex the knees and lower the arms, taking the shoulders to approximately 45° of abduction, with the elbows slightly bent, forearms pronated, wrists in slight extension, and fingers abducted and extended (b). It may help the client to visualize the arms during this movement are like the "wings of a bird". This exercise trains both the upper extremities and lower extremities.

competition form. Tai Chi was introduced into the West during the 19th century, but it was not until the 1970s that it became well known in the United States.[8] Although there are several forms of Tai Chi practiced today in the United States, the most common is Tai Chi Chuan.

Basic Technique

In contrast to most other martial arts, the movements of Tai Chi are slow and flowing in quality. The practitioner strives to remain alert and relaxed, without allowing any body area to become tense or to go limp. Although Tai Chi is rarely used as a martial art, it is known to be highly effective, even lethal, when used in this manner.[8] This is due in part to its basic premises. For example, rather than oppose force with force, Tai Chi movements and postures are used to absorb or deflect an adversary's assault. A traditional Tai Chi saying is that a force of 4,000 pounds can be deflected with a force of four ounces.[107] Hence, the effectiveness of a Tai Chi push or kick relies in part on di-

recting energy generated from the "tan tien" (also known as dantien in Qigong), a point approximately two inches below the navel, rather than on using aggressive, muscular strikes. In recognition of its effectiveness, the Peking or Beijing style of Tai Chi is included in the martial arts division of the modern Asian athletic games.

According to Taoist philosophy, Tai Chi postures are typically carried out in pairs of opposing movements designed to balance the positive (yang) and negative (yin) forces, thereby promoting, restoring, and maintaining the body's energy (*Chi*) in perfect harmony.[8] For example, a movement that begins on the right will typically end with a move to the left. With each position or posture, the client's weight shifts between the right and the left foot, causing the leg muscles to contract and relax, thereby improving the flow of blood and chi throughout the body.[8] The movements themselves are relatively simple and all involve bending and unbending the knees, the transfer of body weight, as well as the raising and lowering of the arms. However, it is the coordination of each movement

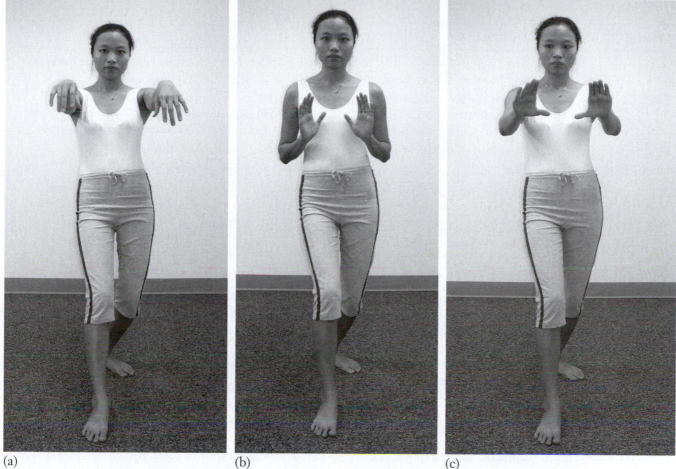

(a)   (b)   (c)

Figure 10.19   Pushing the Wave. The client begins in relaxed standing with one leg pointing forward and the back foot turned 45° out, keeping her body weight shifted toward the back leg. While maintaining this posture, the client lifts both arms to shoulder height (a). While inhaling, she brings the hands toward the chest by flexing the elbows and retracting the scapulae with the palms facing slightly forward. Simultaneously, the client lowers ther body down into a slight squat position (b). As she exhales, she shifts her body weight more toward the front foot while rising up on the toes of the back foot and simultaneously pushing forward with the arms until the front leg is straight (c). This exercise is good for strengthening the musculature surrounding the knee, enhancing balance, and reducing fatigue.

along with its correct breathing pattern that constitutes Tai Chi. The ultimate goal of Tai Chi and its movements and coordinated breathing sequences is to achieve harmony between body, mind, and spirit.[15]

There are many styles of Tai Chi, which are summarized in **Table 10.5**. As noted previously, Tai Chi not only emphasizes self-awareness, but encourages the circulation and balancing of the body's internal energy. Proponents believe that breathing assists the movement of "chi" around the body.[8] For example, as the body inhales, the mind lifts the energy from the solar plexus region, which is considered the central energy source of the body. During exhalation, the energy is directed from the solar plexus to the lower abdomen. The techniques of breathing combined with arm and leg movements alone are not enough to move the Qi throughout the body; they must be combined with the power of concentration. Since Tai Chi is

known to be a powerful centering activity, it may be an effective tool in terms of preparation for vigorous physical or mental activity.[8] In this case, physical movements are used to sustain, support, promote, and guide internal concentration as well as to circulate the chi.

Therapeutic Indications

A client can benefit from the physical components of Tai Chi without understanding its spiritual or energy-based dimensions. In general, from a physical benefit perspective, Tai Chi has been shown to enhance an individual's physical capacity, general health, well being, respiratory function, balance, coordination, and gracefulness.[8] It can enhance muscle toning, thereby building strength and flexibility rather than muscle mass, improve circulation, alleviate pain, improve energy as well as stamina, and provide the

TABLE 10.5   Styles of Tai Chi Chuan

Style	Description
Yang	Most popular, most commonly practiced, gentlest style. Recommended for elderly clients and those with poor baseline fitness levels.
Chen	Oldest form. Characterized by dynamic, physically demanding movements. Clearly demonstrates a polarity of fast vs. slow and small vs. large movements. Recommended for beginners and clients who are seeking a high degree of physical strength and suppleness.
Cheng Man-Ch'ing	Modification of the yang style. Strongly emphasizes softness and relaxation.
Li or Hou	Not widely taught. Uses small stance and smaller steps, encouraging mobility.
Sun	Characterized by small circular movements, high stances, and low energy expenditure. Good for teaching clients to apply Tai Chi to their normal walking posture/position.
Wu	Characterized by a forward lean. Recommended for beginners and for more advanced practitioners.

individual with a sense of body control.[8] Tai Chi can be used to complement traditional exercise programs aimed at improving balance, posture, strength, agility, coordination, flexibility, cardiovascular fitness (i.e., control blood pressure), joint mobility, endurance, and a sense of well being via the release of Beta-endorphins.[8] Cardiovascular indications include heart disease, hypertension, and deconditioning. Tai Chi has demonstrated usefulness as a therapeutic exercise modality to improve cardiopulmonary function, muscular strength, and balance.[107–112] Of particular interest, Tai Chi also appears to improve kinesthetic sense (see Chapter 7), which could indirectly improve movement quality and thus neuromuscular coordination (see Chapter 8).[113]

Emotional benefits of Tai Chi include alleviating anxiety, stress, restlessness, and depression. From a psychosocial perspective, Tai Chi provides socialization and is believed to reduce stress, and maximize physical, spiritual and emotional potential.[114] The greatest potential benefit of Tai Chi may be its use for the prevention of disease and injury and the promotion of health and wellness.[114] It is especially well suited for the elderly and clients who are frail because the movements are slow, controlled, and do not involve direct impact to the joints.

Contraindications

There are no specific dangers to Tai Chi practice.[8,15,114] Movements are slow and gentle and can be performed even by clients with chronic diseases or who are confined to a wheelchair. It is important that clients warm up prior to Tai Chi participation to prevent stretching injuries. As with any physical exercise, clients performing Tai Chi can experience sprains or strains. The rehabilitation clinician should encourage clients to stretch before and after each Tai Chi session (see Chapter 3) and to change positions slowly in order to prevent unexpected injuries. Two other possible complications associated with Tai Chi are falls and fractures, especially while performing single leg stance postures. Again, proper use of stretching and slow movements should lessen the injury risk.

Evidence

The first scientific studies on Tai Chi were published in China in the late 1950s.[115] Compared to sedentary control subjects, experienced Tai Chi practitioners reportedly have less osteoporosis and spinal deformity, better spinal flexibility, greater vital capacity, lower baseline blood pressure, and better cardiovascular responses to exercise.[115] Although there are relatively few scientific articles on Tai Chi in Western peer reviewed journals, the body of evidence has grown in the last 10 years. None of the medical studies reviewed reported any injury resulting from Tai Chi practice. The following is a review of the available medical literature.

Cardiovascular   Many researchers classify Tai Chi as a form of moderate intensity aerobic exercise. The energy cost of Tai Chi has been estimated to be between 4.0 and 4.6 metabolic equivalents (METs) (see Chapter 4).[116,117] Some reports, however, describe the aerobic intensity of Tai Chi as light. Lansheng et al.[118] reported the maximum heart rate during practice of the Tai Chi short form to be less than 100 beats/minute and that pre- and post-exercise blood pressures were identical. In a randomized controlled clinical trial, Tsai et al.[119] investigated the effects of a 12-week Tai Chi Chuan exercise program on blood pressure, lipid profile, and anxiety (State Trait Anxiety Inventory) of 76 clients with high normal or stage I hypertension. The Tai Chi exercise group displayed significant decreases in systolic over diastolic blood pressure, decreased serum total cholesterol levels, decreased trait and state anxiety levels, and increased high-density lipoprotein cholesterol levels compared to the sedentary control group.

Lan et al.[120] conducted a study evaluating the training effect of a one year duration Tai Chi program for clients who had undergone coronary artery bypass surgery and who had participated in a Phase II cardiac rehabilitation program. The Tai Chi group had a higher weekly attendance than the control group. In addition, the Tai Chi group increased 10.3 percent in VO_2 peak and 11.9 percent in peak work rate while the control group demonstrated slight decreases in both VO_2 peak and peak work rate. Other studies[121–123] also found that the practice of Tai Chi involves relatively low energy expenditures but has positive effects on cardiopulmonary response, including heart rate. One study, however, reported that there are differences in energy expenditure between the different styles of Tai Chi, with the Chen style displaying more than twice the energy cost compared to the yang style.[122]

Channer et al.[124] explored the changes in hemodynamic parameters following Tai Chi, aerobic exercise, or non-exercise support group participation among 126 subjects who were recovering from an acute myocardial infarction. Blood pressure and heart rate measurements were taken before and after each training session. The results revealed that over 11 sessions, only the Tai Chi group displayed a trend toward reduced diastolic blood pressure values. Significant decreases in systolic blood pressure were seen in both the Tai Chi and the aerobic exercise groups. Of note, the mean heart rate of the Tai Chi group during exercise increased by only two beats per minute, far less than the aerobic exercise group.[124] Young et al.[125] reported a comparable decrease in systolic and diastolic blood pressures in sedentary elderly subjects who performed Tai Chi or moderate intensity aerobic exercise for 12 weeks.

Pulmonary.   The slow, diaphragmatic breathing pattern used during Tai Chi may be more efficient than in other forms of exercise.[124–126] Regular practice of Tai Chi over two years was associated with significantly reduced VO_2 maximum levels of elderly men and women, compared with age-matched sedentary control subjects. Brown et al.[126] reported that the ventilatory frequency and ventilatory equivalent during Tai Chi practice was lower than values observed during bicycle ergometry at the same VO_2 level and that a higher percentage of the minute ventilation was used for alveolar ventilation. Schneider and Leung[127] noted that Tai Chi practitioners, compared with Wing Chun (a form of Kung Fu) practitioners, had a lower ventilatory equivalent. In studies of older sedentary adults, Lai et al.[128,129] reported that at maximum exercise levels, the VO_2, O_2, and work rate of subjects who had been practicing Tai Chi were significantly higher than that of control group subjects. In examining Tai Chi training effects on the maintenance of cardiopulmonary function in 84 community dwelling older adults (64 ± 9 years of age) with no history of significant cardiovascular, pulmonary, or musculoskeletal disease, some of whom had been practicing Tai Chi for many years, Lai[129] reported that males in the Tai Chi group demonstrated a significantly reduced

decline in VO_2 maximum at two years following study initiation compared to a sedentary control group.

Musculoskeletal.   Using a cross sectional study design, Wong et al.[108] investigated the effects of Tai Chi exercises on the postural stability of older subjects. Static postural stability tests included six combinations of vision (eyes open, eyes closed, sway-referenced) and dynamic balance involving three tests of weight shifting (i.e., right-left, forward-backward, multidirectional) at three different speeds were performed using a balance testing system. The results revealed that in static postural control, there was no difference in the simple conditions. However, in more complicated conditions (i.e., eyes closed with sway surface, sway vision with sway surface), the Tai Chi group displayed significantly better results in the rhythmic forward-backward weight shifting test than the control group.

Several studies have reported that practicing Tai Chi improves range of motion, flexibility, and lower extremity strength, especially in older subjects. Lan et al.[109] compared an 18 subject control group (9 males, 9 females) with 20 subjects who participated in the Tai Chi group (9 males, 11 females) ranging in age from 58 to 70 years. In cardiopulmonary function, strength, flexibility, and body fat percentage, both males and females in the Tai Chi group displayed improvements (respectively: 16.1 percent and 20.3 percent increase in VO_2 maximum; 11° and 8° increase in thoraco-lumbar flexibility; 18.1 percent and 20.3 percent improvement in knee extensor muscle strength; 15 percent and 15.9 percent increase in knee flexor muscle strength). The control group demonstrated no significant changes in these parameters.[109]

Song et al.[130] investigated the effects of Sun-style Tai Chi exercises on the physical function of subjects with osteoarthritis. Twenty-two subjects participated in the Tai Chi group and 21 were in a control group that was matched based on demographic data and pre-test measures. The Tai Chi group displayed significantly less perceived pain and joint stiffness and reported fewer difficulties in physical functioning, while the control group showed no change or deterioration in physical functioning. The Tai Chi group also showed significant improvements in balance and abdominal strength. However, significant differences were not observed for flexibility, upper body, or knee muscle strength.

Van Deusen and Harlowe[131] randomized 46 subjects with rheumatoid arthritis to a control group or to a range of motion dance program, which incorporated elements of Tai Chi, guided relaxation, and group discussion. The four-month follow-up evaluation revealed greater shoulder range of motion in the intervention group, greater enjoyment of rest and exercise, and no difference in wrist or lower extremity range of motion compared with controls. Jerosch and Wustner[132] evaluated 32 subjects diagnosed with subacromial pain syndrome who completed a four week program using proprioception training tools (such as the Bodyblade,™ Hymanson, Inc., Marina Del Rey, CA) (**Figure 10.20**), specific Tai Chi movements, sensorimotor training for the glenohumeral joint, and aquatic gymnastics. The results showed significant improvements on Constant and UCLA shoulder scores. Sensorimotor testing showed an increased proprioceptive component, especially in the motion detection test, whereas the angle reproduction test showed only moderate improvement (see Chapter 7). Subjects did not display improved strength scores. Several other studies have reported improved limb strength, proprioception or flexibility among subjects who practiced Tai Chi compared to control group subjects.[109,116,133–136]

Using a case control study design, Qin et al.[137] investigated the potential benefits of Tai Chi exercise on the density of the weight bearing bones of post-menopausal women (age range 50–59 yrs) with 17 participating in a Tai Chi exercise group and 17 serving as non-exercising control group subjects. Lumbar spine, proximal femur, and distal tibia bone mineral density measurements taken at baseline were significantly higher in the Tai Chi group than the control group. At the 12-month follow-up, both groups had bone loss, but decelerated rates of bone loss were observed for the Tai Chi group.

Several studies reported Tai Chi to be beneficial in reducing pain among subjects with various forms of joint disease. For example, Bhatti et al.[138] reported that six weeks of Tai Chi exercise reduced the pain of a subject with chronic low back pain and improved their mood better than conventional care. Lumsdem et al.[139] suggested that Tai Chi exercise enhanced mobility and reduced pain among subjects with osteoarthritis, but it did not affect joint pain.

Koh,[140] in a personal case study report, used Tai Chi to relieve symptoms from moderately severe ankylosing spondylitis. After practicing Tai Chi on a daily basis for 2.5 years, he noted improvements in strength, coordination, balance, chest movement, ability to relax, and overall health as well as a reduction in his flexion spinal deformity. However, he also noted that if the Tai Chi was not continued on a daily basis for a period of one week, his pain, weakness, and general malaise returned.

Neurological. There is a growing body of evidence indicating that learning Tai Chi directly improves balance, promotes postural control, and prevents falls among elderly and brain injured subjects.[141–146] In addition, there is encouraging evidence that training elderly subjects in Tai Chi may also enhance mental concentration and relieve tension, thereby providing emotional benefits.[15,104,117]

The extensive studies by Wolf et al.[142–144] as part of the *Atlanta Frailty and Injuries: Cooperative Study of Intervention Techniques* (FICSIT) trials concluded that moderate Tai Chi training can positively impact biomedical and psychosocial indices of frailty as well as have favorable effects upon the occurrence of falls. Two hundred subjects (162 men, 38 women with a mean age of 76 years) were evaluated regarding the effects of two exercise approaches: Tai Chi and computerized balance training on specific primary outcomes (i.e., biomedical, functional, and psychological indicators of frailty) and secondary outcomes (i.e., occurrence of falls). This study used a prospective, randomized controlled clinical trial with three arms (Tai Chi, balance training, education control) and a 15-week intervention period. Primary outcomes were measured before and after the intervention plus four months later. The second outcome, occurrence of falls, was monitored continuously throughout the study. Biomedical measurements included strength, flexibility, cardiovascular endurance, and body composition. Functional measurements included instrumental activities of daily living. Psychological and psychosocial well being measurements included the Center for Epidemiologic Studies Depression Scale, the Fear of Falling questionnaire, mastery index, and measurements of subject perception of present and future health, perceived quality of sleep, and intrusiveness. The

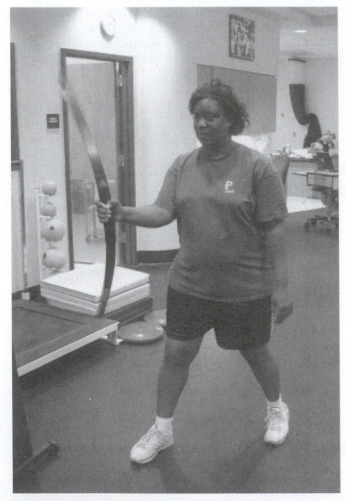

Figure 10.20   Standing weight shifting activity with a Bodyblade.™

results revealed that grip strength declined in all groups and range of motion also showed lower, but statistically significant reductions. Blood pressure was decreased both before and after a 12-minute walk subsequent to Tai Chi training. In addition, Tai Chi training reduced the risk of multiple falls by 47 percent.

Other studies, however, have shown equivocal results in terms of the effects of Tai Chi on postural stability with some showing improved balance among Tai Chi practitioners[113,117] and other studies failing to show statistically significant differences.[142,143] Still other studies have revealed improvement in parameters other than balance, but no statistically significant improvements in balance itself, and so conclude that Tai Chi exercise can be beneficial for clients because of improved confidence and strength, for example, if not necessarily for postural stability.[145-146]

Modified Tai Chi movements have been used in special cases. Shapira[141] reported on the use of Tai Chi with three severely head injured subjects following completion of traditional neurological rehabilitation. They completed two to four years of Tai Chi therapy, first training on a weekly basis and then twice weekly, including one hour a day at home. The initial weeks of Tai Chi training (phase I) were performed only while seated. Emphasis was placed on learning and performing combinations of movement and practicing breathing patterns. The second phase involved having subjects assume a traditional Tai Chi standing position but in a doorway for balance assistance and progressed to teaching them to relax, to shift their weight from side to side, and to complete the movements in the center of the room (without support). For these subjects, the original steps were broken down into much smaller movements. The results indicated that in phase I (sitting), the subject's quality of motion became more controlled and flowing. In phase II (standing) teaching the subject to look forward and not down had a significant impact on improving their balance and confidence level. After several weeks, subjects were able to stand and keep their balance for prolonged periods of time. At the completion of the Tai Chi program, all three subjects could walk without assistance, would rarely fall, and felt more secure while walking. In addition, all subjects reported improved control over themselves, their memory, concentration levels, and their surroundings as well as a decrease in hypertonicity.

Integumentary System.   Wang et al.[147] evaluated the cutaneous microcirculatory function in a group of community dwelling geriatric Tai Chi practitioners. The experimental group consisted of 10 elderly men while the control group consisted of 10 sedentary men who were matched for age and body size. The Tai Chi group had practiced Tai Chi for an average of 11.2 years, approximately five times a week. Each Tai Chi session consisted of 20 minutes of warm-up, 24 minutes of Tai Chi exercise, and 10 minutes of cool down. Although resting heart rate, systolic and diastolic blood pressure, work rate, ventilatory equivalent, and mean arterial pressure did not differ significantly between groups during graded exercise testing, the Tai Chi group displayed a 34 percent greater VO_2 maximum in addition to significantly higher skin blood flow, cutaneous vascular conductance, peak oxygen pulse, skin temperatures and levels of plasma nitric oxide metabolite than the control group both at rest and during exercise. Wang et al.[147] concluded that practicing Tai Chi can be of benefit to the elderly by slowing the progressive decline in peripheral microcirculation associated with natural aging.

Wang et al.[148] also investigated the effects of Tai Chi training on endothelial function in the skin vasculature of older men. Thirty-two men (10 older Tai Chi practitioners, 10 older healthy sedentary subjects, 12 younger healthy subjects) participated in the study. The older men had practiced the yang style of Tai Chi for an average of five times/week for 11 years, whereas the sedentary younger men had not participated in any form of regular exercise for the past five years. Different doses of 1 percent acetylcholine and 1 percent sodium nitroprusside were iontophoretically applied to the skin of each subjects' lower leg. Cutaneous microvascular perfusion responses were determined by laser Doppler measurements. In addition, arterial and venous hemodynamic variables were measured by impedance plethysmography. Results revealed that the younger sedentary group had a higher acetylcholine induced cutaneous perfusion and a higher ratio of acetylcholine to sodium nitroprusside cutaneous perfusion than the two older groups. However, the Tai Chi group subjects showed a higher acetylcholine induced perfusion and a higher ratio of acetylcholine to sodium nitroprusside than the older sedentary group subjects. Wang et al.[148] concluded that regular practice of Tai Chi is associated with enhanced endothelium-dependent dilation in the skin vasculature of older adults. Also, Tai Chi training may delay the age-related decline of venous compliance and hyperemic arterial responses, potentially helping to reduce the effects of orthostatic hypotension.

Psychological (Mood).   Brown et al.[149] has suggested that Tai Chi, with its "mindful" component, when added to a moderate intensity therapeutic exercise program will help to reduce mood disturbances including tension, depression, anger, and confusion among participants. Women participants in the Tai Chi group also reported greater satisfaction with their physical attributes. Jin[104] in studying stress among Tai Chi practitioners who were randomly assigned to one of four activity groups—(brisk walkers, meditation, Tai Chi exercisers, and quiet neutral readers)—found that the effect of participating in Tai Chi exercises evoked physiological changes for reducing stress that were similar to those of moderate intensity exercise.[104]

Kutner et al.[150] in another study associated with the Atlanta FICSIT (*Frailty and Injuries: Cooperative Studies on Intervention Techniques*) trial placed subjects who were 70 years of age or older into three groups—Tai Chi, balance training, or exercise control education—for 15 weeks. Exit interviews regarding perceived benefits of participation revealed that both the Tai Chi and balance training groups had significant increases in confidence in balance and movement. However, only the Tai Chi group reported that their daily activities and overall life satisfaction had been changed as well. Subjects within the Tai Chi group also reported changing their normal physical activity routine to incorporate and continue practicing Tai Chi.

Equipment

To engage in Tai Chi exercise, the rehabilitation clinician and client will need a well lit room, preferably carpeted to provide solid footing, with adequate floor space to permit movements without interfering with anyone else.[8,114] The rehabilitation clinician should instruct the client to wear loose fitting clothing and aerobic sneakers or appropriate non-skid footwear. Fitted slippers are acceptable if they have a non-skid sole. It is the rehabilitation clinician's responsibility to make sure that the client is wearing appropriate footwear in order to reduce the risk of slipping and falling during a Tai Chi session.

Technique

Clients of all ages, sizes, and physical abilities can practice Tai Chi because it relies more on technique than strength.[114] Although the guidance of a knowledgeable rehabilitation clinician or Tai Chi instructor is needed to master Tai Chi, careful practice of the basic steps will still provide many of the physical, mental, and spiritual benefits. Before a client begins a Tai Chi session, the rehabilitation clinician should assess their physical health, specifically the client's balance, mobility, and endurance and should also explain the purpose of the session, emphasize that the movements should be slow and non-stressful, and encourage them to participate to the extent that they feel comfortable, not to the point of pain.[114]

In general, the rehabilitation clinician or Tai Chi instructor should face the client or group and lead them through some simple stretching exercises to loosen their muscles and prevent injury. For the first session, the rehabilitation clinician may want the client to learn only a few postures. Then as the client's confidence, skills, and coordination grows, new movements as well as breathing instructions can be added with each session. The client needs to be reminded to skip any movement that they find too difficult or painful.

Although each style of Tai Chi is distinctive, they all follow the same basic principles. Regardless of the style or form, the client learns a series of rhythmic and coordinated movement patterns, which they then perform slowly and methodically, with one posture and movement leading into the next.[2] The movements have descriptive names, such as Green Dragon Dropping Water, Parry-Punch, Grasping the Bird's Tail, and White Crane Spreads Its Wings. Each movement flows from the previous one, which results in a continuous series of relatively effortless and smooth movements. While the subject practices the postures and movements they should also pay close attention to their breathing, which should be focused on the diaphragm rather than on the intercostals (i.e., the upper chest region).[114] It is abdominal breathing that is believed to enhance the flow of energy (Chi or Qi) throughout the body. It is important to note that gradual mental detachment may occur, since energy is contained in the body and gently released in a systematic manner through movement and breathing.

Most routines take approximately 20 minutes to perform. Tai Chi can be performed independently, with an instructor or rehabilitation clinician, as part of a group, or with a partner. Tai Chi is often performed with a partner to help understand another person's energy. A typical Tai Chi session ends with additional stretching exercises to allow the clients' muscles to cool down. To close the session, the rehabilitation clinician should have the client take a few slow, deep breaths. The rehabilitation clinician should document the session, the techniques used, and the clients' responses to the treatment session in addition to instructing them to stop exercising if they experience pain or shortness of breath.[114]

The progression of Tai Chi movement sequences from slow, controlled movements to fast, complex movement patterns follows basic motor learning theory. Neuromuscular coordination is clearly developed as the complexity of the movement sequences increase (see Chapter 8). In addition, Tai Chi uses knowledge of performance to enhance this motor learning process. Other neuromuscular coordination measurements such as kinematic parameter assessments and electromyographic evaluations of muscle or muscle group activation have not been extensively explored. Since they are invariant components of motor programs, a scaled muscle force increase would be expected in conjunction with a movement speed increase. Regardless, using slow to fast and simple to complex movements, Tai Chi progressions have a beneficial effect on improving movement control.[108] Factors that make Tai Chi beneficial for therapeutic exercise program consideration include the progression of movement speed, knowledge of performance, focusing on external forces, and most important the use of repetitive practice to reinforce these new movement patterns.

Beginning Tai Chi Exercise Program

Most rehabilitation clinicians divide a beginning Tai Chi exercise routine into three segments. Phase I involves double stance exercises such as "Ward Off Right" (**Figure 10.21a–d**). Phase II involves increasing flexibility, range of motion, and coordination of movements, plus good posture, focus, control, precision, mobility, and balance as well as progressing towards single leg stance postures. An example of a phase II or intermediate level exercise is the "White Crane Spreads Its Wings" (**Figure 10.22a–d**). Phase III includes more advanced exercises that combine single leg stance postures with dynamic motions to develop balance, deepening one's consciousness regarding balance awareness, gaining specific tissue-joint mobility, and increasing coordination between the left and right sides of the body. An example of a more advanced, phase III Tai Chi exercise is the "Golden Rooster Stands on One Leg" (**Figure 10.23a–e**). (Section 2, Animation 1)

Practitioner Training

Most forms of Tai Chi can be self-taught. In the past, Tai Chi students became "teachers" if and when their own teacher considered it appropriate.[8] However, new standards are evolving to ensure that Tai Chi instructors are capable of teaching. In the United Kingdom, a proposal is being considered to introduce a five-year teacher training syllabus coordinated by the Tai Chi Union of Great Britain.

> ## Key Point:
> Tai Chi. . . .
> - Combines breathing, meditation, and slow controlled, choreographed movements.
> - Focuses on enhancing the flow of vital life force or energy called *qi or chi.*
> - Consists of six key phases: awareness, mastery of kinematics, awareness of external forces, mastery of movement at various speeds, adjustment of movement flow, and adaptation to environmental changes.
> - Is used to induce relaxation, improve balance, posture, coordination, endurance, strength, and flexibility.
> - Allows the client to assume an active role in health promotion and disease prevention.
> - Can be performed by clients of all ages, abilities, physical conditions, and levels of functional limitation, impairment, or disability.
> - Should be practiced on a daily basis to achieve maximum benefits.
> - Can result in long life, good health, physical and mental vigor, and enhanced creativity.
> - Research has demonstrated the efficacy of this complementary and alternative therapeutic exercise approach in the treatment of a wide variety of physical and psychological conditions.

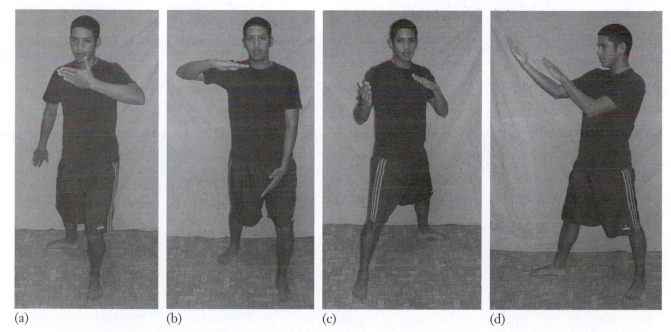

(a)   (b)   (c)   (d)

Figure 10.21   Ward Off Right. While in a relaxed straddle stance, the client shifts his body weight to the front (left) foot (a), rotates the hips to the left (b), and steps forward onto the right leg (bow and arrow stance) (c). At this point, 70 percent of the client's body weight should be on the front (right) leg and 30 percent on the back leg (d). During this exercise, the client may find it helpful to imagine a surge of energy in the form of a wave racing toward the shore, especially while completing the arm motions. The purpose of this movement is to fill the body from the inside with a bouncy, spring-like energy, and to impart feelings of buoyancy, natural strength, and spaciousness. It displays two contrasting aspects: gathering in and expanding out.

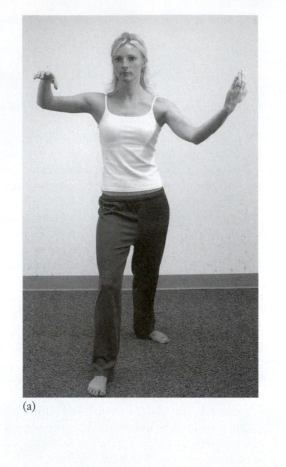
(a)

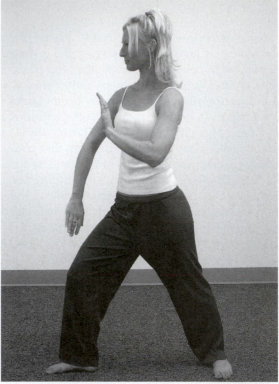
(b)

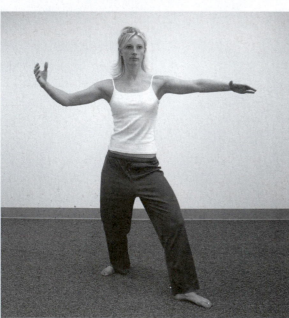
(c)

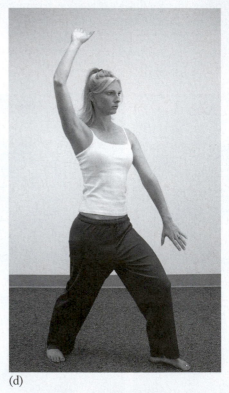
(d)

Figure 10.22   White Crane Spreads Its Wings. While standing, the client transfers most of her body weight onto the left leg while stepping forward with the right foot (a). The hips should be aligned at approximately a 45° angle to the right foot (b). The client then places most of her body weight onto the front (right) foot while the right arm is raised and the left arm arcs to the left in a sweeping motion (c). As the left arm moves downward, the right arm moves up toward the ceiling (d). It may help the client to visualize that she is drawing curtains apart and carefully stepping forward. At the completion of this exercise, 90 percent of the client's body weight should be located at the right (back) leg with the remaining 10 percent on the left (front) leg. This exercise is recommended for enhancing shoulder flexibility, range of motion, and coordination of scapulohumeral rhythm. It also encourages rib cage expansion when used with the correct breathing techniques.

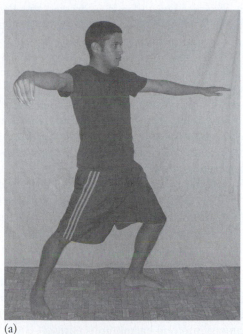

(a)

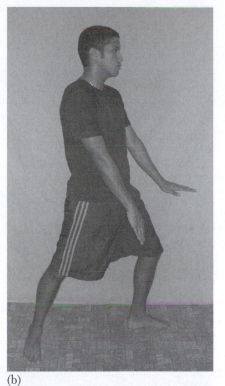

(b)

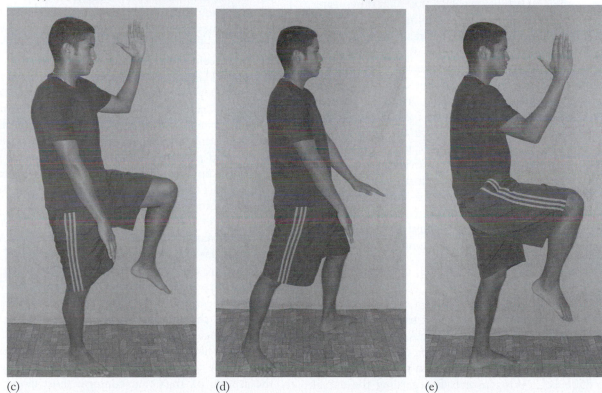

(c)   (d)   (e)

Figure 10.23 Golden Rooster Stands on One Leg. From a relaxed stance, the client abducts both shoulders to approximately 90° (a). He then shifts his body weight toward the front (left) leg while sweeping the arms down toward his sides (b). As the right arm sweeps upward, the right leg is lifted up from the floor (c). From this position, the client steps down and back with the right foot (d). Finally, the client raises the left hand and leg upward (e). To create a more challenging and dynamic posture, during the stork phase of this exercise, the client can sit deeper into the plant leg while simultaneously bringing the lifted knee up to touch the elbow (i.e., left knee to left elbow). The purpose of this exercise is to train and develop balance and good posture. This exercise is good for working on deepening one's consciousness regarding sense of balance. It may be helpful for the client to imagine that his body is a pillar beginning at the foot upon which the rest of the body from the hip to the top of the head balances. It may also be helpful for the client to visualize that although he is standing during this exercise, he is "sitting on the hip", which is solidly grounded to the floor.

YOGA

One of the oldest known health practices, *Yoga* (which means "union," "unity," or "oneness" in Sanskrit) is the integration of physical, mental, and spiritual energies to promote health and wellness.[11,151] Yoga traditionally is a way of life that encompasses ethical conduct, social responsibility, nutrition, and physical health practices. It is based on the Hindu principle of mind-body unity,[11,151] which says, for instance, that a chronically stressed, restless, or agitated mind will result in poor health and reduced or diminished mental clarity. Practitioners believe that practicing Yoga can combat these negative physical and psychological effects and restore good mental, emotional, spiritual, and physical health.[8,11,151] Yoga practitioners also believe that without making any undue demands, a client practicing Yoga can find their body, breathing, brain, and mind working as "one," thereby resulting in higher functional abilities and enhanced performance levels.[11,151]

While practicing specific postures, the client pays close attention to their breathing, exhaling at certain times using the lower abdominal muscles and inhaling using diaphragmatic breathing at others.[11,151] The breathing techniques associated with Yoga are believed to help maintain the postures or positions as well as promote relaxation and enhance the flow of vital energy or life force known as *prana* (similar to the Chinese concept of Qi or Chi).[11] Prana is considered an extension of the same cosmic energy that directs and sustains the universe.[8] Yoga also encompasses the idea of the chakras, or seven wheels, which are considered energy centers that transform universal energy into usable human forms of energy. While there are several schools of Yoga, this section will focus on Hatha Yoga. Hatha Yoga aims to cleanse the body of toxins, energize and realign the body, release muscle tension, increase flexibility, enhance physical strength, maintain physical fitness, and clear the mind.[11,151]

Background

Yoga is an ancient Indian art thought to have originated approximately 4,000 years ago.[152] The *Rig-Veda*, meaning "knowledge of praise," contains definite elements of Yoga, and is one of the oldest texts known in the world, dating back to 2500 B.C. Written records regarding the use of breathing exercises and specific postures for spiritual and physical well being have been found dating from 1500 B.C., with references in other texts in 400 B.C.[8] The first detailed descriptions of the eight limbs of Yoga were written by Patanjali in 300 B.C.[8] Although only a few written versions are still in existence, the hymns of the *Rig-Veda* were passed down orally by Hindu priests for hundreds of years.[152] Despite its age, Yoga is timeless, transcending cultures, philosophies, and eras. Over the centuries it has offered guidance on living a long and healthy life.

Yoga was first brought to the United States in 1893 when Swami Vivekandanda addressed the Parliament of Religions.[152] In the beginning, Yoga in the United States was philosophical in nature. Over the next few years, several swamis came to the United States to teach Americans the principles and philosophies associated with various Yoga forms.[152] By the 1920s, Hatha Yoga was introduced as a physical fitness movement.[8] During the 1960s, Eastern philosophy was introduced to Americans, largely through pop culture figures such as the Beatles and Ravi Shankar, and Hindu ways, music, and practices, including Yoga, became popular.[152]

Two of the most widely practiced aspects of Yoga are Hatha Yoga, consisting of a physiological based program, and Raja Yoga, which is based on mental mastery for the sake of well being. Hatha ("ha" means sun and "tha" means moon) Yoga is often a stepping stone to Raja Yoga, as *Hatha Yoga* focuses on gaining control of the body while *Raja Yoga* focuses on gaining control of the mind. These opposites parallel the yogic belief of unification of the individual energy of self and the universal energy of the environment into one harmonious entity.

Although the practice of Hatha Yoga was originally intended for achievement of this control over the physical body, spiritual fitness, and balance attributes, many people choose to concentrate on strength, flexibility, and relaxation through Hatha Yoga. The spine plays a major role in keeping the body upright, provides mobility and stability with functional activities, and provides a vital channel for the nervous system.[153] Hence, keeping the spine flexible and working the spinal and trunk muscles effectively forms a central part of Yoga postures. The result is believed to be a supple and strong spine as well as enhanced digestive and organ function, neural enhancement, and effective breathing patterns which influences brain activity.[153]

There are many schools of Yoga (**Table 10.6**), which grew or were developed from different teachers and traditions. There are also several branches of Yoga that focus on different aspects or goals of practice (**Table 10.7**). Finally, there are several limbs, or principles, of Hatha Yoga (**Table 10.8**), the pursuit of which provides the total lifestyle that Yoga is traditionally known for. We will focus the discussion here on Hatha Yoga and the principles of *asana* (posture) and *pranayama* (breathing) because they are the aspects of Yoga that conform most closely with physical fitness and therapeutic exercise as they are understood in the West.[9,11,151–153]

The purpose of Hatha Yoga is to enable the client to balance their prana, thereby allowing it to ascend through all of the chakras until it emerges from the crown chakra (at the top of the skull), and to achieve self-realization.[8] The ultimate aim of Hatha Yoga is to prepare the client for a spiritual experience by purifying the body. No single posture is adequate to cleanse or purify a person. Hence, it is important that the client be aware of Yoga's eight limbs

TABLE 10.6 Schools of Yoga[8,9,11,151–153]

School	Description
Hatha	Purpose is balance of *prana*, thereby allowing it to ascend through all of the chakras until it emerges from the crown chakra (at the top of the skull), and to achieve self-realization. See text for further discussion.
Ashtanga	Power yoga. Vigorous, fast-paced series of poses performed in a continuous flow (Vinyasa), designed to condition the body and realign the spine, as well as improve concentration and meditative ability.
Kripalu	Known as a compassionate and introspective yoga. Can be practiced at any level of intensity.
Rising Phoenix	Developed from Kripalu yoga. One form of an individualized yoga training program. Focuses on aiding clients in releasing physical and emotional tensions.
Integral	Developed for the busy urban dweller to assist in relaxation and centering.
Iyengar	Developed by BKS Iyengar. Emphasizes precision and attention to anatomy and alignment. Maintains a highly developed correlation between specific poses and the medical conditions for which they are thought to be beneficial.
Viniyoga	Gentle and individualized approach focusing on the particular needs of the client. Emphasizes that there is some aspect of Yoga that can be beneficial, regardless of physical, emotional, or mental limitations.
Therapeutic Yoga	Geared especially toward those with back problems. Uses props, especially ropes, to assist in maintaining a pose for longer than might be comfortable otherwise.

TABLE 10.7 Branches of Yoga

Branch	Description
Raja Yoga	Classic yoga, yoga of the mind, meditation yoga or the Royal Path. Focus is on training the mind through meditation to serve the spirit. Meditation, concentration, and breath control are paramount. Religious orders and spiritual communities often dedicate themselves to this branch.
Kriya and Karma Yoga	Yogas of action. *Kriya* (spiritual action) involves the practice of quieting the mind through self-study, breathing techniques, mantras, and meditation. Breathing and meditation help to bring the energy up the spine. *Karma* is the path of service yoga. Emphasis is on selfless action, transcending concerns of success, egoism, and selfishness.
Bhakti Yoga	Path of devotion or yoga of the heart. It involves devotion, reverence, and perpetual remembrance of whatever is meaningful to the client. All intellectual concerns, unsettled mind, and the material world fall away, and empathy, compassion, love, and thoughts of the divine take over.
Jnana Yoga	Path of the mind or the path of wisdom. Purpose is to seek and walk the path of knowledge and wisdom as well as discern what is real from unreal. It encourages one to temporarily question everything one thinks, believes, feels, and knows by inquiring deeply within oneself via questioning, meditation, and contemplation until all that remains is the person, the universe, the elimination of illusion, and the presence of true knowledge.
Tantra Yoga	The place where opposites meet and become one. Involves the study of sacred writing and rituals to eliminate obstacles to enlightenment. Teaches that there is no difference between infinite and finite or divine and the divinity.
Mantra Yoga	The study of potent and sacred sounds. Centers on the principle that sound can affect consciousness by clearing the mind, allowing the client to attain higher states of consciousness, and encouraging spiritual awakening.
Kundalini Yoga	The study of energy movement along the spine. It involves techniques meant to awaken the energy at the base of the spine, which is released through breath and specific Hatha yoga movements.

TABLE 10.8   Eight limbs (Principles) of Hatha Yoga

Principle	Description
Yama	Do good. Five commandments focused on moral conduct, ethical standards, sense of integrity, and health guidelines:
Ahimsa	• True nonviolence, freedom of anger and fear.
Satya	• Truth in thought, word, and deed.
Asteya	• Not claiming what belongs to others.
Brahmacharya	• Transcendence of all desire.
Aparigraha	• State of not being attached.
Niyama	Self-discipline and spiritual observance. Five rules focus on being good and give the ground rules for self-discipline and inner awareness:
Saucha	• Physical and spiritual cleanliness and purity.
Samtosa	• Contentment.
Tapas	• Desire to reach a pristine state (i.e., chastity).
Swadhyaya	• Study of oneself.
Ishwarapranidhana	• Devotion and surrender to higher infinite power.
Asana	Physical postures and exercises to facilitate concentration and keep the body healthy, keep the mind calm, and create an atmosphere in which the spirit can flow freely.
Pranayama	Regulation of life force. Focuses on understanding the link between breath, mind, and body by encouraging the client to control the breath in order to enhance the flow of energy throughout the body.
Pratyahara Dharana Dhyana Samadhi	The final four principles deal with attaining a higher state of concentration, enhancing the senses, and the mind. They focus on meditation, which is the process of quieting or controlling the constant waves of thoughts.

and their branches. The limbs and branches are systematically arranged to outline detoxification regimens, hygiene, lifestyle, physical, and psychological practices.

Posture (Asana) and Breathing (Pranayama)

The word asana means "ease" in Sanskrit and is concerned with body control.[11,152] There are two main types of asana, meditative and therapeutic. *Meditative asanas* improve the alignment of the spine and head, promote proper blood flow throughout the body, and instill a state of relaxation and stillness that facilitates increased concentration during meditation. They are believed to help keep the glands, lungs, and heart properly energized. *Therapeutic asanas*, such as the spinal twist and shoulder stand, are geared toward improving health and physical well being and are commonly prescribed for clients with back, neck, and joint pain. Originally, therapeutic asanas were designed simply to create a condition of ease in the body as a prelude to meditation. It has only been within the past century that Yoga postures have been applied to specific physical disorders.

Asanas are a unique combination of physical postures and exercises to facilitate concentration and keep the body healthy, keep the mind calm, and create an atmosphere in which the spirit can flow freely.[152,154] The goal of a properly executed asana is to create a healthy body with a balance between movement and stillness[11,151] that allows a client to develop the habit of discipline and the ability to concentrate.[8] Although many of the asanas require little movement, they require the mind to concentrate on the body's position, postures, and movements. Yoga practitioners note that with practice and meditation, a client can learn to regulate their autonomic functions (i.e., heartbeat, respiration rate) and reduce both physical muscular tensions and psychological stressors.[11,151]

In terms of prevention, therapeutic exercise, or athletic preparation (in season or off season), asanas can play a valuable role. For example, asanas can be used as a form of supplemental exercise training to help to correct muscle imbalances, speed up recovery between training sessions, increase or decrease general body or specific muscle group activation, as a warm-up exercise to enhance concentration and neuromuscular coordination, and as a cool-down exercise.[154] Postures may be modified for clients who do not have the strength or flexibility to perform and/or maintain them. Assistive devices such as ropes, blocks, and folded blankets are used as needed to maintain a pose. As the client becomes more adept at performing and holding the postures, assistive devices can be discarded. All demographic groups can practice Hatha Yoga.

Pranayama, meaning regulation of prana or life force extension, involves breathing exercises and focuses on the link between breath, mind, and body by encouraging the client to control the breath in order to enhance the flow of energy throughout the body.[8,30,154] Yoga teaches that prana, like Chi or Qi, circulates through the body in a system of approximately 72,000 delicate nerves. In Yoga, these nerves are referred to as *nadis*.[30] When the flow of prana is interrupted through stress, improper diet, or toxins, one's physical, emotional, and mental health is impaired.[11,30,152-154] Pranayama yogic techniques claim to alleviate conditions such as asthma, bronchitis, colds, sinus infections, neurosis, insomnia, headache, obesity, constipation, and nicotine addiction.[8,11,152,153]

If the breath is calm and controlled, the mind can be settled at rest and yet focused.[30] If the mind is calm and focused, the breathing will be steady, deep (diaphragmatic), and rhythmic. If the mind is restless and agitated, breathing will be shallow (intercostal), rapid, and agitated. A fundamental aspect in yogic breathing is the elimination of any jerkiness, unevenness, or awkwardness in the breathing motion itself.[30] Instead, yogic breathing practices advocate the unconscious maintenance of smoothly flowing breath, the use of consistent breathing patterns, and the use of full, even (right to left), deep (diaphragmatic) breathing motions. This correlates with subsequent smoothness in the flow of thoughts, making yogic breathing exercises useful in calming the restlessness of the mind and creating clarity, focus, and heightened energy.[30] Therefore, pranayama is often implemented as a technique to prepare for meditation.

Therapeutic Indications

Yoga has been used successfully for pain management programs.[155] Yoga has also been found to be effective in the treatment of hypertension, cardiovascular conditions[156–161] (i.e., heart disease), heart arrhythmia, bone marrow depletion, thyroid disorders, and other physical ailments[155,157]; a variety of musculoskeletal ailments (i.e., low back pain, osteoarthritis, carpal tunnel syndrome[151,162–164]; various pulmonary conditions and diseases (asthma, bronchitis),[165–169] multiple sclerosis and cerebrovascular accidents[170,171] and premenstrual tension, menstrual problems, labor pain, and symptoms of menopause.[155,172,173] Finally, Yoga has also been claimed to be a useful form of treatment for migraine headaches, sexual dysfunction, diabetes, cancer, gastrointestinal problems (ulcers, hemorrhoids), anxiety, and improved athletic performance, as well as other medical conditions (i.e., obsessive-compulsive disorder, diabetes, mental retardation, insomnia, and memory impairments).[155–178] Numerous studies have demonstrated Yoga 's effectiveness as a complementary therapy for addictions such as tobacco and alcohol.[11,179] Yoga techniques can fit the needs of clients five years of age and older who are in almost any physical condition. Clients who cannot perform some of the more physically demanding postures can still benefit from the breathing and meditation techniques.[11]

Contraindications

Some of the more physical aspects of Yoga can cause musculoskeletal injury if they are not performed properly or if the client tries to force their body into difficult positions.[8,11] For example, a client with diagnosed sciatica should not try to perform Yoga exercises that involve intense stretching, especially in forward flexed positions. Also, women who are actively menstruating should not participate in inverted poses. Pregnant women should not do breath retentions, breath suspensions, or inverted poses. In addition, clients suffering from glaucoma, hypertension, or diagnosed cervical conditions (i.e., instability, disc herniation, spondylosis, or vertebral artery syndrome) should not do breath retentions or inverted poses.[8] Clients should be advised to consult their physician before undertaking a Yoga program. Rehabilitation clinicians should also advise beginning clients to attempt new Yoga postures slowly and cautiously. It is also important to remind clients that very few individuals can perform all the postures and movements in the beginning.

Evidence

Since the early 1970s, there have been over 1,000 studies of meditation and Yoga that report on their effectiveness in alleviating stress and anxiety, reducing blood pressure and heart rate, decreasing respiratory rate, improving memory and intelligence, relieving pain, improving motor skills, relief from addictions, heightening visual and auditory perceptions, enhancing metabolic and respiratory functions, and producing brain wave activity associated with relaxation.[155–168, 174–179] The breath control aspect of Yoga has also been shown to aid digestion, regulate cardiac function, and reduce the frequency of asthma attacks.[11] Below is a selected review of the literature concerning the efficacy of Yoga as a therapeutic exercise intervention.

Cardiovascular System.   Medical literature confirms that Yoga has beneficial effects on the cardiovascular system. Schell et al.[158] evaluated the effects of Yoga practice among young healthy women. Subjects who participated in regular Yoga practice displayed lower heart rates compared to a control group, but these changes were only evident during the Yoga practice sessions. Examination of blood pressure in the same study revealed no significant changes. Sundar et al.[159] monitored the mean systolic and diastolic blood pressures of 25 subjects with essential hypertension. The study reviewed usage patterns of anti-hypertensive medications. Subjects were taught yogic techniques that were performed over a six-month period. Results revealed decreases in both systolic and diastolic blood pressures during the study time period. Furthermore, anti-hypertensive medication usage decreased in the five subjects that had been using them prior to using yogic techniques. The blood pressure levels of subjects who left the Yoga practice group during the study returned to pre-study levels.

Manchanda et al.[160] performed a prospective randomized, controlled trial of 42 men with coronary atherosclerotic disease. The experimental group was treated with Yoga, control of risk factors, diet control, and moderate aerobic exercise. The control group was managed by conventional methods of risk factor control and the American Heart Association Step I diet. At one year post intervention, the Yoga group displayed significant reductions in anginal episodes per week, improved exercise capacity, and decreased body weight compared to the control group. Repeat coronary angiography at one year post-intervention showed a greater percentage of lesion regression and a lower percentage of lesion progression in the experimental group.

Musculoskeletal System.

In a randomized, controlled study, Garfinkel et al.[162] reported on the influence of Yoga on subjects with osteoarthritis of the hands. In their initial study outcome variables included pain, strength, motion, joint circumference, tenderness, and hand function using the Stanford Hand Assessment questionnaire. The Yoga group participated in eight 60-minute sessions, one per week for eight weeks, with one instructor. The Yoga instruction included traditional postures, or asanas, as well as instruction in breathing control. The results showed that compared to a control group, the Yoga group displayed statistically significant improvement in finger joint tenderness, pain with hand activity, and finger range of motion.[162] The remainder of the variables, although showing improvement, did not reach statistical significance. They concluded that Yoga was effective in providing relief in subjects with osteoarthritis of the hand.[162] A randomized, single-blind study by Garfinkel et al.[163] investigated the effects of Yoga on 42 subjects with carpal tunnel syndrome (22 in the Yoga group and 20 in the standard treatment group). Outcome measurements included grip strength, pain intensity; sleep disturbance, Phalen's sign, Tinel's sign, and median nerve motor and sensory conduction times. Subjects in the Yoga based intervention group received a program focused on upper body postures: improving flexibility; correcting alignment of hands, wrists, arms, and shoulders; stretching; and increasing awareness of optimal joint position during use. The control group used a wrist splint in conjunction with standard care. Results revealed a statistically significant increase in grip strength and decreased pain intensity in the Yoga group. The other variables showed no significant change.[163]

Pulmonary / Respiratory System.

Respiratory function has been among the most frequently measured variables in scientific evaluations of Yoga primarily because of the emphasis Yoga places on breathing, especially *pranayama* breathing exercises, and breath control. Studies have shown that Yoga has a beneficial effect on the respiratory system, with results ranging from lowered breathing rates to increased lung capacity, and a reduction in the frequency of asthma attacks.[30,165-169,176]

Nagarathna and Nagendra[169] performed a controlled study of subjects afflicted with bronchial asthma who were divided into two comparison groups: one that practiced Yoga (experimental) and another that used medication (control). Subjects in the Yoga (experimental) group were taught varying techniques, which included specific postures, slow breathing techniques, and meditation, over a two-week period. The Yoga group was instructed to practice the learned material for 65 minutes daily. Both groups were matched for age, sex, and type and severity of asthma. Significant results in the Yoga group compared to the control group was improved peak flow rates, decrease in number of asthmatic episodes per week, and decrease in amount of medication used.[169]

Vedanthan et al.[166] explored the effects of Yoga on clients with asthma. In this study, 17 adult subjects with asthma, ranging from 19 to 52 years of age, were divided into two groups. Nine were taught Yoga techniques, including pranayama, asanas, and meditation; the remaining eight subjects served as controls. The test group was taught Yoga three times a week for 16 weeks. All clients maintained logs of symptoms and medication use. Samples of both morning and evening peak flow readings (amount of air the subject could expire; low levels indicating airway obstruction) were collected throughout the study. They found that the test group reported a higher degree of relaxation, more positive attitudes, better tolerance to exercise, and less use of beta-adrenergic inhalers compared to the control group. Pulmonary function did not differ significantly between groups, but the authors concluded that Yoga techniques did appear to prevent exacerbation of asthma attacks.[166]

Khanam et al.[167] investigated the efficacy of a short term Yoga program (one week) on nine subjects who were diagnosed with bronchial asthma. The researchers reported that both pulmonary and autonomic function was significantly improved. Subjects did not show improvement in their volumes or expiratory flow rates, but did demonstrate improvement in pulmonary ventilation by way of relaxation of voluntary inspiratory and expiratory muscles.[167] Behera,[168] in studying the effect of Yoga on the lung function of 15 subjects with chronic bronchitis, reported improved dyspnea as measured by a visual analog scale, and improved lung function parameters including vital capacity following the four week duration intervention.

Nervous System. One aspect of Yoga that distinguishes it from other forms of traditional therapeutic exercise is its focus on the health of the nervous and endocrine systems. Both of these systems are believed to be stimulated and toned by Hatha Yoga movements, postures, breathing exercises, and practices. This is believed to occur via two methods. First, asanas produce increased circulation to the endocrine glands and the various nerve plexuses. For example, when a client assumes the cobra position (bhujangasana), they contract the lumbosacral region musculature that in turn increases the circulation to the lumbosacral plexus. Or if a client has moved into a shoulder-stand position, which is an advanced Yoga posture, the effects of gravity results in increased circulation to the thyroid gland.[30] A second way in which Hatha Yoga practices support the health of the nervous system is by means of the breathing exercises (pranayama). During inhalation, deep breathing expands 24 ribs, two lungs, and moves the diaphragm down, slowly filling up the abdominal cavity, lower thoracic cavity, and the chest. Upon exhalation, the ribs and lungs compress, the abdominals contract, the diaphragm rises. It is this manipulation of the breathing system that is believed to have a highly beneficial effect on the nervous system. The body of evidence exploring the efficacy of Yoga directly to nervous system function however is minimal.[163]

Endocrine System. Jain et al.[174] investigated the efficacy of Yoga for non–insulin dependent diabetes. In this study, 149 subjects with non–insulin dependent diabetes participated in Yoga for 40 days. Results revealed that 70 percent of the subjects displayed both a reduction in the need for drugs to maintain normal blood sugar levels as well as decreases in their incident of hyperglycemia. Using positron emission tomography, to study eight members of a Yoga meditation group, Herzog et al.,[180] reported that the ratios of frontal vs. occipital regional cerebral metabolic rate of glucose metabolism were significantly elevated during Yoga meditation, suggesting a change in brain function during the meditative state.

Additional Benefits. Goyeche[181] expounded on the psychosomatic effects of Yoga, reporting favorable outcomes from studies of subjects who suffered from conditions of anxiety, depression, hypochondriasis, obsessive disorders, and phobias. Indian literature also reports a benefit of Yoga with acute and chronic pain management, although these studies are not available in western journals. As noted previously, Schell et al.,[158] in studying the effects of Yoga on healthy women, reported that although cortisol, prolactin, and growth hormone levels did not differ between the Yoga practicing group and a control group; the Yoga group showed higher life satisfaction, as well as lower scores in excitability, aggressiveness, emotionality,

and somatic complaints. Shannahoff-Khalsa and Beckett,[175] in studying the effect of a specific Yoga breathing pattern for helping eight adults with obsessive-compulsive disorder, reported that by alleviating anxiety, most of the subjects were able to either reduce to discontinue their medication.

Research involving Yoga and memory has revealed that Yoga breathing increases spatial memory scores by 84 percent in trained subjects, but did not increase verbal scores.[178] In a controlled clinical study, Telles et al.[182] assessed the relationship between Yoga training on visual focusing among 60 subjects who were between 18 and 42 years of age. After one month, 86 percent of the Yoga group displayed a significant decrease in degree of optical illusion, whereas the control group showed no change between pre- and post-study values.

A review of the literature by Telles and Naveen[176] reported that mentally retarded children who practiced Yoga benefited in the areas of general mental ability, coordination, social adjustment, and behavior. In a study that compared Yoga training for five hours per week over one academic year among 45 children with mental retardation with 45 age and sex matched mentally retarded control group subjects, Uma et al.[177] reported a "highly significant" improvement in IQ and social adaptation among the treatment group.

Yoga has also been reported to be effective in reducing anxiety in visually impaired children; decreasing substance abuse including tobacco and alcohol addictions; improving the general sense of well being among individuals who are HIV positive; and significantly improving the appetite, sleep, and general sense of well being among prisoners.[176] In a randomized clinical trial of subjects who were in outpatient methadone maintenance treatment programs for substance abuse, Shaffer et al.[179] reported similar effectiveness between Yoga exercise therapy and conventional psychotherapy intervention with methadone.

Equipment

Minimal equipment is needed to practice Yoga. A quiet, private environment that is free from distractions should be available, and there should be enough room for the client to move around freely without touching or distracting those nearby.[11,152,153] The client should wear loose, lightweight clothing, preferably made of cotton. Some clients prefer to wear shoes or slippers, while others prefer to be barefoot. The client should use a mat (called a sticky mat), small blanket, or large towel for some of the postures to provide extra cushioning. Rolls, cubes or bolsters can also be used for some of the postures to assist the client with maintaining proper alignment or to enhance the difficulty of certain postures. Some clients like to bring a pillow to sit on and a lightweight shawl or blanket for covering during meditation or deep relaxation exercises.

Technique

Yoga training usually is performed in a class situation, but can also be undertaken on an individual level. A serious student of Yoga practices on a daily basis between classes. A typical Yoga class begins with stretching and centering postures (poses). Each class is tailored to the needs of the population and the philosophy of the style being practiced. Emphasis is placed on self-care, attention to one's own limitations, and the dynamic interaction between neuromuscular, cardiopulmonary, and emotional function while holding a pose. Advocates of Yoga emphasize that physical strength, flexibility, relaxation, and smooth flow of energy, or prana, are attained while maintaining a pose. The instructor uses verbal direction in addition to hands-on assistance. A portion of a class or session always is devoted to relaxation. There are many styles of Hatha Yoga, ranging from very vigorous and athletic to gentler forms for disabled populations. Yoga classes are also available for specific populations (clients with back problems, cardiovascular conditions, rheumatoid arthritis, cancer survivors, multiple sclerosis, etc.).

Although Yoga postures may involve very little movement, the mind is involved in the performance of every asana, to provide discipline, awareness, and a relative openness. This discipline and awareness helps maintain the posture, relaxation and openness, needed to stimulate the circulation of prana (life energy), allowing the client to experience Yoga's full benefits. A properly executed asana creates balance between movement and stillness, exertion and surrender, which is precisely the state of a healthy body.[30] The client learns to regulate autonomic functions like heartbeat and breathing, while physical tensions fade into relaxation.

Example Yoga Program

While some specific Yoga asanas can help particular health conditions, the safest and most reliable way to use Hatha Yoga therapeutically is to follow a balanced program of postures to achieve an overall normalizing and health enhancing or inducing effect. It is best for the beginner to start with a simple program of basic postures. A beginning Yoga program can be performed in approximately 30 minutes.[8,11,30] An initial structured class or instruction is suggested as a foundation prior to performing more advanced exercises.

The first posture, called the corpse, or Shavasana (**Figure 10.24**), is an excellent posture to start a Yoga program, as it focuses on relaxation and diaphragmatic breathing. It is important to remember that relaxation is the opposite of activity and is a process of observation without intervention. Throughout this exercise, the client should feel their muscles relaxing, tension falling away, their breathing and heart rate becoming slower, and the mind becoming more quiet and peaceful. The corpse po-

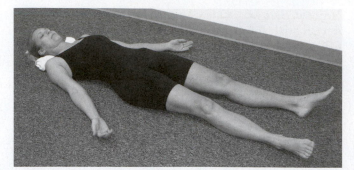

Figure 10.24   Corpse, or Shavasana. While in supine position, the client relaxes and takes slow, deep diaphragmatic breaths, allowing the abdomen to expand with each inhalation and contract using the lower abdominal muscles with each exhalation.

sition has many suggested benefits, including: 1) aiding circulation and improving nervous system function; 2) helping to relax the skeletal muscles, enabling one to go further into the postures while reducing the likelihood of injuries; and 3) to help relax and prepare the mind for the next posture in the sequence, and at the conclusion of the program to help reduce fatigue. Every Yoga session ends with a relaxation exercise. For beginners, this relaxation period is typically 5–10 minutes and can be gradually increased to 15–20 minutes.

The Child's Posture exercise (**Figure 10.25**) is believed to relax the back and promotes healing of back injuries by taking pressure off the intervertebral disc and providing a mild and natural form of traction; and relieve pain in the lower back that may be caused by other postures, therefore it can be used as a bridge between various asanas if lower back pain persists.

This posterior stretch exercise is purported to provide the following benefits: 1) Stimulates the peristaltic move-

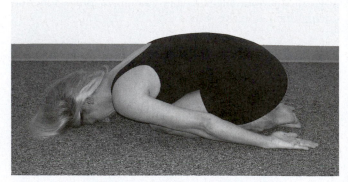

Figure 10.25   Child's Posture, or Balasana. From a kneeling position, while exhaling, the client bends forward slowly from the hips until the stomach and chest rest on the thighs and the forehead touches the floor in front of the knees.

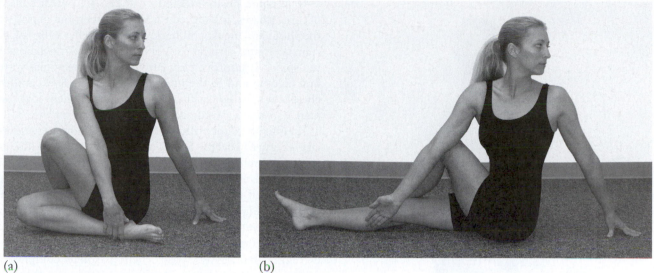

(a)   (b)

Figure 10.26   Half spinal twist. While in a short-seated position with a leg crossed over the opposite thigh, the client rotates her trunk in the opposite direction while keeping her back straight (a). An advanced form of this exercise is performed in a long sitting position (b).

ment (wave-like contractions) of the digestive tract and prevents constipation; 2) stimulates the entire abdominal area: kidneys, liver, stomach, spleen, and pancreas; 3) relieves indigestion and poor appetite; 4) may be therapeutic in the treatment of diabetes; 5) stretches the hamstring muscles of the thighs and the muscles and ligaments of the back; and 6) gently mobilizes the intervertebral discs; develops flexibility of the spinal column.

The half spinal twist exercise (**Figure 10.26a–b**) is believed to: 1) provide segmental motion throughout the spinal column; 2) stretch and lengthen spinal muscles and ligaments; 3) keep the spine elastic and healthy; 4) alternately compress each half of the abdominal region, mobilizing the internal organs, and promote improved circulation through the abdominal cavity; and 5) ease constipation, reduce fat, and improve digestion.

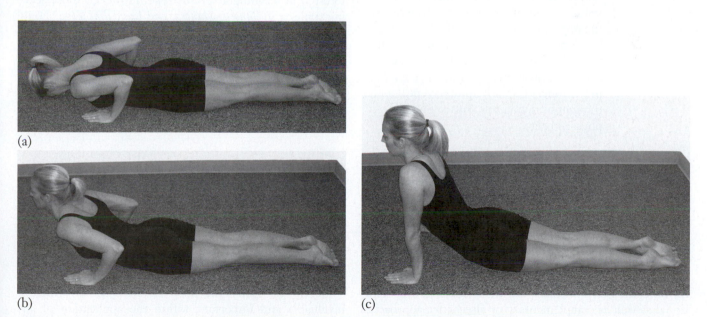

(a)

(b)   (c)

Figure 10.27   Cobra position. The client begins in a prone position with the palms on the floor and near her sides (a). While inhaling, she slowly raises her head and upper trunk upward (b). Without solely using upper extremity strength to push the body off the floor, the client continues to slowly raise the shoulders and chest using only the muscles of the back (c). The client's navel should remain on the floor, keeping both the feet and legs together and relaxed.

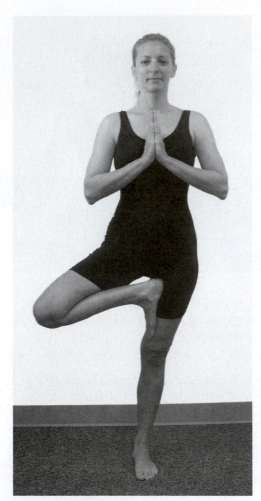

Figure 10.28   Simple Tree, or Vrikshansana. While standing, the client places one foot up on the opposite while letting the hip move into external rotation and abduction. She then places the hands together on the chest and closes her eyes. Some Yoga practitioners find it helpful to repeat a thought or saying to enhance mental and physical balance.

The cobra position (**Figure 10.27a–c**), which consists of three phases, is believed to: 1) strengthen the muscles of the shoulders, neck, and back; 2) develop flexibility of the spinal column, cervical vertebrae, and correct deviations of the spine; 3) improve circulation around the spinal vertebral column and to the intervertebral discs; 4) expand the chest and develop elasticity of the lungs; 5) help low back pain, constipation, stomach pains, and gas pains.

The final exercise illustrated is the standing tree exercise (**Figure 10.28**). Some clients may need to do the standing stretch exercise before performing this exercise, which involves coordinating diaphragmatic breathing with stretching of the arms over the head as if picking apples. The standing tree exercise can be performed once the standing stretch is mastered. This Yoga exercise is believed to: 1) provide a deep stretch to the posterior lower extremity (hamstrings, gastrocnemius-soleus complex) as well as the plantar fascia; 2) rejuvenate and train the anterior lower extremity musculature; 3) revitalize the nerves in the pelvis and hip region; and 4) improve balance.

Practitioner Requirements

There are several forms and schools of Yoga available in the West, with each emphasizing a different aspect of the body/mind/spirit relationship.[8,152,153] There are presently no national certification, licensing, or regulation requirements for Yoga instructors. Training is available in a wide range of Yoga schools and philosophies with each offering instructor certification classes for individuals who are interested in teaching a specific type. However, those seeking training in *Tantra*, *Mantra*, and *Kundalini* Yoga should seek the guidance of a qualified master teacher, as these three limbs of Yoga require an additional level of emotional, mental, and moral preparation.

Summary

No single sport or therapeutic exercise regimen gives a client's body everything it needs to functional optimally. As rehabilitation clinicians, we must consider the traditional as well as complementary or alternative approaches to rehabilitating our clients, enhancing their performance, and preventing injury. Research to date has been extensive. However, as Ives and Sosnoff[14] mentioned earlier, more scientifically rigorous prospective, randomized, clinical trials are needed to validate the limits of the usefulness of many of these alternative approaches. There are those who subscribe to the idea that the scientific knowledge somehow dampens our deep intuitive sense, which is invaluable and important within the application of any complementary or alternative therapy. A balance must somehow be found between the intuitive and the scientific in order to fully prove the true value of complementary and alternative approaches to client care.

References

1. Kessler HH. *The Knife Is Not Enough.* New York: Norton, 1968.

2. Shiflett SC. Overview of complementary therapies in physical medicine and rehabilitation. *Phys Med Rehabil Clin N Am.* 1999:10:521–529.

3. Eisenberg DM, Kessler RC, Foster C, et al. Unconventional medicine in the United States: Prevalence, costs, and patterns of use. *New Engl J Med.* 1993;328:246–252.

4. Eisenberg DM, Davis RB, Ettner SL, et al. Trends in alternative medicine use in the United States, 1990–1997. *JAMA.* 1998;280:1569–1575.

5. *A Nationwide Telephone Survey of 1,000 Americans.* Stanford Center for Research in Disease Prevention: Online report. Stanford University, Palo Alto, CA.

6. Shiflett SC, Krauss HH, Godfrey C, et al. Predictors of usage of alternative therapies in the physically disabled. *Ann Beh Med.* 1999:21:5089.

7. Trivieri L. Jr. *The American Holistic Medical Association Guide to Holistic Health.* New York: John Wiley & Sons, 2001.

8. Kuhn MA. *Complementary Therapies for Health Care Providers.* Philadelphia, PA: Lippincott, Williams & Wilkins, 1999.

9. Gingerich BS. *Complementary Medicine Modalities: Teaching and Assessment Tools.* Gaithersburg, MD: Aspen Publishers, 2002.

10. Jonas W. Complementary and alternative medicine at the NIH. Office of Alternative Medicine. Advisory Council Address. 1996;3:1.

11. *Nurse's Handbook of Alternative and Complementary Therapies.* Springhouse, PA: Springhouse Corporation, 1998.

12. Sierpina VS. *Integrative Health Care: Complementary and Alternative Therapies for the Whole Person.* Philadelphia,: F.A. Davis Co., 2001.

13. Kibler WB, Herring SA, Press JM (eds). *Functional Rehabilitation of Sports and Musculoskeletal Injuries.* Gaithersburg, MD: Aspen Publishers Inc., 1998.

14. Ives JC, Sosnoff J. Beyond the mind-body exercise hype. *Physician Sportsmed.* 2000;28(3):67–8, 70, 75–6.

15. Charman RA. *Complementary Therapies for Physical Therapists.* Oxnard: Butterworth–Heinemann, 2000.

16. Simpson L. *The Book of Chakra Healing.* New York: Sterling Publishing Co. Inc., 1999.

17. McPartlend J, Miller B. Bodywork therapy systems. *Phys Med Rehabil Clin N Am.* 1999;10(3):583–602.

18. Cohen SO, Walco GA. Dance/movement therapy for children and adolescents with cancer. *Cancer Practice* 1999;7(1):34–42.

19. Lewis RN, Scannel ED. Relationship of body image and creative dance movement. *Percep Motor Skills.* 1995;81:155–160.

20. Heber L. Dance movement: A therapeutic program for psychiatric clients. *Perspect Psych Care.* 1993;29:22–29.

21. Hanna JL. The power of dance: Health and healing. *J Alt Compl Med.* 1995;1:323–331.

22. Serlin I, Frances B, Vestevich K, et al. The effect of dance/movement therapy on women with breast cancer. *Altern Ther Symposium Abstrs.* 1997;3:103.

23. Kudlacek S, Pietschmann E, Bernecker P, et al. The impact of a senior dancing program on spinal and peripheral bone loss. *Am J Phys Med Rehabil.* 1997;76:477–481.

24. Berrol C. Dance/movement therapy in head injured rehabilitation. *Brain Injury.* 1990;4:257–265.

25. Goldberg W, Fitzpatrick J. Movement therapy with the aged. *Nurs Res.* 1980;29:339–346.

26. Hamburg J, Clair AA. The effects of a Laban-based movement program with music on measures of balance and gait in older adults. *Activities Adapt Aging.* 2003;28(1):17–33.

27. Jonas WB, Levin JS. *Essentials of Complementary and Alternative Medicine.* Philadelphia, PA: Lippincott, Williams & Wilkins, 1999.

28. Feldenkrais M. *Awareness Through Movement.* New York: Harper & Row, 1972.

29. Davis CM. *Complementary Therapies in Rehabilitation: Holistic Approaches for Prevention and Wellness.* Thorofare, NJ: Slack Incorporated, 1997.

30. Trivieri L, Anderson JW. *Alternative Medicine: The Definitive Guide,* 2nd ed. Berkeley, CA: Celestial Arts, 2002, pp. 122–124.

31. Jackson O. The Feldenkrais Method: A personalized learning model in contemporary management of motor control problems. *Proceedings of the II Step Conference.* Alexandria, VA: Foundation for Physical Therapy, 1991, pp 131–135.

32. Ruth S, Kegerreis S. Facilitating cervical flexion using Feldenkrais Method: Awareness through movement. *J Orthop Sports Phys Ther.* 1992:16:25–29.

33. Kerr GA, Kotynia F, Kolt GS. Feldenkrais awareness through movement and state anxiety. *J Bodywork Movement Ther.* 2002;6(2):102–107.

34. Malmgren-Olsson E, Armelius B, Armelius K. A comparative outcome study of body awareness therapy, Feldenkrais, and conventional physiotherapy for patients with nonspecific musculoskeletal disorders: Changes in psychological symptoms, pain, and self-image. *Physiother Theory Pract.* 2001;17(2):77–95.

35. Smith AL, Kolt GS, McConville JC. The effect of the Feldenkrais method on pain and anxiety in people experiencing chronic low back pain. *N J Physiother.* 2001;29(1):6–14.

36. Kolt BS, McConville JC. The effects of a Feldenkrais Awareness Through Movement program on state anxiety. *J Bodywork Movement Ther.* 2000;4(3):216–220.

37. Lundblad I, Elert J, Gerdle B. Randomized controlled trial of physiotherapy and Feldenkrais interventions in female workers with neck-shoulder complaints. *J Occup Rehabil.* 1999;9(3):179–194.

38. James M, Kolt G, McConville J, Bate P. The effects of a Feldenkrais program and relaxation procedures on hamstring length. *Aust J Physiother.* 1998;44(1):49–54.

39. Johnson SK, Frederick J, Kaufman M, Mountjoy B. A controlled investigation of bodywork in multiple sclerosis. *J Altern Complement Med.* 1999;5(3):237–243.

40. Wildman F. *The Intelligent Body: Awareness Through Movement Lessons* (vols. I, II). Berkeley, CA: Frank Wildman, PhD, 1983.

41. Isaacs B, Kobler J. *The Nickolaus Technique.* New York: Viking Press, 1978.

42. Robinson L, Fisher H, Knox J, Thomson G. *The Official Body Control Pilates Manual.* London: MacMillan Publishing Ltd., 2000.

43. Selby A, Herdman A. *Pilates' Body Conditioning: A Program Based on the Techniques of Joseph Pilates.* Hauppauge, NY: Barron's Educational Series, Inc., 2000.

44. Pilates JH, Miller WJ. The Complete Works of Joseph Pilates' Return to Life Through Contrology and Your Health. In Joseph H. Pilates, William J. Miller (eds.) *A Pilates Primer: The Millenium Edition* (2000). Incline Village, NV: Presentation Dynamics, Inc.

45. Karter K. *The Complete Idiot's Guide to the Pilates Method.* Indianapolis, IN: Alpha, 2001.

46. Schroeder JM, Crussemeyer JA, Newton SJ. Flexibility and heart rate response to an acute Pilates Reformer session. *Med Sci Sports Exerc.* 2002:34(5): S258.

47. McLain S, Carter CL, Abel J. The effect of a conditioning and alignment program on the measurement of supine jump height and pelvic alignment when using the Current Concepts Reformer. *J Dance Med Sci.* 1997;1:149–154.

48. Hutchinson MR, Tremain L, Christiansen J, Beitzel J. Improving leaping ability in elite rhythmic gymnastics. *Med Sci Sports Exerc.* 1998;30(10): 1543–1547.

49. Lange C, Unnithan V, Larkham E, Latta PM. Maximizing the benefits of Pilates-inspired exercise for learning functional motor skills. *J Bodywork Movement Ther.* 2000;4(2):99–108.

50. Fitt S, Sturman J, McClain-Smith S. Effects of Pilates-based conditioning on strength, alignment, and range of motion in university ballet and modern dancers. *Kinesiol Med Dance.* 1994;16:36–51.

51. McMillian A, Proteau L, Lebe R. The effect of Pilates-based training on dancers' dynamic posture. *J Dance Med Sci.* 1998;2(3):101–107.

52. Exercise: Pilates incorporates mind and body. *Harvard Women's Health Watch.* 2000;7(6):6.

53. Duschatko DM. Certified Pilates and gyrotonics trainers . . . frozen shoulder. *J Bodywork Movement Ther.* 2000:4(1):13–19.

54. Brown SE, Clippinger K. Rehabilitation of anterior cruciate ligament insufficiency in a dancer using the clinical reformer and a balanced body exercise method. *WORK.* 1996;7(2):109–114.

55. Loosli AR, Herold D. Knee rehabilitation for dancers using a Pilates-based technique. *Kinesiol Med Dance.* 1992;14:1–12.

56. Dolan AM, Hutchinson MJ, Fraser RD. The Pilates based exercise programme in the management of low back pain. *J Bone Joint Surg.* 2001:83B (Suppl 1): 82.

57. Hall DW. *The Effects of Pilates Based Training on Balance and Gait in an Elderly Population.* Unpublished thesis. San Diego, CA: San Diego State University, 1998.

58. Mallery LH, MacDonald EA, Hubley-Kozey CL, et al. The feasibility of performing resistance exercise with acutely ill hospitalized older adults. *BCM Geriatrics.* 2003:3:3.

59. Kish RL. *The Functional Effects of Pilates Training on College Dancers.* Doctoral dissertation: California State University–Fullerton, 1998. ISBN 0-599-11072-4.

60. Rydeard RA. *Evaluation of a Targeted Exercise Rehabilitation Approach and its Effectiveness in the Treatment of Pain, Functional Disability, and Muscle Function in a Population with Longstanding, Uunresolved Low Back Pain.* Doctoral dissertation, Queen's University at Kingston, Canada, 2001. ISBN 0-612-59398-3.

61. Bryan M, Hawson S. The benefits of Pilates exercise in orthopedic rehabilitation. *Tech Orthop.* 2003:18:126–129.

62. Anderson BD, Spector A. Introduction to Pilates-based rehabilitation. *Orthop Phys Ther Clin North Am.* 2000;9(3):395–410.

63. Porterfield JA, DeRosa C. Treatment of Lumbopelvic Disorders. *In Mechanical Low Back Pain: Perspectives in Functional Anatomy.* Philadelphia, PA: W. B. Saunders, 1991.

64. Farrell SJ, Ross AD, Sehgal KV. Eastern movement therapies. *Phys Med Rehabil Clin N Am.* 1999;10: 617–629.

65. Dorcas A, Yung P. Qigong: Harmonizing the breath, the body and the mind. *Complement Ther. Nurs. Midwifery.* 2003;9(4):198–202.

66. Sancier K. Medical applications of Qigong. *Altern Ther Health Med.* 1996;2:40–46.

67. Watkins A. (ed). Successsful aging. In *Mind Body Medicine: A Clinician's Guide to Psychoneuroimmunology*. London:Churchill-Livingstone, 1997.

68. Eisenberg D, Wright TL. *Encounters with Qi—Exploring Chinese Medicine*. New York: Marlow, 1983.

69. Cohen K. *The Way of Qigong*. New York,: Ballantine Books, 1997.

70. Takahashi M, Brown S. *Qigong for Health*. Tokyo: Japan Publication, 1986.

71. Tse M. *Qigong for Health & Vitality*. London: Piatkus, 1998.

72. Huang Z. Effect of Qigong on heart function. Paper presented at Second World Conference for Academic Exchange of Medical Qigong, Beijing, 1993.

73. Wang C, Xu D, Qian Y, Shi W. Effects of Qigong on preventing stroke and alleviating the multiple cerebro-cardiovascular risk factors: A follow-up report on 242 hypertensive cases over 30 years. Proceedings from the Second World Conference for Academic Exchange of Medical Qigong; Beijing China, 1993, pp. 123–124.

74. Mou FF, Yen ZF, Li CY, Chao GL. Study of Qigong's bi-directional regulation and its mechanism. *Chin J Mod Dev Trad Med*. 1991;10:353–356.

75. Lee MS, Lim HJ, Lee MS. Impact of qigong exercise on self-efficacy and other cognitive perceptual variables in patients with essential hypertension. *J Altern Complement Med*. 2004;10(4):675–680.

76. Tsai TJ, Lai, JS, Lee SH, et al. Breathing coordinated exercises improves quality of life in hemodialysis patients. *J Am Soc Nephrol*. 1995;6:1392–1400.

77. Wang C, Xu D, Qian Y, et al. The beneficial effects of Qigong on the ventricular function and microcirculation of deficiency in heart energy hypertensive patients. *Chin J Intern Med*.1995;1:21–23.

78. Wang CX, Xu DH, Qi YH, Kuang AK. The beneficial effect of Qigong on the hypertension incorporated with coronary heart disease. *J Gerontol*. 1988;8:83.

79. Hetzler RK, Knowlton RG, Kaminsky LA, Kamimori GH. Effect of warm-up on plasma free fatty acid responses and substrate utilization during submaximal exercise. *Res Q Exer Sport*. 1986;57:223–228.

80. Wang CX, Xu DH. Influence of qigong therapy upon serum HDL-C in hypertensive patients. *Zhong Xi Yi Jie He Za Zhi*. 1989; 9:516,543–544.

81. Wang C, Xu D, Qian Y. Medical and healthcare Qigong. *J Trad Chin Med*. 1991;11:296–301.

82. Wang C, Xu D, Qian Y, Kuang A. *The beneficial effects of Qigong on hypertension and heart disease*. Proceedings from the Third International Symposium on Qigong; Shanghai, China: Shanghai Institute of Hypertension, 1990, p.40.

83. Xie HC. *The Scientific Basis of Qigong*. Beijing China: Beijing Institute of Technology, 1988.

84. Kuang AK, Wang CX. Research on the "anti-aging" effect of breathing exercises (qigong). *Chung Hsi I Chieh Ho Tsa Chih*. 1987;7(8):455–458, 451.

85. Ruether I, Aldridge D. Qigong Yangshen as a complementary therapy in the management of asthma: A single case appraisal. *J Altern Complement Med*. 1998;4:173–183.

86. Lim YA, Boone T, Flarity JR, Thompson WR. Effects of Qigong on cardiorespiratory changes: A preliminary study. *Am J Chin Med*. 1993;21:1–6.

87. Liu GL, Cui RQ, Li GZ, et al. Changes in brainstem and cortical auditory potentials during Qigong meditation. *Am J Chin Med*. 1990;18:95–103.

88. Zhang JZ, Li JZ, He QN. Statistical brain topographic mapping analysis for EEG's recorded during Qigong state. *Int J Neurosci*. 1988;38:415–425.

89. Zhang JZ, Zhao J, He QN. EEG findings during special psychical state (Qi Gong state) by means of compressed spectral array and topographic mapping. *Comp Biol Med*. 1988;18(6):455–463.

90. Ryu H, Lee HS, Shin YS, et al. Acute effect of Qigong training on stress hormonal levels in man. *Am J Chin Med*. 1996;24:193–198.

91. Skoglund L. The Use of Qigong as a Method of Reducing Stress Amongst Computer Operators. Are Stress Levels and/or Psychosomatic Symptoms Influenced by Qigong Training? MSc paper. Sweden; Karoliinska Institute, 1998.

92. Kuang A, Wang C, Xu D, Qian Y. Research on anti-aging effect of Qigong. *J Trad Chin Med*. 1991; 11:153–158, 224–227.

93. Omura Y, Beckman SL. Application of intensified (+) qigong energy, (a) electric field, magnetic field, electric pulse, strong shiatsu massage or acupuncture on the accurate organ representation areas of the hands to improve circulation and enhance drug uptake in pathological organs. *Acupunct Electrother Res*. 1995;20:21–72.

94. Omura Y, Lin TL, Debreceni I, et al. Unique changes found on the qigong master's and patient's body during qigong treatment. *Acupunct Electrother Res*. 1989;14:61–89.

95. Zhang QC, Hsu HY. *AIDS and Chinese Medicine*. Long Beach, CA: OHAI Press, 1990.

96. Lee RH (ed). *Scientific Investigations into Chinese Qigong*. San Clemente, CA: China Healthways Institute, 1992.

97. Wu WH et al. Effects of qigong on late stage complex regional pain syndrome. *Altern Ther Health Med*. 1999;5:45–54.

98. Sancier K. Anti-aging benefits of Qigong. *J Int Soc Life Info Sci*.1996;14:12–21.

99. Guo B. Introducing Qigong: Turn back the clock and rejuvenate. *J Complementary Med*. 1994;45: 14–17.

100. Xu D, Wang C. Clinical study of delaying effect on senility of hypertensive patients by practicing yang jing yi shen gong. Proceedings of the Fifth International Symposium on Qigong. Shanghai, China: 1994, p.109.

101. Hu SH, Shen YM. An observation of senior qigong practitioners' bone density. *Qigong.* 1992;13: 99–100.

102. Ye M, Zhang RH, Wu XH, et al. Relationship among erythrocyte superoxide dismutase (RBC-SOD) activity, plasma sexual hormones (T, E2), aging, and qigong exercises. Third International Symposium on Qigong. Shanghai, China, 1990.

103. Lee MS, Hong SS, Lim HJ, et al. Retrospective survey on therapeutic efficacy of qigong in Korea. *Am J Chin Med.* 2003;31(5):809–815.

104. Jin P. Efficacy of tai chi, brisk walking, meditation, and reading in reducing mental and emotional stress. *J Psychosom. Res.* 1992;36:361–370.

105. Zhou MR, Lian MR. Observation of Qigong treatment in sixty cases of pregnancy induced hypertension. *Chin J Mod Dev Trad Med.* 1989;9:16–18.

106. Jang HS, Lee MS. Effects of qi therapy (external qigong) on premenstrual syndrome: A randomized placebo-controlled study. *J Altern Complement Med.* 2004;10(3):456–462.

107. Farrell SJ, Ross AD, Sehgal KV. Eastern movement therapies. *Phys Med Rehabil Clin N Am.* 1999:10: 617–629.

108. Wong AM, Lin YC, Chou SW, et al. Coordination exercise and postural stability in elderly people: Effect of Tai Chi Chuan. *Arch Phys Med Rehabil.* 2001;82:608–612.

109. Lan C, Lai JS, Chen SY, Wong MK. 12-month Tai Chi training in the elderly: Its effect on health fitness. *Med Sci Sports Exerc.* 1998;30:345–351.

110. Lan C, Lai JS, Chen SY, Wong MK. Tai Chi Chuan to improve muscular strength and endurance in elderly individuals: A pilot study. *Arch Phys Med Rehabil.* 2000;81:604–607.

111. Tsang WW, Hui-Chan CW. Effect of a 4- and 8-wk intensive Tai Chi training on balance control in the elderly. *Med Sci Sports Exerc.* 2004;36(4):648–657.

112. Tsang WW, Hui-Chan CW. Effects of exercise on joint sense and balance in elderly men: Tai chi versus golf. *Med Sci Sports Exerc.* 2004;36(4):658–667.

113. Jacobson BH, Chen HC, Cashel C, Guerrero L. The effect of T'ai Chi Ch'uan training on balance, kinesthetic sense, and strength. *Percept Mot Skills.* 1997;84:27–33.

114. Luskin FM, Newell KA, Griffith M, et al. A review of mind/body therapies in the treatment of musculoskeletal disorders with implications for the elderly. *Altern Ther Health Med.* 2000;6(2):46–56.

115. Shengwen X, Zhenhua F. Physiological studies of t'ai chi chuan in China. *Med Sports Sci.* 1988;28: 70–80.

116. Lan C, Lai JS, Wong MK, Yu ML. Cardiorespiratory function, flexibility, and body composition among geriatric T'ai Chi Chuan practitioners. *Arch Phys Med Rehabil.* 1996;77:612–616.

117. Tse SK, Bailey DM. T'ai chi and postural control in the well elderly. *Am J Occup Ther.* 1992;46: 295–300.

118. Lansheng G, Jianan Q Jisheng Z, et al. Changes in heart rate and electrocardiogram during t'aijiquan exercise. *Chin Med J.* 1981;94:589–592.

119. Tsai JC, Wang, WH, Chan P, et al. The beneficial effects of Tai Chi Chuan on blood pressure, lipid profile, and anxiety status in a randomized controlled trial. *J Altern Complement Med.* 2003:9: 747–754.

120. Lan C, Chen SY, Lai JS, Wong MK. The effect of T'ai Chi on cardiovascular function in patients with coronary artery bypass surgery. *Med Sci Sports Exer.* 1999; 31:634–638.

121. Chao YF, Chen SY, Lan C, Lai JS. The cardiorespiratory response and energy expenditure of Tai Chi Qui-Gong. *Am J Chin Med.* 2002:30:451–461.

122. Zhuo OI, Shephard RL, Plyley MI, Davis GM. Cardiorespiratory and metabolic responses during T'ai Chi ch'uan exercise. *Can J Appl Sport Sci.* 1984;9:7–10.

123. Vaananen J, Xusheng S, Wang S, et al. Tai Chi Quan acutely increases heart rate variability. *Clin Physio Funct Imaging.* 2002:22:2–3.

124. Channer KS, Barrow D, Barrow R, et al. Changes in haemodynamic parameters following T'ai Chi Ch'uan and aerobic exercise in patients recovering from acute myocardial infarction. *Postgrad Med J.* 1996;72:349–351.

125. Young DR, Appel LJ, Jee S, Miller ER. The effects of aerobic exercise on T'ai chi on blood pressure in older people: Results of a randomized trial. *J Am Geriatr Soc.* 1999;47(3):277–284.

126. Brown DD, Mucci WG, Hetzler RK, et al. Cardiovascular and ventilatory responses during formalized T'ai Chi Ch'uan exercise. *Res Q Exerc Sport.* 1985;60:246–250.

127. Schneider D, Leung R. Metabolic and cardiorespiratory responses to the performance of wing chun and t'ai chi ch'uan exercise. *Int J Sports Med.* 1991; 12:319–323.

128. Lai JS, Wong MK, Lan C, et al. Cardiorespiratory responses of t'ai chi chaun practitioners and sedentary subjects during cycle ergometer. *J Formos Med Assoc.* 1993;92:894–899.

129. Lai JS, Lan C, Wong MK, Teng SH. Two-year trends in cardiorespiratory function among older t'ai chi chuan practitioners and sedentary subjects. *J Am Geriatric Soc.* 1995;43:1222–1227.

130. Song R, Lee EO, Lam P, Bae SC. Effects of Tai Chi exercise on pain, balance, muscle strength, and perceived difficulties in physical functioning of older

women with osteoarthritis: A randomized clinical trail. *J Rheumatol.* 2003;30:2039–2044.

131. Van Deusen J, Harlowe D. Efficacy of the ROM dance program for adults with rheumatoid arthritis. *Am J Occup Ther.* 1987;40:90–95.

132. Jerosch J, Wustner P. Effect of a sensorimotor training program on patients with subacromial bursitis. *Unfallchirurg.* 2002:105:36–43.

133. Hong Y, Li X, Robinson D. Balance control, flexibility, and cardiorespiratory fitness among older t'ai chi practitioners. *Br J Sports Med.* 2000;34:29–34.

134. Christou EA, Yang Y, Rosengren KS. Taiji training improves knee extensor strength and force control in older adults. *J Gerontol A Biol Sci Med Sci.* 2003;58:763–766.

135. Li F, Harmer P, McAuley E, et al. An evaluation of the effects of Tai Chi exercise on physical function among older persons: A randomized controlled trial. *Ann Beh Med.* 2001;23:139–146.

136. Yan JH. Tai Chi practice reduced movement force variability for seniors. *J Gerontol A Biol Sci Med Sci.* 1999;54:M629–M634.

137. Qin L, Au S, Choy W, et al. Regular Tai Chi Chuan exercise may retard bone loss in postmenopausal women: A case controlled study. *Arch Phys Med Rehabil.* 2002;83:1355–1359.

138. Bhatti TI, Gillin JC, Atkinson JH, et al. T'ai Chi Chih as a treatment for chronic low back pain. *Altern Ther Health Med.* 1998;4:90.

139. Lumsden DB, Baccala A, Martire J. T'ai Chi for osteoarthritic: An introduction for primary care physicians. *Geriatrics,* 1998;53:84,87–88.

140. Koh TC. T'ai Chi and ankylosing spondylitis: A personal experience. *Am J Chin Med.* 1982;10: 59–61.

141. Shapira MY, Chelouche M, Yanai R, et al. Tai Chi Chuan Practice as a tool for rehabilitation of severe head trauma: Three case reports. *Arch Phys Med Rehabil.* 2001;82:1283–1285.

142. Wolf SL, Barnhart HX, Kutner NG, et al. Reducing frailty and falls in older persons: An investigation of T'ai Chi and computerized balance training. *J Am Geriatr Soc.* 1996;44:489–497.

143. Wolf SL, Sattin RW, O'Grady M, et al. A study design to investigate the effect of intense Tai Chi in reducing falls among older adults transitioning to frailty. *Control Clin Trials.* 2001;22:689–704.

144. Wolf SL, Barnhart HX, Ellison GL, Coogler CE. The effect of T'ai Chi chuan and computerized balance training on postural stability in older subjects. Atlanta FICSIT Group. *Phys Ther.* 1997;77: 371–381, (discussion) 382–384.

145. Wu G, Zhao F, Zhou X, Wei L. Improvement in isokinetic knee extensor strength and reduction of postural sway in the elderly from long-term Tai Chi exercise. *Arch Phys Med Rehabil.* 2002;83: 1364–1369.

146. Mak MK, Ng PL. Mediolateral sway in single leg stance is the best discriminator of balance performance for Tai Chi practitioners. *Arch Phys Med Rehabil.* 2003:84:683–686.

147. Wang JS, Lan C, Wong MK. Tai Chi Chuan training to enhance microcirculatory function in healthy elderly men. *Arch Phys Med Rehabil.* 2001;82: 1176–1180.

148. Wang JS, Lan C, Chen SY, Wong MK. Tai Chi Chuan training is associated with enhanced endothelium-dependent dilation in skin vasculature of healthy older men. *J Am Geriatr Soc.* 2002;50: 1024–1030.

149. Brown DR, Wang Y, Ward A, et al. Chronic effects of exercise and exercise plus cognitive strategies. *Med Sci Sports Exerc.* 1995;27:765–775.

150. Kutner NG, Barnhart H, Wolf SL, et al. Self-reported benefits of t'ai chi practice by older adults. *J Gerontol B Psychol Sci Soc Sci.* 1997;52:242–246.

151. Anonymous. Yoga gets into a popular position: Once a spiritual journey for the few, yoga is now just a good workout for the many. *Harvard Health Lett.* 2003;29(2):4–5.

152. Budilovsky J, Adamson E. *The Complete Idiot's Guide to Yoga,* 2nd ed. Indianapolis, IN: Alpha Books, 2001.

153. Kent H. *Yoga Made Easy.* Singapore: MetroBooks, 2002.

154. Kogler A. *Yoga for Athletes: Secrets of an Olympic Coach.* St. Paul, MN: Llewellyn Publications, 1999.

155. Nespor K. Pain management and yoga. *Int J Psychosom.* 1991;38:1–4:76–81.

156. Stancak A Jr., Kuna M, Novak P, et al. Observations on respiratory and cardiovascular rhythmicities during yogic high-frequency respiration. *Physiol Res.* 1991;40:345–354.

157. Brownstein AH, Dembert ML. Treatment of essential hypertension with yoga relaxation therapy in a USAF aviator: A case report. *Aviation Space Envir Med.* 1989;60:684–687.

158. Schell FJ, Allolio B, Schonecke OW. Physiological and psychological effects of Hatha-Yoga exercise in healthy women. *Int J Psychosom.* 1994;41:46–52.

159. Sundar S, Agrawal SK, Singh VP, et al. Role of yoga in management of essential hypertension. *Acta Cardiol.* 1984;39:203–208.

160. Manchanda SC, Narang R, Reddy KS, et al. Retardation of coronary atherosclerosis with yoga lifestyle intervention. *J Assoc Phys India.* 2000;48: 687–694.

161. Bharshankar JR, Bharshankar RN, Deshpande VN, et al. Effect of yoga on cardiovascular system in subjects above 40 years. *Ind J Physiol Pharmacol.* 2003;47(2):202–206.

162. Garfinkel MS, Schumacher HR, Husain A, et al. Evaluation of a yoga based regimen for the treatment of osteoarthritis of the hands. *J Rheumatol.* 1994; 21:2341–2343.

163. Garfinkel MS, Singhal A, Katz WA, et al. Yoga-based intervention for carpal tunnel syndrome: A randomized trial. *JAMA*. 1998;280:1601–1603.

164. Galantino ML, Bzdewka TM, Eissler-Russo JL, et al. The impact of modified Hatha yoga on chronic low back pain: A pilot study. *Altern Ther Health Med*. 2004;10(2):56–59.

165. Singh V, Wisniewski A, Britton J, Tattersfield A. Effect of yoga breathing exercises *(pranayama)* on airway reactivity in subjects with asthma. *Lancet*. 1990;335(9702):1381–1383.

166. Vedanthan PK, Kesavalu LN, Murthy KC, et al. Clinical study of yoga techniques in university students with asthma: A controlled study. *Allergy Asthma Proc*. 1998;19:3–9.

167. Khanam AA, Sachdeva U, Guleria R, Deepak KK. Study of pulmonary and autonomic functions of asthma patients after yoga training. *Ind J Phys & Pharm*. 1996; 40:318–324.

168. Behera D. Yoga therapy in chronic bronchitis. *J Assoc Phys India*. 1998; 46:207–208.

169. Nagarathna R, Nagendra HR. Yoga for bronchial asthma: A controlled study. *Br Med J*. 1985;291:1077–1079.

170. Oken BS, Kishiyama S, Zajdel D, et al. Randomized controlled trial of yoga and exercise in multiple sclerosis. *Neurology*. 2004;62(11):2058–2064.

171. Bastille JV, Gill-Body KM. A yoga-based exercise program for people with chronic poststroke hemiparesis. *Phys Ther*. 2004;84(1):33–48.

172. Miller C. Making a difference: Yoga in pregnancy. *Birth Gazette*. 1996;13:34–35.

173. Gaffney L, Smith CA. Use of complementary therapies in pregnancy: The perceptions of obstetricians and midwives in South Australia. *Australian NZ J Obstetr Gynaecol*. 2004;44(1):24–29.

174. Jain SC, Uppal A, Bhatnagar SO, Talukdar B. A study of response pattern of non–insulin-dependent diabetics to yoga therapy. *Diabetes Res Clin Pract*. 1993;19:69–74.

175. Shannahoff-Khalsa DS, Beckett LR. Clinical case report: Efficacy of yogic techniques in the treatment of obsessive compulsive disorders. *Int J Neurosci*. 1996; 85:1–17.

176. Telles S, Naveen KV. Yoga for rehabilitation: An overview. *Indian J Med Sci*. 1997;51:123–127.

177. Uma K, Nagendra HR, Nagarathna R, et al. The integrated approach of yoga: A therapeutic tool for mentally retarded children—A one year controlled study. *J Ment Defic Res*. 1989; 33:415–421.

178. Naveen KV, Nagarantha R, Nagendra HR, Telles S. Yoga breathing through a particular nostril increased spatial memory effects without lateralized effects. *Psychol Rep*. 1997;81:555–561.

179. Shaffer H, LaSalvia T, Stein J. Comparing Hatha Yoga with dynamic group psychotherapy for enhancing methadone maintenance treatment. *Altern Ther Health Med*. 1997;3:57–66.

180. Herzog H, Lele VR, Kuwert T, et al. Changed pattern of regional glucose metabolism during meditative relaxation. *Neuropsychobiol*. 1990–91;23(4):182–187.

181. Goyeche J. Yoga as therapy in psychosomatic medicine. *Psychother Psychosom*. 1979;31:373–381.

182. Telles S, Nagarathna R, Vani PR, Nagendra HR. A combination of focusing and defocusing through yoga reduces optical illusion more than focusing alone. *Indian J Physiol Pharmacol*. 1997;41(2):179–182.

11

Therapeutic Exercise Program Design Considerations: "Putting It All Together"

THOMAS W. MILLER

JOHN NYLAND

WENDY WORMAL

Objectives
The reader will be able to:

- Describe future models of health information processing, care pathways, and practice guidelines.
- Describe the paradigm shift in therapeutic exercise program development.
- Develop intervention strategies to improve client compliance with therapeutic exercise programs and facilitate the development of positive health behaviors.
- Define the concept of quality of life and discuss its relevance to therapeutic exercise program intervention.

- Describe the similarities and differences between health locus of control and self-efficacy.
- Explain the relationship between aging, osteoarthritis, surgical interventions, and therapeutic exercise program modifications.
- Create individualized, functionally relevant treatment goals.
- Relate the usefulness of functional performance tests and self-reported client outcome data to return to activity decision making.

Outline

INTRODUCTION TO HEALTH INFORMATION PROCESSING

The development of a therapeutic exercise program requires consideration of client needs and desires, psychophysiological interactions, exercise and exercise volume selections, and the potential risks and benefits of the selected program. In addition to this, considerable attention must be given to the capacity of the client to understand and process the educational component of the therapeutic exercise program.

How a client processes health information is of great concern to the rehabilitation clinician. Traditional health education materials contain information that is the same for every client, a kind of "one size fits all" approach. With the advent of new computer technologies, a different approach to constructing health education materials has emerged: Materials are not mass produced, but generated one at a time by computers and tailored to the individual client. Psychosocial and behavioral data are gathered and entered into a computer program that determines which health messages from among a library of possibilities are most appropriate for each client.

The *Elaboration Likelihood Model* (ELM)[1] provides a theoretical rationale for tailored communication. According to this model, clients are more likely to actively and thoughtfully process information by engaging in what the authors refer to as central-route processing if they perceive it to be personally relevant. The ELM is based on the premise that under many conditions, clients are active information processors—considering messages carefully, relating them to other information they have encountered, and comparing them with their own past experiences. Studies have shown that messages processed in this way (i.e., elaborated upon) tend to be retained for a longer time and are more likely to lead to permanent behavioral changes than messages that are not elaborated upon.[2]

Evidence based decision making in the clinical design of a therapeutic exercise program suggests that the tailored educational materials elicit: 1) greater attention, 2) greater comprehension, 3) greater likelihood of discussing the content with other people, 4) greater intention to change the behaviors addressed by the content, and 5) greater likelihood of actual behavior change.[3] Sev-eral research studies suggest that the design and composition of a rehabilitation clinician's message is more likely to be read and remembered,[4] saved,[5] discussed with other people,[6] and perceived by readers as interesting,[7] personally relevant, and having been written especially for them[6] if it is tailored to the individual needs of the client.

Bull et al.[8] assessed the relative effects of tailoring and personalization in adult primary care clients who were randomly assigned to one of three groups that received physical activity materials or to a usual care control group. Findings showed that the tailored and personalized materials were perceived as being more personally relevant than the general materials, whether personalized or not, and those clients that received the personalized tailored materials increased their physical activities of daily living (e.g., work in the home, doing yard work) more than the other experimental groups or the control group. In most cases, the general, personalized materials were rated least favorably, suggesting it is unlikely that personalization alone accounted for the tailoring effects observed in previous studies.

Kreuter et al.[9] studied 198 overweight men and women who were randomly assigned to receive either tailored or non-tailored printed educational materials on weight loss. Participants completed a brief survey about their weight-related goals, beliefs, and behaviors, and then received one of three types of weight loss materials. The first was tailored specifically to their responses on the survey. The second was a generically prepared brochure on weight loss, produced by the American Heart Association. The third covered the same content as the second, but was formatted to look exactly like the tailored materials. Inclusion of this latter condition provided a mechanism for assessing whether it was the content or some other attribute of the tailored messages that led to the outcomes realized in the study. Results suggested that the ELM model is a central-route cognitive process (very efficient), displaying superior results when tailored rather than non-tailored materials were used for educational purposes.[9] Re-analysis of the data from the weight loss study confirmed this predication.[10] All participants who received non-tailored information were classified into one of three categories based on how well the content fit with their individual needs. On a variety of cognitive, affective, and behavioral measures (e.g., attention given to the materials, positive cognitive responses, choosing low-fat foods), "well fitting" non-tailored materials had outcomes as good as or even better than the outcomes for tailored materials. At the same time, moderate and poor fitting non-tailored materials were usually inferior to the other approaches overall.

Care pathways, algorithms, and practice guidelines have been employed by the health care industry to provide a standard flowchart of the evidence-based diagnostic and treatment methods to be provided for a spectrum of diseases and disorders.[11] There is considerable evidence in the health care literature[12–14] that the use of care path-

---

Key Point:

Educational materials that are tailored for the client elicit greater attention, greater comprehension, greater likelihood of discussing the content with others, greater intention to change the behaviors addressed by the content, and greater likelihood of behavioral change.

ways based on clinical research will help in standardizing client care and will provide the necessary ingredients for effective diagnostic and counseling interventions. The goal is to make the client management guideline the accepted professional behavior and a reward in itself.[15] To the extent that this is successful, five components occur: 1) The guideline is widely used and becomes habitual, 2) multidisciplinary healthcare professionals can use it to anticipate care events, 3) rehabilitation clinicians can use it as a shorthand or outline to guide their decisions and their communications to others, 4) the logistics for delivering the guideline components are convenient and reliable, and 5) the guideline defines the measure of performance and incorporates information collected that can be used for its evaluation and improvement. The individualized plans that rehabilitation clinicians develop also contribute information for guideline revision.

> ## Key Point:
> The goals of client management guidelines are for them to become widely used and habitual, provide multidisciplinary healthcare professionals a way of anticipating care events, serve as a decision making guide and communication medium for rehabilitation clinicians, help increase the convenience and reliability of healthcare delivery, and serve as a method of measuring performance.

Rehabilitation clinicians such as physical therapists recognize the importance of standards of care and standardized models of evaluation and intervention. Examined here is a care pathway guideline developed to ensure consistency in the evaluation and treatment offered where the spectrum of symptoms are identified in the course of screening and counseling clients.

CARE PATHWAYS ALGORITHM DEVELOPMENT

Algorithms are developed and used to provide case management. In today's world, accountability is a top priority for all professionals. Case management through algorithms presents a systematic perspective. Algorithms try to answer the question, "What is the best way to systematically handle this problematic condition?" Algorithms have a problem solving orientation coupled with specific functional actions or critical pathways to be followed. If desired results are produced, the problem was managed effectively. If the desired results are not produced, adjustments can be made to achieve the desired results.

The point to be made is that rehabilitation clinicians must be creative problem solvers who can translate relevant research into functional interventions. Intervention approaches must be managed to ensure relevant results. Thus, the rehabilitation clinician must have a process skill that is dynamic yet organized around solid principles and practices. This is not to imply that this is an easy process. The critical pathways that algorithms provide take time and energy to develop, but they also provide a systematic methodology that can prove effective in dealing with critical problematic areas for the rehabilitation clinician as they develop a therapeutic exercise program.

Steps in Building an Algorithm

1. Define the problem. Specify the client's condition and the individualized or tailored needs of the client.

2. Review the flow process of the condition, all possible causes of the condition, and alternative strategies for diagnosis, client education, management and intervention, and follow-up or re-evaluation.

3. Present diagnostic, therapeutic, or management steps in the following order:
   a. Rule out any emergency or urgent conditions.
   b. Rule out the most common conditions in order of frequency.
   c. Rule out the less frequent causes of the condition.
   d. Review flow chart accuracy regarding conditions that have been ruled out (e.g., referred pain syndrome as a cause of arthritic symptoms.)
   e. Relegate unlikely causes of the condition to a footnote.

4. Alternately sequence decision boxes and intervention boxes.

5. Present the interventions in detail, including:
   a. Formulate steps to monitor or confirm diagnosis or condition.
   b. Specify interventions.
   c. For clinical cases, specify evidence based interventions.
   d. Define end points of intervention (e.g., level of functioning; discharge; referral to a specialist).

6. Purpose of annotations and footnotes:
   a. Elaborate on the algorithm and/or define terms used in the algorithm (e.g., the high risk client).
   b. Explain what should be excluded in the algorithm and what is relevant but does not add to the clinical management process.
   c. Clarify a clinical rationale, using evidence based citations (**Table 11.1**).
   d. Detail information about the problem intervention and/or decisions made in the algorithm.

TABLE 11.1 Levels of evidence for primary research question

	Types of Studies			
	Therapeutic studies: Investigating the results of treatment	**Prognostic studies: Investigating the outcome of disease**	**Diagnostic studies: Investigating a diagnostic test**	**Economic and decision analyses: Developing an economic or decision model**
Level I	1. Randomized controlled trial a. Significant difference b. No significant difference but narrow confidence intervals 2. Systematic review[2] of Level I randomized controlled trials (studies were homogeneous)	1. Prospective study[1] 2. Systematic review[2] of Level I studies	1. Testing of previously developed diagnostic criteria in a series of consecutive clients (with universally applied reference gold standard) 2. Systematic review[2] of Level I studies	1. Clinically sensible costs and alternatives; values obtained from many studies; multiway sensitivity analyses 2. Systematic review[2] of Level I studies.
Level II	1. Prospective cohort study[3] 2. Poor-quality randomized controlled trial (e.g., <80% follow-up) 3. Systematic review[2] a. Level II studies b. Nonhomogeneous Level I studies	1. Retrospective study[4] 2. Study of untreated controls from a previous randomized controlled trial 3. Systematic review[2] of Level II studies	1. Development of diagnostic criteria on basis of consecutive clients (with universally applied reference gold standard) 2. Systematic review[2] of Level II studies	1. Clinically sensible costs and alternatives; values obtained from limited studies; multiway sensitivity analyses 2. Systematic review[2] of Level II studies
Level III	1. Case-control study[5] 2. Retrospective cohort study[4] 3. Systematic review[2] of Level III studies		1. Study of nonconsecutive patients (no consistently applied reference gold standard) 2. Systematic review[2] of Level III studies	1. Limited alternatives and costs; poor estimates 2. Systematic review[2] of Level III studies
Level IV	Case series (no, or historical, control group)	Case series	1. Case-control study 2. Poor reference standard	No sensitivity analyses
Level V	Expert opinion	Expert opinion	Expert opinion	Expert opinion

1. *All clients were enrolled at the same point in their disease course (inception cohort) with greater than or equal to 80 percent follow-up of enrolled clients.*

2. *A study of results from two or more previous studies.*

3. *Clients were compared with a control group of clients treated at the same time and institution.*

4. *The study was initiated after treatment was performed.*

5. *Clients with a particular outcome ("cases" with, for example, a failed total hip arthroplasty) were compared with those who did not have the outcome ("controls" with, for example, a total hip arthroplasty that did not fail).*

This chart was adapted from material published by the Centre for Evidence-Based Medicine, Oxford, UK. For more information, please see www.cebm.net.
From http://www.ejbjs.org/misc/public/instrux.shtml#levels.

Basic Clinical Algorithm Construction

Clinical algorithms are composed of three differently shaped boxes:

1. The oval describes a clinical problem or entity.

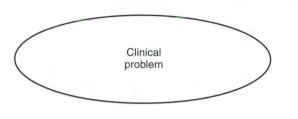

2. The rectangle describes an action to be taken or intervention to be provided.

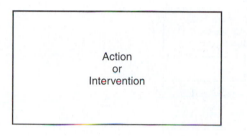

3. The hexagon describes what clinical question has emerged leading to an evidence based decision.

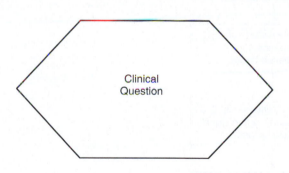

There are always two possibilities that follow the decision box. Each decision box must have two branches attached to it for a Yes and a No decision. Based on this decision, options for each must be included in the decision making process and should be summarized in the algorithm.

CARE PATHWAY GUIDELINES FOR REHABILITATION CLINICIANS

Care pathway guidelines delineate specific information and timelines in which diagnosis, treatment, and follow-up should occur. They further address the decision mak-ing process, the who, what, and when of various actions relevant to the client and the client's condition, the clinical services offered, and the potential interactions among interdisciplinary health care professionals and providers for the specific needs of the individual client who is referred. Clinical information systems capable of supporting the functional requirements of a comprehensive critical pathway also provide direction to the development and implementation of care pathways appropriate for change.[16] The care pathways for clients who need a therapeutic exercise program involve several stages. Sometimes the client will present with symptoms. The pathway then moves through the history and systems review, identification of symptoms, and diagnostic criteria for acute and/or chronic conditions. In addition to symptoms, it also considers specific treatments, and supportive care, and how the rehabilitation clinician can reassess and monitor the clinical condition over time. A standardized flowchart that assists the rehabilitation clinician in completing a thorough diagnostic and intervention model is shown in **Figure 11.1.**

The care pathway delineates the specific timelines in which assessment and treatment or interventions must occur. Note with specificity the importance of the diagnostic and treatment responsibilities for the condition. Specific emphasis here is on evidence based decision making, both diagnostically and therapeutically. In addition, specific information is related to clinical management for clients who present with specific problems unique to their case. These become the critical ingredients to be considered in a care pathway that would provide standardized care and treatment for the client who is in need of a therapeutic exercise program. **Table 11.2** provides a sample care pathway that addresses what activity should be completed at various stages in the provision of treatment interventions.

PARADIGM SHIFTS IN THERAPEUTIC EXERCISE PROGRAMS

From traditional models, rehabilitation clinicians, physicians, and others have become part of a network of health-care professionals who contract with multi-skilled specialists to provide rehabilitation services. Future shifts in these networks will be driven by cost containment, capitation, and contracts for services that focus on efficiency and use of financial incentives to replace what has come to be known as fees for services by clinicians.

As we approach the challenges of the next decade, rehabilitation clinicians should consider issues raised by Covey et al.,[17] who encourage us to understand our unique endowments. The endowments Covey et al.[17] discuss for clinicians are *self-awareness*, which is our capacity to stand apart from our wins and losses and examine our thinking, our understanding of the whole client and our motives and commitment to healthcare. The second human

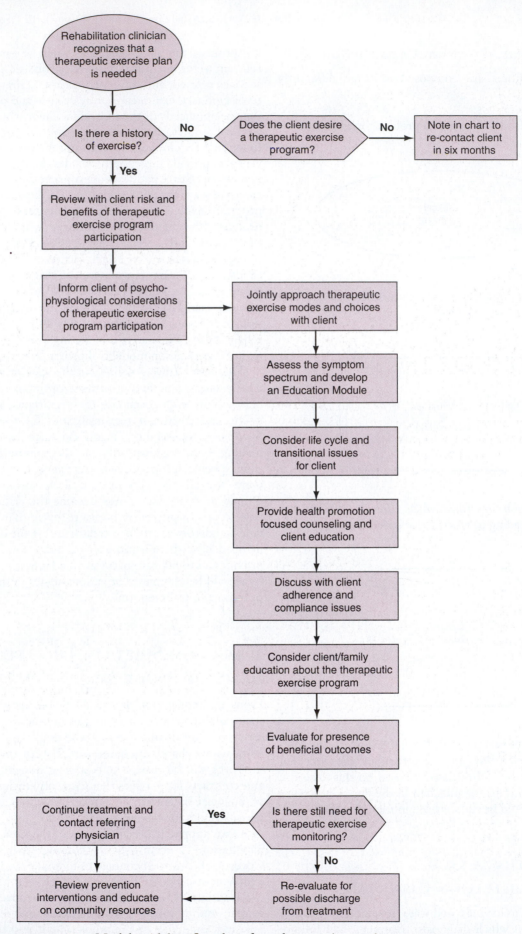

Figure 11.1 Model guideline flowchart for a therapeutic exercise program.

TABLE 11.2   Integrated sample care pathway for therapeutic exercise program

Activity	Visit 1	Visit 2	Visits 3–7	Visit 8
Assessment	Screening for therapeutic exercise program participation	Review results of screening	PRN assessment of client	Re-assess therapeutic exercise program intervention (particularly educational goals)
Intervention	Therapeutic exercise program is reviewed with the client	Education module focused on components of the client's therapeutic exercise program	Provide gradients of intervention (modifications, etc.) for the client's therapeutic exercise program	Consideration for further therapeutic exercise programs needs (modifications, maintenance)
Consults/ assessments considered	Internist Psychologist Orthopedic surgeon	Consider referral as needed	Integrate consultation recommendation into the therapeutic exercise program	Review the need for further consultation
Client/family education	Consider involving family or significant others in the client's therapeutic exercise program	Meet with significant others to review the client's therapeutic exercise program	Review with client and family the importance of a supportive environment for the client's therapeutic	Encourage continued client and family support for maintaining therapeutic exercise program participation

endowment is well recognized in the clinician's personal development and addresses the Jungian concept known as *conscience*. Covey et al.[17] argue that conscience connects us with the wisdom of the ages and the understanding of human potential. It adds an ethical component to what we bring to the clinical encounter. The third endowment is that of *independent wealth*, which is seen as our ability as clinicians to recognize all that we are capable of being, and to act in the best interest of our clients. The fourth endowment is *imagination*, which is the power to envision creative innovation as clinicians and the direction for which we can provide our clients with creative and tailor made therapeutic exercise programs and other interventions.

Rehabilitation clinicians must engage fellow professionals and consumers through effective interpersonal skill development; new models of diagnostic and therapeutic management; creation of quality tools for a spectrum of interventions including therapeutic exercise management; and clinical research that measures the effectiveness of the interventions we provide (such as an evaluation of a client's understanding after the initial intervention (**Figure 11.2**). All of these shifts are within the repertoire of the rehabilitation clinician. *Diagnosis* is the term that identifies the primary dysfunction toward which the rehabilitation clinician directs the treatment.[18] Medical diagnosis is not solely sufficient to direct the practice, education or research of the rehabilitation clinician, or to determine the efficacy of the intervention. Information regarding the client's medical diagnosis, condition, pathology, injury, impairment, func-

tional limitations, and disability level is synthesized during the history taking process. Impairment information is determined via specific clinical tests and measurements such as manual muscle testing, goniometry, isokinetic dynamometry, etc. However, information regarding the client's functional limitation are determined via specific functional tests such as the Timed Up and Go, the Single Leg Hop, the Berg Balance Scale, and the Six-Minute Walk Test.[19] We must begin to recognize that client expectations and clinical outcomes must be the result of mutually discussed and agreed upon dimensions of interdisciplinary clinical services (**Figure 11.3**).

One might ask, What are the significant changes that will emerge over the next decade in the field of rehabilitation?

- Rehabilitation clinicians will require a cutting edge understanding of the *genetic interface* (including the information provided by genetic analysis as it pertains to the diagnostic and prognostic aspects of client health) with traditional treatment plans.
- Diagnostic evaluation, as we have known it, will be replaced by a more complex analysis of a system of networks that will analyze how genetic factors that influence motivation and behavior in clients are affected by intellectual and personality markers that result in patterns of compliance.
- Rehabilitation clinicians will, by necessity, need to be multi-skilled specialists providing a spectrum of clinical services to clients.

**Client Health Education
EVALUATION
Anterior Cruciate Ligament Injury**

Directions: Indicate in the column on the left what your knowledge of the injury is currently based upon the following criteria:

1 = Not familiar
2 = Somewhat familiar
3 = Familiar
4 = Very familiar

Evaluation prior to consultation	Objectives	Evaluation after consultation
_____	1. Where is the anterior cruciate ligament (ACL) located?	_____
_____	2. Do you know what caused the ACL to tear?	_____
_____	3. Is surgery required or are there other options?	_____
_____	4. What will happen if this condition goes on untreated?	_____
_____	5. Are there any changes in living conditions or behavior that will result from this condition?	_____
_____	6. How long is the period of rehabilitation for this injury?	_____
_____	7. Is there a high likelihood that you will return at top level to your sport next year?	_____
_____	8. Will the condition of your knee worsen over time?	_____
_____	9. What is your plan for treatment and rehabililitation?	_____
_____	10. Do you know what you need to do in order to manage this injury and maintain the health of your knee after the period of rehabilitation?	_____
_____		_____
Total points		Total points

Figure 11.2   Client educational evaluation.

■ Breakthroughs in technology, including new diagnostic models and intervention techniques, will impact treatment planning.

■ Therapeutic exercise "super centers" will feature multi-disciplinary medical and rehabilitative health care, specialists (including therapists, dieticians, exercise physiologists and technicians, athletic trainers, physicians, rehabilitation nursing specialists) all under one roof—a clinical health care "mall."

■ New alliances in rehabilitation medicine, education, psychology, and science will emerge with rehabilitation clinicians as significant partners in treating client health care needs.

■ Databases will hold key information in addressing patterns of therapeutic exercise performance and compliance that can be expected of clients influenced by physical, psychological, genetic, and biochemical characteristics.

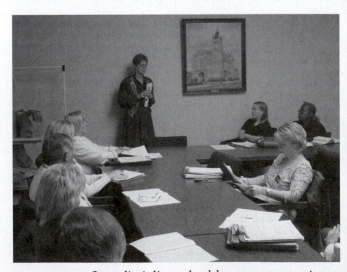

Figure 11.3   Interdisciplinary healthcare team meeting.

- Education and information, awareness and understanding become critical ingredients in addressing quality of life issues for clients, with rehabilitation clinicians providing a key role in this process.

Some of the anticipated shifts that rehabilitation clinicians might encounter are summarized in **Table 11.3**.

Key Point:

Future directions in healthcare will include greater emphasis on psychophysiological, multidisciplinary intervention (with greater consideration of genetic markers) and client education from an evidence based decision making perspective.

Success of health promotion and prevention programs, as well as intervention strategies, will depend on rehabilitation clinicians making fundamental use of clinical models of assessment and intervention in cases of clients who are in need of a therapeutic exercise program.

IMPROVING CLIENT COMPLIANCE AND ACHIEVING POSITIVE BEHAVIORAL CHANGE

According to Guccione,[20] the term *compliance* implies that the client must do as the rehabilitation clinician instructs in order for the intervention to be successful. The term *adherence* is sometimes preferred because it implies freedom of choice and action on the part of the client. Throughout this section, we will use the terminology employed by the cited work. Cardiovascular system training adaptations are known to occur more slowly in older people.[21] However, Sheldahl et al.[22] reported that healthy men between 60 and 71 years of age show a time course and magnitude of physiologic changes within six months of endurance training similar to that achieved by healthy men between 35 and 50 years of age. They also reported that a higher percentage of older (71 percent) than middle-aged (45 percent) clients continued to participate in a high intensity therapeutic exercise program for an additional six months following study completion. One reason for this difference might be more available time for participation

TABLE 11.3   Anticipated shifts in therapeutic exercise program delivery

	Present	Future
Organizational paradigm	Traditional models of methods with some specialization in therapeutic exercise	Networks and alliances of specialists contracting through integrated systems of therapeutic exercise programs at all levels
Communication and information systems	Paper records, individual developed profiles, record systems, local networks accessibility, limited access	Electronic profiling and clustering clients by learning styles, genetic predisposition, on-line support systems, e-mail, electronic files, Web pages by conference with rehabilitation, medical, and health-related information systems
Assessment systems	Limited measures and assessment procedures for clients, paper and pencil screening; basic physiological assessment	Integrated networks of assessment that address genetic, physiological biochemical markers; learning and cognitive styles through components-based integrated assessment systems
Interventions	Individualized assessment and interventions addressing stepwise interventions and motivation styles of clients; traditional text role approaches to therapeutic exercise program intervention	Integrated interventions based on genetic and biochemical markers using virtual reality models in diagnosis and training, and treatment with applications in therapeutic exercise programs
Prevention and wellness focus	Few incentives for prevention-based initiatives for the client	Wellness; prevention interventions, incentives for clients, greater use of behavioral medicine and genetic counseling in health promotion

among the older group, due to retirement. However, there appears to be a higher injury potential for older clients who participate in high intensity training programs.[22] Kohrt et al.[23] reported an approximately 50 percent incidence of orthopedic injuries for older clients who participated in a high-intensity therapeutic exercise program.

The *transtheoretical model* has been applied to subject initiation and compliance with cardiovascular endurance exercise programs.[24–28] The model suggests that a client changes a behavior (stops smoking, begins exercise) by progressing through five stages: 1) *precontemplation* (no real intention to change behavior); 2) *contemplation* (true intention to change behavior, but no action yet taken); 3) *preparation* (intermittent starting and stopping to display true behavioral changes); 4) *action* (consistent behavioral change for six months or less); and 5) *maintenance* (sustained behavior change for longer than six months).

> ## Key Point:
> The five stages of the transtheoretical model are precontemplation, contemplation, preparation, action, and maintenance.

Initial health behavior changes are typically not all or none, but tend to be characterized by frequent stops and starts. Concurrently, a client can become stuck in any stage, can regress to an earlier stage, or can progress to a later stage. Many rehabilitation clinicians are probably effective at designing a therapeutic exercise program for clients who are in the action stage. However, the majority of our non-compliant clients are in the pre-contemplative or contemplative stages. This is a problem, because therapeutic exercise programs designed for clients in the action stage have not been shown to be successful for clients who are in the pre-contemplative or contemplative stages.[27]

Marcus et al.[25] suggests that successful therapeutic exercise program initiation and compliance would be more effective if the intervention differed according to the client's behavioral stage. The reason for this is that there is a strong relationship between behavioral stage and how a client perceives the relative importance of benefit and barriers or the pros and cons of engaging in the changed behavior. Possible barriers include secondary gains with the current behavior (workman's compensation benefits, litigation, etc.), the time needed to participate in the therapeutic exercise program, fear, pain expectations, embarrassment, feeling fatigued, and belief that the program will not help. Benefits may include pain free function, increased confidence and independence with activities of daily living, increased body awareness, and enhanced quality of life. To progress through all five stages, the client's perception of the relative importance of benefits and barriers needs to change. In the pre-

contemplative and contemplative stages, clients tend to place greater importance on barriers than benefits. In the preparatory stage, the benefits and barriers are of almost equal importance, and in the action and maintenance stages, the benefits increasingly outweigh the barriers leading to a more likely positive health behavior change.[27] With behavioral changes such as smoking cessation, a multifaceted approach that includes educational, behavioral, and motivational strategies seems to have the best chance for success. These same concepts may help the rehabilitation clinician's client progress through these behavioral stages, particularly when the program is largely home program based. Future research needs to better delineate the diverse and highly individualized benefits and barriers perceived by our clients as they consider participating in a therapeutic exercise program. Conceivably, some form of pre-treatment survey may provide sufficient feedback to the rehabilitation clinician regarding the individual client's perception of benefits and barriers, setting the stage for them to better verify these factors during the history taking process (**Figure 11.4**) and helping to direct discussions as to ways to increase their perception of program benefits and decrease their perception of associated barriers.

In today's health care environment, self-treatment in the form of home therapeutic exercise program intervention is playing an ever-increasing role. A reliance on this form of treatment when the client is in the pre-contemplative and contemplative stages could be detrimental if steps have not been taken to monitor program effectiveness, and positive changes in client's perceptions and behaviors.

Sluijs et al.[29] suggested that the true efficacy of therapeutic exercise programs can only be established when clients comply with the program. Jette,[30] however, reported that up to 45 percent to 60 percent of clients with arthritis do not follow prescribed therapeutic exercise regimens. Dutch physical therapists have estimated that approximately 64 percent of their clients comply with short

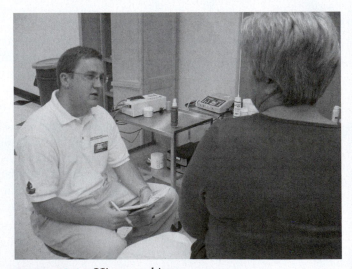

Figure 11.4   History taking.

term therapeutic exercise regimens but only 23 percent persevere with their program in the long run.[29] Client beliefs and attitudes relate strongly to their level of program compliance.[31,32] The problems that a client perceives with being compliant are strongly associated with non-compliant behaviors. These problems or costs as defined by various theories of decision making and perceived barriers as defined in the *health belief model* play strong roles in both illness and health behaviors.[33,34] When the client experiences an illness that is linked with a higher disability level and perceives the illness to be very serious, they tend to be more compliant with therapeutic exercise program interventions than do clients who have a less severe illness. Clients with chronic or long term illnesses, however, tend to be less compliant with therapeutic exercise program intervention than clients with more acute illnesses. Conceivably, the expected recovery from acute illnesses may motivate the client to adhere to the prescribed therapeutic exercise program regimen. Litt et al.[35] reported that the initial adoption of positive therapeutic exercise behaviors was best predicted by the client's readiness to change. Sociological research suggests that clients make reasoned and rational decisions about adherence depending on their own belief systems, personal experiences, and the information available to them.[36] Rosenstock[37] hypothesized that for clients to behave in ways that would help them to avoid a disease or condition they would have to believe four things: 1) that they were susceptible to the disease or condition, 2) that the disease or condition would have serious consequences, 3) that taking a particular course of action would be beneficial, and 4) that the action would not entail overriding barriers to therapeutic exercise program participation such as cost, convenience, and pain.[37]

pervision. Oldridge[40] reported a program adherence drop from 59 percent with a supervised therapeutic exercise program to 29 percent adherence after six months of unsupervised programming. When rehabilitation clinicians provide instructions that are unclear and/or fail to explain their rationale, unintended non-compliance can arise from the client either forgetting or misinterpreting the instructions. When the rehabilitation clinician fails to connect the prescribed therapeutic exercise program with the client's own ideas and perceptions about health and illness, non-compliance is likely.[40–43] Henry et al.[43] devised a scoring system to evaluate the effectiveness of home therapeutic exercise performance (**Figure 11.5**). A close or trusting relationship between the client and the rehabilitation clinician generally leads to greater satisfaction and improved therapeutic exercise program adherence. The three primary factors related to non-compliance with therapeutic exercise programs are the barriers that the client perceives, a lack of positive feedback, and their perception of helplessness.[29] Based on data from studies that have been conducted in supervised therapeutic exercise settings, the factor most likely to influence physical activity behaviors and therapeutic exercise program compliance are perceived barriers to exercise, benefit expectations, self-efficacy, self-motivation, past exercise history/activity level/program participation, exercise group cohesion, social support from family, and actual or perceived exercise facility access.[43] Knowledge, however, is only one component in the dynamic process of behavior modification. Education was once perceived to be the universal remedy for behavioral change, but actual behavioral change involves a complex intrinsic process that dramatically alters the way that clients view the necessary changes expected of them.[44]

Key Point:

Clients are more likely to implement positive behavioral changes if they believe that they are susceptible to the disease or condition, if they believe that the disease or condition will have serious consequences, if they believe that taking a particular course of action will be beneficial, and if that action will not entail barriers such as cost, inconvenience or pain.

Key Point:

The three primary factors related to therapeutic exercise program non-compliance are the barriers that the client perceives, the lack of positive feedback, and their perception of helplessness. Of these, perceived barriers are the strongest factors associated with non-compliance.

Clients tend to be more compliant with relatively simple therapeutic exercise program regimens than complex ones. Additionally, compliance is less likely when the therapeutic exercise program is not tailored or individualized to the client's situation or daily routine. The ability for the rehabilitation clinician to provide prolonged supervision is a strong factor in therapeutic exercise program compliance.[38,39] Clients whose compliance is being monitored and who receive feedback about their efforts and progress tend to comply better than clients who do not receive su-

Perceived barriers are the strongest factor associated with non-compliance. Barriers specifically associated with therapeutic exercise programs include the time required for program participation, the lack of program tailoring to the situation of the individual client, and the design of a program that does not effectively fit the client's daily routine. Rehabilitation clinicians should be careful to not overlook the real and perceived problems that their clients encounter when they attempt to change their behaviors or lifestyles. Unless these real or perceived barriers are identified, the

Name _____   Exercise# _____

The performance score will be the sum of the 3 components. A maximum of 12 points is possible for each exercise.

I. Cueing

1	2	3	4
Relied on exercise sheet, or maximum verbal and/or manual cueing	Moderate verbal and/or manual cueing	Minimum verbal and/or manual cueing	No cueing

II. Alignment

1	2	3	4
Alignment never established	Correct alignment maintained <50% of exercise	Correct alignment maintained >50% of exercise	Alignment maintained throughout exercise

III. Exercise quality

1	2	3	4
Lacks control, coordination, and/or rhythm during exercise	Controlled, coordinated, and continuous <50% of exercise	Controlled, coordinated, and continuous >50% of exercise	Controlled, coordinated, and continuous throughout exercise

TOTAL = _____

Figure 11.5   Evaluation of appropriate therapeutic exercise technique. (From KD Henry, C Rosemond, LB Eckert. Effect of number of home exercises on compliance and performance in adults over 65 years of age. *Phys Ther.* 1999; 79(3):270–277.)

client's problems cannot be effectively managed. Rehabilitation clinicians should carefully inquire about the kinds of problems or barriers that each client may encounter.[30] When a rehabilitation clinician perceives a client to be non-compliant, they should not assume that they completely understand the reason(s) for the client's non-compliance. There is a strong association between a client's feeling of helplessness and non-compliance. Long term compliance with a therapeutic exercise program is often desired for primary or secondary prevention, but research has shown that clients are unlikely to maintain compliance with purely preventative interventions.[29]

A motivated client is more likely to comply with therapeutic exercise program intervention. *Motivation* is a complex interaction of wants, beliefs, and perceived rewards vs. costs of the behavior.[43]

> **Key Point:**
>
> Client motivation is a complex interaction of wants, beliefs, and perceived rewards vs. costs of a particular behavior.

Older clients may display decreased therapeutic exercise program compliance because of multiple pathologies,[29] but if this information is appreciated early during program de-

velopment, compliance may improve. The client's living conditions may also influence their compliance level. Lorenc and Branthwaite[45] reported that clients over 65 years of age that live alone were less compliant with prescription medication usage than younger adults.

Martin and Dubbert[46] reported that therapeutic exercise program compliance decreased when the client attempted to perform the program at inconvenient locations. Clinic or health club hours that do not fit the client's lifestyle may increase non-compliance. Haynes et al.[47] reported that interventions that require more than one step or task produced a higher non-compliance rate. Essentially, as program complexity increased, compliance decreased. There is presently no reliable method of assessing client compliance with therapeutic exercise program intervention. Although client self-reports tend to overestimate compliance they are still the most cost-effective, feasible, and frequently used method available for assessing therapeutic exercise program compliance.[43,47]

> **Key Point:**
>
> Consideration of underlying pathologies, use of easy-to-perform tasks, and use of facilities with convenient locations and hours of business will improve therapeutic exercise program compliance.

Ultimately, healthy lifestyle modifications require a long term commitment from clients, adequate social reinforcement, and attainable goals.[48] Therapeutic exercise intensity level is inversely related to program participation, but may be a useful factor for determining whether clients will eventually adopt exercise as a component piece of their lifestyle.[49] *Self-efficacy* (belief in one's ability to organize and execute the actions required to manage prospective situations) and perceived effort are associated with therapeutic exercise program adherence, however attendance is lower in higher intensity exercise groups.[50] This suggests lower client self-confidence in their ability to perform at that level of exercise with a higher intensity target being perceived as too challenging.[51]

It seems irrational to provide expensive therapeutic exercise intervention if no significant changes in client behaviors will result.[52] Therefore, when populations undergo therapeutic exercise program intervention, regardless of the diagnosis, attention to program adherence and identification of factors that may negatively affect adherence seems warranted.[52] McAuley et al.[53] reported that clients who received maximum information regarding their therapeutic exercise capability were more likely to adhere to program recommendations than those who did not receive such information. Hartigan et al.[52] recommended providing focused coaching of and problem solving for clients who reported more significant barriers to therapeutic exercise program adherence. Each individualized program should include the creation of a physiologically adequate, practical, low tech, low cost, and minimally time-consuming post-treatment maintenance regimen.[52]

Dorn et al.[54] reported that lower client education levels, blue collar occupations, unemployment, smoking, and female gender all related to a lower participation rate in an exercise based cardiac rehabilitation program with a precipitous drop off by the third year of intervention (**Figure 11.6**). The influence of client age on program participation has displayed contrasting results, with both younger[55] and older[56] clients displaying high dropout rates. Psychological traits identified as being associated with poor cardiac rehabilitation program compliance include depression, anxiousness, and hypochondriasis.[57] Increased compliance has been associated with social support, particularly family encouragement.[58] Cues to exercise and severity of disease threat have been identified as health belief model factors that influence cardiac rehabilitation program compliance.[56] While more frequent cures have been linked with increased program compliance, clients with a greater perception of disease severity tend to be more non-compliant.[56] Factors that negatively influence cardiac rehabilitation program enrollment and compliance include additional illnesses or medical conditions, transportation difficulties, lack of health insurance coverage, and low levels of previous physical activity.[56,58,59] Among cardiac rehabilitation program participants, transition from a controlled laboratory setting to a less tightly controlled gymnasium or aquatic therapy setting may have discouraged participation.[54] In a study that

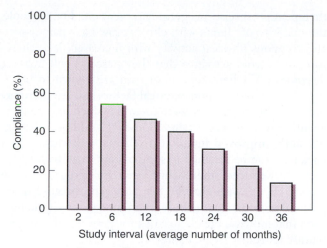

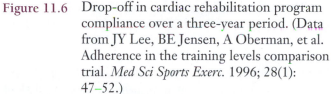

Figure 11.6   Drop-off in cardiac rehabilitation program compliance over a three-year period. (Data from JY Lee, BE Jensen, A Oberman, et al. Adherence in the training levels comparison trial. *Med Sci Sports Exerc.* 1996; 28(1): 47–52.)

compared attendance rates between cardiac rehabilitation program clients who were randomized to either a low (50 percent VO_{2max}) or a high (85 percent VO_{2max}) intensity exercise program, Lee et al.[51] reported that the low intensity group had a significantly better average participation rate over the first year of program participation. It appeared that cardiac rehabilitation program compliance decreased over time, and clients who were at the highest risk for repeat events were the ones who were most likely to display poor compliance.

Research has consistently shown that up to 50 percent of all clients do not follow their prescribed drug regimen.[36,60–64] Issues related to client non-compliance have been relatively neglected in physical therapy, even though it is the recommended first line therapy for many clients with chronic and acute musculoskeletal disorders, including osteoarthritis of the knee.[60] Poor client compliance to prescribed treatments, diets and therapeutic exercise programs continues to be the single greatest barrier to controlling diseases such as diabetes and preventing the serious long term complications associated with the disease.[65] Schneider et al.[66] suggested that a lifestyle management program including client education, nutrition counseling, and therapeutic exercise training is a high priority over the initial six months of a program for clients with diabetes mellitus, but attrition rates at 3 and 12 months were approximately 50 percent and 90 percent, respectively.

Chronic Pain and Behavioral Change

Although acute pain warrants a drastic reduction in activity level and immediate treatment, clients with chronic pain represent a different consideration regarding therapeutic exercise program intervention. For example, the majority of clients with chronic low back pain associate strenuous physical activity with increased pain; therefore, they avoid activities that they perceive will increase discomfort.[67] Client reports of pain are known to be affected by numerous non-physical factors and are therefore not a reliable or valid measurement on which to base therapeutic exercise recommendations.[67–73] Additionally, significantly improved function in clients with chronic low back pain can be attained in spite of continued pain symptoms.[74] Reduced therapeutic exercise program goals among clients with chronic low back pain because of reports of pain may contribute to an unnecessary sedentary state that increase the client's risk for poor health and premature mortality (see Chapter 1).[75–77]

Chronic low back pain is a major medical and social problem in industrialized countries.[78] In the early 1990s in the United States, the direct medical and indirect costs associated with treating low back pain were estimated to be more than $50 billion per year.[79] Considering the socioeconomic impact of low back pain, there is an obvious need for effective prevention strategies and treatments, especially in occupational healthcare. Currently, however, there is only limited evidence for the effectiveness of therapeutic exercise with respect to primary prevention of low back pain (i.e., intervening before the onset of disease) and there is no evidence that any other intervention effectively prevents the onset of low back pain.[80,81]

From both a societal and scientific perspective, there are important questions concerning the cost effectiveness of various return to work interventions.[78] Of the 19 return to work interventions for clients with low back pain that were evaluated by Staal et al.[78], 17 included therapeutic exercise, 15 included an education module, 7 included behavioral treatments, but only 3 included ergonomic measures.[78] The prevailing component combinations included therapeutic exercises, behavioral treatment, and client education. Behavioral treatment included coping skills training[82] to set up more realistic goals and to change client attitudes toward their pain sensations.[83] Operant behavioral approaches are believed to eliminate or reduce pain behaviors (such as prolonged inactivity and over-medication) and substitute behaviors that are inconsistent with a sickness role.[82]

Key Point:

Although evidence is quite limited, successful inventions for clients with chronic pain should include therapeutic exercises in combination with behavioral training and education. Each component should address focused and measurable goals.

Relaxation training may also help to modify the subjective experience of pain.[82] Lindstrom et al.[84,85] reported on the effects of graded therapeutic exercise interventions

with an operant conditioning approach on physical fitness variables reporting improved cardiovascular fitness, and improvements in lumbar range of motion at one year follow-up compared to traditional care. Mannion et al.[86] and Kaser et al.[87] studied the effects of three types of active therapy on back muscle structure and function (conventional physical therapy, muscle re-education using exercise devices, or low impact aerobics). At three months post-intervention, there were no differences among groups for back muscle performance, with all groups displaying significant improvements in trunk strength, lateral bending, axial rotation and erector spinae muscle electromyographic activation during isometric back extension tests.

Lessons learned from other chronic pain populations may be useful in managing the health care of clients with osteoarthritic conditions at lower extremity joints. Therapeutic exercise intervention alone without education and the attainment of true behavioral changes (decreased high impact activities, reduced body weight, optimized joint range of motion and strength, and adequate nutrition and rest) will lead to less than optimal results. Additionally, appropriate, more individualized interventions by the rehabilitation clinician early during therapeutic exercise program performance may help to prevent medical conditions from becoming chronic.

Quality of Life

Across all disciplines of healthcare, client perspectives are being formally included in the process of selecting among treatment options and in evaluating the effectiveness of the intervention.[88–91] Improving the client's quality of life lies at the forefront of the rehabilitation clinician's decision making process. Quality of life has a variety of different meanings and interpretations (socioeconomic status, employment status, housing, etc.) and is an evolving health care concept. Similar to the World Health Organization's definition of health, quality of life considers optimized physical, mental, and social well being, not merely the absence of disease or infirmary.[92,93] No longer is mortality alone considered to be an appropriate outcome measurement.[93] The chronic nature of certain illnesses like heart disease and cancer demand that quality of life issues be assessed to determine how the client really is doing. Quality of life assessment is client based, focusing more on the subjective or "softer" scientific measurements of outcome and not on what the physician or rehabilitation clinician believes is important.[94] Quality of life includes the clients' perceptions of their own physical and occupational function, psychological state, social interaction, and somatic sensation.[95,96] The concept of quality of life encompasses a broad range of physical and psychological characteristics and limitations which describe a client's ability to function and to derive satisfaction from doing so. The vital message to the rehabilitation clinician is that the concept of quality of life is centered on the individual client, not on the thoughts or opinions of the health care provider.

> **Key Point:**
>
> Quality of life encompasses the client's perception of their physical and occupational function, psychological state, social interaction and somatic sensation. Quality of life is centered on the individual client, not on the thoughts or opinions of the health care provider.

Stewart and King[97] observed a positive relationship between therapeutic exercise participation and enhanced quality of life, a finding that was corroborated by a recent review on aging and physical activity for both non-impaired and impaired populations.[98] Strength training has been described as a bridge to independence among the elderly[99] and exercise has been shown to improve the balance of older clients, reducing their risk of sustaining physically disabling falls.[100] There continues to be a need for determining the optimal, adequate and minimal doses of exercise sufficient to get a target response and improve various indices of disability.

Health Locus of Control and Self-Efficacy

Locus of control is the degree to which the client perceives having control over the environment.[101] There are two types of control, internal and external, which anchor a continuum that approximates a normal distribution.[101] Clients are said to have an internal locus of control when they believe that reinforcements are contingent upon their own behavior or stable personal characteristics. External locus of control is evident when clients believe that reinforcements are due to luck, fate, or powerful others outside of their control. The American Medical and Nursing Associations have concluded that "a sense of purpose and control over one's life is integral to the health of the aged."[102] Reports have indicated that elderly clients with internal locus of control beliefs are more active, alert, and have lower mortality rates than those with external beliefs.[103–105] Giving older adults more control results in similar benefits.[106]

The other social learning construct, *self-efficacy*, is defined as clients' judgments of their capabilities to organize and execute a course of action required to attain designated types of performance.[107] Self-efficacy can be distinguished from locus of control in that locus of control centers around the causal beliefs clients have about the relationship between their actions and particular outcomes. Self-efficacy, however, pertains to personal judgments clients make about their competence in performing the behaviors that may lead to the desired outcome.

> **Key Point:**
>
> While health locus of control centers around causal beliefs, self-efficacy pertains to personal judgments the client makes about their ability to perform the behaviors that may lead to the desired outcome.

Activities as simple as giving nursing home residents the responsibility to care for a plant or to determine when to watch a movie have been shown to have a dramatic effect on residents' psychosocial adjustment, presumably by increasing their sense of control.[102,104] Interventions that decrease an elderly client's anxiety while performing a task, or that provide vicarious learning by observing a fellow resident perform a task, may be useful to help increase the self-efficacy expectations of nursing home residents.[108] Johnson et al.[108] reported that older adults with increased self-efficacy and internal health locus of control made more successful adjustments to a nursing home environment.

Self-efficacy and internal health locus of control are significant predictors of compliance with home therapeutic exercise programs. An enhanced internal health locus of control with greater compliance or client engagement might occur if rehabilitation clinicians encourage greater participation from clients in treatment planning, problem solving, and goal setting. The clients' sense of control may also be enhanced if rehabilitation clinicians attempt to decrease the possible barriers to compliance, such as fear from lack of knowledge, or the family members' lack of understanding for the importance of their support. Strategies to improve client self-efficacy for management of a home therapeutic exercise program may also help treatment outcomes, such as teaching clients to set realistic weekly goals to ensure success.[109] Clients who display an external locus of control (belief that health and illness depend little on their own behavior) appear to be less compliant than those with an internal health locus of control.[29] Clients with a more internal health locus of control generally possess a stronger generalized expectancy that reinforcement is contingent upon their own behavior; they tend to be more active, alert, and self-directed in attempting to control and manipulate their environment than are clients with a more external health locus of control.[110] Clients with an internal health locus of control are generally better at assembling environmental cues and internalizing them to their advantage for strategically performing a task or solving a problem. In contrast, clients with an external health locus of control perform better with external guidance and direction. The more cognitively loaded a motor task or sport happens to be, the more important the role of internal or external locus of control becomes in determining a client's response to situational cues within the environment. Clients with an external health locus of control are more dependent on additional extrinsic reinforcement, such as praise or positive reinforcement from the rehabilitation clinician, while clients with an internal health locus of control perform just as well without. Clients with an external health locus of control pay more attention to social stimuli during task performance, tending to have a greater desire to please others, potentially leading to greater anxiety, less confidence, and greater uncertainty during the initial stages of task performance.

COUNSELING AND EDUCATION SKILLS

It is essential that rehabilitation clinicians develop appropriate counseling and education skills so that they will be able to deliver it to clients in a sensitive and caring manner. Toward that goal, there are a number of important considerations that they should incorporate into their training.

Fundamental skills for counseling by rehabilitation clinicians should include 1) a basic understanding of various counseling theories, fundamental communication skills training and counseling techniques; 2) an ability to assess a client's educational needs and transform those into a counseling plan; and 3) an appreciation and understanding of different learning and teaching styles, and the skills to create and implement an *Individualized Education Plan* (IEP). In addition, rehabilitation clinicians need to 1) understand both the theory and the practice of self-management skills needed to educate the client for therapeutic exercise program compliance; 2) understand the theory and practice of being able to integrate counseling, teaching, and self-management skills into a useful program for clients based on the stage of change at which the clients may be currently functioning, per the transtheoretical model;[27] 3) plan and implement an effective therapeutic exercise program geared to the unique needs of the individual client; 4) evaluate the effectiveness of the therapeutic exercise program that has been developed for the client; and 5) provide knowledge of the resources necessary for maintenance of the program by the client.

COGNITIVE BEHAVIORAL MODELS FOR THERAPEUTIC EXERCISE PROGRAM INTERVENTION

One example of a self-management program is the *SMARTS* program, developed by Miller.[111] SMARTS stands for Self Management Approach for Responsible Treatment Sucess. The SMARTS program includes goal selection, targeting behaviors, self monitoring, developing a plan for change, self-contracting, and evaluating the plan for change. The SMARTS program consists of a 15-week self-management program that combines self-monitoring, self-reward, self-contracting, and stimulus control. These strategies have been applied successfully to many client populations with differing problems, such as anxiety, depression, obesity, and pain.

Through self-management assessment and intervention, behavioral change can be brought about by teaching clients to use coping skills in problematic situations. Generalization and maintenance of client outcomes are enhanced by encouraging them to accept the responsibility for carrying out these strategies on a daily basis. In self-management programs, clients make decisions concerning specific behaviors that they want to control or change, such as obesity or overeating. Clients frequently discover that a major reason they do not attain their goals is the lack of certain skills. A self-directed approach can provide both the needed guidelines for behavioral change and a plan that will lead to change.

Five characteristics of an effective self-management program have been identified by Cormier and Cormier:[112]

- A combination of several self-management strategies is usually more effective than following a single strategy.
- Consistent use of these strategies is essential. If self-management strategies are not regularly used over a sustained time, their effectiveness will be limited, and significant positive behavioral changes may not be observed.
- Realistic goals must be established and re-evaluation should be performed to see if they are being met.
- The use of self-reinforcement strategies is an important component of self-management programs.
- Environmental support is necessary to maintain positive behavioral changes that result from a self-management program.

Based on the Watson and Tharp[113] model designed for self-directed change, the SMART program is designed to address four key stages based on the findings of several studies.[112–115] The four key stages are:

- **Selecting goals.** The initial stage begins with specifying what behavioral changes are desired. Goals should be established one at a time, and they should be measurable, attainable, positive, and significant for the client. If the goal is not perceived to be significant by the client, the program has a real possibility of failing.
- **Translating goals into target behaviors.** Next, the goals selected in the initial stage are translated into target behaviors. To that effect, questions such as the following are relevant: "What specific behaviors do I want to increase or decrease? "What chain of actions is needed for my goal to be achieved?"
- **Self-monitoring.** A major first step in self-directed change is the process of self-monitoring, which consists of deliberately and systematically observing one's own behavior.[115] This monitoring presumably leads to awareness, focusing on concrete, observable behaviors

rather than on historical events. Keeping a behavioral diary is one of the simplest methods of observing and monitoring one's behavior. The occurrence of a particular behavior is recorded, in addition to comments about the relevant antecedent cues and consequences. For example, if the client desires to change eating habits, the behavioral diary will contain entries of what is eaten, events and situations that occur before eating or snacking, meal frequency, the types of food eaten, and so forth. Total counts can be transferred at the end of each day or week to a chart, providing a visual illustration of progress (or lack of it) toward self-selected goals. Cormier and Cormier[112] maintain that self-monitoring is indispensable as a measuring device to define problems and to collect evaluative data. Although self-monitoring is necessary and useful for many clients, it is often not sufficient unless it is used in conjunction with other self-management procedures, such as stimulus control, self-reward and self-punishment, and self-contracting (discussed later).

■ **Working out a plan for change.** This stage begins with a comparison between the information obtained from self-monitoring and the client's own standards for a specific behavior. After clients evaluate the behavioral changes that they would like to acquire, they need to devise an action program to bring about actual change. Plans help to gradually replace an unwanted action with a desirable one or to increase a desirable action. Such a plan of action entails some type of self-reinforcement system and the negotiating of a working contract.

An essential part of the plan for change is *self-reinforcement* such as participating in activities that the client perceives as pleasurable. *Self-praise* is a useful reinforcer, because it can easily be applied after a target behavior occurs. The use of reinforcement to change behavior is the cornerstone of modern behavior therapy. It is important to choose appropriate rewards, meaning ones that are perceived by the client as being personally motivating. Watson and Tharp[113] suggest that the purpose of *self-reinforcement* is to make desired behavior so successful that the natural consequences of daily life will sustain it. In other words, self-reinforcement is a temporary strategy to be used until the client can implement new behaviors in their everyday life. *Self-contracting* is another facet of a plan for change that involves determining in advance the external and internal consequences that will follow the execution of the desired or undesired action. Such contracts can help clients keep their commitment to carry out their action plan with some degree of consistency.

Evaluation of the plan for change is essential to determine the degree to which clients are achieving their goals. After a plan of action is set forth, it must be modified as clients learn other ways to meet their goals. This evaluation is an ongoing process rather than a one-time occurrence. Watson and Tharp[113] advise that a completely perfect plan for

any problem does not exist; however, successful plans generally have these characteristics:

■ Rules that state which behaviors and techniques for change will be used in various situations.
■ Explicit goals and sub-goals.
■ A system of getting feedback on one's progress, derived largely from self-observation.
■ A comparison of feedback with one's goals and sub-goals to measure progress.
■ Adjustments in the plan as conditions change.

> ## Key Point:
> Identify the problem, list ideas to solve the problem, select one method to try, assess the results, modify the plan by substituting another idea if the first one did not work, utilize other resources, own the problem and solve it now.

SMARTS Program

Becoming a Self-Manager. Like any new skill, self-management must be learned and practiced by the client. The rehabilitation clinician should help the client during this process. Self-managers must:

■ Decide what they want to accomplish.
■ Look for alternative ways to accomplish the goal.
■ Start making short term plans by contracting or making an agreement with themselves.
■ Carry out their contracts.
■ Check the results.
■ Make changes as needed.
■ Remember to reward themselves.

Deciding What One Wants to Accomplish. Deciding what one wants to accomplish may be the most difficult part. The client must be realistic and very specific. The rehabilitation clinician should have the client make a list of three goals and place an asterisk (*) next to the goal that they would like to work on first.

Next, the client should write the list of options for the main goal, and then put an asterisk (*) next to the two or three options they would like to work on.

The list might look like this:

Goals.
1. Lose 10 pounds of bodyfat
2. Be able to walk 2 miles in 30 minutes without having to stop to rest*

3. Be able to climb 2 flights of stairs without having to stop to rest

4. Be able to carry a full laundry basket from the laundry room up two flights of stairs without experiencing low back pain

Options.

1. Get up at 6:00 A.M. and walk for 1 mile down the beach and back in 30 minutes, 4 times a week.*

2. Perform 30 minutes of continuous walking and active range of motion exercises in a swimming pool 3 times a week.

3. Walk up one flight of stairs, then around the apartment complex, down one flight of stairs back to apartment in 15 minutes, twice, 3 times a week.

Prepare. First, the rehabilitation clinician should help the client make sure that the goals that they have developed are behavior specific. That is, rather than just deciding "to relax," the goal should include information regarding the mechanism of relaxation, such as "listening to my muscle relaxation tapes." Next, the client should develop a specific plan. This is the most difficult and important part of making a contract. Deciding what one wants to do is worthless without a plan to do it. The rehabilitation clinician should have the client consider the following questions and answer them specifically in the plan:[111]

- **Exactly what am I going to do?** How far will I walk, how will I eat less, what breathing techniques will I practice?

- **How much will I do?** Will I walk around the block, walk for 15 minutes, not eat between meals for three days, practice breathing exercises for 15 minutes?

- **When will I do this?** Before work? At lunchtime? After dinner? Again, this must be specific.

- **How often will I do the activity?** There are a couple of rules for writing the contract that may help the client achieve success. First, they should start where they are, or start slowly. Second, they should give themselves some time off. All clients will have days when they they do not feel like doing anything. That is good reason for saying that they will do something three times a week instead of every day. That way, if they don't feel like walking one day, they can still meet the obligations of the contract.

Once clients have developed the contract, they should ask themselves the following question: "On a scale of 0 to 10, with 0 being totally unsure and 10 being totally confident, how confident am I that I can complete this contract?"

If they answer 7 or above, this is probably a realistic contract. They should be congratulated, and should congratulate themselves, for doing good work. If their answer is less than 7, they should re-assess the contract, ask them-

selves why they are not confident, and identify the problems that they foresee. Then they should see if they can either solve the problems or change the contract accordingly to make themselves more confident of success. Once they have made a contract they are happy with, they should write it down and post it where they will see it every day. They should keep track both of how they are doing and the problems they encounter. The basics of a successful contract are presented in **Table 11.4.** A sample contract form is presented in **Table 11.5.**

As part of the SMARTS program, an individualized education plan is developed for the client based on the transtheoretical model.[27] It becomes important for the rehabilitation clinician to know at what stage of change the client is currently functioning. Based on that determination, goals and measurable objectives should be developed for the individual client. Examples of individualized education plan goals and objectives based on the transtheoretical model appear in **Table 11.6.**

Bio-Behavioral Approaches to Treatment

Bio-behavioral approaches to treatment for clients needing the services of a rehabilitation clinician may include the following options:

- Bio-behavioral therapy helps clients to unlearn self-defeating patterns of behavior and habits in their lives. It also teaches new, healthy skills, and ways of positively reacting to situations that trigger maladaptive behavior and lifestyles. Behavioral strategies may include progressive muscle relaxation techniques, changing breathing patterns (see Chapter 10), positive and negative reinforcement, and learning empowering ways to live more effective lives.

TABLE 11.4 Basics of a successful client self-management contract

The rehabilitation clinician should help the client to . . .

1. Plan something that they want to do and is achievable.
2. Be reasonable.
3. Be behavior specific.
4. Provide answers to these questions: What? How much? When? and How often?
5. Achieve a confidence level of 7 or more.
6. Prepare to initiate the contract.
7. Confront the commitment.
8. Cope with failure and modify the contract if needed.
9. Self-reinforce success.
10. Complete the program.

TABLE 11.5   Sample client self-management contract form

In writing the contract, the client should be sure it includes:

1. What they are going to do.
2. How much they are going to do.
3. When they are going to do it.
4. How many days a week they are going to do it.

   For example: This week, I will walk (what distance, pace, etc.) around the block (how much, laps, etc.) at (when, before or after lunch, etc.) for (how many, three times per week).

This week I will _____ (what)
_____(how much)
_____(when)
_____(how many)

How confident are you of your ability to effectively honor the contract? (0 = not at all confident, 10 = totally confident)_____

	Check off completion	Comments
Monday		
Tuesday		
Wednesday		
Thursday		
Friday		
Saturday		
Sunday		

- Cognitive therapy assumes that by changing self-defeating thought patterns and transforming them into more successful belief systems, clients can improve their lives. Cognitive therapy teaches clients to change emotions and behaviors by changing self-defeating thoughts such as all or nothing beliefs, negative assumptions, labeling, and catastrophising.

- Cognitive-behavioral therapy, or CBT, is a combination approach that uses both cognitive and behavioral therapy. Cognitive and behavioral therapies complement each other. When used together, they stimulate areas of growth that are difficult to achieve using either by itself. Cognitive-behavioral therapy is commonly used to address the thoughts and behaviors that promote and perpetuate anxiety.

- Medication can be a helpful adjunct in bio-behavioral treatment by reducing physical symptoms, but it is not a cure-all. Used alone, it does not address any of the several root causes of symptoms and does not pro-mote healthy lifestyle changes. Medications are often used in combination with other treatment options such as cognitive-behavioral therapy. Rehabilitation clinicians need to become familiar with these medications and their possible influence on the client's ability to effectively participate in a therapeutic exercise program.

Key Point:

Medication alone does not address the root causes of maladaptive behaviors and does not promote healthy lifestyle changes. Medications used for cognitive-behavioral problems are most effective when they are combined with treatment options such as cognitive-behavioral therapy.

TABLE 11.6   Individualized education plan

	Goal	Objectives
Precontemplation	Lose weight	1. Elicit reasons for not losing weight and perceived barriers to losing weight 2. Provide simple educational information on losing weight 3. Be open (talk about a program when the client is ready)
Contemplation	Stop smoking	1. Motivate by describing the benefits of stopping smoking and define the specific goals, involve the client's family or other support if possible. 2. Elicit client commitment.
Preparation	Increase strength	1. Identify specific goals 2. Start plans (date, equipment, etc.) 3. Follow-up
Action	Increase endurance	1. Review specific goals 2. Suggest coping strategies (for fatigue, discomfort, etc.) 3. Follow-up
Maintenance	Present mood	1. Review coping strategies 2. Reassess goals 3. Advise on prevention

Resource Information: Useful Websites

Websites that provide useful counseling, education skill, and behavioral aspects of healthcare include www.mentalhealth.com, the UCLA Neuropsychiatric Institute www.npi.ucla.edu, the Nemours Foundation for Children at www.kidshealth.org, and the Department of Veterans Affairs at www.va.gov.

AGE, OSTEOARTHRITIS, ARTHROPLASTY, AND THERAPEUTIC EXERCISE

Buskirk et al.[116] reported that continued physical activity and fitness are directly related to the maintenance of long term health and longevity. Both *morbidity* (the quality or state of being diseased) and *mortality* (the quality of being mortal, death rate) have been shown to be favorably impacted by regular exercise performance (**Table 11.7 and Table 11.8**).[17–119]

Key Point:

Both client morbidity and mortality are favorably impacted by regular participation in an appropriately designed therapeutic exercise program.

With the percentage of clients who are over 65 years of age expected to increase dramatically over the next two decades, health related issues facing older adults are an important focus for rehabilitation clinicians both in practice and research.[108] Although aging is a predictable and inevitable process, the biological and environmental changes associated with growing older can affect a client's perceived range of controllable situations and competence in implementing the behaviors necessary to control events.[120] Rowe and Kahn[121] have suggested that clients who are able to minimize these negative effects undergo successful aging while those who become impaired undergo usual aging. As mentioned earlier, two constructs from social learning theory, locus of control[101] and self-efficacy,[50,107] may help to explain why some clients undergo successful aging while others undergo usual aging.

Osteoarthritis is one of the most common causes of chronic joint pain and disability in adults, imposing enormous personal, social, and economic burdens.[122] Hurley[122] described the effects of cognitive restructuring and exercise on the psychosocial consequences of clients who have osteoarthritis (**Figure 11.7**). Several controlled studies have supported the efficacy of therapeutic exercise for clients with osteoarthritis.[123–125] Benefits include improved function through improved joint range of motion, flexibility, muscle strength, endurance and power, gait, pain control, and ability to perform activities of daily living. Appropriate therapeutic exercise intervention en-

TABLE 11.7   Facts about U.S. activity behaviors

More than 60 percent of U.S. adults do not engage in the recommended amount of activity

Approximately 25 percent of U.S. adults are not active at all

Physical inactivity is more common among:

- Women than men
- African American and Hispanic adults than whites
- Older than younger adults
- Less affluent than more affluent people

Social support from family and friends has been consistently and positively related to regular physical activity.

People with disabilities are less likely to engage in regular moderate activity than people without disabilities, yet they have similar needs to promote their health and prevent unnecessary disease.

(From U.S. Department of Health and Human Services (1996), Physical Activity and Health: A Report of the Surgeon General. U.S. Dept. of Health and Human Services, Centers for Disease Control and Prevention, National Center for Chronic Disease Prevention and Health Promotion. Atlanta, GA.)

hances joint health and also helps prevent the secondary effects of osteoarthritis such as decreased mobility, which can be more disabling than the medical condition itself.[126] Therapeutic exercise helps decrease the risk of poor health and its resulting disability through improved weight control, cardiovascular health, enhanced psychosocial health, and social participation.[127] For example, during aquatic based therapeutic exercise, joint pain is diminished due to the reduced joint compression associated with buoyancy and the increased sensory input from the moving water, and its pressure and temperature, in addition to the mental stimulation that serves as a distraction from pain (see Chapters 4 and 5).[128–130] In a randomized controlled trial of 24 clients with rheumatoid arthritis or osteoarthritis, those who participated in an aquatic exercise therapy program reported improved aerobic capacity, endurance, disease activity, and function compared to those who performed a home based range of motion and isometric exercise program.[131]

In the 1990s in the United States alone, it was estimated that more than 218,000 hip and knee arthroplasties

are performed each year.[132] Older persons are being encouraged to exercise and increase their activity levels as a preventative health measure.[133] Several studies have shown that total joint replacements have a higher incidence of loosening and failure in younger, more active clients.[134,135] Client education to achieve the appropriate match of therapeutic exercise activity intensity and frequency of performance is essential to enhancing their fitness level and quality of life while preventing the progression of osteoarthritis or prosthesis loosening. Healy et al,[136] Vail et al,[137] and Nicholls et al.[138] have provided sporting activity recommendations for clients who have undergone total joint arthroplasty, derived from Mayo Clinic recommendations (**Table 11.9**), surveys of the Hip and Knee Society (**Table 11.10**), and those of Duke University based on impact loads (**Table 11.11**) and upon anatomic location of the arthoplasty (**Table 11.12**).

Measurable health benefits can be derived from a total joint replacement.[138] Macnicol et al.[139] reported that clients who had undergone total hip arthroplasty displayed increases in maximal walking speed, stride length,

TABLE 11.8   Benefits of physical activity

- Reduces the risk of dying from coronary heart disease and of developing high blood pressure, colon cancer, and diabetes
- Can help people with chronic, disabling conditions improve their stamina and muscle strength
- Reduces symptoms of anxiety and depression, improves mood, and promotes general feelings of well being
- Helps control joint swelling and pain associated with arthritis
- Can help reduce blood pressure in some people with hypertension

(From Centers for Disease Control (CDC), National Physical Activity Initiative. Atlanta, GA: U.S. Dept. of Health and Human Services, Centers for Disease Control and Prevention, 1996.)

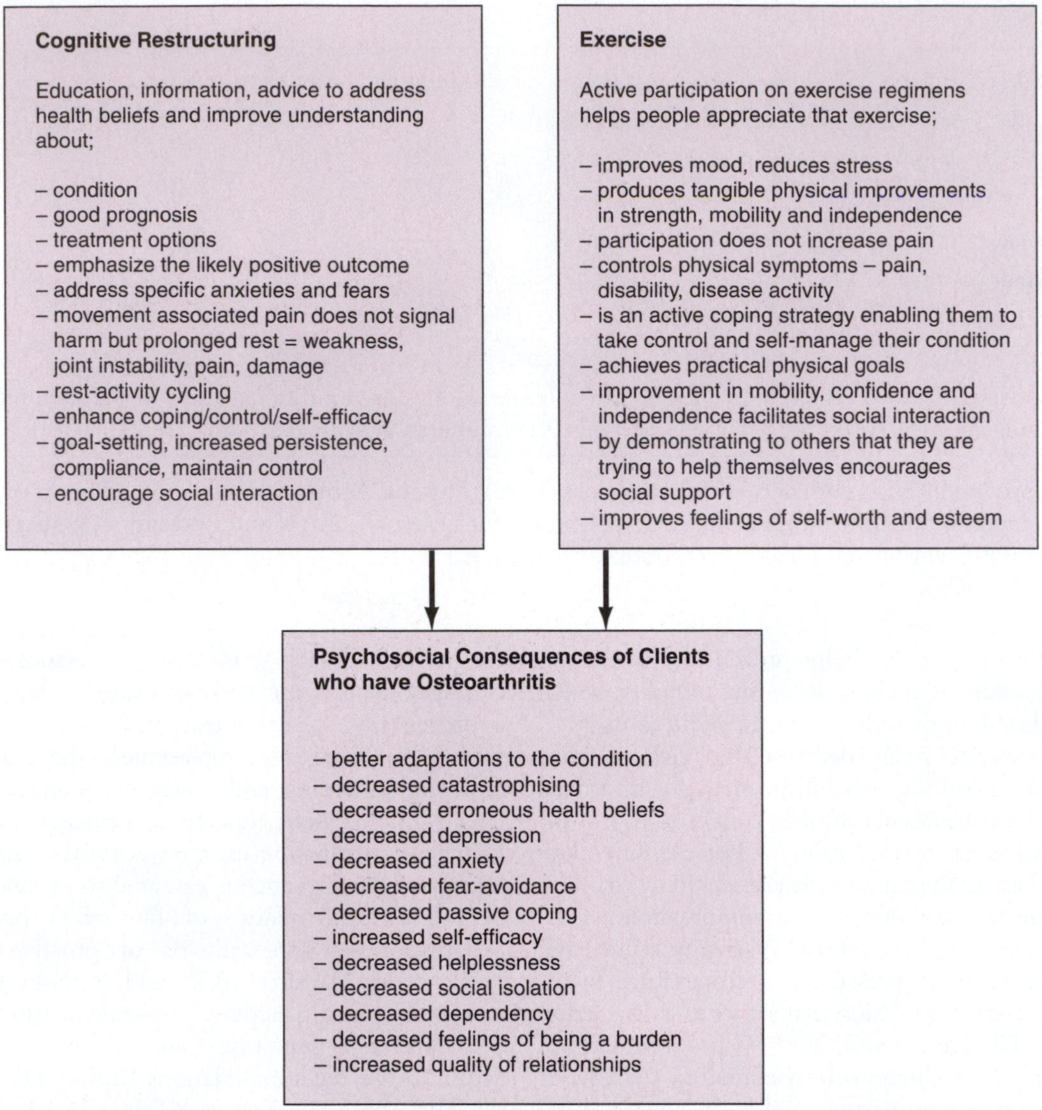

Cognitive Restructuring

Education, information, advice to address
health beliefs and improve understanding
about;

– condition
– good prognosis
– treatment options
– emphasize the likely positive outcome
– address specific anxieties and fears
– movement associated pain does not signal
  harm but prolonged rest = weakness,
  joint instability, pain, damage
– rest-activity cycling
– enhance coping/control/self-efficacy
– goal-setting, increased persistence,
  compliance, maintain control
– encourage social interaction

Exercise

Active participation on exercise regimens
helps people appreciate that exercise;

– improves mood, reduces stress
– produces tangible physical improvements
  in strength, mobility and independence
– participation does not increase pain
– controls physical symptoms – pain,
  disability, disease activity
– is an active coping strategy enabling them to
  take control and self-manage their condition
– achieves practical physical goals
– improvement in mobility, confidence and
  independence facilitates social interaction
– by demonstrating to others that they are
  trying to help themselves encourages
  social support
– improves feelings of self-worth and esteem

**Psychosocial Consequences of Clients
who have Osteoarthritis**

– better adaptations to the condition
– decreased catastrophising
– decreased erroneous health beliefs
– decreased depression
– decreased anxiety
– decreased fear-avoidance
– decreased passive coping
– increased self-efficacy
– decreased helplessness
– decreased social isolation
– decreased dependency
– decreased feelings of being a burden
– increased quality of relationships

Figure 11.7   Effects of psychosocial interventions and exercise on the psychosocial consequences of osteoarthritis. (From MV Hurley, HL Mitchell, N Walsh. Osteoarthritis, the psychosocial benefits of exercise are important as physical improvements. *Exerc Sports Sci Rev.* 2003;31(3):138–143.)

and cadence (see Chapter 9). Additionally, oxygen consumption returned to normal values and mean power output during stair climbing doubled. An increase in participation in recreational activities such as walking, cross country skiing, cycling, and swimming after total hip arthroplasty have also been reported.[140]

The rehabilitation clinician should recommend low impact, low contact activities that are performed in moderation for clients with osteoarthritis or those who have undergone lower extremity arthroplasty. Clients should expect to be active enough to pursue routine cardiovascular health but should not pursue participation in competitive sports activities or conditioning. Client education regarding the risks of activities after total joint arthroplasty and in-

volvement with the decision making process will lead to a more satisfying client–rehabilitation clinician interaction.[138]

Similar interventions along the continuum of surgical and nonsurgical management of lower extremity osteoarthritis such as realignment osteotomies, unicompartmental knee

Key Point:
Following diagnosis of osteoarthritis it is essential to restrict or modify client activities on an individualized basis according to activity impact loads, frequency, and client desires.

TABLE 11.9   Mayo Clinic recommendations for resumption of sporting activities after hip or knee replacement

	Sports
Recommended	Golf
	Swimming
	Cycling
	Bowling
	Sailing
	Scuba diving
Intermediate	Hiking
	Speed walking
	Backpacking
	Ice skating
	Singles/doubles tennis
	Aerobics
	Volleyball
	Softball
	Alpine skiing
Not recommended	Handball
	Racquetball
	Running
	Hockey
	Baseball
	Water skiing
	Karate
	Basketball
	Soccer
	Football

(From WL Healy, R Iorio, M Lemos. Athletic activity after joint replacement. *Am J Sports Med.* 2001;29:377–388.)

joint arthroplasty, or joint injection with sodium hyaluronate derivatives should also be considered.[141]

TREATMENT GOAL DOCUMENTATION

In establishing client goals, the rehabilitation clinician should distinguish between the client's impairments, functional limitations, and disabilities (as discussed in Chapter 1). As a reminder . . .

- **Impairment:** Loss or abnormality of physiological, psychological, or anatomical structure or function.

- **Functional limitation:** Restriction of the ability to perform at the level of the whole person a specific physical action, task, or activity in an efficient, typically expected and competent manner.

- **Disability:** Inability to engage in age specific, gender related, or sex specific roles in a particular social context and physical environment.

After this definition is arrived at, the rehabilitation clinician should attempt to relate the impairments to the client's functional limitations and disabilities for each problem that has been identified. It is essential that each goal be written so that it can be observed and measured, reflecting the role of the rehabilitation clinician in the health care team approach. When writing treatment goals, it is also important to provide a timetable for the expected achievement of each goal, remembering that the goals merely represent observable and measurable points in the process, not the process (for example, "Improve range of motion" is not a goal, but a means toward the goal). Goals should also be refined toward specific functions that help to minimize the client's disability level. Merely increasing a client's strength or range of motion is not very meaningful if it does not result in improved function.[142,143] As you review the cases that follow this chapter, you will have an opportunity to develop short and long term treatment goals for several clients, in addition to making diagrams of decision making algorithms.

> ***Key Point:***
> Treatment goals that link impairment based measurements to functional limitations and client disability increase the likelihood that the rehabilitation clinician will direct their therapeutic exercise program design toward targets that are vital to the client's quality of life.

Both short and long term goals generally begin with a problem list that summarizes history and clinical examination findings. From these data, the rehabilitation clinician attempts to sort out and list the impairments, functional limitations, and disability problems. Written goals attempt to reflect the inter-relationship between impairment—functional limitation—disability with long term goals representing the perceived endpoint of the plan of care, and the short term goals representing achievement expectations at an earlier interval. Some identified problems will require referral to other health care specialists. When writing client progress notes at the end of short term goal intervals, the rehabilitation clinician should always refer to the original short and long term goals.

TABLE 11.10   Recommendations for activity after total hip or knee replacement according to Hip and Knee Society surveys

	Sport		Sport
Recommended	Stationary bicycling	**Not recommended**	High impact aerobics
	Croquet		Baseball
	Ballroom dancing		Basketball
	Golf		Football
	Horseshoes		Gymnastics
	Shooting		Handball
	Shuffleboard		Hockey
	Swimming		Jogging
	Doubles tennis*		Lacrosse
	Walking		Racquetball
	Low impact aerobics**		Squash
	Bowling**		Rock climbing
	Horseback riding**		Soccer
Allowed with experience	Doubles tennis**		Singles tennis
	Low impact aerobics		Volleyball
	Road bicycling	**No conclusion**	Ice skating
	Bowling		Roller/in-line skating
	Canoeing		Rowing
	Hiking		Speed walking
	Horseback riding		Downhill skiing
	Cross country skiing		
	Ice skating**		
	Rowing**		
	Speed walking**		

*After hip arthroplasty only.

**After knee arthroplasty only.

(From WL Healy, R Iorio, M Lemos. Athletic activity after joint replacement. *Am J Sports Med.* 2001;29:377–388.)

Key Point:

When an impairment based measurement such as limited knee joint range of motion is linked to a functional limitation such as an inability to drive a truck and a disability such as an inability to participate in family functions or work activities, both the client and the rehabilitation clinician are more likely to appreciate the relevance of the therapeutic exercise program and the importance of developing an effective relationship.

THE REHABILITATION–CONDITIONING TRANSITION: ACHIEVING FUNCTIONAL READINESS

The human body consists of multiple systems that must function in harmony. This section introduces a series of basic steps and natural progressions that are essential to preparing the client for either a return to athletic activities or to a physically challenging vocation. This process begins with preparing the core region of the body for the stabilization demands of intense activities. The process ends with athletic movement challenges designed to test the client's capacity for maintaining appropriate three dimensional dynamic joint stabilization when confronted

TABLE 11.11   Sports participation of clients with joint replacements based upon level of impact loading

Impact level	Examples	Recommendations
Low	Stationary cycling	• Can improve general health
	Calisthenics	• Desirable for most clients, but may increase rate of wear
	Golf	• Orthotics and activity modifications can reduce impact loads
	Stationary skiing	• Concentration on conditioning and flexibility rather than strengthening
	Swimming	
	Walking	
	Ballroom dancing	
	Water aerobics	
Potentially low	Bowling	• Desirable for most clients, but may increase rate of wear
	Fencing	• Requires pre-activity evaluation, monitoring and development of guidelines by surgeon
	Rowing	
	Isokinetic strength training	• Balance and proprioception must be intact
	Sailing	• Orthotics and activity modifications can reduce impact loads
	Speed walking	• Emphasize high number and repetitions with minimal resistance
	Cross country skiing	
	Table tennis	
	Jazz dancing and ballet	
	Bicycling	
Intermediate	Free weight lifting	• Appropriate only for selected clients
	Hiking	• Requires pre-activity evaluation, monitoring and development of guidelines for participation by surgeon
	Horseback riding	
	Ice skating	• Excellent physical condition is necessary
	Rock climbing	• Orthotics, impact-absorbing shoes and activity modification are frequently necessary
	Low impact aerobics	
	Tennis	
	In line skating	
	Downhill skiing	
High	Baseball/softball	• Should be avoided
	Basketball/volleyball	• Significant probability of injury and need for revision
	Football	
	Handball/racketball	
	Jogging/running	
	Lacrosse	
	Soccer	
	Water skiing	
	Karate	

(From TP Vail, WJ Mallon, RA Liebelt. Athletic activities after joint arthroplasty. *Sports Med Arthroplasty Rev.* 1996;4:298–305.)

TABLE 11.12   Sports participation for clients with joint replacements based upon anatomic location of arthroplasty

Sport	Acceptable	Possible	Not recommended
Ballet dancing	Shoulder	Hip, knee	
Ballroom dancing	Hip, knee, shoulder		
Baseball/softball			Hip, knee, shoulder
Basketball			Hip, knee, shoulder
Bicycling	Hip, knee, shoulder		
Bowling	Hip, knee	Shoulder	
Calisthenics		Hip, knee, shoulder	
Cross country skiing	Hip, knee, shoulder		
Downhill skiing	Shoulder	Hip, knee	
Fencing		Hip, knee	Shoulder
Football			Hip, knee, shoulder
Golf	Hip, knee, shoulder		
Handball/racketball		Shoulder	Hip, knee
Hiking	Shoulder	Hip, knee	
Horseback riding	Hip, knee, shoulder		
Ice skating	Hip, knee, shoulder		
In line skating	Hip, knee, shoulder		
Jazz dancing	Shoulder	Hip, knee	
Jogging/running	Shoulder	Hip, knee	
Karate			Hip, knee, shoulder
Lacrosse			Hip, knee, shoulder
Low impact aerobics	Hip, knee, shoulder		
Rock climbing		Hip, knee, shoulder	
Rowing	Hip, knee	Shoulder	
Sailing	Hip, knee, shoulder		
Soccer		Shoulder	Hip, knee
Speed walking	Hip, knee, shoulder		
Stationary cycling	Hip, knee, shoulder		
Stationary skiing	Hip, knee, shoulder		
Swimming	Hip, knee	Shoulder	
Table tennis		Hip, knee, shoulder	
Tennis		Hip, knee, shoulder	
Volleyball			Hip, knee, shoulder
Walking	Hip, knee, shoulder		
Water aerobics	Hip, knee, shoulder		
Water skiing		Hip, knee	Shoulder

(From TP Vail, WJ Mallon, RA Liebelt. Athletic activities after joint arthroplasty. *Sports Med Arthroplasty Rev.* 1996;4:298–305.)

with spontaneous cues during the performance of functionally relevant, activity specific movement patterns. Positive reinforcement by the rehabilitation clinician is considered to be essential to developing the client's confidence level.

Since at this phase in treatment the rehabilitation clinician generally does not see the client as frequently, developing a trusting relationship is essential to achieving adequate program compliance, particularly with the avoidance of over-training (see Chapter 5). When the client is attempting to return to an athletic activity in the middle of the competitive season, they will need to develop a conditioning base to meet the demands of the activity prior to any consideration of being released to a competitive situation. An initial short term goal may be to complete a 30-minute run covering 3.5 miles with sprint intervals (see Chapter 4), or perhaps to complete an obstacle course that incorporates a mix of lower extremity strength, agility, and dynamic stabilization demands over a designated time (see Chapters 5 and 9). Once the rehabilitation clinician understands the goals and objectives of the client, they can begin to design a conditioning program that will enhance the client's return to activity readiness.

Phase I. Core Muscle Activation

The first step in this process begins with teaching the client to activate core muscles. Activation of the core musculature should precede every movement pattern the client performs. Ultimately, the client will only be as strong as the weakest link along the kinetic or kinematic chain. For most clients, that weak link, particularly after recovering from upper or lower extremity joint injury or surgery, is strength in the core region of the body. Many clients have low back pain or have experienced abdominal, hip flexor, or groin muscle strains. Strong upper and lower extremities with a weak core represent an injury waiting to happen. Virtually all upper and lower extremity movements are initiated from and supported by musculature in the core region.

The *core* includes all of the musculature of the lumbopelvic region and all muscles that make attachment on the pelvis. A strong core goes considerably beyond just having a visible abdominal muscle "six pack." Having a strong core represents the capacity to dynamically stabilize the lumbopelvic and hip regions during three dimensional movement challenges.

> ## *Key Point:*
> A strong core represents the capacity to dynamically stabilize the lumbopelvic and hip regions during three dimensional movement challenges.

Abdominal muscle activation begins by actively drawing in the navel toward the lumbar spine. This simple action activates all of the low back region musculature, creating a dynamically stable base for movement with reduced lumbar spine stress. While performing this movement the client should also activate the hip musculature to stabilize the pelvis maintaining a slight, but not excessive, anterior pelvic tilt, maintaining the natural curvature of the lumbopelvic region. This foundational posture essential to dynamic stabilization of the lumbopelvic region should be assumed prior to performance of every movement and maintained until the movement is completed.

Phase II. Assessment

The second step in achieving functional readiness for return to activities includes a series of simple maneuvers that enables the rehabilitation clinician to assess the existing conditioning level of the client to help decide on what intensity level would be appropriate to achieve a positive training effect without risking injury. The maneuvers that are selected will depend on the client's specific injury and current conditioning level. Assessing balance, joint flexibility, musculotendinous extensibility, core strength, and endurance should be considered when selecting these tests and measurements. It is important for the client to understand the purpose of the tests and realize how progress and eventual release to full activity depends directly on on their ability to perform the selected maneuvers effectively.

As an example, let's consider a female college soccer player, Holly, who is nine months post-anterior cruciate ligament (ACL) reconstruction surgery at her right knee. Her goal is be fully functional for the fall competitive soccer season. To do this, she will need to demonstrate multi-directional speed and agility, "explosive" movements, muscular (anerobic) and aerobic endurance, and total body strength. The first test selected might be a postural analysis to look for asymmetry in shoulder and iliac crest heights; excessive lumbar spine lordosis or kyphosis; asymmetrical muscle hypertrophy or lower extremity alignments; and any other asymmetrical postural alignments that might contribute to knee joint re-injury. Detailed observation may identify muscular strength and extensibility imbalances and areas of restricted joint function that necessitate immediate attention prior to implementation of an intense conditioning program. In addition to a static postural examination, evaluating Holly during a slow jog, with exaggerated or reverse or retro motions, may further help to delineate problems that need attention. Key components to look for during the jog activities include:

■ Core stabilization—neutral pelvic tilt (sagittal plane)
■ Symmetrical stride length (sagittal plane)
■ Appropriate upper body rotation (transverse plane)
■ Balanced arm and leg swing (sagittal plane)

- Patella tracking with the second metatarsal of the foot (frontal plane)
- Symmetrical joint range of motion and musculotendinous extensibility (sagittal and frontal planes)
- Good overall posture with retracted shoulders (sagittal and frontal plane)

Key Point:

Both static and dynamic postural evaluations should be performed prior to intensive pre-activity conditioning program participation.

The second series of tests include a sit and reach flexibility test (see Chapter 3) and a vertical jump test (see Chapter 5). These tests will evaluate Holly's composite lower extremity and low back joint flexibility and musculotendinous extensibility and lower extremity power, respectively. Incorporating lower extremity power training and dynamic stretching are essential conditioning program elements to prepare Holly for the stresses of competitive athletic activities.

Holly's aerobic conditioning level at baseline can be evaluated by having her perform a timed two-mile run or a similar distance on a stationary bicycle. Running is preferred because it is more specific to soccer, but the identification of strength or musculotendinous extensibility imbalances may necessitate a substitute method of evaluating her aerobic condition. Whenever possible, the rehabilitation clinician should attempt to evaluate baseline conditioning levels with consideration of sport, position, and style of play (fast break or pressing vs. set-up style) specificity versus generic, non-specific conditioning. Other tests that can be used to determine aerobic and anerobic system baseline conditioning include beep tests (progressively shorter interval repeats with verbal cueing), interval sprints, and a 300 yd shuttle run) (see Chapters 5 and 9). Regardless of which particular tests are selected, they should be consistently employed across the course of the conditioning program.

Key Point:

Conditioning level tests should be used consistently across the course of the conditioning program so the client and rehabilitation clinician can effectively assess improvements over time.

Coaches of differing sports have specific tests that they prefer to use to evaluate the conditioning level of their athletes. Some tests have been developed for sport specific conditioning (the beep test for soccer, line drills for basketball) and some coaches prefer more traditional methods

such as the timed mile. Depending on Holly's injury history, her existing conditioning level, mutually established goals, and knowledge of the competitive environment to which she will be returning, the rehabilitation clinician should choose the tests that they deem to be most appropriate. Remember, testing standards will vary on a client to client basis. The focal point for functional readiness testing is proper execution of the selected maneuvers. For example, can Holly maintain appropriate technique during repetitive single leg bounding? If not, the test should be terminated and bounding technique and strength training should resume. This is a common sign that the client is not ready for progression to the next step.

The final series of tests include methods of evaluating Holly's muscular strength and dynamic joint stability. Dynamic tests such as walking lunges (**Figure 11.8**), step-ups with a unilateral dumbbell press (**Figure 11.9**) (● **Section 3, Animation 1**), barbell squats (**Figure 11.10**) (● **Section 3, Animation 2**), power cleans (**Figure 11.11**) (● **Section 3, Animation 3**), deadlifts (**Figure 11.12**) (● **Section 3, Animation 4**) and single leg squats (**Figure 11.13**) will provide excellent indicators of functional lower extremity strength. These tests necessitate that Holly display dynamic joint stability and balance without the assistance of machines or other supports. The rationale for this is that she will not be able to rely on machines or other supports after returning to the playing field. It is critical that proper lifting techniques be used while performing these strength tests. Critical points to observe during the performance of these maneuvers are dynamic core stabilization, patella–second metatarsal tracking, knee over ankle (not foot), and evenly distributed, well balanced force distribution.

When performing the strength tests with submaximal or body weight resistance, Holly should be able to pause (3 to 6 seconds) at any point during the movement. For example, while executing body weight squats (**Figure 11.14**) periodically ask her to pause at different points

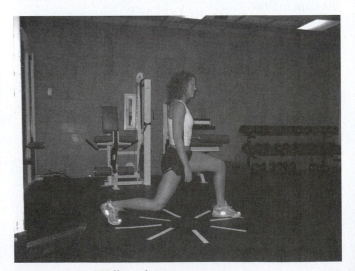

Figure 11.8   Walking lunges.

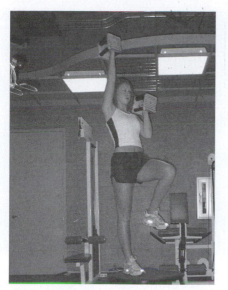

Figure 11.9   Dumbbell step-ups with unilateral press.

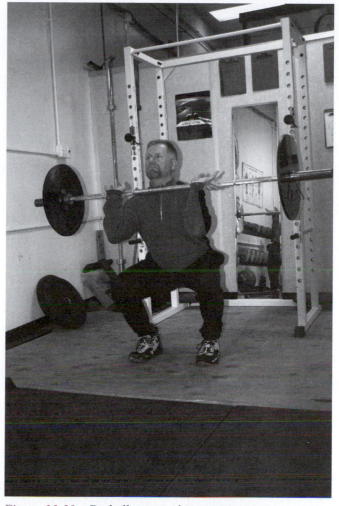

Figure 11.11   Barbell power clean.

during the movement and attempt to maintain an isometric muscle contraction at that point. The pause is effective for several reasons: It creates an opportunity for the rehabilitation clinician to instruct in proper technique or to give positive feedback; it forces Holly to keep her dynamic core stabilizers activated in order to maintain balance; and it enables her to train at weak points in the range of motion and eventually develop a sense of safety during the movement. If she is not able to pause, her technique is incorrect, she is using too much resistance, or she does not have adequate strength to perform the maneuver.

Key Point:

Pausing during body weight or low resistance movements at a specific point in the range of motion is an excellent method of instructing the client in proper technique, providing positive feedback, increasing endurance of the muscles that provide dynamic stability to the core, working at weak points in the range of motion, and increasing the client's confidence in their ability to perform the movement.

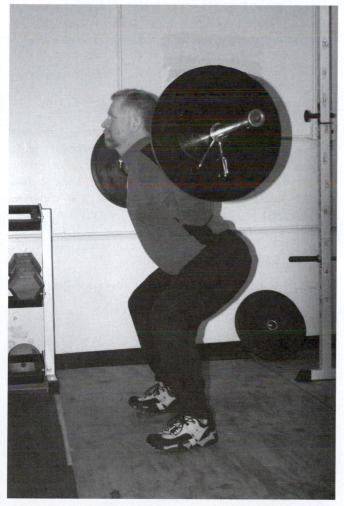

Figure 11.10   Barbell squat.

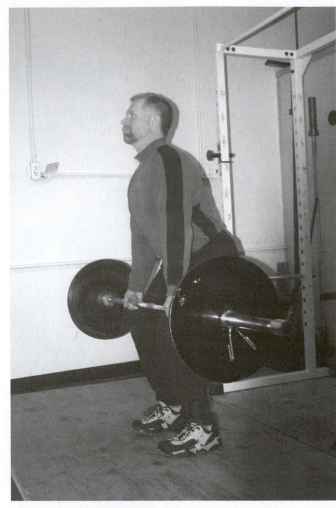

Figure 11.12   Barbell deadlift.

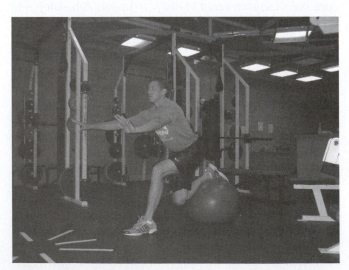

Figure 11.13   Single leg squat with stability ball.

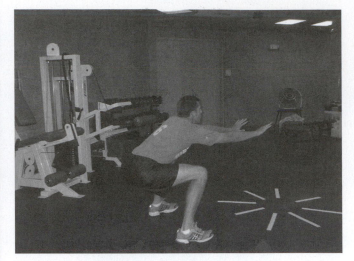

Figure 11.14   Body weight squat.

If Holly still cannot perform the maneuver correctly even with only body weight resistance, the rehabilitation clinician may need to select less intense maneuvers to gradually develop the functional strength needed to hold the pause. The pause technique is also helpful during basic running drills like "high knees," butt kicks, and assorted agility maneuvers (see Chapter 9). Once the testing has been completed the rehabilitation clinician can begin to design an individualized conditioning program for Holly. Remember that Holly's goals are a priority during program development.

Phase III. Program Development

The "nuts and bolts" of developing a functional strength and conditioning plan include many of the key elements identified during the testing process. The plan should consist of, but not be limited to, the elements that follow. The rehabilitation clinician is reminded that creativity should be used to develop sports specific tasks, and appropriate technique is paramount to whatever tasks are selected. The key components of a functional readiness conditioning program are as follows:

- Dynamic warm-up and stretch
- Core stabilization with proper transfer of motion
- Movement efficiency
- Balance and flexibility
- Running technique and speed
- Strength training
- Agility training
- Plyometric training
- Conditioning
- Holistic ideas

A sample program will now be discussed for our collegiate soccer athlete, Holly.

Dynamic Warm-Up and Stretch.   The environment selected for Holly to perform conditioning program activities will depend largely on her existing level of conditioning. Ideally, most of these activities will be performed on a soccer field with her wearing running shoes and/or rubber soccer cleats. This variable training surface will provide a greater challenge and will enhance the specificity of the program. All dynamic warm-up drills will be performed over a 20-yd distance. Beginning maneuvers will include jogging, skipping, running with "high knees," running with "butt kicks," and the "grapevine" or carioca. Each maneuver will be performed forwards, backwards, sideways, and diagonally (see Chapter 5). As Holly performs several repetitions of each maneuver, her heart rate will begin to increase and her body temperature will rise (see Chapter 3). This provides an excellent opportunity to stretch her major muscles groups in a dynamic setting versus stretching cold muscles in a stationary setting. This warm-up with dynamic stretching is similar to the pre-practice or pre-competition activities that Holly will perform when she rejoins the soccer team. This form of stretching is particularly useful in conditioning bi-articular lower extremity muscles.[144,145] As the warm-up continues, low intensity plyometric activities such as forward, backward, and lateral double leg hopping movements are performed with soft, quiet landings (see Chapters 5 and 6). This technique initiates body control and dynamic knee joint stabilization, which is imperative to prevent further injury (see Chapters 6 and 7). Another key factor to incorporate into the dynamic warm-up is the pause. For example, as Holly executes a forward running drill with high knees, she will be cued to pause every third step while maintaining perfect balance and technique, necessitating immediate dynamic core stabilization. This pause provides an opportunity for the rehabilitation clinician to check for proper posture, joint alignment and running technique, and provide feedback. As Holly comes out of the pause, she is forced to integrate motion from the core region to composite body function. Again, the pause technique should be used in all movement directions as Holly's strength and stability improves.

Depending on a client's existing conditioning level, the dynamic warm-up is sometimes used for the entire conditioning program merely by extending activity duration and decreasing rest periods. The rehabilitation clinician is reminded, however, to avoid subjecting Holly to excessive fatigue where appropriate technique is no longer maintained. Once Holly is completely warmed up and all muscles have been actively stretched, more intensive conditioning maneuvers can be performed.

> ## Key Point:
> Proper movement technique must be maintained throughout all aspects of functional readiness training.

Agilities and Plyometrics.   According to Gambetta,[146] agility is the ability to decelerate, accelerate, and change direction quickly while maintaining body control without decreasing speed (see Chapter 9). The creativity level of the rehabilitation clinician is the limiting factor when developing agility and plyometric drills. Low intensity levels should be used at first with progressive increases as ability improves. Speed of execution should also begin slowly and increase with confidence and ability. Key factors to watch for while performing agility drills include movement efficiency and proper transfer of motion. *Efficiency of movement* simply means performing the tasks with as few extraneous movements as possible (making sharp cuts without extra steps), maintaining forward motion with appropriate postural alignment of all body parts, and basic core stabilization. Proper *transfer of motion* is detectable by watching the arms and legs move with respect to the torso or core. If Holly appears to be unbalanced or uncoordinated during these tasks, the problem usually lies with a lack of dynamic core stabilization. When this occurs the rehabilitation clinician needs to re-assess the difficulty of the task and possibly go back to incorporating a pause in the movements to encourage her to reconnect with the center or core. A sample qualitative method of evaluating frontal and sagittal plane performance during single or double leg hopping or jumping tasks is presented in **Table 11.13**. Holly should be able to perform each activity with precision before moving to the next level, otherwise bad habits and injury will likely occur.

Some common agility drills include the pro agility drill, dot drills (**Figure 11.15**) , speed ladder drills, various cone courses, and simple running patterns (see Chapters 5 and 9). Many variations exist, but the "magic" agility drill does not, so the rehabilitation clinician is advised to create drills to fit the needs of the individual client. Reaction time drills are also important when focusing on agility training. During actual sporting events, many potentially injurious movement patterns are performed as spontaneous reactions. It is prudent to put Holly "on the spot" and force her to process visual and auditory cues as she attempts to maintain speed during sudden directional changes (see Chapters 8 and 9). This can be simulated during training sessions by using a whistle, handclap, flashing light, or silent hand movements. Sample drills include stop and go progressions during straight, lateral, diagonal, or backward running drills. The stopping pattern may be a double leg hop stop or a simple jump stop followed by a tuck jump. Reaction drills are a good indoor training alternative if bad weather prevents outdoor activities. Agility and reaction drills can be performed daily. Due to the repetitious eccentric loads and delayed onset muscle soreness associated with plyometric drills, they should not be performed daily. Additionally, the rehabilitation clinician is advised to use caution and a keen eye when determining the appropriate level of difficulty and volume of plyometric activities. Plyometric exercises should be performed no more than two to

TABLE 11.13   Sample qualitative scoring form to grade frontal and sagittal plane jumping landing technique

	Frontal plane			Sagittal plane		
	2	**1**	**0**	**2**	**1**	**0**
Eye and head alignment	Head centered, eyes looking forward	Head to one side, eyes looking forward	Head to one side, eyes looking down at feet	Head up, eyes looking forward	Head slightly down, eyes looking down at feet	Head down, eyes looking down at feet
Trunk alignment	Well centered trunk	Slight trunk lean during landing	Excessive trunk lean during landing	Slightly flexed, chest over knees	Excessively flexed, chest collapse with landing	Extended, not using hip extensors
Arm alignment	Symmetrical with slight, controlled arm-swing (abduction), with low guard	Symmetrical with moderate, controlled arm-swing (abduction), with low guard	Asymmetrical with poorly controlled arm-swing (abduction) with high guard	Symmetrical with slight, controlled arm-swing (flexion) with low guard	Symmetrical with moderate controlled arm-swing (flexion) with low guard	Asymmetrical with poorly controlled arm-swing (flexion) with high guard
Hip-thigh alignment	Symmetrical with alignment over feet without excessive adduction or abduction during controlled, soft landing	Symmetrical with moderate adduction or abduction during controlled, soft landing	Asymmetrical adduction or abduction, knees touch or flare outward (extreme coxa varus or valgus) noted during a poorly controlled landing	Symmetrical with moderate hip flexion during controlled soft landing	Symmetrical with excessive hip flexion during controlled soft landing	Asymmetrical or with excessive or minimal hip flexion during poorly controlled landing

Knee-leg alignment

Symmetrical alignment over feet without visible wobble or sway during controlled, soft landing	Symmetrical abduction or adduction, slight wobble or sway noted during controlled, soft landing	Asymmetrical abduction or adduction, knees touch or flare outward (extreme genu valgus or varus) noted during a poorly controlled landing
2	1	0
Symmetrical with moderate knee flexion during controlled soft landing	Symmetrical with excessive knee flexion during controlled soft landing	Asymmetrical or with excessive or minimal knee flexion during poorly controlled landing
2	1	0

Ankle-foot alignment

Symmetrical with feet aligned with toes pointing forward or slightly toed out during controlled, soft landing	Symmetrical with feet moderately toed out or toed in during controlled, soft landing	Asymmetrical with one or both feet, extremely toed out or toed in, or a secondary hop during a poorly controlled landing
2	1	0
Symmetrical with moderate ankle dorsiflexion during controlled soft landing	Symmetrical with excessive ankle dorsiflexion during controlled soft landing	Asymmetrical or with excessive or minimal ankle dorsiflexion during poorly controlled landing
2	1	0

Total frontal plane score = _____ /12

Total sagittal plane score = _____ /12

Overall qualitative jump landing score = _____ /24 = _____ %

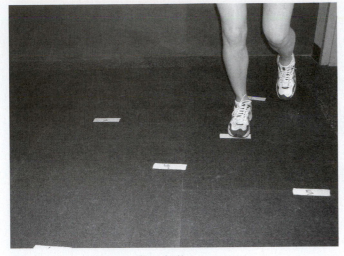

Figure 11.15   Dot agility drill.

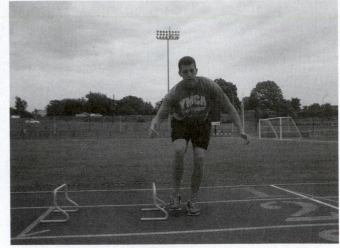

Figure 11.16   Lateral hop plyometric maneuver with a pause.

three times per week, depending on muscle recovery and soreness.[147] It is essential that in the landing phase the client employ soft, quiet, and balanced landings with appropriate postural control and dynamic joint stabilization (see Chapters 5 and 6).

Key Point:

A soft, quiet, well controlled double or single leg landing suggests the presence of appropriate dynamic joint stabilization.

Progression involves beginning with double leg activities moving into single leg activities. It is imperative to control rest periods to allow for proper recovery given the ultimate goal of plyometrics activities, which is to improve power, not endurance. Various forms of plyometric activities include bounding, hopping, jumping, skipping, box jumps, hurdle jumps, depth jumps, etc. Incorporating the pause phase during plyometric activity performance can also aid in facilitating dynamic joint stabilization. For example, Holly might perform a series of double leg jumps through a set of low hurdles while pausing in a squat position between each hurdle (**Figure 11.16**). This allows for maximum core stabilization, provides an opportunity to critique technique, and adds extra strengthening potential. Proper squat technique is imperative, with body weight distributed back toward the heels, knees over the ankle, and chest up in a good posture. The plyometric drills can be performed in all directions and planes, as the dynamic warm-up drills were conducted. During competition, change of direction and power demands are often not predictable; therefore, it is imperative to prepare Holly for these circumstances.

Running Technique and Speed Training.   There are numerous theories on how running technique and speed training should be performed. The specifics of these components are beyond the scope of this chapter, but a great deal of literature has been published regarding both topics and the rehabilitation clinician is advised to review it prior to implementing a program.[144–148,149] These are important components of sport specific training and should be included in Holly's program.

Strength Training.   Applying functional strength training principles into the functional readiness program involves a few gadgets or machines in addition to a creative mind (see Chapters 5, 6, and 7). Effective programs can be designed using only a set of dumbbells, a stability or Swiss ball, and medicine balls of varying resistance. Selected activities should include movements that are applicable to Holly's specific sport or lifestyle. For example, multidirectional lunges can be transferred directly into soccer specific movement. The emphasis for each exercise begins with activating the core muscles and performing the movement with absolute control and balance. When using dumbbells, combining alternating upper and lower extremity movements can be used to challenge Holly to better maintain core stability. For example, she may perform a unilateral dumbbell press in combination with a walking lunge or step-up maneuver (**see Figure 11.9**). Again, another variable to add increasing difficulty and dynamic core stabilization challenge is the pause. Squats (**Figure 11.17**) or lunges (**Figure 11.18**) performed with a pause at the bottom or performed on an unstable surface like a balance disc or wobble board (● **Section 3, Animation 5**) will similarly improve dynamic joint stabilization.[150] Other effective conditioning activities that may be useful when preparing Holly for a return to activity include multidirectional lunges with alternating dumbbell presses, single or double leg straight leg dead lifts, jump squats with a medicine ball

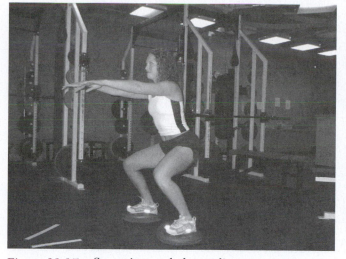

Figure 11.17   Squatting on balance discs.

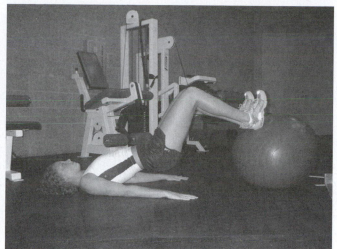

Figure 11.19   Bridge with leg curl.

throw, multidirectional step-ups with alternating dumbbell presses, stability ball leg curls **(Figure 11.19)** (⦿ **Section 3, Animation 6)**, stability ball pike-ups with a trunk twist **(Figure 11.20)** (⦿ **Section 3, Animation 7)**, stability ball bridging **(Figure 11.21)** (⦿ **Section 3, Animation 8)**, supine dumbbell chest presses on a stability ball, chin-ups or pull-ups, push-ups on a stability ball, power cleans, push-jerk and clean-to-jerk movements using dumbbells with alternating arms on the jerk movement.

Conditioning.   Conditioning is a primary facet of athletic performance, as are strength, agility, plyometric training, and flexibility. Sport specificity can also be applied in the conditioning plan. For example, just because Holly can run a sub-five minute mile does not mean she is adequately conditioned to withstand a 45-minute half of a soccer game. It is important to develop a conditioning program based on progressive drills and decreasing recovery periods. In general, the less time Holly needs to re-

cover between exercise sets and sessions, the greater her fitness level. The target energy system will determine the intensity, volume, and recovery time allotted for a drill (see Chapters 2 and 4). For example, to target the aerobic system the intensity of exercise may be at a 70 percent to 80 percent exertion rate for 30–45 minutes with little or no rest. Specific examples include distance runs, *Fartlek training* (speed play or run-spring intervals), or repeat 800-m sprints. Examples of targeting the anaerobic system may include 100-m sprints with a full two to three minutes of active recovery, stadium stair sprints, or a weight training circuit. When considering the fitness needs of a soccer player like Holly, the training emphasis must be placed on speed-endurance. A soccer midfielder may run more than seven miles in one game; however, the game also involves multidirectional sprinting, jogging, walking, powerful running directional changes, jumping and jump stopping movements, and physical contact. Due to these specific circumstances, the conditioning program

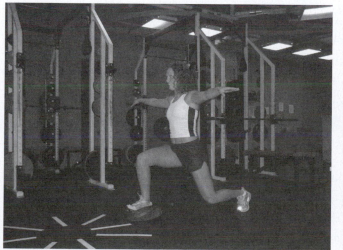

Figure 11.18   Forward lunge on a balance disc.

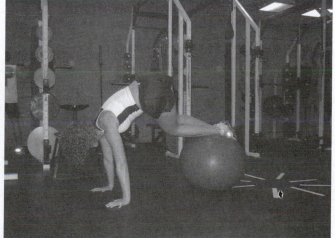

Figure 11.20   Pike-up with torso twist.

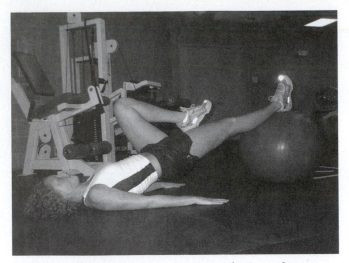

Figure 11.21   Bridge with alternating knee to chest.

must include activities that simulate each of these challenges. A sample week of conditioning for Holly is presented in **Table 11.14.** Intensity, volume, and recovery time will change as Holly gains soccer specific fitness.

Holistic ideas.   Many coaches would be pleased if athletic success were based solely on physiological variables. However, when dealing with human beings, many factors contribute to the corresponding levels of success. Especially in our ever changing world, today's client has become more aware of variables that may influence their athletic or vocational performance. The rehabilitation clinician should remember to help the client develop a positive attitude and self-image and understand proper nutrition (see Chapter 2) and the importance of adequate hydration and

recovery time. Stress management techniques will be discussed later in this chapter.

Return to Competition

How do you determine when Holly is ready to return to full activity? Unfortunately, there is no definite answer to this question. However, there are signs and key factors to look for when making this decision. Once Holly can complete all of the activities previously mentioned in this section, it is time to consider the return to full activity option. It is imperative that Holly display proficiency in the warm-up drills and in agility, plyometric, reaction time, and strength-conditioning activities before being placed in the uncontrolled environment of competitive athletic play. All of the activities previously mentioned in this section while attempting to improve Holly's physiological capacity for returning to play are also intended to develop her mental confidence. Often the client will be physically able to compete, but their mental state will not enable them to perform. If Holly is struggling mentally the rehabilitation clinician must continue to build her confidence through physical activity and positive feedback. Some physical signs to look for when deciding when to return a client to activity are listed in **Table 11.15.** The key factors listed in **Table 11.15** are important to watch for during practice or competition. If a client such as Holly displays more attributes from the left column, competition should be the next step. If a large percent of factors from the right column appear, the client should continue drills in a controlled setting. Provide weekly opportunities for the client to attempt movements in a semi-competitive setting. Transition can occur rapidly, so be aware of progress. Appropriate strength training and conditioning should be a part of the client's life for as long they desire to remain athletically active.

TABLE 11.14   Sample functional readiness training program for Holly

Monday	Tuesday	Wednesday	Thursday	Friday
10 min. dynamic warm-up	10 min. dynamic warm-up	10 min. dynamic warm-up	10 min. dynamic warm-up	10 min. dynamic warm-up
	10 min. agility drills	30 min. interval run		10 min. agility drills
10 min. agility drills	10–15 min. plyometric drills	15 min. interval sprints on stationary bicycle	10 min. agility drills	5 min. reaction drills
5 min. reaction drills				3, 400 m sprints
3 mile run in < 23 min				4, 200 m sprints
Total body weight training	10–50 yd sprints		10–15 min. plyometric drills	6, 100 m sprints
	10–30 yd sprints	Upper body weight training		
	10–20 yd sprints		20–30 min. stadium stair sprints	Lower body weight training
Abdominal exercises	Cool down/stretch	Abdominal exercises	Cool down/stretch	Abdominal exercises
Cool down/ stretch		Stretching		Stretching

TABLE 11.15   Functional readiness indicators

Ready to compete	Not ready to compete
Structural integrity	Loose joints
Dynamic balance	Off balance
Bilateral movement symmetry	Favors one side
Core stability	Out of control
Executes sharp, angular cuts	Performs loopy directional changes
Bilateral hypertrophy	Unilateral hypertrophy
Non-impaired joint mobility	Restricted joint mobility
Endurant muscular function	Early muscular fatigue, sloppy movements
Aerobic fitness	Bent over posture when running, or decides to walk
Decelerates with a low center of gravity	Decelerates with an upright posture
Displays first step quickness with acceleration	Does not move with "explosive" quickness

RETURN TO ACTIVITY DECISION MAKING

The question often asked the rehabilitation clinician is when will a client be ready to return to activity, rather than how are they doing in terms of health, and how will the injury the client sustained affect his or her life down the road? Matheson[151] advises asking the following three alternative questions before attempting to decide on return to activity:

1. What is the medical diagnosis? (without this, there can be no objective discussion of injury management, prognosis, or return to play timetable).

2. What are the best interventions to perform for both the short and long term health of the client? Proper decision making for both the immediate and long-term outcome is what effective health care is all about.[151] Only once the first two questions have been addressed can the final question be addressed.

3. When can the client return to activity? While the first two questions are solely health care related, the final question is related more to return activity environment (recreational athletics, vocation, etc.). Too often the return to activity question gets asked first and the health care team fails to re-sequence the questions, making the mistake of attempting to answer the third question before having answered the first two. From the perspective of the rehabilitation clinician we suggest adding a new second question: What are the physical dysfunctions or movement related impairments experienced by the client? Even when answering the return to activity question it is advisable to use broad recovery times with more concrete information regarding specific functional milestones (range of mo-

tion, strength, power, endurance, etc.) that must be achieved first.

In evaluating the return to athletic activity decision making process following cervical spine injury, Morganti et al.[152] reported a wide variability of physician responses, related to the opinion/personal bias, clinical experience, clinical training, geographic area, and the medico-legal environment of the physician. The return to activity decision can be difficult for all involved in the process, including the client, their family, and their coaches or employer. Potential re-injury risk factors are often not well defined, and the risk to benefit ratio differs depending on the values, biases and opinions of the decision makers.[152] The client, once advised to refrain from activity, may seek a second opinion. Differing recommendations among health care providers can further confuse and distress all involved in the process. This may be particularly true in cases of neck-injured athletes, because the risk of a bad outcome includes catastrophic injury.[152,153] Collision sports and high velocity sports are perceived to hold a greater risk for further cervical spine injury (**Table 11.16**).

Athletes of all ages are reluctant to miss a portion of a season or even a single game due to an injury. Three areas in which rehabilitation clinicians who treat injured athletes need to be particularly careful are: 1) providing treatment designed to enable continued play with an injury before it is fully healed; 2) informing an athlete of the potential health risks of continued athletic activity given their physical condition, and 3) evaluating and advising an athlete concerning their physical ability to resume athletic activity.[154] Courts have held that the failure of health care personnel to fully disclose to an athlete the potential adverse health consequences of proposed treatment or playing with their medical condition creates legal liability. Clients have the right to determine what to do with their

TABLE 11.16   Classification of type of play

	Type of play
1	Collision sports (e.g., football, hockey)
2	Contact sports (e.g., lacrosse, basketball)
3	Noncontact, high velocity sports (e.g., skiing, gymnastics)
4	Noncontact, repetitive load sports (e.g., running)
5	Noncontact, low impact sports (e.g., golf, bowling)
6	No sports

(From C Morganti, CA Sweeney, SA Albanese, et al. Return to play after cervical spine injury. *Spine.* 2001;26(10):1131–1136.)

own bodies and generally rely upon health care personnel to provide them with the information necessary to make a responsible decision regarding proposed health care treatment and activity participation under the circumstances.[154] Along with the referring physician, the rehabilitation clinician should clearly warn an injured client about the known short and long term risks associated with continued participation. The possibility of alternative treatments that may delay a return to play but further a client's medical best interests should also be discussed. Such information should be disclosed in simple language so that the injured client can understand the potential adverse consequences to their health and make responsible decisions about undergoing treatment or returning to activity. There is potential legal liability for providing medically unjustified treatment to enable athletic participation, negligently clearing a client to full activity, or failing to inform a client of the material risks of aggravating an injury or suffering permanent disability or impairment while playing.[155] Although one of the rehabilitation clinician's objectives may be to facilitate an injured client's return to competitive activity, greater concern should be placed on restoring their physical function, non-impaired movement, and their ability to engage in everyday activities of daily living without long term impairment. The rehabilitation clinician is not liable for a good faith error in judgment if they use ordinary care in establishing a rehabilitation program consistent with an injured client's medical best interests.[155]

To determine an injured client's physical ability, the rehabilitation clinician needs a reliable means of evaluating whether or not they are able to satisfy the physical requirements of the activity. Objective criteria and guidelines will assist the rehabilitation clinician in making this determination and provide a basis for a recommendation consistent with a client's physical well being. There are close parallels between industrial rehabilitation and sports physical therapy in that both clients are expected to return quickly to productive levels in their respective arenas.[154]

Decisions to resume participation in sports or work both need to be based on the best available objective data. Rehabilitation clinicians who work in industry currently use functional/physical capacity evaluations to obtain this type of information. By having the worker perform lifting, climbing, pushing, pulling, and other job related activities, objective data can be obtained regarding their ability to fulfill job requirements. Similar approaches are used with athletically active clients. For example, objective criteria for a running back to return to play after an ankle injury may include factors such as his ability to run a specified distance or cut at a particular angle without significant loss of speed due to pain or dysfunction. The client's post-injury speed could be compared to his pre-injury speed.

Some medical organizations have developed guidelines for determining whether an athlete with a physical abnormality or disorder should be medically cleared to play a sport. In a joint effort to protect the health and safety of athletes the American Academy of Family Physicians, American Academy of Pediatrics, American Medical Society for Sports Medicine, and the American Osteopathic Academy of Sports Medicine recently published a monograph establishing guidelines for preparticipation physical evaluation and medical disqualification of young athletes.[156] Along with the need for athletic participation guidelines for pre-existing medical conditions, there is a corresponding need for return to play guidelines following sports injuries.[154] The rehabilitation clinician has a unique opportunity to provide sound counseling to an injured client because of the comparatively larger amount of time they spend with them during the therapeutic exercise process compared to the referring physician.

Functional Performance Tests

Single leg hop tests are commonly used as physical performance measures of function, particularly for clients who are recovering from ACL reconstruction surgery.[157] A variety of hop tests have been described, including forward single leg hops for distance,[158–160] lateral single leg hops for distance,[161] hop and stop,[162] and vertical jump tests.[158,163] Rehabilitation clinicians rely on single leg hop tests to assess their clients' lower extremity muscular power and ability to withstand sudden loading forces during eccentric muscle activations while maintaining postural control and dynamic joint stability. Hop tests have been used in studies to reflect changes in functional status in response to knee rehabilitation programs.[160,164,165] In most studies, the data indicate that hop test performance generally improves concomitantly with improvements in other outcome measurements that are used to identify improved functional status in response to treatment.

Wilson and Gansneder[166] measured activity scores including the 40 m timed walk, 40 m run, figure-8 run, forward single leg hop, cross over hop,[159] and stairs hop,[164] self-reported athletic ability scores, and selective measures of physical impairment as predictors of disability duration in athletes with acute ankle inversion sprains. While impairment measures accounted for approximately one-third of the variance in disability duration, the addition of the activity limitation measurements to the regression equation improved predictions of disability duration to 67 percent, while activity limitation measurements alone accounted for 65 percent of the total variance in the number of days lost due to injury. They concluded that the effect of impairment (ankle sprain) on disability duration (time away from practice or competition) was mediated by functional limitations (hop on one leg, etc.).

Sapega and Nicholas[167] reported that side-to-side musculoskeletal profiling comparisons are only adequate when there is an uninvolved or non-impaired side to use as a comparative standard and when the musculoskeletal parameters in question are normally symmetrical. Additionally, bilateral comparative analysis provides no information on the absolute performance capabilities of the client within their particular sport and competitive level (see Chapter 5). Properly constructed musculoskeletal profiles enable the rehabilitation clinician to overcome these problems because they establish the normal range of values for muscular strength, endurance, power, flexibility, and other physical performance parameters according to the client's age group, gender, sport, competitive level, playing position, and anthropometric characteristics. Profiles also permit more specific interpretations of bilateral test results because they document the normal range of physical asymmetry when it is typically present such as in throwing and racket sports. By profiling appropriate sample populations from specific groups of clients, objective standards or norms for those groups can be defined. When such norms are available, new dimensions for the evaluation and therapeutic exercise program intervention for injured clients will emerge.

Survey Measurements of Function

Clinical research studies are placing an increased emphasis on the perspective of the client with the use of health related quality of life instruments.[168] Client perspectives can be determined by measuring self-reported functional status, the influence of symptoms, and their concern about or satisfaction with treatments.[169,170] Client expectations are important because they are linked to requests for elective and possibly costly therapeutic interventions and are strongly related to their eventual self-assessment of outcome. Clients have many expectations of knee surgery that vary by medical diagnosis, client values, and functional status.[88]

Subjective assessment of treatment outcome can be obtained by interview or by questionnaires completed by the client at various stages in the treatment progress.[171] A questionnaire is a highly structured form of interview designed for systematic collection of data.[171] Although self-

completion of a questionnaire may be seemingly free from any bias, a client's education level will influence their ability to appropriately complete the questionnaire. Errors such as these can be minimized by keeping the questions simple (**Table 11.17**).

The results of clinical research studies are of questionable value if the measure used to evaluate treatment effectiveness was not *reliable, valid, responsive, flexible* and of adequate *range*. (**Table 11.18**). Surveys are often used as primary outcome measures because they accurately reflect symptoms and disabilities that are specific and important to clients.[168] Responsiveness is dependent not only on the instrument but also on the magnitude of change actually experienced by the client. The magnitude of change measured in a cohort of clients is determined by the initial score (lower initial scores enable more room for improvement), the quality of the intervention, the instrument used to measure the health status, and the statistic that is used to calculate responsiveness.[172]

Key Point:

To be effective a survey instrument should be reliable, valid, responsive, achieve an adequate range of scores and be practical to use.

There is a growing recognition among health policy makers that new approaches must be developed to assess the true value of expensive health care services.[173] Appropriate studies of client outcomes are needed to demonstrate

TABLE 11.17   Factors that affect questionnaire completion

Client characteristics	Literacy level
	Language comprehension
	Personality
	Psychological state
	Tick box fatigue
Questionnaire characteristics	Length of questionnaire
	Ease of comprehension
	Relevance of questions
Other factors	Environment
	Influence of family members or caregivers
	Pending compensation
	Secondary gain

(From RR Bindra, JJ Dias, C Heras-Palau, et al. Assessing outcome after hand surgery: The current state. *J Hand Surg Br.* 2003;28(4):289–294.)

TABLE 11.18   Attributes of an effective questionnaire

	Questionnaire attributes
Reliability	A reliable measurement tool is free from random error and will yield the same results when repeated in the given population under the same testing conditions.
Validity	The instrument can measure what it is supposed to measure for a given application.
Responsiveness	A responsive tool has the ability to detect significant changes over time.
Range	The measurements yielded must be distributed throughout the range without accumulation at either end—the so-called "floor and ceiling effect."
Flexibility	The practical effectiveness in applying the measurement tool in clinical practice.

(From RR Bindra, JJ Dias, C Heras-Palau, et al. Assessing outcome after hand surgery: The current state. *J Hand Surg Br*. 2003;28(4):289–294.)

how therapeutic exercise program interventions improve quality of life and that the procedures are, therefore, economically worthy of continued support by government agencies and by private insurance carriers. Published outcomes studies frequently compare postoperative outcomes with preoperative conditions. The outcomes that need to be measured are the effects of the treatment on the health of those who were treated, and the quality of their lives after receiving the treatment. Such outcome measures are relevant to the appropriateness of the reported treatment for all of the clients who have the condition under study. The reader should be provided with enough information to judge whether the anticipated benefits to health outweigh the anticipated negative effects sufficiently to make the treatment generally worthwhile for their clients.

Sgaglione et al.[174] reported that there is no single outcome measurement format that is optimal for measuring client outcomes following ACL reconstruction surgery. Irrgang et al.[170] reported that a complete system for the evaluation of clinical outcomes should include measures of each disability domain (active pathology, impairment, functional limitation and disability) described by Nagi.[175] Active pathology involves an interruption of or interference with normal processes (due to infection, trauma, metabolic imbalance, degenerative disease, or other etiologies) and the simultaneous efforts of the organism to regain a state of normalcy (see Chapter 1). Clinical measurements of musculoskeletal pathology include information regarding the extent of the injury, disease or condition, and the healing status as determined from the client interview, medical history, clinical examination, laboratory and imaging studies, and the surgical intervention. Some of these clinical measurements for musculoskeletal system impairment include range of motion, muscle function and joint stability. Clinical measurements of functional limitations and disability include performance based clinical tests such as one leg hop tests (see Chapter 5) and client reported assessments. Difficulties associated with the use of performance based measures of function in the clinical setting and the dearth of normative data for inter-

pretation of the results has led rehabilitation clinicians to consider alternatives such as client self-reported measures of function. Client reported measures of function include both general and specific measures of health status. General measures of health status that are commonly used for clients with musculoskeletal conditions include the Medical Outcomes Study Short Form 36 (SF-36),[176–178] SF-12[179] and the Sickness Impact Profile.[180].

Key Point:

A complete system of clinical outcome evaluation should include measures of each disability domain (active pathology, impairment, functional limitation and disability).

As each questionnaire is designed for a specific purpose, they have individual advantages and drawbacks. General health questionnaires have been designed to study the effect of disease on the client as a whole, whereas region specific questionnaires restrict the questions to one part of the body. Disease specific questionnaires are designed for a particular clinical condition and are usually restricted for use in that condition alone.[171] General health questionnaires have too wide a focus to be useful and sensitive in specialized areas like hand or knee surgery. They do however serve as a useful complement to a region specific or disease specific questionnaire.

Specific health status measurements are designed to focus on aspects of health that are specific to a primary condition of interest, with the intent of creating a more responsive measure. Examples of client reported measurements that are specific to the knee include the Lysholm Knee Scoring Scale,[181] the Tegner Knee Rating Scale,[160] the Cincinnati Knee Scale[182] and the Knee Injury and Osteoarthritis Outcome Score (KOOS).[183] Instruments such as the guidelines established by the International Knee Documentation Committee (I.K.D.C.),[184] and those developed by the Knee Society[185] and the Hip Society[186] combine self-reported measures of function with measures of functional limitation following ACL reconstruction, total knee arthroplasty, and total hip arthroplasty, respectively.

Irrgang et al.[170] developed the Knee Outcome Survey (KOS) as a self-reported instrument for the measurement of functional limitations commonly experienced by clients with differing knee disorders (ligament or meniscal injury or reconstruction, osteoarthritis, patellofemoral conditions). The Knee Outcome Survey has two separate scales, the Activity of Daily Living (ADL) and the Sports Activity (SAS) scales. The KOS-ADL Scale can be used to assess functional limitations resulting from a wide range of conditions that affect the knee. The KOS-ADL Scale has been shown to be reliable (reproducible), valid (well substantiated) and responsive (effective at detecting real changes) for measurements of function related to pathological disorders or impairments of the knee.[170] In comparing the Harris Hip Score with SF–36, and a test of walking speed and pain during walking among 75 clients who had osteoarthritis, Hoeksma et al.[187] reported that the Harris Hip Score was more responsive than the other tests for evaluating hip function changes.

Health related quality of life (HRQL) is becoming another frequently reported outcome measurement and refers to those aspects of quality of life that relate specifically to a client's health. The effect of intervention on quality of life assumes significant importance in evaluating the outcome of intervention in conditions such as palliative treatment of cancer when it is clear that the treatment will not affect the survival rate.[188] In addition, when a new treatment with unknown toxic side effects is being evaluated, HRQL measurement provides valuable insight into the effect of the intervention on client well being. There are several validated HRQL indices based on the condition being studied that generally follow the three primary dimensions of physical, mental and social well being included in the World Health Organization's definition of health. If relevant to the particular condition that is being evaluated, additional domains such as general health perceptions, global quality of life, fatigue, self-esteem, and others may also be measured.[171]

The Disabilities of the Arm, Shoulder and Hand questionnaire (DASH) is a region specific tool that was designed to measure the outcome of musculoskeletal conditions and disabilities that affect the entire upper extremity.[189] The advantages of the DASH are its sound development methodology and the normative data that are available for many upper extremity conditions that involve the hand, wrist, elbow, and shoulder. The disadvantage of the DASH is that it is not specific to a joint like the shoulder. For more specific outcome assessment of the shoulder, surveys such as the U.C.L.A. shoulder assessment,[190] the Neer shoulder assessment,[191] the Hospi-

tal for Special Surgery shoulder assessment,[192] the Constant shoulder assessment,[193] the American Shoulder and Elbow Surgeons shoulder evaluation form[194] or the Western Ontario Shoulder Instability Index (WOSI)[195] can be used.

A complete outcome assessment should contain both objective and client reported subjective measurements. Objective measurements are easy to select and usually include those factors that are expected to change after treatment. Factors to be considered when selecting a questionnaire include the study population, the type of study, the disease or condition, and the type of intervention.[171] Recommended assessments should include a combination of a general health questionnaire such as the SF-36 or SF-12 along with a region-specific questionnaire such as the WOSI or Knee Outcome Survey. Used in combination, these tools will provide a good indication of the effect of therapeutic exercise intervention on restoring function as well as on the overall improvement in general health status.[171] The transition of the use of outcome assessment measurements from the domain of research and epidemiology to routine clinical practice has been a gradual one. Rehabilitation clinician should stay current with this ever changing area of practice.

STRESS MANAGEMENT

Data suggest that health locus of control may well be a factor in injury proneness and frequency of reported injuries by highly stressed, externally controlled female cross country runners.[196] Nideffer[197] addressed the issue of psychological consequences of injury and described various situations in which injuries followed excessive or improper actions produced by psychological sequelae. Clients who have high anxiety levels, which is a common symptom of stress, were noted by Nideffer[197] to have increased muscle tension, pressure on joints, and narrowing of attention factors essential to effective competitive running. Morgan[198] discussed the impact of high stress on clients and concluded that it affected interpersonal relationships in the home, work and social setting, and that obsessive-compulsive symptoms were often realized by clients who felt compelled to attempt to cope with their anxiety with daily exercise and could not live without the daily recreational running experience. Often, this anxiety and stress are recognized most readily in aberrant behaviors including depression, anxiety, extreme irritability, insomnia, and generalized fatigue. The two most relevant symptoms to reveal themselves are sleep pattern variability and problems with interpersonal relationships, usually manifested by depression, anxiety or irritability. Sanderson[199] discussed the psychological implications of injury, which vary according to personality. The most significant findings in Sanderson's research is that the more stable or internally oriented client does not experience major problems unless the injury is severe and the prognosis is very discouraging.[199] Miller and Vaughn[200] reported that non-stressed runners displayed a more internal health locus of control, and were less apprehensive, having less need of reassurance. Miller and Vaughn[200] proposed a four-module cognitive and behaviorally oriented stress management training program with specific therapeutic tasks and expected outcomes (**Table 11.19**).

Stress management training provides skills in assisting a client to evaluate and develop the coping mechanisms needed to relieve the physical and psychological features of anxiety and stress. The behavioral assessment phase involves the careful analysis of the variety of stress components experienced by the client.

Key Point:

Stress management training provides skills to the client to evaluate and develop the coping mechanisms needed to relieve the physical and psychological features of anxiety and stress.

Significant life events initiate stress reactions in clients mainly because they have some direct impact on their lives. Because of this, it is essential that clients take responsibility for the stress and discomfort they are experiencing by carefully evaluating the circumstances that lead up to the stressful situation and the extent to which they can cope with the stressful situation. The cognitive phase of stress management aims to assess the specific process of cognitively interpreting stressful events. The cognitive appraisal phase recognizes that clients perceive life events in a variety of ways. Clients may display these perceptions by the way they communicate them to others and the way they link them with their own anticipatory anxiety, aspirations, and threats, as they attempt to cope satisfactorily with stressful life events, and pain. This cognitive appraisal has the potential for causing further anxiety. The statements that clients make often emphasize their ability or inability to cope with the given situation. During the cognitive appraisal, changes in the physiological state of the body occur. Some of these responses may include muscle tension, elevated blood pressure, perspiration, or other somatic concerns.

The third module of the program involves education and training. This module teaches four specific ingredients that are essential to the client's preparation for dealing with stress and painful experiences. The initial phase of the third module is to prepare for the anticipated stressful or painful situation. In preparing for this, the client thinks through and carefully evaluates what triggers their pain or stress. Preparing for the triggering event enables the client carefully to think through the options they have in how to deal with it. Simple visual image role playing of the particular situation helps to reduce anxiety. As part of preparing for this stress producing situation, a client can use muscle relaxation skills in conjunction with visual imagery as a method of coping with the anticipated stressful situation. The second phase of the third module is being able to confront the stressful or painful situation by cognitively rehearsing the way in which the client has chosen to deal with this significant life event. Once this rehearsal phase has been completed, the client should be ready to face the triggering event and to use both the cognitive visual imagery and relational skills that will enable them to

---

TABLE 11.19   Stress management training for athletes

Module	Therapeutic tasks	Expected outcome
I. Behavioral assessment	Assess the components of stress experienced by the athlete as it relates to life events.	Athlete understands elements of stress and specific factors that trigger anxiety and result in stress.
II. Cognitive appraisal	Appraise the manner in which the athlete perceives and communicates stress behavior in life stress events.	Athlete understands how they process the perception of stressful situations and use this information to control stress-producing experiences.
III. Education and training	Educate and train the athlete to utilize a four-step model in dealing with stress and pain.	Athlete understands and employs the four-step model in stress management skills training.
IV. Stress management skills	Train the athlete in the use of cognitive imagery and muscle relaxation skills as the medium for reducing stress and pain.	Athlete learns effective use of cognitive coping skills and employs them in the control of anxiety, stress and tension.

(Modified from TW Miller, MP Vaughn, JM Miller. Clinical issues and treatment strategies in stress-oriented athletes. *Sports Med.* 1990; 9(6):370–379.)

TABLE 11.20   Stress management training for athletes using muscle relaxation skills (modified from the Jacobsen Muscle Relaxation Module)

Muscle group	Self-directed activity
Breathing exercises	Slowly inhale, hold and release, repeat 2–3 times.
Right hand and forearm	Tense by making a tight fist. Hold and release.
Left hand and forearm	Tense by making a tight fist. Hold and release.
Biceps and triceps	Tense by bringing elbows in towards the body. Hold and release.
Forehead	Tense by raising eyebrows upward. Hold and release.
Facial muscles	Tense by squinting and wrinkling nose. Hold and release.
Mouth and jaw	Tense by clenching the teeth and lips. Hold and release.
Neck	Tense by pushing head back and rolling in one continuous motion.
Shoulders and chest	Tense by pressing shoulder blades back and together. Hold and release.
Abdomen	Tense by tightening stomach muscles. Hold and release.
Lower back	Tense by arching back. Hold and release.
Thighs	Tense by raising leg (left, then right) off of the ground. Hold and release.
Calves	Tense by pointing toes toward head. Hold and release.
Feet and toes	Tense by curling toes and pointing feet inward. Hold and release.

(TW Miller, MP Vaughn, JM Miller. Clinical issues and treatment strategies in stress-oriented athletes. *Sports Med.* 1990; 9(6):370–379.)

function effectively during this stressful life event. The third phase of the third module emphasizes coping with the stressful situation based on the preparation and cognitive rehearsal phases, reasoning things through and mentally preparing for stressful life events. The fourth and final phase of the third module evaluates the level of satisfaction the client has realized in coping with the particular stressful experience. This phase involves self-statements that support the client's efforts to be in control and to manage the level of control they have realized in the utilization of stress management skills.

The fourth module of the stress management program involves cognitive imagery and muscle relaxation exercises. Relaxation exercises become the physical response that should be experienced in conjunction with cognitive appraisal and coping skills. Relaxation exercises involve tensing and relaxing 14 different muscle groups, summarized in **Table 11.20**.[200] As part of the muscle relaxation training, individuals are asked to listen to an audiotape that leads them through sequential muscle relaxation training. Muscle relaxation training recognizes that anxiety, stress and tension become manifest in various muscle groups of the body. By deliberately tensing the muscle groups that routinely become tense when anxiety, stress and tension are experienced, the client learns to physiologically control muscle tension, thereby enhancing coping skill. Like any new skill, practice is essential. Although stress management techniques are best taught under the direction of a psychologist, once the initial training has taken place the rehabilitation clinician can assist, thereby reinforcing the lessons.

Summary

Rehabilitation clinicians need to process health care information, participate in interdisciplinary care pathway development, facilitate compliance with therapeutic exercise program interventions, and attempt to establish positive health behaviors to improve their clients' quality of life. To do this effectively, they must have a sound understanding of health locus of control and self-efficacy. An aging population who experiences problems associated with osteoarthritis requires considerable therapeutic exercise program focus to minimize functional limitations and disabilities. Developing therapeutic exercise programs that reflect the individuality of each client mandates that treatment goals be directed toward essential components of the client's daily life. Returning the client to high-stress occupational function or athletics depends on the implementation of a functional readiness program in a controlled or semi-controlled environment designed to simulate the physiological and psychological stressors that they will encounter in the uncontrolled, competitive situation. Stress management instructions may help the client deal with the psychological aspects of their return to increased activity levels. Although functional performance testing and survey data will assist the rehabilitation clinician and the referring physician as to the client's readiness for return, it is essential that the client be informed of the possibility for re-injury and how their current condition may impact their life in the future.

References

1. Petty RE, Cacioppo JT. *Attitude and Persuasion: Classic and Contemporary Approaches.* Dubuque, IA: W.C. Brown Publishers, 1981, pp. 312–314.

2. Cacioppo JT, Strathman AJ, Priester JR. To think or not to think: Exploring two routes to persuasion. In S. Shavitt and TC Brock (eds.), *Persuasion: Psychological insights and perspectives.* Boston: Allyn and Bacon, 1994, pp. 112–147.

3. Kreuter MW, Skinner CS. Tailoring: What's in a name? *Health Educ Res.* 2000:15: 1–3.

4. Skinner CS, Campbell MK, Rimmer BK, et al. How effective is tailored print communication? *Ann Behav Med.* 1999;21:290–298.

5. Brug J, Steenhaus I, Van Assema P, De Vries H. The impact of a computer-tailored nutrition intervention. *Prev Med.* 1996;25:236–242.

6. Petty RE, Caciioppo JT. Personal development as a determinant of argument-based persuasion. *J Pers Soc Psychol.* 1991;41:847–855.

7. Miller TW, Vaughn MP, Adams JM. Clinical issues and treatment strategies in stress oriented athletes. *Sports Med.* 1990;9(6):370–379.

8. Bull FC, Kreuter MW, Schariff DP. Effects of tailored, personalized, and general materials on physical activity. *Patient Educ Couns.* 1999;36:181–192.

9. Kreuter MW, Bull FC, Clark EM, Oswald DL. Understanding how people process health information: A comparison of tailored and untailored weight loss materials. *Health Psychol.* 1999;18:487–494.

10. Kreuter MW, Oswald DL, Bull FC, Clark EM. Are tailored health education materials always more effective than nontailored materials? *Health Educ Res.* 2000;15:305–316.

11. Miller TW. Shifts in the health care industry: Assessing critical factors. Invited medical grand rounds. University of Texas Health Science Center, Nov. 20, 1998, San Antonio, TX.

12. Gilgun JF. Methodological pluralism and qualitative family research. In S Steinmentz, M Sussman, & G Peterson (Eds.) *Handbook of marriage and the family* (3rd ed., pp. 147–163). New York: Plenum. 2000.

13. Griffith JR. *Designing 21st Century Healthcare: Leadership in Hospitals and Healthcare Organizations.* Chicago: Administration Press. 1998.

14. Shereer JL. Five trends shaping the future of healthcare. *Hospital Health News.* 1993;67(4):30–35.

15. Naisbitt J. *Megatrends 2000.* New York: Morrow & Company, 1990.

16. Miller TW. The psychologist with 20/20 vision. *Consult Psychol J Pract Res.* 1998;50(1):25–35.

17. Covey ST, Merrill AR, Merrill RR. *First Things First.* New York: Simon and Schuster, 1994.

18. Sahrmann SA. Movement science and physical therapy. *J Phys Ther Educ.* 1993;7(1):4–7.

19. Steffen TM, Hacker TA, Mollinger L. Age- and gender-related test performance in community-dwelling elderly people: Six-Minute Walk Test, Berg Balance Scale, Timed Up & Go, and Gait Speeds. *Phys Ther.* 2002;82(2):128–137.

20. Guccione AA. *Geriatric Physical Therapy.* St. Louis, MO: Mosby-Year Book Inc.; 1993; pp. 331–349.

21. Blumenthal JA, Emery CF, Madden DJ, et al. Effects of exercise training on cardiorespiratory function in men and women > 60 years of age. *Am J Cardiol.* 1991;67:633–639.

22. Sheldahl LM, Tristani FE, Hastings JE, et al. Comparison of adaptations and compliance to exercise between middle-aged and older men. *J Am Ger Soc.* 1993;41:795–801.

23. Kohrt WM, Malley MT, Coggan AR, et al. Effects of gender, age, and fitness level on response of $VO_{2\ max}$ to training in 60–71 year olds. *J Appl Physiol.* 1991;71:2004–2011.

24. Marcus BH, Rakowski W, Rossi JS. Assessing motivational readiness and decision making for exercise. *Health Psychol.* 1992;11(4):257–261.

25. Marcus BH, Selby VC, Niaura RS, Rossi JS. Self-efficacy and the stages of exercise behavior change. *Res Q Exerc Sport.* 1992;63(1):60–66.

26. Marcus BH, Simkin LR. The transtheoretical model: Applications to exercise behavior. *Med Sci Sports Exerc.* 1994;26(11):1400–1404.

27. Prochaska JO, Marcus BH. The trans-theoretical model: The applications to exercise. In RK Dishman (ed.), *Advances in Exercise Adherence.* Champaign, IL: Human Kinetics Publishers, 1994, pp. 161–180.

28. Blanpied P. Why won't patients do their home exercise programs? *J Orthop Sports Phys Ther.* 1997;25 (2):101–102.

29. Sluijs EM, Kok GJ, van der Zee J. Correlates of exercise compliance in physical therapy. *Phys Ther.* 1993;73(11):771–786.

30. Jette AM. Improving patient cooperation with arthritis treatment regimens. *Arthritis Rheum.* 1982; 25:447–453.

31. Ferguson K, Bole GG. Family support, health beliefs, and therapeutic compliance in patients with rheumatoid arthritis. *Patient Couns Health Ed.* 1979; 1:101–105.

32. Heiby EM, Carlson JG. The health compliance model. *J Compliance Health Care.* 1986;1:135–152.

33. Janz NK, Becker MN. The health belief model: A decade later. *Health Educ Q.* 1984;11:1–47.

34. Sonstroem RJ. Psychological models. In RK Dishman, (ed.), *Exercise Adherence: Its Impact on Public Health.* Champaign, IL: Human Kinetics Publishers Inc, 1988.

35. Litt MD, Kleppinger A, Judge JO. Initiation and maintenance of exercise behavior in older women: Predictors from the social learning model. *J Behav Med.* 2002;16:915–929.

36. Donovan JL, Blake DR. Patient non-compliance: Deviance or reasoned decision making. *Soc Sci Med.* 1992;34:507–513.

37. Rosenstock IM. Historical origins of the health belief model. In MH Becker, *The Health Belief Model and Personal Health Behavior.* Thorofare, NJ: Charles B. Slack, 1974; pp. 1–8.

38. Blackwell B. Counseling and compliance. *Patient Couns Health Ed.* 1978;3:45–49.

39. Haynes RB, Wang E, Da Mota Gomes M. A critical review of interventions to improve compliance with prescribed medications. *Patient Educ Couns.* 1987; 10:155–166.

40. Oldridge NB. Adherence to adult exercise fitness programs. In ID Matarazzo, SM Weiss, JA Herd, et al. (eds.), *Behavioral Health: A Handbook of Health Enhancement and Disease Prevention.* New York: John Wiley & Sons Inc, 1984, pp. 467–487.

41. Lazare A, Eisenthal S, Frank A, Stoeckle JD. Studies on a negotiated approach to patient-hood. In JE Stoeckle, (ed.), *Encounters Between Patients and Doctors.* Cambridge, MA: The MIT Press, 1987, pp. 413–432.

42. Leventhal H, Cameron I. Behavioral theories and the problem of compliance. *Patient Educ Couns.* 1987;10:117–138.

43. Henry KD, Rosemond C, Eckert LB. Effect of number of home exercises on compliance and performance in adults over 65 years of age. *Phys Ther.* 1999;79(3):270–277.

44. Buckworth J, Dishman RK. Determinants of physical activity: From research to application. In JM Rippe, (ed.), *Lifestyle Medicine.* Malden, MA: Blackwell Science, Inc., 1999, pp. 1016–1027.

45. Lorenc L, Branthwaite A. Are older adults less compliant with prescribed medication than younger adults? *Br J Clin Psychol.* 1993;32:485–492.

46. Martin JE, Dubbert PM. Exercise applications and promotion in behavioral medicine: Current status and future directions. *J Consult Clin Psychol.* 1982; 50:1004–1017.

47. Haynes BR, Taylor DW, Sackett DL. *Compliance in Health Care.* Baltimore, MD: The Johns Hopkins University Press, 1979.

48. Oldridge NB. Compliance with exercise in cardiac rehabilitation. In RK Dishman (ed.), *Exercise Adherence: Its Impact on Public Health.* Champaign, IL: Human Kinetics, 1988, pp. 283–304.

49. Dishman RK, Sallis JF. Determinants and interventions for physical activity and exercise. In C Bouchard (ed.), *Proceedings of the Second International Conference on Physical Activity, Fitness, and Health.* Champaign, IL: Human Kinetics Publishers, 1994, pp. 214–238.

50. Bandura A. Self-efficacy: Toward a unifying theory of behavior change. *Psychol Bull.* 1977;84:191–215.

51. Lee JY, Jensen BE, Oberman A, et al. Adherence in the training levels comparison trial. *Med Sci Sports Exerc.* 1996;28(1):47–52.

52. Hartigan C, Rainville J, Sobel JB, Hipona M. Long-term exercise adherence after intensive rehabilitation for chronic low back pain. *Med Sci Sports Exerc.* 2000;32(3):551–557.

53. McAuley E, Courneya KS, Rudolph DL, et al. Enhancing exercise adherence in middle-aged males and females. *Prev Med.* 1994;23:498–506.

54. Dorn J, Naughton J, Imamura D, et al. Correlates of compliance in a randomized exercise trial in myocardial infarction patients. *Med Sci Sports Exerc.* 2001;33(7):1081–1089.

55. Oldridge NB, Ragowski B, Gottlieb M. Use of outpatient cardiac rehabilitation services: Factors associated with attendance. *J Cardiopulm Rehabil.* 1992;12:25–31.

56. Oldridge NB, Streiner DL. The health belief model: Predicting compliance and dropout in cardiac rehabilitation. *Med Sci Sports Exerc.* 1990; 22:678–683.

57. Blumenthal JA, Williams RS, Wallace AG, et al. Physiological and psychological variables predict compliance to prescribed exercise therapy in patients recovering from myocardial infarction. *Psychosom Med.* 1982;44:519–527.

58. Lieberman L, Meana M, Stewart D. Cardiac rehabilitation: Gender differences in factors influencing participation. *J Women's Health.* 1998;7:717–723.

59. Schuster PM, Wright C, Tomich P. Gender differences in the outcomes of participants in home programs compared to those in structured cardiac rehabilitation programs. *Rehabil Nurs.* 1995;20: 93–101.

60. Campbell R, Evans M, Tucker M, et al. Why don't patients do their exercises? Understanding non-compliance with physiotherapy in patients with osteoarthritis of the knee. *J Epidemiol Community Health.* 2001;55:132–138.

61. Sackett DL. The magnitude of compliance and non-compliance. In DL Sackett, RD Haynes (eds.), *Compliance with Therapeutic Regimens*. Baltimore, MD: Johns Hopkins University Press, 1976, pp. 9–25.

62. DiMatteo MR. Enhancing patient adherence to medical recommendations. *JAMA*. 1994;271:79–83.

63. Morris LS, Schulz RM. Patient compliance—An overview. *J Clin Pharm Ther*. 1992;17:283–295.

64. Haynes RB, McKibbon KA, Kanani R. Systematic review of randomized trials of interventions to assist patients to follow prescriptions for medications. *Lancet*. 1996;348:383–386.

65. Woodard CM, Berry MJ. Enhancing adherence to prescribed exercise: Structured behavioral interventions in clinical exercise programs. *J Cardiopulm Rehabil*. 2001;21:201–209.

66. Schneider SJ, Khachadurian AK, Amorosa LF, et al. Ten-year experience with an exercise-based outpatient life-style modification program in the treatment of diabetes mellitus. *Diabetes Care*. 1992; 15:1800–1810.

67. Rainville JDK, Ahern K, Phalen L, et al. The association of pain with physical activities in chronic low back pain. *Spine*. 1992;17:1060-1064.

68. Biggs SJ, Spengler DM, Martin NA, et al. Back injuries in industry—A retrospective study: III. Employee-related factors. *Spine*. 1986;11:252–256.

69. Biggs SJ, Battie MC, Spengler DM, et al. A prospective study of work perceptions and psychosocial factors affecting the report of back injury. *Spine*. 1991;16: 1–6.

70. Chan CW, Goldman S, Ilstrup DM, et al. The pain and Waddell's nonorganic physical signs in chronic low-back pain. *Spine*. 1993;18:1717–1722.

71. Greenough CG. Recovery from low back pain: 1–5 year follow-up of 281 injury-related cases. *Acta Orthop Scand*. 1993; 254 (Suppl 64): 1–34.

72. Ransford AL, Cairns OD, Mooney V. The pain drawing as an aid to the psychologic evaluation of patients with low back pain. *Spine*. 1990;15:1325–1332.

73. Uden A, Astrom M, Bergenudd H. Pain drawings in chronic back pain. *Spine*. 1988;13:389–392.

74. Rainville J, Ahern DK, Phalen L. Altering beliefs about pain and impairment in a functionally oriented treatment program for chronic low back pain. *Clin J Pain*. 1993;9:196–201.

75. Paffenbarger RS, Hyde RT, Wing AL, et al. Physical activity, mortality, and longevity. *N Engl J Med*. 1986;314:605–613.

76. Paffenbarger RS, Hyde RT, Wing AL, et al. The association of changes in physical-activity level and other lifestyle characteristics with mortality among men. *N Engl J Med*. 1993;328:538–545.

77. Sandvik L, Erikssen J, Thaulow E, et al. Physical fitness as a predictor of mortality among healthy, middle-aged Norwegian men. *N Engl J Med*. 1993; 328:533–537.

78. Staal JB, Hlobil H, van Tulder MW, et al. Return-to-work interventions for low back pain: A descriptive review of contents and concepts of working mechanisms. *Sports Med*. 2002; 32(4):251–267.

79. Frymoyer JW. Quality: An international challenge to the diagnosis and treatment of disorders of the lumbar spine. *Spine*. 1993;18:2147–2152.

80. Lahad A, Malter AD, Berg AO, et al. The effectiveness of four interventions for the prevention of low back pain. *JAMA*. 1994; 272(16):1286–1291.

81. van Poppel MN, Koes BW, Smit T, et al. A systematic review of controlled clinical trials on the prevention of back pain in industry. *Occup Environ Med*. 1997;54(12):841–847.

82. Altmair EM, Johnson BD. Health-related applications of counseling psychology: Toward health promotion and disease prevention across the lifespan. In SD Brown, RD Lend (eds.), *Handbook of Counseling Psychology*, 2nd ed. New York: Wiley and Sons, 1992, pp. 315–347.

83. Bendix T, Bendix A, Labriola M, et al. Functional restoration versus outpatient physical training in chronic low back pain: A randomized comparative study. *Spine*. 2000;25(19):2494–2500.

84. Lindstrom I, Ohlund C, Eek C, et al. The effect of graded activity on patients with subacute low back pain: A randomized prospective clinical study with an operant-conditioning behavioral approach. *Phys Ther*. 1992;72(4):279–293.

85. Lindstrom I, Ohlund C, Eek C, et al. Mobility, strength, and fitness after a graded activity program for patients with subacute low back pain: A randomized prospective clinical study with a behavioral therapy approach. *Spine*. 1992;17(6):641–652.

86. Mannion AF, Taimela S, Muntener M, et al. Active therapy for chronic low back pain: Part I. Effects on back muscle activation, fatigability, and strength. *Spine*. 2001;26(8):897–908.

87. Kaser L, Mannion AF, Rhyner A, et al. Active therapy for chronic low back pain: Part 2. Effects on paraspinal muscle cross-sectional area, fiber type size, and distribution. *Spine*. 2001;26(8):909–919.

88. Mancuso CA, Sculco TP, Wickiewicz TL, et al. Patients' expectations of knee surgery. *J Bone Joint Surg Am*. 2001;83(7):1005–1012.

89. Iversen MD, Daltroy LH, Fossel AH, Katz JN. The prognostic importance of patient pre-operative expectations of surgery for lumbar spinal stenosis. *Patient Educ Couns*. 1998;34:169–178.

90. Kravitz RL, Callahan EJ, Paterniti D, et al. Prevalence and sources of patients' unmet expectations for care. *Ann Intern Med*. 1996;125:730–737.

91. Wright JG, Rudicel S, Feinstein AR. Ask patients what they want: Evaluation of individual complaints before total hip replacement. *J Bone Joint Surg Br.* 1994;76:229–234.

92. Spitzer WO. State of science 1986: Quality of life and functional status as target variables for research. *J Chronic Dis.* 1987;40:465–471.

93. Ware JE. Conceptualizing and measuring health outcomes. *Cancer.* 1991; 67 (Suppl):774–779.

94. Guyatt GH, Bombardier C, Tugwell PX. Measuring disease-specific quality of life in clinical trials. *Can Med Assoc J.* 1986;134:889–895.

95. Schipper H. Quality of life: Principles of the clinical paradigm. *J Psychosocial Oncol.* 1990;8:171–184.

96. Schipper H, Clinch J, Powell V. Definitions and conceptual issues. In B Spilker, (ed.), *Quality of Life Assessments in Clinical Trials.* New York: Raven Press, 1990: pp. 11–24.

97. Stewart AL, King AC. Evaluating the efficacy of physical activity for influencing quality of life outcomes in older adults. *Ann Behav Med.* 1991;13:108–116.

98. Rejeski WJ, Brawley LR, Ettinger W, et al. Compliance to exercise therapy in older participants with knee osteoarthritis: Implications for treating disability. *Med Sci Sports Exerc.* 1997;29(8):977–985.

99. Work JA. Strength training: A bridge to independence for the elderly. *Physician Sportsmed.* 1989; 17:134–140.

100. Tinetti ME, Mendes De Leon CF, Doucette JT, Baker DI. Fear of falling and fall-related efficacy in relationship to functioning among community-living elders. *J Gerontol.* 1994;49:140–147.

101. Rotter J. Generalized expectancies for internal vs. external control of reinforcement. *Psychol Monogr.* 1966;80:1–28.

102. Rodin J. Aging and health. Effects of the sense of control. *Science.* 1986;233:1272–1276.

103. Brothen T, Detzner D. Perceived health and locus of control in the aged. *Percept Mot Skills.* 1983;56:946.

104. Langer E, Rodin J. The effects of choice and enhanced personal responsibility for the aged: A field experiment in an institutional setting. *J Pers Soc Psychol.* 1976;34:191–198.

105. Waller KV, Bates RC. Health locus of control and self-efficacy beliefs in a healthy elderly sample. *Am J Health Promot.* 1992;6:302–309.

106. Langer E, Rodin J, Beck P, et al. Environmental determinants of memory improvement in late adulthood. *J Pers Soc Psychol.* 1979;37:2003–2013.

107. Bandura A, Wood R. Effect of perceived controllability and performance standards on self-regulation and complex decision making. *J Pers Soc Psychol.* 1989;56(5):805–814.

108. Johnson BD, Stone GI, Altmaier EM, Berdahl LD. The relationship of demographic factors, locus of control and self-efficacy to successful nursing home adjustment. *Gerontologist* 1998;38(2):209–216.

109. Chen C-Y, Neufeld PS, Feely CA, Skinner CS. Factors influencing compliance with home exercise programs among patients with upper-extremity impairment. *Am J Occup Ther.* 1999;53:171–180.

110. Hall EG. The application of locus of control to sport and physical activity. In LK Bunker, RJ Rotella, AS Reilly (eds), *Sports Psychology: Psychological Considerations in Maximizing Sports Performance.* Ann Arbor, MI: McNaughton & Gunn Inc., 1985.

111. Miller TW. *Self Management Approach for Responsible Treatment Success (SMARTS).* Training manual. Lexington, Kentucky: Department of Psychiatry, University of Kentucky, 1993.

112. Cormier WH, Cormier LS. *Interviewing Strategies for Helpers: Fundamental Skills and Cognitive Behavioral Interventions* (3rd ed.), Pacific Grove, CA.: Brooks/Cole Pub. Co. 1991.

113. Watson DL, Tharp RG. *Self-directed Behavior: Self-modification for Personal Adjustment* (6th ed.), Pacific Grove, CA.: Brooks/Cole Pub. Co., 1993.

114. Kanfer F, Gaelick-Buys L. Self-management methods. In Kanfer FH, Goldstein AP. (eds.), *Helping People Change: A Textbook of Methods*, 4th ed. Pergamon General Psychology Series, vol. 52. Pergamon Press, 1991.

115. Kazdin AE. *Behavior Modification in Applied Settings* (5th ed.). Pacific Grove, CA.: Brooks/Cole Pub. Co. 1994.

116. Buskirk ER. Perspectives on exercise and wasting. *J Nutr.* 1999;129:295S–302S.

117. Blair SN, Kohl HW III, Paffenbarger RS Jr, et al. Physical fitness and all-cause mortality: A prospective study of healthy men and women. *JAMA.* 1989;262:2395–2401.

118. Kushi LH, Fee RM, Folsom AR, et al. Physical activity and mortality in postmenopausal women. *JAMA.* 1997;277:1287–1292.

119. Lee I-M, Paffenbarger RS Jr. Do physical activity and physical fitness avert premature mortality? *Exerc Sports Sci. Rev.* 1996;24:135–171.

120. Birren J, Livingston J. *Cognition, Stress and Aging.* Upper Saddle River, NJ: Prentice Hall, 1985.

121. Rowe J, Kahn R. Human aging: Usual and successful. *Science.* 1987;237:143–149.

122. Hurley MV, Mitchell HL, Walsh N. Osteoarthritis: the psychosocial benefits of exercise are important as physical improvements. *Exerc Sports Sci Rev.* 2003;31(3):138–143.

123. Ettinger WH, Burns R, Messier SP, et al. A randomized trial comparing aerobic exercise and resistance exercise with a health education program in older adults with knee osteoarthritis. *JAMA.* 1997; 277:25–31.

124. Minor MA, Hewett JE, Webel RR, et al. Efficacy of physical conditioning exercise in patients with rheumatoid arthritis and osteoarthritis. *Arthritis Rheum.* 1989;32:1396–1405.

125. Van Baar ME, Assendelft WJ, Dekker J, et al. Effectiveness of exercise therapy in patients with osteoarthritis of the hip or knee: A systematic review of randomized clinical trials. *Arthritis Rheum.* 1999;42:1361–1369.

126. Ravesloot C, Seekins T, Young Q-R. Health promotion for people with chronic illness and physical disabilities: The connection between health psychology and disability prevention. *Clin Psychol Psychother.* 1998;5:76–85.

127. Patrick D. Rethinking prevention for people with disabilities: Part I. A conceptual model for promoting health. *Am J Health Promot.* 1997;11:257–260.

128. Hall J, Skevington SM, Maddison PJ, Chapman K. A randomized and controlled trial of hydrotherapy in rheumatoid arthritis. *Arth Care Res.* 1996;9:206–215.

129. McNeal RL. Aquatic therapy for patients with rheumatic disease. *Rheum Dis Clin North Am.* 1996; 16:915–929.

130. Wesby MD. A health professional's guide to exercise prescription for people with arthritis: A review of aerobic fitness activities. *Arthritis Rheum.* 2001; 45(6):501–511.

131. Sanford-Smith S, Mackay-Lyons M, Nunes-Clement S. Therapeutic benefit of aquaerobics for individuals with rheumatoid arthritis. *Physiother Can.* 1998;50:40–46.

132. Praemer A, Furner S, Rice DP. *Musculoskeletal Conditions in the United States.* Park Ridge, IL: American Academy of Orthopaedic Surgeons, 1992.

133. Pollock ML, Wilmore JH. *Exercise in Health and Disease: Evaluation and Prescription for Prevention and Rehabilitation,* 2nd ed. Philadelphia, PA: W.B. Saunders, 1990.

134. Collins DK. Cemented total hip replacement in patients who are less than 50 years old. *J Bone Joint Surg Am.* 1984;66:353–359.

135. Dorr LD, Takei GK, Conaty JP. Total hip arthroplasty in patients less than 45 years old. *J Bone Joint Surg Am.* 1983;65:474–479.

136. Healy WL, Iorio R, Lemos M. Athletic activity after joint replacement. *Am J Sports Med.* 2001;29: 377–388.

137. Vail TP, Mallon WJ, Liebelt RA. Athletic activities after joint arthroplasty. *Sports Med Arthroplasty Rev.* 1996;4:298–305.

138. Nicholls MA, Selby JB, Hartford JM. Athletic activity after total joint replacement. *Orthopedics.* 2002; 25:1283–1287.

139. Macnicol MF, McHardy R, Chalmers J. Exercise testing before and after hip arthroplasty. *J Bone Joint Surg Br.* 1980;62:326–331.

140. Visuri T, Honkanen R. Total hip replacement: Its influence on spontaneous recreation exercise habits. *Arch Phys Med Rehabil.* 1980;61:325–328.

141. Caborn D, Rush J, Lanzer W, et al. A randomized, single-blind comparison of the efficacy and tolerability of hylan G-F 20 and triamcinolone hexacetonide in patients with osteoarthritis of the knee. *J Rheumatol.* 2004;31(2):333–343.

142. Page CG. *Managing Physical Therapy Documentation.* Course notes presented at the Florida Physical Therapy Association Conference, Orlando, FL, March 1999.

143. Page CG. Goal setting. Inservice presentation at Morton Plant-Mease Hospitals, Clearwater, FL, January 10, 2000.

144. Santana JC. Hamstrings of steel: Preventing the pull: Part I. Isolated versus integrated function. *Strength Cond J.* 2000;22(6):35–36.

145. Santana JC. Hamstrings of steel: Preventing the pull: Part II. Training the triple threat. *Strength Cond J.* 2001;23(1):18–20.

146. Gambetta, V. *Building and Rebuilding the Complete Athlete.* Optimum Sports Training, Inc., Sarasota, FL. 2000.

147. Chu, D. *Jumping into Plyometrics.* Champaign, IL: Leisure Press, 1992.

148. Bompa, T. *Theory and Methodology of Training: The Key to Athletic Performance.* Dubuque, IA: Kendall/Hunt Publishing Company, 1985.

149. Plisk P. Speed, agility, and speed-endurance development. In T Baechle, R Earle (eds), *Essential Principles of Strength and Conditioning,* 2nd ed. Champaign, IL: Human Kinetics, 2000.

150. Goldenberg L, Twist, P. *Strength Ball Training.* Champaign, IL: Versa Press, 2002.

151. Matheson GO. First, ask no harmful questions. *Physician Sportsmed.* 2002;30(5):7.

152. Morganti C, Sweeney CA, Albanese SA, et al. Return to play after cervical spine injury. *Spine.* 2001;26(10):1131–1136.

153. Nack W. Was justice paralyzed? *Sports Illustrated,* July 1988; 25 pp. 32–36.

154. Mitten MJ, Mitten RJ. Legal considerations in treating the injured athlete. *J Orthop Sports Phys Ther.* 1995;21(1):38–43.

155. Mitten MJ. Team physicians and competitive athletes: Allocating legal responsibility for athletic injuries. *U Pitt Law Rev.* 1993;55(1):129–169.

156. Swander H. *Preparticipation Physical Evaluation.* Kansas City, MO: American Academy of Family Physicians, American Academy of Pediatrics, American Medical Society for Sports Medicine, American Osteopathic Academy of Sports Medicine, 1992.

157. Fitzgerald GK, Lephart SM, Hwang JH, Wainner RS. Hop tests as predictors of dynamic knee stability. *J Orthop Sports Phys Ther.* 2001;31(10):588–597.

158. Barber SD, Noyes FR, Mangine RE, et al. Quantitative assessment of functional limits in normal and anterior cruciate ligament-deficient knees. *Clin Orthop.* 1990;255:204–214.

159. Noyes FR, Barber SD, Mangine RE. Abnormal lower limb symmetry determined by functional hop tests after anterior cruciate ligament rupture. *Am J Sports Med.* 1991;19:513–518.

160. Tegner Y, Lysholm J, Lysholm M, Gillquist J. A performance test to monitor rehabilitation and evaluate anterior cruciate ligament injuries. *Am J Sports Med.* 1986;14:156–159.

161. Kea J, Kramer J, Forwell L, Birmingham T. Hip abduction-adduction strength and one-leg hop tests: Test-retest reliability and relationship to function in elite ice hockey players. *J Orthop Sports Phys Ther.* 2001;31(8):446–455.

162. Juris PM, Phillips EM, Dalpe C, et al. A dynamic test of lower extremity function following anterior cruciate ligament reconstruction and rehabilitation. *J Orthop Sports Phys Ther.* 1997;26:184–191.

163. Petschnig R, Baron R, Albrecht M. The relationship between isokinetic quadriceps strength test and hop tests. *J Orthop Sports Phys Ther.* 1998;28:23–31.

164. Risberg MA, Ekeland A. Assessment of functional tests after anterior cruciate ligament surgery. *J Orthop Sports Phys Ther.* 1994;19:212–217.

165. Howell SM, Deutsch ML. Comparison of endoscopic two-incision techniques for reconstructing a torn anterior cruciate ligament using hamstring tendons. *Arthroscopy.* 1999;15:594–606.

166. Wilson RW, Gansneder BM. Measures of functional limitation as predictors of disablement in athletes with acute ankle sprains. *J Orthop Sports Phys Ther.* 2000;30(9):528–535.

167. Sapega AA, Nicholas JA. The clinical use of musculoskeletal profiling in orthopaedics. *Physician Sportsmed.* 1981;9(4):80–88.

168. Marx RG, Jones EC, Allen AA, et al. Reliability, validity, and responsiveness of four knee outcome scales for athletic patients. *J Bone Joint Surg Am.* 2001;83(10):1459–1469.

169. Barber-Westin SD, Noyes FR, McCloskey JW. Rigorous statistical reliability, validity, and responsiveness testing of the Cincinnati knee rating system in 350 subjects with uninjured, injured, or anterior cruciate ligament-reconstructed knees. *Am J Sports Med.* 1999;27:402–416.

170. Irrgang JJ, Snyder-Mackler L, Wainner RS, et al. Development of a patient-reported measure of function of the knee. *J Bone Joint Surg Am.* 1998;80:1132–1145.

171. Bindra RR, Dias JJ, Heras-Palau C, et al. Assessing outcome after hand surgery: The current state. *J Hand Surg Br.* 2003;28(4):289–294.

172. Wright JG, Young NL. A comparison of different indices of responsiveness. *J Clin Epidemiol.* 1997;50:239–246.

173. Gartland JJ. Orthopaedic clinical research. Deficiencies in experimental design and determinations of outcome. *J Bone Joint Surg Am.* 1988;70(9):1357–1364.

174. Sgaglione NA, Del Pizzo W, Fox JM, Friedman MJ. Critical analysis of knee ligament rating systems. *Am J Sports Med.* 1995;23:660–667.

175. Nagi SZ. Disability concepts revisited: implications for prevention. In AM Pope, AR Tarlov (eds.), *Disability in America: Toward a National Agenda for Prevention.* Washington, DC: National Academy Press, Appendix A, pp. 309–327, 1991.

176. McHorney CA, Ware JE Jr., Raczek A. The MOS 36-Item Short-Form Health Survey (SF-36): II. Psychometric and clinical tests of validity in measuring physical and mental health constructs. *Med Care.* 1993;31:247–263.

177. McHorney CA, Ware JE Jr., Lu JF, Sherbourne CD. The MOS 36-Item Short-Form Health Survey (SF-36): III. Tests of data quality, scaling assumptions, and reliability across diverse patient groups. *Med Care.* 1994;32(1):40–66.

178. Ware JE Jr., Sherbourne CD. The MOS 36-Item Short-Form Health Survey (SF-36): I. Conceptual framework and item selection. *Med Care.* 1992;30:473–483.

179. Ware JE, Kosinski M, Keller SD. A 12-item short-form health survey: Construction of scales and preliminary tests of reliability and validity. *Med Care.* 1996;34:220–233.

180. Bergner M, Bobbit RA, Carter WB, Gilson BS. The sickness impact profile: Development and final revision of a health status measure. *Med Care.* 1981;19:787–805.

181. Lysholm J, Gillquist J. The evaluation of knee ligament surgery results with special emphasis on the use of a scoring scale. *Am J Sports Med,* 1982;10:150–154.

182. Noyes FR, McGinniss GH, Mooar LA. Functional disability in the anterior cruciate insufficient knee syndrome: Review of knee rating systems and projected risk factors in determining treatment. *Sports Med.* 1984;1:278–302.

183. Roos EM, Roos HP, Lohmander LS, et al. Knee injury and osteoarthritis outcome score (KOOS): Development of a self-administered outcome measure. *J Orthop Sports Phys Ther.* 1998; 28(2):88–96.

184. Hefti F, Muller W, Jakob RP, Staubli HU. Evaluation of knee ligament injuries with the IKDC form. *Knee Surg Sports Traumatol Arthrosc.* 1993;1:226–234.

185. Insall JN, Dorr LD, Scott RD, Scott WN. Rationale for the Knee Society clinical rating system. *Clin Orthop.* 1989;248:13–14.

186. Katz JN, Phillips CB, Poss R, et al. The validity and reliability of a total hip arthroplasty outcome evaluation questionnaire. *J Bone Joint Surg Am.* 1995; 77(10):1528–1534.

187. Hoeksma HL, Van Den Ende CH, Ronday HK, et al. Comparison of the responsiveness of the Harris Hip Score with generic measures for hip function in osteoarthritis of the hip. *Ann Rheum Dis.* 2003;62 (10):935–938.

188. Osoba D, Slamon DJ, Burchmore M, Murphy M. Effects of quality of life of combined trastuzumab and chemotherapy in women with metastatic breast cancer. *J Clin Oncol.* 2002;20(14):3106–3113.

189. Hudak PL, Amadio PC, Bombardier C. Development of an upper extremity outcome measure: The DASH (disabilities of the arm, shoulder and hand). The Upper Extremity Collaborative Group (UECG). *Am J Ind Med.* 1996;29:602–608.

190. Ellman H, Hanker G, Bayer M. Repair of the rotator cuff: End result study of factors influencing reconstruction. *J Bone Joint Surg Am.* 1986;68: 1136–1144.

191. Neer CS II, Watson KC, Stanton FJ. Recent experience in total shoulder replacement. *J Bone Joint Surg Am.* 1982;64:319–337.

192. Warren RF, Ranawat CS, Inglis AE. Total Shoulder Replacement Indications and Results of the Neer Unconstrained Prosthesis. In AE Inglis (ed.), *The American Academy of Orthopaedic Surgeons Symposium on Total Joint Replacement of the Upper Extremity.* St. Louis: CV Mosby, 1982.

193. Constant CR, Murley AH. A clinical method of functional assessment of the shoulder. *Clin Orthop.* 1987;214:160–164.

194. Barrett WP, Franklin JL, Jackins SE, et al. Total shoulder arthroplasty. *J Bone Joint Surg Am.* 1987; 69:865–872.

195. Kirkley A, Griffin S, McLintock H, Ng L. The development of a disease-specific quality of life measurement tool for shoulder instability: The Western Ontario Shoulder Instability Index (WOSI). *Am J Sports Med.* 1998;26(6):764–772.

196. Miller TW, Vaughn MP, Miller JM. Clinical issues and treatment strategies in stress-oriented athletes. *Sports Med.* 1990;9(6):370–379.

197. Nideffer R. *The Ethics and Practice of Applied Sport Psychology.* Ithaca, NY: Movement Publications, 1981.

198. Morgan WP. The 1980 C. H. McCloy Research Lecture: Psychophysiology of self-awareness during vigorous physical activity. *Res Q Exerc Sport.* 1981; 52(3):385–427.

199. Sanderson FH. Personality factors in physical injury. *Br J Sports Med.* 1978;11:56–65.

200. Miller TW, Vaughn MP. Psychological stressors and symptom formation in female cross country runners. Colloquium presentation, Department of Mental Health and Behavioral Sciences, Veterans Administration and University of Kentucky Medical Centers, October 21, 1986.

PART II

Therapeutic Exercise Program Implementation

Introduction to Client Cases

This section presents 10 client cases, each prepared by a different author with a different background and level of experience. These cases provide a guided experience through the therapeutic exercise program management of each of the clients. Each author has used a slightly different style in developing their case so do not expect to see the same questions or tasks presented across all cases. Information obtained from the earlier chapters should be used to formulate a therapeutic exercise program intervention for each case. You may disagree with the care pathway selected by the case author and have other intervention suggestions that are based on sound clinical evidence. Please share your own personal experiences regarding individuals that you know who have had problems similar to those of the clients discussed in these cases. From these shared experiences, it is our hope that you will develop therapeutic exercise program interventions that reflect the diversity and individuality of each client while minimizing their disability levels and enhancing their quality of life.

CLIENT CASE #1

Andrea Gallagher Hoff

History

Client: Kate

Age: 15 years

Height: 5′9″

Weight: 130 lbs

Education: Currently a junior in high school

Occupation: Full time student; works part time at a fast food restaurant

Medical/Surgical History: "Mild" left ankle sprain one year ago

Chief Complaint: Right shoulder pain when serving or hitting a volleyball; feels like it "slips" sometimes

Two weeks ago Kate (**Case Figure 1.1**) was playing in a volleyball tournament and dove after a ball. When she hit the ground, she felt a sharp pain in her right shoulder. Two days later her pediatrician had radiographs taken and performed a clinical examination. The radiographs were negative for any evidence of fracture or dislocation and she was diagnosed with a right shoulder subluxation. She was then referred to you for evaluation and treatment. Since the time of her injury, she has not been participating with her volleyball team. The team that Kate plays for is a USA Volleyball (USAV) Club Team (www.usavolleyball.org) which is quite competitive, and her goals are to return to playing competitive volleyball and participate fully in a regional tournament in 8 weeks. She began playing volleyball at age 12 and is now in her fourth season. The team practices twice a week—Sunday afternoons from 3-5 PM and Wednesday nights from 7-9 PM. Kate's parents have been very supportive of her athletic endeavors and they enjoy attending matches and transporting her to practices. Twice a month the team participates in all-day tournaments and can play as many as 13 games in one day. Kate's primary position is outside hitter, which involves a great deal of overhead upper extremity motion both to spike and block volleyballs at the net. She also plays defense when she is in a rotation that places her on the back row.

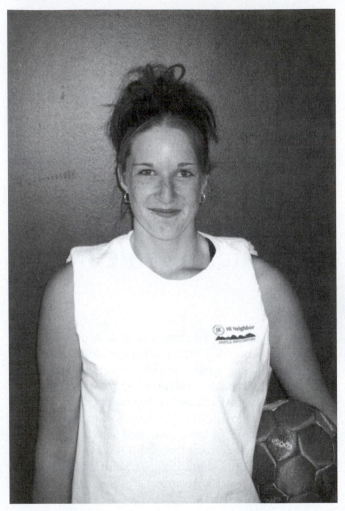

Case Figure 1.1   Kate.

Physical Examination

Musculoskeletal Assessment

Posture: Sits and stands with a slumped posture—forward head, increased thoracic kyphosis, protracted scapulae, internally rotated glenohumeral joints, right shoulder slightly elevated compared to the left. She is able to correct her posture with verbal cues.

Passive Shoulder Range of Motion:[1]

	Right	Left
Flexion	180°	175°
External rotation at 0° abduction	85°	80°
External rotation at 45° abduction	95°	85°
External rotation at 90° abduction	105°	90°
Internal rotation at 90° abduction	60°	70°

Global Ligamentous Laxity: Beighton/Horan Hypermobility Index[2,3] = 8 (see Chapters 3 and 6)

Manual Muscle Testing: Normal strength (5/5) of the anterior deltoid and subscapularis. Good strength (4/5) of the middle deltoid and supraspinatus. Fair strength (3/5) of the middle trapezius, lower trapezius and infraspinatus/teres minor.[4]

Musculotendinous Extensibility: Positive for pectoralis minor muscle and posterior glenohumeral joint capsule tightness[4-6]

Pain: Client rates her current pain level as 0/10 on a Pain Analog Scale (PAS).[7] She rates her worst pain level in the last week at 6/10 and reports that it occurred when trying to throw a ball to her dog two days ago

Special Tests:[8]   Sulcus sign, positive. Relocation test, positive. Hawkins Test, positive. Neer Test, positive. O'Brien's Test, negative. Cross body adduction, negative

Palpation: There is minimal tenderness to palpation at the rotator cuff insertion and the bicipital groove.

Neuromuscular Assessment

Scapulohumeral Biomechanics: With active right shoulder flexion there is excessive scapular elevation during the concentric phase. Additionally, there is an excessive amount of and rapidly occurring downward rotation and slight winging of the right scapula with eccentric lowering from the elevated position.

Cardiopulmonary Assessment

Resting Heart Rate: 63 bpm

Integumentary Assessment

Not applicable

Client Self-Report of Function and Functional Limitations

Global Function Rating:[9]   80% for activities of daily living (ADLs), 50% for sport activities

SF-36:[10]   Norm Based Scoring (NBS)—Physical Component Summary (PCS) = 39.0 (1.1 SD below the mean) and Mental Component Summary (MCS) = 64.4 (1.4 SD above the mean)

Functional Limitations: Has difficulty braiding her hair due to pain. Unable to serve or spike a volleyball without significant pain, which is affecting her

accuracy and ability to positively contribute to her team.

A. Given that Kate is a 15-year-old female, what other information might you want from her or from her physician in creating your intervention plan, as well as counseling her in general health, wellness and injury prevention? Write out your answers on a separate piece of paper. *See Author's Comments A*

B. What would your working diagnosis be? What would be the appropriate Preferred Practice Pattern from the *Guide to Physical Therapist Practice*[11] for Kate? What is the appropriate ICD-9 code? *See Author's Comments B*

We know a lot about Kate from her examination and initial interview, but the picture of her is not complete. When planning a therapeutic exercise program, we need to have a good understanding of the factors that are competing for Kate's time and work with her to find ways to integrate the program into her life as seamlessly as possible. Involving her in the problem solving process will create the best therapeutic exercise "program" integration into her busy schedule. If we expect her to "buy into" the program, she needs to be willing and able to commit to what we are asking her to do (see Chapter 11).

Information About Kate

School
- Honors Student −3.9 GPA
- Skipped 6th grade
- Likes biology, anatomy
- Active on Student Council

Home
- Father is an engineer
- Mother is a part-time teacher
- 2 older sisters
- Lives ½ mile from school

Activities
- Church youth group
- Club Volleyball—currently unable to participate due to shoulder pain
- Works at McDonald's some weekends and during the summer
- JV basketball at school—currently out of season

ADLs
- Has some shoulder pain when trying to French braid her hair
- Walks the family dog in the evenings—occasionally has pain with this

C. All of Kate's activities and interests are linked in some way. What are some of these other aspects that you can use to your advantage when structuring her therapeutic exercise program? What things might have a negative effect? Please write out your answer in table format, with Potential advantages in the right-hand column, and Potential negative effects in the left-hand column. *See Author's Comments C*

D. Review the results of Kate's physical examination and write, in two separate lists, what you feel are her most significant impairments and most significant functional limitations. *See Author's Comments D*

Given the acute nature of her injury and the level of pain that she is still experiencing, Kate's pain is a primary impairment and will need to be addressed early on, even prior to initiating a therapeutic exercise program. This can be done effectively with controlled rest and judicious use of non-steroidal anti-inflammatory drugs (NSAIDs) as prescribed by her physician, in addition to other therapeutic modalities that you deem to be appropriate.

Overhead athletic activities such as volleyball, tennis and baseball place a great deal of fatigue stress on rotator cuff and periscapular musculature. The rotator cuff plays a critical stabilization role for the glenohumeral joint for all activities that involve the shoulder, especially ballistic overhead activities such as volleyball.[12] With the capsuloligamentous laxity that Kate demonstrates, the rotator cuff must be a primary strength and endurance focus during the therapeutic exercise process. She also appears to have poor postural awareness since she displays a slumped forward posture in both sitting and standing. This places the posterior scapular muscles on stretch and can result in a stretch weakness that impairs performance.

Emphasizing the need not only to strengthen but utilize these muscles in daily activities and improved posture also will be vital. Studies have shown that one thing that elite volleyball players have in common is loss of internal rotation range of motion,[13] and that loss of internal rotation and tightness of the posterior glenohumeral joint capsule increases the stress and potential for anterior capsule laxity.

Addressing these issues early in Kate's career is important, both to decrease the chances of recurring impingement, and to prevent long term loss of motion. All of these impairment level problems contribute to the functional limitations that she has, i.e., not being to perform all of the activities that are important to her. Kate's global ligamentous laxity also needs to be considered when designing her treatment program. Intervention should incorporate stability and coordination activities that will also allow her to focus on strength and dynamic control of the scapulothoracic "joint." With rotator cuff weakness and ligamentous laxity at the glenohumeral joint, the role of the scapular stabilizers will be critical in providing a stable scapulothoracic foundation from which the glenohumeral joint can function. It will also be very important to work on stability and control of the entire kinetic chain, including the ankles (she sprained her left ankle 1 year ago), back, hips and knees. Improving her core stability as well as lower extremity strength and power will contribute greatly to decreasing upper extremity loads during her return to aggressive overhead sporting activity.[14]

Prior to starting any sort of intervention, it is important to first establish functional, realistic and measurable short term and long term goals that are focused around the activities that Kate wants to return to (see Chapter 11). When addressing an impairment level problem, the rehabilitation clinician should always be able to relate the goal established to the deficient functional activity. Given that this is a first time injury and that Kate is young and healthy, her short term goals should be those you would expect to be able to achieve in about four weeks, and long term goals in eight weeks.

E. List several short term goals and several long term goals for the therapeutic exercise program that you will develop for Kate's recovery process. *Author's Comments E*

Analyzing the motions and the forces needed to perform an overhead hit of a volleyball will give you a better understanding of what muscle groups and joint motions need to be addressed during Kate's therapeutic exercise program (**Case Figure 1.2a–c**).[15]

F. Look at the pictures of the three phases of a volleyball spike (wind up, cocking, and follow through—not unlike the three phases of a baseball pitch or tennis serve) and give a written analysis of what is happening from (a) to (b) to (c) for the shoulder and back (lumbar spine), two of the most injured sites in volleyball players. *See Author's Comments F*

G. What muscle groups do you think are most active during this transition from (a) to (b)? List them in order from the ankle up to the wrist. Do the same for the (b) to (c) transition. *See Author's Comments G*

Now we have a more complete picture of Kate. We have considered her impairments and functional limitations, the demands imposed on her entire body by the nature of her sport and her lifestyle. At this point you have enough information to decide not only what to include in an independent therapeutic exercise program, but also how much "hands on" intervention this client will need. For an adolescent who has never been injured and has poor dynamic scapular and trunk postural control, it would be advan-

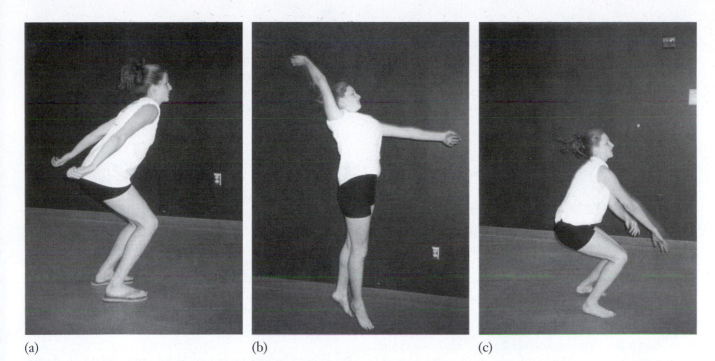

(a)   (b)   (c)

Case Figure 1.2   Hitting a volleyball. (a) wind up; (b) cocking phase; (c) follow through.

tageous and a productive use of time to have her attend several sessions in the clinic initially. The time would best be spent reviewing her therapeutic exercise program and making certain that she is able to perform each with emphasis on proper form. She appears to be a bright young woman who has excelled in her sport and wants to continue to participate for the long term. Utilize those strengths and desires by educating her on why you have selected each exercise and the rationale for each one. If she understands, she will be more likely to comply with the program you develop. With any athlete—particularly a young athlete—it is important to incorporate exercises that closely mimic or can be easily related to their sport of interest. This increases the face validity of your program and should enhance therapeutic exercise program compliance. In addition, you want to make it as much fun and as enjoyable as you can. The more Kate enjoys the exercises and sees how they relate to her end goal, the more devoted she is likely to be.

As you structure your program, remember the therapeutic exercise principles of training for strength (see Chapter 5), joint stability (see Chapter 6) and proprioception (see Chapter 7) endurance (see Chapter 4), and neuromuscular coordination (see Chapter 8).[16,17] Also consider the different types of resistance training and benefits of each (i.e., closed kinetic chain, open kinetic chain, isotonic, isokinetic, plyometrics, use of medicine balls, Swiss balls, etc.). The following paradigm can help as you get started selecting exercises for an initial program and then advancing the program to make it more challenging as Kate improves.

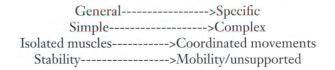

General------------------>Specific
Simple-------------------->Complex
Isolated muscles----------->Coordinated movements
Stability----------------->Mobility/unsupported

Kate has access to elastic bands, Swiss Ball, a medicine ball, free weights and a simple weighted pulley column at school. She also has access to elastic bands, free weights and a Swiss Ball at home.

H. Select no more than 10 appropriate exercises for Kate's initial therapeutic exercise program and arrange them into a table using the following column headings: Exercise order, selected exercise, muscle group/body region trained, and rationale for inclusion. As you select each exercise, make sure that it addresses one or more of the identified impairments or functional limitations from your examination and, conversely, be sure that all identified impairments and functional limitations are being addressed in some way. *See Author's Comments H*

I. Consider the therapeutic exercise volume, intensity, rest-to-work and frequency ratios that are appropriate for Kate, given that she needs work on endurance and control in combination with power. Complete a table for your previously selected exercises using the following column headings: Exercise order, sets/repetitions, intensity level, rest-to-work ratio, and frequency/work. *See Author's Comments I*

J. Now take three of the strengthening exercises you selected and consider how you can take each exercise and advance it to be more complex, regaining greater coordination, and more specific to Kate's needs. Set up a table with the column headings Primary Muscle group, Selected exercise, and Advanced form of same exercise. *See Author's Comments J*

K. List some ways that you could take those same exercises and modify them to incorporate greater trunk/core stability. *See Author's Comments K*

Therapeutic Exercise Program Compliance

For teenagers who perform therapeutic exercises post-injury, establishing program compliance can be a big challenge (see Chapter 11). If Kate is going to be successful, she is going to need to invest some time and energy into the program. As a busy high school student she has many things competing for her time. Once you have been able to establish a relationship with her as an individual, and have shown her that you respect her but also expect some investment from her, she will be more likely to engage in the process and actively participate. The next thing that you need to establish is that it is critical for her to be a part of the decisions about how and when she does her therapeutic exercises, particularly given all of the things in her life that demand her time. It is often helpful to ask, before you ever begin to plan a therapeutic exercise program, how much time a client is willing and able to commit to the program and when the most realistic times would be for her to perform the exercises. This can give you an idea of what barriers she perceives, and you can help her to problem solve ways to discover the time needed to perform the therapeutic exercises on a regular basis.

L. List several ways that Kate might be able to work her therapeutic exercises into other activities that she is already committed to. *See Author's Comments L*

M. When clients are very busy, they sometimes forget whether they have performed their therapeutic exercises on a particular day, or forget to do them at all. List several things that Kate could do to keep track of her exercises and follow through with them more consistently. *See Author's Comments M*

Re-assessment

After four weeks of treatment (two sessions per week) with you in the clinic and daily home exercises, you formally reassess Kate's progress to determine whether she has met her short term goals and make a decision as to whether continuing clinic visits are necessary. Having seen her on a regular basis, you have been able to reinforce the performance of appropriate upper extremity biomechanics and overhead hitting form and the importance of long term injury prevention and shoulder health. This is something that might have been much more difficult if she had merely been doing a home program.

N. What clinical tests would be appropriate to determine Kate's progress toward the short term goals that were established at her initial evaluation? What is the rationale for each? (Refer to your initial evaluation and short term goals if needed.) *See Author's Comments N*

There are many functional clinical outcome measurement tools for the shoulder, but very few evaluate either an athlete's level of sports activity or their self-report of sport function. The Western Ontario Shoulder Instability Index (WOSI) is an excellent tool for evaluating shoulder function in relation to physical symptoms, sports/recreation/work, client lifestyle, and emotions.[18,19] Since impaired sport performance is Kate's primary functional limitation, this would be an appropriate outcome tool to use.

At your four week re-assessment, your examination reveals the following:

Physical Examination

Musculoskeletal Assessment

Posture: Stands with minimally rounded shoulders; right shoulder slightly elevated as compared to the left

Passive Shoulder Range of Motion:[1]

	Right	Left
Flexion	180°	175°
External rotation at 0° abduction	85°	80°
External rotation at 45° abduction	95°	85°
External rotation at 90° abduction	105°	90°
Internal rotation at 90° abduction	70°	70°

Manual Muscle Testing: Normal strength (5/5) of the anterior deltoid and subscapularis. Good strength (4/5) of the middle deltoid and supraspinatus. Good strength (4/5) of the middle trapezius and infraspinatus/teres minor. Fair strength (3/5) of lower trapezius

Global Ligamentous Laxity: Beighton/Horan Hypermobility Index = 8

Musculotendinous Extensibility: Within normal limits at posterior shoulder

Pain: Client rates her current pain level as 0/10 on the Pain Analog Scale (PAS). She rates her worst pain level in the last week at 2/10 and this occurred after she had been participating in a volleyball drill involving light overhead swings at the ball in practice yesterday. No pain with braiding her hair or overhead ADLs

Special Tests:[6]   Sulcus sign, positive. Relocation test, negative. Hawkins test, negative. Neer test, negative. O'Brien's test, negative

Palpation: No tenderness to palpation

Neuromuscular Assessment

Scapulohumeral Biomechanics: Observation of the clients scapulohumeral rhythm with active shoulder flexion reveals slight winging of the right scapula during eccentric lowering from the elevated position

Cardiopulmonary Assessment

Resting Heart Rate: 67 bpm

Integumentary Assessment

Not applicable

Client Self-Report of Function and Functional Limitations

Global Function Rating:[9]   85%
Athletic Shoulder Outcome Rating Scale:[20]   80/100
WOSI:[18,19]   78% (1638 / 2100)
SF-36:[10]   Norm Based Scoring (NBS)—Physical Component Summary (PCS) = 45.7 (.4 SD below the mean) and Mental Component Summary (MCS) = 65.2 (1.5 SD above the mean)

Kate's self-report of function and her improvements in impairment level function have led to an improvement in her ability to perform her sport and activities of daily living with less pain. The changes in her strength, however, are likely not solely from muscular strength changes alone, but also from neuromuscular adaptations, improved muscular activation patterns and coordination. It also appears that she has been able to maintain her cardiopulmonary conditioning, for the most part. You would not expect to observe changes in scores such as the Beighton-Horan Hypermobility index, nor the Sulcus sign, given that these represent underlying capsuloligamentous laxity that she has come by genetically. It is important to recognize and help Kate to understand that her rotator cuff strength and muscular endurance are even more important because of the lack of stability offered by her static or non-contractile joint stabilizers (see Chapters 5 and 6). If Kate is going to be able to continue to play at a high level, she will increase her chances of maintaining a healthy shoulder by maintaining good balance in the muscular

performance and extensibility of her rotator cuff. It will also be critical to share the load with the entire kinetic chain by emphasizing core strengthening in order to decrease the ultimate stress on the weakest link—the shoulder complex.

She is now at a place where her shoulder function and pain are greatly improved and she has reached her short term goals. One of her long term goals is to play in the regional tournament (all day) four weeks from now, so it will be important to structure the next four weeks of her strengthening and return to activity routine to focus on this goal. Keep in mind, however, that if Kate's re-examination had revealed her to have persistent pain and loss of function in spite of your therapeutic exercise program intervention, this would be the appropriate time to recommend to Kate, her parents and her pediatrician a referral to a sports medicine specialist to determine whether there were other underlying mechanical issues preventing her from successful therapeutic exercise progress.

O. What might be a logical return to play progression for an overhead activity (volleyball, in Kate's case) to prepare her for being as close as possible to 100 percent in four weeks? Create and complete a table with the following column headings: week number, activity, intensity, and volume. See Author's Comments O

P. Now that you are comfortable with Kate's progress to date and have thought through a logical, progressive return to sport, you need to turn your attention to modifying and advancing her exercise program, with inclusion of volleyball specific, synergistic exercises. Consider moving from simple exercises with isolated muscle groups to more complex exercises involving the entire kinetic chain. Create and complete a table with the following column headings: exercise order, selected exercise, muscle group/body region, and rationale for inclusion. See Author's Comments P

Q. Complete a table for the exercises you selected using the following column headings: exercise order, volume, intensity level, rest-to-work ratio, frequency/week. See Author's Comments Q.

Case Summary

High school athletes, particularly ones who have underlying musculoskeletal characteristics that may predispose them to certain injuries, can provide a challenging combination of factors to consider when designing a therapeutic exercise program. Not only do you have to consider the

specific impairments that you find on your examination, but you also have the issues related to body image, peer pressure, over or under commitment and desire to return to play as soon as possible. It is important to keep the client's goals at the forefront when designing her program.

If the client can see how her program relates to her goals, she will be more likely to comply (see Chapter 11). By advancing the initial therapeutic exercise program to include more sport specific activities you allow the client's body the opportunity to be gradually stressed more and be able to adapt to the demands imposed. In addition, designing a return to play progression that a client can look at and see how it will help her to work back to her long term goal gives her the freedom to start moving in that direction, while also assuming greater responsibility in the process (see Chapter 11). Helping clients understand what things they can actively work to improve (flexibility, shoulder complex strength and core stability) and how those exercises lend support to the things that they cannot change (i.e., capsuloligamentous laxity, alignment) gives them some of the tools that they need to prevent repeated shoulder injuries or injury to other structures while remaining at a competitive level of athletic performance for many years.

R. On a separate sheet of paper, diagram a decision making algorithm for Kate's case (acute shoulder subluxation, muscular weakness). *See Author's Comments R*

Referring to Chapter 10 for guidance, discuss any alternative or complementary therapeutic exercises that you believe might benefit this client. Provide the rationale for your selection(s).

References

1. Norkin CC, White DJ. *Measurement of Joint Motion: A Guide to Goniometry*, 2nd ed. Philadelphia, PA: FA Davis, 1995, pp. 49–66.
2. Beighton P, Solomon L, Soskolen CL. Articular mobility in an African population. *Ann Rheum Dis.* 1973;32:413–418.
3. Decoster LC, Vailas JC, Lindsay RH, et al. Prevalence and features of joint hypermobility among adolescent athletes. *Arch Pediatr Adolesc Med.* 1997;151:989–992.
4. Kendall FP. *Muscles: Testing and Function*, 2nd ed. Baltimore, MD: Williams and Wilkins, 1993, pp. 268–288.
5. Tyler TF, Roy T, Nicholas SJ, Gleim GW. Reliability and validity of a new method of measuring posterior shoulder tightness. *J Orthop Sports Phys Ther.* 1999;29(5):262–274.
6. Tyler TF, Nicholas SJ, Roy T, Gleim GW. Quantification of posterior capsule tightness and motion loss in patients with shoulder impingement. *Am J Sports Med.* 2000;28(5):668–673.
7. Jensen MP, Karoly P, Braver S. The measurement of clinical pain intensity: A comparison of six methods. *Pain.* 1986; 27(1):177–126.
8. Magee DJ. *Orthopedic Physical Assessment.* 4th ed. Philadelphia, PA. W.B. Saunders, 2002, pp. 245–276.
9. Williams GN, Gangel TJ, Arciero RA, et al. Comparison of the single assessment numeric evaluation method and two shoulder rating scales: Outcomes measures after shoulder surgery. *Am J Sports Med.* 1999; 27:214–221.
10. Ware JE, Snow KK, Kosinski M, Gondek B. SF-36® Health Survey Manual and Interpretation Guide. Quality Metric, Inc. Lincoln, RI, 2000.
11. *Guide to Physical Therapist Practice*, 2nd ed. In *Phys Ther.* 2001;81(1):S1-S738.
12. Rokito AS, Jobe FW, Pink MM, et al. Electromyographic analysis of shoulder function during the volleyball serve and spike. *J Shoulder Elbow Surg.* 1998;7 (3):256–263.
13. Kugler A, Kruger-Franke M, Reininger S, et al. Muscular imbalance and shoulder pain in volleyball attackers. *Br J Sports Med.* 1996;30:256–259.
14. Riegger-Krugh C, Keysor JJ. Skeletal malalignments of the lower quarter: Correlated and compensatory motions. *J Orthop Sports Phys Ther.* 1996; 23(2):164–170.
15. Coleman SG, Benham AS, Northcott SR. A three-dimensional cinematographical analysis of the volleyball spike. *J Sports Sci.* 1993;11:295–302.
16. *ACSM's Guidelines for Exercise Testing and Prescription*, 5th ed. Baltimore: Williams & Wilkins, 1995.
17. McArdle WE, Katch JI, Katch VL. *Exercise Physiology, Energy, Nutrition and Human Performance*, 4th ed. Philadelphia, PA: Williams & Wilkins, 1996.
18. Kirkley A, Griffin S, McLintock H, et al. The development and evaluation of a disease-specific quality of life measurement tool for shoulder instability: The Western Ontario Shoulder Instability Index (WOSI). *Am J Sports Med.* 1998;26(6):764–772.
19. Kirkley A, Griffin S, Dainty K. Scoring systems for the functional assessment of the shoulder. *Arthroscopy.* 2003;19(10):1109–1120.
20. Tibone JE, Bradley JP. Evaluation of treatment outcomes for the athlete's shoulder. In FA Matsen, FH Fu, RJ Hawkins (eds.), *The Shoulder: A Balance of Mobility and Stability.* Rosemont, IL: American Academy of Orthopedic Surgeons, 1993, pp. 519–529.

Author's Comments A

With a young female client, it is always important to know whether she is having regular menstrual cycles, has adequate calcium intake, and has adequate nutritional intake overall. The "female athlete triad" of anorexia nervosa, amenorrhea, and osteoporosis can be catastrophic to young female athletes if they are not adequately counseled and receiving sufficient nutritional support. A young woman Kate's age should have at least 1500 mg of calcium in her diet per day, should be menstruating fairly regularly, and should also have enough protein and carbohydrate intake to support her activity level. If she is not menstruating and does not have adequate calcium intake, she is at higher risk for stress fractures and osteoporosis.

Author's Comments B

The most appropriate diagnosis for Kate would be impingement, or more specifically, inflammation of the rotator cuff tendons and/or subacromial bursa. Using the Preferred Practice Patterns from the *Guide to Physical Therapist Practice*, this would fall into Pattern 4E: "Impaired joint mobility, motor function, muscle performance and range of motion associated with localized inflammation." The appropriate ICD-9 code would be 726.10: "Disorder of bursae and tendons in the shoulder region—unspecified." But bear in mind that an underlying issue is the ligamentous laxity of her shoulder. Sometimes this combination of laxity and resultant impingement will be referred to in the orthopedic community as secondary impingement.

Author's Comments C

Potential advantages	Potential negative effects
1. Appears motivated–good student, active	1. May be overachiever. May overdo her therapeutic exercise program. May have difficulty allowing herself to rest.
2. Supportive family	2. Overextended. Involvement in many things may affect time for exercise.
3. Athletic. Multi-sport athlete	3. Pressure from coaches/ teammates to return too early

Author's Comments D

Impairments:

1. Pain: Rated 6/10 at its worst, which is interfering with activities of daily living (ADLs), instrumental activities of daily living (IADLs), and sport
2. Weakness/impaired muscular performance of her rotator cuff and posterior scapular muscular stabilizers
3. Decreased right shoulder internal rotation
4. Poor posture

Functional Limitations:

1. Inability to serve or hit a volleyball with her desired accuracy (to a specified position on the court)
2. Inability to completely perform all self-care activities

Author's Comments E

Short Term Goals (4 weeks)

1. Perform 60 minutes of non-impact aerobic activity three times per week
2. Improve periscapular and rotator cuff strength to 4/5 measured by MMT to allow spiking a volleyball with 50% effort and 0/10 pain
3. Describe and demonstrate the principles of proper posture
4. Braid hair and do all overhead reaching with 0/10 pain
5. Participate without pain in all non-overhead volleyball drills
6. Demonstrate evidence of compliance with home program

Long Term Goals

1. Play a full day of volleyball with 0/10 pain
2. Maximize and maintain lower extremity strength, abdominal strength, and back flexibility to lend additional support to the kinetic chain
3. Comply independently with a long term preventative and maintenance exercise program

Author's Comments F

Wind up phase

Shoulder: Moves into a extended, horizontally abducted and internally rotated position
Lumbar spine: Flexed

Cocking phase

Shoulder: Moves into a flexed, abducted and maximally externally rotated position
Lumbar spine: Extended and rotated to the ipsilateral side, some side bending to the contralateral side

Swing to follow through phase

Shoulder: Internally rotates, extends and horizontally adducts
Lumbar spine: Flexes and rotates to the contralateral side and goes into some side bending to the ipsilateral side

Author's Comments G

Muscle groups working to move from A to B. Plantar flexors, knee extensors, hip extensors, back extensors and rotators, oblique abdominals, scapular elevators and retractors, shoulder external rotators, and wrist extensors

Muscle groups working from B to C. Hip flexors, rectus abdominus and obliques, shoulder extensors and adductors, elbow extensors and wrist flexors

Author's Comments H

Kate's Initial Therapeutic Exercise Program

Exercise order	Selected exercise	Muscle group/ body region	Rationale for inclusion
1	Warm-up jog	Whole body	Increase core temperature to increase tissue extensibility
2	Static shoulder internal rotation stretch	Shoulder external rotators	Improve external rotator extensibility
3	Trunk stretches: knees to chest, rotations, press up	Low back, thoracic spine	Improve trunk motion/extensibility: prevent back injury and decrease stress on the anterior shoulder
4	Side-lying external rotation with a resistive band or dumbbells (**Case Figure 1.3**) (● **Section 4, Animation 1**)	Posterior rotator cuff	Increase rotator cuff strength and endurance and shoulder muscular balance
5	Standing row with a band or bent over row with dumbbells (**Case Figures 1.4 a–b**)(● **Section 4, Animation 2**) and 1.5)(● **Section 4, Animation 3**)	Trapezius, rhomboids, latissimus dorsi	Increase scapular stabilizer strength and endurance and shoulder muscular balance
6	Forward flexion or elevation with a band or dumbbells (**Case Figure 1.6**)	Anterior deltoid, supraspinatus	Increase rotator cuff and scapular stabilizer strength and endurance
7	Medicine or plyoball sit-up with rotation and diagonal toss against a wall (**Case Figure 1.7a–b**). Could be done sitting on a Swiss ball to promote additional core strengthening	Whole body/ kinetic chain	Core body strength combined with shoulder complex strength; both rotator cuff and scapulothoracic stabilizers in a sport specific pattern
8	Prone trunk extensions holding two lb plyoball in the 90°/ 90° shoulder position (**Case Figure 1.8a–b**). Could also be done prone over a Swiss ball to promote additional core strengthening	Trunk, shoulder complex	Improve back extensor strength for injury prevention and reinforcing shoulder complex stability (rotator cuff and scapulothoracic stabilizers) in a static position
9	Volleyball passing and setting to self or against a wall	Whole body	Maintain skills, keeping coordination sharp using a foam ball that produces less stress on the shoulder
10	Static shoulder internal rotation stretch using a towel or doorknob	Shoulder external rotators	Improve external rotator extensibility following shortening caused by strengthening

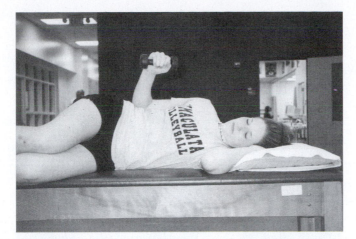

Case Figure 1.3   Side lying shoulder external rotation with a dumbbell.

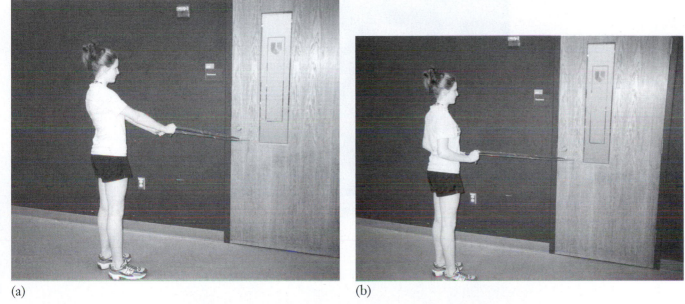

(a)   (b)

Case Figure 1.4   Standing row with elastic band resistance. (a) starting position; (b) finish position.

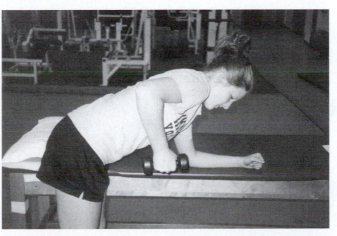

Case Figure 1.5   Bent over row with dumbbell resistance (finish position).

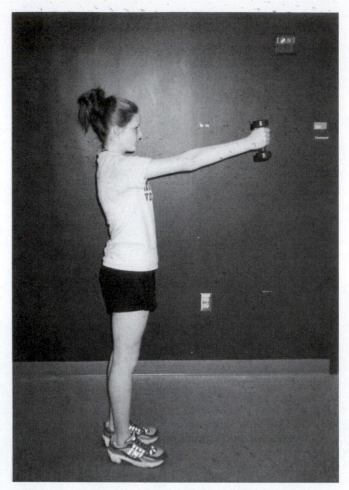

Case Figure 1.6   Forward elevation with a dumbbell.

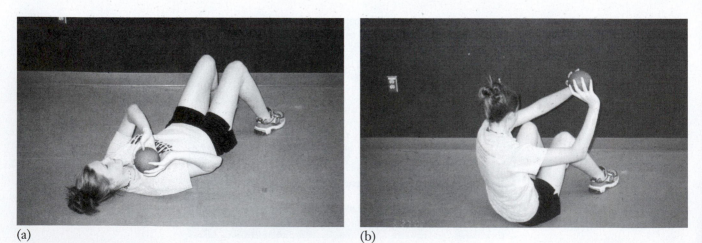

(a)   (b)

Case Figure 1.7   Plyo-ball sit-up with rotation and diagonal toss. (a) starting position; (b) pre-toss finish.

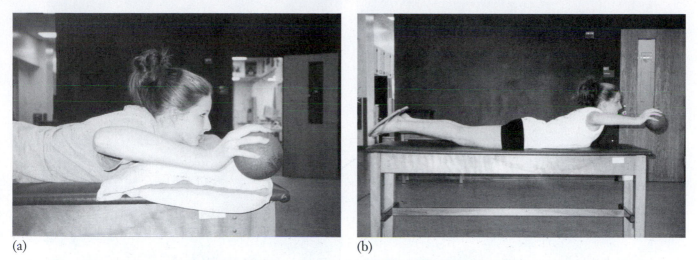

(a)   (b)

Case Figure 1.8   Prone trunk extension holding a two lb plyo-ball. (a) isolated upper torso and shoulder; (b) total body extension.

Author's Comments I

Exercise order	Volume (sets/repetitions/duration)	Intensity	Rest to work ratio	Frequency/ week
1	1 set/10 minutes	Low, enough to break a light sweat	NA	Daily
2	1 set/4 repetitions/20 sec. hold	Low intensity, long duration	1:1	2 × daily
3	1 set/4 repetitions each/20 sec. hold	Low intensity, long duration	Alternate sides where applicable 1:1	Daily
4	3 sets/20 repetitions or fatigue	Low to moderate intensity	2:1	3–5 ×/week
5	3 sets/20 repetitions or fatigue	Low to moderate intensity	2:1	3–5 ×/week
6	3 sets/20 repetitions or fatigue	Low to moderate intensity	2:1	3–5 ×/week
7	3 sets/10–15 repetitions	Low to moderate intensity −4 lb. plyo-ball	2:1	3 ×/week
8	3 sets/10–15 repetitions	Low to moderate intensity −2 lb. plyo-ball	2:1	3 ×/week
9	2 sets/20 repetitions for passing 2 sets/20 repetitions for setting	Low intensity	3:1	3 ×/week
10	1 set/4 repetitions /20 sec. hold	Low intensity, long duration	1:1	After every workout

Author's Comments J

Muscle group	Selected exercise	Advanced form of same exercise
Posterior rotator cuff	Side lying external rotation with a resistive band or dumbbells	Shoulder external rotation in prone with a band or dumbbell with arm at 90° of abduction (**Case Figure 1.9a–b**)
Rhomboids, latissimus dorsi middle trapezeus	Standing row with a resistive band or bent over row with dumbbells	Row with shoulders in 90° abduction moving toward bilateral external rotation (**Case Figure 1.10**)
Anterior deltoid, supraspinatus	Forward flexion or elevation with a resistive band or dumbbell	D2 PNF pattern with a resistive band or dumbbell (see Chapter 6) (**Case Figures 1.11a–b**) and (**Case Figures 1.12a–b**)

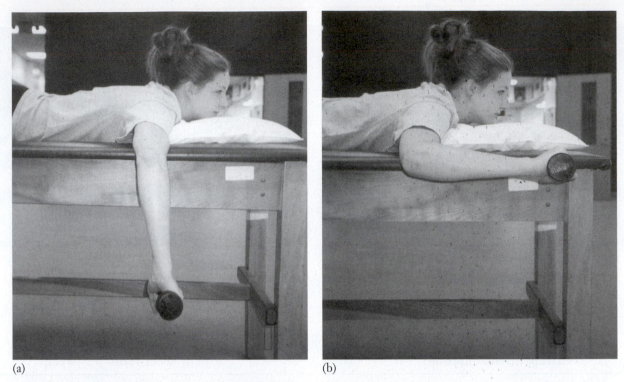

(a)   (b)

Case Figure 1.9   Shoulder external rotation with elastic band or dumbbell resistance with arm at 90° abduction. (a) start position; (b) finish position.

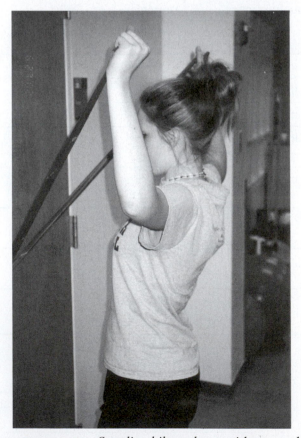

Case Figure 1.10   Standing bilateral row with external rotation shoulder at 90° abduction and trunk extension using elastic band resistance.

Author's Comments K

1. Stand on a balance beam in tandem stance
2. Stand on one foot on a foam half roll, rocker/balance board, or mini-trampoline***
3. Sit on a Swiss Ball*

***While performing the strengthening exercises above.

Author's Comments L

1. Design her therapeutic exercises so that they can be performed during her team's practice times that will keep her involved with the team, while not adding one more thing to fit into her already busy schedule.
2. If she has a gym period at school see if she can substitute her therapeutic exercise program for any part of the gym class that she is not able to participate in because of her injury.
3. If she enjoys a certain weekly television show or listening to music, have her do some of her stretches or strengthening exercises during that time.

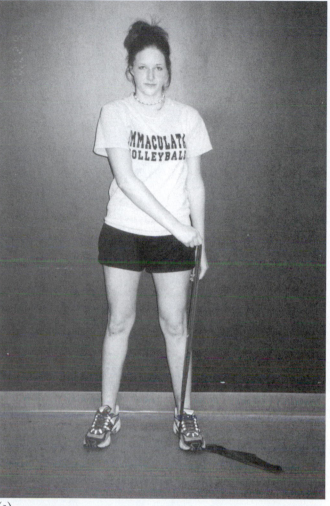
(a)

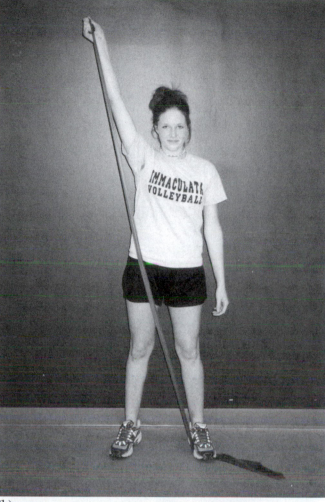
(b)

Case Figure 1.11   D2 PNF pattern with elastic band resistance. (a) starting position; (b) finish position.

Author's Comments M

1. Keep a grid log in a prominent place (mirror at home, gym bag if doing exercises at school/practice) of all therapeutic exercises and check them off each day as they are completed.

2. She could ask one of her siblings or a friend on the team if they would be interested in doing the exercises with her, which would help to motivate her and keep her accountable.

3. Choose a consistent time during daily activities that she does her exercises.

Author's Comments N

Measure	Rationale
Manual muscle testing[2]	Muscle performance
Visual Pain Analog scale[3]	Pain with functional and athletic activities
Goniometric measurement[1]	Range of motion
Athletic Shoulder Outcome Rating scale[18]	Client self-report of level of function
Postural assessment with plumb line	Client's ability to self-correct her posture
Resting heart rate	Maintenance of cardiovascular endurance

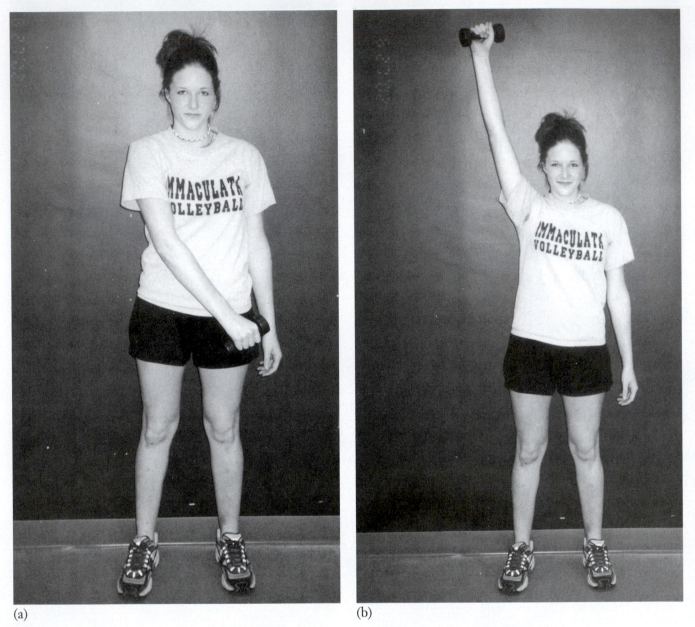

(a)   (b)

Case Figure 1.12   D2 PNF pattern with dumbbell resistance. (a) starting position; (b) finish position.

Author's Comments O

Week	Activity	Intensity	Volume
1	a) Serving overhead b) Hitting at the net	50%	a) Half court distance; half of teammates' repetitions b) Half of teammates' repetitions; flat trajectory
2	a) Serving overhead b) Hitting at the net	75%	a) Three-quarters court distance; three-quarters of teammates' repetitions b) Three-quarters of teammates' repetitions, mid-court trajectory
3	a) Serving overhead b) Hitting at the net	100%	a) Full court distance; repetitions equal to teammates b) Repetitions equal to teammates' angled trajectory
4	a) Serving overhead b) Hitting at the net	100%	Full team scrimmage

Author's Comments P

Kate's Maintenance Therapeutic Exercise Program

Exercise order	Selected exercise	Muscle group/body region	Rationale for inclusion
1	Warm-up jog	Whole body	Increase core temperature to increase tissue extensibility
2	Static shoulder internal rotation stretch	Shoulder external rotators	Improve external rotator extensibility
3	Trunk stretches: knees to chest, rotations, press up	Low back, thoracic spine	Improve trunk motion/extensibility–prevent back injury
4	Isolated shoulder external and internal rotation with pulley or elastic band/tubing resistance	Rotator cuff	Basic rotator cuff stabilization exercise; lend protective support to the static stabilizers of the shoulder
5	Standing pulley trunk rotation and extension with simulated cocking phase external rotation at the shoulder (mimics D2 flexion pattern) (**Case Figure 1.13**)	Whole body	Integration of upper and lower body with core for strength, balance and whole kinetic chain coordination with sport specific motions
6	Standing pulley trunk flexion and rotation with simulated serving/hitting motion (mimics D2 extension pattern) (**Case Figure 1.14**)	Whole body	Integration of upper and lower body with core for strength, balance and whole kinetic chain coordination with sport specific motions
7	Prone trunk extensions over a Swiss ball, with simulated cocking phase using 2 lb. plyoball (**Case Figure 1.15**)	Trunk, shoulder complex	Improve core strength and reinforce shoulder complex strength and coordination with integrated motions
8	"Pepper" warm-up passing, setting and light overhead hitting with a partner	Whole body	Core body strength combined with shoulder complex strength in a sport specific pattern
9	Return to play interval program (see Author's Comments O)	Whole body	Gradual introduction of increased stresses on the shoulder and entire kinetic chain
10	Static shoulder internal rotation stretch	Shoulder external rotators	Improve external rotator extensibility following shortening caused by strengthening activities

Author's Comments Q

Exercise Order	Volume (sets/repetitions/duration)	Intensity determination	Rest-to-work ratio	Frequency/week
1	1 set/10 minutes	Low; enough to break a light sweat	NA	Daily
2	1 set/4 repetitions/20 sec. hold	Low intensity, long duration	1:1	2× daily
3	1 set/4 repetitions each/20 sec. hold	Low intensity, long duration	1:1 Alternate sides where applicable	Daily

(continued)

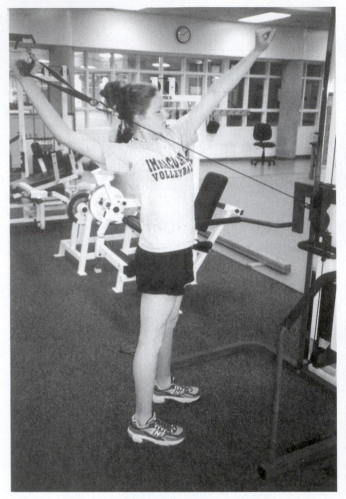

Case Figure 1.13   Standing trunk rotation and extension with weighted cable pulley resistance, while simulating the cocking phase of hitting a volleyball (finish position).

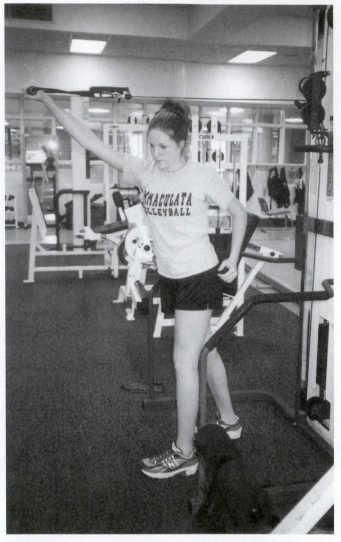

Case Figure 1.14   Standing trunk rotation and flexion with weighted cable pulley, while simulating overhead volleyball hitting (mimics PNF D2 extension pattern).

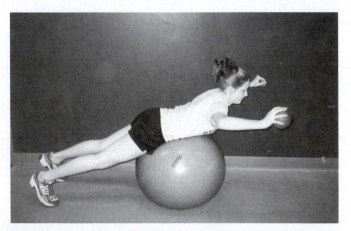

Case Figure 1.15   Prone trunk extension over a Swiss ball with simulated "cocking phase" using a 2 lb plyoball.

Exercise Order	Volume (sets/repetitions/duration)	Intensity determination	Rest-to-work ratio	Frequency/week
4	3 sets to fatigue	All sets to fatigue with 50% of 10 RM	3:1 Alternate sides	5 times/week
5	3 sets/10–15 repetitions	1 set/ 70% 10 RM 1 set/ 80% 10 RM 1 set/ 90% 10 RM	3:1	3–5 times/week
6	3 sets/ 10–15 repetitions	1 set/ 70% 10 RM 1 set/ 80% 10 RM 1 set/ 90% 10 RM	3:1	3–5 times/week
7	3 sets/ 20 repetitions or fatigue	Moderate intensity using 2 lb plyoball	2:1	3–5 times/week
8	10–15 minutes 2 min. rest after 5 min	Low intensity; enough to break a light sweat and loosen shoulder and trunk	1:2	3 times/week
9	See specific interval program outlined	Increasing intensity	1:1	3 times/week
10	1 set/4 repetitions/20 sec. hold	Low intensity, long duration	1:1	After every workout

Author's Comments R

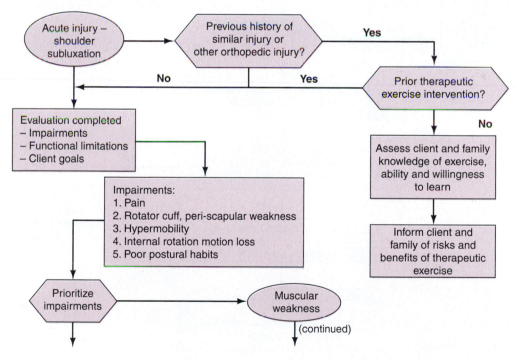

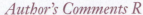

Author's Comments R

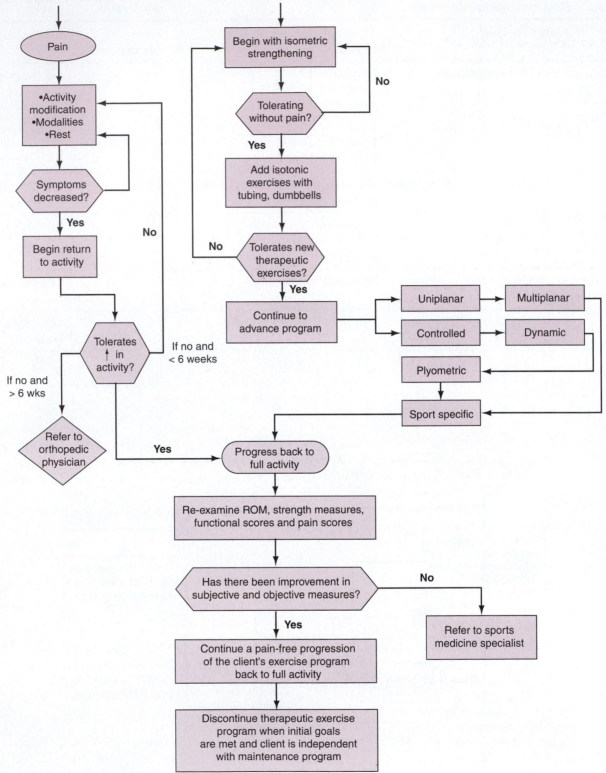

CLIENT CASE #2

Angela M. Corio

History

Client: Dominic

Age: 88 yrs

Height: 5′ 9″

Weight: 178 lbs

Education: High school

Personal: Widowed one month ago; two adult children with two grandchildren (out of state)

Occupation: Retired; formerly owned and operated a small printing business

Medical/Surgical History: History of gout, hypertension and hyperlipidema, laminectomy at lumbar vertebral levels 4 and 5, 10 years ago to resect a herniated disc

Medications: Lipitor® for hyperlipidema; Lopressor® for hypertension

Chief Complaint: Inability to complete daily activities due to fatigue, general decline in physical capabilities, and occasional low back and bilateral knee pain. Would like to be able to resume recreational golf one or two times per week

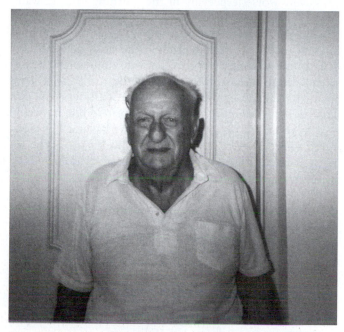

Case Figure 2.1   Dominic.

Dominic (**Case Figure 2.1**) retired and sold his printing business in Manhattan 22 years ago. He and his wife, Theresa, subsequently moved to South Florida to spend their "golden years." They bought a one-story home in Bonita Vista, a planned retirement community in Ft. Lauderdale. Dominic and Theresa participated in all the group activities (e.g., dancing, bingo, sightseeing trips), as well as bowling and golf leagues. Dominic and Theresa also walked regularly together in order to maintain a healthy lifestyle and for enjoyment.

About six months ago Theresa suffered a debilitating stroke. Dominic, along with home health support, cared for Theresa at home. Dominic spent all his time caring for his wife, including her personal care and hygiene, medications, and transportation to and from doctors' offices. Theresa lived six months until she had a second stroke that caused her death. Theresa and Dominic were married for 64 years.

On the advice of his daughter, Dominic visited his doctor for a check-up immediately after Theresa's death, since he had neglected his own health while caring for his ailing wife. At his examination, Dominic told the doctor of the pain in his back and knees from time to time and complained of some shortness of breath when taking the garbage out to the curb. Dominic reported that sometimes he feels unsteady when walking, especially when his knees hurt.

At the doctor's office, Dominic's resting blood pressure was 140/80 mm Hg and his cholesterol level was 140. The doctor also reported that Dominic has some arthritic changes in his knees, along with crepitus and mild inflammation. An x-ray of Dominic's spine showed the prior laminectomy but no other abnormalities besides degenerative changes normal for a man of his age. The doctor prescribed ibuprofen for the knee pain and issued a prescription for 12 visits (two times/week) of therapeutic exercise instruction at your clinic for general conditioning, balance training, and a structured home exercise program (HEP).

Physical Examination

The client reports that he has had pain in both knees "on and off" for the past 10 years. The pain has become progressively worse, especially in the morning or after walking. He also reports that he occasionally feels unsteady. Due to the unsteadiness, he is afraid to return to activities such as golfing or volunteering at the hospital for fear of falling (see Chapter 9). Since his wife's illness and subsequent death, he also feels tired all the time. He worries about having enough energy to make it through the day. His back has begun to hurt him as well. While he would like to return to his prior activities, he has not felt motivated to return to social events without his wife. The activity center within his retirement community includes a fitness gym, but he has never used the facility.

Musculoskeletal Assessment

Upper Extremity Active Range of Motion (UE AROM):   Within normal limits at bilateral upper extremities

Lower Extremity Active Range of Motion (LE AROM):   Left knee flexion 90°, right knee flexion 94° with mild discomfort at end range; remaining LE AROM within normal limits

Trunk Active Range of Motion: Within normal limits with the exception of trunk rotation limited bilaterally: left rotation 25°, right rotation 30°

PROM: Left knee flexion 96°, right knee flexion 100°

Deep Tendon Reflexes: 2+ for bilateral biceps, triceps, patellar, and Achilles tendon

Manual Muscle Testing (MMT):   Upper extremities were grossly 4/5, bilateral hip flexion and extension 3⁺/5, bilateral knee flexion and extension 3⁺/5, bilateral hip abduction and adduction 3⁺/5; remaining lower extremity muscles grossly 4/5

Sensation: Light touch intact and equal bilaterally for upper and lower extremities

Posture: Moderate forward head and rounded shoulders; kyphosis of thoracic spine

Gait: Decreased step length, wide base of support; no assistive devices (see Chapter 9)

Pain: At worst 6/10 on visual analog scale for knees bilaterally when stooping to pick something off the ground or after sustained walking (end range descriptors 0 = no pain, 10 = worst imaginable pain)

Cardiopulmonary Assessment

Resting Blood Pressure: 140/80 mm Hg
Resting Heart Rate: 74 bpm
Respiratory Rate: 16 breaths per minute

Integumentary Assessment

Skin intact; no redness or ulcerations. No symptoms of gout in either foot

Neuromuscular Assessment

Berg Balance Score: 43 out of 56 (a score of below 45 indicates fall risk) (see Chapter 9)

Evaluation

You have taken Dominic's history and completed the physical examination, including several tests and measures. You have a copy of the referring physician's report and you have met and spoken with the client. Now you can begin putting together a plan of care that includes a structured therapeutic exercise program. Before we begin, review the concepts of impairments, functional limitations, and disabilities (see Chapter 1). These concepts will be useful in your career in client evaluation and in developing goals for your client.

According to the *Guide to Physical Therapist Practice*, "Impairments are alterations in anatomical, physiological, or psychological structures or functions that both result from underlying changes in the normal state and contribute to the illness."[1] Impairments are alterations to the norm at the tissue, organ, and/or system level. Examples of impairments would include blood pressure above normal, skin breakdown, muscle strain, or decreased or absent range of motion at a joint.

A. Given Dominic's examination results, list what you think are the most relevant impairments. *See Author's Comments A*

Impairments may or may not result in a restriction of activities. An impairment that effectively restricts a person's physical activity or ability to perform an action in an efficient manner is called a functional limitation.[1] You have to look at what is a "normal" activity for that client. Just as impairments will differ from client to client, functional impairments will also vary. Activities of daily living (bathing, dressing, personal hygiene) and instrumental activities of daily living (balancing a checkbook, grocery shopping, mowing the lawn) can be examples of functional limitations if these are activities that the client can no longer effectively perform due to an impairment.

B. List the functional limitations related to Dominic's case. Keep in mind that there may be many functional limitations. Focus on those that you can do some-

thing about with your therapeutic exercise intervention. *See Author's Comments B*

Numerous components may contribute to a client's disability level, and there are also several disability models in use today (see Chapter 1). The American Physical Therapy Association (APTA) has encompassed several of these components and models in order to come up with their meaning for the word disability. The *Physical Therapist Guide to Practice* defines disability broadly as "the inability or restricted ability to perform actions, tasks and activities related to required self-care, home-management, work (job/school/play), community and leisure roles in the individual's sociocultural context and physical environment."[1] Disabilities have to do with an individual's role in society. Is this person a mother, a father, a worker, a student, a hospital volunteer? These are just a few examples of roles that an individual may have. The concept of disability has to do with these roles and the interactions between the individual within that role and the community.

Let's take an example. A college cross country runner has torn her Achilles tendon. Her impairment is the underlying pathology, a torn tendon, pain, and inflammation. Her functional limitations might include an inability to plantar flex her ankle, inability to walk full weight bearing, inability to climb stairs at her home. Her disability would be her inability to compete as an athlete. It might also include her role as a student. With her injury, she may not be able to reasonably get back and forth across campus for class.

Back to our client . . .

C. What disabilities, if any, may be present for Dominic?[2-9] List and discuss these disabilities. *See Author's Comments C*

Prevention

As both health care providers and as consumers, we have come to realize the value of prevention. By adopting preventative interventions in health care, not only are we able to prevent the onset of a pathology, but we can interrupt the progression from impairment, to functional limitation, and to disability. There are three types of prevention: primary, secondary, and tertiary (see Chapter 1).

D. List some primary prevention, considerations for Dominic that therapeutic exercise intervention might help. *See Author's Comments D*

E. List some secondary prevention, considerations for Dominic that therapeutic exercise intervention might help. *See Author's Comments E*

F. List some tertiary prevention considerations for Dominic that therapeutic exercise intervention might help. *See Author's Comments F*

Preferred Practice Patterns

The APTA, in the *Guide to Physical Therapist Practice*, has developed practice patterns in order to help therapists better develop a plan of care for their clients. There are four main practice patterns: musculoskeletal, neuromuscular, cardiovascular/pulmonary, and integumentary. Each practice pattern is further divided into subcategories based on examination findings, including criteria for exclusion.[1]

G. What practice patterns best apply to Dominic's case? *See Author's Comments G*

H. What is the prognosis for a client like Dominic under your selected practice patterns? Does the expected range of visits for this episode of care coincide with your expected treatment plan or with the referring physician's prescription? *See Author's Comments H*

Plan of Care

You now have the referring physician's note, a completed medical history and physical examination, and you have spoken with the client about his concerns and needs. You have outlined the impairments, functional limitations, and disabilities along with areas of prevention you would like to address with Dominic. You have also looked at several practice patterns that apply to Dominic and can assist you in managing his care. Based on these findings, you can focus your client's therapeutic exercise program. Remember to address the problems that you can directly affect with therapeutic exercise intervention and the problems that are most important to Dominic's physical and mental health and his quality of life.

I. Make a problem list for your client, based on the findings of his case. *See Author's Comments I*

Goals

Given your problem list, how will you solve these problems? By setting some short term and long term goals, you can direct Dominic's plan of care with selected interventions and treatments. Select goals that are reasonable, observable, and written clearly so they are not open to misinterpretation or confusion. Goals should also be related to function. For example, it may be desirable for a client to gain 10 more degrees of elbow flexion; however, it is more important that he be able to bend his elbow far enough to eat, brush his hair, or operate equipment essential to his job. (see Chapter 11)

Dominic was given a prescription for 12 visits to be seen twice a week. We do not know for sure whether or not he will reach the desired goals in 12 visits. He may reach them in fewer than eight visits or he may need more time. We may encounter confounding pathologies that will necessitate modification of the duration of treatment. Nor can we assume that the doctor will extend Dominic's prescription or that Medicare or the insurance provider will pay for further visits. For Dominic's current plan of care, let's set short term goals to be achieved within the first three weeks and long term goals to be achieved by the end of the 12th visit.

J. Make a list of short-term goals that complete this sentence:[6,7,10–18]

In three weeks, the client . . . *See Author's Comments J*

K. Make a list of long term goals that complete this sentence:

In six weeks (at the end of treatment), the client . . . *See Author's Comments K*

Now that you have selected the goals for your client, you can design an individualized therapeutic exercise program. Keep in mind physiological fundamentals, including training principles and energy system considerations. By selectively utilizing these principles and considerations, you will design an effective, well rounded program for your client.

Therapeutic Exercise Program

You will be seeing Dominic twice a week for six weeks. Remember: you are creating a program for an 88-year-old man. The exercises should not be overly complicated or involve difficult or uncomfortable positioning. Especially since we will only be seeing him twice a week, we want to design a program that Dominic can do readily at home. If the exercises are too confusing and/or frustrating, compliance is unlikely (see Chapters 4 and 11). Ultimately, we want to have an exercise program that Dominic can participate in for the rest of his life. We would like him to integrate this program into his daily routine in order to enjoy a healthy lifestyle and an improved quality of life. Elderly clients who regularly participate in exercise programs, including resistance training, have shown documented improvements in strength, flexibility, endurance, functional capacity, and balance.[6, 7, 10–18]

L. Initially, limit the program to 10 or fewer exercises to be performed under your guidance and at home at least twice a week. Make a list of the exercises you have chosen and the body region they involve, placing them in the order in which you would like Dominic to perform them. Also write rationales for your choices.

See Author's Comments L

M. Now that you have selected the exercises, determine the volume of exercise (sets and repetitions), the intensity, the rest-to-work-ratio, and frequency/ week, for each exercise. *See Author's Comments M*

Selection of Exercises and Determination of Sets and Repetitions

Note that we have chosen exercises that are simple and do not require confusing or potentially unsafe positioning. Most of the exercises can be performed at home and are related to daily functions such as stair climbing, squatting, and golf. It would also be wise to provide the client with a written copy of the program that contains illustrations demonstrating proper form.

Given Dominic's age and deconditioned status, we have chosen to begin with one to two sets of exercises with 10 repetitions. This is an appropriate selection not only for Dominic, but also for other beginning clients. Dominic's ability to complete the exercises along with his increased knowledge and confidence with the exercises will determine progression of sets and repetitions (**Case Figure 2.2a–c**) (● **Section 5, Animation 1**), (**Case Figure 2.3a**) (● **Section 5, Animation 2**), (**Case Figure 2.3b**) (● **Section 5, Animation 3**), (**Case Figure 2.4a–b**) (● **Section 5, Animation 4**), and (**Case Figure 2.5a–b**) (● **Section 5, Animation 5**).

Determination of Exercise Intensity

While VO_2 maximum is an ideal way to measure the intensity of exercise and physiologic response, it is not always the appropriate measure for every client. Given Dominic's age and health status, a vigorous VO_2 maximum testing protocol may do more harm than good, given other available measures (see Chapter 4). Plus, many facilities do not have the appropriate equipment necessary for this type of testing.

We have developed a therapeutic exercise program that includes aerobic activity via walking and biking. We would like to provide Dominic with ways to self-monitor his exercise intensity so he can improve his aerobic capacity without exceeding his training threshold. The general rule is, "aerobic capacity improves if exercise is sufficiently intense to increase heart rate to about 70% of maximum."[19] We will use a standard, simple formula for predicting the maximum heart rate for Dominic.

For an 88-year-old man, we would calculate his heart rate maximum at 220 minus his age (88) (see Chapter 4). So Dominic's maximum heart rate is approximately 132 bpm. His training heart rate would be 132 multiplied by 0.70, to equal approximately 92 beats per minute for the minimum of the range. In order to maintain exercising use the aerobic system rather than the anaerobic system, we will advise him to not exercise beyond that level of inten-

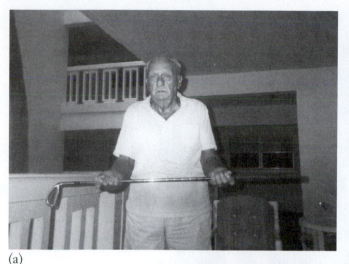

(a)

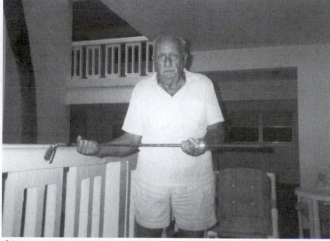

(b)

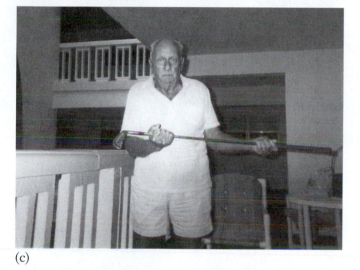

(c)

Case Figure 2.2   Shoulder external-internal roatation using golf club assistance. (a) start, (b) external rotation of right shoulder, (c) internal rotation of right shoulder.

sity (to further simplify, for a 10-second count that would be about 15–16 beats). More important than the heart rate measurement, in Dominic's situation, is that he should never reach an intensity level at which he cannot carry on a conversation while exercising (see Chapter 4). A proper diet, frequent hydration, and participation clearance from a physician is recommended for any older client who decides to begin an exercise program.

Home Evaluation/Inventory

It is worth mentioning that when treating clients who may be at risk for falls, that an assessment of the home may be valuable. We can discuss strategies with our clients for reducing the likelihood of falling as well as available assistive or adaptive devices. While we have included step-up activities in our program, it would be wise to review safe stair-climbing techniques with or without

an assistive device such as a cane or walker. Removing throw rugs that are not secured to the ground is another fall prevention strategy.

As for assistive devices, the placement of a handrail (if there is not one there already) for stairs going into the home is another suggestion. We should discuss with the clients any and all obstacles in the home that may increase the risk of falls and how to address these obstacles for safe transfers and ambulation.

N. Please list any other suggestions you have for helping prevent falls in Dominic's case. *See Author's Comments N*

Re-Assessment

It has been 3 weeks since you began treating Dominic. Below are the results of your re-assessment.

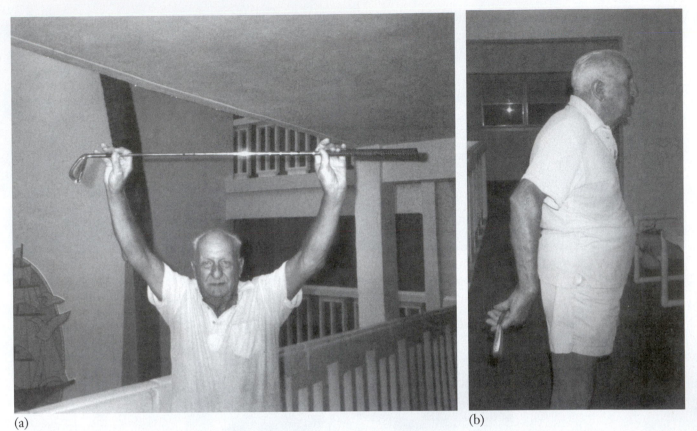

(a)   (b)

Case Figure 2.3   Shoulder flexion (a) and extension (b) with a golf club.

Physical Examination

Client reports that he is feeling much better. He is able to get around better and take walks around the block without pain for up to 45 minutes. He feels steadier when walking and no longer has recurring back pain. He has not returned to golfing or to volunteering at the hospital, but feels that he will be ready soon. Bending and stooping is only mildly painful at times. He reports that he is performing his exercises three to four times a week at home. He has decided that he would like to start going to his community fitness facility to use the exercise equipment and maybe take a group fitness class. Client reports that his pain at worst is a 2–3/10 on a visual analog scale for knees bilaterally when stooping to pick something off the ground or after sustained walking.

Musculoskeletal Assessment

UE AROM: Within normal limits

LE AROM: Left knee flexion 118°, right knee flexion 120° without pain; remaining LE AROM within normal limits

Deep Tendon Reflexes: 2+ for bilateral biceps, triceps, patellar, and Achilles tendon

Manual Muscle Testing: Upper extremities grossly 4+/5, bilateral hip flexion and extension 4/5, bilateral knee flexion and extension 4+/5, bilateral hip abduction and adduction 4/5; remaining lower extremity MMT grossly 4+/5

Sensation: Light touch intact and equal bilaterally for upper and lower extremities

Posture: Mild forward head and rounded shoulders; mild kyphosis of thoracic spine. Able to self-correct posture with cueing

Gait: Normal gait pattern; client demonstrates increased stability and confidence during ambulation

Cardiopulmonary Assessment

Resting Blood Pressure: 135/80 mm Hg

Resting Heart Rate: 70 bpm

Respiratory Rate: 15 breaths per minute

Integumentary Assessment

Skin intact; no redness or ulcerations. No symptoms of gout in either foot.

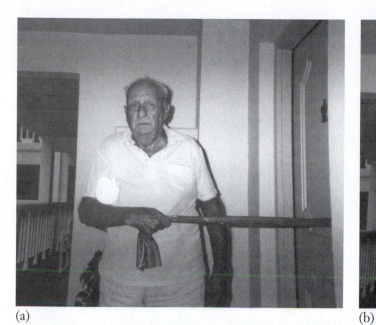
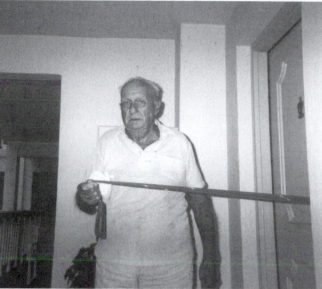

(a)   (b)

Case Figure 2.4   Shoulder external rotation using an elastic resistance band (a) start, (b) finish.

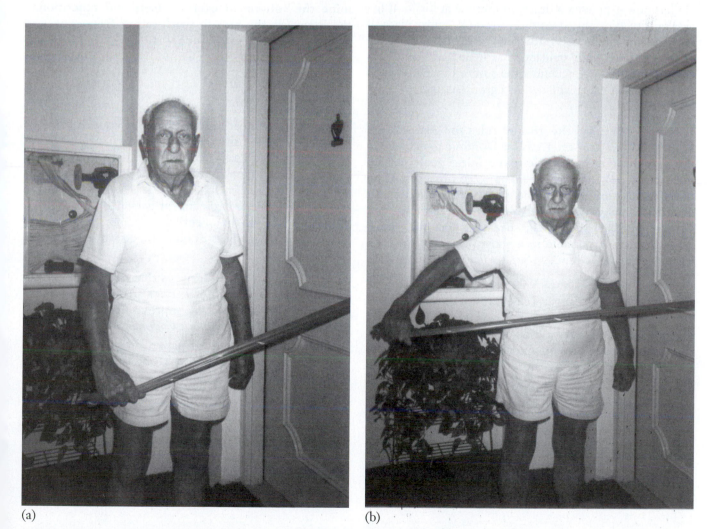

(a)   (b)

Case Figure 2.5   Shoulder abduction using an elastic resistance band (a) start, (b) finish.

Neuromuscular Assessment

Berg Balance Score: 46 out of 56 (a score of below 45 indicates fall risk)

Objective Measurements

The above objective measurements are commonly used in the outpatient clinic.

O. Can you think of other measurements that may be appropriate for a client such as Dominic? Please list them. *See Author's Comments O*

Review of Goals

Dominic has completed 8 of his 12 visits. He has made progress both subjectively through his reports of increased activities and objectively through standard measurements. Assuming we have six more visits until discharge, now is the time to re-address Dominic's goals. He has now expressed a desire to exercise at his local fitness facility. Not only does this provide a regular place of exercise, but it may also further motivate him to continue exercising once your guidance has ended. He may also enjoy the additional benefits of exposure to new types of exercise and/or exercising within a group setting.

P. Keeping in mind the ground rules for goal setting, select a few short term goals for Dominic to achieve in the next three weeks. Review your initial goals. Which goals were met and which goals were not met? If an initial goal was not met, do you need to address it again? Review your updated subjective comments and current measurements. Be sure to select functional goals that are attainable in a short period of time. In three weeks, the client . . . *See Author's Comments P*

We have chosen goals that we believe are the most important to Dominic's function, safety, and quality of life. The increased walking time will allow not only for improved cardiovascular and cardiopulmonary fitness but for him to be able to participate in more recreational activities. It also incorporates the knowledge and practice of exercising within the target heart rate zone.

Since it may be difficult for Dominic to practice balance activities without assistance, we will make this component an important part of our sessions with him. Our last goal is appropriate in that it bridges his therapeutic exercise program from a guided program to independent home and gym activities (see Chapter 11). It also addresses a specific goal for our client to continue exercising at his local fitness facility.

Revised Therapeutic Exercise Program

You now have the options of selecting exercises that can be done at home or at a regular health club facility. It is probably a good idea to select a few exercises for both settings. Remember: Dominic can still perform the exercises that were prescribed during his initial program. You may make use of stationary machines and/or free weights (see Chapters 4 and 5) . You must make sure that the exercise selections and exercise equipment choices you recommend for Dominic are both appropriate and available.

Q. As previously, make a list of exercises, the body region they involve, and your rationale for including them. List them in the order in which you would like Dominic to perform them. *See Author's Comments Q*

R. Now that you have selected the exercises, determine the volume of exercise (sets and repetitions), the intensity, the rest-to-work ratios, frequency, and rationale for each exercise. *See Author's Comments R*

Transition from Guided Therapeutic Exercise Program to Discharge

As our client approaches discharge, we want to continue to facilitate the transition to independence with his therapeutic exercise program. We have created a program that Dominic should be able to perform comfortably at home and at his local health club facility. It is also a good idea to contact the fitness coordinator or personal trainer at Dominic's gym (with the client's permission, of course) so that they can properly assist him with his workout routine.

S. Are there any other services that may be of benefit to Dominic? What other service providers (not limited to health care) could improve his overall health and well being? *See Author's Comments S*

T. On a separate sheet of paper, diagram a decision-making algorithm based on Dominic's impairments, functional limitations, and disabilities. *See Author's Comments T*

Referring to Chapter 10 for guidance, discuss any alternative or complementary therapeutic exercises that you believe might benefit this client. Provide the rationale for your suggestion(s).

Case Summary

You have successfully put together a therapeutic exercise program that addresses your client's impairments, functional limitations, and disabilities. You have addressed areas of prevention and surveyed your client's home and community environment to facilitate Dominic's continued improvement of health and well being. Because you have created a therapeutic exercise program that meets the physiologic and psychologic needs of your client, Dominic is more likely to continue his exercise regimen and to enjoy an active, healthy lifestyle.

Suggested Web sites for information on the elderly and exercise

1. Association of American Retired People. Health and wellness. http://www.aarp.org/health. Accessed December 15, 2004.
2. American College of Sports Medicine. Health and fitness information. http://www.acsm.org/health%2Bfitness/index.htm. Accessed December 15, 2004.
3. National Institute of Health. Medline plus health information. Exercise for seniors. http://www.nlm.nih.gov/medlineplus /exerciseforseniors.html Accessed December 15, 2004.

References

1. *Guide to Physical Therapist Practice*, 2nd ed. In *Phys. Ther.* 2001;81:9–744.
2. Deyle GD, Henderson NE, Matekel RL, et al. Effectiveness of manual physical therapy and exercise in osteoarthritis of the knee. *Ann Intern Med.* 2000;132:173–181.
3. Ettinger WH Jr, Burns R, Messier SP, et al. A randomized trial comparing aerobic exercise and resistance exercise with a health education program in older adults with knee osteoarthritis: The fitness arthritis and seniors trial. *JAMA.* 1997;277:25–31.
4. Fisher NM, Pendergast DR, Gresham GE, Calkins E. Muscle rehabilitation: Its effect on muscular and functional performance of patients with knee osteoarthritis. *Arch Phys Med Rehabil.* 1991;72: 367–374.
5. Fisher NM, Gresham GE, Abrams M, et al. Quantitative effects of physical therapy on muscular and functional performance in subjects with osteoarthritis of the knees. *Arch Phys Med Rehabil.* 1993;74: 840–847.
6. Bemben, MG, Bemben DA, Fields D, Walker L. The effects of 16 weeks of resistance training on strength and flexibility in elderly women. *Issues on Aging.* 1996;19:10–14.
7. Rubenstein LZ, Josephson KR, Trueblood PR, et al. Effects of a group exercise program on strength, mobility, and falls among fall-prone elderly men. *J Gerontol A Biol Sci Med Sci.* 2000;55:M317–321.
8. Perrig-Chiello P, Perrig WJ, Ehrsam R, et al. The effects of resistance training on well-being and memory in elderly volunteers. *Age Ageing.* 1998;27: 469–475.
9. Singh NA, Clements KM, Singh MA. The efficacy of exercise as a long-term antidepressant in elderly subjects: A randomized, controlled trial. *J Gerontol A Biol Sci Med Sci.* 2001;56:M497–504.
10. Berg KO, Wood-Dauphine SL, Williams JI, Gayton D. Measuring balance in the elderly: Preliminary development of an instrument. *Physiother Can.* 1989;41(6):304–311.
11. Berg KO, Wood-Dauphinee SI, Williams JI, Maki B. Measuring balance in the elderly: Validation of an instrument. *Can J Public Health.* 1993;83(2): S7–11.
12. Berg KO, Maki BE, Williams JI, et al. Clinical and laboratory measures of postural balance in an elderly population. *Arch Phys Med Rehabil.* 1992;73: 1073–1080.
13. Bogle-Thorbahn LD, Newton RA. Use of the Berg Balance Test to predict falls in elderly persons. *Phys Ther.* 1996;76:576–585.
14. Shumway-Cook A, Gruber W, Baldwin M, Liao S. The effect of multidimensional exercises on balance, mobility and fall risk in community-dwelling older adults. *Phys Ther.* 1997;77:46–57.
15. Shumway-Cook A, Baldwin M, Polissar NL, Gruber W. Predicting the probability of falls in community-dwelling older adults. *Phys Ther.* 1997;77: 812–819.
16. Steffen TM, Hacker TA, Mollinger L. Age- and gender-related test performance in community-dwelling elderly people: Six-Minute Walk Test, Berg Balance Scale, Timed Up & Go Test, and gait speeds. *Phys Ther.* 2002;82:128–137.
17. Cress ME, Buchner DM, Questad KA, et al. Exercise: Effects on physical functional performance in independent older adults. *J Gerontol A Biol Sci Med Sci.* 1999;54:M242–248.
18. Mueleman JR, Brechue WF, Kubilis PS, Lowenthal DT. Exercise training in the debilitated aged: Strength and functional outcomes. *Arch Phys Med Rehabil.* 2000;81:312–318.
19. McCardle WD, Katch FI, Katch VI. *Exercise Physiology: Energy, Nutrition, and Human Performance,* 4th ed. Baltimore, MD: Williams and Wilkins, 1996.

Author's Comments A

1. Decreased knee flexion bilaterally with pain at end range
2. Decreased strength: Hip flexion/extension/abduction/adduction and knee flexion/extension
3. Poor posture, rounded shoulders/forward head, thoracic kyphosis
4. Poor standing balance, unsteady gait
5. Pain 5/10 with bending activity, walking

Others: Limited trunk rotation, and possible impairments related to hypertension, hyperlipidema, gout

Author's Comments B

1. Unable to bend knees/squat for activities such as sitting into chair, golfing, and stair climbing, without pain
2. Inability to play golf and participate in recreational/social activities
3. Inability to walk long distances/community ambulation
4. Difficulty completing home activities (cleaning, meal preparation, getting in and out of bathtub, etc.)

Author's Comments C

1. Inability to volunteer at hospital
2. Unable to fully participate in family activities such as playing with grandchildren

Dominic's lack of knee flexion contributes to his decreased ability to perform daily activities. This lack of knee flexion is probably due to a number of factors: arthritic changes in the knees, pain, lack of mobility, and decreased leg strength. We cannot reverse the arthritic changes. However, we can address mobility and strength issues, which impede his overall quality of life. Studies have shown that exercise and resistance training can result in functional improvements in those with osteoarthritis of the knee.[2-5]

The poor posture and kyphosis may have developed over time due to spinal changes related to age and habitual behavior. With conditioning and posture training, we may reduce or eliminate Dominic's back pain (see Chapter 11) and help to reduce his balance deficits (see Chapter 9). Participation in a regular exercise program has been associated with a decreased risk of falls in the elderly.[6-7] Upon beginning treatment, we will be able to further evaluate Dominic's gait pattern. If we cannot improve his balance to a level where he is not at risk for falls, he may be a candidate for an assistive device such as a cane or walker. Dominic's current pain level is not only physically limiting, but psychologically limiting. The pain resulting from his impairments can be frustrating and discouraging for someone trying to maintain his independence at home and in the community.

Dominic used to be quite active. Currently, his impairments have significantly restricted or eliminated certain activities that were once routine. Most important, he is most restricted in performing activities related to daily living. He is responsible for maintaining his home and for all his self-care. His physical limitations prevent him from carrying out many of these actions thoroughly and efficiently. His health may further decline if he his not able to maintain his personal hygiene, prepare his meals, or keep a clean living area. If he is not able to care for himself, this will drastically alter his lifestyle. He may come to depend upon others to take care of him or have to relocate to an assisted living facility. Without incorporating physical activity (walking, golfing, bowling) into his daily schedule, he is more likely to develop additional health problems. Given the recent loss of his wife and the lack of family nearby, he is also at risk for isolation and depression. Physical activity, especially group activity, can also improve his sense of self-esteem and overall quality of life.[8-9]

Even though Dominic is retired, he continues to fulfill roles in society. He had been doing volunteer work at a local hospital until his health declined. He is a father and a grandfather. He likely has friends in the community who rely on him for friendship and socialization.

Author's Comments D

1. To prevent the need for use of an assistive device to ambulate
2. To prevent disorders/pathologies related to generalized deconditioning and lack of physical activity (diabetes, pneumonia, heart disease, circulatory problems, etc.)

Author's Comments E

1. To prevent further loss of range of motion and strength
2. To prevent further back pain problems due to poor posture and lack of mobility
3. To prevent further decline in balance and gait abilities
4. To prevent recurrence of gout

Author's Comments F

1. To prevent isolation from friends, family, community
2. To prevent decline in independent functions in order to carry out daily activities (Other areas of prevention may also apply.)

Author's Comments G

1. 4B, Musculoskeletal: Impaired Posture
2. 4C, Musculoskeletal: Impaired Muscle Performance
3. 5A, Neuromuscular: Primary Prevention/Risk Reduction for Loss of Balance and Falling

4. 6A, Cardiovascular/Pulmonary: Primary Prevention/Risk Reduction for CV/Pulmonary Disorders

5. 6B, Cardiovascular/Pulmonary: Impaired Aerobic Capacity/Endurance Associated with Deconditioning

(Others may also apply, but these are the most relevant for Dominic.)

Author's Comments H

With the selected practice pattern above from the Guide to Practice, the expected range of the number of visits was from 1 to 30 visits with a prognosis range of six weeks to six months.[1] So our plan of care consisting of 12 visits over 6 weeks falls within these guidelines. Again, co-morbid pathologies or other unexpected factors may alter the number of visits and prognosis. Later, we can again refer to the Guide to Practice when choosing interventions. We can confirm that the interventions chosen are appropriate for the diagnosis. We may also find other interventions that we overlooked, yet could be beneficial to our client. Checking the Guide to Practice in this manner is also important in preventing reimbursement denials from insurance providers due to unnecessary or unproven interventions.

Author's Comments I

1. Inability to bend knees to 120° or more restricts squatting, kneeling, and impairs gait

2. Decreased lower extremity strength reduces endurance and tolerance for ADLs/IADLs and recreational activities

3. Poor balance/unstable gait puts client at risk for falls and further pathologies

4. Pain prevents client from completing daily activities/responsibilities and activities that are integral to his quality of life

5. Lack of physical activity/general deconditioning puts client at risk for further decline in general health and may prevent continued independent living

6. Lack of client education (body mechanics, transfer techniques, and home exercise program)

Author's Comments J

Short Term Goals

In three weeks, the client . . .
1. Will be able to actively bend his knees bilaterally to 120° or more for functional motions and activities

2. Will be able to walk at self-selected pace continuously for 30 minutes or more pain free

3. Will have increased his MMT grade by ½ or more for hip flexion/extension/abduction and adduction in order to complete home tasks and recreational activities

4. Will have increased his MMT grade by ½ or more for knee flexion/extension in order to complete home tasks and recreational activities

5. Will be able to demonstrate proper posture and body mechanics during balance activities to prevent further injuries and back problems

6. Will be independent in home exercise program

7. Will report decreased pain during squatting or after sustained walking to a 3 or lower on a visual analog scale (VAS).

Author's Comments K

Long Term Goals

In six weeks (at the end of treatment), the client . . .
1. Will improve his Berg Standing Balance Score to 45 or higher to decrease fall risk

2. Will be able to walk 60 minutes or more pain-free

3. Will be able to play nine holes of golf pain-free 1–2 times per week

4. Will have a 4/5 or better MMT grade for all lower extremity muscle groups in order to complete home tasks and recreational activities

5. And the rehabilitation clinician will have reviewed home modifications to facilitate ADLs/IADLs and to decrease the risk of falls

6. Will have increased cardiovascular endurance to be able to return to ½ day volunteer work at the hospital

Any of these goals can be modified to be either a short-term or long-term goal by changing the measurement values. The important thing for the rehabilitation clinician to remember is to create goals that can be measured; goals that are objective; goals that are functional; goals that are realistic; and goals that meet the individual needs and wants of the client. The goals selected here relate to physiologic principles including ROM, strength, balance, and endurance necessary to complete basic daily activities and recreational activities safely and pain-free. We have also selected goals that include specific activities important to Dominic. These activities are vital to maintaining and/or improving his quality of life. (You may have other goals that would be applicable to Dominic.)

Note the Berg Balance instrument was chosen because it is an objective performance-based measure of balance in the elderly; it tests tasks common in everyday life; and is easy to administer. The Berg Balance Scale has also been shown to have strong intrarater and interrater reliability along with evidence to support content, construct, and criterion-related validity.[10–15] However, new research indicates that age-related norms may be appropriate for the Berg Balance Scale in interpreting and evaluating the data in order to make the best clinical judgements[16] (see Chapter 9).

Author's Comments L

Exercise order	Exercise selection	Body region	Rationale for inclusion
1	Stationary bike or treadmill	Whole body	Improve cardiovascular fitness, knee ROM, warm-up for exercises/ stretching
2	Active assisted; heel slides in supine	Knee	Increase knee flexion
3	Straight leg raises, including hip flexion, extension, abduction, adduction	Hip flexors, extensors, abductors, adductors and knee extensors	Increase lower extremity strength in all planes, improve exercise tolerance
4	Supine hip abduction with resistance band/ adduction with therapy ball	Hip abductors/adductors	Increase hip abductor and adductor strength
5	Mini-squats with handrail	Lower extremities	Closed-chain lower extremity strengthening/balance training
6	Step-ups in all directions on four inch step with handrail use	Lower extremities	Increasing lower extremity strength/ endurance; balance training
7	Weight shifting with perturbations from clinician in standing and while seated on a exercise ball	Trunk and upper extremity	Increase core trunk strength; balance
8	Hamstring/heel cord and quadriceps stretching	Lower extremities	Increase hamstring and heel cord extensibility/prevent sore muscles
9	Active shoulder ROM exercises with golf club: flexion, extension, abduction, adduction, internal rotation, external rotation	Upper extremities	Increase AROM at shoulder for functional activities/golfing
10	Shoulder exercises w/resistance band for flexion, extension, abduction, adduction, internal rotation, external rotation, diagonals	Upper extremities	Increase upper extremity strength/ ROM for functional activities/ golfing

Author's Comments M

Exercise order	Sets/ repetitions	Intensity	Rest-to-work ratio	Frequency/ week
1	1 set/ 5–15 min.	Low to medium	N/A	2–3/week
2	1–2 sets/ 10 repetitions	Pain-free range	1:1 Alternate lower extremities	2–3/week
3	1 set/ 10 repetitions; increase resistance as tolerated	Achieve repetition goal with minimal to moderate effort	3:1	2–3/week
4	1 set/10 repetitions; increase resistance as tolerated	Achieve repetition goal with minimal to moderate effort	3:1	2–3/week
5	1–2 sets/10 repetitions	Increase depth of squat and hold times as tolerated with minimal to moderate effort	3:1	2–3/week

Exercise order	Sets/ repetitions	Intensity	Rest-to-work ratio	Frequency/ week
6	1 set/10 repetitions each in each direction	Increase step height as tolerated with minimal to moderate effort	3:1	2–3/week
7	5–10 minutes total with rehabilitation clinician	Increase challenges as tolerated without loss of balance	2:1	2/week
8	3 repetitions of each stretch/30 sec. hold	Low intensity	1:1 Alternate lower extremities	2–3/week
9	2 sets of 10 repetitons in each direction	Low intensity	1:1	2–3/week
10	2 sets of 10 repetitions for each exercise	Achieve repetition goal with minimal to moderate effort	3:1	2–3/week

Author's Comments N

1. Shower chair
2. Handrails by the commode for sit/stand
3. Properly illuminated rooms
4. Raised toilet seat
5. Other cushioning or platform devices that raise seat height
6. Non-skid surface rug/appliqués to prevent slipping in shower or tub
7. Shoes with good support to prevent falls

Author's Comments O

1. Girth measurements to measure edema/effusion/atrophy
2. Volumetrics to measure edema/effusion/atrophy
3. Instrumented or non-instrumented single-leg stand test to measure balance
4. Others may also be appropriate

Author's Comment P

Short Term Goals

In three weeks, the client . . .

1. Will be able to walk 60 minutes or more in his neighborhood or on the treadmill at a self-selected pace, and comfortably in his target heart rate zone for both community ambulation and for improving his cardiovascular fitness
2. Will demonstrate a 47 or higher score on the Berg Balance Scale in order to decrease his risk of falls and to prepare him for returning to golf
3. Will be independent with regular exercise program participation including safe and proper use of exercise equipment at his local health club facility

Author's Comments Q

Exercise order	Exercise selection	Body region	Rationale for inclusion
1	Stationary bike or treadmill	Whole body	Improve cardiovascular fitness, knee ROM, warm-up for exercises/stretching
2	Leg press machine	Lower extremities	Increase quadriceps and hamstring strength
3	Seated knee flexion/hamstring machine	Hamstrings	Increase hamstring strength
4	Seated hip abduction/adduction machine	Hip abductors/adductors	Increase hip abduction/adduction strength
5	Half squats against wall or with Swiss ball	Lower extremities	Weight bearing lower extremity strengthening/balance training
6	Half lunges, alternating legs, using handrail for support (Case Figure 2.6a–b)	Lower extremities	Increasing lower extremity strength/endurance; balance training

(continued)

Exercise order	Exercise selection	Body region	Rationale for inclusion
7	Hamstring/heel cord and quadriceps stretching.	Lower extremities	Increase muscle group extensibility, increase active knee ROM
8	Bicep curls/triceps curls with dumb bells (**Case Figure 2.7 a–b**)	Biceps/triceps	Increase biceps/triceps strength for lifting
9	Low-rows, 90° with resistance band	Upper back	Increase back strength to help improve posture/core strength
10	Wall push-ups	Pectorals, triceps	Improve core strength/increase functional ability (ex. pushing open car door)

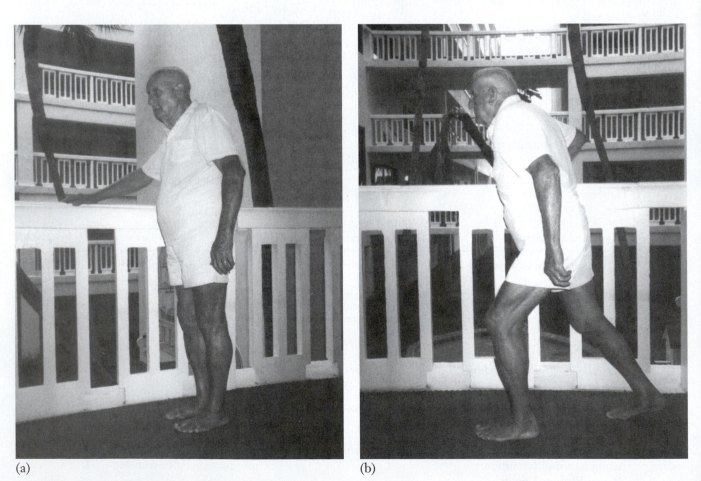

(a)   (b)

Case Figure 2.6   Half lunges, alternating legs, using handrail for support (a) start, (b) finish.

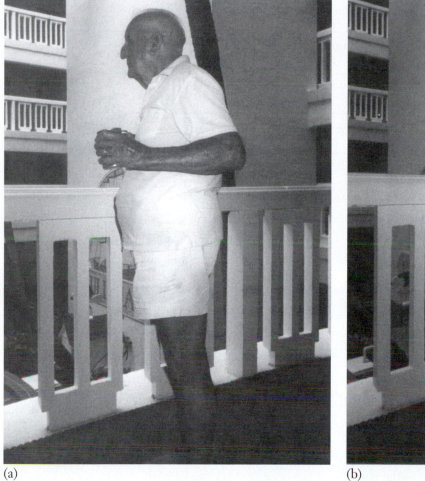 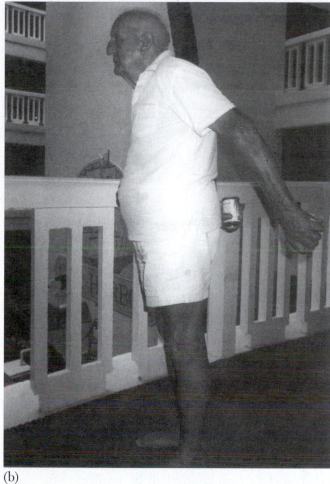

(a)   (b)

Case Figure 2.7   Biceps curls (a) and triceps extensions (b) with "weights" (cans of soup)

Author's Comments R

Exercise order	Sets/repetitions	Intensity	Rest-to-work ratio	Frequency/ Week
1	1 set/ 15–30 min.	Target heart rate	N/A	2–3/week
2	1–2 sets/ 15 repetitions	Subjectively moderate intensity as tolerated	3:1	2–3/week
3	1–2 sets/ 15 repetitions	Subjectively moderate intensity as tolerated	3:1	2–3/week
4	1–2 sets/15 repetitions of each machine	Subjectively moderate intensity as tolerated	3:1	2–3/week
5	2 sets/15 repetitions	Subjectively moderate intensity as tolerated	2:1	2–3/week
6	2 sets/ repetitions 15 each leg	Subjectively moderate intensity as tolerated	2:1	2–3/week
7	3 repetitions at each lower extremity/ 30 sec. hold	Low intensity	1:1 Alternate lower extremities	2–3/week

(continued)

Exercise order	Sets/repetitions	Intensity	Rest-to-work ratio	Frequency/ Week
8	2 sets of 15 repetitions for each exercise	Subjectively moderate intensity as tolerated	3:1	2/3/week
9	2 sets of 15 repetitions for each position	Subjectively moderate intensity as tolerated	2:1	2–3/week
10	2 sets of 15 repetitions	Subjectively moderate intensity as tolerated	3:1	2–3/week

Note that we have selected a combination of exercises that can be performed at home or the gym and some exercises that require gym equipment. We would have to call the facility or make a site visit to determine what equipment is available. Is the selected equipment appropriate for Dominic? Is he able to get in and out of the equipment easily and independently? Will he be able to safely and effectively use the resistance training devices that you have selected?

Prior to discharge, you can demonstrate and then observe Dominic's use of the equipment at your clinic or his community facility. This will increase his confidence about using the equipment safely and properly. You can also make any necessary adjustments in positioning, resistance, and volume to his program.

Again, it is a good idea to provide a written copy of the program along with illustrations (if possible) to the client (see Chapter 11).

Author's Comments S

1. Nutritionist to aid in selection of foods that provide a well rounded diet and help to avoid high cholesterol foods
2. Psychology counselor to assist Dominic in dealing with the loss of his wife
3. The American Association of Retired People (AARP) or other senior citizen organizations. They may have group activities, benefits, or other resources that are available to Dominic at no charge or reduced fees.
4. Others: Personal trainer, massage therapist, Tai-Chi/martial arts groups (see Chapter 10), and transportation providers for the elderly.

Author's Comments T

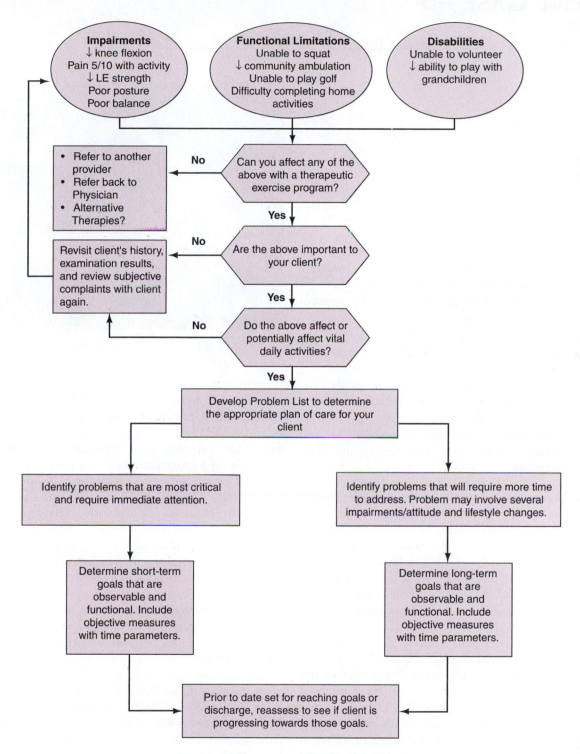

CLIENT CASE #3

Tom Squires

History

Client: Michele

Age: 21 years

Height: 5′ 6″

Weight: 110 lbs

Education: Currently a sophomore in college

Occupation: Full time student, competitive cross country runner

Personal: Client is a highly motivated competitive runner who has many first place finishes and wants to compete in conference championships in less than one month. Client has been treated by university team athletic trainer.

Medical/Surgical History: Right hip injury one year ago, treated as groin strain. Magnetic resonance imaging (MRI) some weeks later revealed a stress fracture of the right femoral neck, which healed in a few months. Medial collateral ligament sprain to knee in high school.

Chief Complaint: Pain in the anteromedial aspect of her right knee with running, after driving, and with climbing stairs.

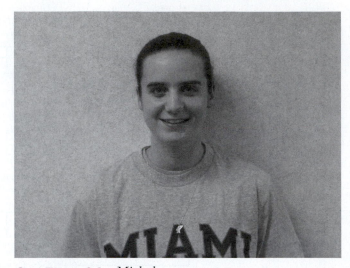

Case Figure 3.1 Michele

Ever since her arrival at the local NCAA Division III University Michele, a 20 year old cross country athlete, had been known as a very hard worker. The work ethic had paid off with several first-place finishes and, combined with a svelte running body with only 8% body fat, had made Michele a force to be reckoned with in the conference as well as nationally. Unfortunately, Michele has grown very familiar with her orthopedic surgeon (**Case Figure 3.1**).

Michele's current complaint is pain in the anteromedial aspect of her right knee with running. She reports that though she is able to "run through the pain" she has had to reduce her mileage and she can only run four or five times per week. It is late September and the conference championships are less than one month away. The pain has worsened since its onset one month ago and now lingers throughout the remainder of the day after she has run, particularly after she has been driving her car and when she ascends and descends stairs. Michele is worried that she will not return to the performance level that she will need to be conpetitive at the conference meet.

This is not the first running related injury for Michele. Last year, when she was a college freshman, she had a right hip injury. At that time she was in the middle of a successful season, particularly for a freshman. According to

Michele, that injury was precipitated by a misstep as she landed on an uneven part of the ground during a meet. Instantly she felt right groin pain, but was able to finish the last 1.5 km of the race. After the injury, she was treated aggressively for a groin strain by the medical staff at the university. During one session with the staff athletic trainer Michele expressed some concern that she had not had a menstrual period for nine months. The athletic trainer told her that it was normal for runners to go a long time without menstruation, so Michele dismissed the issue.

To complete the season, Michele altered her training regimen from running 50–70 miles/week to running 20–30 miles/week with supplements of sessions on a Stairmaster® device (see Chapter 4). She was able to finish the last two meets of the season and the national championship qualifier despite worsening hip pain. The treatment at that time consisted of stretching, therapeutic modalities such as ice, ultrasound and electrical muscle stimulation, over the counter anti-inflammatory medication (ibuprofen), and cross training (See Chapters 4 and 5). Michele did not qualify for the regionals of the Division III Championship, although her times earlier in the year would easily have been good enough. Michele admitted that she just could not keep to the pace that she was accustomed to because of the pain and altered running mechanics.

At the end of the season Michele, under the advice of the university medical staff, took one month off from training to rest the hip so that she could be ready for the indoor track season in January. Michele was compliant. She continued her rehabilitation and avoided running, although she continued an aerobic therapeutic exercise regimen of sessions on a Stairmaster® device and a stationary bicycle 6 days a week for 30–45 minutes per session (**Case Figures 3.2–3.3**). Over the Christmas break, Michele visited a local orthopedic surgeon who had treated her when she experienced tibial stress fractures in high school.

The surgeon ordered a bone scan and hip/pelvis MRI to be performed the day after her consultation. The results revealed a stress fracture at the neck of her right femur. Michele was issued crutches and instructed to be non–weight bearing for four weeks, progressing to partial weight bearing between weeks four to six. The surgeon requested that Michele return for a follow-up bone scan at the beginning of February to determine the healing status of the fracture and wrote a prescription for instruction in a therapeutic exercise program. Michele's first session has been scheduled to begin in one week at your clinic.

A. From the limited information that you have, list some therapeutic exercises that would be appropriate for Michele to perform at this time in her apartment,

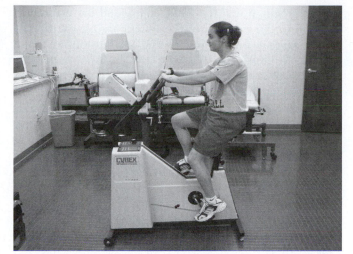

Case Figure 3.3   Stationary cycling.

prior to making her initial visit to your clinic. *See Author's Comments A*

B. As Michele increases her weight bearing, what modes of aerobic exercise would be appropriate, excluding running? Please list these modes in order of progression.[1] *See Author's Comments B*

C. What other concerns might there be for this type of client that have not been addressed?[2–4] Please make a list, with explanations. *See Author's Comments C*

Although Michele experienced a full recovery from her stress fracture, she did not return to competition during the late spring of the same year. Michele felt that she needed a little break from training, but found herself training again by early summer and even entered a few races—"just for fun," she told herself.

By mid-summer of this year, Michele found herself in her old training regimen: running five days a week and training two days per week on a stationary bicycle or Stairmaster® device. Her weekly running mileage totaled 40–45 miles. Ironically, because she feared that she was not back to the competitive level that she was accustomed to, she decided not to join the team training camp in August. Upon returning to campus, she was contacted by the cross country team coach, who convinced her to join the team. Re-joining the team meant that Michele had to increase her mileage to 55 miles per week, exclusively running. Michele reports that about two weeks after her return to the team, she began to experience right knee pain.

Michele reports first noticing the pain after a particularly long training run at a nearby state park on grass, as always. She had a history of a medial collateral ligament (MCL) sprain to her right knee in high school after stepping in a hole during a race. Because the current knee pain was in a similar location and the latest run had been on particularly uneven ground, Michele believed that she had

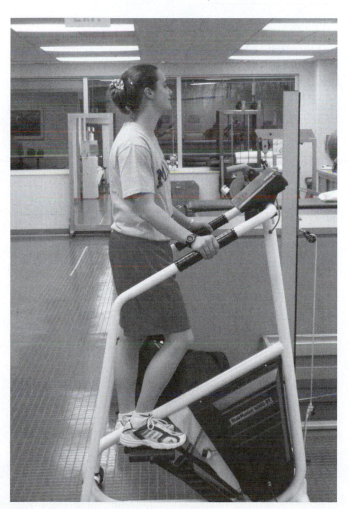

Case Figure 3.2   Vertical stepping machine.

simply re-aggravated the MCL injury and did not report her pain to the coach or to the athletic training staff. The pain continued for the rest of the day, but did not cause Michele to limp. The following day produced no pain in Michele's knee and she was able to run, but she completed a shorter run than the day before. Michele reported that the right knee pain persisted after she ran for the next week. Approximately one week after the onset, Michele noticed that she was experiencing the knee pain during the day when she climbed stairs while going to class, and she noticed increased right knee stiffness when she stood up after sitting in class.

D. Please list some probable contributing factors to Michele's recent onset of knee pain.[5] *See Author's Comments D*

Early Intervention

When Michele noticed this increase in her symptoms, she consulted with the athletic trainer that was working with the team. Together they determined that the injury was not a result of a recent change in training habits, or inappropriate shoe wear. The athletic trainer advised her to spend more time warming up, utilize ice packs after workouts and to implement some cross training whenever possible. As expected, Michele did ice and warm up more, but she did not change her training habits or workout intensity and the pain continued to worsen. Michele reported that her running times were beginning to suffer and she also noticed that she was altering her running style to compensate for the pain.

E. What are some compensatory changes that you might expect to see in a runner with knee pain?[6] Please list them. *See Author's Comments E*

Because Michele was not improving the team physician referred her to a local clinic that was affiliated with the university. The medical diagnosis at the time of referral was patellofemoral syndrome, and an old grade II MCL sprain at right knee. The order requested evaluation and treatment over a four week duration.

Physical Examination

Chief Complaint: Right anteromedial knee pain with running, particularly after 2 miles, after driving or sitting in a car for longer than 10 minutes, and when climbing stairs.

Training Regimen: Run (four to five times/week, 25–35 total miles)—down from 40–55 miles/week; Stairmaster® (two times/week, 30–45 minutes)

Occupation: Full time student

Specific Pain Report: Right knee pain during heel strike and initial loading phase of running

Primary Goal: Run in conference championships (30 days from now) without pain and with normal running style

Musculoskeletal Assessment

Body Type/Size: Ectomorphic, 5′ 6″, 110 lbs. Body fat: 12%[7]

Posture: Spine: Cervical, normal

Thoracic, slightly flexed, flexible

Lumbar, normal

Upper Quarter: Normal

Lower Quarter:

Pelvis, Minimally increased anterior pelvic tilt

Femur, slightly increased medial rotation, hip joint adduction, bilaterally

Knee, slight genu recurvatum bilaterally

Tibia, not remarkable

Feet, slight pes cavus bilaterally

Walking Gait: Noticeable lateral rotation of the hip during initial swing phase bilaterally with significant medial hip rotation from heel strike to midstance. Heel strike on lateral rearfoot bilaterally

Single Leg Stance: Decreased balance at right lower extremity with increased hip adduction. Maintains position for 35 sec. at left lower extremity and 14 sec. at right lower extremity (see Chapter 9)

Step-up: Anteromedial right knee pain when attempting to step up onto a six-inch step. Concurrent increased right hip adduction and medial rotation. Resolution of symptoms with right gluteal facilitation and increased hip abduction and lateral rotation (**Case Figure 3.4a–b**).

Timed Step-Down (120 seconds):   Right: 25 repetitions with poor control. Client unable to complete past 45 seconds due to increasing (7/10) knee pain.

Left: Able to perform 80 repetitions with good control and no knee pain

ROM: Within normal limits and equal bilaterally at hips, knees, ankles and feet

Flexibility: Hamstring, bilaterally, 5° from complete extension beginning in 90°/90° position

Hip flexors, decreased bilateral tensor fascia lata—iliotibial band extensibility in Modified Thomas Test Position[8] (**Case Figure 3.5**).

Gastrocnemius-soleus, active dorsiflexion bilaterally 14°.

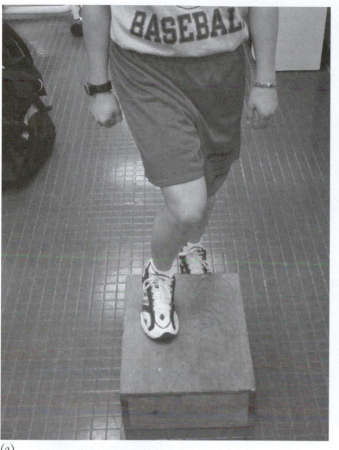 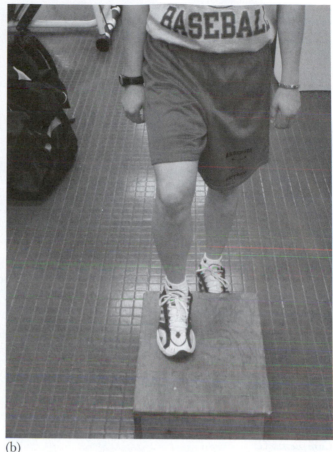

(a)   (b)

Case Figure 3.4   Step-up exercise. With medial hip rotation-adduction (a) and following gluteal facilitation (b).

Ober's Test: Minimally decreased tensor fascia latae/iliotibial band (TFL/ITB) extensibility bilaterally. Reproduction of symptoms at end range on her right side. Resolution of symptoms with manual medial glide of patella (**Case Figure 3.6a–b**)

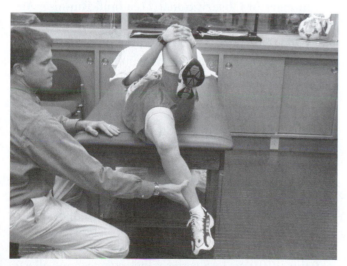

Case Figure 3.5   Modified Thomas Test.

Manual Muscle Testing: 5/5 throughout bilateral lower extremities, with the exception of 3+/5 bilateral posterior gluteus medius strength and strong/painful right quadriceps strength with resisted knee extension

Patellofemoral Joint Examination: Minimal lateral tilt bilaterally

Special Tests: Negative for ligamentous laxity tests and patellar apprehension test. Palpation failed to reveal focal areas of knee joint discomfort.[8]

Pain: Right anteromedial knee pain 2/10 on Visual Analog Scale (VAS) (0 = no pain, 10 = worst pain imaginable) with long sitting, 3/10 with stair climbing, 5/10 with stair descent, and 4/10 during running, particularly during stance phase

F. Please compile an impairment problem list from the case history and examination findings.[9–11] *See Author's Comments F*

G. Develop a list of short and long term goals for Michele. These goals should be functional and help illustrate your expectations of Michele when she returns in two weeks and four weeks.

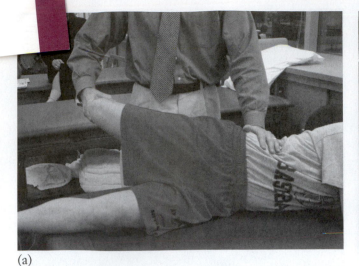
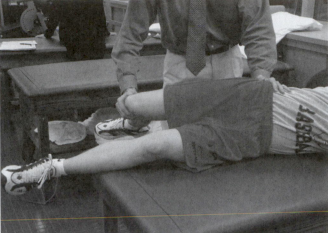

(a)   (b)

Case Figure 3.6 Ober's Test. (a) start position; (b) finish position.

Short Term Goals

By two weeks, the client will . . .

Long Term Goals

By four weeks, the client will . . . *See Author's Comments G*

H. Describe your initial plan of care for Michele for the next two weeks, including frequency of visits and training recommendations. *See Author's Comments H*

I. Exercise Prescription:

Create and complete a table listing no more than 6 home exercises in the order that they are to be performed by Michele. Use column headings of exercise order, selected exercise, daily frequency, and rationale. *See Author's Comments I*

Two-Week Visit

Michele returns to the clinic after spending two weeks following the prescribed plan of care. Prior to the visit, the staff athletic trainer confirmed via telephone Michele's compliance to the plan. Michele reports that she has been asymptomatic for 10 days and is able to perform all of her therapeutic exercises without pain. She has been able to exercise on an elliptical trainer for the last seven days, up to 20 minutes the last session. Michele reports that she has completed the first appointments with the university nutritionist and sports psychologist. Follow-up visits are due in the next two weeks with those specialists. Michele seems very pleased with the resolution of symptoms, but is very anxious to resume running because the conference meet is only three weeks away.

Musculoskeletal Assessment

Single Leg Stance: 35 seconds at left lower extremity, 38 seconds at right lower extremity. Normal balance and dynamic right lower extremity control

Step-up: Pain-free at right lower extremity on six-inch step. Client independently maintains appropriate lower extremity alignment during task performance

Timed Step-down (120 seconds): 55 repetitions with good biomechanics at right lower extremity for first minute of test, but 3/10 pain and decreased dynamic control during the final minute

Ober's Test: Minimally decreased bilaterally. No pain at end range, right knee

Manual Muscle Testing: Bilateral 4/5 posterior gluteus medius strength

Summary of Observational Treadmill Running Assessment:

Duration: Covered 1.5 miles prior to symptom onset

Intensity: Self-regulated by client to mimic training pace

Swing phase: Symmetrical at bilateral lower extremities

Heel strike: Decreased bilaterally, increased toe striking

Midstance: Bilaterally increased hip medial rotation and adduction. Normal midfoot pronation

Terminal Stance/Push-off: Reduced supination at midfoot bilaterally with continued significantly increased bilateral hip medial rotation and adduction

Pain: 0/10 on VAS with six-inch step task and all activities of daily living (ADLs)

J. Compile an updated impairment problem list from the case history and examination findings. *See Author's Comments J*

K. Update Michele's short term goals with a list, as previously. Update Michele's long term goals with a list, as previously. *See Author's Comments K*

L. Make two suggestions for other functional tests that would have been appropriate.[10,11] *See Author's Comments L*

M. List two differences between treadmill running and running on the ground.[12–15] *See Author's Comments M*

N. Considering Michele's symptoms and her desire to return to competitive running in three weeks, please outline a progression for aerobic exercise for the next two weeks. Modes of exercise available to Michele at the university include a stationary bicycle, upper body ergometer (UBE) (Case Figure 3.7), elliptical trainer, vertical stepper (Stairmaster®), running, and swimming. You can have Michele perform more than one mode of exercise/day. Create and complete a table with the following column headings: day, exercise activity, and duration. *See Author's Comments N*

O. Michele has access to the university weight room. Before her injury, she was lifting three times/week with the team. Michele's team is currently performing (sets × repetitions) bench press 3 × 10, lat. pulldown 3 × 15, seated shoulder press 3 × 10, bicep curls 2 × 20, dips 4 × 5, abdominal crunches 2 × 40, leg press 3 × 15, seated knee extentions 3 × 15, knee curls 3 × 15, heel raises 3 × 15. Do you believe that this is a good time for her to return to lifting weights? If so, what exercises should she perform. On a separate

sheet of paper create and complete a table listing the exercises that Michele should perform, and the main muscle group(s) that are targeted. For any exercises that you believe should be avoided, please explain your rationale for exclusion. Make adjustments to sets and repetitions as necessary. *See Author's Comments O*

P. Considering what you have prescribed above, what other specific therapeutic exercises would you prescribe for Michele at this point? Create and complete a table with column headings for: exercise order, exercise selection, daily frequency, and rationale. *See Author's Comments P*

Four-Week Visit

Michele returns to the clinic for her third visit, very pleased with her progress. She has been compliant with all instructions, again verified by the university athletic trainer, and reports no pain during exercise but some soreness after running that lasts for 2–3 hours post-cessation. Michele reports that although the soreness is in the front of her knee, it is not the same as the original pain and appears to be more diffuse. The conference meet is in eight days, with the national qualifications the following week. Michele is convinced that she will be ready to compete if she is given the green light to return to full mileage.

Musculoskeletal Assessment

Step-up: Pain-free at right lower extremity with 10-inch step. Client independently maintains appropriate lower extremity alignment

Timed Step-down (120 seconds): 90 repetitions and able to maintain good dynamic control for 90 seconds at right lower extremity, but displayed fair control with fatigue during last 30 seconds. No knee pain reported during test.

Ober Test: Minimally decreased bilaterally. No pain at end range, right knee

Manual Muscle Testing: Bilateral posterior gluteus medius, 5/5

Q. Please compile a revised impairment problem list from the case history and examination findings. *See Author's Comments Q*

R. Update Michele's treatment goals. *See Author's Comments R*

S. Should Michele be allowed to increase her training and participate in the conference meet? Please state your rationale. *See Author's Comments S*

Case Figure 3.7   Upper body ergometer (UBE).

Case Summary

Because of their high fitness level and motivation, athletically active clients can be very enjoyable to work with. However, they present with their own set of challenges. Recognizing and addressing treatment issues outside the realm of musculoskeletal injury or movement based impairment management is essential to achieving a long lasting recovery. As with most athletes, Michele presented with a high level of function without many physical impairments, despite her injury. The most difficult part of establishing a therapeutic exercise program was not addressing Michele's impairments, but prescribing an appropriate therapeutic exercise regimen that would allow her to reach her primary goal, while not aggravating the injury. Michele will need to be followed closely after the conference meet and through the national championships until the end of the season. Management of Michele's training regimen for the rest of her collegiate career will be necessary to prevent an exacerbation of the anterior knee pain. A long term plan for Michele needs to be carefully developed due to her history of musculoskeletal injuries. A comprehensive team approach that includes Michele, the coach, the team athletic trainer, sport psychologist, nutritionist and the rehabilitation clinician would be appropriate. The outcome of this meeting should include a timeline of follow-up, either directly or via the athletic trainer, for general training guidelines and nutritional habits, and a protocol to follow if new or past pain symptoms reappear. This team approach increases the likelihood of successfully managing the client who participates in competitive athletics.

T. Diagram a decision making algorithm for Michele's case (focus on management of the anterior knee pain that she experiences when running). See Author's Comments T

Referring to Chapter 10 for guidance, discuss any alternative or complementary therapeutic exercises that you believe might benefit this client. Provide the rationale for your selection(s).

References

1. Appell HJ. Skeletal muscle atrophy during immobilization. *Int J Sports Med.* 1986;7(1):1–5.
2. Winters KM, Adams WC, Meredith CN, et al. Bone density and cyclic ovarian function in trained runners and active controls. *Med Sci Sports Exerc.* 1996;28(7):776–785.
3. De Cree C. Sex steroid metabolism and menstrual irregularities in the exercising female: A review. *Sports Med.* 1998;25(6):369–406.
4. Highet R. Athletic amenorrhoea. An update on etiology, complications and management. *Sports Med.* 1989;7(2):82–108.
5. Bennell KL, Malcolm SA, Thomas SA, et al. Risk factors for stress fractures in track and field athletes: A twelve-month prospective study. *Am J Sports Med.* 1996; 24(6):810–818.
6. Novacheck TF. Running injuries: A biomechanical approach. *Instr Course Lect.* 1998;47:397–406.
7. Going S, Davis R. Body composition, In Roitman JL (ed). *ACSM's Resource Manual for Guidelines for Exercise Testing and Prescription*, 3rd ed. Baltimore: Williams & Wilkins, 1998, pp. 378–386.
8. Magee DJ. *Orthopaedic Physical Assessment*, 3rd ed. Philadelphia: W.B. Saunders Co., 1997.
9. Olson BR. Exercise-induced amenorrhea. *Am Fam Physician.* 1989;39(2):213–221.
10. King MB, Judge JO, Whipple R, Wolfson L. Reliability and responsiveness of two physical performance measures examined in the context of a functional training intervention. *Phys Ther.* 2000;80 (1):8–16.
11. Sahrmann S. *Diagnosis and Treatment of Movement Impairment Syndromes.* St. Louis: C.V. Mosby, 2002 (Chapter 8, pg 425).
12. van Ingen Schenau GJ. Some fundamental aspects of the biomechanics of overground versus treadmill locomotion. *Med Sci Sports Exerc.* 1980;12(4): 257–261.
13. Nigg BM, De Boer RW, Fisher V. A kinematic comparison of overground and treadmill running. *Med Sci Sports Exerc.* 1995;27(1):98–105.
14. Stolze H, Kuhtz-Buschbeck JP, Mondwurf C. Gait analysis during treadmill and overground locomotion in children and adults. *Electroencephalogr Clin Neurophysiol.* 1997;105(6):490–497.
15. Van Gheluwe B, Smekens J, Rosen P. Electrodynographic evaluation of the foot during treadmill versus overground locomotion. *J Am Podiatr Med Assoc.* 1994;84(12):598–606.

Author's Comments A

Any therapeutic exercise that maintains the appropriate weight bearing restrictions, is pain free, and does not place abnormal stress on the fracture site would be considered safe for this situation. Chapter 1 described the effects of disuse of the musculoskeletal system, so it is important to continue to stress the body appropriately to maximize physical health during recovery. Possible exercises could include isometric quadriceps and gluteal sets, seated knee extensions, seated leg lifts, side lying leg lifts, and abdominal exercises.

Author's Comments B

The rehabilitation clinician must always attempt to return the client to a level of aerobic exercise that they can safely perform as soon as possible to negate the negative effects of immobility (see Chapter 1). Swimming could be initiated when Michele is allowed partial weight bearing; this could be followed by using a stationary bicycle, Nordic-Track®, elliptical trainer, and/or Stairmaster device (see Chapter 4). This is a natural progression that allows for progressively increased weight bearing and exercise intensity. The elliptical trainer, most notably, will mimic running without placing a significant impact load through the lower extremity.[1]

Author's Comments C

There are often contributing factors to client complaints that are not of musculoskeletal system or movement impairment origin. The fact that Michele has a history of multiple stress fractures combined with amenorrhea should raise an alarm. Significant risk factors for stress fractures have been reported in female athletes, including lower bone mineral density, a history of menstrual disturbance, less lean mass in the lower limb, a discrepancy in leg length, and a low fat diet. Overtraining and poor nutrition can also lead to menstrual disturbances, which leads to an increased risk of stress fractures. Poor nutrition can also lead to a low body fat percentage.[2–4]

Author's Comments D

Realizing contributing factors is critical to successful intervention into a musculoskeletal condition. Resolution of symptoms will only be temporary if the true causes of the condition are not addressed.

1. Overtraining
2. Recent increase in training intensity/distance
3. Different training surface—grass
4. No cross training
5. History of right hip injury

One of the most common causes of musculoskeletal injury in an athlete is overtraining or inappropriate training habits. Often the difference can be subtle between an appropriate amount of exercise and an amount that will cause injury. Getting a thorough training history will often "tease out" the subtle changes of a client's training regimen that could precipitate an injury. Repetitive exercise that does not allow the body to recover between sessions will lead to an increased chance of injury. Cross training is a good alternative that will allow the client to exercise daily while the body recovers from the previous mode of exercise (see Chapter 5). We must also not forget Michele's recent hip injury. Incomplete rehabilitation of the right hip may predispose any part of the right lower extremity to injury.[5]

Author's Comments E

While each runner will have individual characteristics in their stride, there are some common compensations that will result from knee pain:

1. Decreased stance time on the involved lower extremity (see Chapter 9)
2. Increased knee flexion during stance phase
3. Decreased knee flexion during swing phase
4. Flat foot (decreased heel strike) during initial stance
5. Increased trunk side bend toward the side of the injury during stance phase

You will notice that these compensations are very similar to what you would expect during a painful walking gait, but they are usually more pronounced. Most sports medicine experts would agree that once these abnormalities become apparent, the client should stop running because further injury can result, including injury to other adjacent or functionally related structures.[6]

Author's Comments F

Initial Visit Problem List

1. Decreased right posterior gluteus medius strength
2. Decreased right lower extremity balance during single leg stance
3. Right knee pain with poor dynamic control during step-up task
4. Decreased right tensor fascia lata and iliotibial band extensibility with pain with Ober's Test
5. History of stress fracture and right hip injury
6. Low body weight and body fat
7. Increased medial hip rotation and genu recurvatum

It would be a mistake to discount the combination of Michele's history of stress fractures and her body type when addressing her current concern. Even though you have been told that stress fractures have been ruled out for her current condition, it is apparent that overtraining and poor eating habits can lead to other types of musculoskeletal injuries. It is also apparent that Michele aggressively returned to a heavy training regimen. It is important to assess if this behavior is healthy. An unhealthy reason for an aggressive return to sport after injury is if one is driven by an obsessive personality (see Chapter 11). Often this is seen in conjunction with an altered body image, which may be the main driver for the intense training. If you discover that the client may be driven by motivations that can be disruptive to the therapeutic exercise program, it is important to refer to other health care professionals. To address these concerns, the school athletic trainer was consulted and visits with the university nutritionist and sports psychologist were scheduled. By comprehensively treating Michele at this point, we will be much more effective at preventing future musculoskeletal injuries.[2,9]

The other major concerns from the physical examination include decreased balance at the right lower extremity and pain during a step-up maneuver. This problem is objectively measured with asking Michele to perform step-down maneuvers. By tracking the amount of step-downs she can perform before she experiences knee pain, we are able to establish a functionally relevant baseline with which to track Michele's future progress. A runner performs the sport with only one leg in contact with the ground at a time, so functional measures should be in single leg stance to try to assess how the body is behaving during the stance phase. A runner who is not able to balance well during static or slow dynamic tests will not be effective in maintaining proper mechanics during running (see Chapter 9). A contributing factor to the poor single leg mechanics is the decreased strength of the posterior gluteus medius.[10,11]

An interesting dynamic is displayed by the Ober's Test.[8] Many rehabilitation clinicians utilize the Ober's Test to merely assess the length of the TFL-ITB. Often this test will reproduce anterior knee pain symptoms at end range for a client, even though the length test is normal. Simple manual reduction of the patella in a medial direction by the clinician will usually reduce the symptoms. As the TFL-ITB is brought to end range, it pulls the patella laterally via the iliotibial band-lateral patellar retinaculum connection producing symptoms associated with lateral patellar tracking. Recognizing the contribution of the TFL-ITB to the client's symptoms can help guide your treatment.[11]

Author's Comments G

In order to develop effective goals, the rehabilitation clinician must learn to anticipate how a musculoskeletal injury will evolve. Unfortunately, predicting how an injury will progress can be one of the most challenging aspects of a young clinician's practice. Once expectations and goals are formulated, the rehabilitation clinician will be able to form a better initial therapeutic exercise program and be able to confidently make a client more independent with their program without unjustified return visits to the clinic.

Examples of effective short term goals include:

1. The client will be able to descend 25, six-inch steps with no knee pain and with non-impaired dynamic control in two weeks.
2. The client will be able to drive a car and have 0/10 anterior knee pain getting in and out of the car in two weeks.
3. The client will be able to ascend one six-inch step with no anterior knee pain in five days.

4. The client will be able to ride a stationary bike for 30 minutes without anterior knee pain in 10 days.

Long term goals often will focus on achieving the client's primary therapeutic exercise program goals. Examples of long term goals include:

1. The client will be able to run 20 minutes at 75% intensity two days in row without anterior knee pain in four weeks.
2. The client will be able to exercise on the Stairmaster® device for 30 minutes at 75% intensity without anterior knee pain in three weeks.
3. The client will be able to return to full running competition without anterior knee pain during or after exercise in four weeks.

Author's Comments H

The expertise of the sports medicine department at the university should be tapped so that Michele can have her therapeutic exercise program supervised daily by the athletic training staff. This is important for many reasons: it is much more convenient for Michele, it will utilize the many resources available at the university (swimming pool, weight room, aerobic training equipment), it will keep Michele in constant contact with the team and coaching staff, and it will utilize the experience and skills of the athletic training staff. Athletic trainers are skilled in evaluating the functional readiness of an athletic client and are expert in communication with coaching staffs, adjusting training variables, and in maximizing athletic performance with consideration for an injury, particularly during the middle of a competitive season. Because Michele will be performing her therapeutic exercises at the university, regular visits to your clinic may be unnecessary. Communication with the athletic trainer is essential immediately after each clinic visit and whenever there is a change in status with Michele. A return visit two weeks after the initial evaluation is probably the best choice because Michele would not be expected to make significant enough progress to change the treatment plan until then. Cultivating this relationship between your clinic and the university sports medicine department is essential. One of the best ways to accomplish this, besides communicating regularly with the athletic trainer, is to engage the athletic trainer as well as the client in the decision making process. The team approach usually works best when mutual respect and courtesy is practiced.

To decrease her pain level it is critical that Michele not be allowed to run. Equally important is that Michele continue some mode of aerobic exercise so that she can meet her primary goal (see Chapter 4). This is when the expertise of the athletic trainer can be particularly beneficial. General recommendations of low impact, pain free therapeutic exercises that maximally stress Michele's aerobic system should be sufficient.

There are several options the rehabilitation clinician can use to control or diminish anterior knee pain; however, passive modalities used in isolation are usually not the answer. One should be very careful when recommending solely ultrasound, phonophoresis, heat, electrical stimulation, or massage interventions because they give the client the perception that something needs to be done to them for recovery. Cryotherapy is a passive modality used to reduce pain and inflammation after exercise. The use of ice in this instance may not be indicated, as anterior knee pain is generally not an inflammatory condition. Properly selected therapeutic exercises should not produce any pain, so cryotherapy may not be needed for this client. Taping and bracing of the patellofemoral joint can often provide pain relief to allow the client to perform at higher exercise intensity levels without pain.

Author's Comments I

Therapeutic exercise should be prescribed to address the impairments and their associated functional limitations. While the specific exercise may not be critical, it is important that basic exercise principles be followed to treat the client comprehensively.

Order	Exercise	Repetitions	Daily frequency	Rationale
1	Side lying hip abduction and Sahrmann hip abduction-external rotation progression.[11]	2 sets of 30 repetitions	Two	Strengthen the lateral hip stabilizers for better dynamic control during single lower extremity support
2	Partner or individual tensor fascia lata or iliotibial band stretch	6 repetitions, 30 seconds each	Three	Lengthen the structures to reduce the lateral pull on the patella
3	Single leg stance	10 repetitions, 20 seconds each	Two	Enhance single leg balance and dynamic postural control
4	Step-up	2–3 sets of 10–20 repetitions	Two	Enhance single leg balance and control and build lower extremity strength
5	Progressive unilateral leg press	2–3 sets of 10–20 repetitions	Two	Build lower extremity strength

You may have compiled a larger list for Michele and that would have been appropriate because she is very motivated and will follow all instructions. On the other hand, one must be very careful in over-prescribing exercise for two reasons: 1) It is important that the client not lose sight of the critical parts (functional relevance) of the therapeutic exercise program by doing less meaningful exercises (i.e., she will end up going through the motions if the program is too extensive); and 2) to avoid overtraining, less is better so that each exercise is performed maximally rather than effort spread across too many exercises (see Chapter 5). As a rehabilitation clinician, be very precise with the therapeutic exercise program that you would like the client to perform at home. Only prescribe what is needed, and have a specific rationale for each exercise.

The above approach reconciles the few specific muscle strength and length issues found in the exam with the first two exercises. The issue of knee control/balance is addressed in exercises 3 and 4. The leg press is initiated at this point, not so much to gain strength because pain will limit Michele, but to enhance muscular activity without producing pain. The leg press can achieve this because Michele can adjust the resistance level to maximize a workout while avoiding pain. Did you prescribe a knee extension exercise? Be careful when doing so with a client who has anterior knee symptoms. The joint compression stresses can become very high in the patellofemoral joint during the end ranges of knee extension, particularly between 10 and 35° of flexion.[11]

Author's Comments J

As expected, Michele's problems have decreased since her initial examination. Her problems now have become more functional in nature.

1. Decreased ability to perform repeated step-downs compared to the noninvolved lower extremity

2. Decreased involved side dynamic lower extremity control during treadmill running
3. Client not returned to full running regimen

Author's Comments K

Like the goals from the initial visit, the updated goals should remain functional and reflect your expectations of progress in the future. They can include a revision of the past goals or new goals. If not done previously, new goals can include your expectations on Michele's return to competition as well as your performance expectations.

Short Term Goals

1. Client will be able to adhere to prescribed nutrition program from nutritionist in two weeks
2. Client will be able to exercise on the Stairmaster® device and an elliptical trainer without anterior knee pain at 100% intensity for 30 minutes

Long Term Goals

1. Client will be able to participate in the conference meet in three weeks without anterior knee pain during competition

Author's Comments L

The challenge of utilizing functional tests is finding a measure that not only mirrors the function of the client, but that is objective and reproducible. The most direct functional measure for Michele would be to record the amount of time and distance that she can run before pain. We indirectly do this from the history, but clinical testing is limited by space and/or the use of a treadmill. There are also various step tests that can be performed. Although stair climbing and descending is not the same as running, it is a single lower extremity stance activity that stresses the entire lower extremity and often will replicate anterior knee pain symptoms. Further functional tests include a single leg hop, vertical single leg jump, and repeated squats (see Chapter 5 and 11).[10] Further research is needed to improve the validity of functional tests for specific athletically active client populations.

Author's Comments M

Although running analysis on a treadmill can be a very effective assessment tool, rehabilitation clinicians must take caution when making parallels with traditional running. The main difference on a treadmill is that instead of the runner propelling herself forward, the running surface moves under the runner. When a runner is not forced to propel herself forward, the muscle recruitment patterns may change. For example, the hip extensors become less important from midstance to terminal stance. A decreased use of the gluteals during treadmill running may result in

decreased single lower extremity stability during stance phase. Other changes could include decreased step length, increased swing phase, increased heel strike, or altered upper extremity movements (see Chapter 9).[12–15]

Author's Comments N

Allowing Michele to push the limits of her aerobic energy system while not aggravating her condition is very challenging. Assisting Michele and her team athletic trainer develop a specific therapeutic exercise program can help prevent the tendency for Michele to overtrain.

Day	Exercise activity	Duration
1	Bike, Stairmaster®	20 min., 10 min.
2	UBE, bike, elliptical trainer	20 min., 10 min., 10 min.
3	Rest	
4	Bike, Stairmaster®	20 min., 20 min.
5	UBE, elliptical trainer	20 min., 20 min.
6	Rest	
7	Bike, UBE, running	20 min., 10 min., 5 min.
8	Elliptical trainer, Stairmaster®	20 min., 10 min.
9	Bike, UBE, running	15 min., 10 min., 15 min.
10	Rest	
11	Stairmaster®, running	20 min., 20 min.
12	Stairmaster®, elliptical trainer	20 min., 25 min.
13	Elliptical trainer, running	20 min., 20 min.
14	Stairmaster®, elliptical trainer	25 min., 25 min.

UBE = Upper body ergometer.

Although a detailed prescription can help guide the athletic trainer and serve as the limit that Michele should be allowed to train, it should be made clear to the team athletic trainer that they should use their judgment to adjust the modes and times as Michele experiences symptoms. The basic exercise principles followed above include low impact to high impact exercise, cross training within an exercise session, and between exercise sessions, gradual increase in exercise intensity, and adequate time for rest and recovery (see Chapter 4).

Author's Comments O

Exercise	Sets × repetitions	Muscle group	Exclusion rationale
Bench press	3 × 10	Pectoralis major, triceps	
Lat. pulldowns	3 × 15	Latissimus dorsi, biceps, rhomboids	
Shoulder press	3 × 10	Deltoids, triceps, trapezius	
Biceps curls	2 × 20	Biceps, brachialis, brachioradialis	
Dips	4 × 5	Latissimus dorsi, triceps, pectoralis major	
Abdominal Crunches	2 × 40	Rectus abdominis, internal and external abdominal obliques	
Leg press	3 × 25	Gluteals, hamstrings, quadriceps, gastroenemius, soleus	
Seated Knee extensions		Quadriceps	Increased patellofemoral joint stress; if included should only be performed between 90°–45°.
Knee curls	3 × 15	Hamstrings	
Heel raises	3 × 15	Gastrocnemius, soleus	

There are no significant changes that need to be made as Michele resumes her weight training regimen, except for recommending that she avoid seated knee extensions. You should also make sure that she performs the leg press with one lower extremity at a time, for reasons mentioned above.

Author's Comments P

Order	Exercise selection	Sets/repetitions	Daily frequency	Rationale
1	Side lying hip abduction and Sahrmann hip abduction external rotation progression for gluteus medius strength.[11]	2 sets of 30 repetitions	Two	Strengthen the lateral hip stabilizers for dynamic postural control during single lower extremity stance
2	Partner or individual tensor fascia lata, iliotibial band stretch	6, 30 sec. repetitions	Three	Lengthen the tensor fascia lata, iliotibial band to reduce the lateral pull on the patella
3	Step-down, 6–8 inch	2 sets of 30-40 repetitions	One	Enhance single lower extremity dynamic postural control and balance
4	Star pattern step-down maneuver	4 sets, 45 sec. each	One	Endurance, strengthening, neuro-muscular control

Once again, specific exercise prescription is not as important as complying with the original treatment plan of addressing Michele's impairments while challenging her neuromuscular system with functionally relevant, pain-free exercises. Utilizing a functional measure, like the Star pattern step-down test, as a therapeutic exercise can be very useful, but remember that the test results during the following visit will be skewed because of practice.

Author's Comments Q

The problem list at this point is brief, but can include:
1. Client has not returned to full level of competition without pain
2. Client continues to complain of pain after running
3. Client has been unable to train adequately to perform at prior level of performance without risk of injury

Author's Comments R

Final discharge goals should be completed and can include:

1. Client to return to full competition with no pain and equal level of performance to pre-injury level in four weeks
2. Complete transfer of care to university sports medicine staff to take place in one week

Author's Comments S

Although Michele is still symptomatic, it appears that she is mentally and physically ready to increase her training level and compete in the conference meet. Michele's report of no pain with exercise and pain afterwards that is more diffuse than original symptoms is a good sign that she is not exacerbating her injury with the regimen that was prescribed. Michele should be advised to increase her running times and intensity in line with the original therapeutic exercise program. One full day of rest from running the day before the meet should ensure that she is pain free for competition.

Author's Comments T

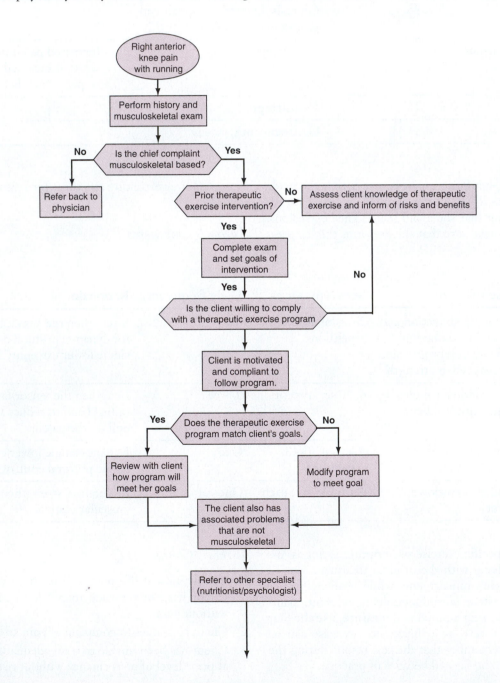

Author's Comments T (con't)

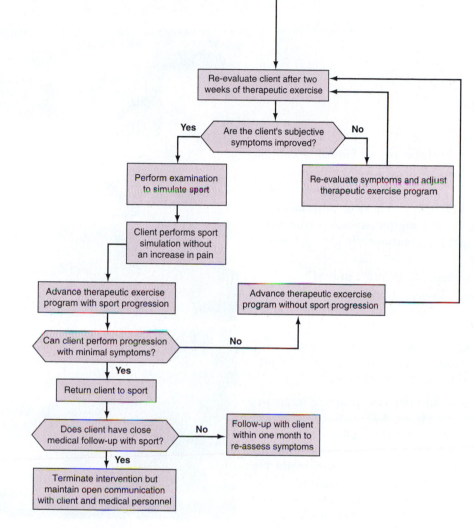

CLIENT CASE # 4

Tony English

History

Patient: Earl

Age: 52 years

Height: 6' 0"

Weight: 280 lbs

Education: BA in business; played football in college

Occupation: Mortgage loan advisor, full time: 7:30 AM–5:30 PM

Medical/Surgical History: Had a myocardial infarction at age 47, and angioplasty was performed at that time; right hip pointer while playing football in college

Current Medications: Celebrex®, Inderal®

Chief Complaint: Weakness and pain in the right hip with walking and descending stairs; limited endurance in walking

Radiographic Examination: Degenerative joint disease noted over the weight bearing area of the right femoral head with no other bony changes

Earl suffered a myocardial infarction resulting in an angioplasty at age 47 (**Case Figure 4.1**). At that time he was advised to begin a low fat diet and a regular exercise program. He has done well on the diet with help from his wife, but he has not been able to exercise consistently. He finds running too difficult and painful; walking is also painful after 30 minutes and he does not "have time to go to a gym or pool." Earl began exercising again when a cardio kick boxing business opened in his neighborhood. Although he enjoys the exercise, he notes limited right hip flexibility and inability to kick effectively with either foot or balance on his right foot when attempting to kick with the left. He also complains of pain in the right hip when trying to kick with the left leg. Earl also reports he becomes very tired and must take frequent rest breaks during the one hour workout. He rests at 15 minutes, 25 minutes, 35 minutes and 45 minutes into the workout for two to four minutes each break.

Earl was referred to you by his family practitioner for examination and treatment of his right hip pain, initiation of a clinic-based therapeutic exercise program and a home

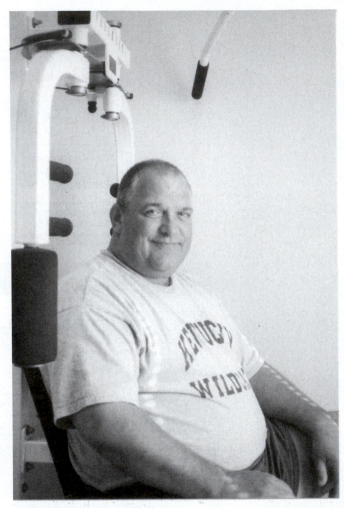

Case Figure 4.1   Earl.

exercise program that he can perform independently when discharged. Earl's primary goal is to walk, ascend and descend stairs, and continue with a regular exercise program without pain and without the feeling of weakness that makes him feel unsafe and in need of a handrail when descending steps at work and when he goes to church. He also enjoys the new kick boxing class and the people he has met there and thinks he will be able to comply with his diet and exercise program better with the support of his new friends (see Chapters 4 and 11).

Physical Examination

Musculoskeletal Assessment

Active Range of Motion (ROM) of the Right Hip: Limited hip flexion, extension and rotation. Flexion 120°, extension 5°, external rotation 70°, internal rotation 30°[1]

Compression/Distraction/Hip Scouring: Compression, slight pain reproduction, distraction. No change in symptoms, hip scouring; pain at 12 o'clock through 5 o'clock[2]

Deep Tendon Reflex Grading: +2 patellar and Achilles tendon reflexes bilaterally[2]

Manual Muscle Testing: 5/5 for upper and lower extremity muscles except right hip abductors = 4−/5, extension = 4−/5, flexion = 4/5, internal rotation = 3+/5, external rotation = 4−/5[3,4]

Timed Single Leg Stance: Left = 30 sec. (considered normal), right = 9 sec.[5]

Musculotendinous Extensibility: FABER Test, left = parallel to the table and measures 10 cm from fibular head to table; right = not parallel and measures 40 cm from fibular head to table. 90°−90° SLR for hamstring flexibility limited as follows: right 40° from full extension, left 20° from full extension. Thomas Test for hip flexor flexibility, right = 25°, left = 20°[1,2]

Sensation: Intact to light touch and equal at bilateral upper and lower extremities.[2]

Pain: Right hip pain of 3/10 with bilateral stance, 5/10 in single leg stance, 7/10 after walking or standing for 30 minutes.[2]

Cardiopulmonary Assessment

Resting Blood Pressure: 126/80 mm Hg[6,7]

Resting Heart Rate: 78 bpm[6,7]

Body Fat Percentage (skin fold caliper assessment): 40 percent

Aerobic Capacity/Endurance: A recent stress test on a treadmill revealed maximum oxygen consumption ($VO_{2\ max}$) of 32 mL/kg/min (see Chapter 4).[6,7]

Neuromuscular Assessment

Standing Balance: Berg Balance Test Score = 52 (out of 56), score reduced due to difficulty with stool stepping, tandem stance, single leg stance, and stand and reach (see Chapter 9).[5]

Integumentary Assessment

Not applicable

A. Given this information about your client, what are your primary concerns regarding musculoskeletal system impairments? Do you have concerns regarding existing or potential cardiopulmonary system impairments? Please list and discuss your concerns. *See Author's Comments A*

Preventing, delaying or minimizing the effects of a disease, illness or impairment is vital to every client. Primary prevention involves general health promotion efforts that focus on preventing disease, illness or impairment. In secondary prevention, the disease, illness or impairment already exists, and the therapeutic exercise program planner's efforts are directed more toward decreasing the duration, severity, and/or sequelae through prompt and appropriate intervention. Tertiary prevention focuses on limiting the disability (and maintaining function) among clients with chronic or irreversible diseases (see Chapter 1).

B. With these considerations in mind, identify the prevention considerations for Earl and provide a rationale for each of your decisions. Create and complete a table with the following column headings: prevention level, preferred practice plan,[8] and the rationale for your decision. *See Author's Comments B*

Although the cluster of identified system impairments provides a foundation for designing our therapeutic exercise program, it does not provide a complete picture of Earl. By learning more about Earl, we can begin to devise a more prescriptive approach to designing the therapeutic exercise program. By acknowledging Earl's unique individual characteristics we will provide for him an individualized intervention plan that will build rapport and confidence in the client–rehabilitation clinician relationship. Looking at Earl as a whole person will provide the catalyst to design a therapeutic exercise program that stimulates his interest, insures adherence and instills lifelong positive behavior modifications (see Chapter 11). In particular we must consider Earl's lifestyle (including social support systems), existing health or fitness interests, instrumental activities of daily living and general activities of daily living.

After considering all factors, you determine that Earl has a good prognosis for functional improvement, provided an effective therapeutic exercise program is designed and followed. Having considered physical examination results, lifestyle (including social support systems), activities of daily living, instrumental activities of daily living, existing health/fitness interests and identified the primary practice patterns,[8] you are ready to generate a list of problems that summarizes the concerns raised by the history and physical examination findings. Focus on problems that you consider critical to Earl's quality of life. One concern is Earl's participation in aerobic kick boxing. His physical condition does not lend itself to participation in this type of activity at a high level. However, the social implications of this class and the fact that Earl has finally found an exercise form he feels he can pursue on a long term basis may benefit you in your planning. Remember that motivating Earl will be important to success. This class could help in the motivational process (see Chapter 11).

C. Based upon the information provided up to this point, list four to six problems that you consider to be critical to Earl's quality of life. *See Author's Comments C*

Having listed problems, you are ready to begin planning the short and long term goals that you would like to help Earl achieve with your therapeutic exercise program. Be sure that the goals you set for Earl are functional, achievable, measurable, objective, understandable, and sustainable (*F-A-M-O-U-S*). Also make sure they are written clearly. Create goals that relate impairments and problems to functional limitations and disability (see Chapter 1). Remember that a goal is a point in the recovery process, not the process (for example "improve strength" becomes a better goal when it is linked to a particular functional activity such as improve strength to be independent descending 10 stairs with ≤ 2/10 pain). For Earl's case, limit your short term goals to those you believe he should be able to achieve after four weeks of complying with the therapeutic exercise program. Base your short term goal achievement expectations on the minimal known times required for musculoskeletal, neuromuscular, and cardiopulmonary physiological system improvements to occur.

D. Based upon the information provided, create three to six short term (≤ four weeks) therapeutic exercise program goals by completing the following statement: By the end of four weeks, the client . . . *See Author's Comments D*

This particular case will also limit your long term goals to those you believe that Earl should achieve after 12 weeks of complying with your therapeutic exercise program. Remember, these goals represent expected achievements by the end of your therapeutic exercise program intervention.

E. Create three to six long term (5–12 weeks) therapeutic exercise program goals by completing the following statement:

By the end of 12 weeks, the client . . . *See Author's Comments E*

Having established the short and long term goals, it is a good idea to review basic exercise physiology fundamentals, including metabolic energy systems (see Chapters 2 and 4) and therapeutic exercise principles (see Chapters 4 and 5) prior to designing a prescriptive therapeutic exercise program for Earl. While no single training principle can be ignored, certain principles may apply more than others to a therapeutic exercise program that is designed for a specific client (such as Earl). Although progressively increased exercise intensity is certainly indicated, so is crossover between his preferred exercise and stair climbing/walking (see Chapters 4 and 5). The weight bearing, alternating limb movements of stairs and walking certainly will help performance in his exercise choice of kick boxing. Likewise, the single leg stance activities of kick boxing should aid in balance and dynamic, eccentric neuromuscular control needed for activities of daily living (ADLs) and to reduce his risk of falls (see Chapter 9). Of similar concern is building on the health and fitness interest Earl has recently developed. He needs cardiovascular and pulmonary system fitness activity because of his history of heart disease and has finally found an exercise mode he enjoys. The problem is, with his newly discovered right hip osteoarthritis, he needs to establish a muscular strength and flexibility foundation that will allow him to exercise regularly with appropriate motor control (see Chapter 8), decrease his weight and percentage of body fat, increase his cardiopulmonary endurance, and perform ADLs safely and without pain.

It is essential to begin the exercise program in a position and at a level that encourages successful improvement while avoiding an increased inflammatory response in the right hip (see Chapter 11). Another consideration is keeping Earl focused on his choice of exercise while establishing foundational joint range of motion, strength, and flexibility[9] (see Chapter 3). He may need to stop kick boxing or be shown how to modify his routine to allow his body to "catch up" to the routine.[10] Earl lives in a neighborhood that has a small swimming pool and clubhouse/exercise room with the following equipment available: multistation isotonic machine, Total Gym® (see Chapter 5), stationary exercise bike, treadmill, elliptical trainer, and paired cuff weights of 3, 5, 7, and 10 lb increments.

F. Using the equipment provided in the neighborhood exercise room, select the exercises that you would like Earl to perform and give a rationale for why each one should be included. List the exercises in the order that you believe they should be performed with consideration for volume (sets, repetitions), how the

desired intensity will be determined, rest-to-work ratios, and frequency. Although some exercises may be performed effectively at home, limit your therapeutic exercise program design to activities performed exclusively at the exercise room. Also limit your exercise options to ≤ 10 tasks. Base your therapeutic exercise program design on five available days (Monday through Friday), with consideration for Earl's work activities. *See Author's Comments F*

Remember that your program may vary considerably from the author's example or from your classmates' example. What should not vary, however, are the links that you establish between key problems, functionally relevant treatment goals, and the scientific rationale used to support your therapeutic exercise variable decision making process.

G. Having initiated the therapeutic exercise program, identify three to six functional tests that you will use in the clinic to verify progress toward short term goal achievement. Provide a rationale for each of the clinical functional tests that you have selected. *See Author's Comments G*

Four weeks have passed and Earl has performed admirably with the therapeutic exercise program you developed. During your four week re-evaluation you take the following clinical functional assessment measurements.

Musculoskeletal Assessment

Manual Muscle Testing: Normal strength at bilateral upper and lower extremities (5/5) except right hip extension of 4+/5[3]

Timed Single Leg Stance: Left = 30 seconds, right = 20 seconds[5]

Functional Assessment: Gait up and down stairs shows reciprocal pattern, slightly less time in stance phase on right, no limp and does not have to use handrail. Client reports he performs cardio kick boxing without kicking and at a reduced intensity for 25 minutes without rest

Musculotendinous Extensibility: FABER, left = 10 cm, right = 20 cm; 90°/90° SLR, right = 20°, left = 20°, Thomas Test, right = 20°, left = 15°[1,2]

Pain: Right hip pain 1/10 in bilateral stance, 3/10 in single leg stance, 5/10 after 30 minutes walking, 2/10 after ascending/descending 10 steps.[2]

Cardiopulmonary Assessment

Resting Blood Pressure: 120/80 mm Hg

Resting Heart Rate: 72 bpm

Body Fat Percentage (skin fold caliper assessment): 36%

Bodyweight: 260 lbs

Neuromuscular Assessment

Standing Balance: Berg Balance Test score = 54; score reduced slightly due to performance of other single leg stance activities.[5]

With the client showing substantial improvement in right hip function, the therapeutic exercise program should be modified to place greater emphasis on the long term goals, particularly returning to modified aerobic kick boxing, walking, and stair climbing. Earl is glad to be able to participate in the aerobic (cardio-) boxing class for an extended period of time and no longer feels like the weakest member of the class. You make note of his obvious enthusiasm, but remind him of the importance of adhering to the intensity and frequency recommendations of a soon to be modified therapeutic exercise program. You also remind Earl of the importance of continuing to perform the exercises paying close attention to proper technique that involves the use of trunk and proximal hip stabilization while exercising.

H. With consideration for therapeutic exercise order determination factors, make a table with a list of your modified exercise selections, the primary body region that the exercise involves, and the rationale for including that exercise in the program. Remember to increase your focus on your long term goals, including more advanced cardio kick boxing. *See Author's Comments H*

I. Following the above exercise selection, document in table format the volume (sets and repetitions), how the intensity of the exercise will be determined, the rest-to-work ratio, and the frequency of exercise performance. *See Author's Comments I*

Remember that your program may vary considerably from the author's example or from your classmates' example. What should not vary, however, are the links that you establish between key problems, functionally relevant treatment goals, and the scientific rationale used to support your exercise variable decision making process.

Case Summary

The modified therapeutic exercise program shifts the focus of the program after the first four weeks from isolated flexibility and stabilization exercises to more total body and functional exercises addressing some of the same concepts. These exercises should address Earl's desire to function daily with less pain and pursue a regular exercise program to assist him with weight reduction, (particularly, body fat reduction), cardiopulmonary performance improvement, and quite possibly decreased stress on the right hip during weight bearing activities. This program has been shifted to a more aggressive walking program combined with functional stair climbing activities and a combination of flexibility and stability activities performed in weight bearing and non–weight bearing positions. The reason for this is to provide a comprehensive program that addresses the key areas of trunk and proximal stability and flexibility which will allow Earl to function daily and increase his participation in his choice of fitness exercise, cardio kick boxing. Earl can continue to use the equipment at his neighborhood fitness room, but will need to have a mechanism for communication with you for program progression, questions that may arise, and any program "troubleshooting." By considering impairments, lifestyle (including social support systems), athletic or fitness interests, instrumental activities of daily living and general activities of daily living, the rehabilitation clinician considers the whole person and not just the limb or joint involved. This will greatly enhance the likelihood that the positive behaviors developed will lend themselves to improving Earl's quality of life.

J. On a separate sheet of paper diagram a decision making algorithm for Earl's right hip weakness with abduction and extension. *See Author's Comments J*

K. On a separate sheet of paper diagram a decision making algorithm for Earl's cardiopulmonary endurance deficit. *See Author's Comments K*

L. On a separate sheet of paper diagram a decision making algorithm for Earl's decreased right hip flexibility. *See Author's Comments L*

M. On a separate sheet of paper diagram a decision making algorithm for Earl's decreased balance during single leg stance. *See Author's Comments M*

N. On a separate sheet of paper diagram a decision making algorithm for Earl's functional limitation in descending and ascending stairs. *See Author's Comments N*

O. On a separate sheet of paper diagram a decision making algorithm for Earl's inability to walk for more than 30 minutes because of right hip pain. *See Author's Comments O*

Referring to Chapter 10 for guidance, discuss any alternative or complementary therapeutic exercises that you believe might benefit this client. Provide the rationale for your suggestion(s).

References

1. Reese NB, Bandy WD. *Joint Range of Motion and Muscle Length Testing.* Philadelphia: W.B. Saunders Co., 2002.
2. Magee DJ. *Orthopedic Physical Assessment.* Philadelphia: W.B. Saunders, 1997.
3. Kendall FP, McCreary EK, Provance PG. *Muscles Testing and Function.* Baltimore: Williams & Wilkins, 1993.
4. Hislop HJ, Montgomery J. *Daniel's and Worthingham's Muscle Testing: Techniques of Manual Examination,* 7th ed. Philadelphia: W.B. Saunders Co., 2002.
5. Shumway-Cook A, Woollacott MH. *Motor Control Theory and Practical Applications.* Philadelphia: Lippincott Williams & Wilkins, 2001.
6. *ACSM's Guidelines for Exercise Testing and Prescription,* 6th ed. Philadelphia: Lippincott Williams & Wilkins, 2000.
7. *ACSM's Resource Manual* for *Guidelines for Exercise Testing and Prescription,* 3rd ed. Baltimore: Williams & Wilkins, 1998.
8. *Guide to Physical Therapist Practice,* 2nd ed. In *Phys Ther.* 2001;81:9–744. Alexandria, VA: American Physical Therapy Association.
9. Bandy WD, Irion JM, Briggler M. The effect of time and frequency of static stretching on flexibility of the hamstring muscles. *Phys Ther.* 1997;77:1090–1096.
10. Sullivan PE, Markos PD. *Clinical Decision Making in Therapeutic Exercise.* Norwalk, CT: Appleton & Lange, 1995.
11. Crosbie WJ, Nimmo MA, Banks MA, et al. Standing balance responses in two populations of elderly women: A pilot study. *Arch Phys Med Rehabil.* 1989;70(10):751–754.
12. Messier SP, Royer TD, Craven TE, et al. Long-term exercise and its effect on balance in older, osteoarthritic adults: Results from the Fitness, Arthritis, and Senior Trial (FAST). *J Am Geriatr Soc.* 2000;48(2):131–138.
13. Riemann BL, Myers JB, Lephart SM. Comparison of the ankle, knee, hip, and trunk corrective action shown during single-leg stance on firm, foam, and multiaxial surfaces. *Arch Phys Med Rehabil.* 2003; 84(1):90–95.
14. Simkin PA, de Lateur BJ, Alquist AD, et al. Continuous passive motion for osteoarthritis of the hip: A pilot study. *J Rheumatol.* 1999;26(9):1987–1991.
15. Arokoski MH, Arokoski JP, Haara M, et al. Hip muscle strength and muscle cross sectional area in

men with and without hip osteoarthritis. *J Rheumatol.* 2002;29(10):2187–2195.

16. Mikkelsen C, Werner S, Eriksson E. Closed kinetic chain alone compared to combined open and closed kinetic chain exercises for quadriceps strengthening after anterior cruciate ligament reconstruction with respect to return to sports: A prospective matched follow-up study. *Knee Surg Sports Traumatol. Arthrosc.* 2000;8:337–342.

17. Anderson T, Kearney JT. Effects of three resistance training programs on muscular strength and absolute and relative endurance. *Res Q Exerc Sport.* 1982;53:1–7.

18. Kraemer WJ, Adams K, Cafarelli E, et al. American College of Sports Medicine Position Stand. Progression models in resistance training for healthy adults. *Med Sci Sports Exerc.* 2002:364–380.

19. Anonymous, American College of Sports Medicine Position stand. The recommended quantity and quality of exercise for developing and maintaining cardiorespiratory and muscular fitness and flexibility in healthy adults. *Med Sci Sports Exerc.* 1998;30:975–991.

20. Chilibeck PD, Calder AW, Sale DG, Webber CE. A comparison of strength and muscle mass increases during resistance training in young women. *Eur J Appl Physiol.* 1998;77:170–175.

21. Carruthers ME, Edwards RH, Pride NB, et al. British pilot study of exercise therapy: I. Middle-aged men. *Br J Sports Med.* 1976;10(2):47–53.

22. Larsen GE, George JD, Alexander JL, et al. Prediction of maximum oxygen consumption from walking, jogging or running. *Res Q Exerc Sport.* 2002;73(1):66–72.

23. Russell WD. On the current status of rated perceived exertion. *Percept Mot Skills.* 1997;84:799–808.

24. Godges JJ, MacRae PG, Engelke KA. Effects of exercise on hip range of motion, trunk muscle performance, and gait economy. *Phys Ther.* 1993;73(7):468–477.

25. Siler WL, Koch NQ, Frese EM. The path utilized affects the distance walked in the 12 minute walk test. *Cardiopul Phys Ther J.* 1999;10(3):80–83.

Author's Comments A

Impairments noted include osteoarthritis in the right hip, history of myocardial infarction and angioplasty and increased body fat percentage. Also noted impairments include pain in the right hip with prolonged stance and a deficit in standing balance and strength on right compared to left. Other factors to consider are his sedentary job and lifestyle, a recent return to a trial of exercise, and his being a former collision sport athlete (see Chapter 11). Earl's combined history of heart disease, angioplasty and right hip osteoarthritis accompanied by pain with walking and stair climbing are critical components of his history. Lifelong exercise is important for cardiopulmonary health and endurance, but Earl has had trouble consistently exercising and now the development of right hip pain may limit him even more.[6,7] No recent history of a specific hip injury is noted, but a history of playing college football, a hip pointer during that time and a gradual onset of right hip pain intensified by weight bearing activities raises concerns about joint integrity, muscular strength and stability. Cardiopulmonary concerns are present due to history and the medications he currently takes for hypertension. These will impact our conditioning exercise program selection. Earl recognizes, now, the importance of exercise to be able to function in his daily life. Ascending and descending stairs is important at home and work, and he believes he will enjoy kick boxing for the exercise and the people he meets. This form of exercise, enjoyable as it may be, requires excellent balance and motor control in the trunk and proximal lower extremity areas. Earl may not be a great candidate for reaching a high performance level in this type of exercise. However, this can be a motivational factor for Earl to work hard at core trunk stability while gradually progressing his kick boxing exercises. It will then be imperative for you to educate Earl in appropriate exercises or maybe modify his exercise of choice to minimize the risk of future injury.

Author's Comments B

Prevention			Preferred practice pattern	Rationale
1	2	3		
	X	X	Musculoskeletal	Right hip osteoarthritis with pain, weakness and decreased functional ability
	X		Neuromuscular	Decreased standing balance with single leg stance activities; decreased proximal stability
		X	Cardiopulmonary	History of myocardial infarction, currently controlled with medications, decreased endurance, increased body fat percentage
			Integumentary	Not applicable

Because of existing right hip osteoarthritis, the therapeutic exercise program planner's efforts are directed more toward decreasing the duration, severity, and/or sequelae of disease through prompt and appropriate intervention (secondary prevention). The right hip osteoarthritis also fits the category of tertiary prevention. Osteoarthritic changes are a primary reason for long term dysfunction in the older adult population. Earl is at an age where degenerative changes may already be limiting his activity level. With his current complaint of right hip pain with weight bearing, we are convinced these changes are causing his current problem and could continue to cause long term dysfunction.

Although the physical examination has revealed early indication for potential neuromuscular impairment, therapeutic exercise intervention for secondary prevention can help prevent further neuromuscular deficits which could lead to further musculoskeletal impairments. Earl's history of cardiopulmonary disease and consistent difficulty managing this process with exercise make it appropriate as a tertiary prevention intervention.[8]

Author's Comments C

1. Right hip weakness, especially in abduction and extension
2. Cardiopulmonary endurance deficit
3. Decreased right hip flexibility
4. Decreased balance in right lower extremity single leg stance
5. Difficulty descending/ascending stairs
6. Unable to walk greater than 30 minutes due to right hip pain

Author's Comments D

By the end of four weeks, the client . . .

1. Will descend 10 steps safely without use of a handrail
2. Will ascend and descend stairs independently with ≤ 2/10 right hip pain
3. Will walk independently for 30 minutes with ≤ 2/10 right hip pain

4. Will independently and appropriately perform the home exercise program
5. Will be able to maintain single leg stance on the right leg for at least 20 seconds
6. Will participate in modified aerobic boxing (no kicking) without rest for 30 minutes

Author's Comments E

By the end of 12 weeks, the client . . .

1. Will ascend/descend stairs with handrail with 0/10 right hip pain
2. Will walk 45 minutes with 0/10 right hip pain
3. Will perform modified cardio kick boxing exercise for 45 minutes without rest, including modified kicks while standing on the right lower extremity
4. Will be able to maintain single leg stance on the right leg for 30 seconds
5. Will decrease body fat by 10% from original score of 40%

Author's Comments F

Earl's history and physical examination indicate a need for improved flexibility, proximal lower extremity stability, hip strength and cardiopulmonary endurance. For this reason, the therapeutic exercise program you design should include all these components. It is noted Earl has a slightly increased risk of falls and pain with repeated single leg activities.[5] For these reasons and because of his past history of cardiopulmonary disease, the exercises chosen should be safe and low intensity. Early in the program the desire is to improve endurance, neuromuscular control, mobility and stability to allow improved and less painful function in the home and at work. Since the activities of aerobic kick boxing, walking, and ascending/descending stairs require various metabolic demands, strengthening alone will not be sufficient to help him regain functional independence. The following program has been proposed.

Exercise order	Exercise selection	Body region	Rationale for inclusion
1	Stationary bike	Whole body	Mobility, increase tissue temperature, warm up
2	Prone hip flexor stretch	Hip/lower extremity	Increase flexibility, mobility and ROM
3	Supine hamstring stretch	Hip/lower extremity	Increase flexibility, mobility and ROM

Exercise order	Exercise selection	Body region	Rationale for inclusion
4	Sitting hip internal rotator/ adductor stretch	Hip/lower extremity	Increase flexibility, mobility and ROM
5	Total Gym®; double leg squats	Whole lower extremity/trunk	Stabilization and strengthening
6	Abdominal sets with curl-up	Trunk	Stabilization and strengthening
7	Prone hip extension	Hip/trunk	Strengthening and proximal stabilization
8	Sidelying hip abduction	Hip/trunk	Strengthening and proximal stabilization
9	Lateral step-ups	Whole lower extremity/trunk	Weight bearing strengthening and stabilization that simulates function
10	Elliptical trainer (**Case Figure 4.2**)	Whole body	Cardiopulmonary endurance and aerobic energy system improvement that substitutes for walking without the impact

Exercise order	Volume (Sets/repetitions)	Intensity determination	Rest-to-work ratio	Frequency/week
1	1 set, 10–15 min.	Low intensity, 8–10 on Borg Perceived Exertion Scale	NA	Each workout
2	1 set, 4 repetitions	Low intensity, 20–30 sec. Hold, mild stretch[7]	Alternate lower extremities	Each workout
3	1 set, 4 repetitions	Low intensity, 20–30 sec. Hold, mild stretch[7]	Alternate lower extremities	Each workout
4	1 set, 4 repetitions	Low intensity, 20–30 sec. Hold, mild stretch[7]	Alternate lower extremities	Each workout
5	3 sets, 12–15 repetitions	1 set each at levels 6, 8, 10	3:1	5 times/week
6	3 sets, 8–12 repetitions	Low to moderate intensity with body weight resistance	One minute between sets	5 times/week
7	3 sets, 12–15 repetitions	Low to moderate intensity with body weight resistance	Alternate lower extremities	5 times/week
8	3 sets, 12–15 repetitions	Low to moderate intensity with body weight resistance	Alternate lower extremities	5 times/week
9	3 sets, 8–10 repetitions	Moderate intensity with body weight resistance	Alternate lower extremities	5 times/week
10	1 set, 20 minutes	Target heart rate using Karvonen formula	Not applicable	5 times/week

Author's Comments G

Functional tests

1. Visual analog pain scale
2. Single leg stance for time (hand held stopwatch)
3. Berg Balance Scale
4. Observational gait analysis on stairs
5. Pre- and post-exercise heart rate/ target heart rate
6. Manual muscle test
7. Borg Scale of perceived exertion
8. Goniometry/ flexibility testing

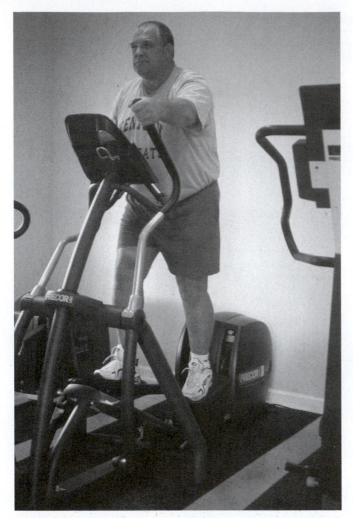

Case Figure 4.2 Exercise on an elliptical trainer.

9. Timed stair climbing
10. 12-minute walk test

Rationales

1. Pain with selected functional activities
2. Balance test under eyes open and closed conditions; also tests lower quarter stability

3. Standing balance with selected functions to assess fall risk
4. Ability to ascend and descend stairs safely
5. Aerobic conditioning
6. Objective measure of muscle strength improvement
7. Objective measure of client's perceived exertion during activity
8. Objective measure of joint ROM and soft tissue extensibility
9. Ability to ascend and descend stairs safely
10. Ability to ambulate at safe speed with adequate endurance

These are examples of appropriate clinical functional tests that are measurable, objective, and fit with the goals selected. Also included are standard objective tests for strength, flexibility, and level of exertion. These tests measure at the impairment level to allow the rehabilitation clinician to assess if progress is being made. Variability is possible with these choices, but remember to use clinical functional tests that are objective, measurable, and meaningful. Tests with strong validity and reliability are good choices, as are those that can be performed quickly and accurately in the clinic. The clinical functional tests should be related to the goals that you and Earl have set.

Author's Comments H

Re-examination has confirmed that Earl has achieved most of the short term goals. The last four weeks of the therapeutic exercise program that focused on hip and lower extremity function has proven successful. Although he has not quite reached expectations for single leg stance capability, musculotendinous extensibility and pain level while walking, he has made substantial progress toward these goals. Additionally, cardiopulmonary assessment measurements suggest that he has maintained his initial level of aerobic fitness and has begun to improve in this area as evidenced by a decrease in body fat and weight.

Exercise order	Exercise selection	Body region	Rationale for inclusion
1	Walking 10–15 min. at low intensity	Total body	Total body (especially lower extremity) warm-up; injury prevention
2	Standing hip flexor stretch	Hip and lower extremities	Increased flexibility, ROM and mobility while working on trunk and lower extremity stability
3	Standing hamstring stretch	Hip and lower extremity	Increased flexibility, ROM and mobility while working on trunk and lower extremity stability

4	Side lunge, bilaterally	Trunk, lower extremity and hip muscles	Increased extensibility of adductors while increasing strength of knee and hip muscles
5	Single leg squats on Total Gym®	Whole lower extremity and trunk	Lower extremity stabilization and strength
6	Standing hip abduction in multi-station machine (**Case Figure 4.3**) (● **Section 6, Animation 1**)	Hip and stance lower extremity	Increased hip abductor strength and endurance; trunk and stance leg stabilization
7	Prone combined upper extremity flexion with trunk and hip extension	Whole body; emphasis on hips and trunk extensors	Increase total trunk stabilization in extension
8	Diagonal trunk curl-ups	Abdominals/trunk	Increase stability and strength
9	Diagonal stepping combined with step-up using resistive bands	Trunk and both lower extremities	Open and closed kinetic chain activity simulating stairs and facilitating trunk rotation and stability
10	Sitting hip internal rotator and adductor stretch (butterfly)	Bilateral hips and lower extremities	Increased extensibility of hip muscles

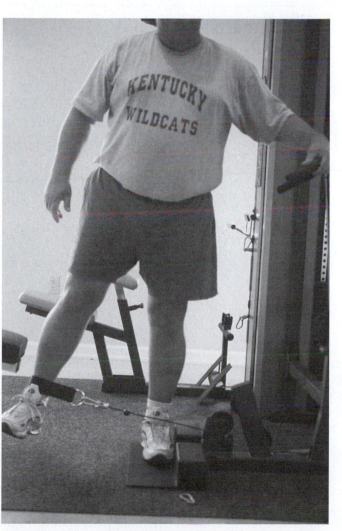

Case Figure 4.3   Standing hip abduction in a multista-tion machine.

Earl's therapeutic exercise program modifications reflect the emphasis on trunk and lower extremity stability in the goals and his functional needs. Key problems continue to be decreased endurance and flexibility that result in limitation in function and recreational exercise. This modified program is a low to moderate intensity workout focused on core proximal stabilization that will allow Earl to ascend stairs, perform his exercise of choice and provide dynamic lower extremity joint stability while avoiding high intensity or high impact exercises that may lead to problems due to his past medical history. Earl should continue to improve and be able to perform all essential ADLs and instrumental ADLs.

Author's Comments I

Exercise Order	Volume (Sets/repetitions)	Intensity determination	Rest-to-work ratio	Frequency/week
1	1 set, 10–15 minutes	Low intensity; 10–12 on Borg perceived exertion scale	NA	Each workout
2	1 set, 4 repetitons/ 20–30 sec.	Low intensity, gentle stretch	Alternate legs	Each workout
3	1 set, 4 repetitons/ 20–30 sec.	Low intensity, gentle stretch	Alternate legs	Each workout
4	2 sets, 10 repetitons	Moderate intensity, focus on form and trunk stabilization	3:1	5 ×/week
5	3 sets, 10 repetitons	Moderate-level 10, focus on form and trunk stabilization	3:1	3 ×/week
6	3 sets, 10 repetitons	Set 1: 50% 10 RM, Set 2: 75% 10 RM, Set 3: 100% 10 RM (RM = repetition maximum)	3:1	3 ×/week
7	1 set, 15 repetitons	Moderate intensity no weights/ focus on breathing	NA	Each workout
8	3 sets, 10 repetitons bilaterally	Moderate intensity focus on breathing	2:1	Each workout
9	3 sets, 10 repetitons bilaterally	Moderate–able to complete without loss of balance	3:1	3 ×/week
10	1 set 4 repetitons/ 20–30 sec.	Low intensity gentle stretch	1:1	Each workout

As you can see from the above program, the modified program still considers Earl's conditioning level and the degenerative changes in the right hip, but increases the level of difficulty. It is important to balance concern for safety and the clients' ability to succeed with the exercise program with appropriate challenges and the clients' goals. Earl really wants to get back to the gym and his exercise class as well as walk and function without pain. Educating Earl in the benefits of a progressive therapeutic exercise program and in the specific relationship of your program to his condition will help develop his confidence in the intervention plan and should aid program adherence. It is also important at this time to educate Earl concerning his full return to the kick boxing class. This is his ultimate goal and he should be advised about the proper way to return to this activity. During the re-examination, Earl stated he had begun doing modified activity in the class. It is now time to advance his participation safely. Since this is not performed at the neighborhood exercise area, the above program does not specifically address this issue. However, it is imperative for the rehabilitation clinician to educate Earl about other interventions meant to prevent a recurrence of his right hip pain and dysfunction.

Author's Comments 7

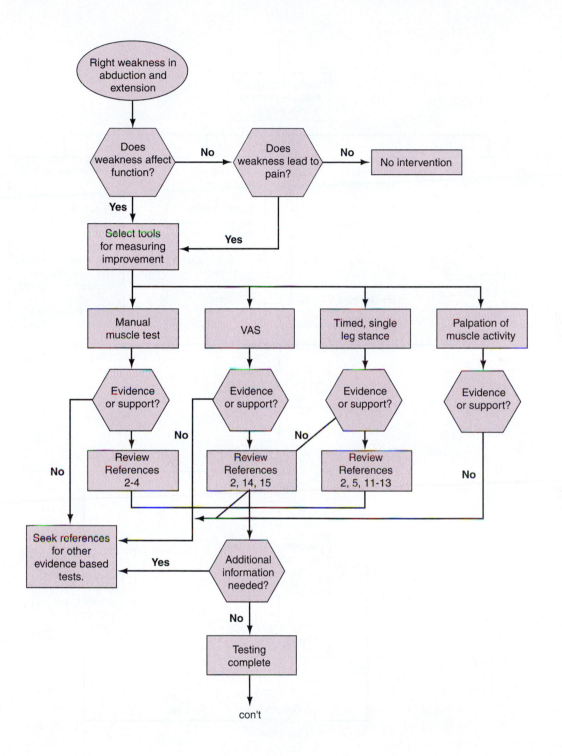

Author's Comments J (con't)

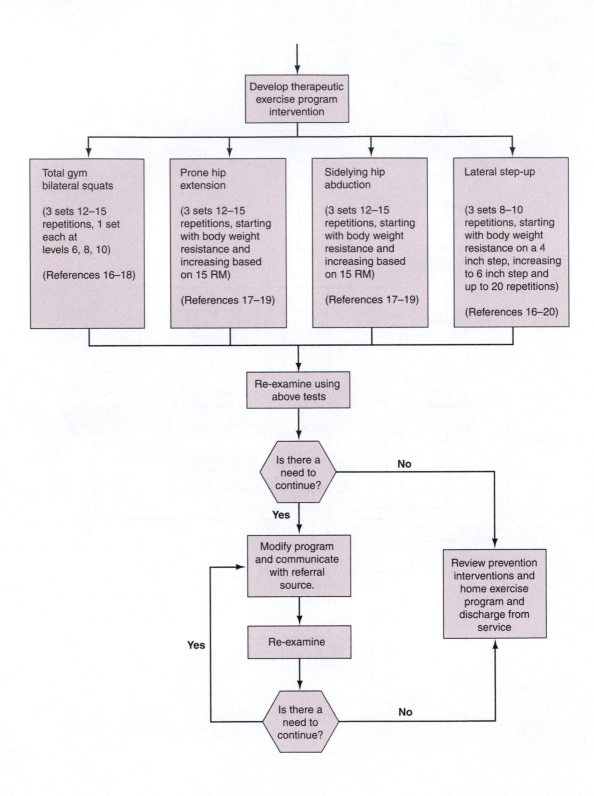

Author's Comments K

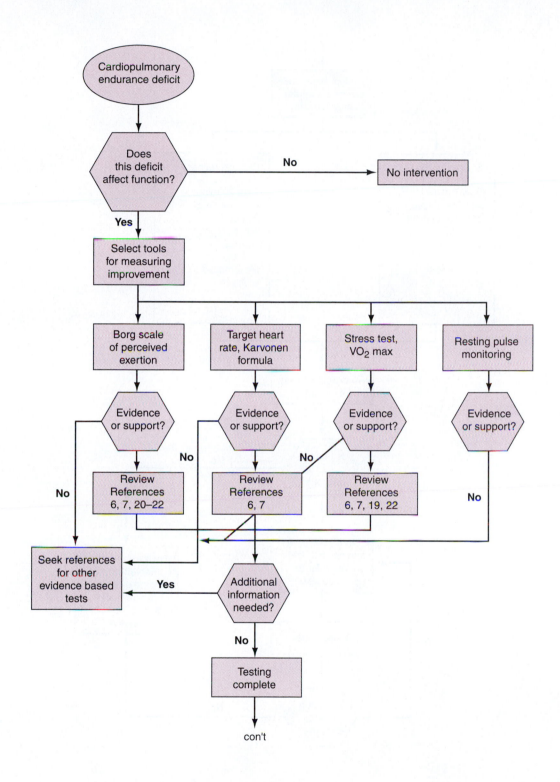

Author's Comments K (con't)

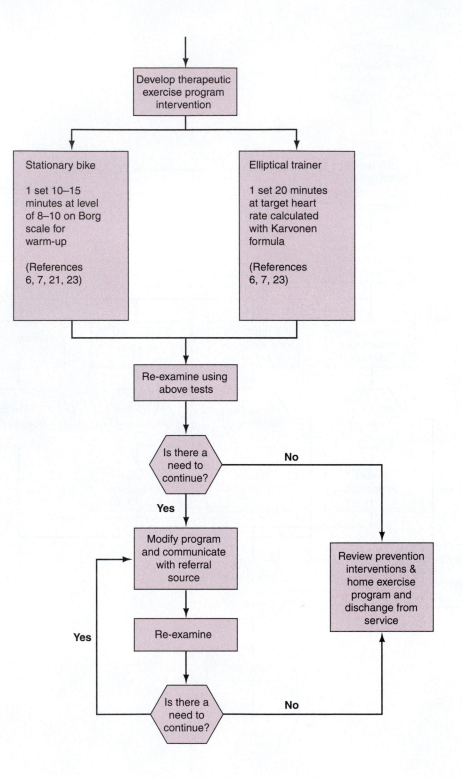

Author's Comments L

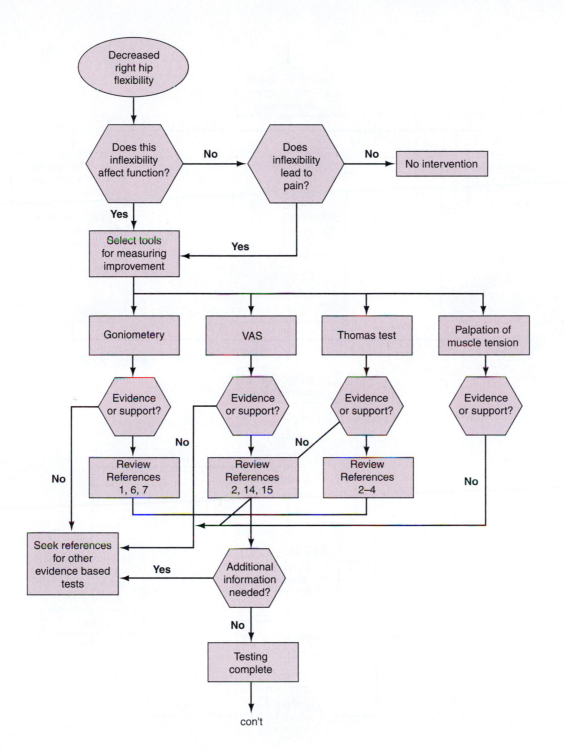

Author's Comments L (con't)

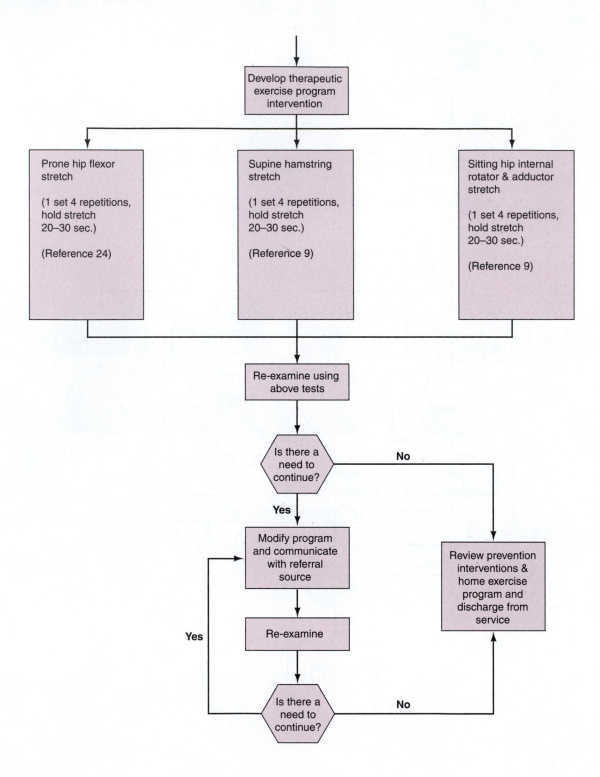

Author's Comments M

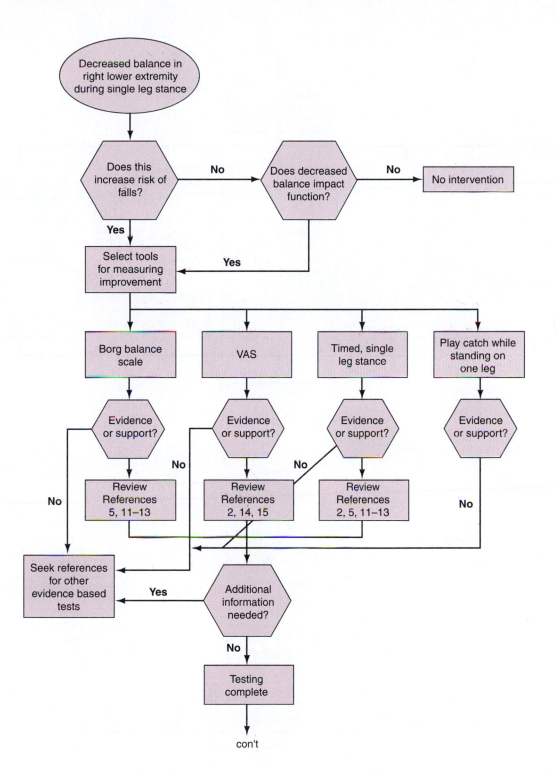

Author's Comments M (con't)

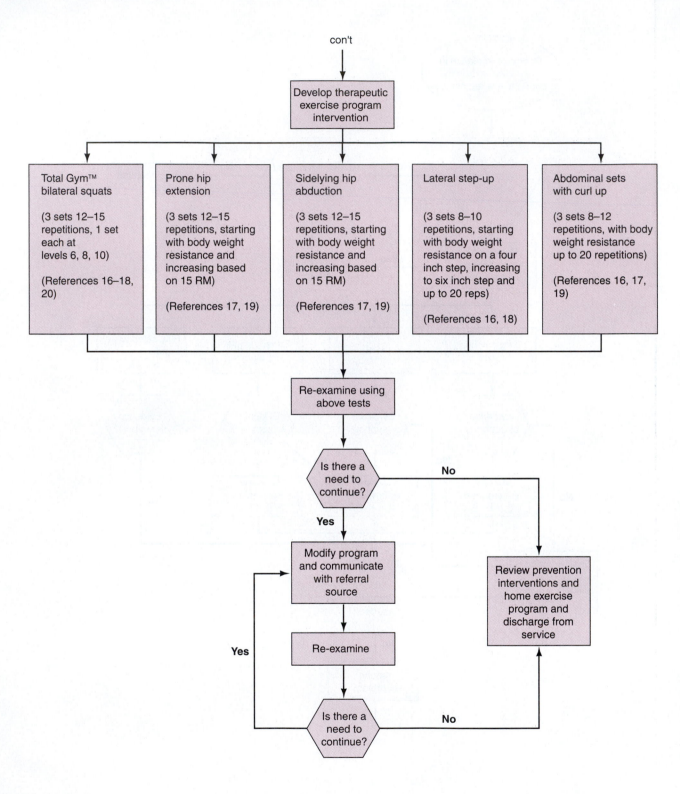

Author's Comments N

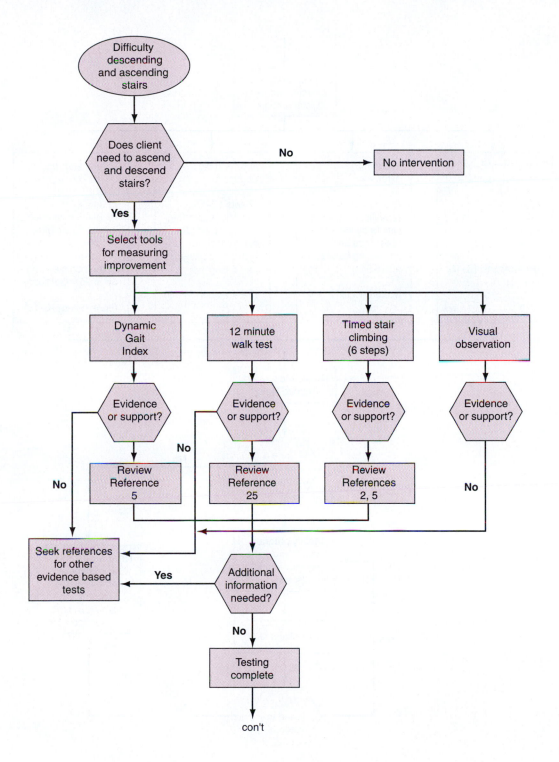

Author's Comments N (con't)

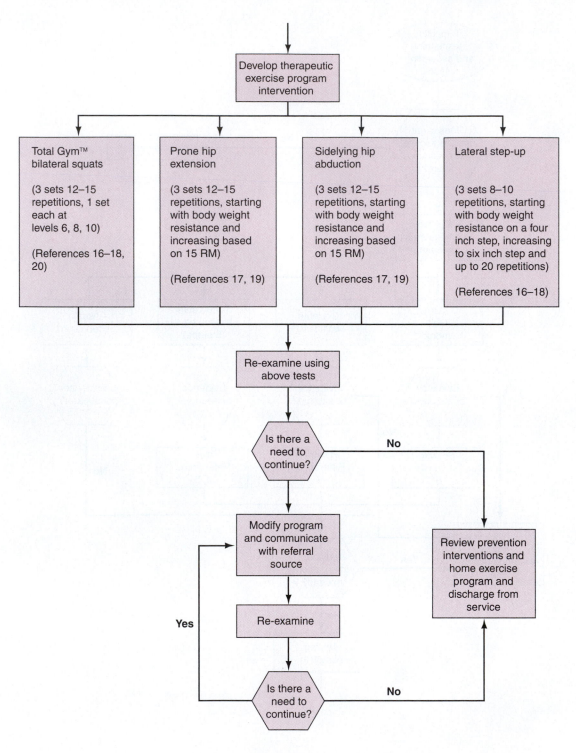

Author's Comments O

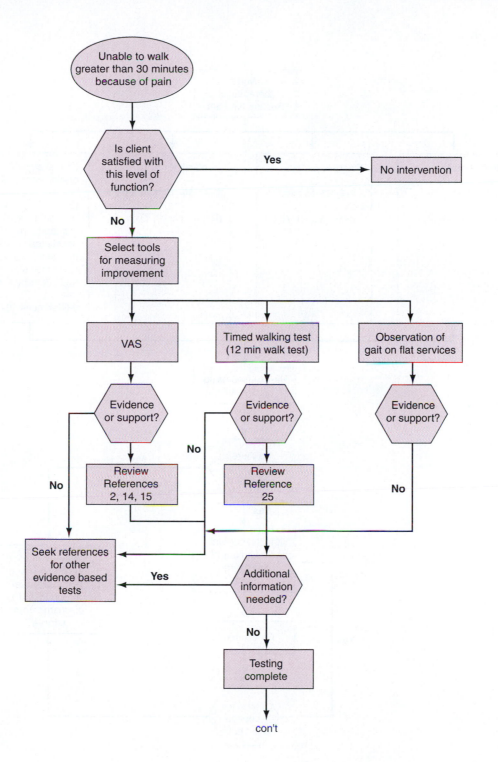

Author's Comments O (con't)

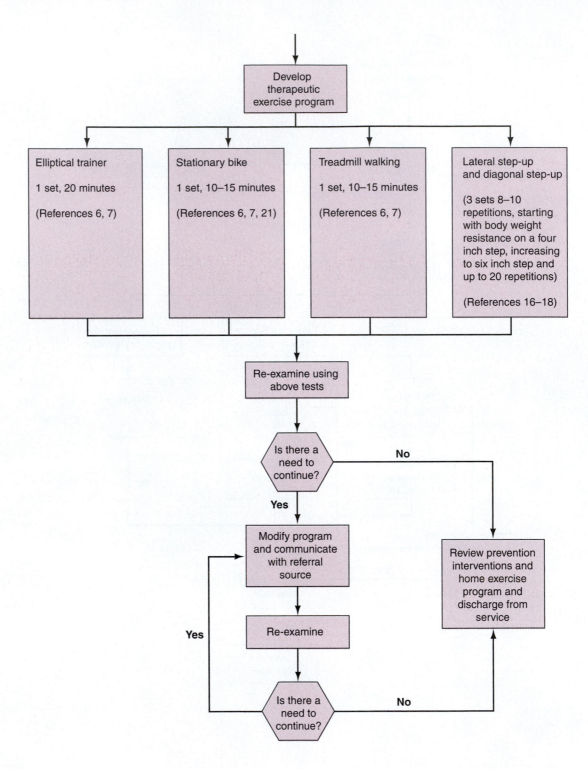

CLIENT CASE #5

Laura Lee (Dolly) Swisher

This case illustrates the importance of a client's individual, social, community, family, and work context for designing an appropriate therapeutic exercise program. Changes in a client's personal, social, or professional life may create significant challenges for them in complying with a therapeutic exercise program. Due to the well documented association between heart disease and a sedentary lifestyle, the client who abandons a therapeutic exercise program as a result of changes at home or work may experience serious health consequences. Major alterations in the client's life may also create physical and emotional stressors that contribute to disease, impairment, and disability (see Chapters 1 and 11). The rehabilitation clinician can play an important role in facilitating client adherence by making appropriate adaptations to therapeutic exercise programs and by providing appropriate referrals to community resources. The ability to make such changes requires professional role flexibility, sensitivity to personal and social changes, knowledge of community resources, and a holistic approach to the life of the client. A client centered model of therapeutic intervention provides a theoretical foundation for viewing their many concerns.

In this case, changes in family situation and health status jeopardize the continued success of a former client's fitness program. Gloria (**Case Figure 5.1**) has been successful in achieving improved physical health, decreased joint pain, an 18 pound weight loss, decreased stress, and improved emotional health. However, she must now care for her aging mother and her teenage son and has recently been diagnosed with rheumatoid arthritis. Between the time required for work and to care for her mother's needs, Gloria feels that she no longer has time to continue with her fitness program. This case also illustrates the importance of the consultant role of the rehabilitation clinician in maintaining an appropriate therapeutic exercise program.

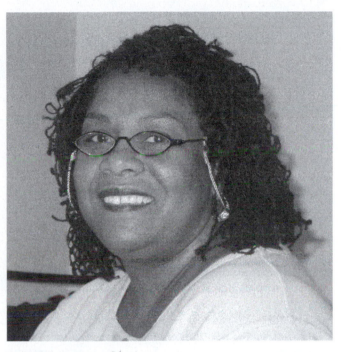

Case Figure 5.1   Gloria

History

Patient: Gloria

Age: 55 years

Height: 5' 6"

Weight: 204 lbs

Education: BS, Business Administration

Occupation: Chief loan officer at regional banking center

Medical History: Recent diagnosis of rheumatoid arthritis, high cholesterol

Surgical: status post hysterectomy (four years ago)

Psychosocial Issues: Mother recently fractured hip and Gloria is now caregiver for mother; single parent for 15 year old son; job requires long hours and elevates her stress level

Chief Complaint: Upper and lower extremity pain, needs help to re-design her therapeutic exercise program

Gloria is a divorced mother of two who works as the chief loan officer at a regional banking center. Gloria's job requires approximately 60 hours of work per week. During her early adult life, Gloria was quite active, participating in a regular exercise program at a health club and playing tennis once or twice weekly. However, when her children were young, the demands of her job and role as mother made it difficult for Gloria to maintain a regular exercise program. Her oldest son is now married and Gloria has a two year old granddaughter. Her youngest son is 15 years old and is just entering high school. After her oldest son graduated from college two years ago, Gloria began a physical fitness program and took up golf. After three months of jogging, Gloria's weight had dropped from 217 to 199 pounds. However, she has begun to experience left knee pain. Her orthopedic surgeon referred her to you

Case Table 5.1

Lifestyle Considerations	
Lifestyle Considerations • Loan officer, works long hours in sedentary job which requires 3–5 hours daily of computer time • Divorced, mother of 15 year old son • Primary caretaker for 80 your old mother • Concern that work performance will be jeopardized by home demands • Concern that performing role as mother/daughter will be jeopardized by work demands • Devout Catholic **Activities of Daily Living** • Difficulty walking up and down stairs **Health, Wellness, Prevention Issues** Increased caregiver responsibilities have resulted in: • Reduced time to exercise	• Less time and energy to devote to cooking healthy meals • Increased stress • Decreased time and energy to receive seek preventative health care **Diagnosis of Rheumatoid Arthritis increased risk of:** • Osteoporosis • Joint Stiffness • Reduced mobility **Instrumental Activities of Daily Living** • Difficulty caring for mother • Difficulty lifting heavy pans/containers to cook • Difficulty doing yard work

with a diagnosis of patellar tendonitis, left knee. Gloria had been happy with her regular fitness program prior to stopping participation three years ago due to restricted time.

Three months ago, Gloria's mother sustained a hip fracture from a fall and required a total hip arthroplasty. Because of this, she is no longer able to care for herself. Due to her mother's limited financial resources, Gloria felt that the only viable alternative was for her mother to live with her. Gloria's 80 year old mother is independent in dressing and ambulating short distances with her walker, but requires assistance with transfers to the bath tub or shower and with lower extremity dressing. Gloria states that the new demands of caring for her mother, in addition to driving her younger son to numerous academic and social events, have made it "almost impossible to even think about exercising, much less do any." She states, "These last few weeks I have spent every minute outside of work driving my mother to doctors' appointments or my son to soccer or band practice, or giving mother injections, or shopping for my mother . . . If I did have any extra time, I really need to try to be there as a mother for my son Jimmy . . . I am so frustrated . . . I feel that I made so much progress on my exercise program, and now I see it all slipping away . . . Now my doctor tells me that I have rheumatoid arthritis . . . my arms hurt all the time . . . I can hardly help Mom get up and down or work at the computer." Your clinical examination reveals the following findings:

History: 55 year old female. Formerly active but has been more sedentary over the last 10 years. Works as loan officer. Job involves significant amount of time sitting. Single mother, lives with her son Jimmy (age 15) and elderly mother. Started a fitness program about two years ago and lost weight; now feels she is unable to participate due to demands of caring for her mother and her son. Reports that she has about one-fourth the amount of time available to exercise that she used to have. Complains of elbow, wrist, hand, and knee pain (left greater than right). Upper extremity pain aggravated by assisting mother out of bathtub, increased household chores, yardwork, and working on computer. Upper extremity pain was 10/10 three weeks ago, and has decreased to 6/10 with Celebrex®. Knee pain worst when going up and down stairs or working in yard. Pain is worse in the right upper extremity, her dominant arm. Would like to continue playing golf about once a week (**Case Table 5.1**).

Chief Complaint: Pain in right arm and knees. Would also like help adjusting fitness program to accomodate her decreased time for the program. "Help me get back on track!"

Personal Medical History: Diagnosed three weeks ago with rheumatoid arthritis. History of high cholesterol, controlled by medication

Surgical History: Status post total hysterectomy four years ago

Family Medical History: Father had a heart attack at age 48. Mother had breast cancer at age 56

Medications: Pravachol®, Celebrex® (physician considering whether she needs additional medications for rheumatoid arthritis [RA])

Review of Systems: See tests and measures

Physical Examination

Musculoskeletal Pattern Tests and Measures

Range of Motion (ROM): Left knee extension, flexion 20°–135° (active) (firm soft-tissue end-feel, pain at end range of flexion); right knee extension, flexion 0°–140° (active)

Right and left elbow ROM, 0°–135° (active, pain free)

Left wrist flexion, 0°–70°; right wrist flexion, 0°–57° (pain at elbow at end range)

Left wrist extension, 0°–60°; right wrist flexion, 0°–52° (limited by pain)

Decreased muscle length/extensibility of hamstrings (lacks 15° of extension in 90°–90° test of hamstring flexibility)

Decreased muscle length/extensibility of right wrist extensors (pain with stretch)

Muscle Performance: Decreased quadriceps and hamstring strength bilaterally (MMT = 4/5), decreased strength of right wrist extensors (MMT = 3+/5)(pain with resistance)[+Cozen's],[1] grip dynamometry (mean of three efforts at position two)[1] right = 18 lbs (pain), left = 25 lbs. Combined score = 43 (poor for her age group)[1]

Joint Integrity: No joint deformities, subluxations, or rheumatoid nodules observed

Posture: Left and right knee slightly increased flexion in standing; left foot moderate increase in pronation

Palpation: Slightly increased warmth noted at wrists and knees; minimal synovial inflammation at bilateral wrists

Cardiovascular/Pulmonary: Blood pressure 125/78 mm Hg, heart rate 78 bpm

Evaluation: Lateral epicondylitis (right), patellofemoral pain (left) aggravated by tight hamstrings and decreased quadriceps strength, risk for osteoporosis, risk for heart disease, risk for joint pain/dysfunction associated with rheumatoid arthritis

Relevant Guide to Physical Therapist Practice Patterns:

Cardiovascular/Pulmonary 6A, Primary Prevention/Risk Reduction for Cardiovascular/Pulmonary Disorders;

Musculoskeletal 4D, Impaired Joint Mobility, Motor Function, Muscle Performance, and Range of Motion Associated with Connective Tissue Dysfunction;

Musculoskeletal 4A, Primary Prevention/Risk Reduction for Skeletal Demineralization;

Musculoskeletal 4E, Impaired Joint Mobility, Motor Function, Muscle Performance, and Range of Motion Associated with Localized Inflammation

A Client Centered Perspective on the Clinical Findings

The patient or client centered model of health care[2] reminds us that *clients* are multi-dimensional beings, with unique psychological concerns embedded in a specific social, community and family context (see Chapter 11) (**Case Figure 5.2**).

By maintaining a client-centered perspective, the rehabilitation clinician may avoid the pitfall of reducing the problem to "Gloria's knee and wrist pain" or "Gloria's lack of conditioning." Gloria's frustration about the limitations of her situation points to the larger social context of the problem. This section of the case provides further background about the psychological, social, and epidemiological context relevant to Gloria's condition. In terms of the present case, it is important to place Gloria's clinical problems within her altered family and professional context. This will mean trying to develop a shorter program that can be accomplished at home, integrating concerns generated by the new diagnosis, and addressing the problem of social support and respite care.

As parents live longer and outlive financial resources or the ability to care for themselves, more adult children may find themselves caring for them. In many cultures, women carry a greater responsibility than men for caregiving. In some cases, women will have some responsibility for the care of aging parents, grandparents, and children. At the same time, women continue to be active in the workplace. Gloria's personal experience of caregiver stress is not unusual. Providing care for a family member may be physically and emotionally stressful, and caregivers may defer personal needs to care for the needs of another. As Gloria's situation indicates, caregivers face unique challenges in maintaining a regular therapeutic exercise program. In a study of family caregivers, Acton[3] found that caregivers scored lower than non-caregivers on health promotion. Similarly, Sisk[4] found that those who perceived the burden of caregiving to be high engaged in fewer health-promoting behaviors. In addition to decreased health promotion activities, those who provide care for another person may also have depression or other psychological reactions to this responsibility.

Etiology, Pathology, Epidemiology, and Clinical Course

Rheumatoid arthritis (RA) is a chronic inflammatory disease that affects multiple joints in a "symmetric" pattern, meaning that the involved joints tend to be affected on both sides. The pathological process in RA involves inflammation of the synovium of the joint with progressive destruction of the cartilage and joint surfaces. Although the exact cause of RA has not been established, some experts believe that its etiology involves an immunological response.[5]

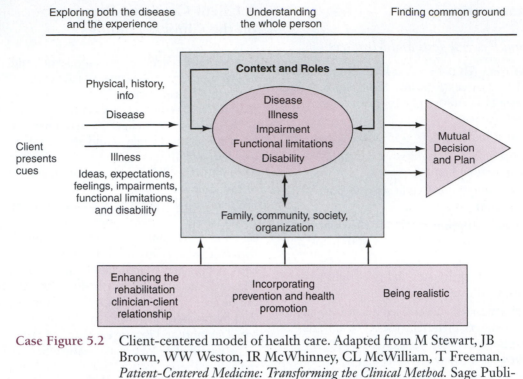

Exploring both the disease   Understanding   Finding common ground
and the experience   the whole person

Case Figure 5.2   Client-centered model of health care. Adapted from M Stewart, JB Brown, WW Weston, IR McWhinney, CL McWilliam, T Freeman. *Patient-Centered Medicine: Transforming the Clinical Method.* Sage Publications, Thousand Oaks, CA: 1995, p. 26.

Some individuals appear to have a genetic predisposition to RA, but environmental factors may also play a role in the disease's development. Approximately 0.8–2 percent[5,6] of the adult population suffers from RA, with three times as many women as men having this condition. The first onset of the disease often occurs between the ages of 35 and 50, but it may occur at any time. Clients typically experience an initial bout of joint swelling and stiffness followed by periods of exacerbation (flares-ups) and remission. The course of the disease varies significantly, with some clients progressing to marked deformity and disability and others having few exacerbations or long-term consequences after the first onset. The joints/regions most affected in RA are the metacarpophalangeal (MCP), proximal interphalangeal (PIP), wrist, elbow, shoulder, knee, hip, cervical spine, and feet. Rheumatoid arthritis may also affect the integumentary, cardiovascular, pulmonary, and gastrointestinal systems and it is best to think of RA as a multi-system pathology. Medical intervention for RA includes anti-inflammatory medications (steroidal and non-steroidal) and disease-modifying anti-rheumatic drugs (DMARDS), and is based on the severity of the disease. Rheumatoid arthritis may also be a risk factor for the development of osteoporosis,[7] especially in the client who requires prolonged use of corticosteriods to control inflammation. Damage to joint surfaces and joint deformities resulting from RA may necessitate surgical interventions, such as total joint arthroplasty.[5–10] **Case Table 5.2** summarizes the features of rheumatoid arthritis.

Although regular exercise is generally regarded as beneficial in the treatment of RA, the fact that RA involves a process of joint destruction has important consequences for Gloria's exercise program. In this regard, it is especially important for Gloria to understand that she should

Case Table 5.2   Features of Rheumatoid Arthritis

Etiology	Genetic predisposition, possible environmental or immunological factors
Epidemiology	Three times more prevalent in women than men
Prevalence	0.8%–2% of the population in the United States[5,6]
Pathology	Inflammation of the synovium; destruction of cartilage and joint surfaces
Signs/symptoms	Morning stiffness lasting more than one hour after arising, fatigue, malaise
Clinical course	Variable from marked disease and deformity to infrequent periods of disease
Primary joints	MCPs, PIPs, wrists, knees, hips, joints of feet, cervical spine

not push herself during flare-ups. The aggressive stretch that could produce soreness in the person without RA has the potential to cause tendon or joint injuries in the person with RA during a period of exacerbation.[8] Similarly, Gloria will need more information about how to help with her mother's care without injuring herself. Principles of joint protection and proper body mechanics will be very important. Education and other appropriate resources (arthritis support groups, agencies, and counseling) can be critical to Gloria's success (**Case Table 5.3**).

Evidence and Therapeutic Exercise for Rheumatoid Arthritis

An appropriate intervention strategy for Gloria should incorporate an understanding of the pathology and medical management of RA. Since Gloria has just recently been diagnosed with RA, the severity of her disease process is not yet known. On one hand, she could experience few exacerbations from the disease, but she could also experience repeated severe debilitating flare-ups. Education about the disease is an important consideration in the treatment of RA. A study of 589 subjects with arthritis found that those who took the Arthritis Self-Management Course had decreased pain, depression, and physician visits.[11] Similarly, a group education program specifically for those with RA resulted in positive outcomes in exercise, sense of self-efficacy, and knowledge, even 14 months after the program.[12] Appropriate educational resources,

such as the self-help program, will enable Gloria to recognize and react to periods of exacerbation. Education will provide the larger context and backdrop for a successful therapeutic exercise program (see Chapter 11).

Another consideration in developing an appropriate program is evidence regarding therapeutic exercise for clients with RA. Given the pathological mechanism of RA, one particular concern is whether it is appropriate for clients with RA to engage in a relatively strenuous program of aerobic exercise, muscle strengthening, and stretching. Although Gloria has been successful in participating in the past, will the same program produce acceleration in joint destruction now that she has been diagnosed with RA? Alternatively, will appropriate modifications to protect Gloria's joints decrease the aerobic effectiveness of the program? A significant body of research indicates that those with RA can participate and benefit from exercise without adverse effects.[13–20] A comparison of exercise strategies in 100 patients with stable RA found that "intensive dynamic exercise" (including stationary cycling at 70 percent to 85 percent of age-predicted heart rate) was more effective than conservative exercise (range of motion, isometric exercise, and home instruction) in increasing aerobic ability, strength, and joint mobility.[13] A subsequent study found that a program of intensive exercise, including isokinetic strengthening, was also more effective than conservative treatment for those who were suffering from active disease.[14] Although neither group who engaged in intensive activity experienced an increase in "disease activity," the researchers did not correlate this

Case Table 5.3   Educational Resources for Rheumatoid Arthritis

Web sites	
Arthritis Foundation	http://www.arthritis.org/default.asp
	This Web site provides a place to enter your zip code in order to get a list of programs and services
WebMDHealth	http://my.webmd.com/webmd_today/home/default.htm
	Provides information about a variety of diseases, tips for patients, and research updates. Use the search function to search alphabetically
National Institute of Arthritis and Musculoskeletal and Skin Diseases	http://www.niams.nih.gov/hi/topics/arthritis/arthexfs.htm#11 Information about types of arthritis. Has a specific section on arthritis and exercise.
Programs	
Arthritis self-help course	A group course available through the Arthritis Foundation to educate about arthritis and strategies to cope with the disease.
Local courses	Local hospitals and organizations sponsor courses and support groups.
Publication	
Primer on the Rheumatic Diseases[23]	

to radiographic evidence of joint destruction. It is important to note, however, that the participants in this study were inpatients who were closely monitored and that activity levels were adjusted based on individual response to the program. A similar study of a 12-week progressive resistance training program found improvements in strength, pain, and fatigue with no increase in disease activity in a sample of those whose disease was controlled.[15] Focusing on women with severe limitations secondary to RA, Harkcom et al.[16] found that exercise durations of 15–35 minutes were effective in improving aerobic capacity; participants experienced improved function and decreased joint pain and fatigue compared to a control group. Beals et al.[17] found that strenuous exercise on a bicycle ergometer did not exacerbate or harm the joints of clients who had arthritis. A systematic review of 30 studies concluded that exercise is effective in improving muscle strength and aerobic capacity without adverse consequences for disease activity or pain; however, the long term effects of exercise on functional activity and progression of radiological indicators have not been established.[18]

The available evidence about exercise suggests that Gloria can benefit from continuing her exercise program and that this program can be more aggressive than a conservative program of isometric and range of motion exercise, especially if she is free of disease exacerbation. In light of the lack of available evidence and existing general knowledge that aggressive exercise with swollen joints can cause joint and tendon damage, caution is indicated during periods of disease activity. A critical factor in developing a therapeutic exercise program for Gloria rests with her answers to the following questions at any time during therapeutic exercise program participation:

■ Does Gloria have a more or less aggressive disease process?

■ Is Gloria currently in a period of exacerbation (flare-up) characterized by more acute inflammation and risk of joint destruction?

If the answer to either of these questions is affirmative, then it is wise to be less aggressive in designing the therapeutic exercise program. Education is an important part of the plan of care for Gloria with the ultimate goal of her being independent in recognizing changes in her disease process and in making appropriate modifications in her regular exercise program.

Given the multiple role demands placed on Gloria, it is especially important that the rehabilitation clinician collaborate with her in designing a therapeutic exercise program that addresses the problems she has identified, works toward her goals, and can be accomplished in a reasonable amount of time. Following a discussion of the available research about therapeutic exercise and RA, you the rehabilitation clinician and Gloria need to agree upon problems and short and long term goals.

A. What do you consider to be Gloria's primary problems? What short term treatment goals would be appropriate for Gloria? What long term treatment goals would be appropriate for Gloria? Make a chart with the problem list on the left and short and long term goals on the right. *See Author's Comments A*

Gloria's need for a shorter duration program is juxtaposed with increased needs to concentrate on maintaining flexibility carried by the new diagnosis of RA. During your discussion, she states that the re-designed therapeutic exercise program will accommodate her needs if she is able to accomplish it at home in no more than 30 minutes at a time. In response to your questions, Gloria also states that she would be able to find 10–20 minutes to stretch at work and that she has the resources to buy a piece of home exercise equipment.

Case Table 5.4   Original Therapeutic Exercise Program

Warm-up:	Low intensity stationary cycling for about 10 minutes' duration, 5 times a week
Hamstring stretches:	One set of four repetitions, each for 20–30 sec. duration, performed bilaterally in alternating pattern (see Chapter 3)
Aerobic conditioning:	Jogging on treadmill at fitness club, for 40-minute duration 5 times a week, monitoring for age-adjusted target heart rate
Stretch cool-down:	Repeat hamstring stretches for 1 set of 4 repetitions as described during warm-up
Strengthening exercises:	3 times per week (3 progressive resistance sets of 8–12 repetitions each) using a cable resistance machine for . . .
	• Bilateral progressive resistance seated knee extension (50, 40, 30 lbs)
	• Bilateral progressive resistance prone knee flexion (40, 30, 20 lbs)
	• Standing unilateral terminal knee extension (50, 40, 30 lbs)
	• Mini-squats with barbell resistance (70, 60, 50 lbs)

B. What are some features that the new therapeutic exercise program should have to accommodate the new diagnosis of rheumatoid arthritis, as well as Gloria's changed life situation? *See Author's Comments B*

Ultimately, the rehabilitation clinician may serve more in the role of consultant, communicating primarily by telephone or e-mail. However, it is important in the early stages of therapeutic exercise program development for regular re-checks to determine Gloria's reaction to increased activity, examining carefully for signs of increased joint inflammation or pain.

The plan of care calls for Gloria to be seen once every other week for four weeks, at eight weeks, and for follow-up at eight months from initiation of treatment. This will allow the clinician to continue to monitor Gloria's reaction to the program and her ability to implement appropriate modifications, if necessary. During the first four weeks, both the rehabilitation clinician and the client will concentrate on education, addressing body mechanics, joint protection, monitoring for joint inflammation, and energy conservation and the client utilizing referrals and general resources about coping with the disease (**see Case Table 5.2**). Gloria's original therapeutic exercise program is displayed in **Case Table 5.4**.

C. Please list the modifications you would recommend making to accommodate Gloria's present concerns? *See Author's Comments C*

Re-examination at Eight Weeks

At the end of eight weeks, Gloria has made good progress toward her goals. Evaluation of her workstation revealed that the unsupported position of her forearms resulted in increased position of wrist extension with increased activity of the wrist extensor muscles (**Case Figure 5.3**). Gloria has modified her workstation, has adapted to a home exercise program, and is able to demonstrate proper body mechanics that she is now using in the care of her mother. She has also identified joint protection measures that she uses in the kitchen to protect her wrists and fingers (such as using smaller, lighter weight pans.) Gloria has met all of the short term goals. As you begin to plan for the future, you introduce the possibility of establishing a measured

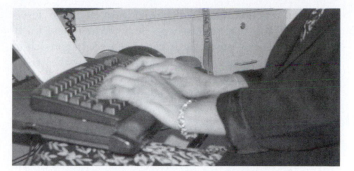

Case Figure 5.3   Workstation prior to modification.

baseline to evaluate possible changes in Gloria's health from RA; she agrees to complete the Arthritis Impact Measurement Scale Short Form (AIMS2-SF)[21,22] before the next session. The AIMS2-SF is a 26-item self-administered questionnaire to evaluate health status using five factors: physical functioning, social interaction, affective experience, symptoms, and role functioning.

At your eight-week appointment, Gloria brings with her the AIMS2-SF, and the results provide an opportunity to evaluate changes in her health and function. On re-examination, she has met all of her goals except that she occasionally has pain of 4/10 in her elbow when doing yard work or assisting her mother in transfers to the bathtub and her grip strength is 22 lbs on the right, 47 lbs combined. She is able to control elbow and wrist pain with the use of ice and correct posture at her workstation. Gloria states that she has had no signs of a flare-up and your physical examination finds no signs of increased joint inflammation. In her opinion, shifting her therapeutic exercise program to the home setting has made it possible for her to care for her mother, comply with her therapeutic exercise program requirements, and adapt her program to this new diagnosis. She has completed an arthritis self-help program offered by a local chapter of the Arthritis Foundation and feels that this has helped her to feel that she can cope, as well as providing some support and new friends. Gloria states, "I feel that I am on track again." In collaboration, you, Gloria, and the physician have agreed that she can continue her therapeutic exercise program independently with a plan of regular appointments with the physician and a yearly follow-up evaluation with you. Gloria agrees to contact you and her physician if she has indications that she is in a period of symptom exacerbation.

Case Summary

Changes in home responsibilities and in health status may be obstacles to adhering to therapeutic exercise program participation. Women frequently face this problem because they are often in the caregiver role. Single parents who have career responsibilities and caregiving responsibility for a parent and/or grandparent may find it difficult to find time for regular therapeutic exercise performance. A diagnosis of

RA may also result in decreased levels of activity or concerns about exercise safety. It is not uncommon for clients to experience challenges to regular therapeutic exercise program adherence from multiple sources: personal, family role, health status, career pressures, and social or health status, to name a few. Given the increased risk of heart disease associated with sedentary lifestyles, it is important for rehabilitation clinicians to collaborate with clients in developing programs that address ways to overcome these many real and perceived obstacles. A client-centered approach to developing therapeutic exercise programs allows the rehabilitation clinician and client to identify the numerous factors that create barriers to the client's ability to adhere to the therapeutic exercise program. The client-centered model requires active listening to their concerns, and engaging in a process of shared decision-making to develop a realistic therapeutic exercise plan.

D. On a separate sheet of paper, diagram a decision making algorithm for Gloria regarding maintenance of cardiovascular/pulmonary health without exacerbating her RA condition. *See Author's Comments D*

E. Additionally, diagram a decision making algorithm that focuses specifically on Gloria's joint protection concerns. *See Author's Comments E*

Referring to Chapter 10 for guidance, discuss any alternative or complementary therapeutic exercises that you believe might benefit this client. Provide the rationale for your suggestion(s).

References

1. Magee DJ. *Orthopedic Physical Assessment*, 4th ed. Philadelphia, PA: W.B. Saunders, 2002.
2. Stewart M, Brown JB, Weston WW, et al. *Patient-Centered Medicine: Transforming the Clinical Method.* Thousands Oaks, CA: Sage, 1995.
3. Acton GJ. Health-promoting self-care in family caregivers. *West J Nurs Res.* 2002;24(1):73–86.
4. Sisk RJ. Caregiver burden and health promotion. *Int J Nurs Stud.* 2000;37(1):37–43.
5. Goodman CC, Boissonnault WG. *Pathology: Implications for the Physical Therapist.* Philadelphia, PA: W.B. Saunders, 1998.
6. Lipsky PE. Chapter 312: Rheumatoid Arthritis. *Harrison's Online.* St. Louis, MO: McGraw-Hill, 2001–2002. Available at www.harrisonsonline.com. Accessed 10/20/04.
7. Brust DG. Update to Chapter 312: Osteoporosis and Rheumatoid Arthritis. *Harrison's Online.* St Louis: McGraw-Hill, 2001–2002. Accessed at www.harrisonsonline.com on 10/20/04.
8. Kisner C, Colby LA. *Therapeutic Exercise: Foundations and Techniques*, 4th ed. Philadelphia, PA: F.A. Davis, 2002.
9. Gornisiewicz, Moreland LW. Rheumatoid arthritis. In L Robbins, ed. *Clinical Care in the Rheumatic Diseases*, 2nd ed. Atlanta, GA: Association of Rheumatology Professionals, 2001; pp. 89–96.
10. Minor MA. Cardiovascular health and physical fitness for the client with multiple joint involvement. *In* JM Walker, A Helewa. *Physical Therapy in Arthritis.* Philadelphia, PA: W.B. Saunders, 1996, pp. 191–209.
11. Lorig K, Holman HR. Long-term outcomes of an arthritis self-management study: Effects of reinforcement efforts. *Soc Sci Med.* 1989;29(2):221–224.
12. Taal E, Riemsma RP, Brus HL, et al. Group education for patients with rheumatoid arthritis. *Patient Educ Couns.* 1993;20(2–3):177–187.
13. van den Ende CH, Hazes JM, le Cessie S, et al. Comparison of high and low intensity training in well-controlled rheumatoid arthritis. Results of a randomised clinical trial. *Ann Rheum Dis.* 1996; 55(11):798–805.
14. van den Ende CHM, Breedveld FC, le Cessie S, et al. Effect of intensive exercise on patients with active rheumatoid arthritis: A randomised clinical trial. *Ann Rheum Dis.* 2000;58:615–621.
15. Rall LC, Meydani SN, Kehayias JJ, et al. The effect of progressive resistance training in rheumatoid arthritis. Increased strength without changes in energy, balance, or body composition. *Arthritis Rheum.* 1996;39(3):415–426.
16. Harkcom TM, Lampman RM, Banwell BF, Castor CW. Therapeutic value of graded aerobic exercise training in rheumatoid arthritis. *Arthritis Rheum.* 1985;28(1):32–39.
17. Beals CA, Lampman RM, Banwell BF, et al. Measurement of exercise tolerance in patients with rheumatoid arthritis and osteoarthritis. *J Rheumatol.* 1985;12(3):458–461.
18. van den Ende CH, Vilet Vlieland TP, Munneke M, Hazes JM. Dynamic exercise therapy in rheumatoid arthritis: A systematic review. *Br J Rheumatol.* 1998;37(6):677–687.
19. Lyngberg K, Danneskjold-Samsoe B, Halskov O. The effect of physical training on patients with rheumatoid arthritis: Changes in disease activity, muscle strength, and aerobic capacity. A clinically controlled minimized cross-over study. *Clin Exp Rheumatol.* 1988;6(3):253–260.
20. Lyngberg KK, Harreby M, Bentzen H, et al. Elderly rheumatoid arthritis patients on steroid treatment tolerate physical training without an increase in disease activity. *Arch Phys Med Rehabil.* 1994; 75(11):1189–1195.
21. Guillemin F, Coste J, Pouchot J, et al. The AIMS2-SF: A short form of the Arthritis Impact Measurement Scales 2. French quality of life in rheumatology group. *Arthritis Rheum.* 1997;40(7):1267–1274.
22. Haavardsholm EA, Kvien TK, Uhlig T, et al. A comparison of agreement and sensitivity to change between AIMS2 and a short form of AIMS2 (AIMS2-SF) in more than 1,000 rheumatoid arthritis patients. *J Rheumatol.* 2000;27(12): 2727–2730.
23. Klippel JH, ed. *Primer on the Rheumatic Diseases*, 11th ed. Atlanta, GA: Arthritis Foundation, 1997.

Author's Comments A

Problems	Goals

1. Pain in both upper extremities due to overuse and lateral epicondylitis, limiting ability to:
 	
• Work at the computer for more than an hour at a time as needed for job
• Assist mother in transfers, ambulation, and activities of daily living
• Cook for her family
• Perform yard work
• Play golf
	Short term:
	By the end of four weeks, Gloria's upper extremity pain will decrease from current range of 6–10/10 on visual analogue scale (VAS) to 3–6/10 during the following activities:
	   • Work for 2 hours at a time at the computer (with short rests)
	   • Assist mother in transfers, ambulation and activities of daily living
	   • Cook for her family
	   • Practice her golf swing for 15 minutes, 3 × a week
	Long term:
	By the end of eight weeks, Gloria's upper extremity pain will decrease from current range of 6–10/10 on visual analogue scale (VAS) to 0–2/10 during the following activities:
	   • Work for 4 hours at a time at the computer (with short rests)
	   • Assist mother in transfers, ambulation and activities of daily living
	   • Cook for her family
	   • Play 9–18 holes of golf once a week

2. Unable to participate in fitness program due to time and inability to go to gym with increased risk for weight gain and diseases associated with decreased physical activity.	Short term: By the end of four weeks, Gloria will be independent in performing a revised fitness program 3–4 times a week. Long term: By the end of eight weeks, Gloria will have gained no additional weight.

3. Left knee pain, limiting ability to:
 	
• Ascend and descend stairs
• Perform yard work
• Play golf
	Short term:
	By the end of four weeks, Gloria's knee pain will decrease from current range of 6–10/10 on visual analogue scale (VAS) to 3–6/10 during the following activities:
	   • Ascending and descending a flight of 12 stairs at work
	   • Performing yard work for 1 hour
	   • Practicing her golf swing for 15 minutes, 2–3 times a week
	Long term:
	By the end of eight weeks, Gloria's knee pain will decrease from current range of 6–10/10 on visual analogue scale (VAS) to 0–2/10 during the following activities:
	   • Ascending and descending a flight of 12 stairs at work
	   • Performing yard work for 2–3 hours
	   • Playing 18 holes of golf a week
	   • Performing a squat

4. Decreased strength and extensibility contributing to upper extremity and knee pain	Short term:
	By the end of four weeks, Gloria will be independent in exercises for increasing strength and extensibility 3–4 times a week.
	Long term:
	By the end of eight weeks, Gloria's strength and extensibility will increase so that:
	   • Quadriceps and hamstring strength have increased from 4/5 to 5/5 on MMT
	   • Hamstring flexibility will increase to lacking less than 10° on 90°–90° measurement
	   • Right wrist flexion will be equal to left and pain-less with stretch
	   • Wrist extensor strength has increased from 4/5 to 5/5 on MMT
	   • Handgrip dynamometer strength has increased to 25 lbs on the right, and 50 lbs combined

(continued)

Problems	Goals
5. Lack of knowledge about RA, body mechanics, ergonomics, workstation, and caregiver stress factors that may contribute to pain and the development of secondary problems (e.g., joint deformity and degeneration, osteoporosis).	Short term: By the end of four weeks, Gloria will be able to: • Describe the main features of rheumatoid arthritis • Verbalize appropriate modifications for her workstation • Verbalize appropriate transfer techniques and correct common errors that can lead to injury • Identify workstation, postural positions, and transfer techniques that contribute to joint pain and injury Long term: By the end of eight weeks, Gloria will be able to: • Describe the indications that she is experiencing a "flare-up" • Modify her exercise routine based on the current status of the RA by choosing the low-impact exercise plan during a "flare-up" • Verbalize and demonstrate joint protection behaviors • Utilize family and community resources to assist with the care of her mother

Author's Comments B

1. The most time consuming exercise (aerobic component) should be performed at home.
2. A low impact alternative such as a stationary bicycle should substitute for higher impact treadmill jogging.
3. Shorter therapeutic exercise session duration should be employed to decrease joint stress.[6,9,10]
4. The total number of therapeutic exercise program sessions may be increased and the number of activities decreased to accommodate Gloria's lifestyle and work commitments.

5. Brief periods of "down time" therapeutic exercise sessions can be performed at work.
6. Flexibility exercises should be employed at joints prone to RA associated stiffness.
7. Since Gloria has been helping her mother exercise, where possible perhaps they can perform some therapeutic exercises together.

Author's Comments C

Original program	Revised program
Warm-up Low intensity stationary cycling About 10 minutes 5 times a week	**Warm-up** Low intensity stationary cycling About 5–10 minutes, 3–4 times a week (Protect wrists and hands when bicycling by changing positions, supporting on forearms, or wearing protective gloves)
Stretch: hamstring (Case Figure 5.4) 1 set of 4 repetitions Duration: 20–30 sec.—each side	**Stretch: Quadriceps and hamstring muscle groups** 1 set of 4 repetitions Duration: 20–30 sec.—each side Intensity: Stretch—not pain! When you have more joint inflammation and pain, be less aggressive in stretching
Aerobic conditioning Jogging on treadmill at fitness club 40 minutes 5 times a week Age-adjusted target heart rate (see Chapter 4)	**Aerobic conditioning** Stationary cycling at home 20–30 minutes (build up to this gradually) 3–4 times a week Age-adjusted target heart rate When you have increased joint inflammation and pain, consider swimming, dividing the exercise into several sessions, or decreasing the total time
Stretch cool-down Frequency: Every workout 1 set of 4 repetitions Duration: 20–30 sec. each side	**Stretch cool-down: quadriceps and hamstring muscle groups** Frequency: Every workout Sets: 1 Reps: 4 Intensity: Be gentle. You should feel stretch—not pain! Duration: 20–30 sec. each side

Strengthen
(Cable resistance machine at local gym)
- Seated knee extension (50, 40, 30 lbs)
- Prone knee flexion (40, 30, 20 lbs)
- Standing unilateral terminal knee extension (50, 40, 30 lbs)
- Standing mini-squats (70, 60, 50 lbs)

Frequency: 3 times per week
Sets: 3
Repetitions: 8–12 each (see Chapter 5)

Strengthen (2 days a week, when you are not bicycling)
Try to do these exercises on days that you are not doing your aerobic exercise Resistive exercise with resistive band and tubing can be performed at home or at work during a lunch break.
- Seated knee extension (**Case Figure 5.5**) (strongest cord)
- Prone knee flexion (medium cord)
- Standing unilateral terminal knee extension (**Case Figure 5.6a–b**) (strongest cord)

Standing mini-squats (strongest cord)
Frequency: 2 times per week
Sets: 1–2
Repetitions: 5–12 each (start with 1 set of 5 repetitions and work up)
(Loop the band around a doorknob—do not hold the cord with your hand)

Exercises to be performed at work or at home

At work
Wrist extensor (**Case Figure 5.7**) and flexor (**Case Figure 5.8**) stretches (do these daily)
Sets and repetitons: 1–2 times a day, 5 repetitions each
Intensity: Be gentle, stretch, but do not elicit pain

Wrist extensor strengthening with lightest cord (loop the band around your palm—do not hold the cord with your fingers or wrists) (**Case Figure 5.9**)
Fix your workstation! Take regular breaks!

At home (before bed or first thing in the morning)
Knee, hip, and back stretches
Intensity: be gentle; you should feel stretch—not pain!

Warning signs that exercise is too intense

Your joints hurt for more than an hour after exercise[7]
A joint that you are stretching has severe pain during the stretch
You have a significant increase in fatigue

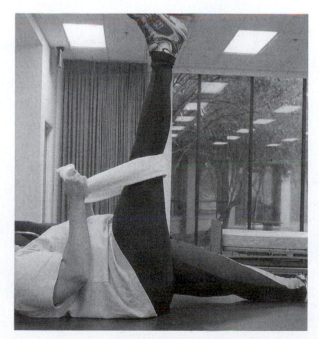

Case Figure 5.4   Supine hamstring stretch with a towel (may substitute doorway as prop during hand-wrist symptom flare-up).

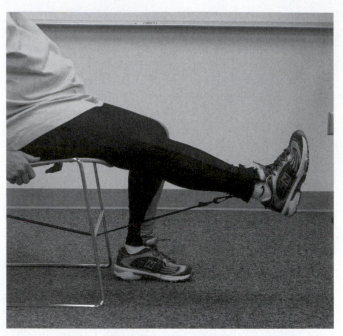

Case Figure 5.5   Seated knee extension with elastic cord resistance.

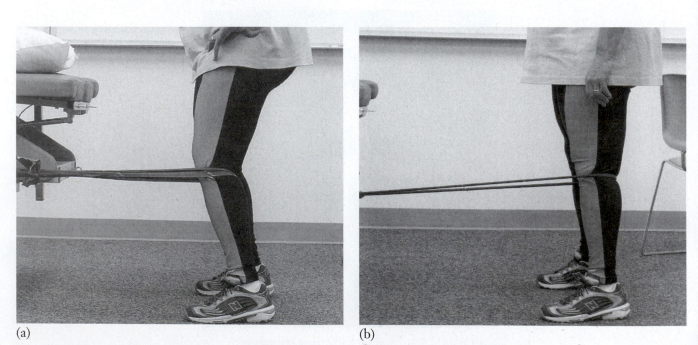

(a)   (b)

Case Figure 5.6   Standing knee extension exercise with elastic band resistance. (a) start; (b) finish.

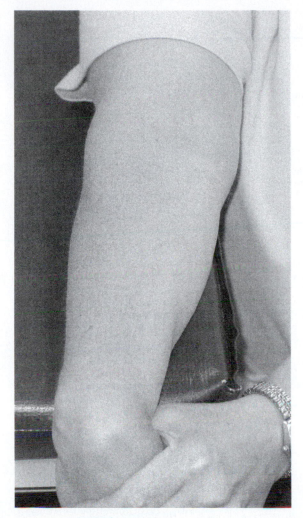

Case Figure 5.7   Wrist extensor stretching.

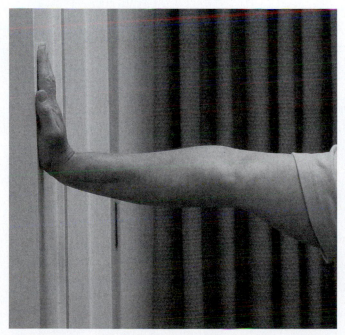

Case Figure 5.8   Wrist flexor stretching against a wall.

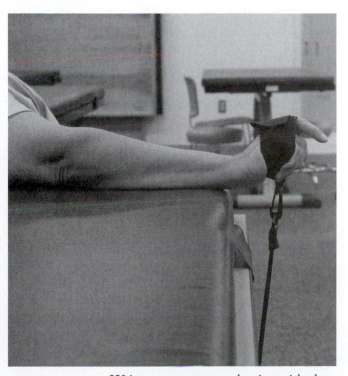

Case Figure 5.9   Wrist extensor strengthening with elastic cord resistance.

Author's Comments D

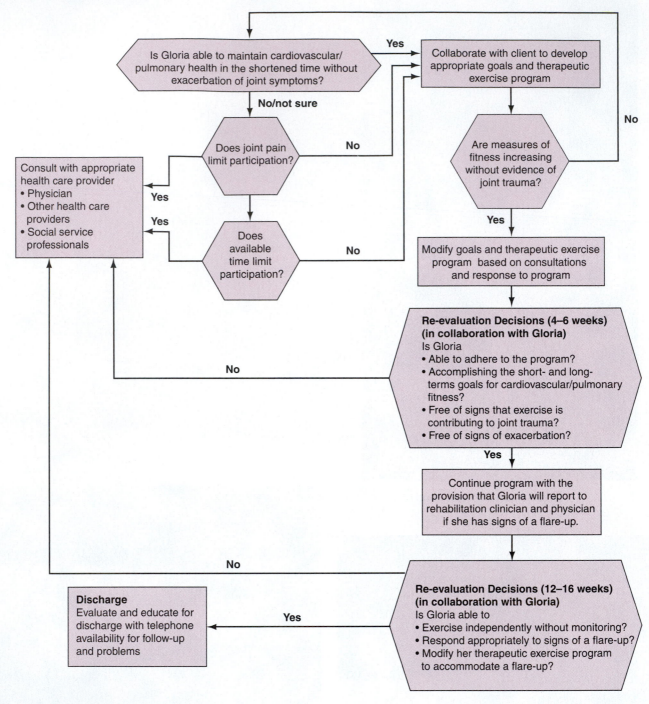

Author's Comments E

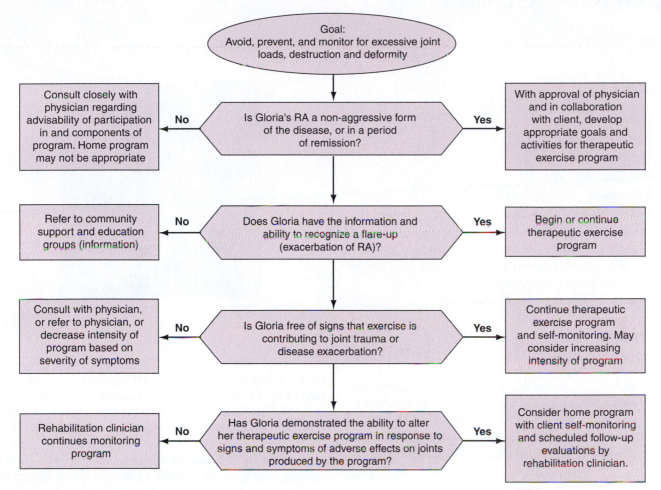

Goal:
Avoid, prevent, and monitor for excessive joint loads, destruction and deformity

No — Consult closely with physician regarding advisability of participation in and components of program. Home program may not be appropriate

Is Gloria's RA a non-aggressive form of the disease, or in a period of remission?

Yes — With approval of physician and in collaboration with client, develop appropriate goals and activities for therapeutic exercise program

No — Refer to community support and education groups (information)

Does Gloria have the information and ability to recognize a flare-up (exacerbation of RA)?

Yes — Begin or continue therapeutic exercise program

No — Consult with physician, or refer to physician, or decrease intensity of program based on severity of symptoms

Is Gloria free of signs that exercise is contributing to joint trauma or disease exacerbation?

Yes — Continue therapeutic exercise program and self-monitoring. May consider increasing intensity of program

No — Rehabilitation clinician continues monitoring program

Has Gloria demonstrated the ability to alter her therapeutic exercise program in response to signs and symptoms of adverse effects on joints produced by the program?

Yes — Consider home program with client self-monitoring and scheduled follow-up evaluations by rehabilitation clinician.

CLIENT CASE #6

Jason Gauvin

History

Patient: TJ

Age: 12 years

Height: 5' 9"

Weight: 135 lbs

Education: Seventh grade student

Sports/Hobbies: Soccer, riding bike, swimming

Medical/Surgical history: 10 days s/p right knee arthroscopically assisted anterior cruciate ligament (ACL) reconstruction using allograft tissue, and partial medial meniscectomy

Chief Complaint: Right knee pain

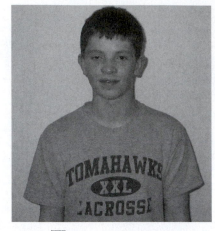

Case Figure 6.1 TJ

Biographic Information about TJ's Parents

Father: 47 years of age. Played high school and Division I college soccer. He received a full scholarship to play for 4 years

Mother: 46 years of age. Played high school soccer and basketball. She played Division III college basketball

Participation in athletics and youth sports has significantly increased over the past 10 years. Injuries have also risen with increased sports participation and has increased the awareness of injury occurence in children. It has been estimated that nearly 45 million children participate in sports annually in the United States.[1] It has also been stated that injuries from sports participation are a significant cause of hospitalization and health care costs in children and adolescents in the United States.[2] Sports related injuries are the second leading cause of emergency room visits for children and the second leading cause of injury in schools.[3] Nearly eight million children seek medical attention for sports related injuries each year.[1] It has been hypothesized that possibly half of these injuries could be prevented and that the reporting of youth injuries may not be completely representative of the actual injury occurrence rates. With the overwhelming growth of youth sports programs nationally, injury rates are expected to continue to rise unless injury prevention programs are implemented across the board. The prevention of injuries in children participating in sports must become a national priority.[4]

The concept of injury prevention is much more of a proactive approach than the concept of treating an injury. The study of injury in children has taken on more focus over the last few years and much research has been conducted on the treatment of the injured adolescent. However, debate continues on what the most effective treatment approach and techniques are for the treatment of the adolescent who has not completed their growth. The following is a case of a young boy who was injured playing youth soccer. Details of his course of treatment will be presented including the surgical and therapeutic exercise interventions, and his eventual outcome.

TJ (**Case Figure 6.1**) injured his right knee while playing forward for his junior high soccer team. He had played soccer since he was five years old. TJ's parents are very involved in youth soccer and his father was the local community college head soccer coach. The parents attended every game and were some of the more "supportive" and vocal of all the youth soccer parents. TJ's injury occurred in the second half of play. TJ was injured while cutting toward the goal (see Chapter 9). He planted his right foot and turned to his left and immediately fell to the ground in pain, holding his right knee. TJ's parents rushed out on the field and quickly transported him to the emergency room of the local hospital. TJ was evaluated by an emergency room physician and diagnosed with a knee sprain and was immobilized in a knee brace locked in full extension and placed on crutches, non–weight bearing (NWB). He was referred to his primary care physician for follow-up. The primary care physician reported that he suspected that TJ had experienced an ACL tear and ordered an MRI of the right knee. The results of the MRI confirmed the diagnosis of a complete midsubstance tear of his right ACL with a concomitant small medial meniscal tear. TJ was referred to an orthopedic surgeon at the university medical center who specialized in pediatric orthopedic surgery. TJ and his parents met with the surgeon, who confirmed the findings and recommended ACL reconstruction surgery and arthroscopic evaluation of the meniscus injury. Four weeks later, TJ underwent an ACL reconstruction using an Achilles tendon allograft with interference screw fixation and partial medial meniscectomy. The ACL reconstruction technique was described as a transphyseal, intra-articular drilling of bone tunnels across the physes of the distal femur and proximal tibia.

TJ presented to your clinic at 10 days post-surgery with the following treatment recommendations and guidelines: NWB × two weeks on crutches, brace locked at 0°, except during rehabilitation. Progressive flexion ROM to 90° by two weeks. Utilize continuous passive motion device (CPM) between 0° and 45° for 6–8 hours a day, progressing ROM by 5–10° each day. No closed kinetic chain (CKC) or weight bearing exercises are to be performed for two weeks and no dynamic open kinetic chain (OKC) or non–weight bearing quadriceps exercises are to be performed with resistance at end-range extension (30° flexion to full extension); "isometric" quadriceps setting is allowed. Begin aquatic therapy as wound allows in neoprene brace with ROM stops set to enable extension to 0° flexion and flexion to 90°. Rehabilitation following ACL reconstruction commonly lasts between four and six months and consists of several phases or stages. These phases are developed with respect to research data on graft strength, fixation strength, healing constraints, and the clinical presentation of the client during regular re-evaluations throughout the therapeutic exercise process. In this case each therapeutic exercise phase will be outlined, but it should be understood that this is intended to serve only as a guideline and not as a protocol.

Our intervention starts the first day of rehabilitation on the tenth post-operative day following suture removal. A complete medical history was taken and initial evaluation was completed, with both parents present. TJ is a very athletic youth who played several sports (other hobbies including baseball, basketball, fishing, camping) up until the past two years, when he began to focus on soccer and going to only soccer camps for extra coaching and instruction. TJ reported that he has never exercised with weights before. TJ's parents reported that he had gone through a growth spurt within the last year. His parents reported that TJ's eating habits were like most boys his age; "he basically eats everything." During the initial evaluation, TJ's father stated that if TJ were going to get a scholarship to play soccer in college, he would have to focus only on playing soccer. TJ's father and mother stated that they were willing to do whatever it took to get TJ back on the field playing soccer again. They volunteered several suggestions, including daily therapeutic exercise, swimming pool workouts, purchasing some exercise equipment for home or hiring someone to personally oversee his program. During the evaluation it appeared that TJ was under an enormous amount of pressure from both of his parents to be the best soccer player he could be. TJ's facial reaction to his parent's comments indicated that he did not appear to be responding positively to his parent's remarks, but he did not say anything. The rehabilitation clinician provided some suggested readings and information sources regarding ACL injury, surgery and recovery to TJ and his parents.

Physical Examination

Post-operative evaluation was limited secondary to surgical restrictions and pain.

Knee ROM: Right knee resting position was in 15° of flexion. Passive right knee flexion to 25° with gentle heel slide. Passive right knee extension to 15° flexion. Left knee full flexion of 135°, 10° of passive knee hyperextension and 7° of active knee hyperextension

Strength: Right quadriceps displays trace activation with attempted isometric quadriceps setting. A superior patellar glide could not be detected with volitional quadriceps activation. TJ was was unable to perform an independent straight leg raise (SLR). Active ankle pump noted. Deferred manual muscle test (MMT) to ankle muscles (5/5) secondary to knee joint pain. Full active quadriceps activation noted with good patellar mobility at the left knee and MMT for all left lower extremity muscles were 5/5

Neurovascular: Sensation was intact at bilateral lower extremities. Negative Homan's sign bilaterally with intact distal pulses

Integumentary: The arthroscopic portal wounds appeared to be healing, minimal bloody drainage was noted and the dressing was intact. Slight bleeding noted from stitch removal. There were no signs of infection. TJ and his parents were instructed to change the dressing as needed; showering was not allowed for 24 hours

ADLs: Client is unable to tie shoelaces with knee immobilized in extension brace

Velcro sneakers were purchased to facilitate independence. Client must use left leg to lift right leg for improved bed mobility. Independent with crutch use, NWB on the right

Knee pain: 8/10 using a visual analog scale (VAS) (0 = no pain, 10 = worst pain possible) during evaluation

4/10 at best with pain medication

8/10 at worst; client cannot sleep well

Special tests: Lachman Test/Anterior Drawer Test deferred because of the stress that they place across the reconstructed ACL. These tests, as well as instrumented arthrometry, should be deferred for 6–10 weeks post-operatively. The attending surgeon may perform the test under their discretion

Knee joint girth measurement not completed for this case

Data collected during the initial evaluation demonstrated that TJ had limited ROM and minimal active quadriceps activation. Pain was limiting his performance of the post-operative therapeutic exercise program that was given to him in the hospital. This program consisted of ankle pumps, quadriceps setting, and straight leg raises. Prior to therapeutic exercise program prescription, TJ, his parents, his surgeon and the rehabilitation team (surgeon, physical therapist, athletic trainer, and strength coach) engaged in an in-depth discussion of the rehabilitation process and the importance of compliance (see Chapter 11). TJ and his parents verbalized understanding and signed a written agreement indicating as such. This agreement was kept on file for future reference. Once this agreement was signed, the parents were asked to leave the room. At that time, TJ was asked several questions. He was asked if he had been having any nightmares, any trouble sleeping, or any troubles in school. He was asked how he felt about sports and in particular soccer. He was asked what his goal was for rehabilitation and if he was looking forward to returning to play soccer when he completed his rehabilitation.

TJ reported he knew that his parents wanted him to play and he liked playing soccer, but he was nervous about playing again after hurting his knee. He stated that the knee really hurt after the injury and that it hurts even worse since surgery. He also reported that all the kids at school looked at him "funny" because he was on crutches and had to wear a knee brace. He was already tired of all the questions and teasing from kids at school. This made him feel uncomfortable and he didn't want to go back to school until he could walk on his own. TJ said he just wanted to have his knee stop hurting and to get off the crutches. He mentioned that he had been having some bad dreams since the injury and has been tired a lot during the day. He said he has not wanted to tell his parents, because he was afraid that they would get upset with him. TJ appeared to be having difficulty coping with his surgery and the pain associated with it. A sports psychology consult was considered, but deferred until more detailed information or consistent behaviors were observed. It is often necessary to consult other disciplines with adolescent injuries because of the emotional concerns that occur following injury and during recovery.

Following evaluation the complex issues associated with this case were addressed in a problem list. Development of a problem list, and short term and long term

goals were completed and discussed with TJ and his family and agreed upon.

A. Please develop a list of problems associated with this case. The development of the problem list will identify concerns and physical limitations. These problems will relate to the development of short term and long term goals. *See Author's Comments A*

B. Make a list of short term goals and include a time frame and function associated with each goal. Begin each goal with: By 6–8 weeks the client will . . . *See Author's Comments B*

C. Make a list of long term goals and include a time frame and function associated with each goal. Begin each goal with: By 6 months the client will . . . *See Author's Comments C*

Scientific Evidence/ Clinical Experience: Treatment and Therapeutic Exercise Prescription

Phase I

The therapeutic exercise progression was discussed with TJ and his parents in the order of importance and relevance to phase I. The rehabilitation clinician should work to achieve all of the treatment goals, but it may be necessary to prioritize what is most important and to logically stage the goals according to their relevance to particular functional milestones over the course of the entire program. The initial therapeutic exercise program consisted of passive knee extension ROM (● **Section 7, Figure 1**), quadriceps setting focusing on active knee hyperextension (● **Section 7, Figure 2**), facilitating a straight leg raise without an extension lag (● **Section 7, Figure 3**) and initiating progressive active flexion ROM. Of note, right knee flexion was restricted to 90° by the surgeon over the initial two weeks following surgery. Regaining full knee extension ROM including full active hyperextension is essential to facilitate a successful outcome following ACL reconstruction. Numerous techniques exist to regain full knee extension. However, passive stretching (if allowed by the surgeon) remains the most effective. Propping the heel off of the treatment table with a small bolster (heel props) (**Case Figure 6.2**) and allowing a low load prolonged stretch for five minutes for several sets is an effective method to regain full extension. Other methods include prone hangs, and passive over pressure applied manually by the rehabilitation clinician with the client in a supine position.

Knee extension loss from immobilization may result in the patella becoming immobile as well as stiffness in the tibio femoral joint. These joints must be mobilized to re-

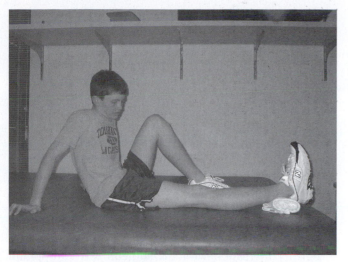

Case Figure 6.2   Bolster use to facilitate full terminal knee extension.

gain normal motion. Numerous complications may result if knee mobility is restricted. Arthrofibrosis, patellofemoral pain, quadriceps weakness and knee stiffness may all result post-operatively following an ACL reconstruction. Clients are often instructed to use a CPM device for 6–8 hours a day if possible. Range from 0° to 45° degrees initially and increasing to 90° gradually over a two week period is commonly prescribed. The most significant patella motions to regain to improve active knee extension and flexion are the superior and inferior glides. Superior (extension) and inferior (flexion) patella mobilizations (grade II–IV) may be performed in combination with active ROM exercises to use treatment time efficiently. The patella should move nearly 1–2 cm superiorly when the quadriceps muscle contracts maximally. Using the index finger and placing it proximal to the superior pole of the patella and seeing if the patella lifts the finger when the quadriceps is activated can confirm this. A knee flexion contracture and a hypomobile patella may compound the effects of a weak quadriceps, resulting in poor active movement.

Regaining quadriceps strength ranks a very close second to regaining knee extension ROM and patella mobility in the prioritization of post-operative therapeutic exercise program goals. Regaining active knee hyperextension (if hyperextension exists at the contralateral knee or existed preoperatively) has proven to be quite important to prevent post-operative complications including limited patella mobility, quadriceps weakness, abnormal gait patterns, knee stiffness, patellofemoral pain syndrome, and patellar tendonitis. Proper performance of quadriceps setting is crucial to achieving improved quadriceps activation. The client is instructed to perform quadriceps setting by attempting to push the posterior as-

pect of their knee flat against the treatment table surface while maximally contracting their quadriceps muscles (**Case Figure 6.3**). Compression forces at the tibio femoral joint limits concern of ACL strain during the quadriceps setting exercise. Emphasis should be placed on not substituting the hamstring or gluteus maximus muscles to achieve solely passive knee extension via active hip extension. Also, attention should be directed to trying to lift the heel off the table (ankle dorsiflexion) while obtaining maximal quadriceps activation and active knee hyperextension.

A trial of biofeedback or electrical muscle stimulation may be appropriate if the client is not able to perform quadriceps setting with the appropriate amount of volitional activation. Occasionally, the client has too much pain in full extension to maximally contract the quadriceps as described above. In this instance, they may benefit from positioning the knee in a minimal amount of flexion while performing the exercise as described above. This may be facilitated by placing a small bolster under the knee and calf, to serve as a fulcum point during the exercise. Caution must be emphasized to avoid the development of a knee flexion contracture when assuming this position. A pillow should never be placed width-wise under the knee for extended periods of time. Phase I therapeutic exercises continued throughout the initial four weeks of treatment.

It seems appropriate to address the high level of emotional stress that TJ appeared to be dealing with. Children may not understand what stress is and may not have any way of coping with the stress associated with challenges in life. Nightmares, failure or difficulty in school, grinding of teeth (bruxism), and insomnia or poor sleeping habits are all possible indicators of stress in children.[5,6] A child may not be able to recognize that they are stressed out, but as rehabilitation clinicians we may be able to gather

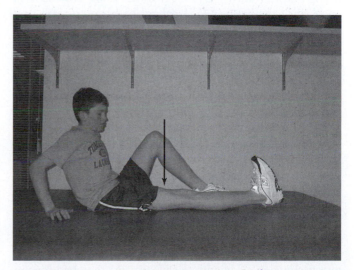

Case Figure 6.3   Quadriceps setting to facilitate active terminal knee extension.

information identifying negative stress or a child's reaction to stress. This information may support your concern that the child may be under stress and having difficulty coping with a situation. Identifying the stressors affecting the child is a key factor to observe during the evaluation. If these stressors are not addressed, the client outcome may be compromised (see Chapter 11).[5,6]

Phase I, Session 2, Week 2

TJ presented the next day for his second formal therapeutic exercise session. The session focused on regaining knee extension, flexion ROM and quadriceps strength. TJ continued to be in a moderate degree of pain reported as a 6/10. He was having difficulty following through with his therapeutic exercises as a result of the pain. He was taking ibuprofen, but with the initiation of exercises, his pain was increased and was not well controlled. TJ presented lacking 15° of knee extension and flexion range to 40°. Continuous passive motion machine use continued six hours a day, but the range of motion could not be increased because of TJ's pain level. It was decided to focus rehabilitation solely on the most important concern, regaining knee extension. Knee extension ROM was emphasized to both TJ and his parents to be the most important factor to having a successful outcome. He was re-instructed in the heel propping and prone hanging methods of regaining knee extension.

Phase I, Session 4, Week 2

TJ presented with a moderately inflamed and swollen right knee (grade 2), and an increased skin temperature was also noted. TJ reportedly returned to school two days prior and had been on his feet much more than he had been since the surgery. TJ's school had been on vacation for a week, which is why he had the surgery at that time, but the school re-convened this week. TJ's attendance had not been discussed previously with the rehabilitation clinician. The parents had discussed TJ's return to school with the surgeon, who allowed TJ to return. TJ's knee appeared to have had a negative reaction to the increased activity; therefore, the activity had to be modified. Discussion with TJ's parents was needed to develop a return to school plan that would not result in any further regression in TJ's condition. It was decided that TJ would attend school on a half-day basis for the rest of the week and he would be re-assessed at the end of the week to determine the school plan for the following week. TJ's parents would contact the school to make the arrangements.

Following the session, TJ's parents pulled the rehabilitation clinician aside and voiced concern they had for not being able to "help" TJ regain his extension. They reported that they could not inflict pain on their son, even if it was "therapeutic." TJ's parents wanted to discuss TJ's pain level and the effect it was having on him and actually on them as well. TJ was continuing to have nightmares and actually fell asleep at school the day before. Of most concern to TJ's parents was the effect that his pain was having on all of them. They found it extremely difficult to "help" TJ regain his knee extension. The rehabilitation clinician suggested that now might be a good time to re-evaluate their focus on TJ's soccer success and the anxiety that TJ feels. TJ's parents agreed to consider this issue and discuss it with the rehabilitation clinician in the future.

Session 4 focused on low intensity active and passive extension ROM activities and ice pack application (**Case Table 6.1**). No range of motion measurements were taken.

Further discussion with the surgeon was appropriate and was facilitated by a phone call placed to his medical office following the evaluation. Discussion with the surgeon provided information on the current research on ACL reconstruction outcomes in pre-pubescent children and the specific surgical procedure used on TJ. The surgeon reported that mid-substance tears are being reported more frequently in the immature athlete, which is most likely related to increased awareness by the medical community and the increased participation of youth in sport.[6–11] The surgeon reported that non-operative treatment was not an option with TJ because of the medial meniscal tear that occurred in association with the ACL tear. The surgeon did not want TJ to risk further or future damage to his knee by completing a non-operative treatment program. He also indicated that the most recent research indicates that non-operative programs may result in poor outcomes.[11–17] The surgeon reported that he had an in-depth discussion with TJ and his family pre-operatively. The surgeon assumed the role of "knee counselor" in educating TJ and his family on the most appropriate treatment plan, including possible risks and outcomes.

Numerous factors should be considered when determining the skeletal maturity of a client. The most appropriate method should be based on the client's chronological age, radiographic age (growth plate closure left hand), secondary sexual characteristics (Tanner staging), family height, evidence of recent growth spurt, athletic goals, and, with minors, the consent of the parents or guardians.[19] The surgeon reported that he performed a complete medical workup including the factors indicated above, and was satisfied that TJ was appropriate for the transphyseal approach to ACL reconstruction using allograft tissue.

D. Perform a literature search and discuss the factors that the surgeon and rehabilitation clinician must take into account when deciding on ACL reconstruc-

Case Table 6.1   Phase I. Therapeutic Exercise Activities

Treatment Program	Type of exercise	Frequency/duration
Passive knee extension	Heel propping, Prone hangs	5 times a day × 5 minutes each
Patella mobilizations	Grade I-III (superior, inferior, medial, lateral)	Once a day for 5 minutes
Quadriceps setting	Facilitating active knee extension	3 times/day × 25–50 repetitons, holding 10 seconds
Straight leg raises (SLR)	Four way (hip flexion, abduction, adduction, extension)	Three times a day × 50 repetitions
Knee flexion ROM	Heel slides, active assisted ROM sitting over the edge of a treatment table	Three times a day × 10–20 repetitions
Continuous passive motion device	Passive range of motion	6 to 8 hours a day as able
Pain and swelling control	Ice, compression, elevation	Multiple times throughout the day (5–6 times)

tion surgery and subsequent therapeutic exercise for an adolescent client.[10–24] *See Author's Comments D*

Both animal model and clinical research have contributed to our understanding of the ACL and its reconstruction since it was first reported in 1917 by Hey Groves.[25] This knowledge has allowed surgeons and rehabilitation clinicians to minimize post-operative complications and improve success rates.

The ideal ACL graft should reproduce the anatomy and biomechanics of the native ACL, have strong initial fixation, incorporate biologically, have minimal donor site morbidity and decrease rehabilitation time. To date no ideal graft exists. However, the most popular choice of graft tissue continues to be the bone-patellar tendon-bone (BPTB) autograft, because it has so many favorable characteristics. The graft tissue has a high tensile load to failure and high stiffness rating, strong bone to bone fixation, good durability, enables relatively early return to sport, low risk of inflammatory reaction, no risk of disease transmission and has been shown to have good long term results.[26,27] However, these advantages do not come without disadvantages. BPTB autografts do run high risks of donor site morbidity and pain, patella tendonitis, quadriceps weakness, knee stiffness, possible arthrofibrosis, patellofemoral pain and occasionally patella fracture.

Development of a therapeutic exercise program for a client with a BPTB autograft is a challenge for the rehabilitation clinician. We must work diligently to prevent the development or increase in donor site pain and patellofemoral pain complications post-operatively in each case. Several authors have reported that the incidence of post-operative patellofemoral pain may be a function of the therapeutic exercise program rather than surgical morbidity from the harvest site.[28–30] Therapeutic exercises can progress rapidly if the client's symptoms allow, but they must often be delayed to control for the symptoms associated with the graft harvest site. Another therapeutic challenge is the treatment of the quadriceps weakness that can persist post-operatively secondary to the disruption in the extensor mechanism and joint effusion. As a result of the high incidence of post-operative complications with BPTB autografts, their use has become less popular with some surgeons. Brown[31] reported at the American Academy of Orthopaedic Surgeons (AAOS) meeting in 2000 that 17–90% of patients who undergo ACL reconstruction using a BPTB autograft develop donor site pain, 13–47% develop patellofemoral pain syndromes, and 10% develop quadriceps weakness. The high incidence of graft site morbidity has pushed surgeons to consider other alternatives.

One option that is being considered is the use of BPTB or Achilles tendon allografts. Fu et al.[27] supported the use of allograft tissue as an alternative for ACL reconstruction. Allograft tissues have many attractive advantages, including: no surgical morbidity from a graft harvest site, less post-operative pain with rehabilitation, less quadriceps atrophy, no disruption of the extensor mechanism, decreased risk of patellofemoral pain, decreased surgery time, improved sterilization and preservation techniques and satisfactory clinical outcomes.[26,27] The outcome studies have shown favorable results for allografts versus autografts, but not superior results. Short term studies[32–35] ranging from three months to three years and long-term studies with five and seven year follow-ups have been reported.[36–39] However, allograft tissue use has disadvantages, including high cost, limited availability, delayed tissue incorporation, risk of graft rejection, risk of chronic inflammation and the most concerning to all the risk of disease transmission.

To increase the likelihood of attaining a positive client outcome following surgery and rehabilitation, the surgeon and the rehabilitation clinician must understand and respect the basic science evidence regarding the biomechanical and histological properties of both the native and reconstructed ACL (see Chapter 3). All biologic tissues, allograft or autograft, undergo similar incorporation once implanted as an ACL graft.[39] The process of incorporation consists of graft necrosis, cellular repopulation, revascularization and collagen remodeling, also referred to as ligamentization. In a well documented study using goat tissue, Jackson et al.[40] reported that the mean maximum load at failure was similar at six weeks post-surgery, but was considerably less at six months in allograft tissue than in autograft tissue.[40] Jackson et al.[40] concluded that histologically the allograft tissue was slower to incorporate and might result in a less robust graft than the autograft tissue in the goat model. On the contrary, Nikolaou et al.[41] demonstrated that in the canine model the allograft and autograft are similar in tissue strength from 8 to 36 weeks post-surgery. Jackson et al.[39] concluded that both tissues demonstrate a loss of overall strength as they mature. Shino et al.[42] reported that human allograft tissue matures at approximately 18 months after implantation. The basic science data continues to be controversial and following a path of "point–counterpoint" made by numerous authors.

Graft fixation strength is an immediate concern during the rehabilitation of the client with an ACL reconstruction. A variety of fixation methods exist and several examples of the most common methods used are the interference screw (both metal and bioabsorbable polymers), staples, crosspins and external buttons. Interference screw fixation currently meets the demands of accelerated rehabilitation and it appears to be the most successful bone-to-bone fixation device for BPTB graft ACL fixation.[43] Biodegradable interference screws are becoming more popular, have been shown to disintegrate over time, and they do not appear to compromise graft incorporation.[44] Brand et al.[43] stated that the weakest link in the early post-operative time frame is graft fixation and unfortunately, no current fixation device matches the strength and stiffness of the native ACL. Fixation methods must be rigid and stiff to allow the accelerated rehabilitation program of early range of motion, progressive therapeutic exercises and early weight bearing.[43] Brand et al.[43] provide an excellent analogy in saying that "the tensile load placed on the graft through its fixation can be described as a chain secured to posts by bungee cords on either end." As a force is applied to the chain the bungee cords, not the chain, will displace under the tensile load.[43] The rigid fix-

ation (bone-to-bone) of the BPTB graft allows less slippage to occur and therefore, theoretically less laxity will develop in the ACL reconstructed knee. Surgeons are encouraged to use anatomic fixation (placing fixation close to the intra-articular joint surfaces) to limit the movement that can occur in the tibial and femoral tunnels.[43] Current data from animal studies suggests that bone-to-bone healing occurs at approximately 6–10 weeks,[44–46] and bone-to-tendon healing may take from 6 to 12 weeks.[44,47] Controversy continues over soft tissue fixation and its effects on accelerated rehabilitation.

Graft strength is also important to the surgeon and rehabilitation clinician in the early post-operative ACL reconstruction client. The ideal graft should approximate the tensile strength of the native ACL both in strength and stiffness. Tissue strength measured by numerous researchers including Wren et al.[48] reported the ultimate tensile load of the fresh-frozen Achilles tendon allograft to be 4617 N and Linn et al.[49] reported Achilles tendon allograft average ultimate tensile load to be 2850 N. This data is compared to the native ACL strength of 2160 N reported previously by Woo et al.[50] and the BPTB autograft strength of 2977 N reported by Cooper.[51] The quadruple hamstring tendon graft has been shown by Hamner et al.[52] to have an ultimate tensile load of 4090 N. Graft strength is less important than graft fixation strength[43] with regard to early and/or accelerated post-operative rehabilitation concerns, however it becomes a primary concern as it relates to long term results (**Case Table 6.2**).

There is no clear gold standard with regard to therapeutic exercise programs for ACL reconstruction using allograft tissues. Concern surrounding fixation and tissue strength suggest that early motion can be allowed, but the graft may need to be protected for 6–12 weeks to allow healing to take place. Others however treat allografts similarly to autografts, using the same ACL protocol with little to no restriction in weight bearing or in therapeutic exercise program progression. Of note, this may be sur-

Case Table 6.2   Ultimate Tensile Loads of the ACL and Commonly Used Grafts

Graft	Ultimate Tensile Load (N)
Normal ACL[50]	2160 ± 157
Achilles tendon allograft (10 mm wide)[49]	2850
Fresh frozen Achilles tendon allograft (10 mm wide)[48]	4617 ± 1107
Quadruple hamstring autograft[52]	4090 ± 295
BPTB autograft (10 mm wide)[51]	2977 ± 516

geon specific and is not meant to be a general treatment suggestion. The current trend clinically appears to be to protect the graft fixation over the initial six weeks, allowing for healing during the "theoretical" weakest time for the graft between four to eight weeks following implantation. Following this time of caution, there is a progressive increase in therapeutic exercises program intensity using both open kinetic chain (OKC) and closed kinetic chain (CKC) exercises (see Chapters 5, 6, and 7). An impact/running progression can be initiated by 12 weeks post-surgery or as determined clinically (see Chapter 9). Impact loading exercises gradually become more intense, placing increased functional demands on the lower extremity. Progressive functional sport specific activities are started by 16 weeks or earlier as able. Return to sport may be as early as 16 weeks or more likely at 24 weeks post-injury, which is more consistent with the national standard of six months. Irrgang and Harner[53] reported that "it is difficult to base rehabilitation strictly on the time required for healing and maturation of the graft." Also adding that "little is known about the graft's ability to withstand loads and strain during healing and maturation, and it is unknown if strain and load on the graft during healing and maturation are beneficial or harmful."[53] Therefore, other considerations must be factored into the development of a therapeutic exercise program.

Rehabilitation following ACL reconstruction should be individualized to the client, otherwise noncompliance is likely to increase and outcomes are likely to decrease[54] (see Chapter 11). As a result, each case must be evaluated independently, assessing the clinical presentation of the client on a regular basis. The rehabilitation clinician should develop the best program based on clinical experience, scientific evidence (preferably from human research) and combine that with the information gained from clinical studies and laboratory tests.[54] However, there are many factors that remain unclear. The current basic science data does not appear to be consistent with the trend to return athletes to full sport activity at four to six months post-injury. Does the graft need to be completely mature in order to provide appropriate stability and control of anterior tibial translation? Does the ACL graft merely function as a robust "rope" to control anterior tibial translation until it reaches full maturity?[55] Through experience, Dillingham[55] suggests that with a durable, strong graft and strong fixation, as is possible with an Achilles tendon allograft, complete ligamentization is less important for return to sport. Agreement exists that clinical assessment and functional evaluation appear to be essential components to facilitate effective therapeutic exercise program progression and a successful transition back to full sports activity. Accelerated rehabilitation, if implemented post-operatively, should control the acute symptoms of pain and swelling and focus on joint range of motion, achieving active knee hyperextension, lower extremity neuromuscular re-education, and normalizing the gait pattern, being sure to protect the graft and fixation sites from excessive stress during the initial healing process.[54]

ACL Allograft Post-operative Management and Rehabilitation Guidelines

Despite all the attractive advantages of allograft tissue, the literature consistently has recommended that allografts be used as an alternative to autografts in cases of multi-ligament reconstructions or ACL revision surgery (**Case Table 6.3**).[26,27] Significant concern exists with regard to allograft tissues including the risk of disease transmission, diminished graft strength and tensile properties, risk of inflammatory reaction, fixation strength, "stretch out" effect, possible delayed incorporation rate and limited published long term results.[26,27] Most concerning to physicians[55] and clients is the risk of HIV transmission, predicted to be 1 in 1,667,600 by Buck et al.[56] Much progress has been made in the processing and preparation of allograft tissues (fresh frozen, gamma irradiation, ethylene oxide, deep freeze with and without drying). The developments may allow for a better, more "ideal" graft in cryopreserved allograft tendons. Several very important steps must be taken to ensure successful and safe allograft use. Viral screening, graft harvesting, sterilization and preservation techniques must all be completed with the utmost care to ensure that a quality graft is supplied. Precise attention to detail during these procedures can minimize the risk of disease transmission and weakening of the graft tissue. Dillingham[55] suggests that some trust must be placed in the tissue bank and their specific processing methods. A risk of transmission certainly exists despite the cryogenic preservation and current sterilization processes. It should be noted that the risk of developing a deep vein thrombosis, pulmonary embolism or knee infection post-surgically for all clients is much higher than HIV transmission.[55,57] Four cases of acquired post-surgical septic arthritis were reported in 2001. Initial reports indicate the septic arthritis was caused by a contaminated ACL allograft (**Case Table 6.4**).[58]

ACL Allograft in Athletes: Outcome Report

Dr. Pier Indelli reported the clinical and functional results of 50 consecutive clients who underwent ACL reconstruction using a cryopreserved or fresh-frozen Achilles tendon allograft at an average of 34 months post-surgery (ranging from 27 to 42 months).[57] Twenty-eight males and 22 females including 5 professional athletes with an average age of 36 years (ranging 17–50 years) participated in the study. The International Knee Documentation Committee (IKDC) Knee Forms were used to standardize data collection (see Chapter 11). Strenuous activity was defined

Case Table 6.3   Post-Operative rehabilitation guidelines for ACL reconstruction using allograft tissues

	Indelli et al.[57] 2003	Harner et al.[38] 1996	Noyes et al.[37] 1996	Peterson et al.[36] 2001 and Shelton et al.,[32] 1997
Early motion	CPM 0°-90°	Early but limited	CPM 0°-90°	Yes, by rehabilitation clinician
Weight bearing	NWB × 2 weeks PWB at 2 weeks	NWB to TDWB × 6 weeks	NWB × 1 week PWB at 1 week FWB by 8 weeks	WBAT × 3 weeks
Crutches	2–4 weeks	10–12 weeks	Not stated but anticipate 6–8 weeks	2 crutches × 3 weeks, 1 crutch × 3 weeks
Exercises	OKC/CKC	Delay quadriceps exercise for 6 weeks	OKC/CKC	CKC early
Post op brace	Yes	Yes	Yes	Not reported
Running	12 weeks	Not reported	10 months	12 weeks
Return to sport	4–6 months	Not reported	12 months	6 months
Bracing	Client choice	Not reported	Not reported	Brace × 1 year

FWB = full weight bearing; NWB = non-weight bearing; PWB = partial weight bearing; TDWB = touchdown or toe touch weight bearing.

Case Table 6.4   Advantages and disadvantages of ACL Grafts

Graft	Advantages	Disadvantages
Ideal Graft	Reproduces anatomy, reproduces bio-mechanics, strong initial fixation, complete biologic incorporation, minimal donor site morbidity, reduced rehabilitation time	The ideal graft would have no disadvantages; *currently no ideal graft exists*
BPTB autograft*	High initial fixation, accelerated incorporation, less risk of tunnel widening	Donor site morbidity 31–79% Patellofemoral pain 13–47% Quadriceps weakness 10% Post-op stiffness
Hamstring autograft*	Less post-operative pain, stiff and strong graft, less donor site morbidity	Donor site pain 6% Hamstring weakness 10% Decreased fixation strength Risk of tunnel enlargement Delayed rehabilitation Neurovascular injury risk
Quadriceps tendon autograft*	Large cross sectional area, less donor site pain than BPTB	Donor site pain Risk of: patellofemoral pain, quadriceps weakness, extensor mechanism dysfunction
BPTB/Achilles tendon allograft**	Strong tissue strength, no donor site morbidity, improved cosmesis, larger grafts available, shorter operative time, useful in difficult cases, shorter rehabilitation time	High cost Limited availability Delayed incorporation Risk of disease transmission Risk of graft rejection Risk of tunnel widening Increased risk of graft stretch-out and re-rupture

Brown,[31] 2000.

**Indelli et al.,[57] 2003.*

as jumping and pivoting and moderate activity included activities like skiing or tennis. Frequency of sport activity was defined as competitive four or more times per week and recreational as one to three times per week. Graft fixation was bone-to-bone for femoral side fixation with an interference screw (either titanium or bioabsorbable) and tibial fixation of the tendon portion of the allograft was performed using a staple or a screw-washer combination. Bone chips from the bone plug of the allograft were inserted into the tibial tunnel to assist in graft-tunnel incorporation. The surgeon has since modified his fixation to interference screws both on the femoral and tibial side to limit graft motion and tunnel widening. Rehabilitation followed pre-established guidelines based on the achievement of key functional milestones. A post-operative brace was used and locked at 0°–30°, progressing to 60° and then to 90° flexion for a total of four weeks. Crutch use was reported as NWB involved side ambulation for two weeks. Progressive weight bearing was then initiated for two more weeks during which time a CKC therapeutic exercise program was started. A jogging and running progression was started after 12 weeks of rehabilitation and a functional CKC strengthening therapeutic exercise program was supervised by the same rehabilitation clinician. IKDC group A (22 subjects) and group B (25 subjects) combined for 94 percent good to excellent results. Forty-six clients returned to their pre-injury athletic level for a 92 percent success rating.

These findings are consistent with Noyes et al.,[59] who reported a 95 percent functional success rate in treating acute ACL ruptures and Noyes et al.,[37] who reported 89 percent good to excellent results with allograft use for chronic ACL deficiency. This data is compared with Shino et al.,[34] who reported on 84 patients treated with tendon allografts resulting in a 94 percent good or excellent outcome at the three year follow up. Other authors who have reported no significant differences in client outcomes following ACL reconstruction using allografts versus autografts are Shelton et al.,[32] Indelicato et al.,[35] Harner et al.,[38] and Stingham et al.[60]

The use of allograft tissue to reconstruct the ACL in athletes may be a new trend in sports medicine. Indelli et al.[57] presented a small sample of active clients, including several professional and many college athletes who chose to have their ACL reconstructed using allograft tissue to preserve their own anatomy. Preliminary results from Indelli et al.[57] are encouraging. The authors reported that Achilles tendon allografts (with interference screw fixation) are a good graft alternative in primary ACL reconstruction and can be used safely with athletic clients. The advantages are good ultimate strength, less donor site morbidity, shorter operative time, shorter rehabilitation time, less post-operative pain and improved cosmesis.[57] Indelli et al.[57] did not report any of the potential problems that have been reported in the literature with

ACL allografts including concerns over a possible stretch out effect causing increased anterior tibial translation, problems with delayed graft incorporation, chronic inflammation or delayed return to sports. The choice of what graft tissue to use is a decision that each client must make. For some, the potential advantages to using an allograft outweigh the risks associated with them, but others find reassurance in using their own tissue as a graft choice for ACL reconstruction.

Surgeons do have some influence in the graft choice selected but should allow the client (and in this case the parents) to make the final decision once all of the advantages and disadvantages (including nonsurgical options) have been adequately discussed. Post-operatively, the therapeutic exercise progression associated with ACL allografts, specifically in the competitive and elite athlete, can progress rapidly because of the limited post-operative symptoms. It should be noted that therapeutic exercise program progressions should not be directed solely by time constraints of healing and graft maturation. However, complete disregard of sound basic science and therapeutic exercise principles in order to hasten recovery should be avoided.[61] It is important for the rehabilitation clinician to stay current with the literature on the structural factors that may contribute to graft failure following ACL reconstruction. In addition to the biological timetable for graft tissue healing, the method of graft fixation and the integrity of the femoral and tibial bone in the region of the tunnel placement warrant consideration.

The rehabilitation clinician should develop the best individualized therapeutic exercise program for each client based on their clinical experience, the client's expectations, and available information gained from clinical studies and laboratory research.[54] Accelerated rehabilitation, if implemented post-operatively, should control the acute symptoms, restore patellar joint mobility and ROM, and achieve active knee hyperextension and muscle control to assist in normalizing the gait pattern, being sure to protect the graft and fixation from excessive stresses during the initial healing process.[54] Future clinical and experimental research is needed to support the use of allograft tissue for ACL reconstruction in the athletic population.

Therapeutic Exercise Program Suggestions

Phase I Therapeutic Exercises (1–4 weeks)

- Immobilization in brace locked at 10° flexion for 3–5 days
- 0°–30° ROM in a brace, followed by 60° at 2 weeks
- 0°–90° ROM in a brace from 2 to 4 weeks as quadriceps activation return allows with controlled weight bearing

- NWB crutch ambulation × 2 weeks, followed by weight bearing as tolerated (WBAT) to 50% body weight over next 1–2 weeks
- CPM day one 0°–40° as tolerated increasing by 5°–10° each day, increasing up to 90°, then cessation of CPM use
- Range of motion exercises (Section 7 Figure 4) (Section 7 Figure 5) (Section 7 Figure 6) (Section 7 Figure 7) (limited until suture removal, progress as symptoms allow and attain passive knee hyperextension if evident at the contralateral non-impaired knee)
- Achieve active knee hyperextension (heel off the table with an isometric quadriceps set, assist with resistance-band as necessary)
- Straight leg raise program performed without an extension lag
- Therapeutic exercises combining both OKC and CKC activities

Phase II Intermediate Therapeutic Exercises (4-8 weeks)

- CKC and limited OKC exercises with increased resistance/difficulty
- Full weight bearing activities (normalized gait pattern)
- Proprioception and balance training
- Full ROM by 8 weeks

Phase III Advanced Therapeutic Exercises (8-16 weeks)

- Isotonic weight training (see Chapter 5)
- CKC and OKC progression
- Proprioception and balance training (see Chapters 6 and 7)
- Jogging progressions
- Functional activity progression, footwork drills, impact and decelerating activities (see Chapters 5, 7-9)

Phase IV Return to Play Preparation (16 weeks plus)

- Sport specific activities (see Chapters 5 and 9)
- Sprint progression
- Transition to controlled and limited supervised practice activities (see Chapter 11)

As stated previously, to facilitate a successful client outcome, the rehabilitation clinician must understand the fundamental research and scientific based principles of ACL reconstruction. Several authors[62,63] have identified advantages of OKC exercises to activate the joint and muscle mechanoreceptors, promote functional activity, and to treat isolated weakness. Disadvantages of OKC exercises are they produce increased distraction and rotational forces, decreased compressive forces and most important to rehabilitation they produce increased shear forces at the knee. Conversely, CKC exercises produce increased joint compressive forces, decreased shear forces, increased joint congruency and dynamic stability, and stimulation of multi-joint proprioceptors. The disadvantage of CKC exercise is that specific weakness may be missed while performing the exercises due to the substitution patterns that may occur. Both CKC and OKC exercises are combinations of complex movement patterns.[62,63] Active knee extension, the most recognized OKC exercise, is a complex movement based on the geometry and kinesiology of a concave structure (tibia) moving on a convex structure (femur) to produce the "screw home" mechanism at terminal knee extension. Anterior gliding occurs with anterior translation of the tibia. The ACL acts as the restraint to the anterior tibial translation. This is an example of the four-bar linkage system of the knee with the ACL, PCL and medial/lateral capsuloligamentous structures acting in concert with each other to control abnormal anterior and posterior tibial translation.[64,65] An example of a CKC exercise is the standing squat, where the convex surface of the femur moves on the relatively stationary concave surface of the tibia. This complex movement results in posterior roll and anterior glide and translation. Increased joint compression is noted secondary to weight bearing. The phenomenon of concurrent shift is in effect where one section of a two joint muscle is working concentrically and the opposite region of the muscle is working eccentrically to control motion. (see Chapter 5).[66] Once again, the four-bar linkage is allowing for normal arthrokinematics at the knee, limiting abnormal accessory rolling and gliding motions. In the presence of an ACL tear the tibia may translate excessively anterior and the femur rolls posteriorly. This excessive motion may cause episodes of giving way which can result in meniscal tears leading to deterioration of the articular cartilage of the knee.

The biomechanical analysis of OKC and CKC therapeutic exercises reveal quite different forces at the knee. CKC exercises tend to produce less anterior tibial displacement compared to OKC exercises. Contact forces during CKC exercises with body weight provide inherent joint stability, allowing for more strenuous strengthening exercises without the excessive shear forces found with OKC exercises (Case Table 6.5).[67]

Sawhney et al.[68] and Grood et al.[69] reported that an isometric quadriceps contraction at 30° and 45° of knee flexion with a 10 pound weight on the ankle caused anterior tibial translation. However, at 60° and 75° of knee flexion, tibial shear was not evident. Lutz et al.[70] also reported decreased shear at 30°, 60°, 90° during CKC compared to OKC exercises, also reporting that peak load on the ACL occurred at 30° knee flexion with 285 ± 120 N during an OKC movement. Daniel et al.[71] referred to the 60–75° angle of knee flexion as the quadriceps neutral angle because isometric exercise at this angle did not ap-

Case Table 6.5   ACL Shear/Strain During Open- and Closed-Chain Exercises: Review of Literature

Author	Subjects	Findings
Sawhney et al.[68]	Non-impaired subjects	Isometric contraction at 30°, 45°, 60°, 75° knee flexion with 10-pound resistance caused tibial translation at 30° and 45° knee flexion
Grood et al.[69]	Cadaveric ACL sectioning	Same as Sawhney et al.
Lutz et al.[70]	Five non-impaired subjects, in vivo	Decreased shear at 30°, 60°, 90° knee flexion with CKC versus OKC ex-ercises. Peak load on the ACL was at 30° knee flexion with 285 ± 120 N in the OKC
Daniel[71]		60°–75° of knee flexion is the quadriceps neutral angle
Voight et al.[72]	ACL-deficient subjects	Minimal anterior tibial translation in the CKC during isometric quadriceps contraction at 30° knee flexion
Arms et al.[73]	19 cadavers	Increased strain on the ACL during simulated quadriceps isometric activation between 0°–45° knee flexion
Renstrom et al.[74]	7 cadavers	Same results as Arms et al.[73] Also, reported minimal ACL strain during passive ROM that decreases from 0° to 45° knee flexion and then increases again, peaking at 120° flexion
Beynnon et al.[75]	10 subjects with non-impaired ACLs	Peak strain on ACL 4.4 percent at 15° flexion during an isometric quadriceps contraction, at 30° flexion was 2.7 percent, no strain at 60° and 90° flexion. Passive ROM produced no ACL strain. Strain during active ROM occurred between 10 and 48°. Isometric quadriceps activation in full extension was < that at 30° flexion
Beynnon et al.[76]	8 subjects following knee anthroscopy	Increased tibial translation and average maximum ACL strain with squats (3.6 percent) and squats with sport cord (4.0 percent) compared to active knee flexion- extension (3.8 percent)
Henning et al.[77]	First in vivo analysis of ACL elongation. Two ACL-deficient subjects participated	Recommended avoidance of OKC exercises for one year post-surgery due to peak strain at 22° knee flexion during isometric quadriceps activation against a 20 N boot. Peak elongation was 87–121 percent of an 80 lb Lachman test. Bicycle and partial squat were deemed acceptable exercises
Beynnon et al.[78]	11 subjects with non-impaired ACLs	ACL strain values are dependent on knee flexion angle and quadriceps activation level. Exercises with low ACL strain values were dominated by the hamstring muscles at any flexion angle and during quadriceps activation at more than 60° of knee flexion
Johnson et al.[79]	Subjects with non-impaired ACLs	Passive ROM no strain on ACL, active ROM 0°–48° = 2.3 percent strain at 20° knee flexion, stairs = 2.69 percent strain, simultaneous quadriceps activation at 15° knee flexion = 2.8 percent strain, active ROM 90°–35° = 2.8 percent strain. Full ROM: Lower ACL shear between 90°–35° knee flexion active ROM with a 45 N boot = 3.8 percent strain, weight bearing = 3.9 percent strain, squatting = 3.6 percent strain, isometric quadriceps activation at 15° knee flexion = 4.4 percent strain
Yack et al.[80]	Studied OKC vs. CKC in 11 subjects with ACL deficiency	Anterior tibial displacement was noted between 64° and 10° of OKC knee extension; authors suggested that this might cause ACL strain. No significant differences were observed in the non-impaired knee.
Jurst & Otis[81]	Studied 15 non-impaired subjects	Anterior tibial displacement increased with distally applied resistance compared to more proximal resistance applications during isometric knee extension between 90° and 30° knee flexion

pear to produce any anterior tibial shear. Numerous authors have reported in the literature that ACL strain significantly increases during the last 30° of terminal knee extension.[68-70,72-75]

Understanding the scientific data is necessary, but it is only one part of the clinical decision making process that every rehabilitation clinician should go through when developing a therapeutic exercise program. Irrgang et al.[65] reported that "developing a rehabilitation program following knee injury or surgery is an imprecise science." Critical thinking is necessary and may assist the rehabilitation clinician in making judgment calls with regards to the appropriateness of a certain therapeutic exercise activity. Breaking the exercise down into its component biomechanical movements, critically analyzing the activity, and relating these thoughts to the client's ability to understand and properly perform the exercise involves clinical reasoning.

Less than optimal client outcomes have stimulated the model of critical thinking/clinical reasoning and scientific based therapeutic exercise programs. Non-compliance of our clients has resulted in accelerated programs and the notion that practice is ahead of medical research. However, scientific data does support the current rationale for accelerated rehabilitation. Researchers have demonstrated that it is generally safer to progress clients quicker in the presence of stronger grafts, improved surgical fixation devices and methods, and improved graft placement by the surgeons. When these other factors exist, even non-compliant clients have displayed improved outcomes when they exceeded the restrictions of conservative therapeutic exercise programs. Concerns still remain over basing program decisions on animal model data and the surgical and rehabilitation practices that always tend to challenge the existing evidence. Rehabilitation clinicians must stay current on existing research in this area and continually question their interventions based on the level of the existing evidence (see Chapter 11).[79-83]

Basic science data indicates that the ACL graft is strongest at implantation during surgery and will become weakest, theoretically at 4–6 weeks,[84] while revascularization occurs between 8–16 wks.[85] The concept of ligamentization[86] is an ongoing process where the tendon tissue transforms into ligament-like tissue. On the contrary, graft fixation may be at its weakest when the graft itself is at its strongest, immediately after surgery. Therefore, rehabilitation clinicians must respect the surgical constraints.

Phase I therapeutic exercises focus on regaining patella mobility, knee ROM, quadriceps neuromuscular control and strength using quadriceps setting, straight leg raises, CKC terminal knee extension (**Case Figure 6.4**) (Section 7 Animation 8), quadriceps setting facilitating active knee hyperextension (**Case Figure 6.5**) (Section 7 Animation 9), calf raises, four-way hip exercises including hip adduction (**Section 7, Animation 10**), hip extension for gluteus maximus and hamstrings (**Section 7, Anima-**

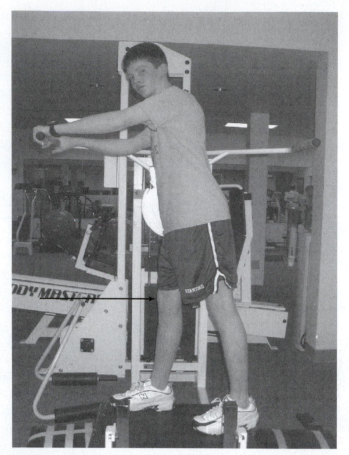

Case Figure 6.4   Weight bearing terminal knee extension exercise on four-way hip device.

tion 11) and for more isolated gluteus maximus activation (**Section 7, Animation 12**), hip flexion (**Section 7, Animation 13**), and hip abduction (**Section 7, Animation 14**), straight leg raises (SLR), isometric quadriceps setting between 90° and 60° of flexion, aquatic therapy in a swimming pool, bicycling for ROM, the use of electrical muscle stimulation to increase quadriceps recruitment, step-downs (Case Figure 6.6)[87](**Section 7, Animation**

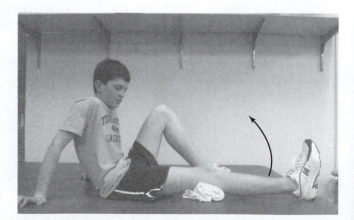

Case Figure 6.5   Active terminal knee extension.

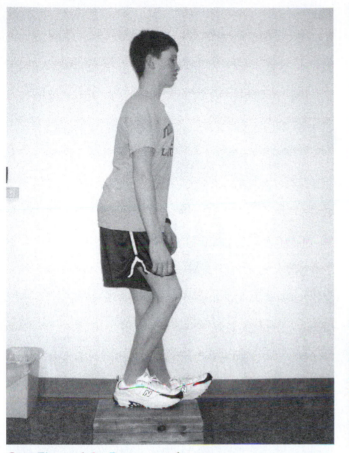

Case Figure 6.6   Retro step-downs.

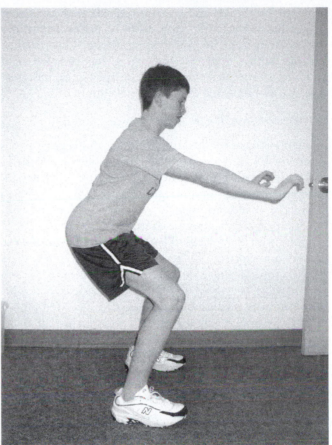

Case Figure 6.7   Mini-squats.

15) and mini-squats between 0° and 60° knee flexion (**Case Figure 6.7**).[88,89] Open kinetic chain exercises such as seated knee extensions are discouraged at this time due to the increased shear they place on the ACL graft. If resistance is to be added to the SLR, knee joint shear forces can be minimized by placing the weight proximal to the knee.[90]

Phase I, Session 6, Week 3

TJ demonstrated independence with the home therapeutic exercise program by session 3. Concern continued over his lack of full right knee extension and mild effusion. He continued to lack 5° of extension at session 6, but had increased his flexion ROM to 90°. TJ was allowed to rock forward and backward on the stationary bike to warm up the knee to facilitate increased ROM prior to other therapeutic exercises. During session 3, TJ was issued a neuromuscular electrical stimulation to use in conjunction with the quadriceps strengthening exercises he was performing at home. The duty cycle of the stimulator was set so that each quadriceps activation lasted 10 seconds, with a 30 second rest period between activations. He was instructed to use the unit for 15 minutes twice a day. His quadriceps function had improved and he was able to perform a SLR independently without assistance.

TJ's knee brace was unlocked and allowed to move 0-30° during ambulation. He was told that at the next session we would open the brace another 30° if he had made good progress over the next two days. TJ was allowed to begin partial weight bearing on his right lower extremity when he met the goal of an independent straight leg raise. TJ was instructed in proper toe touch weight bearing technique with crutches. He demonstrated an understanding of the technique by showing his parents at the end of the session. TJ was instructed in a CKC terminal knee extension exercise using a cable pulley system. The strap was placed behind TJ's right knee and he was instructed to straighten the right knee using the quadriceps and try to avoid substituting with the hamstrings and gluteals. He was also instructed in weight shifting, bilateral standing balance with upper extremity support and quadriceps/ hamstring isometrics co-contractions between 90 to 60° of knee flexion. TJ appeared to be pleased to put some weight on his right leg.

Aquatic therapy continued after each session. TJ's aquatic therapy program consisted of standing weight shifting in chest deep water, walking in chest deep water, SLRs in four directions and mini-squats. All the exercises were performed while wearing a neoprene knee brace with 0-90° stops, primarily to protect the knee during crutch ambulation on the swimming pool deck. The buoyancy provided by the aquatic environment allowed for earlier weight bearing activities than could be performed on dry land without using an unweighting device. TJ secured an ice pack with a compression wrap to his extended right knee for 20 minutes after every therapeutic exercise session. He also repeated this at home five times a day.

Phase I, Session 10, Week 4

TJ demonstrated marked improvement in his gait pattern at session 10. He was weight bearing as tolerated (WBAT) without pain using both crutches per session 8 instruction. TJ was progressed to full weight bearing (FWB) and taken out of the knee brace. Gait training instruction and continuation of his therapeutic exercise program and ROM program were completed. TJ was re-instructed on the use of the stationary bike for ROM. He was able to complete a revolution during session 10. Prior to session 10 he was only capable of partial ROM forward-backward revolutions on the stationary bike because of his limited mobility. TJ was quite satisfied about the progress he had made. The continuous passive motion machine was discontinued at this time. See the ROM summary chart given in Case **Table 6.6** for details of TJ's ROM progression.

Phase II Transition, Session #12, Week 5

At 5 weeks post-surgery, TJ presented with minimal effusion and had regained full knee extension and 125 degrees of flexion by session 12. At this time TJ could perform active knee hyperextension. During session 12, he was progressed completely off of the crutches and demonstrated a mild quad avoidance gait pattern. TJ avoided full extension between the heel contact and mid-stance phases of walking gait (see Chapter 9). Gait training on a treadmill was performed with cueing to encourage increased active knee extension between heel contact and mid-stance. TJ was performing wall slides (**Case Figure 6.8**) (● **Section 7, Animation 16**), unilateral leg presses (**Case Figure 6.9**), terminal knee extensions (TKE), standing balance (unilateral and uneven surfaces), lunges, step-downs, hamstring curls with cuff weights and stationary cycling × 10 minutes. Aquatic therapy was discontinued during session 12 because of TJ's progress.

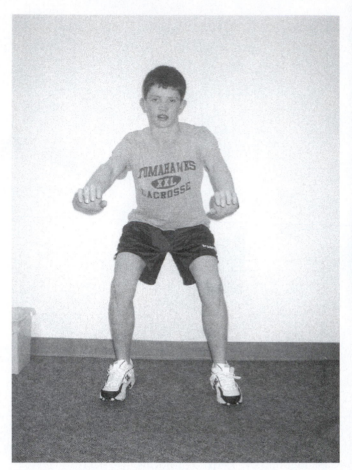

Case Figure 6.8   Wall slides.

E. List some exercises you might incorporate into TJ's therapeutic exercise program. First make a list of early phase I exercises, then a list of late phase I exercises. *See Author's Comments E*

Phase II, Session 15, Week 7

TJ returned ambulating independently without any significant gait asymmetry. He was able to go up and down stairs in a reciprocal style, step-over-step. He demonstrated significant improvement since being advanced to

Case Table 6.6   Range of Motion Summary (Post-operative weeks 1–4)

	Session 1 (week 1)	Session 2 (week 2)	Session 6 (week 3)	Session 10 (week 4)
Extension	Lacked 15°	Lacked 15°	Lacked 5°	Lacked 2°
Flexion	25°	40°	90°	110°
Ambulatory status	NWB	NWB	PWB 2 crutches	FWB 1crutch

NWB = non-weight bearing; PWB = partial weight bearing; FWB = full weight bearing.

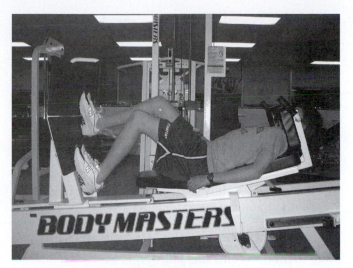

Case Figure 6.9 Unilateral leg press.

Modification of Short Term Goals

1. The client will regain normal balance ability measured by a single leg stance test score of 45–60 seconds with eyes closed on the right lower extremity
2. The client will regain and improve quadriceps muscle voluntary activation to increase muscle strength grade to 4/5 MMT (good) and will display full active knee hyperextension
3. The client will regain flexion ROM to 135 degrees to allow improved performance of the therapeutic exercise program and regain the ability to perform a full ROM active squat without discomfort or compensatory movements
4. The client will regain adequate lower extremity eccentric muscle control demonstrated by having appropriate dynamic hip and knee stability during a step down from a four-inch step to begin therapeutic exercises with increased impact and deceleration demands

Phase II, Session 20, Week 9

At this time TJ was noted to be losing interest in his therapeutic exercise program. He was becoming more frustrated with not being able to play soccer. Several of his friends were starting to ask when he was returning. TJ demonstrated a withdrawal from the rehabilitation staff that had not been observed since program initiation. TJ was asked about this change in behavior. TJ initially responded that he was fine. Following his appointment the rehabilitation clinician asked the parents if they had noticed a change in TJ's attitude and behavior towards his rehabilitation. TJ's parents confirmed the change in behavior. They reported that it had been much more difficult over the last few weeks to get TJ to come in for his therapeutic exercise sessions.

F. Discuss possible reasons for TJ's waning enthusiasm. What could you do to regain and keep his interest during this crucial time period? *See Author's Comments F*

Numerous resources are available to provide to clients and their families as educational materials that support the best clinical practice and recommendations for therapeutic exercise prescription and resistance training in children, including the current position statements of the American Academy of Pediatrics (AAP)[91] and the National Strength and Conditioning Association (NSCA)[92] which support the use of resistance training in children.[91,92] Faigenbaum[93] has reported that resistance training is a safe and effective way for children and adolescents to gain strength and improve their physical appearance. Youth resistance or strength training is becoming

full weight bearing and taken off crutches. His passive ROM was measured at 5° of knee hyperextension and 130° of flexion. The phase II therapeutic exercise program continued with a combination of both OKC and CKC exercises. Step-downs were progressed in height, unilateral leg press resistance was increased and isometric squats were initiated at 90°.

Re-Evaluation

Knee ROM: Right knee resting position was 0° of extension. Right knee passive extension was measured at 5° of hyperextension. Passive right knee flexion was 130°

Strength: Right quadriceps muscle strength was 3+/5 MMT. Full active patella superior glide was noted compared to the contralateral side

Balance: Single leg stance test was performed for 60 seconds duration at each lower extremity with eyes open. With eyes closed test results were 20 seconds for the right leg and 45 seconds for the left leg without upper extremity support or assistance (see Chapter 9)

Swelling: Minimal joint swelling (grade one)

ADLs: Client was able to ambulate independently with normal heel-to-toe gait pattern and step-over-step technique with stair ambulation

Pain: VAS 4/10 during end range over pressure of knee range of motion. Client reported that he did not have any pain at rest and was able to sleep without difficulty or with the use of pain medication

universally accepted as a safe and practical way to improve the strength of children. Clearer definitions and data collection methods have resulted in improved research and understanding that appropriate resistance training in children is safe and can improve strength. Faigenbaum[93] also reported that "despite the contention that strength training was inappropriate or dangerous for young weight trainers, the safety and effectiveness of youth strength training interventions are now well documented," referencing numerous sources[91,92,94,95] and the qualified acceptance of youth strength training by medical and fitness organizations is becoming universal.[91,92,96,97] The AAP[91] position statement on strength training for the prepubescent athlete states that "recent research has shown that short-term programs in which prepubescent athletes are trained and supervised by knowledgeable adults can increase strength without significant injury risk."[91–99] Strength training is defined by the AAP as "weight or resistance training using a variety of methods, including exercise with free weights and weight machines, to increase muscular strength, endurance, and/or power for sports participation or fitness enhancement."[91] Numerous other organizations, including the American Orthopedic Society for Sports Medicine[96] and the American College of Sports Medicine,[97] acknowledge that youth strength training is a safe form of exercise. The NSCA[92] current position is in agreement with the AAP,[91] but provides more specific guidance for strength training program development and supervision criteria. The position of the NSCA[92] is that:

1. A properly designed and supervised resistance training program is safe for children
2. A properly designed and supervised resistance training program can increase the strength of children
3. A properly designed and supervised resistance training program can help enhance the motor fitness skills and sports performance of children
4. A properly designed and supervised resistance training program can help to prevent injuries in youth sports and recreational activities
5. A properly designed and supervised resistance training program can help improve the psychological well being of children
6. A properly designed and supervised resistance training program can enhance the overall "health" of children

A properly designed program should include these components:

1. A proper warm up should include 1–2 sets of light upper and lower body exercises (12–15 repetitions) that are focused on the major muscle groups. Time must be allowed for a proper warm up of 5–10 minutes
2. Proper instruction and supervision must occur
3. The program should be designed from 1–3 sets of 6–15 repetitions performed on 2–3 non-consecutive days of the week
4. Children must demonstrate the appropriate maturity, respect, weight room etiquette, and demonstrate realistic expectations prior to initiating a resistance training program
5. Emphasis must be placed on technique and form, not on the amount of weight lifted

The AAP[91] suggests that prepubescent children should avoid maximal weight lifts but, "At present, there are no justifiable safety reasons to preclude children and adolescents from participating in well-designed strength training programs."[93]

G. Use your clinical reasoning skills to design a phase II ACL therapeutic exercise program. Using a table format, list the exercises in the order in which you think they should be performed, and give numbers of sets and repetitions and the rationale for each exercise. *See Author's Comments G*

Phase II Therapeutic Exercise Program

Scientifically based phase II exercises include the phase I exercises, with the addition of a variety of CKC balance and neuromuscular control exercises. The therapeutic exercise progression in phase II program may include both OKC and CKC exercises, with an increased emphasis on safe neuromuscular control exercises, usually performed while weight bearing. Lunges are initiated with emphasis on keeping the tibia of the surgical leg vertical. The depth of movement and volume (sets, reps, intensity) of lunges, stepdowns, and squatting maneuvers are gradually increased. Rehabilitation clinicians can become more creative at this time with their therapeutic exercise selections with respect to the biomechanical demands of the exercises and the constraints of tissue healing. Other therapeutic exercise suggestions appropriate for this phase include jumping rope, retro treadmill walking with elevation (**Case Figure 6.10**), unilateral balance exercises with lower extremity rotation, diagonal lunges, and numerous weight training techniques that focus on hip function (**Case Figure 6.11**) (see Chapters 5, 6, and 7). Mikkelsen et al.,[100] compared clients who participated in a CKC therapeutic exercise program with clients who followed a CKC program that incorporated OKC isokinetic seated knee extensions at five to six weeks post-operatively performed between 90 and 40° de-

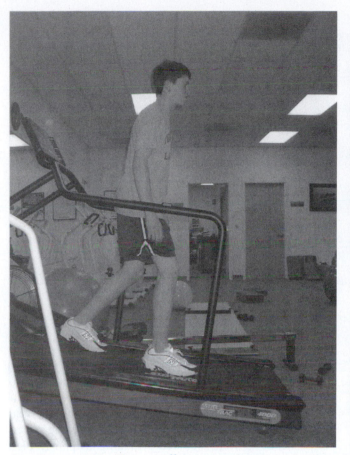

Case Figure 6.10   Retro walking on inclined treadmill.

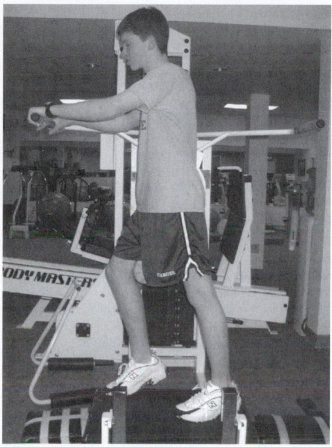

Case Figure 6.11   Four-way isotonic hip strengthening exercises.

grees with an extension progression of 10 degrees/ week. They reported no significant difference in knee joint laxity at six months, less side-to-side difference in knee extension torque, no significant difference in knee flexion torque and the clients who received supplemental OKC exercises returned to sports at the same level, a median of two months earlier than clients who followed the strict CKC program. Sound therapeutic exercise principles would involve a varied environment of rehabilitative exercises. The literature supports a strong emphasis on CKC with a progression to more specific OKC exercises as the graft and the fixation become more secure. Once healing constraints are lifted approximately after 8–12 weeks, increased impact and OKC exercise focus may be initiated.

Phase II, Session 21, Week 9

This session consisted of development and instruction in the weight training program established for TJ. TJ was instructed in one exercise for each associated muscle group. The exercise program for his upper body included push-ups, latissimus pull-downs, rowing, biceps curls and tri-

ceps extensions, abdominal crutches, trunk rotations with medicine balls and lateral raises with dumbbells. The program included 1 set of 12 reps each exercise. The 5-minute warm up was completed on an upper body ergometer. The upper body was stretched out for 5 minutes prior to initiation of the upper body strength training program. Proper supervision was provided by a NCSA certified strength and conditioning specialist. The exercise program followed the criteria noted by the NSCA.[92] Knee rehabilitation followed the weight training program. TJ had demonstrated excellent dynamic lower extremity control during the eccentric or negative phase of active squats, and subsequently was instructed in light squats of 10–15 reps initially just using the weight of the bar. Leg press and single leg step-ups/-downs and lunges continued. Stationary bicycling continued with the addition of the spinner bike for variety (see Chapter 4). TJ began a spin bike workout with sprinting and aggressive pedaling at high revolutions per minute. This exercise focuses on both the quadriceps and the hamstring muscles groups and is an excellent form of cardiopulmonary system training (see Chapter 4) (**Case Tables 6.7–6.8**).

Case Table 6.7   TJ's Weight Trainging Program Summary: Phase II

Weight Training Program	Sets and repetitions (week 1-2)	Sets and repetitions (week 3–4)	Sets and repetitons (week 4+)
Push ups	1 × 10	2 × 10	3 × 10–15
Latissimus pull downs	1 × 10	2 × 10	3 × 10–15
Rowing	1 × 10	2 × 10	3 × 10–15
Biceps curls	1 × 10	2 × 10	3 × 10–15
Triceps extensions	1 × 10	2 × 10	3 × 10–15
Lateral raises	1 × 10	2 × 10	3 × 10–15
Abdominal crunches	3 × 10	3 × 15	3 × 20
Trunk rotations	3 × 10	3 × 15	3 × 20
Cardio-spin bike program	15 minutes: 15 sec. sprint/ 45 sec. steady pace	25 minutes: 30 sec. sprint/ 30 sec. steady pace	35 minutes: 30 sec. sprint/ 30 sec. steady pace

H. Discuss the elements that you would need to consider when designing phase III of TJ's therapeutic exercise program. *See Author's Comments H*

Phase III, Session 25, Week 12

TJ demonstrated excellent dynamic lower extremity control with the step-down and leg press exercises. TJ was instructed to perform light impact jumps with less than body weight on a shuttle trainer (**Case Figure 6.12**) (**Section 7, Animation 17**). He performed sets of 15 jumps with both legs, being sure to weight bear 50% on each leg. With minimal resistance on the shuttle he was also instructed to perform alternating hops on his left and then his right lower extremity. The shuttle exercises progress to full body weight jumping and hopping. Technique was assessed to be sure that TJ was using proper form and avoiding excessive knee valgus and hip internal rotation-adduction (see

Chapters 5 and 11). Proper jumping technique is essential for therapeutic exercise progression and is related to injury prevention. A trampoline was used as a transition from light impact exercises in a gravity alleviated position to more intense impact training exercises. Jumping rope was used to re-educate the lower extremities in plyometric type activities while full weight bearing. Jumping rope techniques can be modified to change the difficulty level for the client. Footwork drills were initiated including skipping, high knees, butt kicks, lateral shuffles, carioca, retro-jogging, forward jogging and gait activities on a treadmill at various elevations both forward and backward (see Chapters 9 and 11). Emphasis was placed on more advanced lower extremity weight training exercises including the leg press, hamstring curl, knee extension between 90 and 40°, squatting and lunges. Plyometric jumps and box jumps were also initiated (see Chapters 5 and 11). OKC isokinetic resistance training programs may be initiated during phase III. TJ was

Case Table 6.8   TJ's Knee Range of Motion Progression

ROM	Session 1 (week 1)	Session 2 (week 2)	Session 6 (week 3)	Session 10 (week 4)	Session 12 (week 5)	Session 15 (week 7)	Session 20 (week 9)	Session 21 (week 9)
Extension	Lacked 15°	Lacked 15°	Lacked 5°	Lacked 2°	Full extension	5° hyper-extension	Full (10°) hyper-extension	Full (10°) hyper-extension
Flexion	25°	40°	90°	110°	125°	130°	Full (135°)	Full (135°)
Post-op	1 week	2 weeks	3 weeks	4 weeks	5 weeks	7 weeks	9 weeks	9 weeks
Ambulation status	NWB	NWB	PWB-2 crutches	FWB-1 crutch	FWB- No crutches		Strength training	

NWB = non-weight bearing; PWB = partial weight bearing; FWB = full weight bearing.

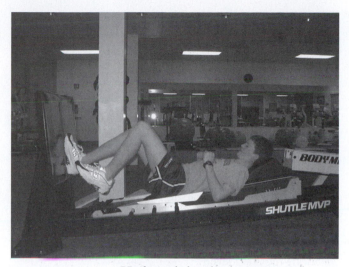

Case Figure 6.12   Unilateral shuttle training.

allowed to return to soccer ball juggling and footwork drills. He was not allowed to run with the ball, cut, or perform running directional changes. His parents were informed of what activities were permitted.

Phase III, Session 30, Week 16

TJ had demonstrated independence in his footwork drills and progressive skipping and jogging activities over the past few sessions. He was jumping rope and performing box drops from a height of 18 inches. Single leg hopping was improved in distance and dynamic eccentric lower extremity control upon landing. He was progressed to full jogging at week 14 and required several sessions of gait instruction and cueing prior to being independent. At week 16 he demonstrated independence and good form with jogging straight ahead. At this time he was allowed to begin jogging on his own. He was instructed in a walk-jog progression, which increased his jogging tolerance and endurance without compromising technique. At this time, TJ was also instructed in single leg hopping in a 45° diagonal pattern. He also was transitioned to a grass surface for some low intensity soccer ball kicking. Kicking included passing and kicking with the instep of each foot. The rehabilitation clinician controlled the intensity and the distance at which TJ was allowed to kick. Initiation of this exercise can be of concern to both the rehabilitation clinician and the client because of the nature of the kicking movement using the instep of the foot and extending the knee (potentially producing high valgus forces). Caution should be placed on this activity and the rehabilitation clinician should get feedback from the client to assist in making decisions regarding progression.

I. What other considerations should the rehabilitation clinician take into account during phase III and the
transition to phase IV for this client's therapeutic exercise program?** *See Authors Comments I*

J. Use your clinical reasoning skills to design a phase III ACL rehabilitation program. In table format, list the exercises you think TJ should perform, in the order in which you would like him to perform them, and give the number of sets and repetitions, and the rationale for inclusion. *See Author's Comments J*

Phase IV, Session 20, Week 20 (5 months post-operative)

TJ continued to make excellent progress. He was now verbalizing a strong desire to return to soccer. TJ was instructed in light cutting maneuvers on the grass field wearing rubber soled gym shoes without cleats. The cutting maneuvers consisted of 45° changes of direction every 10–15 yards, backward stepping, coming toward the ball without passing, and soccer simulation drills of trying to get open for a pass at less than half speed. These drills were progressed in speed as TJ became more confident. TJ was instructed to progress his speed over the next month to full speed wearing his cleats. He was also instructed to increase the angle of his cutting maneuvers from 45° to 90° and 180° over the next month (see Chapter 9). TJ continued the lower and upper extremity resistance exercise program at his junior high school. TJ performed a single leg hop test (see Chapter 5) and triple hop test (see Chapter 11) in preparation for functional testing for clearance to return to sports. He scored above 80% on both the single and the triple hop test at 5 months post-surgery.

Phase IV, Session 25, Week 24 (6 months post-operative)

TJ reported to the clinic having just been re-evaluated by his surgeon. Prior to this visit, TJ had been issued his knee brace and shown how to put it on (don) and take it off (doff). He was to use the brace for all sport activities. TJ reported that his surgeon had "cleared" him to return to playing soccer. The physician's clearance to return to playing soccer was contingent upon TJ passing the functional performance tests (see Chapters 5 and 11). Clinically, TJ had regained full ROM and his strength was continuing to improve. He completed the battery of functional tests[103] including single hop and triple hop tests and an isokinetic evaluation. TJ scored at or above the 90th percentile on the hopping tests and he had regained more than 85% of his quadriceps and hamstring strength at 60°, 180° and 300° per second on the isokinetic test. TJ formally passed all the functional and strength testing for return to play (see Chapter 11).[103] He also demonstrated excellent dynamic lower extremity control during sudden running acceleration and deceleration. TJ did not have any unusual swelling or pain in his knee at 6 months post-surgery. A discharge note was written and faxed to the surgeon. TJ was released from regular supervised therapeutic exercise program attendance. He was asked to return to the clinic on an informal basis and update the rehabilitation clinician on his return to soccer. He agreed to stop by every two weeks to report his accomplishments. The transition to playing soccer was discussed with TJ and his parents. Transition to playing soccer needed to include a progression from "not playing" to "full play", which would include a systematic progression in playing time and intensity allowing skill acquisition (see Chapter 11). TJ's progression back to playing soccer was previously discussed with his coach and TJ, but a meeting was set up to remind them about factors that might influence TJ's return to play readiness (see Chapter 11).

Re-Evaluation

Knee ROM: Right knee AROM and PROM were WNL −5°−0°−135° and equivalent to the left knee

Strength: Right quadriceps muscle was measured at 4+/5 MMT quadriceps contraction. Full active patella superior glide was noted

Balance: Single leg stance tests were bilaterally equal with eyes open (60 seconds) and eyes closed (45 seconds) without upper extremity support/assistance

Swelling: No swelling noted. Client reported that the knee tended to develop a minimal amount of swelling after intense athletic activity but resolved with ice and rest

ADLs: Independent with all daily activities

Pain: No pain reported

Special Tests: Ligamentous Laxity: Lachman Test[65] negative with a firm end-feel bilaterally

Anterior Drawer Test[65] negative with a firm end-feel bilaterally

International Knee Documentation Committee (IKDC)[101] Knee Form scores were rated as normal (unfortunately, the form was not completed prior to surgery and therapeutic exercise program intervention) (see Chapter 11)

Functional Hop Tests: Single Leg Hop for Distance Test,[102] scored 94%, compared to his non-impaired side which is the acceptable range for return to sport

Triple Hop Test,[103] scored 89% compared to his non-impaired side

Crossover Hop Test,[103] scored 90% compared to his non-impaired side

Isokinetic Muscle Strength Testing:[102] Right knee extensor torque was greater than 85% at all test speeds (60°, 180°, 300°/ sec.) compared to his non-

impaired side. Right side knee flexor torque was equivalent to the non-impaired side

Evolution of TJ's Therapeutic Exercise Program Goals

Initial Short Term Goals to be Achieved by 6–8 Weeks

1. The client will protect the healing graft tissue by following his weight bearing restriction and being compliant with the prescribed therapeutic exercise program. Allow healing to occur, protect fixation and ACL graft while limiting the effects of immobilization—goal achieved

2. The client will regain and improve quadriceps muscle activity to improve knee function with an acceptable level graded as 4/5 MMT (good) to achieve full active knee hyper-extension—goal achievement delayed (see below)

3. The client will regain flexion ROM to 120° to allow improved performance of the therapeutic exercise program and regain the ability to ambulate up and down stairs with step-over-step technique without pain or compensatory movements—goal achieved

4. The client will regain full passive extension equal to the opposite knee to facilitate a normal heel-to-toe gait pattern—goal achieved

5. The client will regain non-impaired patella mobility normalizing knee function and performance of the therapeutic exercise program without knee pain—goal achieved

Short-Term Goal Modifications (at re-evaluation during post operative week 7)

1. The client will regain normal balance ability measured by a single leg balance test score of 45–60 seconds with eyes closed on the right leg—goal achieved

2. The client will regain and improve quadriceps contractility to increase muscle function to an acceptable level graded at 4/5 MMT (good) to achieve full active knee hyper-extension—goal achieved

3. The client will regain flexion ROM to 135° degrees to allow improved performance of the therapeutic exercise program and regain the ability to perform a full squat without knee pain or compensatory movements—goal achieved

4. The client will regain dynamic lower extremity eccentric muscle control demonstrated by good hip and knee stability with a step down test to allow impact training and deceleration exercises initiation—goal achieved

Initial Long Term Goals to be Achieved by 6 Months

1. The client will regain full active and passive ROM compared to the non-impaired lower extremity ($-5°-0°-135°$) to allow a safe return to full soccer play—goal achieved

2. The client will regain quadriceps strength of 4+/5 tested by MMT to allow safe and symmetrical return to unrestricted running—goal achieved

3. The client will return to all running and multi-directional cutting activities at full speed, without pain (0/10 VAS) or swelling (<+1) and without compensatory movements—goal achieved

4. The client will display adequate function to begin preparation for returning to competitive soccer—goal achieved (see Chapter 11)

5. The client will perform the single leg hop test and score in the top 15% percentile compared to the opposite lower extremity scores (scores greater than 85%)—goal achieved

K. Use your clinical reasoning skills to design a Phase IV ACL therapeutic exercise program. In table format, list the exercises you think TJ should perform, in the order in which you would like him to perform them, and give the number of sets and repetitions and the rationale for inclusion. *See Author's Comments K*

Case Summary

An ACL injury can be devastating to a client. Injury to the ACL can occur in all active people, but has a higher incidence in athletically active clients, especially females. Physical impairments and functional limitations (see Chapter 1) are the most noticeable effects from a torn ACL, but the client may also suffer emotional distress, loss of sleep, fear of failure, and fear of re-injury. Early during therapeutic exercise intervention the ACL graft must be protected from stretch out or pull out, particularly during the ligamentization process. Therapeutic exercises can generally be advanced after the initial 8 weeks when the surgeon is comfortable with the presentation of the graft's end-feel and the overall presentation of the client's knee. TJ's progress was slow initially, with knee stiffness noted, but progressed well following the cessation of the acute inflammatory response post-surgery. He returned to jogging at 14–16 weeks and was cleared to return to soccer at 6 months post-surgery. He was instructed to wear a functional ACL knee brace during sports participation for one year after surgery.

Following his knee injury and surgery, TJ had significant reservations about returning to soccer. We noted during his rehabilitation, without pressure from those around TJ, he began to become much more interested and excited about playing soccer again, with guidance and encouragement from the rehabilitation clinician. TJ, a 12-year-old boy, was allowed to make his own decision. TJ's parents modified their behavior from being an overzealous and aggressive "soccer mom and dad" to being extremely supportive parents who allowed their child to decide what was best for him.

This case provided in-depth evaluation of the rehabilitative process of a 12-year-old client who sustained a devastating mid-substance ACL tear while playing youth soccer. Injuries similar to this injury can be prevented if early intervention programs are implemented with young athletes (see Chapters 5 and 11). More scientific research is needed to decrease injury rates in this athletic population. The rehabilitation clinician must always remember that the younger population may present with unique issues associated with a musculoskeletal injury. TJ suffered from irregular sleeping patterns post-injury, nightmares, increased stress, parental tensions, fear of rejection from teammates, fear of re-injury, pain induced de-motivation, and a fear of returning to playing sports (see Chapter 11). The rehabilitation clinician will have to make decisions on how to address issues similar to these in their younger clients and decide when appropriate referral to other health care professionals is indicated.

L. On a separate sheet of paper diagram a decision making algorithm for managing TJ's initially poor knee extension ROM. *See Author's Comment L*

M. On a separate sheet of paper diagram a decision making algorithm for managing TJ's initially poor quadriceps muscle activation. *See Author's Comment M*

N. On a separate sheet of paper diagram a decision making algorithm for managing TJ's initially poor knee flexion ROM. *See Author's Comment N*

Referring to Chapter 10 for guidance, discuss any alternative or complementary therapeutic exercises that you believe might benefit this client. Provide the rationale for your suggestion(s).

References

1. Stanitski C. Pediatric and adolescent sports injuries. *Clin Sports Med.* 1997;16:613–633.

2. Smith GS, Gallagher SS, Helsing K, et al. *Sports Injury Hospitalizations: Incidence and coding problems* (abstract). Paper presented at the 115th Annual Meeting of the American Public Heath Association, New Orleans, LA, 1987.

3. Posner M. *Preventing School Injuries: A Comprehensive Guide for School Administrators, Teachers, and Staff.* New Brunswick, NJ: Rutgers University Press, 2000.

4. Micheli LJ, Glassman R, Klein M. The prevention of sports injuries in children. Pediatric and adolescent sports injuries. *Clin Sports Med.* 2000;19(4): 821–834.

5. Metzl JD. Expectations of pediatric sport participation among pediatricians, patients, and parents. *Ped Clin N Am.* 2002;49(3):497–504.

6. Micheli LJ, Rask B, Gerberg L. Anterior cruciate ligament reconstruction in patients who are prepubescent. *Clin Orthop.* 1999;364:40–47.

7. Angel KR, Hall DJ. Anterior cruciate ligament injury in children and adolescents. *Arthroscopy.* 1989; 5:197–200.

8. Brief L. Anterior cruciate ligament reconstruction without drill holes. *Arthroscopy.* 1991;7:350–357.

9. Kellenberger R, von Laer L. Non-osseous lesions of the anterior cruciate ligaments in children and adolescents. *Prog Pediatr Surg.* 1990;25:123–131.

10. Lipscomb A, Anderson A. Tears of the anterior cruciate ligament in adolescents. *J Bone Joint Surg Am.* 1986;68:19–28.

11. McCarroll J, Rettig A, Shelbourne KD. Anterior cruciate ligament injuries in the young athlete with open physes. *Am J Sports Med.* 1988;16:44–47.

12. Aronowitz ER, Ganley TJ, Goode JR, et al. Anterior cruciate ligament reconstruction in adolescents with open physes. *Am J Sports Med.* 2000;28(2): 168–175.

13. Andrews M, Noyes FR, Barber-Westin SD. Anterior cruciate ligament allograft reconstruction in the skeletally immature athlete. *Am J Sports Med.* 1994;22:48–54.

14. Graf BK, Lange RH, Fujisaki CK, et al. Anterior cruciate ligament tears in skeletally immature patients: Meniscal pathology as presentation after attempted conservative treatment. *Arthroscopy.* 1992; 8:229–233.

15. Mizuta H, Kubota K, Shiraishi M, et al. The conservative treatment of complete tears of the anterior cruciate ligament in skeletally immature patients. *J Bone Joint Surg Br.* 1995;77b:890–894.

16. Nottage WM, Matsuura PA. Management of complete traumatic anterior cruciate ligament tears in the skeletally immature patient: Current concepts and review of literature. *Arthroscopy.* 1994; 10: 569–573.

17. Parker AW, Drez D Jr, Cooper JL. Anterior cruciate ligament injuries in patients with open physes. *Am J Sports Med.* 1994;22:44–47.

18. Iobst CA, Stanitski CL. Acute knee injuries. *Clin Sports Med.* 2000;19(4) 621–635.

19. Fehnel DJ, Johnson R. Anterior cruciate injuries in the skeletally immature athlete: A review of treatment outcomes. *Sports Med.* 2000;29(1):51–63.

20. Stadelmaier DM, Arnoczky SP, Dodds J, et al. The effect of drilling and soft tissue grafting across open growth plates: A histological study. *Am J Sport Med.* 1995;23:431–435.

21. Guzzanti V, Falciglia F, Gigante A, Fabbriciani C. The effect of intra-articular ACL reconstruction on the growth plates of rabbits. *J Bone Joint Surg Br.* 1994; 76(6):960–963.

22. Lo IK, Kirkley A, Fowler PJ, Miniaci A. The outcome of operatively treated anterior cruciate ligament disruptions in the skeletally immature. *Arthroscopy.* 1997;13(5): 627–634.

23. Matava MJ, Siegel MG. Arthroscopic reconstruction of the ACL with semitendinosus-gracilis autograft in skeletally immature adolescent patients. *Am J Knee Surg.* 1997;10:60–69.

24. Micheli LJ, Coady CM. Anterior cruciate reconstruction in the pediatric age group. *Sports Med Arthroscopy Rev.* 1997;5:106–111.

25. Hey Groves EW. Operation for the repair of the crucial ligaments. *Lancet.* 1917;674–675.

26. Fu FH, Bennett CH, Lattermann C, Ma CB. Current trends in anterior cruciate ligament reconstruction: Part 1. Biology and biomechanics of reconstruction. *Am J Sports Med.* 1999;27(6): 821–830.

27. Fu FH, Bennett CH, Ma CB, et al. Current trends in anterior cruciate ligament reconstruction. Part 2: Operative procedures and clinical correlations. *Am J Sports Med.* 2000;28(1):124–130.

28. Sachs RA, Daniel D, Stone ML, Garfein RF. Patellofemoral problems after anterior cruciate ligament reconstruction. *Am J Sports Med.* 1989;17: 760–765.

29. Aglietti PA, Buzzi R, Zaccherotti G, De Biase P. Patellar tendon versus doubled semitendinosus and gracilis tendons for anterior cruciate ligament reconstruction. *Am J Sports Med.* 1994;22:211–218.

30. Shelbourne KD, Wilckens JH, Mollabashay A, DeCarlo M. Arthrofibrosis in acute anterior cruciate ligament reconstruction. *Am J Sports Med.* 1991;19: 332–336.

31. Brown CH Jr. Instructional Course. Annual Meeting of the AAOS, Orlando, FL, March 15–19, 2000.

32. Shelton WR, Papendick L, Dukes AD. Autograft versus allograft anterior cruciate ligament reconstruction. *Arthroscopy.* 1997;13(4):446–449.

33. Drez DJ, DeLee J, Holden JP, et al. Anterior cruciate ligament reconstruction using bone-patellar tendon-bone allografts: A biological and biomechanical evaluation in goats. *Am J Sports Med.* 1991;19: 256–263.

34. Shino K, Inoe M, Horibe S, et al. Reconstruction of the anterior cruciate ligament using allogenic tendon: Long term follow up. *Am J Sports Med.* 1990; 18:457–465.

35. Indelicato PA, Linton RC, Huegel M. The results of fresh-frozen patellar tendon allografts for chronic anterior cruciate ligament deficiency of the knee. *Am J Sports Med.* 1992;20:118–121.

36. Peterson RK, Shelton WR, Bomboy AL. Allograft versus autograft patella tendon anterior cruciate ligament reconstruction: A 5-year follow-up. *Arthroscopy.* 2001;17(1):9–13.

37. Noyes FR, Barber-Westin S. Reconstruction of the anterior cruciate ligament with human allograft. *J Bone Joint Surg Am.* 1996;78(4):524–537.

38. Harner CD, Olson E, Irrgang JJ, et al. Allograft versus autograft anterior cruciate ligament reconstruction. *Clin Orthop.* 1996;324;134–144.

39. Jackson DW, Corsetti J, Simon TM. Biologic incorporation of the allograft anterior cruciate ligament replacements. *Clin Orthop.* 1996;324:126–133.

40. Jackson D, Grood E, Goldstein J, et al. A comparison of patella tendon autograft and allograft used for anterior cruciate ligament reconstruction in the goat model. *Am J Sports Med.* 1993;21:176–185.

41. Nikolaou PK, Seaber AV, Glisson RR, et al. Anterior cruciate ligament allograft transplantation: Long-term function, histology, revascularization, and operative technique. *Am J Sports Med.* 1986;14(5):348–360.

42. Shino K, Inoue M, Horibe S, et al. Maturation of allograft tendons transplanted into the knee. *J Bone Joint Surg Br.* 1988;70:556–560.

43. Brand J, Weiler A, Caborn DNM, et al. Graft fixation in the cruciate ligament reconstruction. *Am J Sports Med.* 2000;38(5):761–774.

44. Weiler A, Hoffman RFG, Bail HJ, et al. Tendon healing in a bone tunnel. Part II. Histological analysis after biodegradable interference fit fixation. *Arthroscopy.* 1999;15:548–549.

45. Clancy WG, Narechania RG, Rosenberg TD, et al. Anterior and posterior cruciate ligament reconstruction in rhesus monkeys: A histological microangiographic and biomechanical analysis. *J Bone Joint Surg Am.* 1981;63:1270–1284.

46. Arnoczky, SP. Biology of ACL reconstructions: What happens to the graft? *Instr Course Lect.* 1996;45:229–233.

47. Rodeo SA, Arnoczky SP, Torsilli PA, et al. Tendon-healing in a bone tunnel: A biomechanical and histological study in the dog. *J Bone Joint Surg Am.* 1993;75(12):1795–1803.

48. Wren TA, Yerby SA, Beaupre GS, Carter DR. Mechanical properties of the human achilles tendon. *Clin Biomech.* 2001;16(3):245–251.

49. Linn RM, Fischer DA, Smith JP, et al. Achilles tendon allograft reconstruction of the anterior cruciate ligament-deficient knee. *Am J Sports Med.* 1993;21: 825–831.

50. Woo SL-Y, Hollis JM, Adams DJ, et al. Tensile properties of the human femur-anterior cruciate ligament-tibia complex: The effects of specimen age and orientation. *Am J Sports Med.* 1991;19:217–225.

51. Cooper DE. Instructional course. Annual Meeting of the AAOS, San Francisco, CA, February 28–March 4, 2001

52. Hamner DL, Brown CH Jr., Steiner ME, et al. Hamtring tendon grafts for reconstruction of the anterior cruciate ligament: biomechanical evaluation of the use of multiple strands and tensioning techniques. *J Bone Joint Surg Am.* 1999;21(6):880–886.

53. Irrgang JJ, Harner CD. Recent advances in ACL rehabilitation: Clinical factors that influence the program. *J Sports Rehabil.* 1997;6:111–124.

54. Mangine RE, Noyes FR. Rehabilitation of the allograft reconstruction. *J Orthop Sports Phys Ther.* 1992;15(6):294–302.

55. Dillingham M. Personal communication. 2001.

56. Buck BE, Malinin TI, Brown MD. Bone transplantation and human immunodeficiency virus: An estimated risk of acquired immunodeficiency syndrome (AIDS). *Clin Orthop.* 1989;240:129–136.

57. Indelli PF, Dillingham MF, Fanton GS, Schurman DJ. Anterior cruciate ligament reconstruction using cryopreserved allografts. *Clin Orthop.* 2004;420:268–275.

58. Anonymous. Septic arthritis following anterior cruciate ligament reconstruction using tendon allografts—Florida and Louisiana, 2000. *Morb Mortal Wkly Rep. Surveill Summ.* 2001;50(48):1081–1083.

59. Noyes FR, Barber-Westin SD, Roberts CS. Use of allografts after failed treatment of rupture of the anterior cruciate ligament. *J Bone Joint Surg Am.* 1994;76(7):1019–1031.

60. Stingham DG, Pelmas CJ, Burks RT, et al. Comparison of anterior cruciate ligament reconstruction using patellar tendon autograft or allograft. *Arthroscopy.* 1996;12(4):414–421.

61. Fu FH, Woo SLY, Irrgang JJ. Current concepts for rehabilitation following anterior cruciate ligament reconstruction. *J Orthop Sports Phys Ther.* 1992;15(6):270–278.

62. Jenkins W, Bronner S, Mangine R. Functional evaluation and treatment of the lower extremity, Chap. 6 In B Browstein, S Bronner (eds.), *Functional Movement in Orthopaedic and Sports Physical Therapy.* New York: Churchill Livingstone, 1997, pp. 191–229.

63. Wilk KE, Zheng N, Fleisig GS, et al. Kinetic chain exercises: Implications for anterior cruciate ligament patient. *J Sports Rehabil.* 1997;6:125–143.

64. Muller W. *The Knee: Form, Function and Ligament Reconstruction.* Berlin, Germany: Springer-Verlag, 1983.

65. Irrgang JJ, Safran MR, Fu FH. The knee: Ligamentous and meniscal injuries. In JE Zachazewski, DJ Magee, WS Quillen, eds. *Athletic Injuries and Reha-*

bilitation. Philadelphia, PA: W.B. Saunders Company, 1996, pp. 623–692.

66. Steindler A. *Kinesiology of the Human Body Under Normal and Pathological Conditions.* Springfield, IL: Charles C Thomas, 1977.

67. DeCarlo M. Shelbourne KD, Oneacre K. Rehabilitation program for both knees when the contralateral autogenous patellar tendon graft is used for primary anterior cruciate ligament reconstruction: A case study. *J Orthop Sports Phys Ther.* 1999;29 (3):144–159.

68. Sawhney R, Dearwater S, Irrgang JJ, Fu FH. Quadriceps exercise following anterior cruciate ligament reconstruction without anterior tibial displacement. Presented at the Annual Conference of the APTA. Anaheim, CA, June 1990.

69. Grood ES, Suntay WJ, Noyes FR, Butler DL. Biomechanics of the knee-extension exercise. *J Bone Joint Surg Am.* 1984;66(5):725–734.

70. Lutz GE, Palmitier RA, An KN, Chao EYS. Comparison of tibiofemoral joint forces during open-kinetic-chain and closed-kinetic-chain exercises. *J Bone Joint Surg Am.* 1993;75(5):732–739.

71. Daniel DM, Stone ML, Dobson BE, et al. Fate of the ACL-injured patient: A prospective outcome study. *Am J Sports Med.* 1994;22(5):632–644.

72. Voight M, Bell S, Rhodes D. Instrumented testing of tibial translation during a positive Lachman's test and selected closed-chain activities in anterior cruciate deficient knees. *J Orthop Sports Phys Ther.* 1992;15:49. [abstract]

73. Arms SW, Pope MH, Johnson RJ, et al. The biomechanics of the anterior cruciate ligament rehabilitation and reconstruction. *Am J Sports Med.* 1984; 12(1):8–18.

74. Renstrom P, Arms SW, Stanwyck TS, et al. Strain within the anterior cruciate ligament during hamstring and quadriceps activity. *Am J Sports Med.* 1986;14(1):83–87.

75. Beynnon B, Howe JG, Pope MH, et al. The measurement of anterior cruciate strain in vivo. *Int Orthop.* 1992;16(1).

76. Beynnon BD, Johnson RJ, Fleming BC, et al. The strain behavior of the anterior cruciate ligament during squatting and active flexion-extension. *Am J Sports Med.* 1997;25(6):823–863.

77. Henning CE, Lynch MA, Glick KR. An in vivo strain gage study of elongation of the anterior cruciate ligament. *Am J Sports Med.* 1985;13(1): 22–26.

78. Beynnon BD, Fleming BC, Johnson RJ, et al. Anterior cruciate ligament strain behavior during rehabilitation exercises in vivo. *Am J Sports Med.* 1995;23(1),24–34.

79. Johnson RJ. Instructional course notes. Panther Sports Medicine Symposium, Pittsburgh, PA, 2000.

80. Yack HJ, Collins CE, Whieldon TJ. Comparison of closed and open kinetic chain exercises in the anterior cruciate ligament-deficient knee. *Am J Sports Med.* 1993;21(1):49–54.

81. Jurist KA, Otis JC. Anteroposterior tibiofemoral displacements during isometric extension efforts: The roles of external load and knee flexion angle. *Am J Sports Med.* 1985;13(4):254–258.

82. Wilk KE, Escamilla RF, Fleisig GS, et al. A comparison of the tibiofemoral joint forces and electromyographic activity during open and closed kinetic chain exercises. *Am J Sports Med.* 1996; 24(4):514–527.

83. DeCarlo M, Klootwyk TE, Shelbourne KD. ACL surgery and accelerated rehabilitation: Revisited. *J Sports Rehabil.* 1997; 6:144–156.

84. Butler DL, Noyes FR, Grood ES. Ligamentous restraints to anterior posterior drawer in the human knee: A biomechanical story. *J Bone Joint Surg Am.* 1980;62:259–270.

85. Arnoczky SP, Tarvin GB, Marshall JL. Anterior cruciate ligament replacement using patellar tendon: An evaluation of graft revascularization in the dog. *J Bone Joint Surg Am.* 1982;64:217–224.

86. Snyder-Mackler L, Delitto A, Bailey SL. Strength of the quadriceps femoris muscle and functional recovery after reconstruction of the anterior cruciate ligament. *J Bone Joint Surg Am.* 1995;77:1166–1173.

87. Cook TM, Zimmermann CL, Lux KM, et al. EMG comparison of lateral step up and stepping machine exercises. *J Orthop Sports Phys Ther.* 1992;16: 108–113.

88. Weiss JR. *Electromyographic Analysis of the Minisquat Exercise.* Master's thesis, University of Pittsburgh, 1990.

89. Wilk KE, Andrews JR. Current concepts in the treatment of anterior cruciate ligament disruption. *J Orthop Sports Phys Ther.* 1992;15(6):279–293.

90. Palmitier RA, An KN, Scott SG, Chao YS. Kinetic chain exercise in knee rehabilitation. *Sports Med.* 1991;11(6):402–413.

91. Anonymous. American Academy of Pediatrics Committee on Sports Medicine. Strength training, weight and power lifting, and bodybuilding by children and adolescents. *Pediatrics.* 1994;86(5): 801–803.

92. Faigenbaum A, Kraemer W, Cahill B, et al. Youth resistance training: Position statement paper and literature review. *Strength Cond.* 1996;18:62–75.

93. Faigenbaum AD. Strength training for children and adolescents. *Clin Sports Med.* 2000;19(4):593–619.

94. Falk B, Tenenbaum G. The effectiveness of resistance training in children: A meta-analysis. *Sports Med.* 1996;22:176–186.

95. Payne V, Morrow J, Johnson L, et al. Resistance training in children and youth: A meta-analysis. *Res Q Exerc Sport*. 1997;68:80–89.

96. American Orthopedic Society for Sports Medicine: *Proceedings of the Conference on Strength Training and the Prepubescent*. Chicago, IL: American Orthopedic Society for Sports Medicine, 1988.

97. Faigenbaum AD, Micheli LJ. Preseason conditioning for the preadolescent athlete. *Pediatr Annals*. 2000;29(3):156–161.

98. Sewal L, Micheli LJ. Strength training for children. *J Pediatric Orthop*. 1986;6:143–146.

99. Rians CB, Weltman A, Cahill BR, et al. Strength training for prepubescent males: Is it safe? *Am J Sport Med*. 1987;15:483–489.

100. Mikkelsen C, Werner S, Eriksson E. Closed kinetic chain alone compared to combined open and closed kinetic chain exercises for quadriceps strengthening after anterior cruciate ligament reconstruction with respect to return to sports: A prospective matched follow-up study. *Knee Surg Sports Traumatol Arthrosc*. 2000; 8(6):337–342.

101. Hefti F, Muller W, Jakob RP, Staubli HU. Evaluation of knee ligament injuries with the IKDC form. *Knee Surg Sports Traumatol Arthosc*. 1993; 1: 226–234.

102. Wilk KE, Romaniello WT, Soscia SM, et al. The relationship between subjective knee scores, isokinetic testing, and functional testing in the ACL-reconstructed knee. *J Orthop Sports Phys Ther*. 1994; 20:60–73.

Author's Comments A

Data collected from the initial evaluation resulted in the following list of problems.

1. Graft tissue/fixation vulnerability to injury
2. Poor quadriceps activation and strength
3. Limited knee extension and flexion ROM
4. Decreased patellar mobility
5. Minimal compliance with therapeutic exercise program secondary to pain
6. Minimal understanding of the importance of compliance with therapeutic exercise program and principles
7. Involvement of the parents and their interest in TJ's return to play
8. TJ's concerns about future injury, school, pressure of playing and his painful knee

Author's Comments B

By 6–8 weeks, the client . . .

1. Will protect the healing graft tissue by complying with the weight bearing restriction and with prescribed therapeutic exercises. [Rationale: Allow healing to occur, protect fixation, and ACL graft while limiting the effects of immobilization]
2. Will regain and improve voluntary quadriceps muscle activation to achieve full active right knee hyper-extension.
3. Will regain flexion ROM to 120° to allow improved therapeutic exercise program performance and regain the ability to ambulate up and down stairs using a step-over-step technique.
4. Will regain full passive extension equal to the opposite knee to facilitate a non-impaired heel-to-toe gait pattern
5. Will regain non-impaired patella mobility to participate in activities of daily living and in therapeutic exercise program without right knee pain.

Author's Comments C

By 6 months, the client . . .

1. Will regain full active and passive ROM similar to opposite lower extremity ($-5°-0°-135°$) to allow a safe return to full soccer play
2. Will regain quadriceps strength of 4+/5 tested by MMT to allow safe and symmetrical return to unrestricted running
3. Will return to all running and cutting activities in all planes without pain (0/10 VAS) or swelling (< Grade 1)
4. Will be able to return to playing soccer if he chooses to continue competitive athletics
5. Will perform the single leg hop test and score in the top 15% percentile compared to the opposite leg score (scores ≥ 85%)

Author's Comments D

The literature reports that most conservative treatment programs for ACL deficient knees in children fail and result in frequent episodes of giving way.[11–17] This giving way and repeated injury to the knee may cause damage to the menisci and/or articular cartilage.[18] Therefore, surgical reconstruction has been indicated in this population, specifically when a meniscus tear is diagnosed. Also, literature supports reconstructing the ACL and repairing the meniscus simultaneously to improve the success rate for meniscus healing.[18] A repair of TJ's meniscus tear was not possible because of the radial type and small size. The surgical treatment of the mid-substance ACL tear in the skeletally immature athlete is a topic of considerable debate and controversy within the literature and among surgeons. There appears to be no consensus on what is the most effective and safe reconstruction technique for the skeletally immature athlete. However, the surgeon reported that the current literature supports the use of transphyseal surgical reconstruction of the ACL in prepubescents.[19–21] Surgical timing and technique are concerns to orthopedic surgeons because of the effect that surgery could have on the epiphyseal growth plates of the young client. Surgery-induced growth plate injury could result in abnormal bone growth and subsequent leg length discrepancy. Current research supports the transphyseal reconstruction technique.[10–14,19,22–24] Conversely, Andrews et al.[13] suggested that knee surgeons should avoid drilling through the femoral epiphyseal plate to prevent abnormal growth that may occur during a possible late growth spurt.

As rehabilitation clinicians, we must remember that we need to respect the healing rates and surgical precautions of the ACL reconstruction when developing a therapeutic exercise program for a young client. We must consider the specifics of the type of ACL reconstruction surgery that was performed, including the type of tissue and the method of surgical fixation. The partial meniscectomy will have little effect on the therapeutic exercise program. We must not forget the specific needs of the 12-year-old boy and the stresses associated with the surgery and rehabilitation and his specific needs. We must consider how all of these factors relate to TJ's surgery and therapeutic exercise program. Let's first look at the factors associated with the ACL reconstruction surgery and the use of allograft tissue.

Author's Comments E

Therapeutic Exercise Program—Early Phase I

1. Passive knee extension-ROM (heel props, prone hangs)
2. Patella mobilizations (inferior, superior glides)
3. Isometric quadriceps setting
4. Straight leg raises
5. Knee flexion—ROM
6. Partial ROM revolutions on a stationary bicycle
7. Terminal knee extensions (TKE)
8. Multi-angle quadriceps isometrics between 60° and 90° knee flexion
9. Neuromuscular stimulation—home unit
10. Weight shifting—pre-gait training
11. Aquatic therapy activities in a swimming pool

Therapeutic Exercise Program—Late Phase I

1. Wall slides
2. Wall squats
3. Step downs
4. Hamstring curls
5. Proprioception-Balance—standing balance activities, bilateral/unilateral, even and uneven surfaces
6. Leg press—bilateral/unilateral
7. Lunges

The Phase I therapeutic exercise program continued through session 12. Phase II therapeutic exercises were initiated once the effusion was controlled and the client was able to ambulate independently without a brace or crutches. It must be understood that phases of therapeutic exercise will often blend and the client may be performing exercises and activities that are in two different phases. Irrgang and Harner suggest that the therapeutic exercise progression should not be based solely on healing time frames, but on the clinical presentation of each client.[53]

Author's Comments F

The rehabilitation clinician managing TJ's case believed that he had become frustrated with the daily routine of his program. This is quite common during this post-operative time frame, but it posed a unique problem with TJ because of his lack of maturity and youth. It is essential to keep the client's interest during this time period. Slow and limited progress is usually noted during the strength building period of the phase II rehabilitation program. It was decided to take TJ to a university soccer practice and show him what older athletes go through on a daily basis to be competitive. TJ agreed to the visit. A call was made to the university training room and a visit was set up. The athletic trainer there had an athlete who was going through a similar therapeutic exercise program, so a meeting between the two was arranged.

TJ's level of motivation decreased dramatically during phase II. An intervention was necessary to refocus TJ and maintain his previous high level of dedication. The decision to set up a visit had several objectives. One objective was to show TJ the work ethic needed to succeed in rehabilitation and soccer. It was also important to go to a university soccer practice to see the game played at a high level to see if this would motivate TJ. The trip posed a possible risk that it might negatively affect TJ's attitude and motivation whereby he might come away thinking that he would never get back to playing soccer. The potential benefits were believed to outweigh the risks in this particular case.

Author's Comments G

Therapeutic exercise	Sets and repetitions	Rationale
1. Wall squats	3 × 10	Increase lower extremity strength with co-contraction of quadriceps/hamstrings
2. Step-downs	3 × 25	Improve eccentric and concentric lower extremity strength
3. Unilateral leg press	3 × 10	Increase lower extremity strength
4. Hamstring curls	3 × 10	Increase lower extremity strength
5. Biking	Various	Warm up, cardio, ROM
6. Sport cord resisted dynamic stability exercises	Various	Improve dynamic lower extremity control
7. Retro-treadmill walking	Various	Safe quadriceps exercise, perform in ½ squat position with arched back
8. Single leg balance exercises	Various	Improve balance and dynamic stability

Author's Comments H

Phase III therapeutic exercises include light impact activities, jump rope, hopping drills, and deceleration type activities. These therapeutic exercises are designed to prepare the client to return to jogging and sport simulation training in phase IV. The client must demonstrate a willingness to perform these activities, but more important the rehabilitation clinician must verify the client's progression with a thorough objective functional evaluation. The client must display excellent eccentric quadriceps strength and dynamic lower extremity control prior to the commencement of any impact exercise or activity.

Author's Comments I

The rehabilitation clinician must not lose focus on lower extremity strengthening during phase III. The addition of the more interesting sport simulation activities results in a possible loss of focus regarding performance of the foundational strengthening exercises. This is also a time of increased risk of injury. Clients become more excited with the possibility of returning to sport and become over-zealous, not complying with the therapeutic exercise plan and predisposing themselves to re-injury. Plyometrics may be added during phase III, but close monitoring must occur. The rehabilitation clinician must evaluate each case independently and assess the demands the client will place on their knee and choose the appropriate activities to move the client forward to full activity. Similar reasoning is accurate for the use of jumping rope. Of note: not all clients will be coordinated enough to jump rope. Therefore, the rehabilitation clinician must be aware that adding a jump rope could place the uncoordinated client at increased risk for injury.

Phase IV is the return to play phase. The client should regain and re-learn all the aspects and components during Phase IV to safely be transitioned back to their respective sport (see Chapter 11). Return to sport has been suggested to occur safely between the fourth and sixth month following ACL reconstruction using allograft tissue; however, it may be deferred to 9 to 12 months, and graft maturation takes considerably longer.

Author's Comments J

Therapeutic exercises	Sets and repetitions	Rationale
1. Bike	10 minutes at 60 RPM	General warm-up
2. Jump rope	1 minute for 5 repetitions	Warm-up for skills training
3. Agility program	3, 30 sec. sets	Develop agility, quickness, reaction time
4. Soccer footwork	3, 30 sec. sets	Ball work, quick feet; ask client which soccer components they would like to work on
5. Impact hop program on a foam mat or mini-trampoline	3, 30 sec. sets	Prepare lower extremity to accept impact and develop eccentric lower extremity muscle function

(continued)

Therapeutic exercises	Sets and repetitions	Rationale
6. Shuttle jumps	3 × 15 repetitions, using two to three resistive bands	Progress to full weight bearing
7. Box jumps/drops	3 × 15 repetitions, progressive height (4–18 inches)	Prepare lower extremity to accept impact and develop eccentric lower extremity muscle function
8. Single leg hopping	3 sets of 10–15 repetitions	Prepare lower extremity to accept impact and develop eccentric-concentric lower extremity muscle function
9. Walk-jog-run progression on treadmill	1.5–2 miles (as tolerated)	Return to jogging/running

The rehabilitation clinician initiated phone contact with the surgeon to discuss return to play status. The physician reported that TJ was doing quite well. The surgeon was interested in TJ returning to soccer no sooner than 6 months post surgery. The surgeon also indicated that he wanted TJ to be placed in a functional knee brace for the first full year following the surgery while playing soccer or other sports. The surgeon and the rehabilitation clinician discussed types and styles of braces. Following sizing of TJ's leg, the brace was ordered. TJ's parents were instructed to make an office appointment to see the surgeon in the next few weeks.

Author's Comments K

Therapeutic exercises	Sets and repetitions	Rationale
1. Bike	10 minutes at 60 RPM	Warm up
2. Stretching program	30 sec. hold × 3 repetitions	Increase flexibility
3. Isokinetic program	Multi-velocity spectrum (60°–300°/sec.). 5 sets of 10 repetitions	Increase quadriceps and hamstring muscle strength
4. Advanced single leg balance to simulate soccer activities.	10 sets of 10–30 second duration	Proprioception/kinesthetic awareness
5. Soccer ball kicking program	5, 2 minute duration intervals	Train foundational soccer skill
6. Acceleration/deceleration sprinting program	3, 10, 20 and 40 yard sprints	Train foundational soccer skill (anerobic conditioning)
7. Side step and crossover cutting	3 sets of 10 cuts	Train foundational soccer skill (agility)
8. Single leg hopping	3 sets of 20 foot hopping	Prepare for lower extremity demands of soccer and functional tests
9. Soccer simulation	5, 2 minute duration intervals	Use select soccer drills to train specific deficiencies (anerobic, aerobic conditioning)
10. Foundational strengthening exercises	Continue as before, possibly decrease frequency to avoid overtraining.	Maintain or improve baseline total body conditioning

The decision to return a client back to play must be a team decision. The surgeon should consult the rehabilitation clinician for information regarding the client's strength, functional test scores and capacity for performing activities that replicate the physical demands of the sport. The demands of the sport must be "broken down" into specific therapeutic exercises and activities that will appropriately prepare and transition the client from the therapeutic exercise environment to competitive sports participation. The client must demonstrate competence and confidence with each step of the therapeutic exercise process. The culmination of all of these abilities will prepare the client for a safe return to sport. Therapeutic progression and return to play decisions are based on the client's progression and ability to perform activity specific tasks with appropriate form.

Author's Comments L

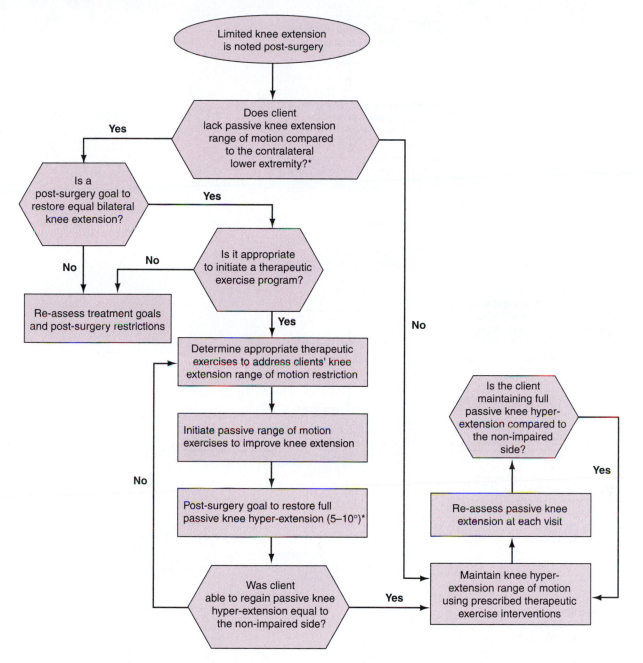

*Do not attempt to achieve > 5°–10° hyper-extension on any post-surgical knee.

Author's Comments M

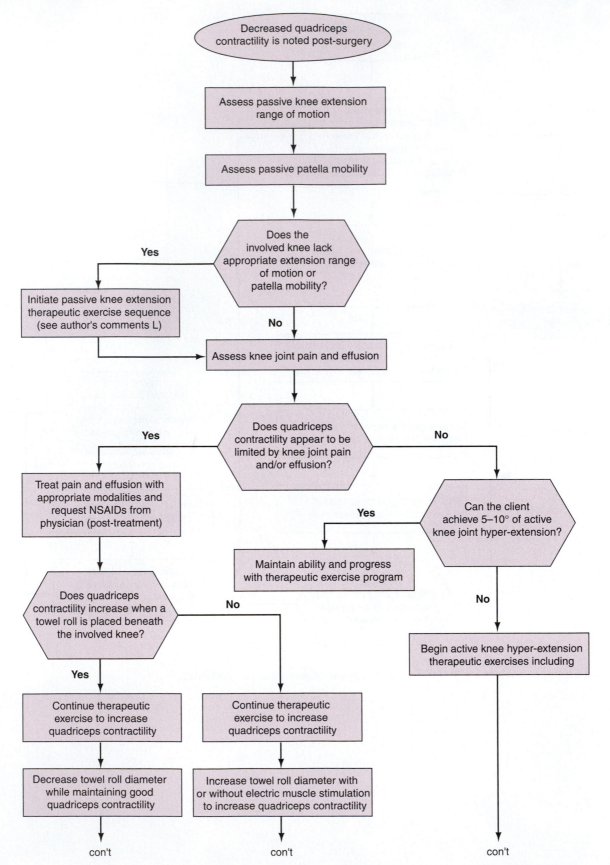

Author's Comments M (con't)

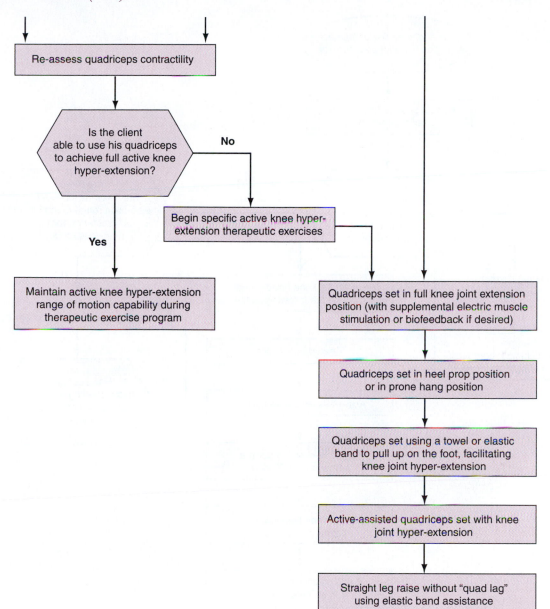

Author's Comments N

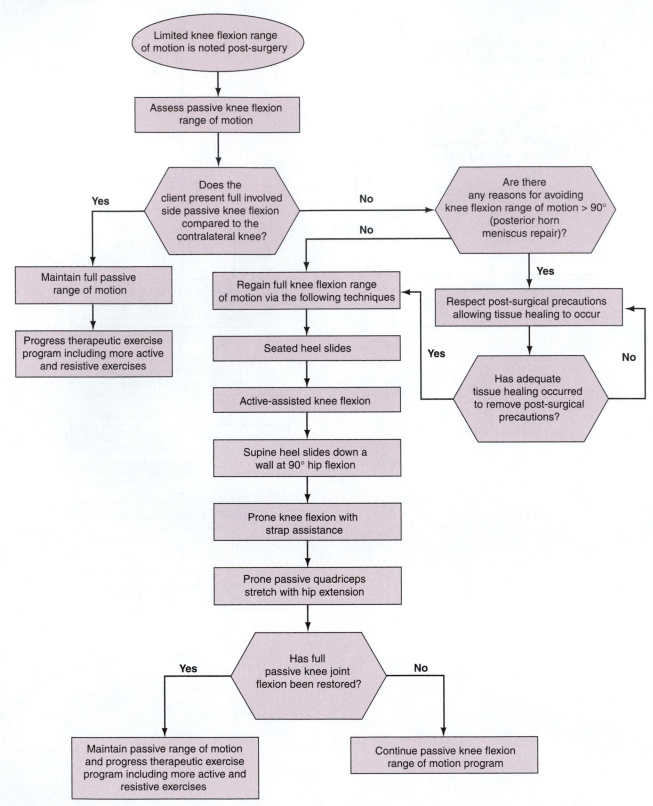

CLIENT CASE #7

Barbara Hoogenboom

History

Client: Susan

Age: 35 years

Height: 5'5"

Weight: 132 lbs (pre-pregnancy weight = 125 lbs.)

Education: College graduate, also has earned an MBA

Occupation: Certified public accountant in a major accounting firm

Medical/Surgical History: Two-week history of patellofemoral pain, recurrent condition last problematic 3 years ago. Client is 9 weeks pregnant

Chief Complaint: Right patellofemoral pain limiting her ability to perform running program and some activities of daily living (ADLs), including sit-to-stand movements, ascending/descending stairs

Case Figure 7.1   Susan.

Susan is an active 35-year-old woman who has been running for her entire adult life, after having run on the cross country team in high school and college (**Case Figure 7.1**). Running is her preferred method of fitness training, but she participates in many other forms of aerobic exercise, including biking, aerobics, spinning and swimming. She runs an average of five days per week, for a usual weekly total of 20–25 miles per week. She competes in 5K road races 4–6 times per year.

Susan has just discovered that she is pregnant for the first time, and she is 9 weeks along. She and her husband are excited about the pregnancy and are eager to have a healthy child. Susan has been referred to you by her obstetrician-gynecologist for exercises for her painful right knee (patellofemoral joint) that has been troubling her over the last two weeks. The physician also would like you to instruct Susan in therapeutic exercise considerations and contraindications related to maternal and fetal health.

Susan began to experience right patellofemoral knee pain approximately three years ago, attributing its onset to an increased level of training. Currently she reports a steady level of training both in terms of mileage and intensity. In the last two weeks she has begun to experience anterior knee pain with running activities as well as with ADLs including sit-to-stand movements (at work desk), and with stair climbing (lives in a two story home). She reports that she occasionally feels as if her right kneecap "slides to the side." Her primary therapeutic exercise program goal is to decrease her right knee pain during ADLs while maintaining a reasonable level of physical fitness throughout her pregnancy. She also desires to continue to run if possible. Potential referral to an orthopedic surgeon may offer more information as to the extent of the patellofemoral pathology. Although not directly related to her right knee condition, consultation services from a dietician for nutrition and weight control information may also be helpful.

Physical Examination

Musculoskeletal Assessment

Posture/Observation: Client has mild genu valgus alignment at bilateral lower extremities, with moderate pes planus at both feet, right > than left. Mild atrophy of the vastus medialis oblique muscle of the right lower extremity was also noted.

Active Knee Range of Motion in Sitting: 135° flexion to complete extension bilaterally with mild complaint of pain at the right patellofemoral joint with full extension

Ligamentous Laxity: Normal and symmetrical for anterior cruciate ligament, posterior cruciate ligament, medial and lateral collateral ligaments

Manual Muscle Testing: Right quadriceps 4/5 with pain (at patellofemoral joint) with resisted testing at

30° flexion and 90° flexion. Difficulty eliciting isometric right vastus medialis oblique muscle activation at full knee extension

Musculotendinous Extensibility: Active hamstring extensibility while in a supine position at 90° hip flexion: right lacks 25° extension, left lacks 20° extension. Positive Ober's test bilaterally, moderate restriction[1]

Patellar Stability: Mildly increased lateral and decreased medial glide at the right patellofemoral joint

Pain: 3/10 (measured using a visual analog scale) during normal ADLs, 6/10 after running distances greater than one mile; 6/10 when stair climbing and occasionally when moving from a sit-to-stand position

Special Test: Equivocally positive apprehension sign at right patellofemoral joint.[1]

Cardiopulmonary Assessment

Resting Blood Pressure: 120/77 mm Hg
Resting Heart Rate: 62 bpm

Neuromuscular Assessment

Sensation/Reflexes: Deep tendon reflexes +2 for patellar and Achilles tendon reflexes, sensation intact to light touch and equal bilaterally at lower extremities

Standing Balance: Single leg stance test (eyes closed) 18 sec left lower extremity, 13 sec right lower extremity

Integumentary Assessment

Not applicable

A. Given this information, what are your primary concerns regarding Susan's musculoskeletal impairments?[2–11] See Author's Comments A

B. What concerns do you have regarding other existing or potential system impairments? See Author's Comments B

C. Preventing, delaying, or minimizing the effects of a disease, illness or impairment is vital to every client. Identify the prevention considerations for Susan and provide a rationale for your decision.[12] Create and complete a table with column headings for prevention level, preferred practice pattern, and rationale. See Author's Comments C

After considering all factors, you determine that Susan has an excellent prognosis for restoring right knee function. Having considered all physical examination data, lifestyle,

ADLs and instrumental activities of daily living, (IADLs) and the client's interests, and having identified the primary practice pattern relevant to Susan, you are ready to generate a list of problems that summarize the concerns raised by the history and physical examination data. Focus on problems that you perceive to be critical to Susan's quality of life.

The identified cluster of signs and symptoms provides a foundation for therapeutic exercise program planning. However, by learning more about Susan, we can devise an appropriate therapeutic exercise program for her musculoskeletal complaints as well as counsel her regarding the ongoing fitness program she participates in throughout her pregnancy. By appreciating the unique attributes of Susan, we can create a personal, meaningful program. By taking a "big picture" look at Susan's life we can design fitness instructions and therapeutic exercises that fit with her personal values and daily routine, thereby stimulating compliance. Of particular concern are her lifestyle and fitness interests, her IADLs, and ADLs.

Lifestyle: Active social life, with friends from work and church. Many of her social contacts revolve around exercise and fitness, as she is a highly motivated, dedicated recreational athlete. Susan is married, and this is her first pregnancy about which she and her husband are very excited. Non-smoker, social drinker (which she has ceased since becoming pregnant).

Health/fitness Interests: Susan is a member of a local running club. Her husband is also an avid runner, very supportive of Susan's wishes to continue running and exercising throughout her pregnancy. General fitness, weight training and aerobic activities are very important to Susan. Susan is also dedicated to good nutrition and wishes to be "smart" about weight gain throughout her pregnancy, while acknowledging the importance of healthy weight gain for a healthy pregnancy.

ADLs: Pain with stair climbing (two story home with bedrooms on the second floor), pain with all squatting tasks (laundry). This concerns Susan because she has not experienced these difficulties before.

IADLs: Sit-to-stand movements are painful at work. She works in an office and must move from sit-to-stand frequently. She also has difficulty performing yard work (squatting). Also of concern to Susan is the potential that these ADL and IADL limitations might continue after her pregnancy, when she will need to perform them with a baby.

D. Based upon the information provided up to this point, list six to eight problems that you consider critical to Susan's quality of life (the ability for Susan to do things that are important to her). See Author's Comments D

Having listed problems, you are ready to begin planning the short and long term goals that you would like to help Susan achieve with your therapeutic exercise program and counseling. Be sure that the goals you set for Susan are observable, realistic, and written clearly and objectively. Create goals that relate impairments and problems to functional limitations and prevention of disability. For Susans case, limit your short term goals to those you believe that she should achieve after four weeks of complying with your therapeutic exercise program. Keep in mind that goals, even for addressing impairments, should have a functional relevance.

E. Based on the information provided create three to six short term (≤ 4 weeks) therapeutic exercise program goals.
"By the end of 4 weeks, the client . . ." *See Author's Comments E*

For this case, be sure to consider several long term educational goals that relate to exercise during pregnancy and modifications that Susan should implement as she moves in to her second and third trimesters.[2,4,9]

F. Create three to six long term therapeutic exercise program goals (5–12 weeks) for Susan to work toward throughout her pregnancy.
"By 6 to 8 weeks, the client . . ." *See Author's Comments F*

The health club where Susan is a member open daily from 6 A.M. to 9 P.M. and has an indoor walking/running track, aerobic exercise equipment (upright and recumbent stationary bicycles, stair-steppers, elliptical trainers, rowing machines and upper body ergometers) as well as a therapeutic pool. Weight training equipment (including Nautilus machines, dumbbells, and cuff weights) is also available. Susan reports that she also has a variety of dumbbells and cuff weights at home ranging in weight from 1 to 5 lbs.

Limit your lower extremity exercise selections to those that she would perform at home. For alternate aerobic interventions, you may choose to utilize equipment at the health club.

G. With consideration for therapeutic exercise order determination factors, create a table listing your therapeutic exercise selections, the primary body region or system that the exercise trains, and your rationale for including that exercise. *See Author's Comments G*
H. Following therapeutic exercise selection, document the volume (sets and repetitions), intensity, the rest-to-work ratio, and frequency in table format.[13–18] *See Author's Comments H*

I. Having initiated your therapeutic exercise program, identify three to six objective clinical measurements you will use to verify progress toward Susan's achievement of the short term goals[1,19–21]: See Author's Comments I

Four weeks have now passed and Susan is doing well with her activities and therapeutic exercises. She has been extremely compliant with the program and is able to show you her progress in all exercises as well in functional activities. She is now 13 weeks into her pregnancy and is beginning her second trimester. Her weight gain is well under control (see re-evaluation data). After these four weeks you re-evaluate and document the following information.

Body Weight: 139 lbs

Musculoskeletal Assessment

Manual Muscle Testing: Normal strength at bilateral lower extremities, with right vastus medialis oblique hypertrophy noted upon observation.
Musculotendinous Extensibility: Active hamstring extension in supine at 90° hip flexed position: (right) 10° from full extension, (left) full extension. Ober's test remains moderately decreased bilaterally
Pain: Right knee pain 1/10 with sit-to-stand movements, 3/10 with stair ascending and descending and 2/10 with attempts to run short distances. Pain is 0-1/10 when taped throughout the day
Patellar Instability: Improved medial patellar glide (increased lateral retinacular extensibility), negative apprehension test with lateral glides, and no complaints of "slipping out" in the last two weeks

Cardiopulmonary Assessment

Resting Blood Pressure: 120/75 mm Hg
Resting Heart Rate: 70 bpm

Neuromuscular Assessment

Standing Balance: Single leg stance test (eyes closed) 20 sec left lower extremity, 20 sec right lower extremity.

Integumentary Assessment

Not applicable

J. With consideration of the above re-examination data and what you know about the progression of your client's pregnancy, list your modified therapeutic exercise program selections in a table providing, exercise order, the exercise selection, and the modification. What additional or ongoing exercises for the knee should Susan continue to perform? What educational issues remain for Susan related to her desire to continue to run?

Remember to focus your interventions on long term goals and primary prevention for a pregnant woman, with consideration for preventing new conditions or the exacerbation of existing conditions. *See Author's Comments J*

Case Summary

Patellofemoral pain and/or instability is not easy to treat in an active runner. Add to this the concurrent condition of pregnancy and its additional physiological, hormonal, musculoskeletal and psychological demands and the treatment targeted at return to function (running) becomes more complex and has more "concerns." Of utmost concern is the health of both the mother and the developing fetus. Contemporary research guides therapeutic exercise selection and fitness activity prescription for pregnant women (ACOG guidelines).

The rehabilitation clinician who treats a client like Susan must address many issues related to her patellofemoral pain and also her fitness/exercise desires throughout pregnancy. The two phases of treatment outlined in this case provide an initial set of interventions to manage her patellofemoral pain/instability and then another phase to address other issues relevant to the active, fitness-oriented pregnant woman. Depending on how her pregnancy progresses in terms of weight gain and other concerns, her physician may allow her to continue running. However, if this becomes difficult, uncomfortable, or medically ill advised, Susan would have many other strategies and options available to her to maintain fitness during the latter portion of her pregnancy.

Susan will also have learned about several strategies to manage signs and symptoms of patellofemoral joint irritation in the future as well. Following completion of her supervised therapeutic exercise intervention, lines of communication should be established for Susan to be able to address general concerns and get answers to new questions regarding her condition. By considering Susan's lifestyle, ADLs, and personal fitness goals, therapeutic exercise interventions provided for her patellofemoral joint problems would have an effect on her quality of life during pregnancy.

K. On a separate sheet of paper, diagram a decision making algorithm for your method of managing the patellofemoral joint pain that Susan experiences. *See Author's Comments K*

Referring to Chapter 10 for guidance, discuss any alternative or complementary therapeutic exercises that you believe might benefit this client. Provide the rationale for your suggestion(s).

References

1. Magee DJ. *Orthopedic Physical Assessment*, 4th ed. Philadelphia, PA: W.B. Saunders, 2002.
2. Calhuneri M, Bird HA, Wright V. Changes in joint laxity occurring during pregnancy. *Ann Rheum Dis.* 1982;41:126–128.
3. Dumas G, Reid J. Laxity of knee cruciate ligaments during pregnancy. *J Orthop Sports Phys Ther.* 1997; 26:1–6.
4. Clapp JF. Exercise during pregnancy. In O Bar-Or, D Lamb, P Clarkson (eds.), *Perspectives in Exercise Science and Sports Medicine: Exercise and the Female—A Life Span Approach.* Carmel, IN: Cooper Publishing Group, 1996.
5. Clapp JF, Little KD. Effect of recreational exercise on pregnancy weight gain and subcutaneous fat deposition. *Med Sci Sports Exerc.* 1995; 27:170–177.
6. Sternfeld B, Quesenberry CP, Eskenazi B, et al. Exercise during pregnancy and pregnancy outcome. *Med Sci Sports Exerc.* 1995; 27:634–640.
7. Clapp JF, 3rd. Exercise during pregnancy. A clinical update. *Clin Sports Med.* 2000; 19(2):273–286.
8. Ireland ML, Ott SM. The effects of pregnancy on the musculoskeletal system. *Clin Orthop.* 2000;(372): 169–179.
9. American College of Obstetricians and Gynecologists (ACOG). ACOG technical bulletin #189: Exercise during pregnancy and the postpartum period. Washington, DC: ACOG Press, 1994.
10. American College of Obstetricians and Gynecologists (ACOG) committee opinion. Exercise during pregnancy and the postpartum period. 2002;267: 37–39.
11. Lindblom L. Exercise during pregnancy. *Physician Sportsmed.* 1997;25:28e, 28i–j, 281.
12. Wang TW, Apgar BS. Exercise during pregnancy. *Am Fam Physician.* 1998;57(8): 1846–1854.
13. *Guide to Physical Therapist Practice.* Alexandria, VA. American Physical Therapy Association, 1999.
14. Crossley K, Bennell K, Green S, McConnell J. A systematic review of physical interventions for patellofemoral pain syndrome. *Clin J Sport Med.* 2001;11(2): 103–110.
15. Herrington L. The effect of patellofemoral joint taping. *Critical Rev Phys Rehab Med.* 2000;12(3): 271–276.
16. McConnell J. The physical therapist's approach to patellofemoral disorders. *Clin Sports Med.* 2002; 21(3):363–387.
17. Salisch GB, Brechter JH, Farwell D, Powers CM. The effects of patellar taping on knee kinetics, kine-

matics and vastus lateralis muscle activity during stair ambulation in individuals with patellofemoral pain. *J Orthop Sports Phys Ther*. 2002;32(1):3–10.

18. Tang SF, Chen CK, Hsu R, et al. Vastus medialis obliquus and vastus lateralis activity in open and closed kinetic chain exercises in patients with patellofemoral pain syndrome: An electromyographic study. *Arch Phys Med Rehabil*. 2001; 82(10): 1441–1445.

19. Witvrouw E, Lysens R, Bellemans J, et al. Open versus closed kinetic chain exercises for patellofemoral pain: A prospective, randomized study. *Am J Sports Med*. 2000; 28(5): 687–694.

20. Rancho Los Amigos National Rehabilitation Center. *Observational Gait Analysis*. Downey, CA: Los Amigos Research and Education Institute, Inc., 2001.

21. Kendall FP, McCreary EK, Provance PG. *Muscles: Testing and Function*, 4th ed. Baltimore, MD: Williams & Wilkins, 1993.

22. Eastlack ME, Arvidson J, Snyder-Mackler L, et al. Interrater reliability of videotaped observational gait-analysis assessments. *Phys Ther*. 1991;71(6): 465–472.

Author's Comments A

Musculoskeletal concerns center around the patellofemoral problems that Susan is experiencing. It appears that she has a positive history for similar complaints. Physical examination has revealed the following impairments: lower extremity biomechanical alignment issues, patellofemoral joint pain/irritability with active knee extension although range of motion is full, vastus medialis oblique atrophy and diminished strength of the right quadriceps, bilateral hamstring extensibility deficits (right more so than left), bilateral iliotibial band extensibility deficits, and possible patellar instability/hypermobility on the right. Her functional deficits include difficulty with sit-to-stand movements, ascending and descending stairs, and running.

Author's Comments B

Given Susan's first trimester pregnancy status, there may be concern regarding her therapeutic exercise prescription. When a woman becomes pregnant, multiple hormonal and physiological changes occur. These changes may facilitate new musculoskeletal complaints (the most common being low back pain) or exacerbate pre-existing conditions. The possibility of increased capsuloligamentous joint laxity in the pregnant client must also be considered. The hormones relaxin and progesterone are believed to contribute to increased joint laxity during pregnancy (see Chapters 3 and 6). Some studies suggest that the majority of joint laxity increases occur early during the pregnancy,[2,3] although no studies to date have been related to

laxity at the patellofemoral joint. Although capsuloligamentous laxity increases during pregnancy[3] there are no published reports of injury related to exercise during pregnancy.[4] In fact, regular exercise during pregnancy has been shown to improve fitness and reduce musculoskeletal complaints due to pregnancy while helping to control maternal weight gain and fat deposition during the later stages.[4–6] Additionally, the combination of a shifting center of mass location and joint laxity may contribute to a neuromuscular balance impairment (see Chapter 9).

Therapeutic exercise recommendations both for aerobic fitness and for Susan's musculoskeletal concerns must be addressed with consideration of changes that occur throughout her pregnancy. Even treatment of a musculoskeletal condition as common as patellofemoral joint pain must take into consideration the potential effects on both the mother and the fetus. Additionally, if the therapeutic exercises selected to maintain her musculoskeletal and cardiopulmonary system fitness also helps her maintain or improve her standing balance, they would be providing another important benefit. Lower extremity therapeutic exercise selections although not considered "weight training" must be chosen with caution in terms of both volume (intensity, frequency) and posture.

Although Susan desires to continue her fitness program throughout the pregnancy, modifications are required. Approximately one-fourth of women planning a pregnancy participate in some form of strenuous activity such as aerobics, running, or stair climbing. Many of these fitness oriented women wish to continue their exercise regimen during pregnancy while following recommended guidelines for safe maternal and fetal participation.[7]

When advising a pregnant woman about therapeutic exercise it is important to first determine her level of fitness before conception.[8] Many physicians used to recommend that females not begin an exercise routine or that they diminish the level of their current routine when they become pregnant. Contemporary reports however suggest that beginning or continuing a regular program of exercise during pregnancy is safe and beneficial for the average, healthy woman.[7] The American College of Obstetricians and Gynecologists (ACOG) provides *Guidelines for Exercise During Pregnancy* that are useful for the rehabilitation clinician who wishes to provide safe therapeutic exercise suggestions to the pregnant female.[9] These guidelines are as follows:

- In the absence of medical or obstetric complications, pregnant women can perform moderate exercise for 30 minutes or more daily.
- Women with uncomplicated pregnancies can remain active, however they should modify their usual exercise routines as medically indicated.
- Pregnant women who exercise should augment heat dissipation by providing adequate hydration, wearing

appropriate clothing, and by selecting an optimal exercise environment (comfortable temperature and humidity.) This is of particular importance during the first trimester.

- Pregnant women who exercise should maintain metabolic homeostasis by ensuring an adequate diet.

- Previously inactive pregnant women and those with medical or obstetric complications should be evaluated before physical activity recommendations are made. Physically active pregnant women with a history of, or risk for pre-term labor or restricted fetal growth should reduce their exercise activities during the second and third trimester.

- After the first trimester, the supine position and motionless standing creates relative obstruction of venous return, which decreases cardiac output and promotes orthostatic hypotension. Pregnant women should avoid performing exercises in the supine position or maintaining a prolonged motionless standing posture.

- Pregnant women should not participate in recreational sports that present a high risk of falling or contact. Morphologic changes during pregnancy should serve as a relative contraindication to exercise in which balance loss could be detrimental to maternal or fetal well being, especially in the third trimester.

- After giving birth, pre-pregnancy exercise programs may be resumed gradually as soon as they are deemed to be physically and medically safe. Stress relieving physical activities performed after pregnancy may help to decrease the incidence of postpartum depression.

Absolute Contraindications	Relative Contraindications	Warning Signs to Terminate Exercise While Pregnant
• Hemodynamically significant heart disease • Restrictive lung disease • Incompetent cervix/cerclage • Multiple gestation at risk for premature labor • Persistent second- or third-trimester bleeding • Placenta previa after 26 weeks of gestation • Premature labor during the current pregnancy • Ruptured membranes • Preeclampsia/pregnancy-induced hypertension	• Severe anemia • Unevaluated maternal cardiac arrhythmia • Chronic bronchitis • Poorly controlled type 1 diabetes • Extreme morbid obesity • Extreme underweight (BMI<12) • History of extremely sedentary lifestyle • Intrauterine growth restriction in current pregnancy • Poorly controlled hypertension • Orthopaedic limitations • Poorly controlled seizure disorder • Poorly controlled hyperthyroidism • Heavy smoker	• Vaginal bleeding • Dyspnea prior to exertion • Dizziness • Headache • Chest pain • Muscle weakness • Calf pain or swelling (need to rule out thrombophlebitis) • Preterm labor • Decreased fetal movement • Amniotic fluid leakage

(Used with permission from the ACOG Committee on Obstetric Practice. Committee Opinion: Exercise during pregnancy and the postpartum period. 2002;267:37–39)

Many of the recommendations from ACOG address cardiopulmonary and thermal concerns with aerobic exercise as well as suggested exercise positions and morphologic changes that occur during pregnancy that could impact both aerobic and anerobic exercise program performance. Extensive cardiopulmonary system changes occur throughout pregnancy. The heart rate of the pregnant female increases 10–15 bpm, average blood volume increases approximately 45%, and cardiac output also increases, being significantly affected by the position of the pregnant client.[8]

Intensity and aerobic exercise mode are important considerations during pregnancy because resting oxygen requirements are increased. Pregnant females display a greater oxygen cost during weight bearing activities compared to non-pregnant females.[11] Therefore, a pregnant woman must adjust her exercise intensity accordingly. In regard to exercise mode, walking is the most popular exercise during pregnancy (43%).[6] Weight bearing exercises that display excessive vertical ground reaction forces, such as running, become more difficult as a woman's body weight increases throughout pregnancy. Most women report greater discomfort with exercise during the later stages of pregnancy.[12] A study of well trained runners demonstrated a decline in all aspects of performance during pregnancy.[5]

Exercise conditions that could cause hyperthermia are also to be avoided during pregnancy. This is due to the fact that hyperthermia increases oxygen demands, and may be associated with neural tube defects that occur early in pregnancy. Pregnant women who exercise must ensure adequate hydration and ventilation to allow for proper heat dissipation.

Author's Comments C

Prevention			Preferred practice pattern (PPP)	Rationale
1°	2°	3°		
	X		Musculoskeletal	Right knee patellofemoral aggravation
			Neuromuscular	
X			Cardiopulmonary	Provide appropriate exercise to avoid stress to mother and fetus during pregnancy
			Integumentary	

Primary (1°) prevention, defined by the *Guide to Physical Therapist Practice*[13] as "preventing a target condition in a susceptible population through such measures as general health promotion," may apply to Susan. We seek to have Susan prevent excessive weight gain and hyperthermic events while utilizing proper techniques and forms of therapeutic exercise throughout her pregnancy. Both of these primary prevention goals can be achieved by educating Susan, who is already very fitness conscious.

Secondary (2°) prevention—PPP 4D, Impaired joint mobility, motor function, muscle performance, and range of motion associated with connective tissue dysfunction.[13] By treating right knee patellofemoral joint dysfunction, we wish not only to decrease the duration and severity of the problem, but to address underlying biomechanical factors in order to prevent functional performance deficits and additional sequelae. The therapeutic exercise program planner's efforts are directed toward decreasing the duration, severity, and/or sequelae of the existing knee pain and recurrent patellofemoral dysfunction, through prompt and appropriate intervention.

Author's Comments D

Problem List

1. Biomechanical malalignment at lower extremities, pes planus feet right > left
2. Right knee vastus medialis oblique atrophy and quadriceps weakness
3. Reduced single leg standing balance (right)
4. Reduced bilateral knee flexor extensibility
5. Reduced bilateral iliotibial band extensibility
6. Right knee patellar hypermobility (lateral)
7. Right knee pain with sit-to-stand movements, ascending and descending stairs, and yard work, particularly squatting
8. Decreased ability to perform desired level of running

Author's Comments E

Short term: By the end of 4 weeks the client should be able to:

1. Run distances of 1.5–2.5 miles, with less than or equal to 3/10 patellofemoral pain when using patellar tape and lower extremity orthotics
2. Demonstrate 5/5 right quadriceps strength to enable pain free sit-to-stand movements and stair ascending and descending
3. Improve bilateral single leg standing balance to 20 second duration to increase safety during locomotion on all surfaces
4. Display pain free sit-to-stand movements and stair climbing while using patellar tape and orthotics
5. Increase bilateral knee flexor extensibility by 15° and iliotibial band extensibility to minimal restriction to decrease anterior knee pain during stair ascending and descending, and running
6. Decrease anterior knee pain during ADLs to 0/10, while using patellar tape and orthotics.

Author's Comments F

Long term: By 6–8 weeks the client should be able to:

1. Describe safe and appropriate alternate therapeutic exercises (i.e., no supine exercise after the 20th week) for later stages of pregnancy.
2. Verbalize the importance of exercising safely in terms of proper hydration and environmental conditions to avoid hyperthermia.
3. Return to running distances of 2–4 miles without right knee pain, and without the use of patellar tape.
4. Maintain a baseline level of aerobic fitness during the duration of her pregnancy with appropriate substitution of low impact aerobic exercises when running becomes difficult.

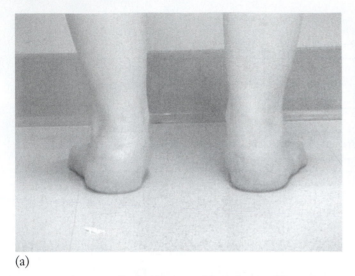

(a)

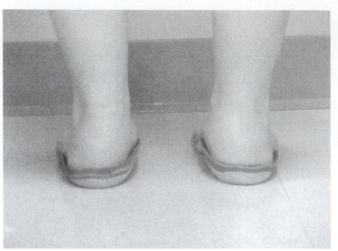

(b)

Case Figure 7.2   Orthotics. pre-(a) and post-(b).

Of particular concern in this section is identifying appropriate therapeutic exercise choices/substitutions that provide both the positive benefits of exercise that Susan is used to, but also maintain an appropriate level of maternal and fetal health throughout her pregnancy. Research on pregnant females suggests that as body weight increases, joint laxity increases, and center of gravity changes occur that affect balance. Less impact during exercise may be required.[2,4,9] For a recreational athlete such as Susan, this decision will be made with her personal physician based on the medical progression of her pregnancy. Switching to walking or swimming/aquatic exercise may be beneficial.

Note: Prior to exercising and activity modifications, I would have Susan fit for custom semi-rigid orthotics to control her arches and assist with maintaining appropriate lower extremity alignment to reduce her patellofemoral joint symptoms (**Case Figure 7.2a–b**). Additionally, I would verify that she is using correct footwear for the sport/activity she is performing; at this point in the case a good cross training or running shoe would be ideal to provide shock absorption and support for her pes planus feet.

Author's Comments G

Exercise order	Exercise selection	Body region	Rationale for inclusion
1	Volitionally low intensity stationary cycling	Whole body	Increase core body temperature for stretching warm-up
2	Static hamstring stretches in supine	Posterior Thigh/Hip	Improve hamstring extensibility
3	Static iliotibial band stretches in sidelying	Lateral Thigh/Hip	Improve iliotibial band extensibility
4	Manual medial patellar glides followed by medial patellar taping. Tape to be worn daily during all waking hours and during therapeutic exercises (**Case Figure 7.3**)(see Chapter 6)	Patellofemoral joint	Improve patellar alignment, stretch lateral retinaculum
5	Seated isometric quadriceps setting exercise with knee positioned in 15° flexion on bolster	Knee joint	Improve isometric quadriceps femoris strength

(continued)

Exercise order	Exercise selection	Body region	Rationale for inclusion
6	Four-way straight leg raise exercise (hip flexion, abduction, adduction, extension)	Hip and knee joints	Improve dynamic hip musculature strength and isometric knee musculature strength
7	Standing mini-squats to approximately 60° knee flexion (● Section 8, Animation 1)	Hip, knee and ankle joints	Improve dynamic hip, knee and ankle musculature strength in weight bearing
8	Multi-directional lunges (star diagram)(Case Figure 7.4a–c)	Hip, knee and ankle joints	Improve dynamic hip, knee and ankle musculature strength in weight bearing
9	Stationary cycling	Whole body	Aerobic system work-out, substitute for jogging*

*Please note: Susan will be allowed to run one mile, 3 times/week if she is completely pain-free. During running activities she will be instructed to use patellar tape and to use orthotics in her running shoes to help control her pes planus foot biomechanics.

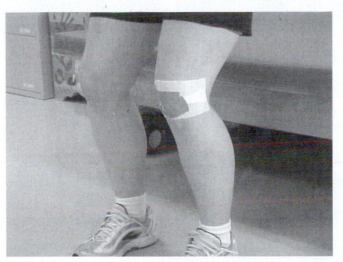

Case Figure 7.3   Use of patellofemoral tape to correct patella alignment during exercise and functional activities.

Author's Comments H

Exercise order	Sets/ repetitions	Intensity	Rest-to-work ratio	Frequency/ week
1	1 set, 8–10 min	Volitional low intensity	Not applicable (warm-up activity)	Daily
2	1 set, 4 repetitions, each for 20 sec. (perform bilaterally in alternating progression)	Low intensity, long duration static stretch	Not applicable (warm-up activity)	Daily

(continued)

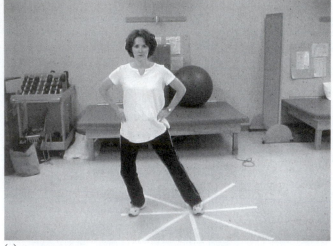

(a)

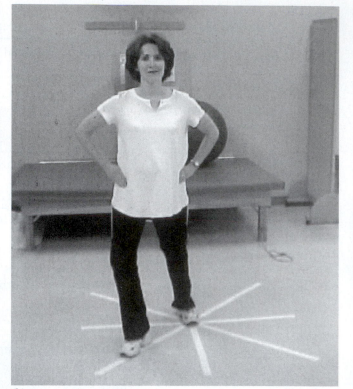

(b)

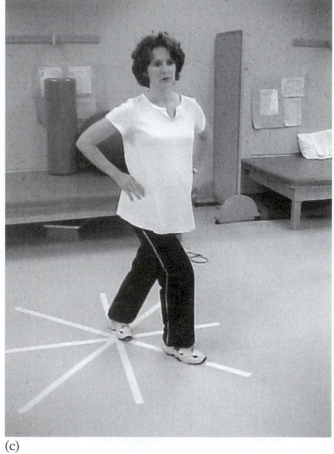

(c)

Case Figure 7.4   Star diagram. (a) side lunge; (b) diagonal lunge; (c) crossover lunge.

Exercise order	Sets/ repetitions	Intensity	Rest-to-work ratio	Frequency/ week
3	1 set, 4 repetitions, each for 20 sec. (performbilaterally in alternating progression)	Low intensity, long duration static stretch	Not applicable (warm-up activity)	Daily
4	1 set, 4 repetitions, eachfor 20 sec. (performbilaterally in alternating progression)	Low intensity, long duration static stretch	Not applicable (warm-up activity)	Daily
5	3 sets of 10 repetitions, each held for 10 sec.	Volitionally maximal effort with concentration on vastus medialis muscle activation	2:1	Daily
6	2 sets of 10 repetitions for each movement	Set 1 = 25% of 1 repetition maximum; set 2 = 50% of 1 repetition maximum	3:1	3 times/week
7	3 sets of 8–12 repetitions	Set 1 = Without additional resistance, hold each repetition for 10 sec.; set 2 = perform with moderate elastic band resistance under both feet; set 3 = perform only with the right lower extremity	3:1	3 times/week
8	1 set of 10 repetitions each direction	Body weight resistance, stepping distance as tolerated with appropriate lower extremity alignment	2:1	Daily
9	25–30 minutes	One set, adjusted to 70% recommended heart rate maximum	1:1	3 times/week

Remember that your program may vary from this example. What should not vary, however, are the links that you establish between key problems, functionally relevant treatment goals, and the scientific rationale used to support your therapeutic exercise prescription. Susan's history and physical examination findings suggest that biomechanical intervention for her pes planus feet is indicated to help improve lower extremity alignment in an effort to improve her patellofemoral joint dysfunction. Significant decreases in patellofemoral pain symptoms have been reported with the use of corrective foot orthotics.[14] Resistance training to strengthen the quadriceps of her right lower extremity is also indicated. Although not completely understood in terms of how it affects the patellofemoral joint, Susan may benefit from McConnell taping of the right patellofemoral joint to decrease the knee pain she experiences during exercise.[15–17] By decreasing her pain, providing alternate sensory input, and modifying the activation timing of the medial and lateral quadriceps, taping may allow her to effectively strengthen the right quadriceps, enabling her to ascend and descend stairs and perform sit-to-stand activities more easily. Much of the current literature suggests that closed kinetic chain or weight bearing activities are helpful for developing quadriceps femoris control, while lessening patellofemoral joint reaction forces compared to open kinetic chain exercises such as the seated knee extension exercise.[18,19]

Activities designed to improve bilateral hamstring and iliotibial band extensibility are also indicated. Exercise tasks that maintain her aerobic energy system capacity are indicated, within guidelines for a pregnant woman. At this stage of her pregnancy, running is acceptable, unless her patellofemoral pain prohibits it. If patellar pain limits Susan's ability to run, substitute aerobic fitness tasks with lesser impact forces (such as cycling, elliptical training, and walking) than those imposed by jogging could be performed. Based on these considerations the following program has been proposed.

Author's Comments I

Several objective clinical measurements that might be utilized to assess Susan:

1. Assess single lower extremity stance and dynamic walking with use of orthotics[20]
2. Manual muscle testing (with or without a handheld dynamometer) or isokinetic test of knee extensor-flexor strength[21]
3. Visual analog scale for pain at rest and during specific functional activities (stair ascending or descending, sit-to-stand movements, running)
4. Ober's test (using a measuring tape to measure the distance between the medial knee joint and the treatment table surface) and hamstring extensibility (measured with a goniometer)[1]
5. Video taped running assessment (frontal and sagittal planes)[22]

Author's Comments J

Re-evaluation has confirmed that Susan has reached most of her short term goals, with the exception of returning to running at the level she desires. With substantial improvements in right lower extremity strength, extensibility and function without pain, the therapeutic exercise program should be modified to address her long term goal of running throughout her pregnancy. Daily patellar taping for all ADLs can be discontinued; Susan will now only tape before she goes running. We must address exercise position (avoidance of supine or prolonged standing positions after the first trimester). Susan remains enthusiastic and committed to running as a form of aerobic exercise during the remaining months of her pregnancy, "until I just feel too big or get too uncomfortable."

In modifying Susan's therapeutic exercise program to include more weight bearing activities and eliminating the supine, or static standing posture activities, we have an opportunity to assist her in returning to her desired level of running as well as providing safe, progressive challenges to standing balance (see Chapter 9) as her body weight increases and her center of gravity changes throughout pregnancy. Based on the progress she has made in the first four weeks of her program she can be given more advanced exercises.

Exercise order	Exercise selection	Modification
1	Static hamstring stretches	Switch position to standing with neutral lumbar spine position
2	Static iliotibial band stretches	Switch position to standing with neutral lumbar spine position
3	Add static gastrocnemius-soleus muscle stretches to maintain extensibility and prevent the calf cramping common to pregnant women (**Case Figure 7.5**).	

(continued)

Exercise order	Exercise selection	Modification
4	Change from horizontal straight leg raise movements to "steamboats" with moderate elastic band or tubing resistance (**Case Figure 7.6a–b**).	Straight leg raises performed in weight bearing that works on neuromuscular strengthening of both the moving and weight bearing lower extremity in addition to dynamic trunk stabilization and standing balance. Susan should discontinue supine position exercises during this phase of her pregnancy
5	Standing unilateral squats on a 6-inch step to approximately 60° knee flexion.	Increased vertical dimension, increased balance challenge. Attempts to maximize quadriceps femoris activation[18]
6	Continued instruction/counseling about proper hydration and alternative lower impact therapeutic exercises foms*	

*Issue written information about alternate exercise possibilities (biking, aquatic exercises, walking) as well as appropriate hydration and hyperthermia prevention. Based on ACOG guidelines and her medical progression throughout her pregnancy, Susan and her physician will decide when running is prohibited. She will have an understanding of possible alternative aerobic exercise alternatives to replace running when it becomes prohibited for her.

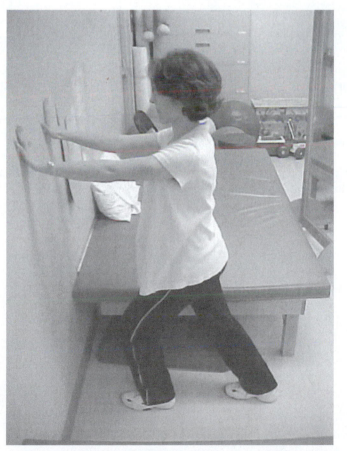

Case Figure 7.5   Standing static calf stretch (bent knee for soleus, straight knee for gastrocnemius).

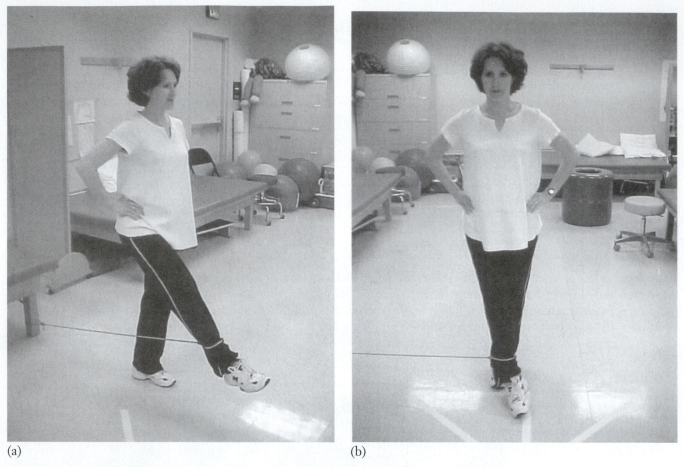

(a)

(b)

Case Figure 7.6   "Steamboat" exercise. hip flexion (a) and hip adduction (b).

Special attention should be paid to hydration issues for Susan as this relates to maintaining proper body temperature. She should ingest water regularly before, during, and after exercise. Additionally, she should be instructed in the differences between indoor and outdoor exercise and the relative influence of each on body temperature (relates to ambient temperature and humidity in the exercise environment) (see Chapter 4).

Author's Comments K

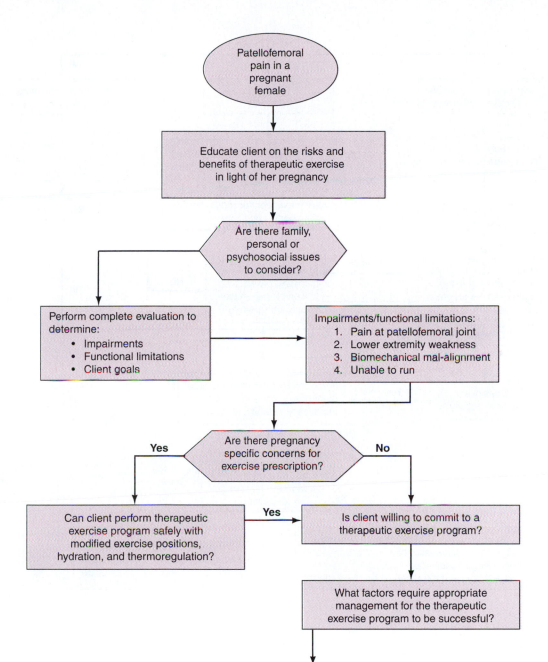

Author's Comments K (con't)

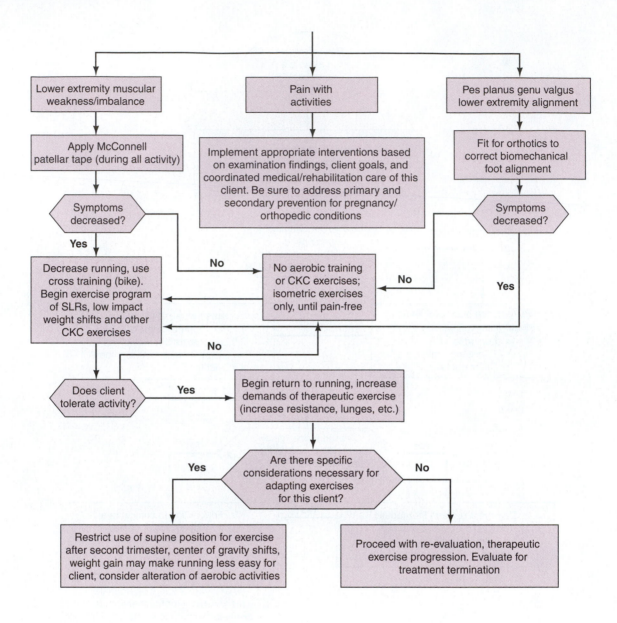

Client Case #8

Ann M. Swartz

History

Client: Matt

Age: 18 years

Height: 5'7 1/2" (172.7 cm)

Weight: 266 lbs (120.5 kg)

Education: High school graduate

Occupation: Student (freshman in college)

Medical/Surgical History: History of obesity, dyslipidemia (high triglyceride levels and low high density lipoprotein cholesterol [HDL-C] levels). *Impaired glucose tolerance* diagnosed (reduced capacity to use glucose, elevated blood glucose levels, related to pre-diabetes mellitus) and *Stage I hypertension* (elevated normal blood pressure) were diagnosed 12 months ago.[1-5] Physician has prescribed diet and therapeutic exercise to improve obesity, *dyslipidemia* (abnormal concentration of lipids or lipoproteins in the blood), impaired glucose tolerance, and hypertension. Non-smoker

Medications: Ibuprofen for pain and inflammation

Exercise/ Activity History: No formal exercise history. Minimal occupational, leisure-time, transportation, or household physical activity. Primary hobby: computers, "surfing" the internet, computer games

Chief Complaint: Chronic pain in his lower back, which prohibits him from participating in certain activities

Matt (**Case Figure 8.1**) went to see his physician last year because his mother was concerned about his health. During the exam Matt expressed to his physician that he was feeling tired all the time and he was stressed at school because he was constantly teased for being "fat." The physician diagnosed him with dyslipidemia (total cholesterol = 210 mg/dL; HDL-C = 28 mg/dL; triglycerides = 388 mg/dL), impaired fasting glucose and impaired glucose tolerance (fasting plasma glucose (FPG) = 106 mg/dL; two-hour glucose level = 180 mg/dL after a 75 g oral glucose tolerance test),[1-4] and stage I hypertension (142/96 mm Hg).[5] His physician was very concerned because he is so young and already developing the metabolic syndrome. The physician recommended he lose some weight and prescribed diet and exercise as his treatment. He provided him with written information on diet and exercise and recommended he come back to see him in a year.

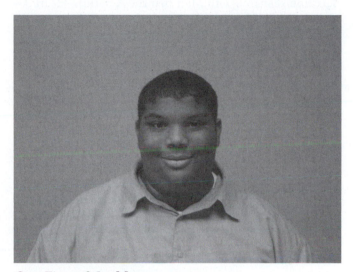

Case Figure 8.1 Matt.

Matt and his mother decided to try to diet together; after all, dieting is easier with a partner. Matt and his mother began to eat healthier, smaller portions, and began to take 45 minute walks together every night. They were doing very well: Matt had lost 25 pounds, he was feeling much better, had more energy and more self-confidence. However, autumn arrived, the weather was turning colder and the holidays were approaching. Over time the walks had stopped, and the diet was forgotten. The weight came back.

A year later, Matt visited his physician again. Little had changed. His weight was up by five pounds and his dyslipidemia, impaired glucose tolerance, and stage I hypertension were still present. In addition, he was complaining of a dull, constant pain in his lower back. He thinks he "pulled a muscle" when moving heavy boxes into his college dormitory room. The physician had x-rays taken and they were negative. The physician referred Matt to you for treatment of his low back pain, and exercise recommendations to aid in weight loss, as well as to help improve his cholesterol, glucose and blood pressure levels. He also referred Matt to a nutritionist on campus for dietary counseling. He warned Matt of all the complications he could encounter if he does not become more active and lose some weight.

Before coming to see you Matt talked with a nutritionist on campus. The nutritionist discussed his current diet with him. He pointed out that Matt was eating far too many high fat foods such as chicken wings, pizza and potato chips. Many of the foods Matt consumes are also high in sodium, which further contributes to high blood pressure. The nutritionist also pointed out how few fruits and vegetables Matt consumed. They talked about the nutritional value of these foods (see Chapter 2), and how important vitamins and minerals are to health. Finally, the nutritionist shared with Matt that the American Heart Association and other health authorities recommend that dietary cholesterol be limited to an average of 300 mg or less per day, and that total fat intake should represent no more than 30% of total daily caloric intake and saturated fat no more than 10% of total daily caloric intake.[6,7] In addition, they discussed the latest Dietary Guidelines for Americans[8,9] and discussed each of the three sections with Matt: 1) aim for fitness, 2) build a healthy base, and 3) choose sensibly. They talked about Matt's current habits compared with the national guidelines, discussed what he needed to change and finally discussed some strategies to make the needed changes.

During the same week, Matt visits your clinic for an evaluation and a therapeutic exercise consultation. When you meet him in the lobby, you notice he winces as he stands up from the chair. You also notice his lack of enthusiasm, and very slow walking pace.

Upon evaluation, you conclude the pain is located in the low back, buttock region and all radicular signs are negative. The quality of pain is described as an ache with three or four slight muscle spasms experienced per day. The pain increases with activity or bending; there is local tenderness and limited spinal motion. Matt is currently taking ibuprofen, as prescribed by his physician to help with the inflammation and pain. His physician told him to keep moving around, not to lie in bed, but to modify his current activities to avoid pain.

Having reviewed the referral from the physician, you decide the evaluation should focus on improving the strength and endurance of the trunk musculature (see Chapters 5 and 6), and increasing activity levels to aid in weight loss. During the initial physical examination the following information is collected:

Physical Examination

Resting Blood Pressure: 144/92 mm Hg

Resting Heart Rate: 84 bpm

Height: 173 cm (5'7 1/2'')

Weight: 120.5 kg (266 lbs)

Body Mass Index score (BMI):   40.3

Body fat (bioelectrical impedance analysis):   46%

Deep Tendon Reflexes: +2, equal bilaterally at patellar and Achilles tendons

Straight Leg Raise Test: Negative bilaterally

Maximal Aerobic Capacity: Not performed due to low back pain.

A. Based on the information noted above, make a list of Matt's current health problems.[1-5] *See Author's Comments A*

B. Given your assessment of his health problems, what is your primary focus for Matt's therapeutic exercise prescription? *See Author's Comments B*

C. What would your secondary focus be for Matt's therapeutic exercise prescription? *See Author's Comments C*

D. Do you have any concerns regarding the back pain that Matt is experiencing? How might it influence your therapeutic exercise prescription? *See Author's Comments D*

E. What are your concerns regarding the existing state of obesity and the therapeutic exercise prescription that you are designing for Matt?[10,11] *See Author's Comments E*

F. What are your concerns regarding existing or potential cardiovascular or cardiopulmonary system impairments and the therapeutic exercise program that you are designing for Matt? *See Author's Comments F*

G. What steps do you plan on implementing to ensure that Matt complies with your therapeutic exercise program, keeping in mind his brief history with exercise?[12] *See Author's Comments G*

H. Based upon the information provided, make a list of three to six short term (≤ 4 weeks) therapeutic exercise program goals by completing the following statement:[13,14]

"By 4 weeks, the client . . ."

Make another list of three to six long term (5–12 weeks) therapeutic exercise program goals by completing the statement
"By 5 to 12 weeks, the client . . ." *See Author's Comments H*

Activity and Exercise Program

This three-stage program (low back pain/dysfunction intervention, lifestyle activity modification, independent therapeutic exercise program participation) will be regularly modified based on Matt's condition and compliance. Remember, this is a program that you want Matt to succeed with whether he is in your clinic, at school, or at home. Therefore, the therapeutic exercises and activities you recommend need to be suitable for your client to perform without special equipment or facilities.

Stage 1

Alleviate back pain and increase strength of abdominal and back muscles (see Chapters 5 and 6). The length of this stage will depend on the presence or absence of any acute pain symptoms that Matt experiences at his low back region. This stage may be as short as 2 weeks in duration or as long as 12 weeks.

I. Based on your decisions, describe the stage I therapeutic exercise program. Create and complete a table with column headings: exercise order, exercise selection, rationale, and repetitions/sets/frequency.

Stage 2

During this stage we would like to increase healthy lifestyle activities. Again, the length of this stage will vary, depending on Matt's condition and compliance. Before continuing to this phase of Matt's therapeutic exercise program, it would be beneficial to perform a graded exercise test to determine safety and cardiovascular, cardiopulmonary, and metabolic responses to exercise (see Chapter 4).

J. What mode of exercise would you choose for the graded exercise test? What type of protocol would you choose? What information do you want before testing Matt? *See Author's Comments J*

The results from the maximal graded exercise test are:

Maximal Heart Rate: 198 bpm
ECG: no significant changes
Maximal Blood Pressure: 204/94 mm Hg

Maximal Rating of Perceived Exertion (RPE):   20
  (on a 6 to 20 scale)
  Comments: Matt complained of leg cramps and he was out of breath at the end of the test

The physician agreed with you that Matt could be cleared for therapeutic exercise program and activity participation.

K. Based on your knowledge, describe the stage 2 activity plan:[3,15,16] *See Author's Comments K*

Stage 3

Formal, more independent therapeutic exercise program. Again, the length of this stage will vary and depend on Matt's condition and compliance.

L. Based on your decisions, describe the stage 3 therapeutic exercise plan. Create and complete a table with column headings: exercise selection (limit to warm-up, 3 exercises and cool-down action), intensity, duration, and frequency.[13,14] *See Author's Comments L*

M. On a separate sheet of paper, diagram a decision making algorithm for Matt's case based on primary and secondary therapeutic exercise considerations. *Author Comment M*

Referring to Chapter 10 for guidance, discuss any alternative or complementary therapeutic exercises that you believe might benefit this client. Provide the rationale for your suggestions.

Case Summary

Throughout the time you are working with Matt, you should re-assess him to ensure that he is getting the most benefit out of his activity/exercise program. It is important to explain theories of progression to him, and encourage him to adjust his program accordingly. However, re-evaluations by you, the rehabilitation clinician, would ideally occur at 4 weeks, 8 weeks, and 12 weeks, 6 months and one year. His program should be constantly evolving. You may find that some things work well, and some do not work at all. Encourage Matt to get more involved in activities on campus and to keep moving!

Useful Web Sites

American Heart Association	www.americanheart.org
Nutrition	www.nutrition.org
American College of Sports Medicine	www.acsm.org
Centers for Disease Control and Prevention	www.cdc.gov/health/physact.htm

References

1. Executive summary of the third report of the National Cholesterol Education Program (NCEP) expert panel on detection, evaluation, and treatment of high blood cholesterol in adults (adult treatment panel III). *JAMA*. 2001;285(19):2486–2497.

2. Executive summary of the clinical guidelines on the identification, evaluation, and treatment of overweight and obesity in adults. *Arch Int Med*. 1998; 158:1855–1867.

3. *ACSM's Guidelines for Exercise Testing and Prescription*, 6th ed. Philadelphia: Lippincott Williams & Wilkins, 2000.

4. Campaigne BN. Exercise and diabetes mellitus. In J Roitman, ed. *ACSM's Resource Manual for Guidelines for Exercise Testing and Prescription*, 3rd ed. Baltimore, MD: Williams & Wilkins, 1998, pp. 267–274.

5. Chobanian AV, Bakris GL, Black HR, et al. The Seventh Report of the Joint National Committee on Prevention, Detection, Evaluation, and Treatment of High Blood Pressure: the JNC 7 report. *JAMA*. 2003; 289:2560–2572.

6. American Heart Association Web site. http://www.americanheart.org.

7. Kris-Etherton P, Eckel RH, Howard BV, et al. Lyon diet heart study benefits of a Mediterranean-style, National Cholesterol Education Program/American Heart Association step I dietary pattern on cardiovascular disease. *Circulation*. 2001;103:1823–1825.

8. Krauss RM, Eckel RH, Howard B, et al. AHA dietary guidelines revision 2000: A statement for healthcare professionals from the nutrition committee of the American Heart Association. *Circulation*. 2000;102:2284–2299.

9. U.S. Department of Agriculture and U.S. Department of Health and Human Services Dietary Guidelines for Americans. Available at www.nutrition.gov. Accessed January 6, 2003.

10. Grilo C, Brownell K. Interventions for weight management. In J Roitman, ed. *ACSM's Resource Manual for Guidelines for Exercise Testing and Prescription*, 3rd ed. Baltimore, MD: Williams & Wilkins; 1998, pp. 570–577.

11. Han T, Schouten J, Lean M, Seidell J. The prevalence of low back pain and associations with body fatness, fat distribution and height. *Int J Obes Relat Metab Disord*. 1997;21:600–607.

12. Miller W, Koceja D, Hamilton E. A meta-analysis of the past 25 years of weight loss research using diet, exercise or diet plus exercise intervention. *Int J Obes Relat Metab Disord*. 1997;21:941–947.

13. Pate R, Pratt M, Blair S, et al. Physical activity and public health: A recommendation from the Centers for Disease Control and Prevention and the American College of Sports Medicine. *JAMA*. 1995;273: 402–407.

14. U.S. Department of Health and Human Services. *Physical Activity and Health: A Report of the Surgeon General*. Atlanta, GA: U.S. Department of Health and Human Services, Centers for Disease Control and Prevention, National Center for Chronic Disease Prevention and Health Promotion, 1996, p. 5.

15. Brubaker PH, Myers J. Cardiorespiratory assessment of high risk or disease populations. In J Roitman, ed. *ACSM's Resource Manual for Guidelines for Exercise Testing and Prescription*, 3rd ed. Baltimore, MD: Williams & Wilkins, 1998; pp.354–362.

16. Noonan V, Dean E. Submaximal exercise testing: Clinical application and interpretation. *Phys Ther*. 2000;80(8):782–807.

Author's Comments A

- Obesity: BMI = 39.4
  - Body mass index (BMI), or Quetelet index (calculated as weight in kilograms divided by height in meters squared [kg/m^2]), is used to assess weight relative to height. Although using BMI to determine classification of obesity is not ideal, this simple tool provides an indication of obesity level. For most individuals, obesity related health problems increase with a BMI of 25 and higher.[3] BMI classifications are as follows: underweight <18.5 kg/m^2; normal 18.5–24.9 kg/m^2; overweight 25.0–29.9 kg/m^2; obesity class I 30.0–34.9 kg/m^2; obesity class II 35.0–39.9 kg/m^2; obesity class III ≥ 40 kg/m^2.[1,3]
  - Dyslipidemia: Total cholesterol = 210 mg/dL; HDL = 28 mg/dL; triglycerides = 388 mg/dL
  - The Third Report of the National Cholesterol Education Program Expert Panel on Detection, Evaluation, and Treatment of High Blood Cholesterol in Adults[1] recommends a desirable total cholesterol level < 200 mg/dL, HDL cholesterol > 40 mg/dL, and triglycerides < 150 mg/dL. We do not have any information on LDL cholesterol, however; ideally, it should be below 100 mg/dL

- Impaired fasting plasma glucose (FPG) and impaired glucose tolerance: FPG = 106 mg/dL; 2-hour glucose = 180 mg/dL
  - Impaired glucose tolerance is now known as prediabetes. Having both impaired fasting plasma glucose and pre-diabetes puts Matt at significant risk for type 2 diabetes mellitus, which is a serious disease with many life-altering side effects
  - Normal fasting plasma glucose < 100 mg/dL; normal glucose tolerance: 2-hour glucose < 140 mg/dL
  - For a definitive diagnosis, either of these findings needs to be recorded on two separate occasions

- Hypertension = 142/96 mm Hg
  - Normal blood pressure: systolic blood pressure < 120 and diastolic blood pressure < 80 mmHg.[5]
  - For a true diagnosis, this finding needs to be recorded on two separate occasions.

- Metabolic syndrome
  - From the information we have on Matt, the metabolic syndrome is most likely in his future.
  - Clinical diagnosis of the metabolic syndrome includes the following risk factors:[1]
    - Abdominal obesity (by waist circumference): men >102 cm, women > 88 cm
    - Triglycerides ≥ 150 mg/dL
    - HDL cholesterol: men < 40 mg/dL, women < 50 mg/dL
    - Blood pressure ≥ 130/ ≥ 85 mm Hg
    - Fasting glucose ≥ 110 mg/dL
- Inactivity:
  - At this point in his life, Matt does not engage in any leisure time physical activity or structured exercise
  - Backache: Matt's chronic backache is preventing him from engaging in any activity. One method of evaluating his back pain is to take him through a number of flexion and extension exercises to determine the positions that reproduce the pain, what aggravates the pain and what does not. Knowing how he responds to the flexion and extension exercises will help you design a more effective therapeutic exercise program.

Author's Comments B

Once the diagnosis and the source of the back pain have been identified, the primary focus of the therapeutic exercise program should be alleviating the back pain and strengthening the abdominal musculature; however, Matt's chronic back condition should not dictate the entire therapeutic exercise program progression (see Chapter 11).

Author's Comments C

The secondary focus of the exercise program should begin after any acute pain symptoms have subsided and are no longer prohibiting Matt from performing activities. This part of the therapeutic exercise program should focus on increasing lifestyle activity levels in order to help improve his health (decrease obesity, improve hypertension, impaired glucose tolerance and dyslipidemia).

Author's Comments D

Further injury and prevention of future injuries. As a rehabilitation clinician, you want to prevent any further injury to the back and also prevent future injuries. Therefore, the back pain will be the first issue considered. After this condition is deemed to be subacute and non-progressive, then therapeutic exercises can be gradually included to increase the strength and endurance of the trunk musculature. In addition, a stretching program (see Chapter 3) will help increase flexibility. In general, thera-peutic exercise programs that facilitate weight loss (see Chapter 4), trunk strengthening (see Chapters 5 and 6), and the stretching of associated musculotendinous structures can also help alleviate low back pain.

Author's Comments E

- Additional weight is a consequence of a complex interaction of cultural, social, genetic, physiological, behavioral, and psychological factors.[10]
- The excess weight may also result in a negative body image. In addition, the inactivity could be the cause or the consequence of obesity. Therefore, the activity program must start slowly and incorporate behavioral change strategies to increase the likelihood of success (see Chapter 11). In addition, realistic goals must be set, starting with short term goals that lead up to a long term goal.
- Carrying around excess weight can increase the strain on joints. Therefore, low impact activity that involves large muscle groups is ideal. This kind of exercise will exert the least amount of stress on the joints while expending a large amount of kilocalories (see Chapters 4 and 5).
- Excess weight has a direct effect on the likelihood of developing low back pain, as well as an adverse effect on recovery from low back pain.[11]

Author's Comments F

Matt has many cardiovascular and cardiopulmonary system risk factors for exercise. Therefore, he should complete a graded exercise test to determine safety of exercise along with physician's clearance, which was already provided. A maximal exercise test should not be completed until his back condition has stabilized.

Author's Comments G

Matt has had very little experience with activity and/or exercise. He has never performed any formal exercise except for the walking program he attempted last year. He has always avoided activity; for example, he takes the bus to class instead of walking the half mile. He was successful with walking for a short while last year. However, in order for this lifestyle change to take place, an exercise or activity routine that Matt can stick with for the rest of his life needs to be implemented. You need to be enthusiastic and positive about the rewards of being active (see Chapter 11).

Matt sees exercise and activity as work, and feels exhausted after the exercise. He does not see exercise as being enjoyable and does not see much benefit in exercising. Emphasize to Matt that exercise is a key component in weight loss programs in which people succeed in keeping off the weight they have lost.[12] In addition, exercise can reduce his cardiovascular and cardiopulmonary system risk factors and thereby prevent his having to take medications in the near future to control his hypertension and dyslipidemia.

Author's Comments H

It is important that you and Matt create these goals together so that he will have some feeling of control and some vested interest in his therapeutic exercise program. It is important to create small, attainable goals.

Short Term Goals (based on initial problems):

By 4 weeks, the client . . .

1. Will decrease or eliminate back pain, so that he can begin to function normally and increase his activity level
2. Will improve his diet by decreasing the consumption of fried foods and junk foods such as potato chips, limiting to one item of junk food or fried food per day
3. Will reduce his caloric intake by 500 calories per day
4. Will reduce his dietary intake of saturated fat, cholesterol and sodium: < 30% of diet should be fat, with < 10% being saturated fat; < 300 mg of cholesterol; < 6 grams of salt per day (2,300 milligrams of sodium)
5. Will increase daily physical activity by walking to class and around campus instead of taking the bus
6. Will demonstrate independent, appropriate performance of initial therapeutic exercises for low back condition

Long Term Goals

By 5 to 12 weeks, the client . . .

1. Will lose one to two pounds per week until he gets to his goal weight (which will be decided on together by the client, rehabilitation clinician, and nutritionist)
2. Will maintain an active lifestyle by always walking to class and other places on campus instead of taking the bus and accumulating 30 minutes of moderate intensity activity on most, if not all, days of the week.[13,14]
3. Will achieve regular, independent participation in a therapeutic exercise program (minimum three days per week)
4. Will decrease resting blood pressure
5. Will improve glucose tolerance and fasting plasma glucose levels
6. Will reduce dyslipidemia indicator levels

Author's Comments I

Stage 1   Alleviate back pain and increase strength of abdominal and back muscles. The length of this stage will depend on Matt's recovery; it may be as short as 2 weeks or as long as 12 weeks. Static stretching should be performed on

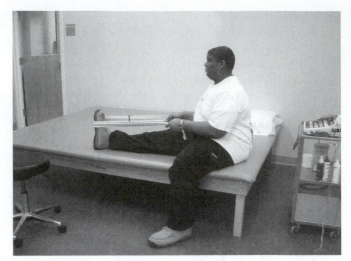

Case Figure 8.2   Long sitting static hamstring muscle group stretching with a strap.

a daily basis and the strengthening exercises should be performed every other day. It is very important that the rehabilitation clinician teach proper technique of each therapeutic exercise that is performed to prevent future injury. To begin a stretch, the client should begin in a relaxed position. Begin the stretch and move until the point in the range of motion where a sensation of mild muscular discomfort is felt. Hold the stretch for 20–30 seconds (see Chapter 3). All lower extremity stretches should be performed at both sides (**Case Figures 8.2–8.3**). If Matt is experiencing any pain that radiates down his lower extremity or if he experiences a loss of sensation, then his technique should be re-evaluated, and the intensity of the stretch may need to be decreased. Repeat experiences of these symptoms may necessitate that the selected stretch movement be discontinued. Additionally, active lumbar mobility exercises performed in a quadruped position may help restore

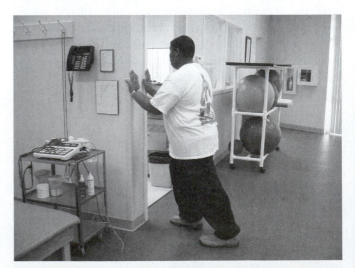

Case Figure 8.3   Standing static calf muscle stretching.

non-impaired pain-free mobility to this region (**Case Figure 8.4a–b**) (● **Section 9, Animation 1**). During these active movements, a hold period of 5 to 10 seconds is sufficient.

Although most of the therapeutic exercises designed to strengthen the low back region are performed on a low mat table, the rehabilitation clinician must be sure that Matt is in a stable body position before beginning the exercise. This initial stability increases the likelihood that Matt will maintain proper positioning throughout the movement. Make sure Matt moves through the full range of motion while performing posterior pelvic tilt exercises to improve abdominal strength and restore low back mobility (**Case Figure 8.5a–b**)(● **Section 9, Animation 2**), progressing to partial curl-ups (**Case Figure 8.6**) (● **Section 9, Animation 3**) and during the trunk extensor strengthening associated with alternating, contralateral upper and lower extremity raises from a quadruped position (**Case Figure 8.7**) (● **Section 9, Animation 4**) (see Chapters 5 and 6). Repetitions should be performed in a slow, controlled manner with proper breathing and body positioning emphasized with each exercise. In addition, watch for signs of muscle soreness, pain, or fatigue during and after each exercise session.

Exercise order	Exercise selection	Rationale	Repetitions/Sets/Frequency
1	Posterior pelvic tilt	Strengthen muscles of lower back and supporting musculature	Hold for 5–10 sec.; perform 3–5 times daily
2	Single knee to chest (single leg trunk flexion exercise)	Stretch muscles of lower back and supporting musculature	Hold for 30 sec.; perform 3–5 times daily
3	Double knee to chest (double leg trunk flexion exercise)	Stretch muscles of lower back and supporting musculature	Hold for 20–30 sec.; perform 3–5 times daily
4	Hamstring stretch	Stretch muscles of hip and posterior thigh	Hold for 30 sec.; perform 3–5 times daily
5	Total body extension in supine ("Superman")	Stretch abdominal muscles and strengthen back muscles	Hold for 5–10 sec.; perform 3–5 times daily
6	Abdominal crunch, partial curl-up	Strengthen abdominal musculature	3 sets of 8 repetitions, daily
7	Diagonal/oblique crunches	Strengthen abdominal musculature	3 sets of 8 repetitions, daily
8	Alternating single leg-arm lift while on hands and knees	Strengthen back musculature	5–10 repetitions; hold each for 5 sec. daily

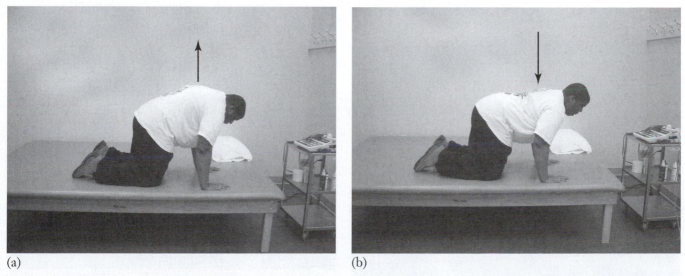

(a)   (b)

Case Figure 8.4   "Cat back – Camel back" exercise to increase active lumbar spine mobility. (a) Cat back phase; (b) Camel back phase.

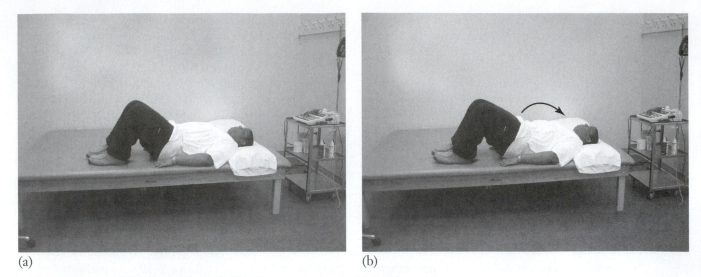

(a)   (b)

Case Figure 8.5   Posterior pelvic tilt. (a) starting position; (b) finish position.

Author's Comments J

Stage 2   Increasing activity levels. Again, the length of this stage will vary and will depend on Matt's compliance and commitment (see Chapter 11). Before continuing onto this phase of Matt's therapeutic exercise program it would be beneficial to perform a maximal graded exercise test to determine safety and cardiovascular, cardiopulmonary and metabolic responses to exercise. A good choice for the maximal exercise test would be a walking test because this is the mode of activity he will partake in the most. A standard protocol such as the Balke-Ware protocol[15,16] would be a good choice because it begins at a low metabolic level and is a walking protocol. Noonan and Dean[16] have also presented a thorough review of submaximal effort graded exercise test options. Information

you would want to collect or compute before testing Matt includes any risk factors. Based on the sixth edition of the American College of Sports Medicine Guidelines for Exercise Testing and Prescription,[3] Matt would be categorized as a "moderate risk" because he meets the threshold for two or more coronary artery disease risk factors and therefore it is recommended that you have a physician present during the test. In addition, you should calculate his estimated maximal heart rate (220−age). This estimation, along with RPE information, will give you an indication of when Matt is approaching his maximal effort. You will also want to record an electrocardiogram (ECG) including heart rate and blood pressures at every stage, or minimally at every other stage, throughout the exercise test. Finally, you will want to monitor Matt closely after the exercise test, recording 12-lead ECG strips and blood

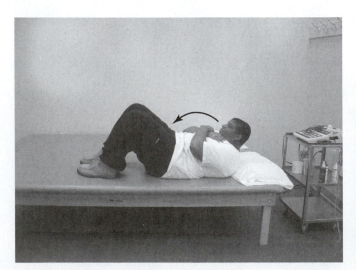

Case Figure 8.6   Partial curl-up exercise.

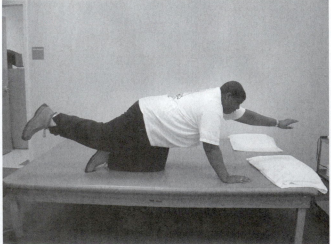

Case Figure 8.7   Alternating contralateral upper and lower extremity lift from a quadruped position.

pressure at one- or two-minute intervals during the recovery period.[3]

Author's Comments K

The therapeutic exercise program for this stage will be based on the American College of Sports Medicine-Center for Disease Control lifestyle recommendation[13,14] that "all adults perform 30 or more minutes of moderate-intensity physical activity on most, and preferably all, days of the week, either in a single session or accumulated in multiple bouts, each lasting at least 8–10 minutes." Therefore, Matt can begin by performing three, 10-minute segments of moderate intensity activity, within the first month, increase to a continuous duration of 30 minutes, and then continue to increase the duration and intensity. It is important to discuss the importance of a warm-up and cool-down before and after activity (see Chapter 3). You may wish to discuss methods of behavior change with Matt, and emphasize that this is a change he needs to make for the rest of his life, to become a more active person (see Chapter 11). Inform him of different techniques and strategies used to aid behavior change, such as scheduling the activity into his daily routine and taking "small steps" towards his ultimate goal. Encourage him to try different strategies to find the best one for him.

Also, mention to him that walking (**Case Figure 8.8**) and stationary cycling (**Case Figure 8.9**) are not his only options; home repair, gardening, yard work, and recreational games played outside are also options. Matt has mentioned that he enjoys walking around campus (**Case Figure 8.10**). So your initial suggestion could include walking to class instead of taking the bus, thereby incorporating the activity into his life. Using the data from the graded exercise test, you explain to Matt what "moderate intensity" activity means (50–69 percent maximal heart rate range = 99–137 bpm).[14] You teach Matt how to take

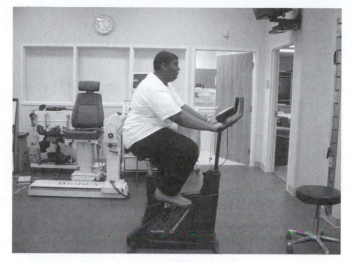

Case Figure 8.9   Stationary bike workout.

his heart rate and also explain alternative, but less precise, methods to determine intensity such as the *talk test* and the RPE scale (moderate RPE = 11–12).[14] Before he begins this section of his lifestyle activity program, you need to make sure he has appropriate shoes for walking exercise. In addition to increasing his activity levels, Matt should continue with the strengthening and stretching exercises performed in stage 1. However, these exercises should be re-evaluated to increase the volume and/or intensity level (sets, repetitions, resistance, duration, etc.) (see Chapters 4 and 5) and provide some more challenging exercises. In addition, you should talk with Matt regarding staying active in the winter, since that is when he stopped walking last year. Since he is on a university campus and has access to the campus recreation center, you can discuss some of the exercise/activity options at the recreational center with him. In addition, proper exercise attire in the cold should be addressed.

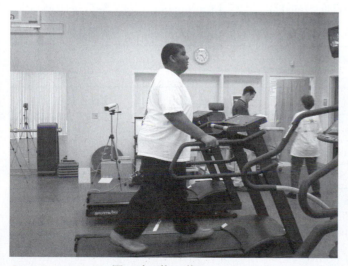

Case Figure 8.8   Treadmill walking.

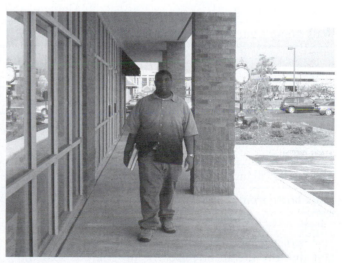

Case Figure 8.10   Walking across campus.

Author's Comments L

You may be asking yourself, "Shouldn't we do another maximal treadmill test?" The answer to that question is "not necessarily." The purpose for doing the maximal exercise test in stage two was to determine if increased therapeutic exercise activities would be safe for Matt. We determined that exercise was safe for Matt. We were able to get a good maximal heart rate from that test, and therefore can base our therapeutic exercise prescription on that data.

Depending on how Matt is doing with the increase in daily physical activity, you can encourage him to begin a formal, more independent therapeutic exercise routine. Encourage him to continue walking to class and performing the strengthening and stretching exercises, but also explain the physiological and psychological benefits of formal regular exercise. You could create a number of different options for Matt to try, and he can chose the one(s) that he likes best. I have provided four possibilities.

Option 1 (Max. HR = maximum heart rate)

Exercise Selection	Intensity	Duration	Frequency
Walk to the recreation center	Light (30–49% Max. HR)	5–10 minutes	3-5 days/week
Stationary Bicycling	Moderate (50–69% Max. HR)	30 minutes	3–5 days/week
Ski machine or rowing machine	Moderate (50–69% Max. HR)	15 minutes	3–5 days/week
Walk home from the recreation center	Light (30–49% Max. HR)	5–10 minutes	3–5 days/week

Option 2

Exercise Selection	Intensity	Duration	Frequency
Walk to the recreation center	Light (30–49% Max. HR)	5–10 minutes	3–5 days/week
Treadmill walking	Moderate (50–69% Max. HR)	30 minutes	3–5 days/week
Stationary Bicycling	Moderate (50–69% Max. HR)	15 minutes	3–5 days/week
Walk home from the recreation center	Light (30–49% Max. HR)	5–10 minutes	3–5 days/week

Option 3

Exercise Selection	Intensity	Duration	Frequency
Walk to the recreation center	Light (30–49% Max. HR)	5–10 minutes	3–5 days/week
Stationary Bicycling	Moderate (50–69% Max. HR)	30 minutes	3–5 days/week
Treadmill walking	Moderate (50–69% Max. HR)	15 minutes	3–5 days/week
Walk home from the recreation center	Light (30–49% Max. HR)	5–10 minutes	3-5 days/week

Option 4

Exercise Selection	Intensity	Duration	Frequency
Walk to the recreation center	Light (30–49% Max. HR)	5–10 minutes	3–5 days/week
Stair stepper	Moderate (50–69% Max. HR)	30 minutes	3–5 days/week
Treadmill walking	Moderate (50–69% Max. HR)	15 minutes	3–5 days/week
Walk home from the recreation center	Light (30–49% Max. HR)	5–10 minutes	3–5 days/week

There are many options for Matt; however, it is important that the therapeutic exercise program be something that he enjoys.

Author's Comments M

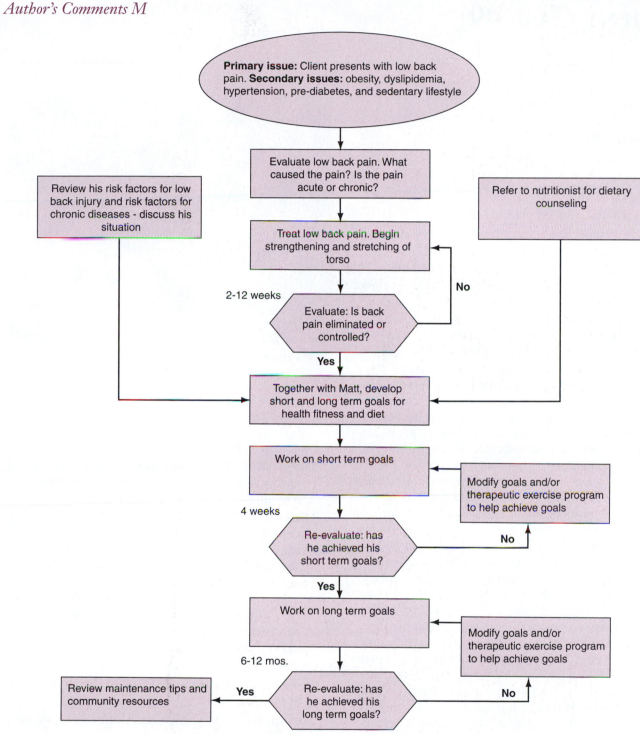

CLIENT CASE #9

Kent J. Adams

History

Client: Mary

Age: 85 yrs

Height: 5′ 0″

Weight: 95 lbs

Education: College graduate (B.S.)

Occupation: Retired teacher. Part-time caregiver to great grandchildren. Church volunteer

Personal: Three children, five grandchildren, seven great grandchildren. Widowed. Lives alone, independently

Medical/Surgical History: Congestive heart failure (CHF) diagnosed eight months ago. Mary's physician considers her CHF to be stable and controlled. No acute flare-ups or exacerbations of CHF have occurred over the last six months. Hypertension has been diagnosed as well and is presently controlled with an angiotensin converting enzyme (ACE) inhibitor (reference #1, p. 278 describes effects on heart rate, blood pressure, ECG), and exercise capacity.[1] Mary (**Case Figure 9.1**) is a non-smoker, but experienced considerable past high exposure to second-hand smoke (late husband smoked for 30 yrs). Mary has a history of a right wrist Colles fracture at age 63. She also has been diagnosed with osteoporosis and has been receiving treament with Alendronate over the last 5 yrs (information regarding medications and osteoporosis available at the National Osteoporosis Foundation (NOF) website [www.nof.org]). Mary has a slight dowager's hump and she has lost 2 inches of height since menopause. Presently she takes a calcium supplement with vitamin D (review www.nof.org for National Academy of Sciences recommendations for calcium and vitamin D consumption). Mary has degenerative osteoarthritis in several lower extremity joints; however, her function is only slightly impaired, primarily during cold weather. Her geriatrician is concerned about *sarcopenia* (loss of lean body mass with aging).[2] Mary recently experienced two falls that resulted in minor bruises. She has increased fear of falling however, since a close friend who recently fell and broke her hip, was subsequently admitted to a nursing home (see Chapter 1) and passed away the following year. Mary's vision is good when she

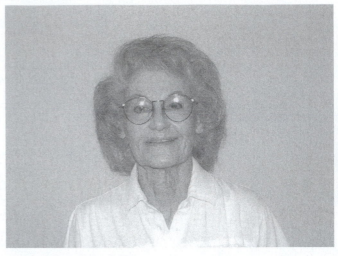

Case Figure 9.1 Mary.

wears her bifocals and she has no signs of macular degeneration. Despite being mentally alert, Mary is feeling increasingly isolated and alone (see Chapter 11).

Diagnosis: Osteoporosis skeletal assessment via dual energy X-ray absorptiometry (DEXA) assessment 6 months prior

Hip (Femoral Neck): T-score = −2.5 (i.e., bone mass is 2.5 standard deviations lower than the average for a healthy young adult woman). This suggests that her fracture risk is > 2 times normal; Z-score = −2.0 (i.e., her bone mass is two standard deviations lower than the average woman Mary's age) (review www.nof.org for guidance on interpretation of bone density tests)

Spine (L2-4): T-score = −2.5; Z-score = −2.0; slight dowager's hump

Wrists: Right wrist, healed Colles fracture, sustained at 63 yrs of age

Medications: ACE inhibitor, Alendronate, calcium with vitamin D

Exercise/Activity History: No formal exercise history. Mary says she always "worked hard at her job" and did not have time to participate in "exercise class." Enjoys walking, gardening, and caring for her great grandchildren. Mary says she "cut back on her gardening" last year and really missed it. She would like to have a big garden again this year. Mary has been "feeling tired lately" and finds it difficult to do all of the things she would like to do. Mary loved to dance when she was young, but has not danced in years. She recently went on a vacation with a church group, but she was very tired by end of the day and did not attend many of their social functions.

- **Chief Complaint:** Mary's concern seems to combine a general decline in her functional ability and an increased fear of falling. These components have contributed to reduce her quality of life (see Chapters 1 and 11). Specifically, her functional decline and fear of falling is affecting her ability to live independently, care for her great grandchildren, and continue to perform volunteer work at the church.

- **Goal:** Mary's goal is to improve her functional fitness and quality of life (i.e., successful aging).[3]

Background

Mary visited her primary care physician 2 weeks ago for an evaluation of her general health. At this exam Mary communicated to her physician that she was having increasing difficulty performing activities of daily living (ADLs), that she had fallen recently, and that she was fearful of losing her independence.

The medical exam revealed nothing new in Mary's medical profile. Secondary prevention appears to be working, as Mary reports that she has had no recent flare-ups of her CHF symptoms. Her heart rhythm is regular; no fluid has collected in her lungs. The doctor asked the nurse to have Mary perform a 6 minute walk test (at the time of CHF diagnosis, the physician conducted a graded exercise test using the Bruce protocol, resulting in an estimated $VO_{2\ max}$ of 14 ml/kg/min, or 4 METS). Results of Mary's six minute walk test performed today was 300 yds (< 20th percentile for her age; rated as "at risk for loss of functional mobility").[4]

The physician noted that Mary's weight had dropped 3 lbs (98 to 95 lbs) over the past 6 months and that she was "looking a bit too thin." He is concerned that Mary's sarcopenia and loss of muscular strength, power, and endurance are related to her decline in functional ability. Worried about the effects of Mary's functional decline, the physician administered a SF-36 questionnaire[5] to assess her general health status.

In addition to referring Mary to a nutritionist for dietary counseling, her physician (keeping with sound secondary prevention strategies) has referred Mary to you for a functional fitness evaluation and therapeutic activity/exercise program recommendations related to musculoskeletal and cardiovascular/pulmonary fitness (see Chapters 4 and 5).[1,4,6–8] No specific contraindications to activity or exercise were noted and the doctor went over CHF warning symptoms again with Mary, but anticipated no problem with increased fitness activities. In fact, her physician notes that in support of tertiary prevention the dangers of inactivity were far greater than any risk from initiating a properly designed and supervised therapeutic exercise program.[7–10] In addition, osteoporosis, controlled hypertension, and arthritis were noted on Mary's referral for treatment.

The next day Mary visits your clinic for an evaluation and therapeutic activity/exercise consultation. When you meet her in the lobby, you observe that she uses her arms to "press" up from her chair (instead of just standing up). Mary's walking pace seems fine, though, as you take her to the assessment room. Having read Mary's referral record, and considering holistic contributors to Mary's general health and well being, you feel that the evaluation should focus on "functional fitness" (i.e., having the capacity to perform normal everyday activities safely and independently without undue fatigue).

You identify the Senior Fitness Test (SFT) battery of Rikli and Jones[4] as a valid, reliable, cost-efficient and easy to use assessment that can later be administered in Mary's home as an on-site follow-up to the therapeutic exercise intervention. Functional fitness is a composite of factors related to muscular and cardiovascular fitness (i.e., muscular strength, power, and endurance; aerobic endurance; flexibility; dynamic balance and agility; and body composition).[4] The SFT[4] assesses these parameters with the following tests: chair stand test, arm curl test, 6-minute walk test, chair sit-and-reach test, back scratch test, 8-foot up-and-go test, and body mass index (BMI).

A. Given the definition of "functional fitness," what physiological parameters do you believe are most important to measure during your assessment? Please list them. *See Author's Comments A*

Physical Examination Results

Resting Blood Pressure: 124/82 mm Hg (noted that Mary had taken her hypertension medication that morning)

Resting Heart Rate: 68 bpm

Height: 5′ 0″ (60 inches)

Weight: 95 lbs

BMI (kg/m²): 18.6 (rated as "underweight—at risk for loss of mobility")*

Skin-Fold Body Fat Percentage (3-site): 22%

Senior Fitness Test (SFT) Results*

Chair Stand Test: 8 stands in 30 seconds (25–30th percentile for her age; rated right at the threshold for "at risk for loss of functional mobility")

Arm Curl Test: 12 curls with a 5 lb dumbbell in 30 seconds (50th percentile for her age; rated in the bottom half of the "normal range")

6-minute Walk Test:* 300 yds (< 20th percentile for her age; rated as "at risk for loss of functional mobility") [performed previously by nurse at doctor's office]

Chair Sit-and-Reach Test: −1.5 inches (35th percentile for her age; rated at the low end of the "normal range" just above "at risk for loss of functional mobility")

Back Scratch Test: −4.5 inches (45th percentile; rated as at the threshold for "at risk for loss of functional mobility")

8-foot Up-and-Go Test: 10 seconds (20th percentile; rated as "at risk for loss of functional mobility")

* SFT norms to interpret results available in reference 4.

Based on the test results and discussion with Mary, the following short and long term goals are developed.

Short Term Goals

By week 4 Mary will be able to:
1. Perform 12 chair stands in 30 seconds (65–70th percentile for her age—within the normal range).
2. Perform 16 arm curls with a 5 lb dumbbell in 30 seconds (85th percentile for her age—above average range).
3. Reach 1 inch past her toes in the Chair Sit-and-Reach test (approximately the 60th percentile for her age—within the normal range).
4. Come within 2.5 inches of touching her fingertips in the Back Scratch test (approximately the 60th percentile for her age—within the normal range).
5. Perform the 8-foot Up-and-Go test in 8 seconds (approximately the 50th percentile for her age—within the normal range).

Long Term Goals

By week 8 Mary will be able to. . .
1. Demonstrate improvement in the above SFT battery, with goal of achieving "above average" performance as compared to age specific norms.
2. Walk 400 yds during repeat 6-minute walk test at her physician's office (approximately the 45th percentile for her age—within the normal range).

B. Given this information, what are your primary focus points for Mary's therapeutic exercise program? *See Author's Comments B*

C. Given this information, what are your primary concerns regarding the musculoskeletal system and your therapeutic exercise program? *See Author's Comments C*

D. Given this information, what are your primary concerns regarding the cardiovascular and cardiopulmonary systems and your therapeutic exercise program? *See Author's Comments D*

E. Given this information, what are your primary concerns regarding achieving a high level of therapeutic exercise program compliance? ("Selling" the overall activity/exercise program to Mary?) *See Author's Comments E*

Background for Therapeutic Activity/Exercise Program

Mary has emphasized that due to transportation issues and comfort, the therapeutic exercise program needs to be home based. Mary's children have offered to make modest purchases of home equipment as needed. You surprise them when you say that all you need is a set of adjustable dumbbells (0–20 lbs) with a stand, 3, 5, and 10 lb paired ankle-wrist weights stored on a waist-high shelf, resistance bands or tubing, a sturdy chair or an adjustable bench, and a wall mirror.

The next day you visit Mary's home "armed with a smile" and the beginnings of her therapeutic exercise program.

Activity/Exercise Prescription

F. Based on the above concepts, describe the various components of your therapeutic exercise program, including warm-up and cool-down. *See Author's Comments F*

G. With consideration for Mary's therapeutic exercise program goals, develop a program to improve her strength. Create and complete a table with column headings: exercise order, exercise selection and body region trained.

With consideration for program goals, please also provide the therapeutic exercise volume parameters for the strength training exercise/activities you selected. Create and complete a table with the following column headings: sets/repetitions, intensity determination, rest-to-work ratio, frequency/week, and rationale. *See Author's Comments G*

H. With consideration for Mary's poor aerobic endurance, describe the mode, intensity, frequency and duration of aerobic training activities that you would select for her. *See Author's Comments H*

I. **What flexibility training intervention should take place to help Mary achieve her goals? Please describe type, frequency, intensity, duration and repetitions.** *See Author's Comments I*

J. **With consideration for Mary's fear of falling, what balance and/or fall prevention therapeutic exercise activities would you add to the program?** *See Author's Comments J*

Re-testing

Re-testing using the SFT[4] can easily be conducted at regular intervals at Mary's home (e.g., at 4, 8, and 12 wks) to assess her progress and to modify the therapeutic exercise program as needed.

Senior Fitness Test (SFT) Results at Week 4*

Chair Stand Test: 13 stands in 30 seconds, exceeding her goal by 1 repetition.

Arm Curl Test: 18 arm curls with a 5 lb dumbbell in 30 seconds, exceeding her goal by 2 repetitions.

Chair Sit-and-Reach Test: "0" (just touched toes), improved by 1.5 inches, but missing her goal by 1 inch.

Back Scratch Test: −3.5 inches, improving by 1 inch, but missing her goal by 1 inch.

8-foot Up-and-Go Test: 7.9 seconds, exceeding her goal by 0.1 seconds.

*SFT norms to interpret results available in Ref. 4.

Re-Evaluate—Set New Goals

Revised Short term Goals

Our therapeutic exercise program is having the desired effects. Gains in flexibility are positive, but did not meet our goals. That is okay. Discuss all results with Mary. Watch her perform all exercises to assess technique. Modify technique as needed to ensure proper form. Pay close attention to flexibility exercises, possibly modifying or changing your intervention with another stretch method that might provide better results. Find out how she feels about her program. Continue with an individualized progression. Add variety to ensure continued progress and enthusiasm with the therapeutic exercise program.

Revised Long Term Goals

As Mary's fitness improves, additional activities can be encouraged such as involvement with community groups (senior water aerobics, senior dance class, activities with great grandchildren, etc.). Refer to Author's Comments section for additional comments about progression, variety and modification of the exercise prescription.

Case Summary

Mary is responding positively to her therapeutic exercise program. Feel good about this, but do not relax. Being enthusiastic, encouraging communication, and addressing Mary as an individual with unique concerns and requirements will help ensure that she sticks with her plan and optimizes her quality of life.

K. **On a separate sheet of paper diagram a decision making algorithm for developing Mary's therapeutic exercise program.** *See Author's Comments K*

Referring to Chapter 10 for guidance, discuss any alternative or complementary therapeutic exercises that you believe might benefit this client. Provide the rationale for your suggestion(s).

References

1. American College of Sports Medicine. *ACSM's Guidelines for Exercise Testing and Prescription*, 6th ed. New York, NY: Lippincott Williams & Wilkins, 2000.

2. Fiatarone MA, Evans WJ. The etiology and reversibility of muscle dysfunction in the aged. *J Gerontol.* 1993;44:77–83.

3. Rowe JW, Kahn RL. *Successful Aging.* New York, NY: Pantheon Books, 1998.

4. Rikli RE, Jones CJ. *Senior Fitness Test Manual.* Champaign, IL. Human Kinetics, 2001.

5. Shephard RJ, Franklin B. Changes in quality of life: A major goal of cardiac rehabilitation. *J Cardiopul Rehabil.* 2001;21:189–200.

6. American College of Sports Medicine. *ACSM's Resource Manual for Guidelines for Exercise Testing and Prescription*, 4th ed. New York, NY: Lippincott Williams & Wilkins, 2001.

7. American College of Sports Medicine. ACSM position stand on exercise and physical activity for older adults. *Med Sci Sports Exerc.* 1998;30:992–1008.

8. National Institute on Aging. *Exercise: A Guide from the National Institute on Aging.* Baltimore, MD. Publication No. NIH 98-4528.

9. Pate RR, Pratt M, Blair SN, et al. Physical activity and public health: A recommendation from the Centers for Disease Control and Prevention and the American College of Sports Medicine. *JAMA*. 1995;273:402–407.

10. Adams KJ. Cardiac rehabilitation and exercise. In CW Bales, CS Ritchie, eds. *Handbook of Clinical Nutrition and Aging*. Totowa, NJ: Humana Press, Inc, 2003.

11. Fiatarone Singh MA (ed.). *Exercise, Nutrition, and the Older Woman*. Boca Raton, FL: CRC Press, 2000.

12. Fleck SJ, Kraemer WJ. *Designing Resistance Training Programs*, 2nd ed. Champaign, IL: Human Kinetics, 1997; pp. 81–115.

13. Nelson ME. *Strong Women, Strong Bones*. New York NY: Penguin Putnam Inc, 2000.

14. Nelson ME, Fiatarone MA, Morganti CM, et al. Effects of high-intensity strength training on multiple risk factors for osteoporotic fractures. *JAMA*. 1994;272:1909–1914.

15. American College of Sports Medicine. ACSM position stand on osteoporosis and exercise. *Med Sci Sports Exerc*. 1995;27:i-vii.

16. National Osteoporosis Foundation. *Physicians Guide to Prevention and Treatment of Osteoporosis*. Washington, DC: NOF, 2003.

17. Fiatarone MA, Marks EC, Ryan ND, et al. High intensity strength training in nonagenarians: Effects on skeletal muscle. *JAMA*. 1990;263:3029–3034.

18. American College of Sports Medicine. ACSM position stand on progression models in resistance training for healthy adults. *Med Sci Sports Exerc*. 2002;34:364–380.

Author's Comments A

Functional fitness is defined as having the capacity to perform normal, everyday activities safely and independently without undue fatigue.[4] Maintaining and improving functional fitness is a critical component of successful aging. Functional fitness is a composite of factors related to muscular and cardiovascular fitness.[4] Therefore, assessments related to muscular strength, power, and endurance; aerobic endurance; flexibility; dynamic balance and agility; and body composition are warranted.[4] The Senior Fitness Test battery (SFT)[4] assesses these parameters with the following tests: chair stand test, arm curl test, 6-minute walk test, chair sit-and-reach test, back scratch test, 8-foot up-and-go test, and body mass index (BMI).

Author's Comments B

1. **Start low, go slow.** Conservative progression is key. The biggest mistake in therapeutic exercise program planning with elderly clients is applying too much stress too soon.[11,12] The best therapeutic exercise program is the one based on the needs and tolerance of the individual client.[1,10,12]

2. **Improvement of Mary's functional fitness and maintenance of independence is paramount.** Per the SFT results,[4] Mary is basically "at risk for loss of functional mobility" in all categories. These categories are primarily related to muscular fitness.[4] Therefore, the priority should be placed on resistance training within Mary's overall therapeutic exercise prescription. Regarding Mary's CHF, based on her SFT results, formal aerobic training i.e., walking ability, stationary biking, etc. will be better tolerated after she has developed a musculoskeletal fitness base through resistance training.[11–14] Lifestyle activities[9] should also be recommended, in addition to formal aerobic training within the first few weeks of Mary's regimen per her stress tolerance and progress. Also, introducing all of the therapeutic exercise program parameters in the beginning may overwhelm Mary and decrease therapeutic exercise program adherence (see Chapters 4 and 11).[1,6]

3. **Fall prevention.** A fracture at this stage of Mary's life—especially a hip fracture—would have devastating consequences to her health and quality of life.[13,15,16] Musculoskeletal fitness parameters, balance, and fall-proofing Mary's environment are all essential (see Chapter 9).[13,16]

4. In addition to acquiring the health benefits of physical activity, quality of life and adherence to the therapeutic exercise plan may be enhanced by incorporating mild to moderate lifestyle activities, such as gardening and dancing, which Mary used to enjoy. Inquiring about community based senior fitness classes, water aerobics, etc. may also add positive social outlets to Mary's daily life.

Author's Comments C

1. **Osteoporosis:** the number one concern is the avoidance of a fracture, specifically a hip fracture. Fall prevention should be addressed in two essential ways: 1) evaluation of the inside and outside of Mary's house for items that may contribute to an increased fall risk (extension cords, throw rugs, slippery steps, no hand rails, etc.); and 2) therapeutic exercises chosen to improve strength, balance, agility, coordination, and flexibility, thereby effectively reducing the likelihood that Mary will fall and sustain a fracture.[15] It is important to note that resistance exercises can simultaneously reduce the risk profile for the multiple contributors to fracture risk.[14]

   Progressive weight bearing (closed kinetic chain) exercise activities both stress and strengthen bone while simultaneously improving muscle strength and balance. To avoid lumbar spine injury Mary should avoid bending and twisting at the waist during exercise.[13,16] She should also avoid bending forward and twisting during daily activities such as vacuuming, raking, coughing, sneezing, and lifting.[13,16] Mary should be instructed in the proper way to get into a lying position on the floor and to get back up for both exercises (such as a posterior pelvic tilt performed on the floor) and daily activities such as getting out of bed.[13,16] Since Mary enjoys gardening, she should understand proper body mechanics for activities such as "weed pulling" and lifting flower pots. Suggest that Mary acquire a knee-pad to kneel on in the garden for stability. Emphasize postural stability during all therapeutic exercises and activities of daily living. Balance training should also be emphasized.[11] The National Osteoporosis Foundation at www.nof.org is an excellent resource to investigate treatment interventions.

2. Sarcopenia is the loss of lean body mass and quality with age.[2] Sarcopenia is highly related to the loss of functional fitness and independence that many clients experience as they age.[3,7,17] Exercise (and appropriate nutrition) that improves muscle quality and mass should be emphasized (e.g., resistance exercise) (see Chapter 5). Resistance exercise will also have the most benefit in appearance—something you have observed Mary takes pride in.

3. Close monitoring of any exacerbation of Mary's arthritis symptoms should take place with modification of therpeutic exercise program variables as needed. Properly administered aerobic and resistance exercises can be safely and effectively performed by clients with arthritis.[1,6]

Author's Comments D

1. **Congestive Heart Failure (CHF).** Mary's CHF is stable and controlled, and her estimated MET capacity is > 3 METs—all important considerations for CHF clients selected for exercise therapy.[1,10] Exertional fatigue and dyspnea with exertion are primary symptoms in clients with CHF. Muscle atrophy and weakness (age-related sarcopenia) are exacerbated by the typical pattern of disuse observed in the population (sedentary lifestyles). Poor nutrition typically contributes to the problem (physician has referred Mary to a nutritionist). In clients who have CHF, maintaining muscle mass and function are essential to independence with ADLs.[10] Therefore resistance exercise is key.

2. **Hypertension (controlled).** Aerobic exercise can be used safely and effectively among individuals with hypertension. Aerobic exercise recommendations for clients with controlled hypertension generally do not vary substantially from those recommended for low risk clients.[1,6] Resistance exercise is also an appropriate and safe component of a well designed therapeutic exercise program.[1,6,10,11,13]

Author's Comments E

Mary has stated that she has no formal exercise history (she "worked hard, with no time for formal exercise class participation"). It is important to "sell" the program to Mary by relating the activity and therapeutic exercise program to her overall quality of life—maintaining independence, playing with great grandchildren, helping others, gardening, feeling good, and being able to meet the challenges of everyday life. Using quotes such as "the goal of life is to die young, as late as possible" (A. Montague), and "if exercise could be put in a bottle it would be the most prescribed medicine in history" (R. Butler) may help. Emphasizing to Mary that it is "never too late" to benefit from a therapeutic exercise program is critical. Emphasize that resistance training is essential to maintaining functional independence as one ages. Consider giving her a copy of Miriam Nelson's book *Strong Women, Strong Bones*[13] to help allay fears of resistance training. Use published data to support your case. Exercise is new to Mary and raises fears, so be enthusiastic in conveying your message. Emphasize the safety and effectiveness of appropriately performed activities and therapeutic exercises among the elderly. In other words, it is more dangerous to do nothing (i.e., remain sedentary) than it is to "get up and move" in a properly designed and supervised therapeutic exercise program. The bottom line is that movement activities and therapeutic exercises are key components of successful aging![3]

Author's Comments F

General Comments. A 5–10 minute warm-up of low intensity activity should begin each session.[1] Remember with Mary, her capabilities are currently low, so a conservative, low intensity warm-up should be employed. Besides basic movement, an effective warm-up incorporates the workout movements at low intensities and pace. In other words, the exercises are "ramped up" in intensity with close monitoring of how Mary feels. A 5–10 minute cool-down period post-workout is important as well.[1] Here, the exercise intensity can be "ramped down," stretching exercises can be employed, and general relaxation initiated (see Chapter 3).

Author's Comments G

General Comments: ACSM guidelines[1,7] suggest performing 8–10 exercises that train the major muscle groups

Exercise order	Exercise selection	Body region
1	Chair squat	Lower extremities
2	Standing leg curl with ankle cuff weight	Hamstrings
3	Heel raise	Calves
4	Ankle dorsiflexion with resistive band	Front shins
5	Wall squat	Quadriceps
6	Front lunge	Lower extremities
7	Stair step-up	Lower extremities
8	Seated row	Upper extremities, scapular retractors
9	Reverse fly with dumbbells	Upper extremities, shoulder horizontal abductors, scapular retractors
10	Wall push-up	Upper extremities, Chest
11	Side lateral raise with dumbbells	Upper extremities, shoulder abductors
12	Overhead tricep extension with a dumbbells	Upper extremities, elbow extensors
13	Bicep curls with dumbbells	Upper extremities, elbow flexors
14	Posterior pelvic tilt	Abdominals

Sets/repetitions	Intensity determination	Rest-to-work ratio	Frequency/week	Rationale
1 set of 10–15 repetitions	Rating of perceived exertion (RPE) = 11–14	3:1	3 sessions/week	Establish proper technique, basic strength

for a minimum of 1 set of 10–15 repetitions, 2–3 times per week for older or frail clients. Typically this will correspond to a score of approximately 11 = fairly light, to 14 = somewhat hard on the Borg Rating of Perceived Exertion category scale (see Chapter 4). This is a good place to start with Mary's progression (each exercise for one set of between 10–15 repetitions, 3 days per week (Monday, Wednesday, Friday for example). Proper breathing, body position and stability, and balance should be emphasized with each movement. Regarding progression, depending on your initial perception, you may start out with only 4–5 exercises the first day, see how Mary responds, and then increase her volume as tolerated to all 8–10 of your therapeutic exercise program recommendations by the second or third therapeutic exercise program session. Remember, a conservative progression is essential. Watch for signs of muscular soreness, cardiovascular or cardiopulmonary system stress, and fatigue. Also, taking the necessary time to teach proper technique is paramount. Once you have established your therapeutic exercise selections (i.e., 8–10 exercises), add another set to select movements, assess tolerance, and progressively increase her volume to 2 sets of between 10–15 repetitions on all exercises, with approximately 1 minute duration rest period between sets. This will probably be attainable during the initial 2–4 weeks. Eventually (within 4–6 weeks), 2–3 sets per exercise $\times$ 10–15 repetitions should be safe and effective. Rapid gains may be possible during this initial period. As training progresses, manipulating the therapeutic exercise program variables (periodization) will become critical to enable continued progress (e.g., 8–12 repetitions at a rating of perceived exertion (RPE) of 15 = hard, to 17 = very hard).[18] Decisions on progressions will be based on parameters of functional fitness (i.e., you may transition into more of a maintenance mode [capping] if function is at the desired level and further fitness increases will take large amounts of time and energy).[12]

These were the considerations I placed on my therapeutic exercise program selections.

Chair Squat: Mary only performed 8 chair stand repetitions in 30 seconds during her Chair Stand

Test. An appropriate modification of the chair squat is to place a phone book (or other appropriate option) on the chair to decrease the depth of the squat. This should allow Mary to do at least 1 set of 10+ repetitions. Once Mary can perform 2–3 sets × 10–15 repetitions at the given height, the phone book can be removed to increase range of motion and stimulus. Soon Mary will be able to perform the chair squats with dumbbells for added resistance (**Case Figure 9.2a–c**).

Standing Leg Curl: I would have Mary use the back of a sturdy chair as a balance support. Ankle cuff weight resistance can be progressively increased, making sure that proper form and balance are maintained. Mary should secure the ankle cuff weight while seated with her foot up on a step stool to avoiding excessive bending at the waist.

Heel Raise: Mary should begin with two-leg heel raises on a level floor. Have her use the back of sturdy chair as a balance support. Once she can tolerate 2–3 sets of two-leg heel raises, progress to one leg at a time, with the eventual addition of a dumbbell for added resistance (remember—keep balance support close (chair or wall).

Ankle Dorsiflexion: This exercise will help to improve the ankle muscle strength and endurance that is critical to balance (see Chapter 9). Have Mary sit in a sturdy chair and use a step stool to attach the resistive rubber band around the forefoot. Perform the desired number of repetitions with the right foot, followed by the left foot.

Wall Squat: During this isometric exercise have Mary begin holding the flexed knee position for about 5–10 seconds as tolerated. Her eventual goal with this exercise is 30 seconds. Additionally, she should begin with approximately 30° knee flexion and progress to 90° knee flexion with parallel thighs (**Case Figure 9.3**).

Forward Lunge: Lunges are a great addition to Mary's therapeutic exercise program for functional strength and endurance, balance, and variety. Mary should begin with body weight resistance, with her hand on a sturdy chair or wall for balance. Eventually, she can progress to free-standing lunges with dumbbell resistance (**Case Figure 9.4a–b**).

Stair Step-Up: Stair step-ups are another great addition to Mary's program. These should begin with 1–2 steps to train the musculoskeletal, cardiovascular, and cardiopulmonary systems. Stair step-ups are a great interval training mode for addressing concerns related to Mary's CHF. Mary should begin this exercise with her hand on a stair rail as needed for support and balance (**Case Figure 9.5a–b**).

Seated Row: With a resistive rubber band attached to a doorknob, Mary grasps each end and with a stable, upright seated posture pull the bands toward her sides, squeezing her shoulder blades together.

Reverse Fly with Dumbbells: While seated in a sturdy chair with her trunk slightly flexed forward and

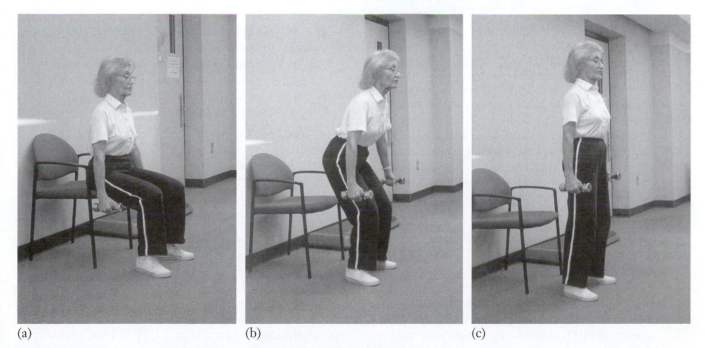

(a)   (b)   (c)

Case Figure 9.2   Chair squats with dumbbells. (a) start; (b) mid-way; (c) finish.

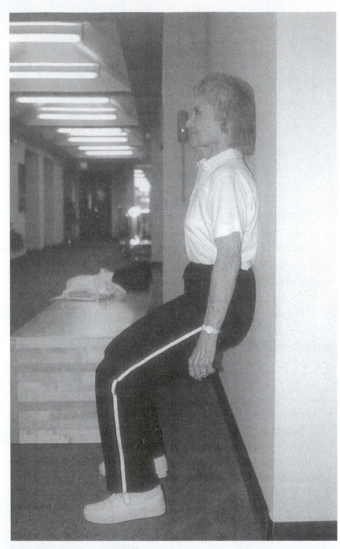

Case Figure 9.3   Wall squats.

keeping her elbows slightly flexed, Mary should raise the dumbbells in a backward arc until the arms are approximately parallel to the ground. At the completion of this movement she should try to squeeze her shoulder blades together (**Case Figure 9.6a–b**).

Seated Shoulder Press with Dumbbells: An overhead seated press designed to increase shoulder and triceps strength (**Case Figure 9.7a–b**).

Wall Push-Up: Positioned with her feet approximately 6 inches away from a wall while standing, Mary slowly extends her elbows as she pushes away from the wall, holds the extended elbow position for 2 seconds and slowly returns to the starting position (**Case Figure 9.8a–b**).

Side Lateral Raise with Dumbbells: Also performed while seated using a sturdy chair. While maintaining an erect seated posture the dumbbells are raised out to the sides until the arms are approximately parallel to the ground (**Case Figure 9.9a–b**).

Overhead Triceps Extension with a Dumbbell: Again seated in a sturdy chair with an upright posture, the upper arm is positioned overhead and stabilized with the opposite hand while Mary slowly extends her elbow overhead. Each arm performs this exercise independently (**Case Figure 9.10a–b**).

Biceps Curls with Dumbbells: Seated dumbbell curls are performed in an alternating manner (**Case Figure 9.11**).

Pelvic Tilt: While positioned in supine with the hips and knees flexed, abdominal muscle activation posteriorly rotates the pelvis and holds this position for 5 sec. As Mary learns this exercise movement the intensity can be gradually increased by incorporating lower extremity and upper extremity movements, or by progressing from a supine to an on knees or half-kneeling position. Mary must pay attention to the technique she employs in getting down into and up from the supine position.

Sample Resistance Training Workout Progression

Day 1:   Warm-up (light activity). Chair squat, standing leg curl, standing two-leg heel raise, seated row, shoulder press, pelvic tilts—each for one set of 12 repetitions. Cool-down with stretching.

Day 2:   Mary feels good. No residual soreness. Warm-up. Chair squat, standing leg curl, two-leg heel raise, seated row, shoulder press, side lateral raise, overhead triceps extension, biceps curl, pelvic tilts—all for one set of 12 repetitions.

Day 3:   Mary was slightly stiff yesterday. Feels good today. Perform same workout as day 2.

Day 4, 5, 6:   Mary is feeling good. Ask Mary to increase repetitions to 15 (one set with each exercise).

Day 7, 8, 9:   Mary is responding well. Increase sets and decrease repetitions (i.e., two sets of 12 repetitions) on all exercises. Keep resistance the same. Allow approximately one minute of rest between sets. Monitor any unusual fatigue per CHF. If day 7 and 8 go well with no adverse symptoms, increase repetitions to 15 on all exercises on day 9.

This completes two weeks of resistance training—during week 3 increase volume to 3 sets of 12 repetitions as tolerated (if any concerns regarding adaptation (e.g., soreness) exist then keep volume at two sets, and resistance the same for this week). Then start increasing resistance (e.g., Mary is performing 3 sets of 12-chair stands with no problem, so you add 2.5 lb dumbbells in each hand and reduce volume to two sets of 10 repetitions, assess tolerance, and increase accordingly over next few workouts to 3 sets of 12 repetitions at a resistance of 2.5 lb dumbbells).

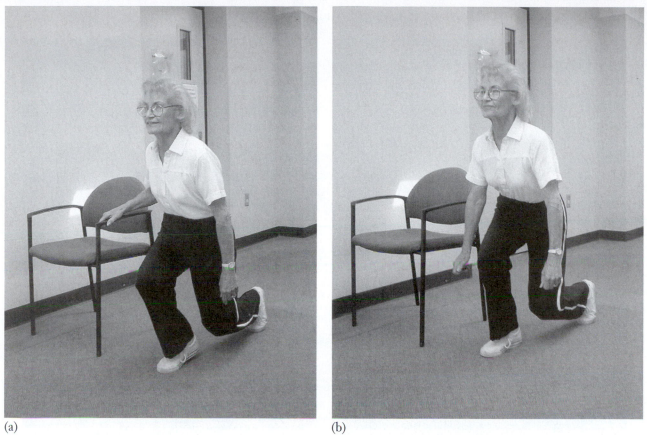

(a)   (b)

Case Figure 9.4   Forward lunge. (a) with chair arm for balance assistance, (b) without balance assistance.

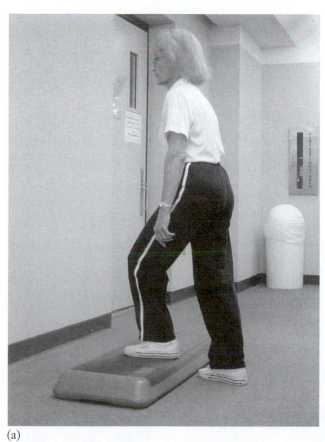
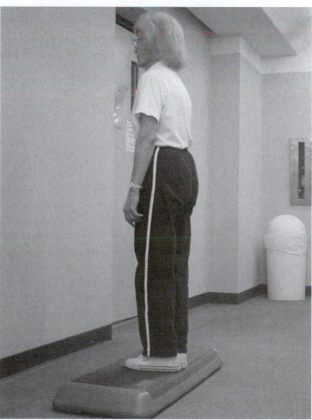

(a)   (b)

Case Figure 9.5   Stair step-up. (a) start, (b) finish.

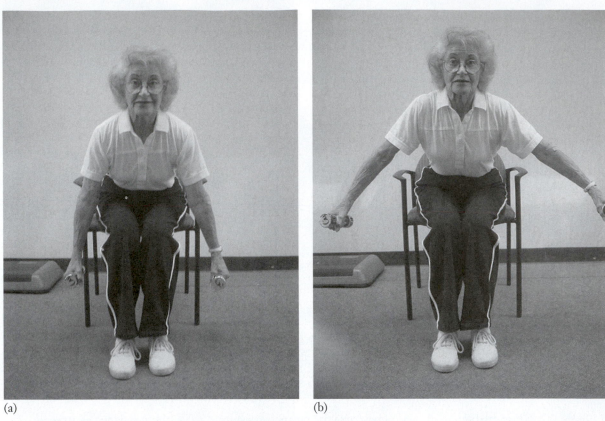

(a)   (b)

Case Figure 9.6   Reverse fly with dumbbells. (a) start, (b) finish.

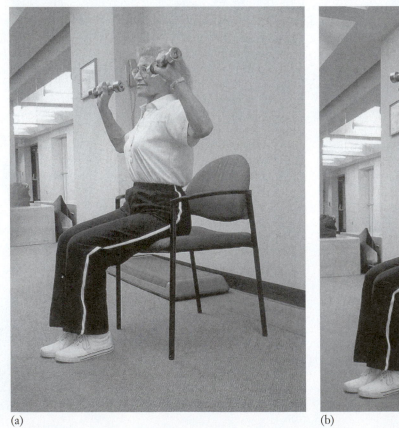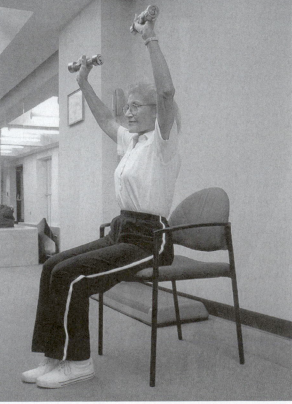

(a)   (b)

Case Figure 9.7   Seated dumbbell press. (a) start, (b) finish.

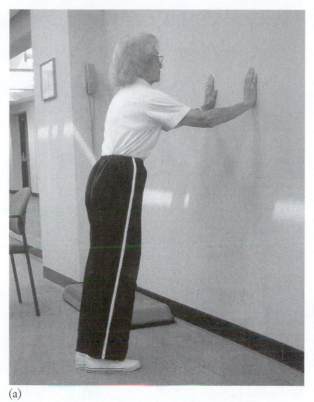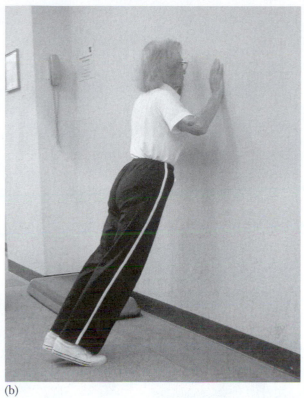

(a)   (b)

Case Figure 9.8   Wall push-up. (a) start, (b) finish.

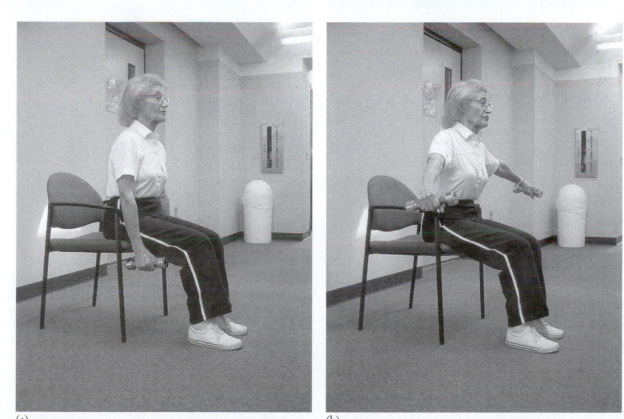

(a)   (b)

Case Figure 9.9   Side lateral raise with dumbbells. (a) start, (b) finish.

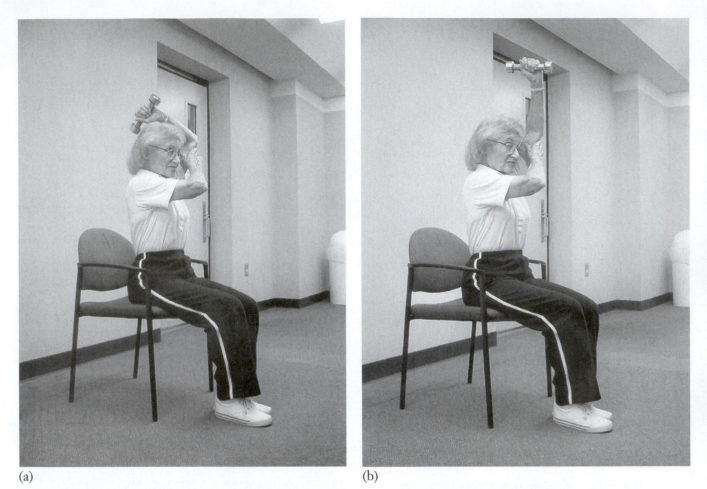

(a)   (b)

Case Figure 9.10   Overhead tricep extension with dumbbell. (a) start, (b) finish.

By the end of week 4, Mary should be seeing dramatic improvements in her strength. Resistance can now be kept in the 8–12 repetition range. Intensity and volume are key to positive changes in bone and muscle mass. More complex exercises can now be added as tolerated (e.g., lunges, one-leg heel raises). Challenges to balance via resistance training can also be increased (e.g., lunges, stair step-ups). Manipulation of acute program variables (periodization) are key to long term progress.[12,18] Recommend employment of both linear and non-linear periodization models targeting strength, power, and muscle endurance.[12,18]

Author's Comments H

As previously stated, the initial phase of training will concentrate on resistance and balance training. Therefore, during early aerobic training, mild to moderate activity should be emphasized. Lifestyle activities[9] where Mary "accumulates" at least 30 minutes of moderate activity (e.g., walking, housework, gardening, etc.) are recommended. As Mary progresses, more formal aerobic prescriptions can be incorporated using set intensity guidelines.[1,7] The physician has stated that cardiovascular

workloads of 45–65% of Mary's maximum heart rate (MHR) are well tolerated. Mary's predicted MHR from the graded exercise test (GXT) at her physician's office is 135 bpm. Therefore her target heart rate (THR) zone is approximately 61 to 88 bpm (ACE inhibitor should have no effect on heart rate during rest or exercise). The physician has also assessed Mary's heart rate response to walking at a safe, controlled pace and found it to be in the acceptable range. On an RPE scale, Mary's should progress to working around a 13 rating (somewhat hard). With improvement in tolerance over time, slightly higher RPE ratings (i.e., 15, hard) may be appropriate. Mary's neighborhood is safe to walk in during good weather, and she happens to have a stationary recumbent bike in her home that she has never used (it was left there by her daughter), which has a heart rate monitor built into the hand grips. Based on the typical aerobic exercise tolerance of clients with CHF, the ACSM[1] suggests aerobic training sessions should initially be short (e.g., 10–20 minutes), and should incorporate work–rest intervals (e.g., four 3-minute bouts of walking, separated by 1-minute rest). You check Mary's shoes and are happy to discover that she has a good pair of walking shoes. In addition to accumulating

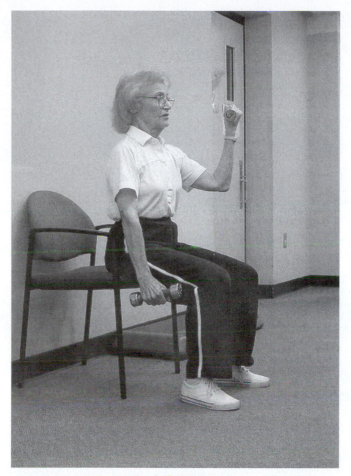

Case Figure 9.11   Seated alternating biceps curls with dumbbells.

30 minutes of general lifestyle activities daily, the following specific parameters will be addressed with the aerobic training prescription at the time of initiation:

Mode: Walking or stationary biking

Frequency: 3 to 5 days per week

Intensity: 45–65% of THR. Rating of perceived exertion per Mary's individual response is useful here as well (usually should progress as tolerated to be in the range of 12, somewhat hard to 15, hard).

Duration: 10–20 minutes at first, progressing to 20–40 minutes as tolerated. Work intervals of 2–6 minutes separated by 1–2 minutes of rest are effective at improving client tolerance.

Sample Aerobic Training Workout Progression

Weeks 1 and 2:   Emphasize accumulation of 30 minutes per day of moderate activity (e.g., walking, housework, gardening, etc.). No formal aerobic ex-

ercise prescription employed yet. Concentrate on the resistance training progression, tolerance, and appropriate technique. Strength and function gains from resistance training should enhance her ability to perform and tolerate aerobic training.

Week 3:   Continue to emphasize accumulation of lifestyle activity. Add walking or stationary biking at low end of Mary's intensity range. Start out at 10 minutes of accumulated work, performed in intervals of 2 minutes with rest breaks of 1 minute. After warm-up, use an interval to "ramp up" intensity to the THR zone—1 minute rest—then use an interval to "ramp down" intensity and move into formal cool-down.

Week 4:   Progressively lengthen aerobic work intervals as tolerance improves. Goal is to achieve 20 to 40 minutes of work per session. Interval work is recommended. Increase volume before intensity. Slowly progress over the next few weeks.

Author's Comments I

Flexibility training can be incorporated into the workout and cool-down periods. Flexibility of the ankle joint is of particular importance, as it relates to balance and falling (see Chapter 9). Exercises such as the wall arch, the standing back bend, the cat stretch, and standing and sitting stretching exercises may all be useful. The ACSM[1] recommends the following flexibility program:

Type: General stretches that target the major musculotendinous structures; static and proprioceptive neuromuscular facilitation (PNF) techniques are recommended

Frequency: At least 2–3 days per week

Intensity: Stretch to a feeling of mild discomfort

Duration: Hold stretch for 10–30 seconds for static stretching; during PNF, hold contraction for 6 seconds followed by a 10–30 second assisted stretch

Repetitions: 3 to 4 for each stretch (see Chapter 3)

Author's Comments J

Weight bearing exercises that improve lower body strength may also help to improve balance.[11,13] The dynamic free weight exercises in this program are especially beneficial. As abilities progress, modifications can be made in the strength exercises, such as holding onto a sturdy chair with only one hand during performance, with eventual progression to no hands. No additional resistance training exercises (or frequency) should be added for balance enhancement. Just modify the supports used during the existing therapeutic exercise movements. Walking heel-to-toe, standing on one foot (with appropriate spotting as needed) (**Case Figure 9.12a–b**) and a standing

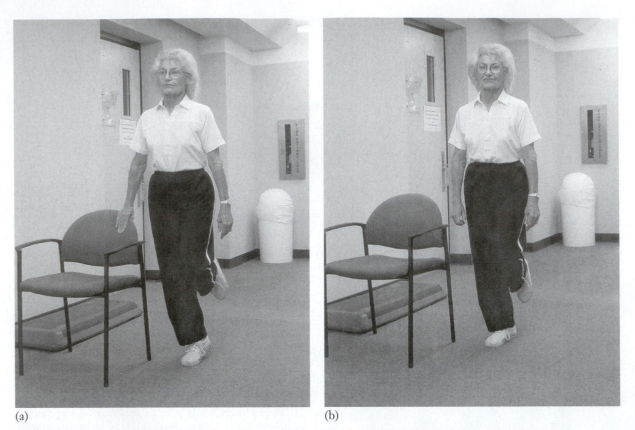

(a)   (b)

Case Figure 9.12   Single leg standing balance training. (a) with chair support, (b) without support.

sway (**Case Figure 9.13**) are also positive additions within the program and can be performed more frequently if desired. Standing hip flexion, extension and side leg raises (**Case Figure 9.14a–b**) can also be incorporated in this progression. If Mary's church offers a community senior dance class, this would offer a fun outlet that incorporates complex movements related to balance, muscular, cardiovascular, and cardiopulmonary fitness (see Chapters 4 and 10). This would be a great goal for Mary to work toward.

Fall-proofing Mary's environment is very important.[11,13,15,16] Perform a safety check of Mary's home. Check for slippery floors and unsecured rugs, clutter such as extention cords, inadequate lighting (night lights, corridor lighting, etc.), stair handrails, non-skid bath and shower mats, grab rails in the shower and tub, and other factors such as unsteady step stools. Suggestions regarding organization of frequently used items to avoid bending and un-safe stretching is also warranted. Caution Mary to avoid walking in socks or slippers. Supportive rubber-soled, low-heeled shoes provide good support and traction. Check outside the home and recommend painting porch steps with gritty, weatherproof paint for traction. Check adequacy of outside lighting to illuminate walkways. Emphasize caution in cold, wet, icy weather. Recommend that Mary keep sand or de-icer readily available for outdoor surfaces.

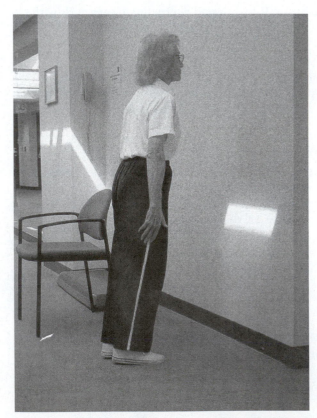

Case Figure 9.13   Standing forward sway.

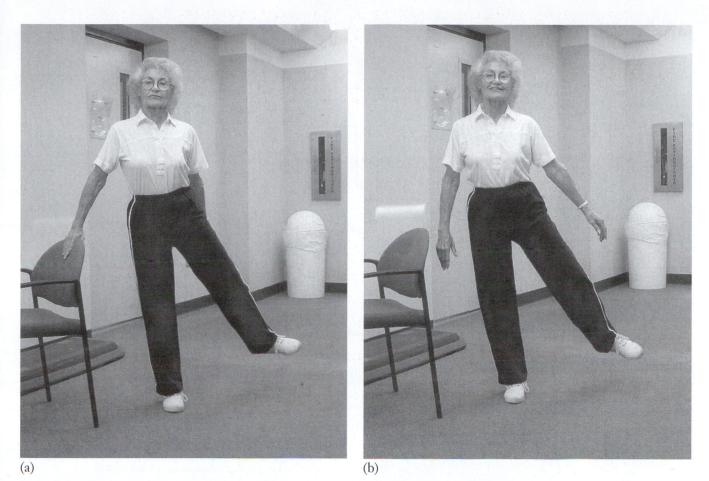

(a)   (b)

Case Figure 9.14   Standing side leg raises. (a) with chair support, (b) without support.

Author's Comments K

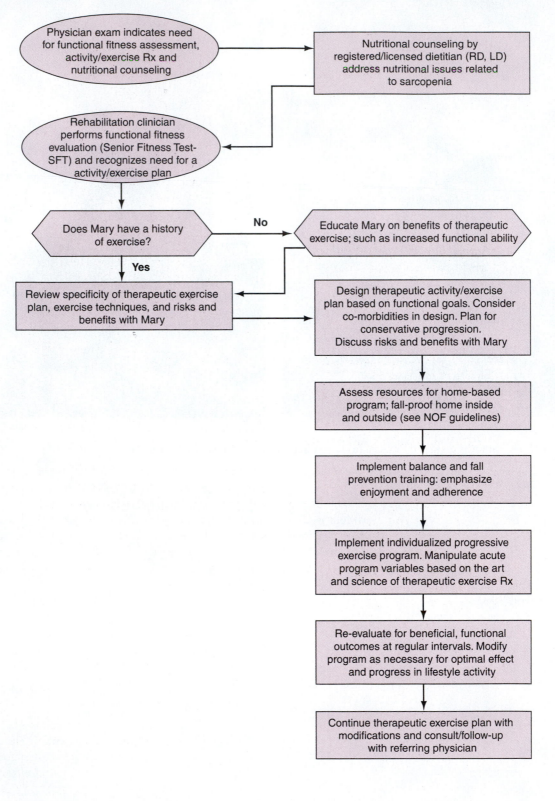

CLIENT CASE #10

Rick W. Wilson

History

Client: Barrett

Age: 75 yrs

Height: 5′ 10″

Weight: 130 lbs

Education: High school graduate

Occupation: Retired retail merchant

Medical/Surgical History: Two months status-post completion of pharmacological androgen ablation therapy and external beam radiation therapy for localized prostate cancer

Chief Complaint: Fatigue, causing inability to participate in accustomed social activities (bridge, gin rummy, golf).

Barrett (**Case Figure 10.1**) moved to a golf and country club community in Florida five years ago following the death of his wife and his retirement from the family's retail appliance business in Michigan. He quickly cultivated a circle of friends among a group of retired businessmen who meet at the club to play cards daily and golf twice each week. Six months ago he was diagnosed with advanced, localized (T3N0M0) carcinoma of the prostate, which was treated with Flutamide and Goserelin Acetate given for two months prior to and during a 70 Gy dose of radiotherapy delivered to the pelvic region over a period of eight weeks.

During the late stages of his treatment, Barrett experienced significant fatigue and weight loss. His oncologist determined that these symptoms were due to anemia and asthenia associated with his cancer treatment and prescribed synthetic erythropoetin. Barrett's physician advised him to resume his normal activities within 4–6 weeks of concluding his course of radiotherapy. However, Barrett gradually withdrew from his social activities during treatment in favor of staying at home to rest. More recently he has also experienced hip and low back pain while

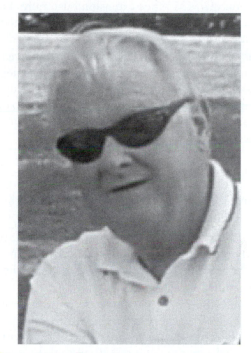

Case Figure 10.1   Barrett.

standing for prolonged periods of time. Subsequent dual emission x-ray absorption (DEXA) and magnetic resonance imaging (MRI) studies revealed the presence of mild osteopenia with a bone mineral density (BMD) 1.2 standard deviations below his age adjusted norm. However, there was no evidence of fractures or focal osteolytic lesions in the lumbosacral spine, pelvis, or proximal femurs.

Aside from his cancer, Barrett has no major health problems. He would like to resume golf and other activities at the club to re-establish social contact with his friends outside the home. However, he believes that increased physical activity will only make him more fatigued and may worsen his prognosis.

Physical Examination

Musculoskeletal Assessment

Posture: Anterior pelvic tilt and an increased lumbosacral lordosis, which is more pronounced in standing than in a seated position. Otherwise unremarkable

Active Range of Motion: Within normal limits for age in all motion planes at the cervical spine and both upper extremities. Decreased lumbar spine flexion observed during forward bending (lacks 10″ of touching finger tips to floor when standing with knees extended). Lumbar side bending is symmetrical and extension is within normal limits. Active range of motion is also within normal limits at both hips, knees, and ankles when assessed in a sitting position

Ligamentous Laxity: Not examined

Manual Muscle Testing: Decreased strength (4/5) at all major muscle groups of both upper and lower extremities

Musculotendinous Extensibility: Active hamstring extensibility while in a supine position at 90° hip flexion was −25° knee extension bilaterally. Thomas test revealed −10° neutral hip extension bilaterally (**Case Figures 10.2–10.3**).

Pain: Complains of backache during prolonged standing (6 out of 10 on modified visual analog scale). Symptoms relieved with sitting or lying down (0 out of 10). Denies numbness/tingling. No other pain complaints. Body Mass Index: 18.6 kg/m^2 (normal range = 20–25 kg/m^2)

Cardiopulmonary Assessment

Resting Blood Pressure: 116/74 mm Hg

Resting Heart Rate: 88 bpm

Hematology Values: Hemoglobin 11.5 g/dL (normal range = 14–17 g/dL); hematocrit 42% (normal range = 38–54%); platelets 150k/μL (normal range = 200–300 k/μL)

Aerobic Capacity/Endurance: A recent symptom-limited graded exercise test performed with open circuit spirometry using a modified Bruce protocol revealed a resting VO$_2$ of 180 ml/min, VO$_2$ at ventilatory threshold of 500 ml/min, and a predicted VO$_2$ peak value of 900 ml/min (approximately 5 METs)

Neuromuscular Assessment

Deep Tendon Reflex Grading: +2 for bilateral biceps, triceps, brachioradialis, patellar, and Achilles tendon reflexes

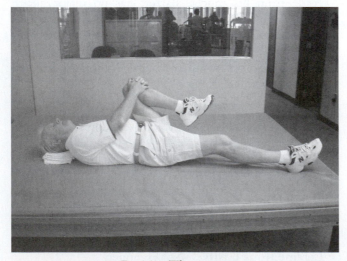

Case Figure 10.2   Positive Thomas test.

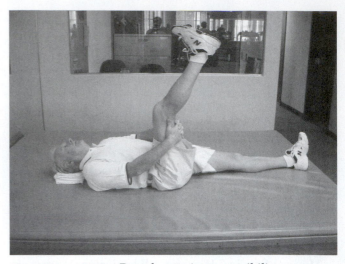

Case Figure 10.3   Poor hamstring extensibility.

Sensory Testing: Intact to light touch at all cervicothoracic and lumbosacral dermatomes.

Integumentary Assessment

Mild erythema and peeling over anterior portion of the lower abdomen. No evidence of excoriation or exudates (see Chapter 1)

A. Given this information, what are your primary concerns regarding musculoskeletal system impairments? *See Author's Comments A*

B. Do you have concerns regarding existing or potential cardiopulmonary system impairments? Please discuss them. *See Author's Comments B*

C. Based upon the information provided up to this point, list four to six problems that you consider to be critical to Barrett's quality of life. *See Author's Comments C*

Having listed the problems, you are ready to begin planning the short and long term goals that you would like to help Barrett achieve with your therapeutic exercise program. Be sure that the goals you set are realistic for Barrett, are observable, and are written clearly. Create goals that relate impairments and problems to functional limitations and disability. Remember that a goal is a point in the recovery process, not the process (for example, "improve range of motion" becomes a better goal when it is linked to a particular functionally relevant event, such as "improve range of motion to be independent climbing stairs").

For Barrett's case, limit your short term goals to those you believe he should achieve after four weeks of complying with your therapeutic exercise program. Base your short term goal achievement expectations on the minimal known times required for musculoskeletal, neuromuscular and cardiopulmonary physiological system improvements to occur.

D. Based upon the information provided, create three to six short term (approximately 4 weeks) therapeutic exercise program goals.
"By four weeks, the client . . ." See Author's Comments D

For this case, limit your long term goals to those you believe that Barrett should achieve after 12 weeks of complying with your therapeutic exercise program. Remember that these goals represent expected achievements by the end of your therapeutic exercise program intervention.

E. Create three to six long term (5–12 weeks) therapeutic exercise program goals.
"By 5 to 12 weeks, the client . . ." See Author's Comments E

Having established the short and long term goals, it is a good idea to review basic exercise physiology fundamentals, including metabolic energy systems and therapeutic exercise principles prior to designing a prescriptive therapeutic exercise program for Barrett (see Chapter 4 and 5). To improve the likelihood of client adherence, limit the number of activities and tasks in your initial therapeutic exercise program. Design your therapeutic exercise program with consideration for Barrett's current energy reserves and his requirements for rest and recovery.

F. Select the exercises (and a rationale for each) that you would like Barrett to perform. List the exercises in the order that you believe they should be performed, the body regions trained, and your rationale for the inclusion. Next, create a table in which the exercises are listed in order to be performed and give the volume (sets, repetitions), how the desired intensity will be determined, rest to work ratios, and frequency for each exercise. See Author's Comments F
G. Now that you have initiated the therapeutic exercise program, identify three to six clinical measurements you will use to verify progress toward short
term treatment goal achievement. *See Author's Comments G*
H. Provide a rationale for each of your clinical measurements. See Author's Comments H

During your 4-week re-evaluation you take the following clinical functional assessment measurements.

Exercise Diary: Barrett has documented 90% compliance with his therapeutic exercise prescription

Musculoskeletal Assessment

Manual Muscle Testing: Normal strength at bilateral upper and lower extremities (5/5)
Musculotendinous Extensibility: Hip extension to neutral alignment (0°) in Thomas test position bilaterally. Hamstrings to $-15°$ extension bilaterally
Pain: Backache during prolonged standing (0 out of 10 on modified visual analog scale). No other pain complaints
Bodyweight: 135 lbs
Body Mass Index: 19.4 kg/m²

Cardiopulmonary Assessment

Resting Blood Pressure: 131/85 mm Hg
Resting Heart Rate: 70 bpm

I. With consideration for exercise order determination factors, list your modified exercise selections, the primary body region that the exercise involves, and the rationale for including that exercise in the program in table format. See Author's Comments I
J. Following exercise selection, document in a table the volume (sets and repetitions), how intensity will be determined, the rest to work ratio, and frequency week. See Author's Comments J

Case Summary

With the therapeutic exercise program design modifications made at the end of the first 4 weeks, the focus has changed from helping Barrett make lifestyle changes incorporating increased physical activity to helping him achieve physical reconditioning levels necessary to resume social and recreational activities (**Case Figure 10.4**). While the biomechanics of the golf swing may impose risks for musculoskeletal injury, discouraging this activity would extinguish one of Barrett's major motivators. More golf-specific training activities at this stage will, if managed properly, reinforce this motivation and improve his ability to perform daily physical activities with less fatigue. This

outcome, together with increased physical activity levels and his eventual return to his accustomed social roles, should have a beneficial effect on Barrett's quality of life.

K. On a separate sheet of paper diagram a decision making algorithm for managing Barrett's cancer-related fatigue condition. See Author's Comments K

Referring to Chapter 10 for guidance, discuss any alternative or complementary therapeutic exercises **that you believe might benefit this client. Provide the rationale for your suggestion(s).**

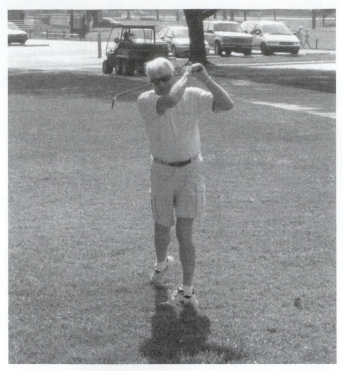

Case Figure 10.4   Barrett's return to golf.

References

1. Devlen J, Maguire P, Phillips P, et al. Psychological problems associated with diagnosis and treatment of lymphomas: 1. Retrospective 2. Prospective. *BMJ*. 1997;295:953–957.

2. Irvine DM, Vincent L, Bubela N, at al. A critical appraisal of the research literature investigating fatigue in the individual with cancer. *Cancer Nurs*. 1991;14:188–199.

3. Nail LM, Jones LS, Greene D, et al. Use and perceived efficacy of self-care activities in patients receiving chemotherapy. *Oncol Nurs Forum* 1991;18:883–887.

4. Schwartz AL. Patterns of exercise and fatigue in physically active cancer survivors. *Oncol Nurs Forum*. 1998;25:486–491.

5. Smets EM, Garssen, B, Schuster-Uitterhoeve AL, de Haes JC. Fatigue in cancer patients. *Br J Cancer*. 1993;69:220–224.

6. Portenoy RK, Miaskowski C. Assessment and management of cancer-related fatigue. In Berger A, Portenoy RK, Weissman DE, eds. *Principles and Practice of Supportive Oncology*. Philadelphia: Lippincott-Raven Publishers, 1998:109–118.

7. Aistars J. Fatigue in the cancer patient: A conceptual approach to a clinical problem. *Oncol Nurs Forum*. 1987;14:25–30.

8. Kaempfer SH, Lindsey AM. Energy expenditure in cancer: A review. *Cancer Nurs*. 1986;9:194–199.

9. St Pierre BA, Kasper CE, Lindsey AM. Fatigue mechanisms in patients with cancer: effects of tumor necrosis factor and exercise on skeletal muscle. *Oncol Nurs Forum*. 1992;19:419–425.

10. Piper BF, Lindsey AM, Dodd MJ. Fatigue mechanisms in cancer patients: Developing nursing theory. *Oncol Nurs Forum*. 1987;14:17–23.

11. King KB, Nail LM, Kreamer K, et al. Patients' descriptions of the experience of receiving radiation therapy. *Oncol Nurs Forum*. 1985;12:55–61.

12. Greenberg DB, Sawicka J, Eisenthal S, et al. Fatigue syndrome due to localized radiation. *J Pain Symptom Manage*. 1992;7:38–45.

13. Nail LM. Coping with intracavitary radiation treatment for gynecologic cancer. *Cancer Pract*. 1993;1:218–224.

14. Larson PJ, Lindsey AM, Dodd MJ, et al. Influence of age on problems experienced by patients with lung cancer undergoing radiation therapy. *Oncol Nurs Forum*. 1993;20:473–480.

15. Fobair P, Hoppe RT, Bloom J, et al. Psychosocial problems among survivors of Hodgkin's disease. *J Clin Oncol*. 1986;4:805–814.

16. Piper BF, Rieger PT, Brophy L, et al. Recent advances in the management of biotherapy-related side effects: Fatigue. *Oncol Nurs Forum*. 1989;16(6 Suppl):27–34.

17. Haeuber D. Recent advances in the management of biotherapy-related side effects: Flu-like syndrome. *Oncol Nurs Forum*. 1989;16(6 Suppl):35–41.

18. Mattson K, Niiranen A, Ivananien N. Neurotoxicity of interferon. *Cancer Treat Rep*. 1983;67:958–996.

19. Courneya KS, Friedenreich CM. Physical exercise and quality of life following cancer diagnosis: A literature review. *Ann Behav Med*. 1999;21:171–179.

20. Cella D, Peterman A, Passik S, et al. Progress toward guidelines for the management of fatigue. *Oncology*. 1998;12:369–377.

21. Demark-Wahnefried W, Winer EP, Rimer BK. Why women gain weight with adjuvant chemotherapy for breast cancer. *J Clin Oncol*. 1993;11:1418–1429.

22. Dimeo F, Bertz H, Finke J, et al. An aerobic exercise program for patients with haematological malignancies after bone marrow transplantation. *Bone Marrow Transplant*. 1996;18:1157–1160.

23. Jenney ME, Faragher EB, Mortis-Jones PH, Woodcock A. Lung function and exercise capacity in survivors of childhood leukemia. *Med Pediatric Oncol*. 1995;24:222–230.

24. Morrow GR, Dobkin PL. Anticipatory nausea and vomiting in cancer patients undergoing chemotherapy treatment: Prevalence, etiology, and behavioral interventions. *Clin Psychol Rev*. 1988;8:517–556.

25. Pelletier C, Lapointe L, LeBlanc P. Effects of lung resection on pulmonary function and exercise capacity. *Thorax*. 1990;45:497–502.

26. Pihkala J, Happonen J, Virtanen K, et al. Cardiopulmonary evaluation of exercise tolerance after chest irradiation and anticancer chemotherapy in children and adolescents. *Pediatrics*. 1995;95: 722–726.

27. Segal R, Reid R, Johnson D, et al. Pilot study of physical fitness and quality of life in patients with breast cancer. In *Proceedings of the Annual Meeting of the American Society of Clinical Oncology*, 1996, p. 142.

28. Young-McCaughan S, Sexton DL. A retrospective investigation of the relationship between aerobic exercise and quality of life in women with breast cancer. *Oncol Nurs Forum*. 1991;8:751–757.

29. Hann DM, Jacobsen PB, Azzarello LM, et al. Measurement of fatigue in cancer patients: Development and validation of the fatigue symptom inventory. *Qual Life Res*. 1998;7:301–310.

30. Hann DM, Denniston MM, Baker F. Measurement of fatigue in cancer patients: Further validation of the fatigue symptom inventory. *Qual Life Res*. 2000;9:847–854.

31. Mendoza TR, Wang XS, Cleeland CS, et al. The rapid assessment of fatigue severity in cancer patients: Use of the Brief Fatigue Inventory. *Cancer*. 1999;85:1186–1196.

32. Piper BF, Dibble SL, Dodd MJ, et al. The revised Piper Fatigue Scale: Psychometric evaluation in women with breast cancer. *Oncol Nurs Forum*. 1998; 25:677–684.

33. Schwartz AL. The Schwartz Cancer Fatigue Scale: Testing reliability and validity. *Oncol Nurs Forum*. 1998;25:711–717.

34. Cella D. *Manual of the Functional Assessment of Chronic Illness Therapy (FACIT) Scales*, Version 4. Evanston, IL: Evanston Northwestern Healthcare, 1997.

35. Cella DF, Tulsky DS, Gray G, et al. The functional assessment of cancer therapy scale: Development and validation of the general measure. *J Clin Oncol*. 1993;11:570–579.

36. McNair D, Lorr M, Droppelman L, et al. *Profile of Mood States*. San Diego, CA: Educational and Industrial Testing Service, 1971.

37. Hays RD, Sherbourne CD, Mazel RM. The RAND 36-item health survey 1.0. *Health Econ*. 1993;2: 217–227.

38. Hays RD, Morales LS. The RAND-36 Measure of Health-Related Quality of Life. *Ann Med*. 2001;33: 350–357.

39. Reich SG: The tired patient: Psychological versus organic causes. *Hosp Med*. 1986;22:142–154.

40. Cella D, Davis K, Breitbart W, et al. Cancer-related fatigue: Prevalence of proposed diagnostic criteria in a United States sample of cancer survivors. *J Clin Oncol*. 2001;19:3385–3391.

41. Radloff LS. The CES-D scale: A self-report depression scale for research in the general population. *Appl Psychol Meas*. 1977;1:385–401.

42. Spielberger CD. *Manual for the State-Trait Anxiety Inventory (Form Y)*. Palo Alto, CA: Consulting Psychologists Press, 1983.

43. Buysse DJ, Reynolds CF, Monk TH, et al. The Pittsburgh Sleep Quality Index: A new instrument for psychiatric practice and research. *Psych Res*. 1988;28:193–213.

44. Hanks GE, Krall JM, Hanlon AL, et al. Patterns of care and prostate cancer by conventional radiation therapy: An analysis of RTOG studies in prostate cancer. Long-term survival, hazard rate long-term outcome. *Int J Radiat Oncol Biol Phys*. 1995;32: 287–292.

45. Burnham TR, Wilcox A. Effects of exercise on physiological and psychological variables in cancer survivors. *Med Sci Sports Exerc*. 2002;34:1863–1867.

46. Dimeo FC, Stieglitz RD, Novelli-Fischer U, et al. Effects of physical activity on the fatigue and psychologic status of cancer patients during chemotherapy. *Cancer*. 1999;85:2273–2277.

47. Friendenreich CM, Courneya KS. Exercise as rehabilitation for cancer patients. *Clin J Sport Med*. 1996;6:237–244.

48. Johnson JB, Kelly AW. A multifaceted rehabilitation program for women with cancer. *Oncol Nurs Forum*. 1990;17:691–695.

49. Mock V, Burke MB, Sheehan P, et al. A nursing rehabilitation program for women with breast cancer receiving adjuvant chemotherapy. *Oncol Nurs Forum*. 1994;21:899–907.

50. Mock V, Pickett M, Ropka ME, et al. Fatigue and quality of life outcomes of exercise during cancer treatment. *Cancer Pract*. 2001;9: 119–127.

51. Segal R, Evans W, Johnson D, et al. Structured exercise improves physical functioning in women with stages I and II breast cancer: Results of a randomized controlled trial. *J Clin Oncol*. 2001;9: 657–665.

52. Winningham ML. Walking program for people with cancer: Getting started. *Cancer Nurs*. 1991;14: 270–276.

53. MacVicar MG, Winningham ML. Response of cancer patients on chemotherapy to a supervised exercise program. *Cancer Bull*. 1986;13:265–274.

54. Dimeo F, Tilmann MHM, Bertz H, et al. Aerobic exercise in the rehabilitation of cancer patients after high dose chemotherapy and autologous peripheral stem cell transplantation. *Cancer*. 1997;79: 1717–1722.

55. Winningham ML, Nail LM, Burke MB, et al. Fatigue and the cancer experience: The state of the knowledge. *Oncol Nurs Forum*. 1994;21:23–36.

Author's Comments A

Musculoskeletal Findings: Bilateral hip flexion contractures; mechanical low back pain. Lumbar spinal osteopenia by history. Given Barrett's history of androgen ablation therapy and radiotherapy, there is an underlying concern for his ability to improve or even maintain his current muscle mass and bone mineral density if he maintains his current sedentary lifestyle. Furthermore, the possible presence of metastatic bone disease must be considered during the differential diagnosis of Barrett's back pain.

Author's Comments B

Hematology Findings: Hemoglobin, hematocrit, and platelet count are near the lower limits of their respective reference ranges following radiation therapy but not sufficiently low to warrant a diagnosis of anemia. Diminished oxygen uptake and aerobic work capacity may limit Barrett's tolerance of aerobic exercise except at very low levels of intensity and duration.

Author's Comments C

Problem List

1. Cancer-related fatigue
2. Reduced aerobic work capacity (impaired energy systems)
3. Reduced muscle mass (sarcopenia) secondary to prostate cancer and testosterone ablation therapy
4. Bilateral hip flexion contractures
5. Low back pain
6. Localized osteopenia; at risk for pathological fractures

Barrett's chief complaint is fatigue. Fatigue is documented as the most commonly reported symptom following diagnosis and treatment for cancer, affecting approximately 2 out of 3 (range 40–90 percent) patients and survivors.[1–5] The exact pathogenesis is unclear, but symptoms of cancer related fatigue (CRF) have been postulated to result from physical deconditioning, psychoemotional stress, and the secondary effects of surgery, chemotherapy, radiotherapy, and biotherapeutic agents.[6–18]

Although fatigue is frequently an expected, temporary side effect of treatment, the problem may persist if other factors continue to be present. For many clients, cancer-related fatigue is severe, imposing limitations on daily activities and diminishing quality of life (QOL). Researchers report that physical and functional effects accompanying CRF include impaired cardiovascular function, reduced pulmonary function, decreased strength, diminished lean body mass, weight loss, sleep disturbances, nausea and vomiting, and pain.[19–28]

A variety of instruments have been developed to assess fatigue, including the Fatigue Symptom Index,[29–30] Brief Fatigue Inventory,[31] Piper Fatigue Self-Report Scale,[32] and the Schwartz Cancer Fatigue Scale.[33] Fatigue may also be assessed using relevant subscales from multidimensional quality-of-life instruments such as the Functional Assessment of Cancer Therapy Fatigue subscale (FACT-F),[34,35] the Profile of Mood States Fatigue/Inertia subscale,[36] and the Fatigue/Vitality subscale of the RAND 36-Item Health Survey,[37,38] but there is currently no universally accepted standard for the measurement of cancer-related fatigue.

An impressive proportion of cancer survivors complaining of fatigue also experience psychological or emotional distress, particularly depression and anxiety.[39] The presence of depression, characterized by loss of interest, difficulty concentrating, lethargy, and feelings of hopelessness can compound the physical causes for fatigue and may persist long past the time when physical causes have resolved.[40] Anxiety associated with the diagnosis of cancer alone may trigger fatigue. Consequently, it is important to distinguish physiological fatigue from depression and anxiety. Mental health professionals may be able to diagnose these conditions using standardized measures such as the Center for Epidemiological Studies-Depression scale (CES-D)[41] or the state version of the State Trait Anxiety Inventory (STAI-S), a widely used self-report measure that assesses the severity of current (state) anxiety.[42] Disrupted sleep, decreased nighttime or excessive daytime sleep or inactivity may be a causative or contributing factor in cancer-related fatigue (CRF). Clients with less daytime activity and more nighttime awakenings were noted to consistently report higher levels of CRF. The Pittsburgh Sleep Quality Index[43] is a widely used self-report measure of sleep patterns and sleep-related difficulties that may be used to identify and document changes in sleep disturbances.

A major challenge for the therapeutic exercise program designer in Barrett's case is to balance the potential risks and physiological costs of exercise against its potential benefits to the client. To balance the health risks and energy costs imposed by exercise, this client's potential for functional improvement with exercise must also be great. The magnitude of functional improvement can be expressed in terms of life expectancy and quality of life. Actuarial data indicate that a 75-year-old man has about a 50 percent chance of surviving to age 85. Long-term studies of cancer survivorship show that men with stage T3 prostate cancer treated with radiotherapy can expect 10 year survival rates of 35–45 percent.[44] In Barrett's case, it would appear that his cancer has reduced his chances of living to age 85 by only 5–15 percent. While there is no known evidence that exercise increases life expectancy for people diagnosed with cancer, preliminary studies have demonstrated the beneficial effects of exercise on the quality of life of cancer patients.

A number of small trials conducted predominantly with breast cancer survivors[45–52] suggest that light to moderate intensity (40–60 percent heart rate reserve (HRR)) walking programs have the potential to improve quality of life for these clients. The benefits shown in these studies and observed in clinical settings include improved physical energy, appetite stimulation, and/or enhanced functional capacity, with improvement in quality of life, and improvements in many aspects of psychologic state, including fatigue, anxiety, and depression.

Barrett's compromised cardiopulmonary/vascular and musculoskeletal systems require the therapeutic exercise program designer to ration and prioritize his limited energy reserves available for exercise. Any changes in daily routine require additional energy expenditure. For this reason, it may be advisable to divide the therapeutic exercise prescription and perform strengthening activities and aerobic conditioning/flexibility activities on alternate days. Barrett's recent history of cancer treatment and his sedentary lifestyle may contribute to his fatigue and make it unlikely that he would be able to tolerate 20–30 minutes of sustained exercise at 40–80 percent of his age-predicted HRR. Several researchers have shown that dividing the daily dose of exercise over several bouts of 5–10 minute durations can be an effective strategy for patients receiving treatment for cancer.[46,49,53,54] Individuals with cancer should also be advised about setting priorities and maintaining a reasonable schedule. Sleep hygiene, including avoidance of lying in bed at times other than when they want to sleep, shortening naps to no more than one hour, avoiding distracting noise (TV, radio) during sleep hours, and other measures may improve sleep and activity cycles.

Resistance exercise may not be a low risk intervention for Barrett. His history of treatment for prostate cancer places him at increased risk for pathological hip fractures, spinal compression fractures, and fibrosis of muscles in the areas exposed to radiation (lower anterior abdomen and pelvis). In this situation, high intensity mechanical forces applied to flexed portions at the lumbo-sacro-pelvic region could reasonably be assumed to have the potential to cause internal derangement or mechanical failure of bone matrix at the anterior vertebral bodies. Even low impact aerobic exercise can be a high energy cost option in situations where impaired energy delivery (borderline anemia) and utilization capacity (asthenia; impaired resting VO_2 and VO_2 reserve) are responsible for limiting the client's quality of life. These factors suggest that a therapeutic exercise program featuring relatively low loads and high repetitions would be appropriate. This strategy is also consistent with Barrett's need to improve his aerobic conditioning and reduce his level of fatigue during normal activities of daily living (ADLs).

Barrett's ongoing androgen ablation therapy also mitigates against a strategy that imposes high resistive loads on musculoskeletal tissues. In the absence of testosterone and related anabolic hormones, he may have difficulty increasing muscle mass. This makes it unlikely that the possible benefit of low repetition, high resistance training for this purpose would outweigh the risk of musculoskeletal injury.

Author's Comments D

By four weeks, the client . . .

1. Will demonstrate adherence to an aerobic training program by engaging in 20 minutes of continuous physical activity in the training heart rate zone (40–60 percent HRR) per day at least three times/week. (If Barrett is unable to sustain continuous activity for 20 minutes initially, he may divide the 20 minutes into shorter sessions conducted over the course of the day, for example, two 10-minute sessions or four 5-minute sessions. The object here is not necessarily to effect a change in physiological parameters but to change sedentary behaviors and establish a pattern of increased physical activity.)

2. Will demonstrate adherence to a regular walking program

3. Will increase bilateral hip extension ROM > 10°

4. Will decrease low back pain by 2/10 during ADLs

5. Will participate in social activities outside the home one to two times/week

Author's Comments E

By 5 to 12 weeks, the client . . .

1. Will return to playing nine holes of golf with a cart once each week without excessive fatigue

2. Will increase BMI to at least 20 kg/m^2

3. Will improve oxygen uptake at ventilatory threshold to 5 METs

4. Will maintain bone mineral density at current levels to prevent spinal compression fractures.

Author's Comments F

While no single training principle can be ignored, certain principles may apply more than others to a therapeutic exercise program that is designed for a specific client. By complying with a regular walking program and initiating a light resistance training program for the upper extremities, Barrett stands to improve his aerobic capacity and muscle mass, particularly in muscle groups stressed during golf. Although progressively increased exercise intensity is certainly indicated, of greater concern for Barrett is the current state of physical de-conditioning exacerbated by his abnormally low level of physical activity, complaints of fatigue, and increased risk of spinal compression fracture. The crossover benefits of aerobic conditioning and upper extremity movements that are common to golf may also help improve Barrett's capacity for performing self-care and ADLs.

The importance of re-establishing social contacts cannot be overemphasized in this case. As a widower, Barrett's golf and card-playing groups may be his primary social support systems. Taking walks with members of these groups may improve program adherence, encourage additional opportunities for socialization, and improve the likelihood of achieving successful rehabilitation.

Respecting his increased risk for musculoskeletal tissue failure and his history of low levels of physical activity that predates his cancer diagnosis, Barrett will be initiating his therapeutic exercise program at very low levels of intensity and duration. Special attention must be paid to posture and positioning during exercise performance to avoid excessive anterior compression and shear forces to the lumbar spine.

Although exercise tasks intended to maintain or improve aerobic energy system capacity and increase bone mineral density provide the core of the intervention plan, the biomechanical stresses imposed by the golf swing on de-conditioned musculoskeletal tissues suggest that aerobic training alone may be insufficient to safely prepare Barrett to resume this activity. Barrett's history and physical examination findings suggest that resistance training exercises to strengthen his trunk and shoulder girdle musculature are also indicated. The overarching goal and challenge of any therapeutic exercise program initiated for this sedentary client is to achieve a pattern of program adherence and increased physical activity. Consequently, the principle that "less is more" applies. Based on these considerations, the following therapeutic exercise prescription has been proposed. To improve the likelihood of client adherence while respecting Barrett's current energy reserves and his requirements for rest and recovery, the number of activities and tasks in the initial therapeutic exercise program has been limited to three per day.

Exercise order	Exercise selection	Body region	Rationale for inclusion
1	Low intensity resistive (rubber tubing) exercises	Shoulders (all planes) and wrist extensors/flexors	Musculoskeletal pre-conditioning for injury prevention during golf
2	Low intensity (spinal stabilization) exercises vs.gravity in supine position (**Case Figure 10.5**) (Section 10, Animation 1)	Lumbosacral spine extensors/rotators and flexor/rotators	Strengthen core lumbo-pelvic region
3	Partial sit-ups	Rectus abdominis	Strengthen core lumbo-pelvic region
4	Walking	Lower extremities	Cardiovascular and cardiopulmonary fitness and energy utilization intervention for fatigue
5	Iliopsoas stretch		Injury prevention during walking program and golf
6	Hamstring stretch (Section 10, Animation 2)		Injury prevention during walking program and golf

Exercise order	Volume (sets/repetitions)	Intensity Determination	Rest-to-work ratio	Frequency/ week
1	1 set/8–10 repetitions	Volitional fatigue	As tolerated	2–3 ×/week
2	1 set/8–10 repetitions	Volitional fatigue	As tolerated	2–3 ×/week
3	1 set/8–10 repetitions	Volitional fatigue	As tolerated	2–3 ×/week
4	20–30 minutes	40–60% HRR	N/A	3–4 ×/week
5	3 times each	20–30 seconds	N/A	2–3 ×/week
6	3 times each	20–30 seconds	N/A	2–3 ×/week

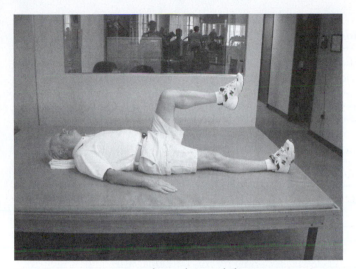

Case Figure 10.5   Lumbo-pelvic stabilization exercise.

An important goal of treating the client with cancer is to facilitate self-care. A shift in responsibility for control of side effects from the rehabilitation clinician to the client is important. It is imperative that clients with cancer be educated to develop the self-care abilities necessary to cope with fatigue. Specific techniques for the management of fatigue include the following:[55]

- Differentiation of fatigue from depression
- Assessment for the presence of correctable correlates or causes of fatigue (e.g., dehydration, electrolyte imbalance, dyspnea, anemia)
- Evaluation of patterns of rest and activity during the day as well as over time
- Encouragement of activity/planned therapeutic exercise programs within individual limitations; making goals realistic by keeping in mind the state of the disease and treatment regimens
- Education of clients and families about fatigue related to cancer and its treatment
- Helping clients with cancer and their families to identify fatigue-promoting activities, and to develop specific strategies to modify these activities
- Suggesting individualized environmental or activity changes that may offset fatigue
- Maintaining adequate hydration and nutrition
- Scheduling important daily activities during times of least fatigue, and eliminating non-essential, stress producing activities
- Addressing the negative impact of psychologic and social stressors, and how to avoid or modify them
- Evaluating the efficacy of fatigue interventions on a regular and systematic basis

Remember that your therapeutic exercise program may vary considerably from this example. What should not vary, however, are the links that you establish between key problems, functionally relevant treatment goals, and the scientific rationale used to support your decisions.

Author's Comments G

1. Diary/record of therapeutic exercise activity
2. Hip ROM (goniometry)
3. Visual Analogue Pain Scale scores during ADLs
4. Height–weight measurements
5. Work capacity during aerobic exercise

Author's Comments H

1. Document adherence to home exercise program
2. Hip flexion contracture, possibly contributing to mechanical low back pain
3. Low back pain with selected functional activities
4. Low BMI
5. Poor cardiopulmonary fitness and energy utilization

Author's Comments I

The initial 4 weeks of a therapeutic exercise program that emphasized aerobic conditioning and included posterior lumbopelvic muscle stretching and shoulder girdle muscle strengthening has proven successful. Barrett, with the support of his peers, has stuck with his therapeutic exercise program fairly regularly. This is a major change in his activity pattern and this behavioral change can be the most difficult obstacle for many clients initiating an exercise program to overcome (see Chapter 11). He is now able to sustain 20–30 minutes of continuous activity at 40–60 percent of his heart rate reserve and reports less fatigue during normal activities. The therapeutic exercise program should be modified to allow progression to higher intensities and longer duration of activity. To maintain Barrett's motivation, greater emphasis may be placed on the long-term goals, particularly returning to golf.

In modifying Barrett's therapeutic exercise program to include more golf specific activities, we have an excellent opportunity to continue to systematically increase his upper extremity and lumbopelvic extensibility and strength. Increasing the intensity and duration of his walking program will crossover to help improve functional capabilities with activities of daily living and instrumental activities of daily living. Based on the progress he has made with the initial therapeutic exercise program and the motivation he has expressed for golf, more advanced golf-related components should be prescriptively included in his program in a manner that will facilitate long term goal achievement.

Exercise order	Exercise selection	Body region	Rationale for inclusion
1	Low intensity resistive (rubber tubing) exercises (**Case Figure 10.6a–b**)	Shoulders (all planes) and wrist extensors/flexors	Musculoskeletal pre-conditioning for injury prevention during golf
2	Low intensity (spinal stabilization) exercises vs. gravity in supine position	Lumbosacral spine extensors/rotators and flexor/rotators	Strengthen core lumbo-pelvic region
3	Partial sit-ups	Rectus abdominis	Strengthen core lumbo-pelvic region
4	Walking	Lower extremities	Injury prevention during walking program and golf
5	Iliopsoas stretch		Injury prevention during walking program and golf
6	Hamstring stretch		Injury prevention during walking program and golf
7	Golf club stretches	Hip and trunk rotators	Injury prevention during walking program and golf
8	Pitch and putt (< 25 yards to start)		Sports or activity specific training

Author's Comments J

Exercise order	Volume (sets/repetitions)	Intensity Determination	Rest-to-work ratio	Frequency/ week
1	1 set/10–15 repetitions	Volitional fatigue	As tolerated	2–3 ×/week minimum
2	1 set/10–15 repetitions	Volitional fatigue	As tolerated	2–3 ×/week minimum
3	1 set/10–15 repetitions	Volitional fatigue	As tolerated	2–3 ×/week minimum

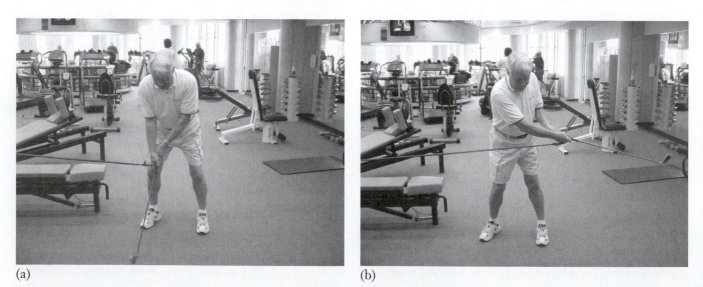

(a)   (b)

Case Figure 10.6   Golf swing simulation using elastic resistance bands. (a) starting position, (b) finish position.

Exercise order	Volume (sets/repetitions)	Intensity Determination	Rest-to-work ratio	Frequency/ week
4	30–40 minutes (total time may be broken up in multiple shorter sessions to start)	40–60% HRR	N/A	3–4 ×/week
5	Three times each	20–30 seconds		2–3 ×/week
6	Three times each	20–30 seconds		2–3 ×/week
7	Three times each	20–30 seconds		2–3 ×/week
8	1 set/10–15 repetitions	Volitional fatigue	As tolerated	2–3×/week

Remember that your program may vary considerably from this example. What should not vary, however, are the links that you establish between key problems, functionally relevant treatment goals, and the scientific rationale used to support your decisions.

Author's Comments K

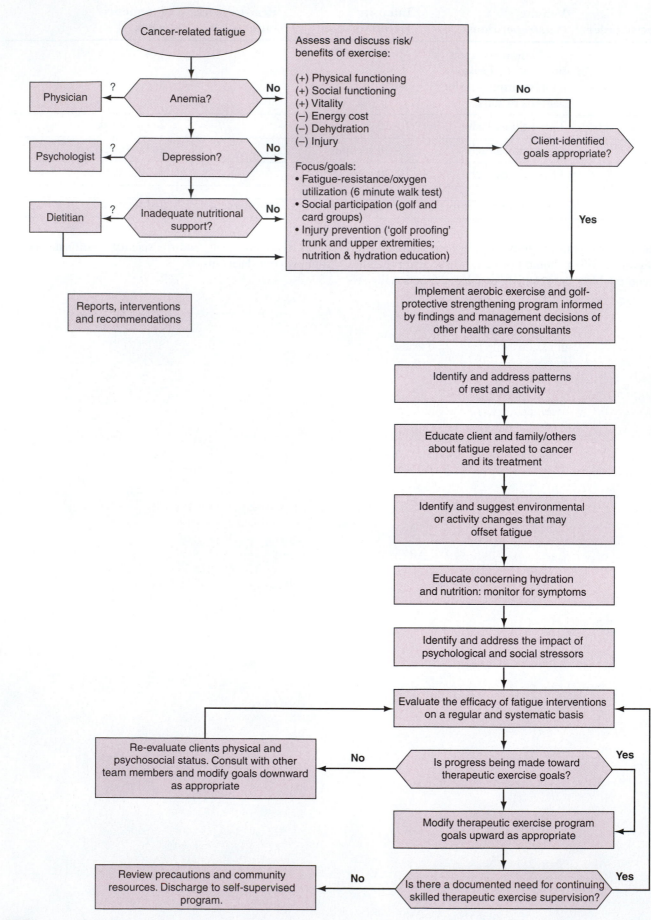

Cancer-related fatigue

Physician — ? — Anemia? — No

Psychologist — ? — Depression? — No

Dietitian — ? — Inadequate nutritional support? — No

Reports, interventions and recommendations

Assess and discuss risk/benefits of exercise:

(+) Physical functioning
(+) Social functioning
(+) Vitality
(−) Energy cost
(−) Dehydration
(−) Injury

Focus/goals:
• Fatigue-resistance/oxygen utilization (6 minute walk test)
• Social participation (golf and card groups)
• Injury prevention ('golf proofing' trunk and upper extremities; nutrition & hydration education)

Client-identified goals appropriate? — No / Yes

Implement aerobic exercise and golf-protective strengthening program informed by findings and management decisions of other health care consultants

Identify and address patterns of rest and activity

Educate client and family/others about fatigue related to cancer and its treatment

Identify and suggest environmental or activity changes that may offset fatigue

Educate concerning hydration and nutrition: monitor for symptoms

Identify and address the impact of psychological and social stressors

Evaluate the efficacy of fatigue interventions on a regular and systematic basis

Is progress being made toward therapeutic exercise goals? — No / Yes

Re-evaluate clients physical and psychosocial status. Consult with other team members and modify goals downward as appropriate

Modify therapeutic exercise program goals upward as appropriate

Is there a documented need for continuing skilled therapeutic exercise supervision? — No / Yes

Review precautions and community resources. Discharge to self-supervised program.

Index

VHI PC-Kits Exercise Software

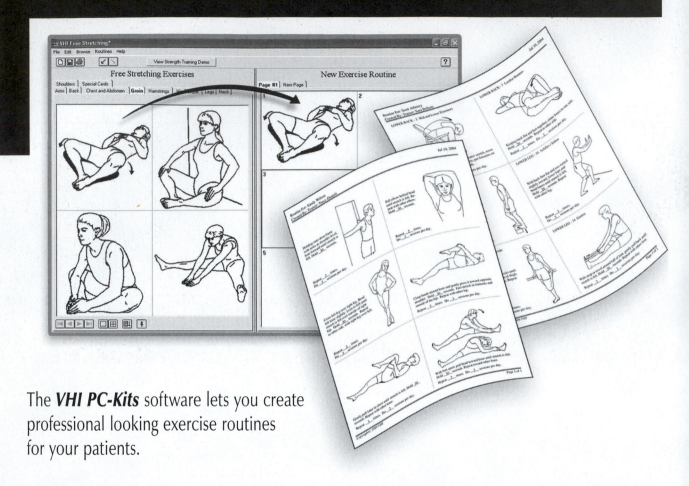

The **VHI PC-Kits** software lets you create professional looking exercise routines for your patients.

This program lets you:

- Edit the text
- Save routines you give to patients
- Save your favorite routines for later recall

...and much more!

A demo of the software can be downloaded at *www.vhikits.com* or one can be sent to you by calling *1-800-356-0709*.

VHI
Visual Health Information

www.vhikits.com or **1-800-356-0709**